ENDOCRINOLOGY
ADULT AND PEDIATRIC

ENDOCRINOLOGY

ADULT AND PEDIATRIC 6TH EDITION

NEUROENDOCRINOLOGY AND THE PITUITARY GLAND

Volume Editor

Shlomo Melmed, MD
Senior Vice President, Academic Affairs and Dean of the Faculty
Cedars Sinai Medical Center
Los Angeles, California

ELSEVIER
SAUNDERS

1600 John F. Kennedy Blvd.
Ste 1800
Philadelphia, PA 19103-2899

Endocrinology, Adult and Pediatric: Neuroendocrinology & the Pituitary Gland   ISBN: 978-0-323-22155-9
POD ISBN: 978-0-323-24062-8

Notice

Knowledge and best practice in this field are constantly changing. As new research and experience broaden our knowledge, changes in practice, treatment, and drug therapy may become necessary or appropriate. Readers are advised to check the most current information provided (i) on procedures featured or (ii) by the manufacturer of each product to be administered to verify the recommended dose or formula, the method and duration of administration, and contraindications. It is the responsibility of the practitioner, relying on their own experience and knowledge of their patients, to make diagnoses, to determine dosages and the best treatment for each individual patient, and to take all appropriate safety precautions. To the fullest extent of the law, neither the Publisher nor the authors, contributors, or editors assume any liability for any injury and/or damage to persons or property arising out of or related to any use of the material contained in this book.

The Publisher

Content for this eBook is derived from a book that may have contained additional digital media. Media content is not included in this eBook purchase.

Library of Congress Cataloging-in-Publication Data
Endocrinology / senior editors, Leslie J. De Groot, J. Larry Jameson ; section editors Ashley Grossman ... [et al.].—6th ed.
    p. ; cm.
Includes bibliographical references and index.
ISBN-13: 978-1-4160-5593-9 (v.1 & v.2: hardback: alk. paper)
ISBN-13: 978-9996074479 (v.1: hardback: alk. paper)
ISBN-10: 9996074471 (v.1: hardback: alk. paper)
ISBN-13: 978-9996074417 (v.2: hardback: alk. paper)
[etc.]
1. Endocrine glands–Diseases.   2. Endocrinology.   I. De Groot, Leslie J.   II. Jameson, J. Larry.
[DNLM: 1. Endocrine System Disease.   2. Endocrine Glands.   3. Hormones.   WK 140 E5595 2010]
RC648.E458 2010
616.4—dc22

Acquisitions Editor: Helene Caprari
Developmental Editor: Mary Beth Murphy
Publishing Services Manager: Anne Altepeter
Project Manager: Jennifer Nemec
Design Direction: Ellen Zanolle

Transferred to Digital Printing in 2013

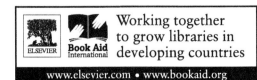

Senior Editors

J. Larry Jameson, MD, PhD

Professor of Medicine, Dean
Northwestern University Feinberg School of Medicine
Northwestern University
Chicago, Illinois

David de Kretser, AO, FAA, FTSE, MD, FRACP

Emeritus Professor
Monash Institute of Medical Research
Monash University
Clayton, Melbourne, Victoria, Australia

Ashley Grossman, BA, BSc, MD, FRCP, FMedSci

Professor of Neuroendocrinology
Endocrinology
St. Bartholomew's Hospital
London, United Kingdom

John C. Marshall, MD, PhD

Andrew D. Hart Professor of Internal Medicine
Director Center for Research in Reproduction
Department of Medicine
University of Virginia School of Medicine
Charlottesville, Virginia

Shlomo Melmed, MD

Senior Vice President, Academic Affairs and Dean of
  the Faculty
Cedars Sinai Medical Center
Los Angeles, California

Leslie J. De Groot, MD

Research Professor
Cellular and Life Sciences
University of Rhode Island, Providence Campus
Providence, Rhode Island

John T. Potts, Jr, MD

Jackson Distinguished Professor of Clinical Medicine
Harvard Medical School;
Director of Research and Physician-in-Chief Emeritus
Department of Medicine
Massachusetts General Hospital
Boston, Massachusetts

Gordon C. Weir, MD

Head, Section on Islet Transplantation and Cell Biology
Diabetes Research and Wellness Foundation Chair
Joslin Diabetes Center;
Professor of Medicine
Harvard Medical School
Boston, Massachusetts

Harald Jüppner, MD

Professor of Pediatrics
Endocrine Unit and Pediatric Nephrology Unit
  Massachusetts General Hospital and Harvard Medical
  School
Boston, Massachusetts

Contributors

Paolo Beck-Peccoz, MD
Professor of Endocrinology
Department of Medical Sciences, University of
Milan
Fondazione Policlinico IRCCS
Milan, Italy

Glenn D. Braunstein, MD
Professor and Chairman, Department of Medicine
The James R. Klinenberg MD Chair in Medicine
Cedars-Sinai Medical Center
Los Angeles, California

Marcello D. Bronstein, MD
Professor of Endocrinology
Chief, Neuroendocrine Unit
Division of Endocrinology and Metabolism
Department of Internal Medicine
Hospital das Clinicas
University of Sao Paulo Medical School
Sao Paulo, Brazil

Paolo Cappabianca, MD
Professor and Chairman of Neurological Surgery
Department of Neurosurgery
Università degli Studi di Napoli Federico II
Naples, Italy

**David Carmody, MB, BCh, BAO, LRCP, SI,
MRCP(UK)**
Doctor
Department of Endocrinology and Diabetes
Beaumont Hospital
Dublin, Ireland

Luigi M. Cavallo, MD, PhD
Department of Neurological Sciences
Division of Neurosurgery
Università degli Studi di Napoli Federico II
Naples, Italy

David R. Clemmons, MD
Director Diabetes Center for Excellence Kenan
Professor of Medicine
Department of Medicine
University of North Carolina School of Medicine
Chapel Hill, North Carolina

Georges Copinschi, MD, PhD
Professor Emeritus of Endocrinology
Laboratory of Physiology
Faculty of Medicine, Université Libre de Bruxelles;
Formerly Chief
Division of Endocrinology, Hôpital Universitaire
Saint-Pierre;
Formerly Chairman
Department of Medicine, Hôpital Universitaire
Saint-Pierre
Brussels, Belgium

Leona Cuttler, MD
William T. Dahms Professor of Pediatric
Endocrinology Chief
Division of Pediatric Endocrinology, Diabetes, and
Metabolism
Director, The Center for Child Health and Policy
at Rainbow
Rainbow Babies and Children's Hospital Case
Western Reserve University
Cleveland, Ohio

Mehul Dattani, FRCP, FRCPCH, MD
Professor of Paediatric Endocrinology
Developmental Endocrinology Research Group,
Clinical and Molecular Genetics Unit
UCL Institute of Child Health London
London, United Kingdom

Oreste de Divitiis, MD
Associate Professor
Department of Neurological Science, Institute of
Neurosurgery
Università degli Studi di Napoli Federico II
Naples, Italy

Leslie J. De Groot, MD
Research Professor
Cellular and Life Sciences
University of Rhode Island, Providence Campus
Providence, Rhode Island

Felice Esposito, MD, PhD, FACS
Department of Neurological Sciences
Division of Neurosurgery
Università degli Studi di Napoli Federico II
Naples, Italy

Bruce D. Gaylinn, PhD
Research Assistant Professor
Department of Medicine, Division of
Endocrinology
University of Virginia
Charlottesville, Virginia

Karen A. Gregerson, PhD
Associate Professor of Physiology
Division of Pharmaceutical Sciences
James L. Winkle College of Pharmacy
University of Cincinnati
Cincinnati, Ohio

**Ashley Grossman, BA, BSc, MD, FRCP,
FMedSci**
Professor of Neuroendocrinology
Endocrinology
St. Bartholomew's Hospital
London, United Kingdom

Mark John Hannon, MD, MRCPI
Doctor
Academic Department of Endocrinology
Beaumont Hospital/RCSI Medical School
Dublin, Ireland

**Peter Hindmarsh, BSC, MD, FRCP,
FRCPCH**
Professor of Paediatric Endocrinology
Developmental Endocrinology Research Group
University College London, Institute of Child
Health
London, United Kingdom

Ken K.Y. Ho, MD
Professor of Medicine
Head, Department of Endocrinology, St. Vincent's
Hospital
Head, Pituitary Research Unit, Garvan Institute of
Medical Research
Sydney, New South Wales, Australia

Nelson D. Horseman, PhD
Professor
Department of Molecular and Cellular Physiology
University of Cincinnati
Cincinnati, Ohio

J. Larry Jameson, MD, PhD
Professor of Medicine, Dean
Northwestern University Feinberg School of
Medicine
Northwestern University
Chicago, Illinois

Márta Korbonits, MD, PhD
Professor of Endocrinology and Metabolism
William Harvey Research Institute
Barts and London School of Medicine and
Dentistry
London, United Kingdom

John J. Kopchick, PhD
Goll-Ohio Professor of Molecular Biology
Edison Biotechnology Institute and Department of
Biomedical Sciences
Ohio University
Athens, Ohio

Paul Lee, MBBS, FRACP
Endocrine Fellow
Department of Endocrinology
St. Vincent's Hospital and Garvan Institute of
Medical Research
Sydney, Australia

Gabriel Á. Martos-Moreno, MD, PhD
Pediatrician
Assistant Professor of Pediatrics
Edison Biotechnology Institute
Ohio University;
Department of Pediatric Endocrinology
Hospital Infantil Universitario Niño Jesús;
Department of Pediatrics
Universidad Autónoma de Madrid;
CIBERobn
Instituto de Salud Carlos III
Madrid, Spain

Shlomo Melmed, MD
Senior Vice President, Academic Affairs and Dean
of the Faculty
Cedars Sinai Medical Center
Los Angeles, California

Madhusmita Misra, MD, MPH
Assistant Professor of Pediatrics, Harvard Medical
School
Pediatrics
MassGeneral Hospital for Children and Harvard
Medical School
Boston, Massachusetts

Damian G. Morris, MBBS, PhD, FRCP
Department of Diabetes and Endocrinology
The Ipswich Hospital
Ipswich, Suffolk, United Kingdom

Ralf Nass, MD
Research Assistant Professor
Division of Endocrinology and Metabolism
University of Virginia
Charlottesville, Virginia

Lynnette K. Nieman, MD
Senior Investigator
Intramural Research Program on Reproductive and
Adult Endocrinology
The Eunice Kennedy Shriver National Institute of
Child Health and Human Development
(NICHD), National Institutes of Health
Bethesda, Maryland

Luca Persani, MD, PhD
Associate Professor of Endocrinology
Dipartimento di Scienze Mediche, Istituto
Auxologico Italiano
Università degli Studi di Milano
Milan, Italy

Michael G. Rosenfeld, MD
HHMI, Department of School of Medicine
UCSD
La Jolla, California

Dorota Skowronska-Krawczyk, PhD
HHMI, Department of School of Medicine
University of California San Diego
La Jolla, California

Peter J. Snyder, MD
Professor of Medicine, University of Pennsylvania
School of Medicine
Department of Medicine
University of Pennsylvania
Philadelphia, Pennsylvania

**Richard Stanhope, BSc, MD, DCH, FRCP,
FRCPCH**
Consultant Paediatric Endocrinologist
The Portland Hospital Consulting Rooms
London, United Kingdom

Adam Stevens, PhD
Research Associate
School of Clinical and Laboratory Sciences
University of Manchester
Manchester, United Kingdom

Chris Thompson, MB, ChB, MD, FRCPI
Professor of Endocrinology
Academic Dept of Endocrinology
Beaumont Hospital/RCSI Medical School
Dublin, Ireland

Michael O. Thorner, MB, BS, DSc, MACP
David C Harrison Medical Teaching Professor of
Internal Medicine
Medicine
University of Virginia
Charlottesville, Virginia

Cristina Traggiai, MD
Pediatrician
Department of Neonatal Intensive Care Unit,
University of Genoa
IRCCS G. Gaslini
Genoa, Italy

Fred W. Turek, PhD
Charles E. and Emma H. Morrison Professor of
Biology
Director, Center for Sleep and Circadian Biology
Department of Neurobiology and Physiology
Northwestern University
Evanston, Illinois

Eve Van Cauter, PhD
Professor
Department of Medicine
The University of Chicago
Chicago, Illinois

Gary Wand, MD
The Alfredo Rivière and Norma Rodriguez de
Rivière Professor of Endocrinology and
Metabolism Director, Endocrine Training
Program
Medicine
The Johns Hopkins University School of Medicine
Baltimore, Maryland

Anne White, PhD
Professor of Endocrine Sciences
Faculties of Life Sciences and Medical and Human
Sciences
University of Manchester
Manchester, United Kingdom

Preface

Endocrinology, Adult and Pediatric, is now in its fortieth year and sixth edition, and it continues to evolve. After all, evolution to fit a changing environment is a law of nature that applies equally well to medical publishing as it does to the biological systems we seek to understand. Indeed, the rapid changes in information dissemination are necessary to keep pace with progress in science and medicine. In the sixth edition, we have retained the founding goals of this text while responding to the innovative means by which students, practicing clinicians, and researchers now acquire information. Accordingly, publication of this derivative eBook monograph focusing specifically on neuroendocrinology and the pituitary gland provides a distinctive enduring educational tool within the scope of the highest quality *Endocrinology* tradition.

A striking feature of our field is the explosion of knowledge ranging from the discovery of new hormones and drugs to the impact of genomics, proteomics, and metabolomics on how we classify diseases and conceptualize signaling pathways. These advances are all the more reason to seek information sources that synthesize and prioritize subject matter relevant to scientific and clinical readers. We are proud to work with the most accomplished international authorities who have succeeded in keeping pace with the latest advances in their specialty areas.

Accordingly, we now provide a comprehensive monograph devoted to understanding the fundamental cellular and physiologic functions of the neuroendocrine system, the mechanisms underlying clinical disorders, and approaches to managing patients harboring disorders of the hypothalamus and pituitary.

This novel monograph provides a comprehensive, contemporary mini-textbook of neuroendocrinology structured in both the traditional differentiated, gland-based approach and an emphasis on multihormonal integration of endocrine function with the master conductor of the endocrine orchestra, the pituitary, perhaps a prime example of "systems biology." Important components of this approach are the comprehensive descriptors, integrating endocrine cell ontogeny, hormonal control of growth and maturation processes, and childhood and young adult pathophysiology with maturation and aging processes.

We are grateful to the many authors who have balanced their numerous other obligations to prepare truly masterful presentations for the sixth-edition derivative eBook.

Shlomo Melmed, MD

Contents

Chapter 1

DEVELOPMENT OF THE PITUITARY

DOROTA SKOWRONSKA-KRAWCZYK and MICHAEL G. ROSENFELD

Advancement in genetic and molecular biology techniques has significantly increased our understanding of mechanisms underlying the development of the pituitary gland. The pituitary gland serves as an intermediary between the brain and the peripheral systems. By means of multiple feedback control mechanisms, the pituitary gland integrates incoming signals from the peripheral and central nervous systems and responds with regulation of production and secretion of critical regulatory hormones to target organs. The pituitary gland facilitates many critical functions, including metabolism, growth, reproduction, circadian rhythm, and stress responses. The functional regulation of gene transcription, pituitary hormone synthesis and secretion, and hormone cell proliferation is critical to homeostasis.

Anatomy and Histology

The pituitary gland, also termed the *hypophysis,* situates in a depression on the upper surface of the sphenoid bone, the *sella turcica.* It is composed of anatomically and functionally distinct entities: the *adenohypophysis,* including the intermediate and anterior lobes, and the *neurohypophysis,* also called the *posterior lobe.* The functional anterior pituitary contains five main cell types. (1) Somatotrope cells produce growth hormone (GH) and regulate linear growth and metabolism; (2) lactotrope cells produce prolactin (PRL), which regulates milk production in females; (3) thyrotrope cells produce thyroid-stimulating hormone (TSH), which controls the secretion of thyroid hormone from the thyroid gland; (4) gonadotrope cells produce gonadotropins (follicle-stimulating hormone [FSH] and luteinizing hormone [LH]), which regulate reproductive development and function; and (5) corticotrope cells produce adrenocorticotropic hormone (ACTH), a product of precursor pro-opiomelanocortin (POMC) cleaved by proteolytic processing, which regulates metabolic function through stimulation of glucocorticoid synthesis in the adrenal cortex. TSH, LH, and FSH are heterodimeric glycoproteins consisting of a common alpha subunit (αGSU) and a specific beta subunit. In the adult pituitary, GH-producing somatotrope cells occupy most of the gland, which weighs less than 1 gram in humans. The size of the pituitary gland and the proliferation of each pituitary cell type are regulated according to physiologic conditions indicated by feedback regulation.[1]

These five anterior pituitary cell types are present at birth (Table 1-1). Initial expression of distinct pituitary hormone genes marks the terminal differentiation events of the cell types, which derive from a seemingly common primordia and are the results of internal programming of the pituitary, as well as a consequence of its interaction with surrounding organs during development. Evidence suggests the internal programming is dictated by the expression of transcriptional regulators, including a cascade of homeodomain transcription factors and additional cell type–restricted transcription factors. The mechanisms that

Table 1-1. Onset of Adenohypophyseal Hormone Expression

Hormone	Human (weeks)	Mouse (dpc)	Chick (dpc)	Zebrafish (hpf)
GH	8	15.5	4.5	42
FSH/LH	8	16	4	—
ACTH	8	12.5	7	24
TSHβ	13	13.3	6.5	42
PRL	13	17.5	6	22

dpc, Days post coitus; *hpf*, hours post fertilization.

control the temporal and spatial expression of these transcription factors include diffusible signals from the developing hypothalamus at the dorsal aspect and factors from surrounding structures. These spatially distributed signals and gradients of signaling molecules are critical in establishing positional pituitary cell–type commitment events.[2,3] Disruption of these apparently evolutionarily conserved events underlying proper development of the pituitary gland can result in morphologic abbreviation and pituitary dysfunction. Through analysis of the expression of pituitary hormone genes in human cases of hypopituitarism, as well as in genetic models of pituitary defects (particularly in mouse models of pituitary dwarfism), a significant amount of knowledge has been accumulated regarding the molecular mechanisms underlying proper development of the pituitary gland.

Pituitary Development

ORIGIN

Phylogenetic studies in several vertebrate species led to the conclusion that the pituitary gland arises from oral epithelia. Fate-mapping experiments conducted in these animal species trace the origins of the pituitary gland back to the neural plate. In studies of grafting quail chick chimeras, the origin of the pituitary was localized to the midline of the anterior neural ridge. By means of surgical ablation performed in chick embryos, the rostral ridge of the neural plate was identified as the source of cells that give rise to pituitary tissue.[4-6] In amphibians, tracing experiments have confirmed the neural origin of pituitary gland[7,8] and similar conclusions have been reached about zebrafish.[9,10] Additionally, by focalized application of a carbocyanin dye, DiI, into the rostral end of the neural plate at the open neurula stage (9.5 days postcoitus) in rats, labeled cells could be identified in Rathke's pouch, and they could develop into the secretory cells of the adenohypophysis in 7 additional days.[11] Thus evidence indicates that the anterior neural ridge is the origin of Rathke's pouch, which eventually gives rise to cells of the pituitary gland. Subsequent to the folding of the embryonic head, the anterior neural ridge is displaced ventrally to form the portion of the oral epithelium that later gives rise to the roof of the mouth and additional structures, including the pituitary gland. Consistent findings in many species make it apparent that the process of pituitary development is, for the most part, evolutionarily conserved from lower vertebrates to higher mammals.

ONTOGENY

In humans, the anterior lobe of the pituitary gland originates from an invagination of the stomodeal epithelium termed *Rathke's pouch.*[12] The stomodeal epithelium that contains the pituitary primordium is formed by the third fetal week, and the invagination of stomodeal epithelium occurs dorsally to form Rathke's pouch by the fourth week. The formation of Rathke's pouch is complete and disconnected from the oral epithelium by the end of the sixth week of fetal life.[13] In parallel, the hypothalamus is the first region of the forebrain to differentiate. From 4 weeks, the hypothalamic sulcus, chiasmatic plate, and mammillary bodies are recognizable. These two organs, hypothalamus and pituitary, develop interdependently.[14]

Similar to the ontogeny observed in humans, Rathke's pouch in mice is derived from an anlage that arises as an upgrowth from the lining of the oral cavity's roof. At its earliest stage, the murine pituitary primordium is defined as an intimate point of contact between the neural ectoderm and the oral roof ectoderm on embryonic day 8.5 postcoitus (e8.5), which marks the first event in the pituitary's development. Organogenesis of the adenohypophysis begins as the cells of the pituitary placode in the oral ectoderm thicken and invaginate to form the nascent pituitary. In the e9.5 mouse embryo, this anlage can be seen located rostrally to the oropharyngeal membrane. Dorsal movement of the epithelial layer from the roof of the mouth induces a cone-shaped intrusion dorsally as Rathke's pouch, or the adenohypophyseal pouch. Before the formation, a developmentally important molecular marker, Sonic hedgehog (Shh), is expressed uniformly in the oral epithelial layer. The expression of *Shh* is excluded before the intrusion of pituitary anlagen can occur in the e9 mouse embryo.[15] Rathke's pouch thickens as development proceeds and elongates dorsally relative to the oral cavity by the stomodia-adenohypophyseal channel. By e10.5 in the mouse, Rathke's pouch has formed as a rudimentary structure and separated from the ventral pharyngeal epithelium.

At the time Rathke's pouch is pinched off at e11 in mice, the first round of accelerated mitotic activity is initiated in the anlagen.[16,17] In the ensuing patterning period, mitotic activity is observed most prominently in the rostral part of Rathke's pouch, with several buds emerging and enveloping areas of vascularized mesenchyme. Progenitors of the hormone-secreting cell types arise from the ventral proliferation of cells, and this region of rostral Rathke's pouch eventually gives rise to the anterior lobe, or the *pars distalis.* The dorsal aspects of Rathke's pouch, in contact with the descending infundibulum processes and rostroventrally with the hypophyseal cleft, remain thin and form the intermediate lobe, or the *pars intermedia.* Anterior pituitary cell types are positionally determined as they initially emerge from proliferation zones,[15,18] with the somatotrope/lactotrope cells arising caudomedially, gonadotrope cells more rostroventrally, corticotrope cells ventrally, and melanotrope cells dorsally. This pattern of pituitary development is generally similar in most mammals.

CELL LINEAGE DETERMINATION

Endocrine pituitary cell types in the adenohypophysis are derived from a single population of cells. The initial expression of pituitary hormone genes marking the terminal differentiation events of individual cell types occurs in a sequential manner. In mice, *POMC* gene expression emerges as the first pituitary marker at e11.5 and can be detected in the anterior pituitary by e13.5. However, the fate of cells that will give rise to those five different anterior pituitary cell types is determined prior to the initial pituitary *POMC* expression. In tissue-culture experiments where pituitary anlagen were taken and placed in a culture away from the influence of the diencephalons, pituitary anlagen taken at

Table I-2. Transcription Factors in Pituitary Hormone Deficiency

| Human | | | Model System | | |
Gene	Chr.	Inheritance	Hormone Deficiency	Mutation	Pituitary Phenotype
Pit1	3p11	Recessive/dominant	GH, PRL, and variable TSH	Snell	Gh, Prl, and Tsh
Prop1	5q35	Recessive	GH, PRL, TSH, FSH/LH, and ACTH	Ames	Gh, Prl, Tsh, and Fsh/Lh
Lhx3	9q34	Recessive	GH, PRL, TSH, and FSH/LH	K.O.	Gh, Prl, Tsh, and Fsh/Lh
Lhx4	1q25	Dominant	GH, TSH, and ACTH	K.O.	Reduction of all anterior cell types
Hesx1	3p21	Recessive/dominant	Variable hormone deficiency	K.O.	Pouch bifurcations, pituitary absence
Pitx2	4q25	Dominant	GH, PRL, TSH, and FSH/LH	K.O.	Gh, Prl, Tsh, and Fsh/Lh
Tbx19	1q23	Recessive	POMC	K.O.	Pituitary Pomc transdifferentiation

Chr., Chromosome location; *K.O.,* targeted deletion in mouse.

e11 were capable of generating cells expressing all five anterior pituitary hormone genes, while anlagen taken at e9.5 required additional growth factors, with the exception of corticotrope, which always differentiates regardless of the culture medium.[19] Critical events occur at the time pituitary anlagen become committed to developing into pituitary precursors that will subsequently express pituitary genes that become regulated in a cell-autonomous fashion.[20] The timing of this commitment event is coincidental with the formation of Rathke's pouch.

As an anlage, Rathke's pouch is the source of all endocrine pituitary cell types. In mice, after the initial appearance of corticotrope, expression of *GH* gene can be detected by e15.5, followed by *thyrotropins, gonadotropins,* and *PRL.* Gene expressions of all anterior pituitary hormones are detectable by e17.5, with the exception of *PRL,* which can be consistently seen by the time of birth (e19 in the mouse). Another early marker of Rathke's pouch is αGSU, and the transcripts are detected throughout Rathke's pouch by e9,[21] although they are confined to the rostral tip of the anterior lobe by e12.5 and ultimately restricted to thyrotrope and gonadotrope from late gestation through adulthood. Following proliferation and early organ expansion, a series of different cell types arise in a distinct spatial and temporal fashion. Table 1-1 provides a time line of the initial expression of pituitary hormone genes in several species.

Transcription Factors and Pituitary Development

Parallel to the sequential emergence of pituitary cell types, a series of homeodomain family transcription factors are expressed as the adenohypophysis is becoming committed. With improved molecular genetic techniques, functional studies of these transcription factors in animal models, particularly in mouse models, have established molecular mechanisms underlying development of the pituitary gland. The expression profiles of *Hesx1, Lhx3, Lhx4, Pitx1/2, Prop1,* and *Pit1* homeodomain factors, in addition to the expressions of *Tbx19* and *GATA2,* dictate the commitment, determination, and differentiation events of the pituitary gland. These genes were initially studied in animal model systems that arose either from naturally occurring mutations or were created by reverse genetic techniques. Without exception, phenotypes observed in each animal model system are also observed in human cases with defects in the corresponding orthologous genes (Table 1-2). The phenotypes observed in human cases range from single pituitary hormone deficiency to combined pituitary hormone deficiency (CPHD) affecting several pituitary hormones in addition to GH. Study of the development

of the pituitary gland serves as a model of progressive restriction in gene expression, and the pituitary gland has become a prototypic model organ system to study organogenesis, cell type determination, and differentiation.

PIT1 GENE

The *Pit1* gene (POU domain, class 1, transcription factor 1 [*POU1F1*]) encodes a 33-kD, 291-amino acid transcriptional activator that is capable of DNA binding and transactivation, and it was initially isolated by its ability to bind to the responsive element of the GH gene promoter.[22,23] *Pit1* is expressed exclusively in the pituitary gland. In mice, the initial expression of the *Pit1* gene transcripts can be detected by e13.5, exclusively in the anterior ventral pituitary (Fig. 1-1). The expression of *Pit1* persists in adults and co-localizes with expression of *GH, PRL,* and *TSHβ* genes. Further studies revealed that the product of the *Pit1* is capable of binding to responsive elements in the promoters of the *GH* gene,[24] the growth hormone–releasing hormone receptor (*GHRHR*) gene,[25] the *PRL* gene,[26] and the *TSHβ* gene. The Pit1 protein is also capable of binding to the responsive elements of the *Pit1* gene itself and is required for the continued transcription of the *Pit1* gene.[27] The structure of the *Pit1* gene is evolutionarily conserved and is found in mouse, human, and all other vertebrate animals examined, although *Pit1* may play diverse functional roles in different physiologic pathways in individual species.

Animal Model

Snell mice[28] are a well-studied animal model of pituitary function, which arises from a spontaneous single nucleotide mutation in the *Pit1* gene that results in the substitution of W261C in the homeodomain, rendering the mutant gene product incapable of DNA binding and hence unable to activate potential target genes.[29] Mice heterozygous for this mutation are phenotypically normal. The homozygous offspring of this mutation are dwarf and infertile, and they exhibit loss of three pituitary hormone cell types, GH, PRL, and TSHβ; whereas the gonadotrope and corticotrope cells are unaffected, suggesting that the *Pit1* is required for terminal differentiation of the somatotrope, lactotrope, and thyrotrope cell types. In the *Pit1*^Snell^ animal model where the *Pit1* gene is functionally defective, the initial activation of the *Pit1* is unaffected, while the later transcription of the *Pit1* gene is altered, resulting in the failed expression of the *Pit1* in the adult animal and a dwarf phenotype.[29,30] The *Pit1* lineage can be converted to alternative fates before e17.5 but exhibits a cell-autonomous commitment after e17.5, when *Pit1* gene regulation shifts from a *Pit1*-independent early enhancer to a *Pit1*-autoregulated later enhancer.[31] *Pit1*^Jackson^ is a second mouse model with a defect in the *Pit1* gene. The genomic structure of the *Pit1*

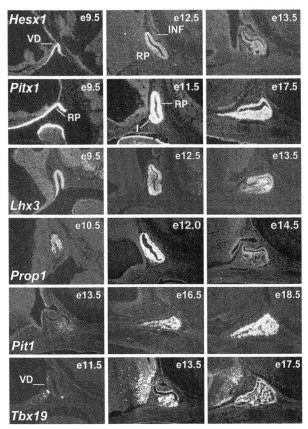

FIGURE 1-1. Expression of selected transcription factors in pituitary development by insitu hybridization. Expression of *Hesx1*, *Pitx1* and *Lhx3* are detected in Rathke's pouch (RP) at mouse embryonic stage e9.5 and are maintained at e12.5, after which *Hesx1* expression is rapidly extinguished while *Pitx1* and *Lhx3* continue to be expressed. *Prop1* expression initiates at e10.5, reaches maximum intensity at e12.5, and attenuates at e14.5. *Pit1* expression initiates at e13.5 and is maintained throughout pituitary development and adulthood. Initial *Tbx19* expression can be observed in the ventral Rathke's pouch and ventral diencephalon (VD) at e11.5, and its expression is maintained.

gene, located on chromosome 16, is grossly rearranged in mutant *Pit1*^Jackson mice, with a phenotype very similar or identical to that of the *Pit1*^Snell mice.[29] In addition, *Pit1* mutations result in decreased activity of the *insulin/IGF1* pathway, which may result in physiologic homeostasis consequences that favor longevity[32,33] (for reviews see refs. 34-36).

Related Diseases

The human *Pit1* gene has been mapped to chromosome 3. Lesions in *Pit1* have been identified as an etiology of CPHD (see Table 1-2). Initial study has revealed a homozygous nonsense mutation R172X in the *Pit1* gene in a patient of consanguineous parents with cretinism due to deficiency of GH, PRL, and TSHβ.[37] Many cases of CPHD with *Pit1* defects have since been reported. It appears that the inheritance of *Pit1* mutations in humans is complex, ranging from autosomal recessive to autosomal dominant to imprinting with variable phenotypic penetrance.[38] Pituitary gonadotropins and corticotropins are normal in *Pit1*-defective patients. Deficiency of GH is consistently observed in all *Pit1* patients, and deficiency for PRL is observed in most patients, whereas TSHβ deficiency usually has a delayed onset and incomplete penetrance (see Table 1-2). Different backgrounds may be the major contributing factor to the TSH phenotypic variation. Alternatively, however, there exists an

embryonic population of thyrotrope termed *rostral tip thyrotrope*. The expression of this embryonic TSH is not *Pit1* dependent, and consequently it may be a contributing element to the TSH phenotypic variation observed in *Pit1* patients. The presentation of patients with *Pit1* disorders varies considerably. At infancy, they usually have a protruding forehead, depressed facial structures, and a saddled nose, although CPHD is generally not diagnosed until growth retardation due to the deficiencies of GH and thyroid hormone becomes obvious.[39,40]

Mechanism

The modular structure of the Pit1 protein can be divided into the transactivation and the DNA-binding domains. The transcriptional activation domain is located in the first 80 amino acids, followed by a POU DNA-binding domain at the C terminus. The POU domain is further divided into a 75-amino acid POU-specific domain, which is conserved among various POU-domain proteins, and a 60-amino acid POU homeodomain with a linker region between them. The POU homeodomain by itself is sufficient for low-affinity DNA binding, although both the POU-specific domain and POU homeodomain are required for specific high-affinity DNA binding of the *Pit1*-responsive elements. Pit1 protein is able to bind as a monomer in solution to the consensus (A/T)(A/T)TATNCAT site, where N may be any nucleotide; in most cases, however, Pit1 binds DNA as a dimer.[41] Analysis of data derived from a cocrystal study of the Pit1 protein and the PRL proximal promoter Pit1-binding element reveals that the Pit1 protein binds to DNA in a parallel dimer form.[42,43] Pit1 protein wraps around the DNA molecule, with the POU-specific domain and the POU homeodomain binding to the DNA molecule in a perpendicular angle in opposite orientation. The POU-specific domain of one Pit1 molecule interacts with the C terminus of the POU homeodomain of the other Pit1 molecule in a dual composition. In addition, the spacing between the DNA contacts made by the POU-specific domain and the POU homeodomain of each monomer is critical. Compared to the Pit1 binding site in the PRL minimum promoter sequences, two additional base pairs spacing are needed to direct restricted GH gene transcription based on elements of two Pit1 binding sites on the proximal promoter of rat *GH* locus.[44]

This dimerization interface is a "hot spot" for debilitating mutations. Additional mutations, like in the *Pit1*^Snell mice, a G-to-T mutation results (W261C) in the third helix of the POU homeodomain, eliminating its DNA-binding ability by altering the contact point of the mutant gene product with the major groove of the responsive elements, causing a dwarf phenotype in an autosomal-recessive fashion. Similarly, several mutations observed in human cases could affect the stability and specificity of this protein-DNA interface.[45,46]

As a transcription factor, Pit1 exerts its effects as a component of a transcriptional complex regulated by coactivator and repressor elements. The Pit1 POU domain can associate with coactivator complex of CBP/p300 and P/CAF, both of which possess histone acetylase activity. N-CoR, acting as a corepressor, can bind to the homeodomain of Pit1 and actively suppress transactivation by Pit1; this suppression depends on Sin3, SAP30, and histone deacetylase. Thus the transcriptional activity of Pit1 may be regulated by the competing binding of complexes mediating either acetylation or deacetylation events, resulting in activation or repression, respectively.[47]

In addition to Pit1, the determination of individual pituitary cell types may require other molecules. The estrogen receptor has been implicated in synergistic activation of the *PRL* gene.[48,49]

Members of the ETS family of transcription factors can bind to Pit1 binding sites in the PRL promoter and mediate signals from growth factors and the Ras/mitogen-activated protein kinase pathway.[50] The transcription factor GATA2 appears to be required for the formation of both thyrotrope and gonadotrope cells; the presence of Pit1 represses the gonadotropic phenotype and promotes the thyrotrope phenotype. Pit1 can inhibit binding of GATA2 to cognate DNA sites important for generation of the gonadotrope phenotype. In contrast, Pit1 leads to synergistic activation with GATA2 on promoters that contain both Pit1 and GATA2 sites.[51]

PROP1 GENE

Prop1 (Prophet of Pit-1) is a homeodomain-containing transcription factor that is capable of binding to its cognate DNA site and activating its target genes. The expression pattern of the *Prop1* gene has been examined in mice and is detected only in Rathke's pouch. *Prop1* expression is detected initially at e10 in the mouse, when the structure of Rathke's pouch has been established. The expression initially is observed dorsally but subsequently involves most cells in Rathke's pouch. Expression of *Prop1* reaches a maximum level of intensity at e12 in Rathke's pouch, with the signal diminishing by e14.5[52] (see Fig. 1-1). It has been shown recently that Notch signaling is required for maintaining high levels of *Prop1* expression at e12.5, which is mediated by Rbp-J protein bound to the evolutionary conserved site within the first intron of the *Prop1* gene.[53] Expression of the *Prop1* gene is required for activation of the downstream *Pit1* gene.[54,55] The integrity of *Prop1* is necessary for full-scale manifestation of pituitary gonadotrope cells, as well as the generation of somatotrope, lactotrope, and thyrotrope cells (see Table 1-2). Mutations in the *Prop1* gene have been identified as the leading cause of familial CPHD, resulting in short stature as a consequence.

Animal Model

The *Prop1* gene was initially identified by a positional cloning strategy in the naturally occurring Ames mouse mutant. The mutant *Prop1* allele at the *Prop1*[Ames] locus harbors a point mutation that results in a single amino acid substitution (S83P) in the second helix of the homeodomain, causing altered progression of nascent pituitary gland and subsequent failed expression of *Pit1*.[52] Phenotypes of the *Prop1*[Ames] mice are transmitted in an autosomal-recessive fashion; heterozygous mutant mice are normal. Homozygous mutant mice are born grossly normal but develop a proportional dwarfism by the time of weaning.[56] The adult mutant mice are about half the size of the wild-type animals. The *Prop1*[Ames] mutation caused dysmorphogenesis of Rathke's pouch at e12.5, with convolution of the lumen and a failure of expression of the *Pit1* lineage. The appearance of gonadotrope was delayed, but corticotrope appeared as expected. In contrast to the complete absence of somatotrope, lactotrope, and thyrotrope cells in the *Pit1*[Snell] mouse, the *Prop1*[Ames] mouse pituitary gland contains a small number (<1%)[54,57] of the normal complement of somatotrope cells, as well as a few lactotrope and thyrotrope cells.[57] *Prop1*[Ames] dwarf mice live twice as long as their wild-type littermates.[58]

Related Diseases

The human *Prop1* coding region has three exons separated by two introns and maps to chromosome 5q34. The *Prop1* gene encodes a polypeptide of 226 amino acids and contains a short N terminus, a 60-amino acid homeodomain, and a transactivating C terminus. Compared to the mouse homologue, the human Prop1 homeodomain is highly conserved, with only two amino acid substitutions.

Initial reports identified mutations in the human *Prop1* gene in patients with short stature in several families. Direct sequencing of polymerase chain reaction (PCR) products of the *Prop1* gene revealed that all the affected patients were harboring mutations in both alleles of the *Prop1* gene, and their parents were heterozygous for the respective mutations, suggesting that the mutations in the *Prop1* gene act in an autosomal-recessive manner, causing CPHD in these patients. All of the affected individuals in this study failed to respond to GHRH, thyrotropin-releasing hormone, and LH-releasing hormone stimulation, suggesting a defect in hormone-secreting cells of the pituitary gland.[59] Subsequent reports have revealed that *Prop1* mutation is a common cause of familial CPHD. These alternations in the *Prop1* gene range from point mutation to deletions, affecting structure and integrity in the homeodomain of the *Prop1* gene. A 2-bp A301G302 deletion, leading to a frame-shift and the loss of DNA-binding homeodomain and C-terminal transactivation domain of the *Prop1* gene product, is the most frequently encountered mutation among these *Prop1* patients, representing a mutational "hot spot."[60] Individuals with various *Prop1* mutations invariably display severe deficiencies for pituitary gonadotropins in addition to the defects of GH, PRL, and TSH levels. In human cases with *Prop1* mutations, many adult patients express ACTH at a normal level; however, there are reported cases with a late onset of corticotropin deficiency (see Table 1-2). The expression of ACTH phenotypes is highly heterogeneous; differences in genetic background in these patients may contribute to the discrepancy of this phenotype.[61,62]

Mechanism

The *Prop1* gene product exerts its actions through binding to the responsive elements of target genes, with the helix-turn-helix motif of the homeodomain providing the contact point for protein-DNA interactions. The fact that most of the naturally occurring mutations of the *Prop1* gene are located in the homeodomain suggests that the Prop1 homeodomain is critical for Prop1 function.

In *Prop1*[Ames] mice, examination of the mutant Rathke's pouch revealed severe dysmorphogenesis, but the pituitary precursor cells were generated. The precursor cells of Rathke's pouch failed to migrate to form the nascent pituitary gland, leading to an expansion of the luminal structure and lack of expression of a late pituitary differentiation marker, the *Pit1* gene. However, proliferation of the mutant precursor cells in the Ames mice continued, resulting in normal-sized pituitary glands.[52,63] In addition to Pit1, both Wnt and Notch pathways are affected in the *Prop1*[Ames] mice.[64,65] Later, persistent expression of *Prop1* under control of the α*GSU* promoter caused decreased gonadotrope differentiation and increased adenomatous hyperplasia,[66,67] indicating that properly extinguishing *Prop1* also may be an important later step in paired-like homeodomain-mediated organogenesis.

Prop1 can bind to its site and activate target genes via the C-terminal transactivation domain, whereas the N terminus and the homeodomain of Prop1 possess repression function,[52,68] suggesting that Prop1 can act as a transcriptional activator as well as a repressor. Recent studies of the pituitary-specific inactivation of the β-catenin gene reveal that a Prop1/β-catenin complex acts as transcriptional activator for *Pit1* and as a repressor for *Hesx1*, depending on the associated co-factors.[69]

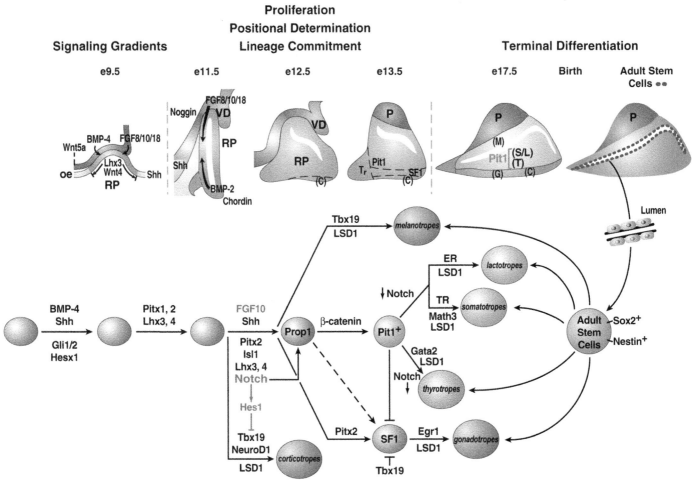

FIGURE 1-2. Ontogeny of signaling molecules and selected transcriptional factors during mouse pituitary organogenesis. Ventral diencephalon, which expresses BMP4, FGF8/10/18, and Wnt5, makes direct contact with oral ectoderm and induces the formation of Rathke's pouch. *Shh* is expressed throughout the oral ectoderm, except in Rathke's pouch, creating a boundary between two ectodermal domains of *Shh*-expressing and nonexpressing cells. The opposing dorsal BMP4/FGF and ventral BMP2/Shh gradients convey proliferative and positional cues by regulating combinatorial patterns of transcription factor gene expression. Pit1 is induced at e13.5 in the caudomedial region of the pituitary gland, which ultimately gives rise to somatotropes (S), lactotropes (L), and thyrotropes (T). Rostral tip thyrotropes (Tr) are Pit1 independent. Corticotropes (C) and gonadotropes (G) are differentiated in the most ventral part of the gland. The dorsal region of Rathke's pouch becomes the intermediate lobe, containing melanotropes (M). The infundibulum grows downward and eventually becomes the posterior lobe (P). A number of transcription factors and cofactors regulating the lineage commitment and terminal differentiation of distinct cell types are illustrated in a genetic pathway. (Modified from Zhu X et al: Signaling and epigenetic regulation of pituitary development. Curr Opin Cell Biol 19(6):605–611, 2007.)

Phenotypic comparisons have been made between the *Prop1*-defective patient and the *Prop1*-mutant *Prop1^Ames* mouse. Deficiencies of GH, PRL, and TSH are consistently observed in both species. All the patients with *Prop1* mutations eventually develop gonadotropin deficiency in their adult lives. In the *Prop1^Ames* mice, the expression of gonadotropin is observed at birth, but the level of expression of the gonadotropin is reduced to one quarter of that of the wild-type animals.[52] The expression of ACTH is apparent during development in the *Prop1^Ames* mouse pituitary, and the level of ACTH in the blood is normal in adults. In human *Prop1* patients, cortisol levels are normal at birth, but some patients develop cortisol deficiency later in life.[70-72] The *Prop1* mutation may affect all the major cell types in the anterior pituitary gland, including the gonadotrope and the corticotrope (see Table 1-2).

HESX1 GENE

Hesx1 (homeodomain gene expressed in ES cells) is a paired-class homeodomain transcription factor that is capable of binding to its cognate DNA site and regulating its target genes. Mutations in the *Hesx1* gene have been identified in septo-optic dysplasia and CPHD. In mice, the earliest expression of the *Hesx1* gene can be detected at the embryonic stem cell stage. High levels of expression can be detected in the ectoderm, subsequently at the anterior extreme of the rostral neural folds, and finally restricted to the ventral diencephalon and to the thickened layer of oral ectoderm, which will give rise to Rathke's pouch at e9.0 in the mouse.[73,74] *Hesx1* gene expression can be observed for 2 more days but only in Rathke's pouch, with diminishing intensity at a time that coincides with the rise of *Prop1* gene expression (Fig. 1-2; also see Fig. 1-1). In humans, strong expression of *Hesx1* in Rathke's pouch can be detected in a 7-week-old embryo. Hesx1 is the earliest molecular marker for the definitive pituitary primordium.

Animal Model

The mouse *Hesx1* gene is located on chromosome 14, and targeted deletion of *Hesx1* resulted in mice that exhibited variable anterior central nervous system defects with reduced prosencephalon and defective olfactory development.[75] Hesx1 mutants also have defects in the pituitary gland, with bifurcations in Rathke's pouch in most cases. By e12.5, multiple oral ectoderm invaginations reflecting pituitary glands are observed in most Hesx1 embryos. Between e13.5 and e15.5, Hesx1 mutants are characterized by a dramatic cellular over-proliferation of all the hormone-producing cell types, leading to a failure of the underlying mesenchyme to condense and form the sphenoid cartilage that separates the pituitary from the oral cavity. In the late stages of pituitary development, the terminal differentiation of the hormone-producing cell types appear normal in most Hesx1 mutants, with overexpression of αGSU, TSHβ, GH, POMC, and Pit1 by e16.5. Earlier in development, there is a delay in the onset of POMC expression both in Rathke's pouch and in the developing hypothalamus at e12.5, and there also appears to be a dual induction of αGSU expression on both the rostral and caudal sides of Rathke's pouch. Strikingly, in occasional Hesx1 gene–deleted mice, the initial thickening of oral ectoderm and minimal activation of Lhx3 are observed at e12.5, but the embryos exhibit a complete arrest of pituitary development, and the pituitary gland is absent by e18.5. The discrepancy of incomplete phenotype penetrance in Hesx1 mutants is likely influenced by the actions of the linked modifier genes.[76,77]

Related Diseases

The human Hesx1 gene contains four exons separated by three introns, and it maps to chromosome 3p21. The Hesx1 gene encodes a highly conserved polypeptide of 185 amino acids with a 60-amino acid homeodomain at its C terminus. Initial analyses of the Hesx1 mutations carried out in kindreds with septo-optic dysplasia identified a nucleotide transition that resulted in the substitution of R160C (in the third helix of the homeodomain) in two children with CPHD born to a highly consanguineous family. Magnetic resonance imaging revealed an ectopic/undescended posterior pituitary associated with a hypoplastic anterior lobe in these two affected siblings.[75] None of the heterozygote parents exhibited features of septo-optic dysplasia, consistent with an autosomal-recessive inheritance. Additional mutations (e.g., Q6H, S170L, T181A, I26T, and 306/307InsAG-X) have been found in the coding region of the Hesx1 gene and are associated with variable phenotypes, including hypopituitarism, ranging from isolated GH deficiency to CPHD. It is clear from these reported cases that mutation in the Hesx1 gene can cause pituitary hormone deficiency with variable phenotypes and with incomplete penetrance.[78,79]

Mechanism

The Hesx1 gene product can bind to either dimer or monomer DNA sites with high affinity in transient transfection assays.[80,81] Modular structure analysis revealed that in addition to the DNA-binding homeodomain, Hesx1 contains two sequences in the N terminus; one is similar to the eh1 motif found in Drosophila engrailed, and one is similar to the WRPW motif found in several helix-loop-helix proteins, both of which are capable of recruiting the Groucho class of corepressors.[82,83] Both the N-terminal and homeodomain regions of Hesx1 can independently act as repressors. Hesx1 is a strong transcriptional repressor that acts by recruiting the mSin3A/B, HDACs 1 and 2, and the Brg1 complexes to its homeodomain and the TLE corepressor to its eh1 domain. The strong association between Tle1 and Hesx1 is mediated by a highly conserved helical motif (FXLXXIL) present in the Hesx1 N terminus, which can also be found in Nkx, Six, and certain Pax homeodomain factors' family members.[84] These recruitments are required and sufficient for the repressive actions of Hesx1 in vivo. Forced persistent expression of Hesx1 and Tle1 resulted in the loss of the Pit1 lineage and a Prop1^{Ames}-like dysmorphogenesis, while the expression of Prop1 and POMC remained. The mutation in human Hesx1 (R160C) has a dominant negative effect both in vitro and in vivo. This dominant negative activity requires the eh1 repression domain, which is also required for full-length recombinant Hesx1 dimerization in solution. This dominant transcription repressor activity may help to explain the heterozygous phenotypes observed in Hesx1 patients.[80] Recent identification of a homozygous mutation in the eh1 motif (I26T) in a patient with CPHD has further underlined that Tle association is an integral mechanism for Hesx1 function in vivo.[85]

Hesx1 and Prop1 share a conserved DNA-recognition site. The repression domain in Hesx1 can suppress the transcription activation activity of Prop1. The Hesx1 repressor can heterodimerize with Prop1 and can bind to the palindromic site as homodimers or heterodimers, with Prop1 acting as an activator and Hesx1 as a repressor, to inhibit Prop1 activation function. The expression of Prop1 is elevated in Hesx1-mutant mice, suggesting not only that Hesx1 can repress Prop1 activation function but also that it is required for proper Prop1 expression.[76] Forced early expression of Prop1 to the uncommitted oral ectoderm blocks the formation of Rathke's pouch, which results in absence of the anterior pituitary gland with no initial induction of Lhx3 expression, demonstrating that premature expression of Prop1 can block the pituitary organogenesis that phenocopies the effects of Hesx1-gene deletion,[15] in contrast to the Hesx1/Tle1 transgenic mouse with a Prop1^{Ames}-like phenotype, suggesting that the antagonistic repressor complex can suppress Prop1 activation of expression.[76] The sequential repression and activation of a common set of regulatory genes may prove to be an underlying strategy in the temporal code of pituitary organ development, with initial repression required for organ commitment and proliferation and subsequent activation required for commitment of specific cell lineages.[69]

LHX3 AND *LHX4* GENES

Lhx3 (LIM homeo box gene 3) is a LIM-type homeodomain transcription factor. In addition to a C-terminus homeodomain, Lhx3 contains two tandem repeats of LIM zinc-binding motifs, each composed of 50 to 60 amino acids with a conserved pattern of cysteine and histidine residues that form a pair of zinc fingers, separated by a linker of 2 amino acids. Expression analysis revealed that mouse Lhx3 mRNA can be detected in the developing nervous system and accumulates in Rathke's pouch beginning at e9.5 (see Fig. 1-1). Lhx3 remains expressed in the entire pouch, and its expression is maintained through e15.5; the expression is particularly strong in the anterior and intermediate lobes of the adult pituitary. In addition, Lhx3 is expressed bilaterally along the spinal cord and the hindbrain at early stages of development.[86]

Structurally, Lhx4 (LIM homeodomain gene 4) is closely related to Lhx3. The Lhx gene family consists of at least 12 members; many of them are expressed in the pituitary during development, including Isl1, Isl2, Lhx2, Lhx3, and Lhx4. Lhx3 and Lhx4 have been genetically defined as required elements for both the early stages of pituitary determination and the later differentiation of pituitary cell types. By insitu hybridization, the Lhx4 gene is found to be expressed transiently in ventrolateral regions of the neural tube and the hindbrain of the developing mouse.

During pituitary development, *Lhx4* is expressed throughout the invaginating Rathke's pouch at e9.5. At e12.5, *Lhx4* expression becomes restricted to the future anterior lobe of the pituitary gland, and by e15.5, *Lhx4* expression diminishes. In the adult pituitary, *Lhx4* is found in the anterior and intermediate lobes at a much lower level than that of *Lhx3*.[87]

Animal Model

Employing a reverse genetic approach, mice with a targeted disruption in the *Lhx3* gene were generated. Mice heterozygous for the mutation are apparently normal and fertile, whereas homozygous individuals are stillborn or expire within 24 hours of birth. In these homozygous mice, the hindbrain, spinal cord, and pineal gland are grossly normal, as is the posterior lobe of the pituitary, but the anterior and intermediate lobes of the pituitary are absent. During embryonic development, the mutant animal exhibits a lack of growth in Rathke's pouch, and pituitary-gland development does not progress beyond the Rathke's pouch stage. With the exception of residual corticotrope, other anterior pituitary cell types are absent, indicating that *Lhx3* is required for the appearance of the somatotrope, lactotrope, thyrotrope, and gonadotrope cell types.[88]

Mice homozygous for the targeted deletion of the *Lhx4* gene exhibit an early postnatal death due to a failure of pulmonary maturation.[87] *Lhx4*-deleted mice have a well-formed Rathke's pouch but display incomplete pituitary development following this stage, and the differentiation of pituitary cell types is perturbed. Consequently, by e12.5, there exists a miniature Rathke's pouch, and by e14.5, the nascent pituitary structure has progressed to a larger pouch, but the anterior lobe is discernible only as a slight thickening in the ventral region. This hypocellularity of the anterior lobe is caused by failure of pituitary precursor cells to survive; large numbers of apoptotic cells are evident throughout the pituitary primordia of *Lhx4*-mutant mice at e12.5.[89] In later gestation stages, Rathke's pouch is hypoplastic, with an enlarged lumen resulting from reduced proliferation of the precursors, and the anterior lobe of the pituitary is reduced in size. Expression analyses have revealed residual amounts of LH- and GNRHR-positive cells at e18.5. Thus, *Lhx4* is not required for specification of gonadotrope cells, but it does support the expansion of the cell population. Similarly, all five anterior pituitary–specific cell lineages are present in the *Lhx4*-mutant pituitary but in dramatically reduced numbers. By contrast, the intermediate-lobe melanotrope cells are undisturbed.

Mice with double deletion of *Lhx3* and *Lhx4* demonstrated that both genes direct formation of the pituitary gland.[90] The early formation of the Rathke's pouch rudiment from pituitary primordium does not depend entirely on the function of either *Lhx3* or *Lhx4* alone, but together these genes redundantly control the formation of the definitive pouch. *Lhx3* also controls a subsequent step of pituitary fate commitment, and in these early stages, *Lhx4* appears to act upstream of the *Lhx3* and *Isl1* genes and is required for expansion of Rathke's pouch. Therefore, *Lhx3* and *Lhx4* dictate pituitary gland identity by controlling decision points of organogenesis and regulation of the proliferation and differentiation of pituitary-specific cell lineages.

Related Diseases

Human *Lhx3* shares a high degree of homology with its mouse orthologue, exhibiting 94% identity at the amino acid level. *Lhx3* is located on human chromosome 9q34 and spans a genomic fragment of at least 6 kb that includes 6 exons.[91,92] In a candidate-gene screen based on pituitary phenotypes observed in a reces-

sive lethal mutation in mice, two mutations in the *Lhx3* gene were identified in two unrelated consanguineous pedigrees that display CPHD.[93] In one family, affected individuals are homozygous for a Y116C mutation located in the highly conserved LIM2 domain of Lhx3, a domain critical for protein-protein interactions. In the second family, affected individuals are homozygous for a 23-base-pair deletion in an intragenic region, predicting a severely truncated protein that lacks the entire homeodomain and rendering it incapable of DNA binding. Lhx3-defective patients have deficiencies in GH, TSH, PRL, FSHβ, and LHβ, but they display intact levels of ACTH, similar to the endocrine profiles observed in *Prop1* patients (see Table 1-2). In addition, these Lhx3-defective patients displayed a rigid cervical spine that restricted their head rotation. More recently, novel 6 mutations have been found in the coding region of the *Lhx3* gene.[94,95] All of them are associated with variable phenotype of hypopituitarism. *Lhx3* mutations are a rare cause of CPHD involving deficiencies for GH, prolactin, TSH, and LH/FSH in all patients. Whereas most patients have a severe hormone deficiency manifesting after birth, milder forms can be observed, and limited neck rotation is not a universal feature of patients with *Lhx3* mutations.

The human *Lhx4* gene encodes a 390-amino acid protein that contains two LIM domains and a homeodomain that shares 99% sequence identity with its mouse orthologue. Genomic analysis revealed that the human *Lhx4* gene contains 6 exons and is mapped to chromosome 1q25.[96] In a large consanguineous pedigree of three generations, a G-to-C substitution in the intron preceding exon 5 of *Lhx4* generates a mutant protein with perturbed homeodomain, which affects its DNA-binding function. Patients with this disease have short stature with CPHD, which affects GH, thyroxine, and cortisol, as well as cerebellar defects and abnormalities of the sella turcica. This mutant allele is transmitted in a dominant fashion, affecting only the maternal side of the kindred with a high phenotypic penetrance.[96] More recently, three novel mutations in the *Lhx4* gene have been mapped.[97] All of them affect the DNA-binding domain, and all of them are associated with CPHD.

Mechanism

LIM homeodomain proteins are transcription factors and exert their effects by regulating target gene expression. Lhx3 binds with high affinity to AT-rich DNA sequences (including minor groove interaction) and bends the DNA molecule to an angle of 62 degrees in a model system.[92] Lhx3 can activate the regulatory regions of pituitary genes, including αGSU, PRL, TSHβ, and Pit1. *Lhx3* expression is partially regulated by the *Lhx4* gene during pituitary development. At e12.5, only a few cells express *Lhx3* in the dorsal-most aspect of the pouch in the *Lhx4* mutants. However, the normal pattern of *Lhx3* expression, including the dorsal-ventral gradient, is established in *Lhx4* mutants by e14.5.[89]

Genetic analysis revealed that *Lhx4* interacts with *Prop1* to stimulate anterior pituitary lobe expansion. Neither gene is essential for initiating corticotrope specification. However, no POMC or αGSU expression is detected in double-mutant mice at e14.5, suggesting that *Prop1* and *Lhx4* have overlapping roles in corticotrope and gonadotrope development.[89] In *Hesx1*-deleted mutants, the domains of *Lhx3* and *Prop1* expression are increased, as well as those of *FGF8* and *FGF10* in the infundibulum, which become expanded rostrally.[76] These findings indicate that *Hesx1* is required for maintaining the proper expression of *FGFs*, consistent with the notion that *Lhx3* expression can be regulated by FGF signaling.

TBX19 GENE

Tbx19 is a T-box transcription factor family member (the T-box in the mouse T [*Brachyury*] gene) that encodes a 448-amino acid protein.[98] Functional identification of *Tbx19* was established after the observation of elements in a critical *cis*-acting sequence in the POMC promoter. Transcripts of *Tbx19* can be found only in the anterior and intermediate pituitary and brain (see Fig. 1-1); *Tbx19* is specifically required for continued *POMC* transcription.[99,100]

Animal Model

Mice with targeted disruption of the *Tbx19* gene have been generated. Mice heterozygous for the mutation are apparently normal. Adult mice homozygous for the mutation have very few ACTH-positive cells in the pituitary, although initial expression of the *POMC* gene is undisturbed at the Rathke's pouch stages. These cells are born in normal quantities in mutants but are lost or fail to expand appropriately, suggesting *Tbx19* is not required for corticotrope cell commitment but is later important for *POMC* lineage differentiation. The intermediate-lobe melanotropes in mutant mice are populated by gonadotrope and some Pit1-independent thyrotrope, also indicating that *Tbx19* normally represses pituitary gonadotrope differentiation.[101,102]

Related Diseases

The human *Tbx19* gene shares 94% amino acid identity with that of mouse *Tbx19* and maps to chromosome 1q23-q24. Several cases of isolated ACTH deficiency were identified with a nonsense mutation C-to-T transition in exon 6 in *Tbx19*, resulting in a truncated gene product (R286X).[103] The transmission of this mutation appears to be recessive. In another case of isolated ACTH deficiency, a heterozygous C-to-T transition in exon 2 of the *Tbx19* gene was identified, resulting in a conserved amino acid S128F mutation, suggesting a dominant negative inheritance.[99] More recent study revealed new mutation in the *Tbx19* gene (missense M86R) that did not affect monomer DNA-binding activity per se, but it impaired DNA binding with other DNA-bound proteins, including itself (homodimers) and Pitx1, resulting in congenital isolated ACTH deficiency.[104] Additional mutations in the *Tbx19* gene have been shown to be a cause of neonatal death due to neonatal-onset isolated ACTH deficiency.[103] *Tbx19* defects result in POMC deficiency in both humans and mice, establishing *Tbx19* as the gene required for effective *POMC* expression in vivo.[101,102]

Mechanism

Tbx19 is a transcriptional regulator, recognizing target genes through its T-box DNA-binding domain. In response to signals elicited by the hypothalamic hormone corticotrope-releasing hormone, Tbx19 functions as an activator of transcription by recruiting SRC/p160 coactivators to its cognate DNA target in the POMC promoter.[105] Tbx19 can synergize with orphan nuclear receptor NGFI-B, serving as part of the transcription regulatory complex on the POMC promoter in response to hormonal stimulation.[106] Transgenic expression of *Tbx19* in non-POMC-producing regions of the pituitary gland can cause ectopic *POMC* expression,[99] and *Tbx19* is an inhibitor of αGSU expression in rostral tip cells, gonadotrope, and thyrotrope, and of TSHβ production in caudomedial thyrotrope.[100] *Tbx19* deficiency is permissive for transdifferentiation of cells normally destined to be corticotrope and melanotrope into alternative cell fates, namely, gonadotrope and rostral tip thyrotrope, suggesting a determina-

tive role of *Tbx19* in cell lineage specification. *Tbx19* defects have no effect on differentiation of *Pit1*-dependent cell lineages (see Figs. 1-1 and 1-2, and Table 1-2).[101,102]

PITX1 AND *PITX2* GENES

Pitx1 and Pitx2 represent two of the bicoid-related Pitx homeodomain transcription factors. They display distinct but overlapping patterns of expression and are critical in the development of several organs, including the pituitary, with Pitx1 required for the gonadotrope, thyrotrope, and *POMC* gene expression[107,108] and Pitx2 required for the earliest phases of pituitary development for the patterning and proliferation events within Rathke's pouch.[109-111] Genetic studies have shown that they are required for cell proliferation, survival, and differentiation in a dosage-sensitive manner, with Pitx2 playing a more prominent role than Pitx1. They both function redundantly in controlling *Lhx3* expression.[111-113]

Animal Model

Inactivation of Pitx1 results in defects in hindlimb development and craniofacial morphogenesis.[108,114] The anterior pituitaries of mutant mice exhibit mild defects with decreased expression of FSHβ, LHβ, and TSHβ and increased expression of POMC. *Pitx2*-/- mice display multiple developmental defects, including failure of body-wall closure, right pulmonary isomerism, and defects in heart, tooth, eye, and pituitary organogenesis.[109,115-117] In the pituitary, a definite pouch forms with induction of Lhx3, Hesx1, Pitx1, and αGSU. However, the gland fails to progress further, with no Pit1 induction and only a few POMC-positive corticotrophes. Transgenic mice overexpressing *Pitx2* in the cornea manifest ocular defects similar to Rieger's syndrome, suggesting that excess Pitx2 activity can be as deleterious to eye development as a loss of function.[118] Overexpression of *Pitx2* during mouse forelimb development results in severe tendon, muscle, and bone anomalies.[119] A small fraction of *Pitx2*-heterozygous mice display some aspects of Rieger's syndrome.

Related Diseases

The *Pitx2* gene was initially identified as the gene responsible for human Rieger's syndrome type I, an autosomal dominant condition characterized by variable defects, including anomalies of the anterior chamber of the eye, dental hypoplasia, a protuberant umbilicus, mental retardation, and isolated growth hormone deficiency.[110] Most of the mutations in *Pitx2* cause defects in DNA binding, transactivation, or both, whereas a single hypermorphic allele of *Pitx2* (V45L) leads to a reduced DNA-binding but an enhanced transactivation activity.[120,121] To date, no mutations within *Pitx1* have been described in humans.

Mechanism

Pitx1 was identified on the basis of its ability to interact with the N-terminal transactivation domain of Pit1[122] and to bind POMC promoter.[123] Synergistic interactions between Pitx1 and Pit-1 activate the *PRL*[122] and the *TSHβ* genes; those with the dimer NeuroD1/E47[124] and Tbx19[99] activate *POMC* expression; and those with SF-1[125] and Egr-1[126] activate the *LHβ* gene. Pitx1 is also able to stimulate the expression of genes coding for the gonadotropin-releasing hormone receptor (GRHR) and Pit-1.[127]

OTHER TRANSCRIPTION FACTORS

Transcription factors act as activators and repressors and often are expressed in a coordinated fashion, mediating organogenesis and cell type specification in the pituitary gland (see Figs 1-1 and 1-2). During the early commitment stage, expression of *Pitx1/2* and *Hesx1* are found in the anterior neural plate stages and in the invagination of Rathke's pouch. *Lhx3* is expressed on e9.5 in the nascent RP and is required for initial organ commitment and growth[88] and for cell proliferation, together with *Lhx4*.[89] *Prop1* appears on e10.5 and is required for determination of four ventral cell types, including the *Pit1*-dependent lineages (somatotrope, lactotrope, and thyrotrope) and the gonadotrope.[52,59] Sequential expression of this cascade of homeodomain genes represents a model system of transcription control of organogenesis and cell type determination and differentiation in mammals. Phenotypic comparisons in these pituitary loci in both mice and humans suggest that the developmental pathways in determination of the pituitary gland are highly conserved.

Some of these factors express transiently in Rathke's pouch, and their reduced expression is likely to be required for the progression of specific cell types, as evident in the *Prop1*[Ames] mutant, where the temporal patterns of *Hesx1, Prop1,* and *Brn4* gene expression are extended. As the lineage-determining transcription factor Pit1 appears, certain transcription factors that characterize earlier stages of development are gradually eliminated, including Hesx1, Pfrk,[15] GATA-2,[51] Pax6,[128] and Brn4.[129]

The list of pituitary-expressed transcription factors implicated in the developing pituitary gland is constantly expanding. Several families of factors, including homeodomain factors (Isl1, Isl2, Oct1, Otx2, Pax6, Pitx3, Six1, Six3, and Six6), zinc-finger (Krox24, Gli1, GATA2, Nzf1, Sp1, Sp3, Zfhep, and Zn16), nuclear receptor (T3R, SF1, ERa, ERb, and Dax), basic HLH domain (AP2, NeuroD, Mash1, Nhlh2, and Math3) and other (Gli2, AP1, Ets1, Foxl2, CBf, Cp1, Rb, Men1, Preb, and Tef) (see reviews [130,131]). Multiple members of the Six family (*Six1, Six6, Six2,* and *Six3*) are also expressed in the pituitary. Six6, acting as a strong tissue-specific repressor in association with dachshund (Dach) corepressors, directly represses cyclin-dependent kinase inhibitors, including the p27[Kip1] promoter, and regulates early progenitor cell proliferation in retinogenesis and pituitary development.[132] Six1 exhibits synergistic genetic interactions with the eyes absent (Eya) family of protein phosphatases and is required to regulate genes that encode growth control and modulate precursor cell proliferation. The phosphatase activity of Eya converts the function of Six1-Dach from repression to activation, causing transcriptional activation through recruitment of coactivators.[133] Evidence suggests that Six3 acts upstream of the Wnt pathway, and deletion of *Six3* in mice resulted in failure of development of the ventral diencephalon and, consequently, development of the pituitary.[134] GATA2 is involved in establishing molecular memory of signaling gradients during pituitary development in conjunction with *Pit1*, and loss of *GATA2* is associated with failure to differentiate into gonadotrope.[51,111] The orphan nuclear receptor steroidogenic factor 1, Sf1, is essential for pituitary gonadotrope.[135] Mice with simultaneous inactivation of both *Gli1* and *Gli2* have very severe defects in pituitary gland development; about half of these mutants completely lack a Rathke's pouch at e12.5. In these mutants, the domains of expression of *Shh* and *Nkx2.1* are abnormal, and the loss of Shh signaling boundary in the oral ectoderm could be a cause of this defect.[136] Gli2 is an upstream regulator of Lhx3 (see Fig. 1-2). One consequence of the *Gli2* defect in *yot*-mutant Zebrafish embryos was the absence of *Lhx3* expression in the anterior part of the adenohypophysis anlage.[137] In the mouse, absence of *Lhx3* results in failure of development of Rathke's pouch into the adenohypophysis.

Otx1 is expressed in the postnatal pituitary gland. Cell culture experiments have shown that *Otx1* may activate transcription of GH, FSHβ, βLH, and αGSU. Analysis of *Otx1*-null mice indicates that at the prepubescent stage, they exhibit transient dwarfism and hypogonadism due to low levels of pituitary GH, FSHβ and LHβ hormones, which in turn dramatically affect downstream molecular and organ targets. Nevertheless, *Otx1*-/- mice gradually recover from most of these abnormalities, showing normal levels of pituitary hormones with restored growth and gonadal functions at 4 months of age. Since the patterns of expression of hypothalamic hormone-releasing hormones (GHRH, GnRH) and their pituitary receptors (GHRHR, GnRHR) are unchanged, it seems that ability to synthesize GH, FSHβ, and LHβ, rather than the number of cells producing these hormones, is affected.[138]

Because *Otx2*-null mice exhibit early embryonic lethality,[139] Otx2 protein has been only recently shown to play a role in pituitary development. Clinical study of one patient has revealed a new heterozygous *Otx2* mutation that is affecting the transactivation domain of *Otx2* and subsequent lack of activation of *Hesx1* and *Pit1* promoters in cell culture transfection assay.[140] Heterozygous *Otx2* knockout mice have highly variable brain and ocular phenotypes, and although pituitary structure and function have not been studied, this recent study might implicate more attention for the role of Otx2 protein in the pituitary.

Although pituitary cell types in the adult anterior lobe do not appear to be stratified, initial appearance of these cell types follows a ventral-dorsal pattern. With the Rathke's pouch cleft as the dorsal reference, GH, PRL, and TSHβ of *Pit1* lineages are located dorsally, whereas gonadotrope cells appear ventrally. Several transcription factors display vertical gradients, including Pax6, which exhibits a dorsal-to-ventral expression gradient; *Pax6*-mutant mice exhibit increased numbers of ventral thyrotrope and gonadotrope, at the expense of the more dorsal somatotrope and lactotrope cell types.[128] Thus *Pax6* may functionally oppose Shh signaling to specify a dorsal rather than ventral cell fate. Another pituitary transcription factor displaying an initial dorsal-ventral gradient is Prop1 (see Fig. 1-1). *Prop1*-mutant mice lose dorsal cell types of the *Pit1* lineage, while ventral cell types of corticotrope and gonadotrope are less affected.

The induction of expression of transcription factors in spatially overlapping patterns in the developing pituitary may act as a molecular memory of prior signals in the positional determination of specific cell types. The signaling pathways that dictate expression patterns of transcription factor are the focus of current research application, with several classes of early morphogenic gradients of broadly expressed signaling molecules likely to be critical elements of pituitary cell type determination and differentiation.

Signaling Pathways in Pituitary Development

Vertebrate organogenesis events are coordinated through the interplay of highly organized signaling pathways, and these developmental signaling systems have proved to be remarkably conserved throughout evolution.[141] Extrinsic signals, in the form of secreted morphogens, create local environments for organ patterning and progenitor cell type determination. These signals are interpreted through the functions of cell type–restricted transcriptional regulators, resulting in various intrinsic or cell-autonomous determination events.[142] Numerous extrinsic signaling molecules have been implicated, including members of the Hh, transforming growth factor-beta (TGFβ)/bone morphogenic protein (BMP), Wingless/Wnt, and fibroblast growth factor (FGF) superfamilies, the Notch pathway, and others (reviewed in ref. 143).

Influenced by the growth of the forebrain structures, the midline anterior neural ridge cells ultimately responsible for the origin of the pituitary gland are displaced and eventually become located immediately ventral to the diencephalons. The initial extrinsic signaling of murine pituitary development requires signals from both the ventral diencephalon and the oral ectoderm. Organogenesis of the anterior pituitary gland begins at e9 in the mouse as the cells of the anterior pituitary placode in the oral ectoderm thicken and invaginate to form the nascent pituitary of Rathke's pouch.[19] Shh, seemingly uniformly expressed in the oral epithelia at the time, is excluded from the pituitary placode prior to initiation of the invagination.[144] The presumptive ventral diencephalon provides Bmp4, the first known dorsal signal required for the initial formation of Rathke's pouch.[18] Immediately following formation, the dorsal portion of Rathke's pouch directly contacts the midline ventral diencephalon, which evaginates at e10 and acts as a key organizing center for the patterning and commitment of Rathke's pouch. Opposing dorsal FGFs/Bmp4 and ventral Shh/Bmp2 gradients provide positional and proliferative signals to the pituitary progenitor field, acting to positionally establish cell types through the induction of overlapping patterns of transcription factor expression.[15,18] Initial proliferation and determination is controlled by sequential cascades of exogenously and endogenously restricted combinatorial signaling, with subsequent attenuation of specific signal events required for establishment of the cellular environment permissive for terminal differentiation (see Fig. 1-2).[2]

SONIC HEDGEHOGS

Shh, one of three vertebrate homologues of the Drosophila-secreted protein Hh, plays an important role in embryo patterning, as well as in the specification of different cell types and in the control of proliferation of numerous cell types.[145] In the early embryo, it is expressed in Hensen's node, the floor plate of the neural tube, the posterior of the limb buds, and throughout the notochord. The mouse, zebrafish, and human Shh homologues are highly conserved,[146] suggesting conserved functional properties. The human Shh gene encodes a predicted protein that is 92.4% identical to its mouse homologue and is mapped to chromosome 7q. Many Shh mutations, including nonsense and missense, deletions, and insertion mutations, are identified throughout the gene in patients with holoprosencephaly, the most common forebrain defect in humans.

Mouse mutants homozygous for a disrupted Shh gene, similarly to the mutations in human patients, revealed defects in the establishment of maintenance of midline structures such as the notochord, floor plate, and cyclopia.[147] In mice, Shh is expressed in ventral diencephalons and throughout the oral ectoderm on e8 but is excluded from the invaginating Rathke's pouch. The Hh receptor Patched1 is expressed in the developing pituitary, indicating that pituitary progenitors respond to the Hh signaling. Transgenic overexpression of hedgehog-interacting protein (HIP), which acts to attenuate Hh function, specifically blocks Hh signaling in the oral ectoderm and Rathke's pouch within the head region, affecting both proliferation and cell type determination, and this results in an absence of ventral cell type markers in Rathke's pouch.[144] In contrast, a gain-of-function transgenic

approach to overexpress Shh in Rathke's pouch results in a phenotype of the expansion of ventral cell types, with modified levels of Lhx3 gene expression. This phenotype is consistent with results derived from an animal cap explant culture with banded Hh in Xenopus laevis, in which the expression domains of pituitary-restricted factor Hesx1 are expanded,[148] supporting a role for Shh signaling in control of proliferative events in pituitary development.[9]

Three related zinc finger transcription factors, Gli1, Gli2, and Gli3, acting downstream of the Shh pathway, are expressed in the developing Rathke's pouch.[149] In zebrafish, Shh produced by neuroectoderm instead of notochord or oral ectoderm is crucial for the initial patterning of the pituitary placode.[150] Mutations that disrupt Hh signaling, like smoothened[smu] and gli2[yot], result in the development of lens tissue from the presumptive pituitary. In addition, in gli2[yot] mutants, the rostral expression domains (analogous to the ventral domains in mice) of pituitary-specific transcription factors such as LIM3 (Lhx3) and Six3 are lost, and other pituitary-restricted factors such as nk2.2 are absent.[137] This observation is consistent with the sequential and cooperative interaction Bmps and Hh exert in limb and neural-tube development,[151] in which Shh acts to induce the expression of Bmps. Overexpression of Shh in zebrafish results in expanded adenohypophyseal expression of lhx3, expansion of nk2.2 into the posterior adenohypophysis, and an increase in PRL- and somatolactin-secreting cells. In addition, Hh signaling is necessary between 10 and 15 hours post fertilization for induction of the zebrafish adenohypophysis, a time when Shh is expressed only in adjacent neural tissue. These results suggest multiple and distinct roles for Hh signaling in the formation of the vertebrate pituitary gland and also suggest that Hh signaling from neural ectoderm of ventral diencephalons is necessary for induction and functional patterning of the vertebrate pituitary gland.[9,150]

FIBROBLAST GROWTH FACTORS

Fibroblast growth factors represent a large family of secreted molecules. Upon binding to their cognate receptors, FGFs activate signal transduction pathways which are required for multiple developmental processes.[152,153] Functions of FGFs are mediated by four distinct FGF-receptor tyrosine kinase molecules. FGF activity and specificity are further regulated by heparan sulfate oligosaccharides with tissue-specific modifications, in the form of a trimolecular complex with receptors.[154,155] The FGF system plays significant roles in many biologic events, including pattern formation in many tissues during vertebrate embryogenesis. Several members of the FGF family are expressed in the infundibulum and provide proliferative and positional cues to Rathke's pouch. FGF8 and FGF10 are expressed in a temporally and spatially overlapping manner within the infundibulum as an evagination of ventral diencephalon makes direct contact with the dorsal portion of Rathke's pouch following Bmp4 induction.

In mice null for FGF10 or the FGFR2 (IIIb) isoform, which presumably would abolish FGF signaling including that of FGF10,[156,157] Rathke's pouch forms but rapidly undergoes apoptosis, with the pituitary becoming completely absent by e14.5, suggesting a critical role in FGF10 signaling for the continued proliferation of the pouch ectoderm. A similar observation has been made in transgenic mice expressing a dominant negative form of FGFR2(IIIb), suggesting that FGF10 signaling is essential for cell survival and proliferation.

FGF8 is expressed in the primitive streak of the gastrulating mouse embryo, as well as in the visceral endoderm. Mice null for *FGF8* lack all embryonic mesoderm- and endoderm-derived structures and do not survive beyond e9.5.[158,159] Therefore, function of *FGF8* in pituitary development is largely drawn from studies of transgenic animals and in-vitro organ culture. In mice null for a homeodomain gene *Nkx2.1*, which is normally expressed in the ventral diencephalons but not in Rathke's pouch, *FGF8* fails to be expressed in the ventral diencephalons, leading to a loss of the infundibulum and consequently a loss of *Lhx3* expression in Rathke's pouch and the loss of all three lobes of the pituitary gland.[160] In transgenic mice misexpressing *FGF8* in the ventral regions of the pituitary under control of the regulatory sequences for the *αGSU* gene, most ventral and intermediate cell types are absent, with dysmorphogenesis of Rathke's pouch and hyperplasia of corticotrope and melanotrope observed, consistent with a role in the positional determination of dorsally arising pituitary cell types and pituitary progenitor cells.[15] In mice null for *Hesx1*, the most severely affected embryos exhibit a complete arrest of pituitary development after the initial induction of Lhx3 on e9.5, with *FGF8* and *FGF10* ectopically expressed in the oral ectoderm to mirror the normal expression in the overlying neural ectoderm. In *Hesx1* mutants with less severe pituitary defects, *FGF* expression is abnormally extended rostrally, causing formation of multiple Rathke's pouches. This is potentially significant because transgenic misexpression of *FGF8* in the oral ectoderm well before the initial invagination of Rathke's pouch produces an identical blockage of pouch formation, and *Hesx1* fails to be expressed in the *Lhx3*-positive rudiment that does form in the transgenic embryos. Thus the dynamic interplay between boundaries of *Hesx* and *FGF8/10* expression[76] could suggest a model of reciprocal feedback regulation. This is in keeping with the role of FGFs in committing oral ectoderm to the Rathke's pouch fate.[160] These genetic data, in conjunction with tissue co-culture evidence, where the infundibulum is both required and sufficient for the induction of *Lhx3* gene expression in cultured pouch and infundibulum activity, can be replaced with FGF8 or FGF2 and inhibited by the FGF receptor antagonist, suggest an instructive role for FGF8 signaling in pituitary development.[2,18,161]

TRANSFORMING GROWTH FACTORS AND BMPs

The transforming growth factor-beta superfamily of secreted signaling molecules, which includes several Bmps, has been demonstrated to play critical roles in patterning and cell type specification in several species.[162] At least two members of the Bmp family, Bmp2 and Bmp4, participate in the development of the anterior pituitary. During the early stages of pituitary development, *Bmp4* is expressed in the ventral diencephalons as the infundibulum makes direct contact with Rathke's pouch at e9.0. Functional evidence with dual explants culture of embryonic diencephalon and Rathke's pouch suggests that Bmp4 is one of the early signaling factors required for the initial commitment of a subpopulation of oral ectodermal cells to form the pituitary gland.[15,18] Deletion of the *Bmp4* gene causes embryonic death at about e10, in which the initial invagination of Rathke's pouch fails to occur.[160] Similarly, driven by the regulatory sequences of the *Pitx1* gene to target the *Bmp2/4* antagonist *Noggin* expression to the oral ectoderm, including Rathke's pouch, pituitary development is arrested at e10, with a failure of the ventral proliferation of cells from the pouch beginning at e11.5 and an absence of pituitary cell types.[15] The phenotype observed in *Pitx1-Noggin* transgenic mice is similar to the phenotype observed in mice with a targeted disruption of the *Lhx3* gene critical for the determination of most pituitary cell types,[88] suggesting a requirement

of Bmp4 signaling for the continued organ development after pouch formation. Together with the ventral diencephalic FGFs, Bmp4 is required for initial pituitary commitment and for continued cell proliferation and progression.

Expression of *Bmp2* is initially detected at the ventral boundary between Rathke's pouch and *Shh*, intrinsic to the pouch in the most ventral aspect of the invaginating gland at e9.5, and in a ventral-dorsal gradient at e10.5.[15] *Bmp2* expression expands throughout the pouch by e12.5. *Bmp2* expression is also detected in the ventral juxtapituitary mesenchyme, along with *Bmp2/4* antagonist Chordin in the caudal mesenchyme, potentially serving to maintain a ventrodorsal Bmp2 gradient. After the closure of Rathke's pouch, *Bmp2* is expressed in mesenchyme adjacent to the pituitary cells expressing ventrally the transcription factors GATA2, Isl1, and the hormone subunit αGSU. Similarly, cultivation of Rathke's pouch explants in Bmp2 is sufficient for the induction of expression of ventral markers such as Isl1 and αGSU.[18] In the developing pituitary expression of *Bmp2* decreases dramatically after e14-e15. Overexpression of *Bmp2/4* under the control of αGSU regulatory elements in ventral mouse pituitary initially leads to a dorsal expansion of the ventral lineage markers Isl1 and Msx1 with induction of *GATA2* gene expression. Proper expression of *Bmp2* is therefore critical for the initiation of the cell fate determination process, however, Bmp2 signaling has to be attenuated to achieve terminal differentiation.[15] These studies suggest that pouch-intrinsic and ventral signals, including Bmp2, contribute to the establishment of the positional identity of ventral pituitary cell types of thyrotrope and gonadotrope marked by αGSU expression.

Another way to study Bmp signaling is to address the role of Bmp antagonists during development. In a recent study, three antagonists—follistatin-like 1, *Nbl1*, and noggin—expression pattern—have implied a possible role of these proteins during pituitary development.[163] Out of three, *noggin-/-* embryos have pituitary defects that range from a lack of a morphologic Rathke's pouch to the formation of secondary pituitary tissue. Noggin attenuates the Bmp4 signal emanating from the ventral diencephalon during the induction and early patterning of Rathke's pouch, but it does not play a role in cell specification in the anterior lobe.[163]

NOTCHs

The Notch signaling pathway is an evolutionarily conserved mechanism that controls cellular differentiation, proliferation, and death in a broad spectrum of developmental systems.[164,165] Multiple ligands and effectors of the Notch signaling pathway were shown to be expressed in the developing pituitary, and a series of recent studies have shown the importance of the pathway in pituitary development.[53,65,166,167] First, *Notch2* expression is almost entirely absent in the *Prop1* mutant mice pituitary, suggesting that the Notch signaling pathway may play a role in the commitment and lineage-specific differentiation of progenitor cells in the embryonic pituitary—in particular, Prop1-dependent cell lineages.[65] Accordingly, conditional inactivation of *Rbp-J*, central mediator of the Notch signaling, using the transgenic Cre line under the control of *Pitx1* regulatory sequences, leads to premature differentiation of progenitor cells, as well as a conversion of the *Pit1* lineage into the coricotrope lineage. Premature progenitor differentiation is phenocopied in the mice deleted for the *Hes1* gene, while the later phenotype is largely due to the significant down-regulation of *Prop1* at e12.5. It has been shown that Rbp-J directly binds to the evolutionary conserved recognition site in the first intron of *Prop1* gene, and it is recruited to this region during pituitary development. Hence Notch signaling directly regulates *Prop1* transcription.[53]

The function of the Notch signaling pathway in pituitary development has also been investigated in *Hes1*-deficient mice and in mice conditionally deleted for both *Hes1* and *Hes5* in Rathke's pouch and the ventral diencephalon, using the *Emx1*-Cre mouse line.[53,166,168] In addition to premature corticotrope differentiation, which is consistently observed in *Rbp-J* conditional KO,[53] these mutant embryos lack both the intermediate and posterior lobes of the pituitary gland, which is in sharp contrast to the enhanced intermediate-lobe melanotrope differentiation detected in *Rbp-J*-conditional KO. The discrepancy might be explained by the different targeting approaches of these studies. Signals emanating from the ventral diencephalon are probably a key aspect of this discrepancy: in mice with *Rbp-J* conditionally inactivated using the *Pitx1*-Cre transgene, the ventral diencephalon remains intact, whereas in *Hes* mutants, it is also targeted because both *Hes1* and the *Emx1*-Cre are both expressed in the diencephalon.

Two independent studies have shown that down-regulation of Notch signaling is necessary for terminal differentiation of distinct cell lineages in the later phases of pituitary development.[53,167] Consistently, persistent expression of *Hes1* in pregonadotropes and prethyrotropes prevents their differentiation.[166] Since there is a feedback loop between Notch signaling and Prop1, it would be very interesting to find out what factor downregulates the Notch pathway during cell differentiation in the developing pituitary gland.

WNTs

The Wnt proto-oncogene family contains at least 19 known members.[169] As classical morphogens, the Wnt family of signaling molecules induces various cellular responses from proliferation to cell fate determination and differentiation. The canonic Wnt pathway stated that Wnt ligands bind to the Frizzled family of seven-transmembrane domain receptors, leading to the stabilization and accumulation of β-catenin, which interacts with members of the TCF/LEF family of DNA-binding transcription factors and changes them from repressors to activators of transcription, primarily by displacing the Groucho/Tle corepressor to influence target gene expression.[170,171]

Several Wnt-signaling molecules are expressed during the development of pituitary.[15,69,172] So far, two of them, Wnt4 and Wnt5a, have been reported to be specifically associated with the developmental events in the anterior pituitary. *Wnt4* is expressed in the ventral diencephalon, and *Wnt5a* is expressed in the cells of Rathke's pouch. In *Wnt4*-mutant mice, the pituitary is mildly hypocellular, with the ventral cell types showing normal differentiation but incomplete expansion. Additionally, cultivation of Rathke's pouch with Wnt5a and Bmp4 can induce expression of the early cell type marker αGSU.[15] *Wnt5a* mutants have expanded domains of *FGF10* and *Bmp* expression in the ventral diencephalon and a reduced domain of *LHX3* expression in Rathke's pouch. As a consequence, *Wnt5a-/-* mice have a morphologically distorted pituitary with an enlarged intermediate lobe and increased numbers of POMC cells.[172,173] Double *Wnt4/Wnt5s* knockout mice display an additive pituitary phenotype of dysmorphology and mild hypoplasia of the anterior lobe and hyperplasia of the intermediate lobe.[172] The phenotype suggests independent roles of those two factors. *Wnt6* is expressed near the pituitary gland during critical times in development; however, examination of embryos deficient in Wnt6 showed no obvious pituitary malformation.[172] The effects of deficiencies of Wnt4, 5a, or 6 seem

unlikely to account for the consequences of deficiencies in the known, critical, β-catenin-regulated transcription factors in the pituitary gland. Rather that Wnt signaling affects the pituitary gland via effects on ventral diencephalon signaling. Other Wnt molecules (Wnt2b, Wnt11, Wnt16)[172] are also expressed during pituitary development, although their role in this process awaits further investigation.

In *Pitx2*-deficient mice, mutant embryos fail to survive to term and exhibit developmental arrest of early determination events in the anterior pituitary gland.[109,113,115,174] *Pitx2a* has been demonstrated to be acting downstream of the Wnt signal, and Lef1 and β-catenin have been demonstrated to physically occupy the *Pitx2a* promoter in the context of a pituitary cell line. *Pitx2*-mutant pituitary glands contained decreased numbers of proliferating cells, whereas transgenic overexpression of *Pitx2* in the anterior pituitary led to increased cell numbers.[113] Also, *Pitx2c* isoform has been shown to be regulated directly by Wnt signaling.[175] In a subtraction expression profiling analysis of *Prop1*[Ames]-mutant pituitary, several members of the Wnt signaling pathway are identified, including the frizzled2 receptor, APC, β-catenin, Groucho, and Tcf7l2.[64] This genetic evidence suggests critical roles for the Wnt pathway in pituitary cellular proliferation and in cell type determination and differentiation.

Other components of the Wnt/β-catenin signaling pathway, including frizzled1-6, frizzled8, Lef1, Tcf3, Tcf4, and others have been reported to be expressed in the developing pituitary.[64,69,172,176] *Tcf4* is detectable in the early pituitary, as well as in surrounding tissues; it is markedly down-regulated by e13.5.[64,177,178] Targeted inactivation of *Tcf4* results in hyperplasia of the anterior lobe, probably caused by the expansion of FGF and BMP expression in the ventral diencephalon, with a concomitant increase in the number of progenitor cells that form Rathke's pouch. Thus Tcf4 may play a role as a repressor to regulate growth of Rathke's pouch by influencing Bmp and FGF signaling.[178] *Lef1* exhibits biphasic expression, initially transiently at e9.0 in Rathke's pouch and later appearing at e13.5 in the anterior and intermediate lobes of the gland. Targeted deletion of *Lef1* leads to elevated expression of *Pit1*, as well as GH and TSHβ, consistent with the role of Lef1 in inhibiting Prop1/β-catenin-mediated *Pit1* activation.[69] Those recent studies have shown yet another role of β-catenin and Wnt signaling during pituitary development. Targeted inactivation of β-catenin in pituitary cells using a *Pitx1*-Cre transgenic line results in a smaller gland with no *Pit1* expression, absence of all three Pit1 lineages, and reduced numbers of gonadotropes. Surprisingly β-catenin does not exert its role through binding with its canonical Tcf/Lef partners. Induction of *Pit1* is mediated by direct interaction between β-catenin and Prop1, through evolutionary conserved *Pit1* early enhancer.[52,69,179] Moreover, Prop1/β-catenin complex is also acting as a transcriptional repressor for *Hesx1*, ensuring differentiation of the progenitors. Genetic studies have demonstrated that proper spatio-temporal activation of Wnt/β-catenin signaling is essential for proper pituitary development, because premature activation of β-catenin leads to *Hesx1* repression and pituitary agenesis.[69]

INTERACTIONS BETWEEN DIFFERENT MORPHOGENIC FACTORS

Opposing BMPs and FGFs Signaling Gradients

Analogous to the combinatorial signal regulation in organogenesis observed in many organs, physically opposing dorsal-to-ventral Fgf8/10/18 and ventral-to-dorsal Bmp2 gradients appear to be associated with the positional determination of specific pituitary cell types.[180] The ability of the infundibulum or FGFs to induce *Lhx3* gene expression correlates with the restricted expression of the Bmp2-induced genes *Isl1* and *αGSU* distal to the source of the FGF signaling.[18] The ability of ventralized expression of *FGF8* to prevent the appearance of ventral cell types in vivo can be attributed to the inhibition of ventral Bmp2 signaling.[15] Conversely, while cultivation of Rathke's pouch with Bmp2/4 initiates the expression of the ventral markers Isl1 and αGSU, it inhibits the expression of more dorsal cell type markers such as ACTH in vitro[18] and Pit1 in vivo.[15] Thus antagonistic and opposing dorsal-to-ventral Fgf8 and ventral-to-dorsal Bmp2 gradients appear to be associated with the positional determination of dorsal and ventral cell types.[2,180]

Independent Hh and FGF Signaling in Pituitary Organogenesis

FGF and *Shh* exhibit complementary expression patterns near the developing anterior pituitary. Studies of zebrafish have shown that graded loss of *Hh,* but not *FGF,* led to ectopic midline lens formation, with either one or two lenses forming, depending on the level of Hh signaling. Moreover, the results suggest that Hh and FGF signaling act independently to induce the pattern of endocrine cell fates along the anterior/posterior axis of the zebrafish anterior lobe, with high doses of Hh signaling required for the induction of the anteriorly located pars distalis and high doses of FGF signaling required for the induction of the posterior pars intermedia.[181]

OTHER POTENTIAL MORPHOGENETIC FACTORS

Extrinsically derived signals that possibly affect Rathke's pouch, arising from ventral mesenchyme beneath the developing pituitary gland, include Indian Hedgehog (IHh), Wnt4, and Bmp2; whereas caudal mesenchyme is a source of a Chordin signal capable of opposing the function of Bmp2.[182] Recently it has been found that blocking EGF/TGFa signaling, by the expression of a dominant negative form of EGF receptor, has a profound stage-specific effect. Expression of mutated EGF receptor in GH-producing cells of embryonic pituitary results in dwarfism and pituitary hypoplasia, with reduced numbers of lactotropes and somatotropes.[183] In addition, little is known about the contribution of cytokines, despite the potent ability of cytokines such as leukemia inhibitory factor (LIF) to maintain mouse embryonic stem cells in an undifferentiated state. A potential role for LIF in pituitary development investigated in pituitary-derived cell lines is that LIF can activate synthesis of ACTH in combination with the hypothalamic peptide corticotropin-releasing hormone.[184] In transgenic animals that express LIF under control of αGSU regulatory information, most cell types fail to properly differentiate, and the pituitary is characterized by the formation of ciliated cysts of Rathke's pouch and corticotrope hyperplasia,[185] suggesting that LIF may contribute to the identity establishment of dorsal-cell phenotypes.

In addition to the dorsal and ventral structures, another organizer signaling center, the notochord, is located just posterior to the developing pituitary gland. The proximity of these two structures, albeit from different origins, suggests a role for the notochord in the initial invagination of Rathke's pouch, as indicated by tissue explant experiments.[19]

Pituitary and Epigenetics

Deep knowledge of physiology and multiple genetic studies performed on the pituitary gland made the pituitary an excellent system for studying details of the regulation of transcription of pituitary-specific genes (for review see [186]). Using genetic models, it is possible not only to detect the important elements in promoter regions to drive expression of the gene in the specific cell type but also to detect the hierarchy of importance of those regions and detailed molecular mechanisms of activation. Here we will provide several examples of how the pituitary gland served to elucidate the regulation of transcription of the specific genes on the molecular level.

PIT1 LOCUS—MULTIPLE ENHANCERS COORDINATE EXPRESSION OF THE GENE

Transgenic studies revealed that 14.8 kb of 5'-flanking sequence of the *Pit1* gene was sufficient to direct the robust expression of a reporter in an identical spatial and temporal pattern as endogenous *Pit1,* whereas its minimal promoter (−327 bp to −13 bp) was insufficient to drive detectable reporter expression in transgenic mice.[31] A distal enhancer located at −10.2 kb from the *Pit1* transcription start site and containing multiple functional Pit1-binding sites was shown to be involved in autoregulation. This element also contains a vitamin-D receptor binding site and a retinoic acid response element that confers Pit1-dependent RA induction.[31] However, the early activation of the *Pit1* gene at e13.5 in the anterior pituitary requires the cooperation of Prop1 and Wnt/β-catenin signaling and is mediated by early enhancer located between at −7.8 kb upstream of the transcription start site[69] in cooperation with ATBF1—giant, multiple homeodomain and zinc finger family factor—to the −5.8 kb enhancer element.[187] Thus proper spatio-temporal expression of the *Pit1* gene is assured through the cooperation of different enhancer elements and require Pit1 protein itself. In the dwarf mice, *Pit1* expression is activated normally, but because Pit1 protein is defective, *Pit1* expression declines and becomes extinguished in the perinatal period.[31]

Biochemical approaches such as chromatin immunoprecipitation (ChIP) on chromatin isolated from developing gland or pituitary cell lines allow detection of changes in chromatin status of regulatory regions of the *Pit1* gene as the pituitary gland develops.[69] At e11.5, the 2mH3K4, 3mH3K4, and AcH3K9 marks of activation are absent, but 2mH3K9 is present on Pit1 regulatory elements, consistent with an active repression of the *Pit1* gene at this time. By e12.5, 2mH3K4 mark is selectively present at early enhancer. At e13.5, marks associated with active promoters[188] are present on *Pit1* promoter (2mH3K4, 3mH3K4, and AcH3K9) and −7.8 kb enhancer (2mH3K4). In the adult, the *Pit1* gene promoter harbors the histone marks of gene activation (3mH3K4, and AcH3K9), with 2mH3K4 now present on both the late and early enhancers, showing the temporal progression of histone modifications on regulatory regions of the *Pit1* gene.

GROWTH HORMONE LOCUS—LCR, BOUNDARY, AND HISTONE CODE

The growth hormone (*GH*) gene provides a well-studied transcription unit that is highly suited for defining how specific chromatin modifications might be responsible for the spatial and temporal order of lineage specification events in the developing pituitary gland. This region is well studied in human and mouse subjects, but important differences can be noted between the species.

The human *GH* locus is represented by a cluster of five *GH*-related genes and their cell type–specific expression is regulated by a Pit-1-dependent locus control region (LCR). Expression of pituitary-specific *GH* gene (hGH-N) is ensured by −500 bp promoter that contains binding sites for Pit1, Sp1, and zinc finger proteins and is required for efficient expression of the gene. The LCR is necessary for proper spatio-temporal expression of hGH-N transgene.[189] Dissection of the hGH-N LCR revealed the existence of two Pit1-dependent DNaseI hypersensitive sites (HSI and HSII) that are sufficient to activate hGH transgene expression.[190,191] The hGH LCR and the hGH-N promoter are encompassed within a 32-kb domain of acetylated histones H3 and H4 in pituitary chromatin, with highest levels of acetylation at HSI,II.[192] Although the 3mH3K4 modifications at the active hGH transgene locus in the mouse pituitary paralleled PolII distribution, they extended through the LCR and adjacent CD79b region and were separated from the hGH-N promoter by an intervening gap of unmodified chromatin.[193] In mouse transgenic models, selective deletion of the pituitary-specific HSI results in the loss of both histone acetylation and methylation throughout the LCR and a marked decrease in hGH-N transcription.[193,194] This recent study revealed also that HSI plays an essential role in the establishment of a complex domain of intergenic transcription 5′ to the hGH cluster.[194] Insertion of an exogenous transcriptional terminator within this domain selectively blocked a subset of downstream LCR transcripts and repressed hGH-N transcription without markedly affecting histone acetylation and methylation within the locus.[193,194] More recent studies showed pituitary-specific interactions between the HSI,II region and the hGH-N promoter, suggesting that noncoding transcripts in the LCR region are essential and a probable prerequisite to looping and gene activation.[193]

Studies of the *cis*-acting elements of the rat growth hormone gene have shown that the minimal information required for the specific expression in somatotropes but not lactotropes resides in the proximal 320 bp of the promoter, with the proximal 180 bp capable of targeting the reporter in vivo.[195] This region contains binding sites for Pit1, thyroid hormone receptor (TR), Sp1, a zinc finger protein (Zn-15), and a recently identified zinc finger–homeodomain transcriptional repressor (Zeb1).[196] Extensive analyses of transgenic mice have revealed that multiple factors are essential to mediate *GH* gene activation in somatotropes (Sp1), others for repression in lactotropes (Zeb1), while TR and Pit1 are required for both activation and repression. Interestingly, mutational studies have shown that replacing GH-specific Pit1 binding sites with the PRL-specific Pit1 site results in a loss of restriction from the lactotropes without affecting expression in somatotropes.[44] Comparative analysis of the cocrystal structure of the Pit1 POU domain dimer bound to either GH-specific or PRL-specific sites has revealed that the spacing between the DNA contacts made by the POU-specific domain and the POU homeodomain of each monomer is increased by 2 bp on the GH-specific site. Deletion of these 2 bp in this promoter leads to a lack of the effective restriction of the reporter gene expression from lactotropes. These data suggest that the Pit1 protein conformation is critical for its specific activity. The transcriptional repressor Zeb1 is bound to the *GH* promoter only in the lactotropes in the sumoylation-dependent manner, and it is not recruited to the *GH* promoter in somatotropes. Together with the other two components of the CtBP-CoREST-LSD1 complex, Zeb1 assembles an LSD1-containing corepressor complex on the *GH* promoter in lactotropes. Earlier in development, LSD1 is present at the *GH* promoter in the MLL1-containing complex in the somatotropes, which is required for activation of the gene.[196] Thus machinery controlling chromatin status (e.g., methylation of histones) is involved in developmental processes such as differentiation.

Another level of complexity of *GH* regulation in somatotropes comes from studies performed in mice. The murine *GH* genomic locus is found on mouse chromosome 11 and encompasses five genes. In contrast to the human locus, the mouse locus does not contain tandem duplications of the *GH* gene, and there is no known murine LCR. The proximal regulatory sequences are very well conserved between mouse and rat. However, specific activation of the endogenous murine *GH* gene also appears to require a boundary element imposed by an upstream SINE B2 repeat.[197] This SINE B2 repeat is able to produce short, overlapping Pol II and Pol III-driven transcripts that are both necessary and sufficient for its enhancer-blocking activity in cultured cells enhancer-blocking assay. Interestingly, the Pol II-driven transcript appears in a temporally regulated manner during pituitary development, concomitantly with translocation of the *GH* locus from condensed heterochromatin territory (marked by H3K9me3) to a euchromatic area (marked by H3K9me2). These studies suggest that active transcription of repetitive sequences may represent one of the strategies for the establishment of functional chromatin domains to control gene expression.

Many mechanisms such as long-range interactions (*hGH, Pit1*), use of multiple enhancers (*Pit1, GH*) and histone modifications have been shown to be implicated in regulation of the expression of genes during pituitary development. DNA methylation represents another layer of complexity in regulation of the gene expression. To date, only the *POMC* promoter has been described as having the particular DNA methylation code that *allows* expression of the gene in tissues where its promoter is not methylated and *prevents* gene expression when the promoter DNA is methylated. The regulatory mechanism of this process, however, is not yet understood.[198]

Adult Pituitary Stem Cells

Existence of tissue-specific stem cells is documented in a growing number of organs by their molecular expression profile and their potential for self-renewal, multipotent differentiation and tissue regeneration. Whether or not the adult pituitary gland also contains a pool of stem cells that drive homeostatic, plastic, and regenerative cell ontogenesis remains unknown. However, adult pituitary has a remarkable ability to adapt the number of each of its cell types in response to changing physiologic demands. For example, the number of somatotropes doubles during puberty, whereas the number of lactotropes expands several-fold during pregnancy, lactation, and weaning.[199] Nevertheless, it is not clear if those changes in numbers of differentiated cells are the result of maturation of uncommitted cells, transdifferentiation of other cell types, mitotic divisions of differentiated cells, or any combination of these mechanisms.

Several different cell types, including folliculostellate cells, rapidly dividing nestin-expressing cells, and side population cells of the anterior pituitary, have been recently proposed to constitute stem cells (reviewed extensively in ref. 200). However, there is no evidence that any of the proposed candidates are able to generate all differentiated cell types and participate in cell renewal in the anterior pituitary gland in vivo.

Recently, two independent in-vivo studies have attempted to identify stem-cell populations in the adult pituitary gland[201,202] (see Fig. 1-2). Fauquier and colleagues have shown that a small (0.03 to 0.05%) population of cells in the adult pituitary gland expresses Sox2, a marker of several early embryonic progenitor and stem cell types. In vitro, Sox2+ cells are able to form pituispheres that can proliferate and self-renew into secondary spheres; under differentiating conditions, some proportion of these cells can differentiate into all-pituitary cell types. During progression towards the differentiated state, cells lose expression of *Sox2* and start expressing *Sox9* and *S100b*. At that stage, the cells were no longer able to form secondary pituispheres and thus were proposed to represent a transition phase from uncommitted to committed progenitor cells. The authors propose that this population of cells corresponds to marginal cells and folliculostellate cells expressing *Sox9* and *S100b* in vivo and represents actively dividing progenitors which are, at a later stage, committed towards differentiation.

In the second report,[202] authors applied a genetic approach to identifying stem cell populations in the adult pituitary. Using a GFP reporter whose expression is driven by the regulatory region of the nestin gene, authors identified a small population of cells in the adult pituitary which retained expression of the marker. Nestin-positive cells are located mostly in the perilumenal region of the gland, which had been previously proposed to be a niche for stem cells. Expression of nestin coincided with expression of *Sox2* and *Lhx3,* suggesting a histogenetic relation to the endocrine cell types of the pituitary. During the first postnatal week, a large fraction of nestin-GFP–expressing cells, both in the glandular zone and in the perilumenal area, was positive for Ki67, a marker of dividing cells, suggesting that these cells participate in the second wave of pituitary gland growth. Supporting this observation, lineage-tracing experiments have shown that the number of GFP-positive cells in nestin-Cre/ROSA-lsl-GFP mice increases during the life of an animal from 2% in the newborn to 15% to 20% at 5 months of age. GFP expression was found in all six terminally differentiated pituitary endocrine cell types. Further supporting the notion of a separate adult stem cell lineage, the differentiation choices differed between the embryonic and adult stem cell–derived progeny. For instance, in females, the ratio of lactotropes to somatotropes was 1.8 times higher for GFP-expressing cells (i.e., cells derived from the presumptive adult stem cells) than for all of the cells of the gland (a mix of embryonic- and adult-generated cells), whereas in males it was 0.7 times lower for the GFP-expressing cells as compared with all cells of the gland. Finally, nestin-positive cells were able to self-renew multiple times in an in-vitro culture and spontaneously differentiate into all pituitary lineages (see Fig. 1-2). Recently in the new study[203] GRFa2 and Prop1 have been shown to be expressed by putative stem cells in the luminal niche of the pituitary gland.

Although these studies strongly suggest the existence of stem-cell-like cells in the adult pituitary, further analysis is necessary to extend the detailed characterization of these cells. One of the issues would be to demonstrate that a particular cell is capable of giving rise to all pituitary cell types. Equally importantly, it remains to be elucidated which extrinsic and/or intrinsic cues are critical in directing those cells towards a particular fate.

Summary

Coordinated regulation of cell type determination, differentiation, and cell proliferation is a central feature in the development of all organs. Organogenesis is controlled by sequential and spatially distributed morphogens of four major families of signaling molecules, including Wnt, Shh, TGF/BMP, and FGF. The distal targets of regulatory signaling pathways are cell-autonomous transcription regulators, including many tissue-restricted transcription factors which act to mediate crucial steps in organogenesis. The downstream effects of the signaling pathways result in the preprogramming of target cells. Pituitary development has become a model system, ideal for demonstrating the principles underlying organogenesis (see Fig. 1-2).

Continued advancement in genomic and genetic applications, particularly genome-based mutagenesis screens in mice and in nonmurine model organisms, will identify novel genes and pathways that influence the signaling and cell-determination events. Biochemical approaches, including proteomics techniques, will define the signaling-induced alterations in protein-protein interactions and phosphorylation/methylation/acetylation essential to these events. Identification of required cofactors and their downstream targets using genome-wide approaches, including complementary studies in epigenetic regulation of chromatin organization and nuclear architecture, will help determine what molecular mechanisms underlie pituitary development. The description of developmental events leading to the formation of the pituitary gland will be described increasingly in molecular terms as the molecular mechanisms are elucidated. For further information, please refer to the many comprehensive recent reviews of pituitary development in the references.[3,186,204-206]

Acknowledgments

We would like to thank members of Rosenfeld's laboratory for helpful discussions, in particular Drs. Chijen Lin, Kathleen Scully, and Xiaoyan Zhu. We also thank Janet Hightower for figure preparation. We apologize to our many colleagues whose contributions could not be cited based on the limitation of references in this format, which also precluded detailed discussions of the impact of hormone receptor systems in development of the pituitary gland. DSK is supported by Swiss National Foundation. MGR is an investigator with the Howard Hughes Medical Institute. Studies cited from MGR laboratory are supported by grants from the NIDDKD.

REFERENCES

1. Melmed S: Mechanisms for pituitary tumorigenesis: the plastic pituitary, J Clin Invest 112(11):1603–1618, 2003.
2. Rosenfeld MG, et al: Multistep signaling and transcriptional requirements for pituitary organogenesis in vivo,

Recent Prog Horm Res 55:1–13; discussion 13–14, 2000.
3. Savage JJ, et al: Transcriptional control during mammalian anterior pituitary development, Gene 319:1–19, 2003.

4. elAmraoui A, Dubois PM: Experimental evidence for the early commitment of the presumptive adenohypophysis, Neuroendocrinology 58(6):609–615, 1993.
5. Levy NB, et al: Is there a ventral neural ridge in chick embryos? Implications for the origin of adenohypophy-

seal and other APUD cells, J Embryol Exp Morphol 57:71–78, 1980.

6. Takor TT, Pearse AG: Neuroectodermal origin of avian hypothalamo-hypophyseal complex: the role of the ventral neural ridge, J Embryol Exp Morphol 34(2):311–325, 1975.

7. Eagleson GW, Harris WA: Mapping of the presumptive brain regions in the neural plate of Xenopus laevis, J Neurobiol 21(3):427–440, 1990.

8. Eagleson GW, Jenks BG, Van Overbeeke AP: The pituitary adrenocorticotropes originate from neural ridge tissue in Xenopus laevis, J Embryol Exp Morphol 95:1–14, 1986.

9. Herzog W, et al: Adenohypophysis formation in the zebrafish and its dependence on sonic hedgehog, Dev Biol 254(1):36–49, 2003.

10. Liu NA, et al: Pituitary corticotroph ontogeny and regulation in transgenic zebrafish, Mol Endocrinol 17(5):959–966, 2003.

11. Kouki T, et al: Developmental origin of the rat adenohypophysis prior to the formation of Rathke's pouch, Development 128(6):959–963, 2001.

12. Rathke H: Ueber die Entstehung der glandula pititaria, Arch Anat Physio Wissened 482–485, 1838.

13. Ikeda H, et al: The development and morphogenesis of the human pituitary gland, Anat Embryol (Berl) 178(4):327–336, 1988.

14. Treier M, Rosenfeld MG: The hypothalamic-pituitary axis: co-development of two organs, Curr Opin Cell Biol 8(6):833–843, 1996.

15. Treier M, et al: Multistep signaling requirements for pituitary organogenesis in vivo, Genes Dev 12(11):1691–1704, 1998.

16. Han KS, Iwai-Liao Y, Higashi Y: Early organogenesis and cell contacts in the proliferating hypophysis of the developing mouse, Okajimas Folia Anat Jpn 75(2–3):97–109, 1998.

17. Ikeda H, Yoshimoto T: Developmental changes in proliferative activity of cells of the murine Rathke's pouch, Cell Tissue Res 263(1):41–47, 1991.

18. Ericson J, et al: Integrated FGF and BMP signaling controls the progression of progenitor cell differentiation and the emergence of pattern in the embryonic anterior pituitary, Development 125(6):1005–1015, 1998.

19. Gleiberman AS, Fedtsova NG, Rosenfeld MG: Tissue interactions in the induction of anterior pituitary: role of the ventral diencephalon, mesenchyme, and notochord, Dev Biol 213(2):340–353, 1999.

20. Dasen JS, Rosenfeld MG: Signaling and transcriptional mechanisms in pituitary development, Annu Rev Neurosci 24:327–355, 2001.

21. Kendall SK, et al: Enhancer-mediated high level expression of mouse pituitary glycoprotein hormone alpha-subunit transgene in thyrotropes, gonadotropes, and developing pituitary gland, Mol Endocrinol 8(10):1420–1433, 1994.

22. Bodner M, et al: The pituitary-specific transcription factor GHF-1 is a homeobox-containing protein, Cell 55(3):505–518, 1988.

23. Ingraham HA, et al: A tissue-specific transcription factor containing a homeodomain specifies a pituitary phenotype, Cell 55(3):519–529, 1988.

24. Mangalam HJ, et al: A pituitary POU domain protein, Pit-1, activates both growth hormone and prolactin promoters transcriptionally, Genes Dev 3(7):946–958, 1989.

25. Lin C, et al: Pit-1-dependent expression of the receptor for growth hormone releasing factor mediates pituitary cell growth, Nature 360(6406):765–768, 1992.

26. Crenshaw EB, 3rd, et al: Cell-specific expression of the prolactin gene in transgenic mice is controlled by synergistic interactions between promoter and enhancer elements, Genes Dev 3(7):959–972, 1989.

27. Chen RP, et al: Autoregulation of pit-1 gene expression mediated by two cis-active promoter elements, Nature 346(6284):583–586, 1990.

28. Snell GD: Dwarf, a new Mendelian recessive character of the house mouse, Proc Natl Acad Sci U S A 15(9):733–734, 1929.

29. Li S, et al: Dwarf locus mutants lacking three pituitary cell types result from mutations in the POU-domain gene pit-1, Nature 347(6293):528–533, 1990.

30. Camper SA, et al: The Pit-1 transcription factor gene is a candidate for the murine Snell dwarf mutation, Genomics 8(3):586–590, 1990.

31. Rhodes SJ, et al: A tissue-specific enhancer confers Pit-1-dependent morphogen inducibility and autoregulation on the pit-1 gene, Genes Dev 7(6):913–932, 1993.

32. Bartke A, et al: Prolonged longevity of hypopituitary dwarf mice, Exp Gerontol 36(1):21–28, 2001.

33. Flurkey K, et al: Lifespan extension and delayed immune and collagen aging in mutant mice with defects in growth hormone production, Proc Natl Acad Sci U S A 98(12):6736–6741, 2001.

34. Bishop NA, Guarente L: Genetic links between diet and lifespan: shared mechanisms from yeast to humans, Nat Rev Genet 8(11):835–844, 2007.

35. Kenyon C: The plasticity of aging: insights from long-lived mutants, Cell 120(4):449–460, 2005.

36. Sinclair DA: Toward a unified theory of caloric restriction and longevity regulation, Mech Ageing Dev 126(9):987–1002, 2005.

37. Tatsumi K, et al: Cretinism with combined hormone deficiency caused by a mutation in the PIT1 gene, Nat Genet 1(1):56–58, 1992.

38. Parks JS, et al: Heritable disorders of pituitary development, J Clin Endocrinol Metab 84(12):4362–4370, 1999.

39. Pfaffle RW, et al: Combined pituitary hormone deficiency: role of Pit-1 and Prop-1, Acta Paediatr Suppl 88(433):33–41, 1999.

40. Wu W, Anderson B, Rosenfeld MG: PIT1 transcription factor and diseases. In Wiley Encyclopedia of Molecular Medicine, Chinchester, UK, 2002, John Wiley & Sons, p 2501.

41. Holloway JM, et al: Pit-1 binding to specific DNA sites as a monomer or dimer determines gene-specific use of a tyrosine-dependent synergy domain, Genes Dev 9(16):1992–2006, 1995.

42. Jacobson EM, et al: Structure of Pit-1 POU domain bound to DNA as a dimer: unexpected arrangement and flexibility, Genes Dev 11(2):198–212, 1997.

43. Jacobson EM, et al: Crystallization and preliminary X-ray analysis of Pit-1 POU domain complexed to a 28 base pair DNA element, Proteins 24(2):263–265, 1996.

44. Scully KM, et al: Allosteric effects of Pit-1 DNA sites on long-term repression in cell type specification, Science 290(5494):1127–1131, 2000.

45. Andersen B, Rosenfeld MG: POU domain factors in the neuroendocrine system: lessons from developmental biology provide insights into human disease, Endocr Rev 22(1):2–35, 2001.

46. Cohen LE, et al: A "hot spot" in the Pit-1 gene responsible for combined pituitary hormone deficiency: clinical and molecular correlates, J Clin Endocrinol Metab 80(2):679–684, 1995.

47. Xu L, et al: Signal-specific co-activator domain requirements for Pit-1 activation, Nature 395(6699):301–306, 1998.

48. Day RN, et al: Both Pit-1 and the estrogen receptor are required for estrogen responsiveness of the rat prolactin gene, Mol Endocrinol 4(12):1964–1971, 1990.

49. Simmons DM, et al: Pituitary cell phenotypes involve cell-specific Pit-1 mRNA translation and synergistic interactions with other classes of transcription factors, Genes Dev 4(5):695–711, 1990.

50. Bradford AP, et al: Functional interaction of c-Ets-1 and GHF-1/Pit-1 mediates Ras activation of pituitary-specific gene expression: mapping of the essential c-Ets-1 domain, Mol Cell Biol 15(5):2849–2857, 1995.

51. Dasen JS, et al: Reciprocal interactions of Pit1 and GATA2 mediate signaling gradient-induced determination of pituitary cell types, Cell 97(5):587–598, 1999.

52. Sornson MW, et al: Pituitary lineage determination by the Prophet of Pit-1 homeodomain factor defective in Ames dwarfism, Nature 384(6607):327–333, 1996.

53. Zhu X, et al: Sustained Notch signaling in progenitors is required for sequential emergence of distinct cell lineages during organogenesis, Genes Dev 20(19):2739–2753, 2006.

54. Andersen B, et al: The Ames dwarf gene is required for Pit-1 gene activation, Dev Biol 172(2):495–503, 1995.

55. Gage PJ, et al: Anterior pituitary cells defective in the cell-autonomous factor, df, undergo cell lineage specification but not expansion, Development 122(1):151–160, 1996.

56. Buckwalter MS, Katz RW, Camper SA: Localization of the panhypopituitary dwarf mutation (df) on mouse chromosome 11 in an intersubspecific backcross, Genomics 10(3):515–526, 1991.

57. Gage PJ, et al: Ames dwarf mice exhibit somatotrope commitment but lack growth hormone-releasing factor response, Endocrinology 136(3):1161–1167, 1995.

58. Brown-Borg HM, et al: Dwarf mice and the ageing process, Nature 384(6604):33, 1996.

59. Wu W, et al: Mutations in PROP1 cause familial combined pituitary hormone deficiency, Nat Genet 18(2):147–149, 1998.

60. Deladoey J, et al: "Hot spot" in the PROP1 gene responsible for combined pituitary hormone deficiency, J Clin Endocrinol Metab 84(5):1645–1650, 1999.

61. Mody S, Brown MR, Parks JS: The spectrum of hypopituitarism caused by PROP1 mutations, Best Pract Res Clin Endocrinol Metab 16(3):421–431, 2002.

62. Wu W, Rosenfeld MG: Prop1 gene. In Wiley Encyclopedia of Molecular Medicine. Chichester, UK, 2002, John Wiley & Sons, p 2597.

63. Ward RD, et al: Role of PROP1 in pituitary gland growth, Mol Endocrinol 19(3):698–710, 2005.

64. Douglas KR, et al: Identification of members of the Wnt signaling pathway in the embryonic pituitary gland, Mamm Genome 12(11):843–851, 2001.

65. Raetzman LT, et al: Developmental regulation of Notch signaling genes in the embryonic pituitary: Prop1 deficiency affects Notch2 expression, Dev Biol 265(2):329–340, 2004.

66. Cushman LJ, et al: Persistent Prop1 expression delays gonadotrope differentiation and enhances pituitary tumor susceptibility, Hum Mol Genet 10(11):1141–1153, 2001.

67. Vesper AH, Raetzman LT, Camper SA: Role of prophet of Pit1 (PROP1) in gonadotrope differentiation and puberty, Endocrinology 147(4):1654–1663, 2006.

68. Showalter AD, et al: Differential conservation of transcriptional domains of mammalian Prophet of Pit-1 proteins revealed by structural studies of the bovine gene and comparative functional analysis of the protein, Gene 291(1–2):211–221, 2002.

69. Olson LE, et al: Homeodomain-mediated beta-catenin-dependent switching events dictate cell-lineage determination, Cell 125(3):593–605, 2006.

70. Agarwal G, et al: Adrenocorticotropin deficiency in combined pituitary hormone deficiency patients homozygous for a novel PROP1 deletion, J Clin Endocrinol Metab 85(12):4556–4561, 2000.

71. Lamesch C, et al: Adrenocorticotrope deficiency with clinical evidence for late onset in combined pituitary hormone deficiency caused by a homozygous 301–302delAG mutation of the PROP1 gene, Pituitary 5(3):163–168, 2002.

72. Pernasetti F, et al: Impaired adrenocorticotropin-adrenal axis in combined pituitary hormone deficiency caused by a two-base pair deletion (301–302delAG) in the prophet of Pit-1 gene, J Clin Endocrinol Metab 85(1):390–397, 2000.

73. Hermesz E, Mackem S, Mahon KA: Rpx: a novel anterior-restricted homeobox gene progressively activated in the prechordal plate, anterior neural plate and Rathke's pouch of the mouse embryo, Development 122(1):41–52, 1996.

74. Thomas P, Beddington R: Anterior primitive endoderm may be responsible for patterning the anterior neural plate in the mouse embryo, Curr Biol 6(11):1487–1496, 1996.

75. Dattani MT, et al: Mutations in the homeobox gene HESX1/Hesx1 associated with septo-optic dysplasia in human and mouse, Nat Genet 19(2):125–133, 1998.

76. Dasen JS, et al: Temporal regulation of a paired-like homeodomain repressor/TLE corepressor complex and a related activator is required for pituitary organogenesis, Genes Dev 15(23):3193–3207, 2001.

77. Thomas PQ, et al: Heterozygous HESX1 mutations associated with isolated congenital pituitary hypoplasia and septo-optic dysplasia, Hum Mol Genet 10(1):39–45, 2001.

78. McNay DE, et al: HESX1 mutations are an uncommon cause of septooptic dysplasia and hypopituitarism, J Clin Endocrinol Metab 92(2):691–697, 2007.

79. Rainbow LA, et al: Mutation analysis of POUF-1, PROP-1 and HESX-1 show low frequency of mutations in children with sporadic forms of combined pituitary hormone deficiency and septo-optic dysplasia, Clin Endocrinol (Oxf) 62(2):163–168, 2005.

80. Brickman JM, et al: Molecular effects of novel mutations in Hesx1/HESX1 associated with human pituitary disorders, Development 128(24):5189–5199, 2001.

81. Quirk J, Brown P: Hesx1 homeodomain protein represses transcription as a monomer and antagonises transactivation of specific sites as a homodimer, J Mol Endocrinol 28(3):193–205, 2002.

82. Jimenez G, Paroush Z, Ish-Horowicz D: Groucho acts as a corepressor for a subset of negative regulators, including Hairy and Engrailed, Genes Dev 11(22):3072–3082, 1997.

83. Tolkunova EN, et al: Two distinct types of repression domain in engrailed: one interacts with the groucho corepressor and is preferentially active on integrated target genes, Mol Cell Biol 18(5):2804–2814, 1998.

84. Eberhard D, et al: Transcriptional repression by Pax5 (BSAP) through interaction with corepressors of the Groucho family, EMBO J 19(10):2292–2303, 2000.

85. Carvalho LR, et al: A homozygous mutation in HESX1 is associated with evolving hypopituitarism due to impaired repressor-corepressor interaction, J Clin Invest 112(8):1192–1201, 2003.

86. Zhadanov AB, et al: Expression pattern of the murine LIM class homeobox gene Lhx3 in subsets of neural and neuroendocrine tissues, Dev Dyn 202(4):354–364, 1995.

87. Li H, et al: Gsh-4 encodes a LIM-type homeodomain, is expressed in the developing central nervous system and is required for early postnatal survival, EMBO J 13(12):2876–2885, 1994.

88. Sheng HZ, et al: Specification of pituitary cell lineages by the LIM homeobox gene Lhx3, Science 272(5264):1004–1007, 1996.

89. Raetzman LT, Ward R, Camper SA: Lhx4 and Prop1 are required for cell survival and expansion of the pituitary primordia, Development 129(18):4229–4239, 2002.

90. Sheng HZ, et al: Multistep control of pituitary organogenesis, Science 278(5344):1809–1812, 1997.

91. Schmitt S, et al: Genomic structure, chromosomal localization, and expression pattern of the human LIM-homeobox3 (LHX 3) gene, Biochem Biophys Res Commun 274(1):49–56, 2000.

92. Sloop KW, Dwyer CJ, Rhodes SJ: An isoform-specific inhibitory domain regulates the LHX3 LIM homeodomain factor holoprotein and the production of a functional alternate translation form, J Biol Chem 276(39):36311–36319, 2001.

93. Netchine I, et al: Mutations in LHX3 result in a new syndrome revealed by combined pituitary hormone deficiency, Nat Genet 25(2):182–186, 2000.

94. Pfaeffle RW, et al: Four novel mutations of the LHX3 gene cause combined pituitary hormone deficiencies with or without limited neck rotation, J Clin Endocrinol Metab 92(5):1909–1919, 2007.

95. Rajab A, et al: Novel mutations in LHX3 are associated with hypopituitarism and sensorineural hearing loss, Hum Mol Genet 17(14):2150–2159, 2008.

96. Machinis K, et al: Syndromic short stature in patients with a germline mutation in the LIM homeobox LHX4, Am J Hum Genet 69(5):961–968, 2001.

97. Pfaeffle RW, et al: Three novel missense mutations within the LHX4 gene are associated with variable pituitary hormone deficiencies, J Clin Endocrinol Metab 93(3):1062–1071, 2008.

98. Yi CH, et al: Identification, mapping, and phylogenomic analysis of four new human members of the T-box gene family: EOMES, TBX6, TBX18, and TBX19, Genomics 55(1):10–20, 1999.

99. Lamolet B, et al: A pituitary cell-restricted T box factor, Tpit, activates POMC transcription in cooperation with Pitx homeoproteins, Cell 104(6):849–859, 2001.

100. Liu J, et al: Tbx19, a tissue-selective regulator of POMC gene expression, Proc Natl Acad Sci U S A 98(15):8674–8679, 2001.

101. Pulichino AM, et al: Human and mouse TPIT gene mutations cause early onset pituitary ACTH deficiency, Genes Dev 17(6):711–716, 2003.

102. Pulichino AM, et al: Tpit determines alternate fates during pituitary cell differentiation, Genes Dev 17(6):738–747, 2003.

103. Vallette-Kasic S, et al: Congenital isolated adrenocorticotropin deficiency: an underestimated cause of neonatal death, explained by TPIT gene mutations, J Clin Endocrinol Metab 90(3):1323–1331, 2005.

104. Vallette-Kasic S, et al: The TPIT gene mutation M86R associated with isolated adrenocorticotropin deficiency interferes with protein: protein interactions, J Clin Endocrinol Metab 92(10):3991–3999, 2007.

105. Maira M, et al: The T-box factor Tpit recruits SRC/p160 co-activators and mediates hormone action, J Biol Chem 278(47):46523–46532, 2003.

106. Maira M, et al: Dimer-specific potentiation of NGFI-B (Nur77) transcriptional activity by the protein kinase A pathway and AF-1-dependent coactivator recruitment, Mol Cell Biol 23(3):763–776, 2003.

107. Marcil A, et al: Pitx1 and Pitx2 are required for development of hindlimb buds, Development 130(1):45–55, 2003.

108. Szeto DP, et al: Role of the Bicoid-related homeodomain factor Pitx1 in specifying hindlimb morphogenesis and pituitary development, Genes Dev 13(4):484–494, 1999.

109. Lin CR, et al: Pitx2 regulates lung asymmetry, cardiac positioning and pituitary and tooth morphogenesis, Nature 401(6750):279–282, 1999.

110. Semina EV, et al: Cloning and characterization of a novel bicoid-related homeobox transcription factor gene, RIEG, involved in Rieger syndrome, Nat Genet 14(4):392–399, 1996.

111. Suh H, et al: Pitx2 is required at multiple stages of pituitary organogenesis: pituitary primordium formation and cell specification, Development 129(2):329–337, 2002.

112. Charles MA, et al: PITX genes are required for cell survival and Lhx3 activation, Mol Endocrinol 19(7):1893–1903, 2005.

113. Kioussi C, et al: Identification of a Wnt/Dvl/beta-Catenin –> Pitx2 pathway mediating cell-type-specific proliferation during development, Cell 111(5):673–685, 2002.

114. Lanctot C, et al: Hindlimb patterning and mandible development require the Ptx1 gene, Development 126(9):1805–1810, 1999.

115. Gage PJ, Suh H, Camper SA: Dosage requirement of Pitx2 for development of multiple organs, Development 126(20):4643–4651, 1999.

116. Kitamura K, et al: Mouse Pitx2 deficiency leads to anomalies of the ventral body wall, heart, extra- and periocular mesoderm and right pulmonary isomerism, Development 126(24):5749–5758, 1999.

117. Lu MF, et al: Function of Rieger syndrome gene in left-right asymmetry and craniofacial development, Nature 401(6750):276–278, 1999.

118. Holmberg J, Liu CY, Hjalt TA: PITX2 gain-of-function in Rieger syndrome eye model, Am J Pathol 165(5):1633–1641, 2004.

119. Holmberg J, et al: PITX2 gain-of-function induced defects in mouse forelimb development, BMC Dev Biol 8:25, 2008.

120. Lines MA, et al: Characterization and prevalence of PITX2 microdeletions and mutations in Axenfeld-Rieger malformations, Invest Ophthalmol Vis Sci 45(3):828–833, 2004.

121. Priston M, et al: Functional analyses of two newly identified PITX2 mutants reveal a novel molecular mechanism for Axenfeld-Rieger syndrome, Hum Mol Genet 10(16):1631–1638, 2001.

122. Szeto DP, et al: P-OTX: a PIT-1-interacting homeodomain factor expressed during anterior pituitary gland development, Proc Natl Acad Sci U S A 93(15):7706–7710, 1996.

123. Lamonerie T, et al: Ptx1, a bicoid-related homeo box transcription factor involved in transcription of the pro-opiomelanocortin gene, Genes Dev 10(10):1284–1295, 1996.

124. Poulin G, et al: Specific protein-protein interaction between basic helix-loop-helix transcription factors and homeoproteins of the Pitx family, Mol Cell Biol 20(13):4826–4837, 2000.

125. Tremblay JJ, et al: Ptx1 regulates SF-1 activity by an interaction that mimics the role of the ligand-binding domain, EMBO J 18(12):3431–3441, 1999.

126. Tremblay JJ, Drouin J: Egr-1 is a downstream effector of GnRH and synergizes by direct interaction with Ptx1 and SF-1 to enhance luteinizing hormone beta gene transcription, Mol Cell Biol 19(4):2567–2576, 1999.

127. Tremblay JJ, Lanctot C, Drouin J: The pan-pituitary activator of transcription, Ptx1 (pituitary homeobox 1), acts in synergy with SF-1 and Pit1 and is an upstream regulator of the Lim-homeodomain gene Lim3/Lhx3, Mol Endocrinol 12(3):428–441, 1998.

128. Kioussi C, et al: Pax6 is essential for establishing ventral-dorsal cell boundaries in pituitary gland development, Proc Natl Acad Sci U S A 96(25):14378–14382, 1999.

129. Rosenfeld MG, et al: Transcriptional control of cell phenotypes in the neuroendocrine system, Recent Prog Horm Res 51:217–238; discussion 238–239, 1996.

130. Zhu X, et al: Signaling and epigenetic regulation of pituitary development, Curr Opin Cell Biol 19(6):605–611, 2007.

131. Zhu X, et al: Genetic control of pituitary development and hypopituitarism, Curr Opin Genet Dev 15(3):332–340, 2005.

132. Li X, et al: Tissue-specific regulation of retinal and pituitary precursor cell proliferation, Science 297(5584):1180–1183, 2002.

133. Li X, et al: Eya protein phosphatase activity regulates Six1-Dach-Eya transcriptional effects in mammalian organogenesis, Nature 426(6964):247–254, 2003.

134. Lagutin OV, et al: Six3 repression of Wnt signaling in the anterior neuroectoderm is essential for vertebrate forebrain development, Genes Dev 17(3):368–379, 2003.

135. Zhao L, et al: Steroidogenic factor 1 (SF1) is essential for pituitary gonadotrope function, Development 128(2):147–154, 2001.

136. Park HL, et al: Mouse Gli1 mutants are viable but have defects in SHH signaling in combination with a Gli2 mutation, Development 127(8):1593–1605, 2000.

137. Kondoh H, et al: Zebrafish mutations in Gli-mediated hedgehog signaling lead to lens transdifferentiation from the adenohypophysis anlage, Mech Dev 96(2):165–174, 2000.

138. Acampora D, et al: Transient dwarfism and hypogonadism in mice lacking Otx1 reveal prepubescent stage-specific control of pituitary levels of GH, FSH and LH, Development 125(7):1229–1239, 1998.

139. Acampora D, Gulisano M, Simeone A: Genetic and molecular roles of Otx homeodomain proteins in head development, Gene 246(1–2):23–35, 2000.

140. Dateki S, et al: OTX2 Mutation in a Patient with Anophthalmia, Short Stature, and Partial GH Deficiency: Functional Studies Using the IRBP, HESX1, and POU1F1 Promoters, J Clin Endocrinol Metab 93(10):3697–3702, 2008.

141. Edlund T, Jessell TM: Progression from extrinsic to intrinsic signaling in cell fate specification: a view from the nervous system, Cell 96(2):211–224, 1999.

142. Ashe HL, Briscoe J: The interpretation of morphogen gradients, Development 133(2):385–394, 2006.

143. Tabata T, Takei Y: Morphogens, their identification and regulation, Development 131(4):703–712, 2004.

144. Treier M, et al: Hedgehog signaling is required for pituitary gland development, Development 128(3):377–386, 2001.

145. Ingham PW, Placzek M: Orchestrating ontogenesis: variations on a theme by sonic hedgehog, Nat Rev Genet 7(11):841–850, 2006.

146. Marigo V, et al: Cloning, expression, and chromosomal location of SHH and IHH: two human homologues of the Drosophila segment polarity gene hedgehog, Genomics 28(1):44–51, 1995.

147. Chiang C, et al: Cyclopia and defective axial patterning in mice lacking Sonic hedgehog gene function, Nature 383(6599):407–413, 1996.

148. Ekker SC, et al: Distinct expression and shared activities of members of the hedgehog gene family of Xenopus laevis, Development 121(8):2337–2347, 1995.

149. Hui CC, et al: Expression of three mouse homologs of the Drosophila segment polarity gene cubitus interruptus, Gli, Gli-2, and Gli-3, in ectoderm- and mesoderm-derived tissues suggests multiple roles during postimplantation development, Dev Biol 162(2):402–413, 1994.

150. Sbrogna JL, Barresi MJ, Karlstrom RO: Multiple roles for Hedgehog signaling in zebrafish pituitary development, Dev Biol 254(1):19–35, 2003.

151. Laufer E, et al: Sonic hedgehog and Fgf-4 act through a signaling cascade and feedback loop to integrate growth and patterning of the developing limb bud, Cell 79(6):993–1003, 1994.

152. Ornitz DM, Itoh N: Fibroblast growth factors, Genome Biol 2(3):REVIEWS3005, 2001.

153. Thisse B, Thisse C: Functions and regulations of fibroblast growth factor signaling during embryonic development, Dev Biol 287(2):390–402, 2005.

154. Allen BL, Rapraeger AC: Spatial and temporal expression of heparan sulfate in mouse development regulates FGF and FGF receptor assembly, J Cell Biol 163(3):637–648, 2003.

155. Lin X: Functions of heparan sulfate proteoglycans in cell signaling during development, Development 131(24):6009–6021, 2004.

156. De Moerlooze L, et al: An important role for the IIIb isoform of fibroblast growth factor receptor 2 (FGFR2) in mesenchymal-epithelial signalling during mouse organogenesis, Development 127(3):483–492, 2000.

157. Min H, et al: Fgf-10 is required for both limb and lung development and exhibits striking functional similarity to Drosophila branchless, Genes Dev 12(20):3156–3161, 1998.

158. Chi CL, et al: The isthmic organizer signal FGF8 is required for cell survival in the prospective midbrain and cerebellum, Development 130(12):2633–2644, 2003.

159. Meyers EN, Lewandoski M, Martin GR: An Fgf8 mutant allelic series generated by Cre- and Flp-mediated recombination, Nat Genet 18(2):136–141, 1998.

160. Takuma N, et al: Formation of Rathke's pouch requires dual induction from the diencephalon, Development 125(23):4835–4840, 1998.

161. Norlin S, Nordstrom U, Edlund T: Fibroblast growth factor signaling is required for the proliferation and patterning of progenitor cells in the developing anterior pituitary, Mech Dev 96(2):175–182, 2000.

162. Zhao GQ: Consequences of knocking out BMP signaling in the mouse, Genesis 35(1):43–56, 2003.

163. Davis SW, Camper SA: Noggin regulates Bmp4 activity during pituitary induction, Dev Biol 305(1):145–160, 2007.

164. Artavanis-Tsakonas S, Rand MD, Lake RJ: Notch signaling: cell fate control and signal integration in development, Science 284(5415):770–776, 1999.

165. Louvi A, Artavanis-Tsakonas S: Notch signalling in vertebrate neural development, Nat Rev Neurosci 7(2):93–102, 2006.

166. Raetzman LT, Cai JX, Camper SA: Hes1 is required for pituitary growth and melanotrope specification, Dev Biol 304(2):455–466, 2007.

167. Raetzman LT, et al: Persistent expression of Notch2 delays gonadotrope differentiation, Mol Endocrinol 20(11):2898–2908, 2006.

168. Kita A, et al: Hes1 and Hes5 control the progenitor pool, intermediate lobe specification, and posterior lobe formation in the pituitary development, Mol Endocrinol 21(6):1458–1466, 2007.

169. Miller JR: The Wnts, Genome Biol 3(1):REVIEWS3001, 2002.

170. Clevers H: Wnt/beta-catenin signaling in development and disease, Cell 127(3):469–480, 2006.

171. Huang H, He X: Wnt/beta-catenin signaling: new (and old) players and new insights, Curr Opin Cell Biol 20(2):119–125, 2008.

172. Potok MA, et al: WNT signaling affects gene expression in the ventral diencephalon and pituitary gland growth, Dev Dyn 237(4):1006–1020, 2008.

173. Cha KB, et al: WNT5A signaling affects pituitary gland shape, Mech Dev 121(2):183–194, 2004.

174. Briata P, et al: The Wnt/beta-catenin–>Pitx2 pathway controls the turnover of Pitx2 and other unstable mRNAs, Mol Cell 12(5):1201–1211, 2003.

175. Ai D, et al: Nuclear factor 1 and T-cell factor/LEF recognition elements regulate Pitx2 transcription in pituitary development, Mol Cell Biol 27(16):5765–5775, 2007.

176. Burns CJ, et al: Investigation of Frizzled-5 during embryonic neural development in mouse, Dev Dyn 237(6):1614–1626, 2008.

177. Brinkmeier ML, et al: TCF and Groucho-related genes influence pituitary growth and development, Mol Endocrinol 17(11):2152–2161, 2003.

178. Brinkmeier ML, et al: TCF4 deficiency expands ventral diencephalon signaling and increases induction of pituitary progenitors, Dev Biol 311(2):396–407, 2007.

179. DiMattia GE, et al: The Pit-1 gene is regulated by distinct early and late pituitary-specific enhancers, Dev Biol 182(1):180–190, 1997.

180. Ohkubo Y, Chiang C, Rubenstein JL: Coordinate regulation and synergistic actions of BMP4, SHH and FGF8 in the rostral prosencephalon regulate morphogenesis of the telencephalic and optic vesicles, Neuroscience 111(1):1–17, 2002.

181. Guner B, et al: Graded Hh and Fgf signaling independently regulate pituitary cell fates and help establish the PD and PI of the zebrafish adenohypophysis, Endocrinology 149(9):4435–4451, 2008.

182. Anderson RM, et al: Chordin and noggin promote organizing centers of forebrain development in the mouse, Development 129(21):4975–4987, 2002.

183. Roh M, et al: Stage-sensitive blockade of pituitary somatomammotrope development by targeted expression of a dominant negative epidermal growth factor receptor in transgenic mice, Mol Endocrinol 15(4):600–613, 2001.

184. Bousquet C, Ray DW, Melmed S: A common pro-opiomelanocortin-binding element mediates leukemia inhibitory factor and corticotropin-releasing hormone transcriptional synergy, J Biol Chem 272(16):10551–10557, 1997.

185. Yano H, et al: Pituitary-directed leukemia inhibitory factor transgene causes Cushing's syndrome: neuro-immune-endocrine modulation of pituitary development, Mol Endocrinol 12(11):1708–1720, 1998.

186. Zhu X, Gleiberman AS, Rosenfeld MG: Molecular physiology of pituitary development: signaling and transcriptional networks, Physiol Rev 87(3):933–963, 2007.

187. Qi Y, et al: Atbf1 is required for the Pit1 gene early activation, Proc Natl Acad Sci U S A 105(7):2481–2486, 2008.

188. Kouzarides T: Chromatin modifications and their function, Cell 128(4):693–705, 2007.

189. Jones BK, et al: The human growth hormone gene is regulated by a multicomponent locus control region, Mol Cell Biol 15(12):7010–7021, 1995.

190. Bennani-Baiti IM, et al: DNase I-hypersensitive sites I and II of the human growth hormone locus control region are a major developmental activator of somatotrope gene expression, Proc Natl Acad Sci U S A 95(18):10655–10660, 1998.

191. Shewchuk BM, et al: Pit-1 binding sites at the somatotrope-specific DNase I hypersensitive sites I, II of the human growth hormone locus control region are essential for in vivo hGH-N gene activation, J Biol Chem 274(50):35725–35733, 1999.

192. Ho Y, et al: A defined locus control region determinant links chromatin domain acetylation with long-range gene activation, Mol Cell 9(2):291–302, 2002.

193. Ho Y, et al: The juxtaposition of a promoter with a locus control region transcriptional domain activates gene expression, EMBO Rep 9(9):891–898, 2008.

194. Ho Y, et al: Locus control region transcription plays an active role in long-range gene activation, Mol Cell 23(3):365–375, 2006.

195. Lira SA, et al: Identification of rat growth hormone genomic sequences targeting pituitary expression in transgenic mice, Proc Natl Acad Sci U S A 85(13):4755–4759, 1988.

196. Wang J, et al: Opposing LSD1 complexes function in developmental gene activation and repression programmes, Nature 446(7138):882–887, 2007.

197. Lunyak VV, et al: Developmentally regulated activation of a SINE B2 repeat as a domain boundary in organogenesis, Science 317(5835):248–251, 2007.

198. Newell-Price J: Proopiomelanocortin gene expression and DNA methylation: implications for Cushing's syndrome and beyond, J Endocrinol 177(3):365–372, 2003.

199. Levy A: Physiological implications of pituitary trophic activity, J Endocrinol 174(2):147–155, 2002.

200. Vankelecom H: Stem cells in the postnatal pituitary? Neuroendocrinology 85(2):110–130, 2007.

201. Fauquier T, et al: SOX2-expressing progenitor cells generate all of the major cell types in the adult mouse pituitary gland, Proc Natl Acad Sci U S A 105(8):2907–2912, 2008.

202. Gleiberman AS, et al: Genetic approaches identify adult pituitary stem cells, Proc Natl Acad Sci U S A 105(17):6332–6337, 2008.

203. Garcia-Lavandeira M, et al: A GRFa2/Prop1/stem (GPS) cell niche in the pituitary, PLOS ONE 4(3):e4815. doi:10.1371/journal.pone.0004815, 2009.

204. Kerr J, Wood W, Ridgway EC: Basic science and clinical research advances in the pituitary transcription factors: Pit-1 and Prop-1, Curr Opin Endocrinol Diabetes Obes 15(4):359–363, 2008.

205. Quentien MH, et al: Pituitary transcription factors: from congenital deficiencies to gene therapy, J Neuroendocrinol 18(9):633–642, 2006.

206. Scully KM, Rosenfeld MG: Pituitary development: regulatory codes in mammalian organogenesis, Science 295(5563):2231–2235, 2002.

Chapter 2

PROLACTIN

NELSON D. HORSEMAN and KAREN A. GREGERSON

Prolactin (PRL) was the first of the pituitary hormones to be biochemically identified and purified,[1,2] and hyperprolactinemia caused by hormone-secreting tumors is the most common human pituitary disease. Only recently, however, have the physiology and biochemistry of prolactin actions yielded to contemporary analytic methods to reveal a biology that is at once elegantly simple and sublimely complex. PRL has been identified in the pituitary glands of members of all vertebrate classes, and it has diverse effects on osmoregulation, metabolism, reproduc-tion, metamorphosis, migratory behavior, parental behavior, and lactation.[3-6] In most species, especially mammals, PRL has a specialized role in the postmating phase of reproduction. The predominant mammalian actions of PRL are stimulation of lacta-tion and maternal behavior, and inhibition of reproductive func-tion. Associated with the specialization of PRL in mammals, novel genes that encode placentally derived lactogens have evolved. PRL does not perform any indispensable function for the survival of the individual, but gestation and lactation lie at the core of the mammalian life cycle, and they place extreme demands on physiology. Adaptations in the control of PRL secre-tion and its physiologic actions have therefore been integral to the biology of all mammals, and abnormalities of PRL secretion are a relatively common cause of endocrine disease. The deepen-ing understanding of PRL actions on both physiologic and molecular levels has facilitated improved therapeutic approaches to diseases of PRL secretion and has opened opportunities to use the physiology of PRL and lactation in new ways.

The Evolutionary Biology of Prolactin

THE PROLACTIN FAMILY

PRL and growth hormone (GH) are related at the primary amino acid sequence level.[7] PRL has been identified in all of the verte-brate classes, and it has been inferred that the PRL and GH genes arose from a duplication of an ancestral gene at least 400 million years ago, at about the time of the origin of vertebrates.[8] Deeper relationships with other hormones are less certain, but erythro-poietin shares substantial primary sequence similarity, as well as three-dimensional structural features, with PRL and GH, suggest-ing that all three of these hormones share an ancient common ancestry. In addition to PRL and GH, which have been conserved in all vertebrate lineages, a wide variety of derivative genes have appeared in specific vertebrate groups by duplication of the PRL or GH gene. The most familiar of these are the various mam-malian placental lactogens.[9,10]

PLACENTAL LACTOGENS

Placental lactogens (PLs) are synthesized during pregnancy in most, but not all, eutherian mammals. Species that apparently do not produce any placental lactogens are distributed among many mammalian families and include familiar species such as pigs, horses, and dogs.[11] Primates (including humans) synthesize a PL that is encoded by a gene duplicated within the GH locus.[8]

The GH locus in humans encompasses five genes spanning a region of about 50 kb on the long arm (q22-24) of chromosome 17. This locus includes two PL or, preferably, chorionic somato-mammotropin (CS) genes (ICSH-1 and ICSH-2). The ICSH-1 and ICSH-2 genes, although slightly divergent at the nucleotide sequence level, encode identical proteins, and the genes are coexpressed in the placenta during gestation. In nonprimates (e.g., rodents, ruminants), the PLs have descended evolutionarily from duplications of the PRL gene.[8] Multiple PL genes and non-lactogenic PRL-like genes have evolved from PRL. In mice, pla-cental lactogen-I (PL-I) is synthesized early during gestation, appearing immediately after implantation. PL-I expression is extinguished at about midgestation and is replaced by PL-II. Both of the mouse PL genes are synthesized in trophoblast giant cells. In species that synthesize PLs, including humans, the major stimulus to mammary gland development during pregnancy is presumably PLs, rather than pituitary PRL. PL levels generally rise in correlation with placental growth, and their secretion is controlled by both positive and negative regulators.[12] Loss of PLs and placental steroids at parturition is accompanied by elevation of pituitary PRL secretion, and a corresponding shift to pituitary-dominated regulation of mammary gland function during lacta-tion. The importance of this shift is that pituitary PRL is strongly regulated by a suckling-induced neuroendocrine reflex, which allows nursing activity to determine directly the lactational stim-ulus to the mammary glands.

NONLACTOGENIC PROLACTIN RELATIVES

Nonlactogenic members of the PRL gene family are synthesized by the placenta of nonprimates. Although the physiologic activi-ties of these PRL-related proteins have not yet been established, the expression patterns for some of these proteins are tightly regulated during gestation,[10] and this has been interpreted to indicate that the proteins are functionally important. In mice and rats, at least six nonlactogenic PRL-like proteins (PLP-A through PLP-F) are present. In addition, mice synthesize two proteins, namely, proliferin and proliferin-related protein, which have been proposed to act as regulators of angiogenesis.[13] Nonlacto-genic PRL-like protein genes have also been extensively charac-terized in cattle.[14] One curious feature of the PRL-like gene family is the apparently rapid evolutionary divergence of members of this family. These proteins generally share less than 25% sequence identity with PRL, but all share two pairs of cysteine residues that are conserved throughout the PRL and GH super-family.[10] Information regarding receptors for the nonlactogenic PRL-related proteins is scant. Proliferin binds to the mannose-6-phosphate insulin-like growth factor-2 (IGF-2) receptor.[15] In mice, some of the non-lactogenic PRL relatives are essential for preventing fetal death during physiologic stresses, such as hypoxia.[16,17] Therefore, the species specificity of PRL relatives may reflect the reproductive stresses that were relevant during the evolutionary divergence of different mammalian groups.

EXTRAPITUITARY PROLACTIN

Many mammalian tissues, including the human mammary gland and uterine decidua, express the PRL gene. In addition, various tissues metabolize PRL to alternative forms that may be biologi-cally active. PRL is synthesized by both the decidua and the uterine myometrium in humans.[18] High concentrations of PRL are present in the amniotic fluid; these can be traced to both decidually synthesized hormone and plasma PRL that is trans-ported across the placenta into the amniotic fluid. The synthesis of human PRL in extrapituitary sites is controlled by a promoter

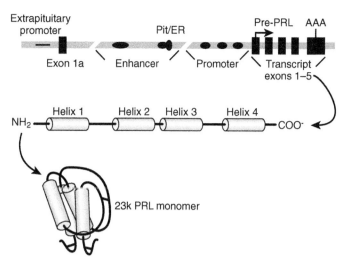

FIGURE 2-1. Biosynthesis of prolactin (PRL). The PRL gene is depicted at the top of the figure as consisting of five exons *(black rectangles)* encoding the structural gene for preprolactin (pre-PRL). The translation start site in exon 1 is marked by an *arrow,* and the polyadenylation site in exon 5 is marked *AAA.* The region labeled *promoter* includes multiple binding sites for the pituitary-specific transcription factor-1 (Pit-1; *black ellipses),* but only three are depicted in the diagram. The line that depicts the DNA sequence is broken by two interruptions to indicate that the upstream regula-tory regions are separated from the promoter by several thousand base pairs. A distal regulatory region (enhancer) includes binding sites for Pit-1 and other factors, includ-ing a complex site that binds both Pit-1 and the estrogen receptor (Pit/ER). Exon 1a is transcribed in extrapituitary tissues and is controlled by a distinct "extrapituitary promoter." After transcription and translation, the PRL protein consists of four α-helical regions, which are labeled *helix 1 through 4,* and intervening β-strand regions. The protein spontaneously folds into a globular structure in which three disulfide bridges connect β-strand regions, and this mature structure is depicted as the 23k PRL monomer.

that is distinct from the pituitary PRL promoter. Human extra-pituitary PRL messenger RNA (mRNA) has a distinct 5′ untrans-lated sequence corresponding to an additional exon (exon 1A)[19] (Fig. 2-1). Exon 1A and the promoter elements associated with it are located about 8000 base pairs (bp) distal to the initiation site for pituitary PRL transcription. In rodents, the evidence for a distinct extrapituitary PRL promoter is less certain than in the human. It is conceivable that rodents use other mechanisms, such as growth factors that control the conventional pituitary PRL promoter, to provide for regulation of PRL synthesis in extrapituitary tissues. The mammary gland is an important site of PRL synthesis and secretion. PRL is present in significant concentrations in milk, and milk PRL is absorbed by the neonatal gut and causes changes in the maturation of the hypothalamic neuroendocrine system.[20] Pituitary PRL is transported out of the circulation, across the mammary epithelium, and into the alveo-lar lumen, and locally synthesized PRL is secreted into milk.[18] To date, no disease states have been connected to dysregulation of extrapituitary PRL secretion. The lack of any clear proof that symptoms are present that are caused by either hypersecretion of extrapituitary PRL—say, from a PRL-secreting ectopic tumor—or loss of extrapituitary PRL gene expression makes it difficult to surmise the normal functional roles of extrapituitary PRL in humans. It has been suggested that locally synthesized PRL in the mammary gland might act as a growth factor for both normal breast epithelium and breast cancer cells.[21] In mice, decidual PRL prevents fetal loss late in pregnancy by inhibiting the expression of multiple genes that are detrimental to pregnancy, including inflammatory cytokines.[22] A recent pilot study reports a lack of endometrial PRL expression in some women with unexplained infertility and patients with repeated miscarriages.[23]

The Biochemistry of Prolactin

Human PRL is synthesized as a prehormone that is encoded by an mRNA with an open reading frame of 684 bases. The native gene for PRL is divided into five exons, and the initiation site for translation is in exon 1[24] (see Fig. 2-1). Preprolactin (pre-PRL) is 227 amino acids in length, with a deduced molecular weight of nearly 26,000. Cleaving the signal peptide from the N-terminus of pre-PRL results in a mature polypeptide that is 199 residues in length and has a molecular weight of nearly 23,000 (23k PRL). On the basis of the fact that the bacterially synthesized recombinant 23k PRL monomer binds to the PRL receptor (PRL-R) and transduces functional signals, it is clear that no additional modifications are essential for the core functions of PRL. PRL folds itself into a tertiary structure that includes three intrachain disulfide bridges, two of which are conserved in all members of the PRL-GH family, and one that links residues 4 and 11 in the N-terminus, which is unique to PRL and its closest relatives.[7] Four α-helical domains in PRL are arranged so that helices 1 and 2 run antiparallel to helices 3 and 4. This general molecular architecture of PRL has been conserved with GH and other homologous proteins and also has evolved independently in several families of cytokines.[25] The convergent evolution of hormone and cytokine ligand architecture apparently has been driven by the properties of receptors that bind these hormones and transduce signals to the intracellular space.

A variety of biochemical variants of 23k PRL, which appear to have altered functions, have been identified. PRL has a tendency to aggregate and form intermolecular disulfide bridges spontaneously when in solution at high concentrations. High-molecular-weight variants (sometimes referred to as "big" PRLs) may arise by virtue of multimerization, glycosylation, or cross-linking with other proteins. Only a small fraction of human PRL is glycosylated, whereas in some other species, such as swine, glycosylated PRL represents a large portion of both pituitary and plasma hormone.[26] Glycosylation may alter the relative potency of PRL by changing its receptor-binding characteristics or by modifying its pharmacokinetic properties in the animal (plasma half-life, partitioning between plasma and interstitial compartments, etc.). PRL is metabolized by tissue uptake and by proteolysis in the circulation or in cells. Proteolysis also produces a 16kDa PRL fragment that has been proposed to have antiangiogenic bioactivity.[27]

Recent studies implicate the cathepsin-cleaved 16kDa PRL as causative of postpartum (or peripartum) cardiomyopathy (PPCM). PPCM is the acute onset of heart failure in women during late-stage pregnancy or the first several months post partum. Hilfiker-Kleiner and colleagues discovered that PPCM developed in mice with selective deletion of the *STAT3* gene in cardiac myocytes.[28] *STAT3* has been shown to be a critical factor modulating cardiac angiogenesis, an important part of the normal cardiac hypertrophy that occurs during pregnancy.[29] In a series of elegant studies, they demonstrated that the absence of *STAT3* led to increased production of reactive oxygen species, upregulation of cathepsin-D, and elevation of the 16kDa fragment of PRL. Treatment of these mice with bromocriptine, which reduces secretion of 23kDa PRL from the pituitary, resulted in enhanced cardiac function and prevention of postpartum mortality. Preliminary studies have shown that circulating levels of 16kDa are barely detectable in healthy nursing women but are elevated in some women with PPCM.[28] A few clinical case reports have found that women with PPCM may respond favorably to treatment with bromocriptine.[28,30,31]

Phosphorylated PRL has reduced potency in standard bioassays, and it antagonizes the actions of the predominant unphosphorylated form.[32] Actions of kinases or phosphatases in either the pituitary or individual target tissues may have an important effect on the bioactivity of PRL in vivo.

The Ontogeny and Physiology of Prolactin Secretion

DEVELOPMENT OF LACTOTROPHS

PRL is synthesized by lactotrophs, which are acidophilic cells that represent 20% to 50% of the anterior pituitary cell population. The lactotrophs are the last of the pituitary cell types to fully differentiate and, coincidentally, the most likely to give rise to pituitary adenomas. Pituitary PRL mRNA synthesis begins at 12 weeks in human gestation and is preceded by GH synthesis by at least 4 weeks.[8,33] In rodents, the pattern is similar, with the GH gene being expressed several days before PRL, and with dual-functioning somatolactotrophs being observed before fully differentiated lactotrophs.[34] Control of pituitary development and lactotroph differentiation depends on the orchestrated expression of a series of intrinsic, tissue-specific regulatory molecules that act as "molecular switches" to induce the sequence of developmental changes that lead up to full pituitary differentiation. Many of the intrinsic factors that have been implicated in pituitary development are evolutionarily related to "homeotic mutation" genes, which were first identified by their dramatic effects on development in fruit flies.[33] Some genetic diseases of the pituitary, pituitary tumors, and physiologic states of hormone deficiency or excess can be attributed to dysfunction of these regulatory molecules.

The homeobox transcription factors are a diverse class of developmental regulatory proteins that share sequence similarities in their DNA-binding regions and are sequentially activated during organogenesis. Two pituitary homeobox proteins (Ptx1 and Ptx2) are expressed in multiple anterior (head and face) tissues before the development of Rathke's pouch, and they continue to be expressed in some differentiated pituitary cells. Rathke's pouch homeobox protein (Rpx) is expressed first in neural structures associated with the head region and then in Rathke's pouch. During the formation of Rathke's pouch, a subgroup of LIM-related homeobox proteins are synthesized (P-LIM, Lhx3, and Lhx4), and these genes continue to be expressed in specific regions of the pituitary throughout life. Properly timed extinction of expression is, for certain genes, as important during development as is their appropriate induction. Rpx must be turned off after Rathke's pouch has been formed, so that genes that are specific to later stages of pituitary differentiation can be turned on. The transcription factor that downregulates Rpx expression is PROP-1 (Prophet of Pit-1). PROP-1 turns off Rpx and turns on Pit-1, leading to differentiation of some of the hormone-producing cells of the pituitary gland, including lactotrophs.[35]

In the adult pituitary gland, a population of stem-like cells provides new progenitors for all of the hormone-secreting cells, including lactotrophs.[36]

Pit-1 is essential for differentiation of both PRL- and GH-secreting cells, hence its alternative name, GH factor-1 (GHF-1).[37] An early developing subpopulation of thyrotrophs is also dependent on Pit-1. The Pit-1 protein shares close sequence similarity with two other transcription factors within regions referred to as the POU (Pit, Oct, Unc)-specific domain, and the POU-homeodomain.[38] Pit-1 expression in the developing pituitary gland precedes the synthesis of hormones and is necessary for the expression of GH, PRL, and thyroid-stimulating hormone (TSH) in fetal pituitaries. Variant forms of Pit-1 are encoded by alternatively spliced mRNAs and may differentially control expression of individual hormones. Pit-1 binds not only to DNA sequences in the GH, PRL, and TSH genes, but also to autoregulatory sites in the Pit-1 promoter. Autoactivation of Pit-1 transcription is one means of preserving phenotypic stability in differentiated pituitary cells. The factors that act after Pit-1 to drive the differentiation of lactotrophs from somatotroph progenitors are not known. Estrogen receptors synergize with Pit-1 to induce PRL, but not GH, gene expression. Estrogen therefore may be one of the factors that drive the ultimate differentiation of lactotrophs.[39-42]

Several extrinsic factors are involved in lactotroph differentiation. Estrogen is an important positive regulator of lactotroph development. Lactotrophs are greater in number and contain more PRL per cell in females during their reproductive years. Estrogen acts directly on lactotrophs to stimulate PRL synthesis and cell proliferation. Estrogen-induced galanin secretion from lactotrophs is an important mediator of these estrogen actions[43,44] and involves signaling through the classic estrogen receptor isoform alpha (ERα).[45] Paracrine factors produced by other anterior pituitary cell types include basic fibroblast growth factor (B-FGF or FGF-2), which has a specific positive stimulatory effect on lactotrophs.[46] Likewise, epidermal growth factor (EGF) stimulates lactotrophs and may act as a developmental regulatory factor as well as a physiologic stimulator of PRL secretion.[47] As will be presented in subsequent sections, the same factors that drive vectorial differentiation of pituitary cells can participate in regulating the tides of hormone secretion on a physiologic time scale and in disorders of hormone secretion.

REGULATION OF PITUITARY PROLACTIN SYNTHESIS AND SECRETION

In mammals, PRL secretion is normally restrained by the action of dopamine (DA), which is secreted from the hypothalamus.[48] Although the levels of other pituitary hormones are modulated by inhibitory secretagogues such as somatostatin, PRL is the only such hormone that is secreted at unrestrained high levels when completely isolated from the positive trophic influences of the hypothalamus. This unconventional situation is unique to mammals. Control of PRL secretion in birds and other nonmammals is more conventional in the sense that positively acting secretagogues are the predominant regulators of PRL secretion.[49,50] Lactotrophs are excitable cells in that they display spontaneous membrane depolarizations associated with calcium ion influx, and their resting membrane potential is influenced by neurotransmitters and peptide neuromodulators.

The normal secretory pattern of PRL is a series of daily pulses, occurring every 2 to 3 hours, which vary in amplitude so that the bulk of the hormone is secreted during rapid eye movement (REM) sleep. REM sleep is the dominant organizer in men and nonparous women and occurs mostly during the latter half of the sleep phase. Thus, the highest levels of PRL generally occur during the night in humans.[51] In nocturnal rodents, the relationship to the light cycle is reversed, so higher PRL secretion occurs during the daytime, which is the inactive phase. It is unclear how REM and PRL secretion are linked. Infusion of PRL increases

REM activity in the electroencephalogram (EEG),[52,53] suggesting that it is PRL that induces REM sleep, and not vice versa.

In lactating women, suckling is a potent stimulator of PRL secretion. This classic neuroendocrine reflex originates with the stimulation of sensory nerve endings in the nipple and is transmitted via the spinal cord and brain stem, ultimately to the hypothalamus. Stress and sexual orgasm are also potent stimulators of PRL secretion. Stress-induced PRL secretion varies with the duration, degree, and modality of the stressor. The relative contributions of PRL-releasing (PRF) and PRL-inhibiting factors to these PRL secretory events remain controversial.

DOPAMINE

As was mentioned earlier, the major regulatory input to lactotrophs is inhibitory, provided in the form of DA produced within the hypothalamus. The primary PRL-regulating DA neurons are the tuberoinfundibular dopaminergic (TIDA) cells, which have their cell bodies in the arcuate nucleus of the hypothalamus; they release DA in the median eminence and the pituitary stalk (Fig. 2-2). A secondary tuberohypophysial dopaminergic system has cell bodies in the rostral caudate and paraventricular nuclei, and these neurons release DA in the posterior pituitary.[48] The type 2 isoforms (D_2) of the DA receptor mediate the direct inhibitory actions of DA on PRL secretion, synthesis, and cell proliferation. Targeted disruption of the D_2 receptor in mice leads to a phenotype of PRL hypersecretion and lactotroph proliferation.[54]

Dopamine is synthesized by a two-step reaction in which tyrosine conversion to levodopa is catalyzed by tyrosine hydroxylase, and levodopa is converted to DA by the action of aromatic amine decarboxylase. As is the case for catecholamine synthesis in other cells, the momentary rate of DA synthesis in the TIDA neurons is determined by the activity of tyrosine hydroxylase. The negative feedback mechanism for controlling PRL release is to increase tyrosine hydroxylase activity in the TIDA neurons, thereby increasing the amount of DA available for release from the median eminence. PRL receptors are located in both the arcuate nucleus (site of the TIDA perikarya) and the median eminence.[55] Therefore, circulating PRL may feed back on TIDA neurons at their terminals, which lay outside the blood-brain

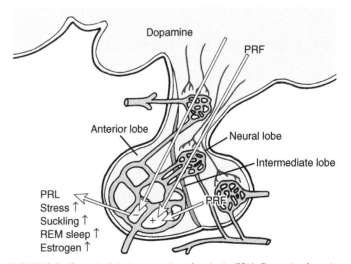

FIGURE 2-2. Control of pituitary secretion of prolactin (PRL). Dopamine from the hypothalamus is the predominant inhibitory regulator of pituitary PRL secretion. Multiple factors act as PRL-releasing factors (PRF; see text), and these come from both the hypothalamus and the posterior pituitary. Physiologic states that stimulate PRL release are listed on the figure. *REM*, Rapid eye movement.

barrier, or systemic PRL may enter the cerebrospinal fluid via the choroid plexus. The choroid plexus expresses high levels of a short isoform of the PRL-R, which may serve to transport PRL across the blood-brain barrier. Levels of PRL in the cerebrospinal fluid reflect changes in PRL in the systemic circulation.[56] Isolated PRL deficiency resulting from targeted gene disruption in the mouse causes decreased DA in the median eminence but does not affect DA levels in other regions of the hypothalamus.[57]

Activation of D_2 receptors in lactotrophs has at least two main actions that result in inhibition of PRL. D_2 receptors are members of the heptahelical G protein–coupled receptor superfamily, and they activate the α_i subunits, which leads to inhibition of cyclic adenosine monophosphate (cAMP) synthesis.[48] In addition, D_2 receptors activate a G protein–coupled, inwardly rectifying potassium channel, which instantaneously causes hyperpolarization of the lactotroph membrane and closes voltage-gated calcium channels.[58] Cytoplasmic calcium levels fall because of decreased influx of extracellular calcium, and the reduction in cytosolic free calcium decreases the exocytosis of secretory vesicles.

Dopamine-induced membrane hyperpolarization opposes the actions of some stimulatory factors such as thyrotropin-releasing hormone (TRH), which acts predominantly to increase influx of extracellular calcium by depolarizing the lactotroph membrane. Inhibition of cAMP by DA also opposes the actions of stimulatory factors such as vasoactive intestinal peptide (VIP), which acts via a positive effect on cAMP. This action decreases PRL release in the short to intermediate term. Second, because cAMP is mitogenic in lactotrophs, as well as in other pituitary cells, activation of G_i signaling by DA is antimitogenic. Lactotroph proliferation is important for physiologic elevation of PRL release during lactation. The proliferative action of cAMP on lactotrophs is understood to be an important promoter of pituitary tumor growth, thereby contributing to pathologic hyperprolactinemia.[35]

Other hypothalamic factors, as well as DA, and local pituitary peptides can inhibit PRL secretion. Somatostatin inhibits PRL secretion and acts through both cAMP-dependent and cAMP-independent mechanisms.[59] Calcitonin has been shown to inhibit PRL secretion and may be secreted from the hypothalamus.[60] Endothelin-1 is produced by lactotrophs and inhibits PRL secretion; transforming growth factor-β_1 can act as a paracrine inhibitor of PRL.[61,62] The biologic significance of these factors in pituitary development and physiology has not yet been established.

PROLACTIN-RELEASING FACTORS

A wide variety of stimulatory PRL secretagogues have been identified over the years, and it is likely that additional PRFs will be identified in the future. Known stimulators of PRL secretion include, but are not limited to, steroids (estrogen[63]), hypothalamic peptides (TRH, oxytocin, VIP,[64,65] pituitary adenylate cyclase activating peptide [PACAP],[66] and galanin[67]), and local pituitary factors (growth factors such as EGF[68] and FGF-2,[69] angiotensin II,[70] and, again, PACAP[71] and galanin[43]).

TRH is a potent and rapid stimulator of PRL release in vitro via a set of calcium-mediated pathways activated by a G_q-coupled receptor. However, the relative contribution of TRH to physiologic control of lactotrophs is not clear. VIP acts through cAMP to stimulate PRL synthesis and release on an intermediate to long-term basis. The importance of VIP as a positive lactotrophic factor is supported by two types of evidence. With the use of antibodies against VIP, the secretion of PRL can be inhibited to a very low level.[47] In addition, VIP appears to be the primary PRF in birds and other nonmammals,[72,73] suggesting that this

positive mechanism may have been in place before the evolution of the dopaminergic inhibitory system in mammals. Oxytocin secretion is tightly coupled with PRL secretion during lactation, and both are secreted in response to nipple stimulation. The potential role of oxytocin as a PRF, given that it can reach the anterior pituitary through the short portal system, has remained controversial. Oxytocin antagonism partially suppresses PRL secretion,[48] so this peptide is likely to provide some portion of the physiologic stimulus for PRL release. PACAP stimulates PRL synthesis and release. Galanin is synthesized in both the pituitary and the hypothalamus. In the pituitary, it colocalizes with PRL in lactotroph secretory granules and acts by autocrine and paracrine mechanisms to stimulate lactotrophs.[43]

A putative PRL-releasing peptide (PrRP) from the hypothalamus was identified by searching for ligands that activate an orphan pituitary G protein–coupled receptor. The mature peptide that was identified from bovine hypothalamus is a 20 amino acid molecule that originally was reported to cause rapid secretion of PRL from isolated pituitary cells.[74] However, subsequent studies have failed to confirm that PrRP acts on lactotrophs to stimulate PRL release.[75] Rather, PrRP may act within the hypothalamus to indirectly elevate PRL by inhibiting DA release. Antagonists of serotonin or opioid receptors inhibit PRL secretion under physiologically meaningful stimuli. Conversely, antidepressants that inhibit serotonin reuptake (fluoxetine [Prozac], etc.) may increase PRL secretion in humans and in laboratory animals. Serotonin and opioids are important indirect regulators of PRL by virtue of their actions on DA and releasing factor secretion in the hypothalamus.

Lactotrophs display a large degree of functional heterogeneity within the anterior pituitary. This heterogeneity is manifested as differences in morphology (i.e., secretory granule size and density), basal hormone release, electrical activity, and response to releasing and inhibiting factors. Assay of hormone release from single cells has revealed not only substantial cell-to-cell variations in function, but also marked temporal variations in a single cell.[76]

Transcription regulators that control the development of the anterior pituitary lactotrophs also participate in controlling PRL synthesis during adult life. Prominent among these factors is the Pit-1 protein. Pit-1 binds to two regions of the human PRL gene, the proximal promoter (within 250 bp of the transcription start) and a distal enhancer (beyond −1300 bp) (see Fig. 2-1). Multiple Pit-1–binding sites are present in each of these regions. Transcription regulators such as cAMP and estrogen receptors can control PRL gene expression by influencing Pit-1 activity.[39,63]

Pathophysiology of Prolactin Secretion

Normal plasma PRL concentrations in women who are neither pregnant nor lactating range from 4 to <20 ng/mL. In men, the values, on average, are several units lower. Late pregnancy and lactational levels normally range from 100 to 200 ng/mL, and the highest levels occur following active bouts of nursing. PRL is normally measured by radioimmunoassay (RIA). Although glycosylation and other chemical modifications of PRL can affect its immunoreactivity and therefore can lead to aberrant RIA results,[26] pathologic levels generally are readily detected by RIA. The original method for bioassay of PRL involved measuring the growth of the pigeon crop sac mucosal epithelium.[77] This method still is used occasionally and serves as the basis for the international standardization of PRL bioactivity. However, the method has been largely supplanted by a simpler bioassay that takes advantage of the ability of PRL to stimulate the proliferation of rat Nb2 lymphoma cells in culture.[78]

PROLACTIN DEFICIENCY

When PRL deficiency occurs, it is normally one component of a combined pituitary hormone deficiency. However, a few cases of PRL deficiency without evidence of other pituitary defects have been reported in women. Isolated PRL deficiency results in lactational failure and reproductive difficulty with no other obvious problems.[79-82] No cases of isolated PRL deficiency have been reported in men. These results in a few humans are consistent with the phenotype of mice in which the PRL gene has been disrupted by a targeted mutation. In mice with disruptions of either PRL or its receptor genes, mammary gland development is defective; the females fail to reproduce, but the males do not have any overt symptoms.[57,84,85] The concordance of these results from humans and mice is remarkable, given the possible differences between PRL physiology in humans and rodents. One important difference is that progesterone secretion in the rodent corpus luteum requires PRL, but in the human, it does not. This difference in luteal control probably explains why women who have isolated PRL deficiency are merely subfertile,[79-82] whereas PRL-deficient mouse females are completely infertile.[84,85]

Mice with a targeted mutation of the PRL gene develop pituitary hyperplasia[57] and adenomas[86] that are more severe in females. Mice with targeted disruption of the PRL receptor gene also exhibit this lactotroph hyperplasia and prolactinoma development.[87] Loss of PRL feedback in both of these genetic models leads to decreased hypothalamic DA, and the deficiency of DA leads to poorly restrained pituitary growth. Some forms of combined pituitary hormone deficiency have been identified in which PRL, GH, and TSH are hyposecreted as a consequence of mutations in important developmental factors. Familial inheritance of defects in the Pit-1 gene or PROP-1 results in individuals who fail to develop lactotrophs, somatotrophs, and thyrotrophs, and consequently are dwarfed and hypothyroid, as well as PRL deficient. Two spontaneous mutations that cause dwarfism in mice have been shown to correspond to these human conditions. In Snell dwarf mice, a mutation of the Pit-1 gene occurs, and in Ames dwarfs, the PROP-1 gene is mutated.[35,88,89]

HYPERPROLACTINEMIA

Hypersecretion of PRL is among the most common of pituitary disorders. Medications that elevate PRL secretion and may cause hyperprolactinemia include commonly used antiemetics, antipsychotics, antidepressants, and narcotics. These medications alter PRL secretion by antagonizing DA action, or by elevating serotonin or endorphin bioactivity. Reserpine and methyldopa increase PRL secretion as a result of DA depletion. DA receptor antagonists, such as haloperidol and phenylthiazines, increase PRL secretion. Serotonin reuptake inhibitors, such as fluoxetine, elevate serum PRL.[48] It is uncommon for any of these medications to cause clinical signs of hyperprolactinemia, because the levels of PRL seldom reach more than 30 to 50 ng/mL with these drugs. One might imagine that subtle hormonal effects may be noted after long-term treatment.

Hyperprolactinemia that manifests clinical symptoms is most commonly a consequence of a lactotroph adenoma. These tumors may secrete high levels of PRL alone or of both PRL and GH. Any intracranial mass or trauma that causes compression or disruption of the pituitary stalk can cause hyperprolactinemia because of the loss of dopaminergic tone from the hypothalamus.

Pituitary adenomas have been discovered to be much more common than was once believed, with more than 20% of individuals harboring tumors measuring at least 3 mm at autopsy.[35] Tumors that do not hypersecrete hormones are usually of gonadotroph or lactotroph origin. Some symptoms of prolactinomas may be caused by tumor mass effects. These include visual field defects, associated with pressure on the medial aspect of the optic chiasm, and alterations in temperature regulation, feeding patterns, or other effects caused by hypothalamic compression. However, effects associated with the physiologic actions of the hormone are the more common presenting symptoms.

Galactorrhea (breast milk secretion in an individual who is not postpartum) and amenorrhea are the result of PRL actions directly on the breast and the hypothalamic-pituitary-ovarian axis. In men, galactorrhea and impotence are the most common presenting symptoms of a hypersecreting prolactinoma. The causes of impotence in hyperprolactinemia, whether hormonal or neurogenic, are unclear. Hyperprolactinemia is treated medically by administration of DA agonists, including bromocriptine and cabergoline, or surgically by resection of the tumor tissue.

Prolactin Receptors and Signal Transduction

RECEPTORS

The PRL-R is a member of the type 1 cytokine receptor family,[90] and its nearest relative is the GH receptor. Several hematopoietic cytokine receptors, such as those for erythropoietin, most interleukins, and granulocyte-macrophage colony-stimulating factor, are also very similar to PRL and GH receptors. Other receptors, such as those for the interferons, are members of a broader superfamily of proteins that includes cell adhesion proteins. Features that define the type 1 cytokine receptor family include two signature motifs in the extracellular domain and one in the intracellular domain. Four cysteine residues in the extracellular domain are absolutely conserved among all of the type 1 cytokine receptors, and they form two disulfide bridges that are essential for the proper tertiary folding of the ligand-binding domain. A short sequence, which includes a tandem repeat of tryptophan-serine interrupted by a single amino acid (the WSXWS motif), is the second signature motif in the extracellular domain. This sequence is highly conserved near the base of the extracellular domain, but the function of these residues has not yet been proven with any degree of certainty. The structure of the PRL-R extracellular domain, like that of the GH and other cytokine receptors, has been analyzed extensively by x-ray crystallography, as well as by biochemical methods.[91] This domain comprises two 100 amino acid subdomains, which are structurally related to the type III repeats of fibronectin. Each of the type III subdomains includes a conserved series of seven β-strands folded into two β-sheets that run in an antiparallel orientation. These type III subdomains are connected by a short, flexible hinge peptide, and residues that contact the ligand span this connector to include amino acids in each of the type III subdomains. Across the vertebrate lineages, substantial conservation of the major features of the PRL-Rs is evident, with some notable exceptions. In birds (pigeons, chickens), the extracellular domain has duplicated and diverged, and in cattle, the distal C-terminus has been truncated, thus eliminating a tyrosine residue that is conserved

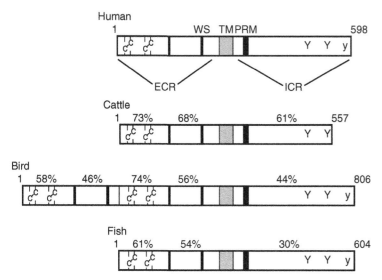

FIGURE 2-3. Prolactin receptor structure and function. Schematic diagram of the linear sequences of representative prolactin receptors. Pertinent structural features are two pairs of cysteines, the flexible hinge *(double line)*, and the WS × WS repeat in the extracellular region (ECR). The transmembrane-spanning sequence (TM) marks the separation between the ECR and the intracellular region (ICR). In the ICR, the conserved motifs are the proline rich box 1 motif (PRM) and conserved tyrosine residues. The uppercase Y indicates ubiquitously conserved tyrosines, and the lowercase y is a tyrosine that is conserved in all known species except cattle. The percentage of identical amino acid residues in each region, compared with the human receptor, is labeled above each receptor.

in other lineages (Fig. 2-3). Neither of these evolutionary changes appears to have functional significance.[92,93]

Within the intracellular region of the PRL-R an 8 amino acid proline-rich motif, referred to as box 1, is the third conserved signature motif that characterizes type 1 cytokine receptors. These amino acids interact directly with the tyrosine kinases that are activated on ligand binding to the extracellular domain, and mutations in box 1 completely disable PRL-R signaling.[5] Multiple PRL-R isoforms vary in terms of length and amino acid sequence of the intracellular domain. The long isoform, which has been identified in all species to date, has an intracellular domain that is about 350 amino acids in length. Short isoforms (<100 intracellular residues) have been identified in rodents, humans, and several other mammalian species. The short forms of the PRL-R include box 1 but lack other regions of the intracellular domain that are required for signal transduction. In particular, conserved tyrosine residues in the distal portion of the long form of the receptor are phosphorylated after ligand binding, and these tyrosines are required for normal signal transduction.

Mutations of the conserved tyrosines indicate some degree of functional redundancy among these residues, but at least one of the conserved tyrosines must be present to allow normal receptor signal transduction. A mutant PRL-R isoform in rat Nb2 lymphoma cells has a large deletion between box 1 and the distal conserved tyrosines, and this receptor is able to transduce all of the known signaling functions of the long form. Multiple short isoforms of the PRL-R have been discovered in a variety of mammalian species. The functional significance of the short isoforms is not completely known. Although these could provide for signaling diversity, they may act as decoy receptors and/or transport molecules. The possibility that the short PRL-R isoforms act as PRL transporters is supported by the observation that the choroid plexus and the liver have a preponderance of short-form receptors. The most likely function of the receptors in these tissues is to transport PRL across membranes. It is also conceivable that short PRL-R isoforms, acting as decoy receptors in some tissues, protect those cells from exaggerated PRL signaling during pregnancy and lactation.

Ligand binding appears to facilitate conformational changes or dimerization of the PRL-Rs as the first step toward signal transduction. The first evidence favoring dimeric receptor interactions as a physiologically important step in PRL signaling was derived from experiments in which antibodies were used to artificially induce receptor dimerization and consequent signaling in PRL-responsive cells. Results from this creative experimental approach were ultimately proved to be correct when hormone-receptor complexes for human GH and PRL receptors were biochemically and crystallographically mapped.[5,91,94,95] Formation of 1:2 complexes of the hormone with its receptor (Fig. 2-4) appears to be the essential first step in the transmission of the biologic signal within target cells. Transcriptional activation requires homodimerization of the long-form PRL-R. Heterodimers of short and long receptors, or short homodimers, do not mediate normal signal transduction.[96]

The PRL-R gene, which is located on the long arm of human chromosome 5 (p13-14), is composed of at least 10 coding exons. Multiple transcripts, reflecting alternative splicing variants and transcription start sites, account for some of the variability in PRL-R structure and tissue distribution.[5]

A human mutation in the PRL-R gene was identified in patients with benign multiple fibroadenomas.[97] The mutation encodes a constitutively active form of the receptor.

TYROSINE KINASE ACTIVATION

JAK2 (Janus kinase-2) is a protein kinase that is associated with the PRL-R through binding to the box 1 motif. Its activation is the first intracellular event in a complex and incompletely understood web of interactions that mediate PRL effects within its target cells (Fig. 2-5). JAK2 has been shown to be the essential PRL-regulated protein kinase by both biochemical and genetic experiments,[98,99] but this kinase is also essential for signaling by other cytokines.[100] Although it is presumed today that JAK2 binds directly to the PRL-R, it remains possible that another protein could mediate this association. This possibility is raised by the observation that JAK2 is associated with unliganded PRL-Rs, whereas in the case of GH signaling, in which JAK2 is also the important receptor-activated kinase, ligand binding is necessary before the kinase can bind to the GH receptor. On ligand-induced dimerization of PRL-Rs, JAK2 phosphorylates specific tyrosine residues on the receptor intracellular domain and autophosphorylates residues within the kinase. These phosphotyrosines serve as docking sites for additional signal transduction proteins. The actions of the kinase are counteracted by multiple tyrosine phosphatases, which rapidly dephosphorylate specific proteins and maintain the steady-state level of tyrosine phosphorylation at a very low level in the absence of hormonal stimulation.

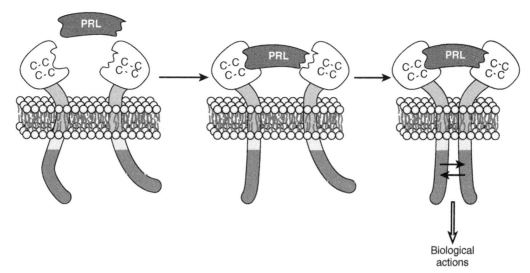

FIGURE 2-4. Dimerization and conformational changes in the prolactin (PRL) receptor cause activation. Based on studies described in the text, PRL is understood to cause receptor interaction between the receptors and associated proteins, leading to activation of appropriate biological actions.

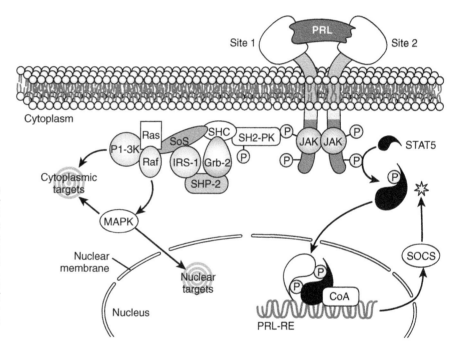

FIGURE 2-5. Intracellular signal transduction by prolactin (PRL). Janus kinase 2 (JAK2) is associated with the PRL receptor and becomes active after receptor dimerization. A signal transducer and activator of transcription protein (STAT5) is phosphorylated (P), dimerizes, associates with Co-activators (Co-A), and binds to appropriate genes through prolactin response elements (PRL-RE). Activation of the JAK2-STAT5 pathway is inhibited (*asterisk*) by suppressors of cytokine signaling proteins (SOCS). JAK2 also activates other Src-related protein kinases (SH2-PK), and these couple with an array of signaling molecules that can activate cytoplasmic or nuclear target molecules, including mitogen-activated protein kinases (MAPK).

In addition to the signal transduction and activators of transcription (STAT)-dependent events triggered by JAK2 activation, other STAT-independent signaling pathways can be activated when PRL binds to its receptor, as shown in Figure 2-6. Src-family kinases may be involved in PRL signaling by virtue of their ability to couple to multiple signaling intermediates. Phosphotidylinositol-3'-kinase, mitogen-activated protein kinases (MAPKs), and protein kinase C have each been observed to be activated by PRL in some systems.[5] The tyrosine phosphatase short heterodimer partner (SHP)-2 is essential for PRL signaling.[100]

STAT-independent pathways have been proposed for PRL signaling, but the physiologic relevance of such mechanisms is not yet clear. It has been suggested that STAT-independent signaling mediates the mitogenic actions of PRL.[101] This action would be consistent with findings in other cytokine-signaling systems, where STAT activation determines certain differentiation-related effector functions, whereas other pathways, such as MAPK activation, are involved in mitogenic signal transduction. However, it is unclear whether this analogy can be extended to PRL. In tissues where PRL has a growth-stimulating action, such as mammary gland or pigeon crop sac, it is not established whether the growth stimulus is direct or is mediated by local synthesis of growth factors other than PRL. The rat Nb2 lymphoma cell line, for which PRL acts as a direct mitogen, expresses a mutated form of the PRL-R, which may transduce an unbalanced set of intracellular signals. The role of specific signal transducers in the proliferative response of Nb2 cells has not yet been established.

TRANSCRIPTIONAL REGULATION

Analysis of PRL-induced genes led, in 1994, to the identification of *cis*-acting elements that bind members of the STAT family of transcription factors.[25,103] PRL-regulated genes were shown to

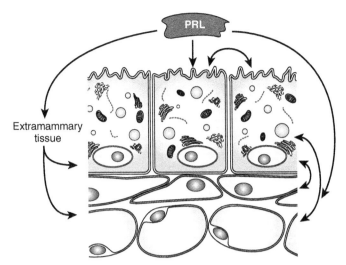

FIGURE 2-6. Mammary gland regulation by prolactin. Acting directly on mammary epithelial cells, and indirectly through extramammary tissues such as the ovaries and other cells within the mammary glands, prolactin causes growth and functional differentiation of the epithelium. Interactions among the cell types may be supportive for prolactin-induced functions or homeostatic negative feedbacks.

include conserved DNA motifs in their promoter regions, and these sequences were bound to STAT proteins.[104] A novel STAT protein (STAT5) was cloned from lactating sheep mammary glands.[105] Mammals synthesize two STAT5 proteins encoded by closely related genes. Genetic studies, making use of targeted gene disruption in mice, have made it clear that both STAT5a and STAT5b are partially responsible for mediating the primary PRL effects in the ovaries and mammary glands. STAT5a is more important in the mammary glands, whereas STAT5b is more important in the ovaries.[106-108] The mouse genetic studies also have revealed a remarkable degree of concordance of the characteristics of animals that lack genes for the ligand (PRL), its receptor, or the PRL-regulated STAT5 transcription factors.[84,85] The concordance among these studies convincingly demonstrates that known PRL-R and STAT5 proteins are the primary mediators of the physiologic actions of PRL. However, subtle differences are seen among the various animal models, which suggest that the STAT5-dependent mechanism might not be the only component of PRL signaling in mammalian cells. STAT5 is phosphorylated by JAK2 on an essential tyrosine residue in its C terminus.[109] After its tyrosine phosphorylation is complete, STAT5 dimerizes through interactions between phosphotyrosine and src homology 2 (SH2) domains. Dimeric STAT complexes translocate into the nucleus, where they interact with specific sites in the promoters of PRL-regulated genes, leading to an increase in the rate of transcription of those genes. The exact mechanism by which STAT5 is transported into the nucleus is not known, nor is it known how this inducible transcription factor interacts with basal transcription machinery during activation of gene expression. Good evidence suggests that the glucocorticoid receptor (GR) collaborates with STAT5 during milk protein gene induction.[110] This positive interaction depends on occupancy of the GR by its ligand.

STAT activation by PRL is regulated inside the cell by a negative feedback mechanism. CIS (cytokine-inducible SH2 protein) and SOCS (suppressor of cytokine signaling) are members of a class of proteins that are transcriptionally regulated by activated STAT proteins. These proteins feed back on the receptor complex to inhibit the coupling of JAK to either receptor or to STAT.[111]

Whereas STAT5 appears to be the exclusive mediator of the primary physiologic PRL actions in mammals, other STAT proteins, such as STAT1, may be activated in response to PRL in certain pathophysiologic or pharmacologic conditions. In a rat T lymphoma cell line (Nb2), PRL induces the expression of the interferon response factor-1 (IRF-1) gene. This effect of PRL is mediated by STAT1 and, paradoxically, is inhibited by STAT5.[112] Although IRF-1 gene regulation probably is not involved in the normal functions of PRL, the regulation of this gene through STAT1 in Nb2 cells provides important lessons regarding potential derangements in PRL signaling that can mediate pathologic changes. Other experimental models in which the normal pathways of PRL signaling are subverted will provide additional important insights.

The Physiology and Pathophysiology of Prolactin Actions in Mammals

MAMMARY GLANDS

PRL is essential for lactation in all mammals, although the precise temporal dimensions of its actions vary among species. The first step in mammary gland organogenesis is the prenatal establishment of the mammary ductal rudiment. Parathyroid hormone-related peptide (PTHrP) is essential at this first stage of mammary gland development, but PRL is not.[83,85,113] The epithelial rudiment and the fat pad grow isometrically until puberty, at which time the epithelial ductal system expands rapidly under the influence of estrogen, GH, and IGF-1.[114,115] During the latter stages of puberty, lobular buds branch off from the ductal system under the influence of PRL and progesterone. As a consequence of the regular cycles of estrous or menstrual hormone surges, the complexity of mammary ductal branching increases progressively, and the epithelial cells undergo cyclic changes. If the female becomes pregnant before lobule budding and maturation are complete, these processes occur during the first pregnancy. As a general rule, progesterone induces ductal arborization, whereas PRL induces the formation of alveolar progenitors. However, the relative roles of progesterone and PRL in the adolescent development of the mammary glands have not been completely resolved at the organ level, and the genes that are induced by each of these hormones during development are not completely known.

During pregnancy, the lobuloalveolar epithelium undergoes extensive proliferation under the influence of PRL, PLs, progesterone, and local growth factors such as RANK-ligand and IGF-2[116-118] (see Fig. 2-6). During and after parturition, progesterone, estrogen, and PLs fall precipitously, and PRL rises. This combination of hormone changes leads to functional lactogenesis and lactation. The lobuloalveolar epithelium is converted to a secretory phenotype, and the full complement of milk proteins and lactogenic enzymes is synthesized. At the end of lactation, involution of the lobuloalveolar system occurs in response to milk stasis and falling systemic lactogens.[119] According to this scheme of development, PRL and PLs, each of which binds to the PRL-R, act during three stages of mammary gland development: lobule budding during organogenesis, lobuloalveolar expansion during pregnancy, and lactational differentiation after parturition.

Pioneering studies using surgical ablation of endocrine glands and hormone replacement established specific roles for estrogen and GH in ductal development, and for PRL, progesterone, and corticosteroids in lobuloalveolar development and lactogenesis.[120] Transgenic and gene disruption techniques have added to our knowledge of hormone actions in mammary gland development in vivo. In laboratory mice, complete PRL deficiency results in the arrest of mammary organogenesis at an immature pubertal state. In this arrested developmental state, the epithelial component of the gland consists of a basic ductal system and terminal end buds, but none of the lobuloalveolar system.

PRL induces the differentiation and growth of alveolar progenitor cells from the ductal epithelium.[121,122] This development of alveoli from precursor cells in the ductal epithelium may involve both clonal growth from committed precursors and induction of phenotypic changes in cells that are near specialized "organizer" cells. PRL is also an essential survival factor for lobuloalveolar cells during both pregnancy and lactation.[123-126] During lactation, PRL regulates several secreted milk proteins, including the caseins, lactoglobulin (except in rodents), lactalbumin, and whey acidic protein. Enzymes such as lactose synthetase, lipoprotein lipase, and fatty acid synthase, which are essential for milk synthesis, are induced by PRL in the mammary gland.

FEMALE REPRODUCTIVE TISSUES

PRL has two general types of actions on female reproduction in mammals. First, high levels of PRL inhibit gonadal activity by actions at the hypothalamus, pituitary, and ovary. These antigonadal effects are manifested during lactation in humans and in clinical hyperprolactinemia. Second, PRL is an essential luteotropic hormone in rodents, although not so in humans or most other mammals.

PRL inhibits reproductive function by decreasing the hypothalamic drive for pulsatile luteinizing hormone (LH) secretion,[127,128] inhibiting ovarian folliculogenesis,[129] and inhibiting granulosa cell aromatase activity, which leads to lower estradiol synthesis.[130,131] Elevated DA levels in the hypothalamus, secondary to high PRL levels, are one mechanism for the antigonadal effects of PRL. PRL contributes to the breakdown of the corpus luteum in many mammalian species, including humans. In rodents, however, PRL is essential to corpus luteum maintenance in early pregnancy. One of the well-characterized mechanisms of the luteotropic action of PRL is inhibition of 20α-hydroxysteroid dehydrogenase activity.[132] This action prevents the conversion of progesterone to 20α-hydroxyprogesterone and therefore increases progesterone secretion from the corpus luteum.

The maintenance of early pregnancy in rodents depends on the establishment of a stereotypic pattern of twice-daily surges of PRL, which are established after coital stimulation of the cervix. In laboratory rodents, the luteal phase of the estrous cycle is transient, and implantation cannot occur unless the corpus luteum is maintained by high levels of PRL. The cervical stimulus drives a hypothalamic reflex, which alters the secretion of a variety of regulatory factors, including DA, opioids, and various putative PRFs. Although it is clear that diurnal and nocturnal PRL surges in early pregnancy are controlled by different sets of factors,[133] neither the exact circuitry nor the essential hypophysiotropic factors that are responsible for each of the surges are yet known.

Lactational infertility is one consequence of high PRL secretion in women who are breastfeeding. Suckling-induced elevation of PRL can decrease gonadotropin-releasing hormone (GnRH), LH, and estrogen secretion and can cause persistent amenorrhea. If ovulatory cycles occur in women who are breastfeeding, the luteal phase defect caused by luteolytic actions of PRL can prevent conception. Although breastfeeding has been promoted as a natural means of contraception, it is very unreliable for most women. Most studies have pointed out that frequent bouts of nursing, especially during the nighttime, are essential to successful lactational contraception. In some societies, where children sleep with the mother for many months, birth spacing has been strongly influenced by lactational infertility.

MALE REPRODUCTIVE TISSUES

High levels of PRL are inhibitory to male reproductive function, much the same as they are to female function. Common presenting symptoms of human hyperprolactinemia in males are loss of libido and impotence. These symptoms may or may not be associated with galactorrhea. PRL inhibits GnRH and LH secretion in males as well as in females.[134] PRL increases LH and follicle-stimulating hormone receptors in the testis, as well as androgen receptors in the prostate.[135] The antigonadal actions of PRL are the most widely conserved PRL actions among mammals and nonmammalian vertebrates.

Male mice with a targeted disruption of either the PRL gene itself or the PRL-R gene are completely fertile.[84,85] Consistent with this, no reports in the literature describe human males with isolated PRL deficiency. The prostate gland of PRL-deficient mice is smaller (by about 30%) than that of normal mice, and high levels of PRL cause prostate hyperplasia in mice.[136] PRL secretion therefore may be a contributing factor in human prostate disease, although no data specifically addressing this possibility are yet available.

ION BALANCE AND CALCIUM METABOLISM

PRL is an essential freshwater survival hormone in many species of fish and amphibians, and it has effects on all of the osmoregulatory epithelia in these species. Its actions include decreasing water permeability in the gills and skin and increasing salt reabsorption in the kidney and urinary bladder (which is evolutionarily homologous with the collecting ducts of the mammalian kidney).[3] Similar actions have not been proved in mammals, which is not surprising, since the osmoregulatory challenges facing terrestrial mammals are not at all similar to those confronted by freshwater fishes. PRL does increase the absorption of a variety of minerals in the intestine of mammals,[137] and this effect may be physiologically important during pregnancy and breastfeeding, which place large demands on water and solute homeostasis.

PRL may have important physiologic actions on calcium metabolism in mammals, and these actions directly relate to changes in calcium balance during pregnancy and lactation. In the mammary gland, PRL induces the secretion of PTHrP, which can act as a local or systemic effector of calcium homeostasis.[138]

Hyperprolactinemia in humans has been associated with decreased bone density, which is normalized when elevated PRL levels are corrected medically. Decreased estrogen, due to the antigonadal effects of PRL, may explain part of the bone loss in hyperprolactinemia, but there appears to be a component of bone loss that is due to direct actions of PRL independent of estrogen loss.[139,140] Recent genetic evidence has shown that the PRL-R is essential to normal bone formation and calcium homeostasis.[140] PRL-R–deficient mice displayed reductions in bone mineral density and bone mineral content, as well as a deceleration in the apposition rate for new bone. Plasma total calcium and parathyroid hormone (PTH) were each higher in the receptor-deficient mice. The phenotypic characteristics of bone growth and calcium homeostasis in PRL-R–deficient mice argue that there must be multiple sites of PRL action that influence calcium metabolism, including both direct effects on bone cells and systemic actions on other hormones or carriers.[141] PRL-R mRNA levels are very high in bone during development,[142] and PLs, as well as PRL per se, could contribute to prenatal control of bone growth.

BRAIN AND BEHAVIOR

The vertebrate brain is a target tissue for numerous PRL actions, many of which are related directly to the parental care of offspring. The first evidence that PRL is a brain-regulating hormone was seen in birds, where systemic or intracranial PRL infusion stimulates behaviors associated with brooding and migration.[3,73] In rats, PRL infusions increase the intensity of parental attendance to offspring or shorten the time required for inexperienced adults to begin showing parental behaviors.[143] Mice that lack the PRL-R are profoundly deficient in maternal behaviors.[144] The neuroanatomic and neurochemical substrates that mediate the PRL-regulated parental behaviors in mammals are not yet known. However, sensory stimuli are clearly important cues for these behaviors and elevated PRL, such as that seen during pregnancy, stimulates neurogenesis in the olfactory lobe of mice.[145]

Whereas stereotypic maternal behavior patterns in animals such as birds, mice, and rats have been quantified and studied objectively, it has not been possible to characterize such behaviors in humans in a way that would allow one to determine whether PRL has a similar role in human parenting. Human PRL increases DA turnover in the nucleus accumbens, corpus striatum, and median eminence, but it decreases DA turnover in the substantia nigra, ventral tegmentum, and cingulate nucleus. It has been proposed that human hyperprolactinemia can be one component of an organic response to psychologic trauma (particularly deprivation from parental attention), and that the behavior patterns associated with high PRL levels (a "maternal subroutine") may be an adaptive psychologic response.[146]

Behavioral actions of PRL that are not directly related to parenting, but may be indirectly supportive, include stimulation of appetite (orexia) and analgesia and increases in REM sleep activity.[52,53,147-149] The analgesia caused by PRL is blocked by naloxone, indicating that the effect occurs through an opioid pathway.

HEMATOPOIESIS AND IMMUNOREGULATION

Several laboratories have made a strong case for an important immunoregulatory role of PRL. PRL-Rs are found on most immune precursor and effector cells in each of the major hematopoietic organs (bone marrow, spleen, thymus). PRL can potentiate the growth and effector functions of lymphoid and myeloid cells, and hematopoietic cytokine receptors and signal transducers are closely related to those used by PRL. The Nb2 cell line, grown from an estrogenized male rat lymphoma, is exquisitely sensitive to growth-promoting and antiapoptotic effects of PRL and has been widely used as a model of PRL actions on immune cells.

In humans, PRL secretion is correlated with disease severity in systemic lupus erythematosus, an autoimmune disease that affects primarily women of child-bearing age.[150] In a rat model of immunosuppression following acute hemorrhagic shock, PRL stimulates immune effector cell functions as well as normal cytokine secretion.[151] Whereas PRL can act as a positive stimulus for immune cells when given to animals by injection or to cells in culture, PRL deficiency does not significantly impair immune function or hematopoiesis.[84] Elevated PRL can block lymphocyte apoptosis, and PRL secretion during stress, pregnancy, and lactation may be sufficient to affect immune cells.[152] It is also conceivable that the higher level of PRL secretion in females compared with males is one factor that contributes to a sexual difference in immune responses.

METABOLISM

PRL-Rs are present in the liver, gut, pancreas, and adipose tissue.[5] PRL causes splanchnomegaly (gut growth) and accelerates liver regrowth after partial hepatectomy.[153,154] Bile acid secretion and taurocholate transport in liver are elevated by PRL during lactation.[155] PRL and placental lactogens stimulate growth of pancreatic β cells during pregnancy and lactation. Beta cell proliferation is both a direct response to PLs and PRL[156] and an adaptive response to gestational insulin resistance. In general, the actions of PRL on organs that control whole-body metabolism are consistent with the metabolic alterations that support successful gestation and lactation. Many hormones in addition to PRL contribute to these metabolic adjustments.

Summary

PRL, along with PLs in many species, plays a central role in ensuring successful reproduction by acting after fertilization to promote a variety of developmental, metabolic, and behavioral adaptations (Fig. 2-7). Hypothalamic DA inhibits PRL secretion and is the dominant PRL regulator in mammals but not in other species. The specialization of the mammalian life cycle to include not only maternal gestation but also postpartum nurturing of offspring has been accompanied by a wide range of physiologic adaptations. Breast milk secretion in mammals, as well as milk-like secretions that occur in certain nonmammalian vertebrates, are direct responses to PRL. PRL suppression of gonadal development and sexual drive in males and females is mediated both centrally and peripherally. The physiologic actions of PRL are pathologically exaggerated in human hyperprolactinemia.

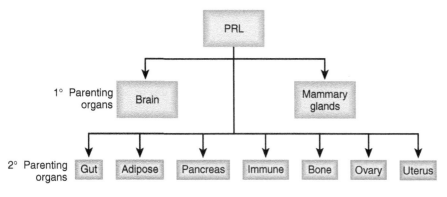

FIGURE 2-7. Prolactin target tissues support parenting. Prolactin has direct effects both on the primary organs associated with parenting (brain and mammary glands) and on a variety of organs that support parenting through secondary physiologic processes.

REFERENCES

1. Riddle O, Bates RW, Dykshorn SW: The preparation, identification and assay of prolactin: A hormone of the anterior pituitary, Am J Physiol 105:191, 1933.

2. Stricker P, Grueter F: Action du lobe antérior de l'hypophyse sur la montée laiteuse, C R Seances Soc Biol Fil 99:1978, 1928.

3. Horseman ND: Models of prolactin action in nonmammalian vertebrates. In Rillema JA, editor: Actions of Prolactin on Molecular Processes, Boca Raton, FL, 1987, CRC Press, p 41.

4. Bern HA, Nicoll CS: The comparative endocrinology of prolactin, Recent Prog Horm Res 24:681, 1968.

5. Bole-Feysot C, Goffin V, Edery M, et al: Prolactin (PRL) and its receptor: Actions, signal transduction pathways and phenotypes observed in PRL receptor knockout mice, Endocr Rev 19:225, 1998.

6. Nicoll CS: Physiological actions of prolactin. In Knobil E, Sawyer WH, editors: Handbook of Physiology, Section 7: Endocrinology, Washington, DC, 1974, American Physiology Society, p 253.

7. Li CH: The chemistry of prolactin. In Li CH, editor: Hormonal Proteins and Peptides, vol 8, New York, 1980, Academic Press, p 2.

8. Cooke NE, Liebhaber SA: Molecular biology of the growth hormone-prolactin gene system, Vitam Horm 50:385, 1995.

9. Soares MJ, Faria TN, Roby KF, et al: Pregnancy and the prolactin family of hormones: Coordination of anterior pituitary, uterine, and placental expression, Endocr Rev 12:402, 1991.

10. Soares MJ, Muller H, Orwig KE, et al: Uteroplacental prolactin family and pregnancy, Biol Reprod 58:273, 1998.

11. Talamantes F, Ogren L, Markoff E, et al: Phylogenetic distribution, regulation of secretion, and prolactin-like effects of placental lactogens, Fed Proc 39:2582, 1980.

12. Handwerger S: Clinical counterpoint: The physiology of placental lactogen in human pregnancy, Endocr Rev 12:329, 1991.

13. Jackson D, Volpert OV, Bouck N, et al: Stimulation and inhibition of angiogenesis by placental proliferin and proliferin-related protein, Science 266:1581, 1994.

14. Kessler MA, Schuler LA: Purification and properties of placental prolactin-related protein-I, Placenta 18:29, 1996.

15. Lee SJ, Nathans D: Proliferin secreted by cultured cells binds to mannose 6-phosphate receptors, J Biol Chem 263:3521, 1988.

16. Ain R, Dia G, Dunmore JH, et al: A prolactin family paralog regulates reproductive adaptations to a physiological stressor, Proc Natl Acad Sci USA 101:16543, 2004.

17. Ho-Chen JK, Bustamante JJ, Soares MJ: Prolactin-like protein-F subfamilty of placental hormones/cytokines: Responsiveness to maternal hypoxia, Endocrinology 148:559, 2007.

18. Ben-Jonathan N, Mershon JL, Allen DL, et al: Extrapituitary prolactin: Distribution, regulation, functions, and clinical aspects, Endocr Rev 17:639, 1997.

19. Gellerson B, Dimattia GE, Friesen HG, et al: Prolactin (PRL) mRNA from human decidua differs from pituitary PRL mRNA but resembles the IM-9-P3 lymphoblast PRL transcript, Mol Cell Endocrinol 64:127, 1989.

20. Kacsóh B, Veress Z, Tóth BE, et al: Bioactive and immunoreactive variants of prolactin in milk and serum of lactating rats and their pups, J Endocrinol 138:243, 1993.

21. Clevenger CV, Furth PA, Hankinson SE, et al: The role of prolactin in mammary carcinoma, Endocr Rev 24:1, 2003.

22. Bao L, Tessier C, Prigent-Tessier A, et al: Decidual prolactin silences the expression of genes detrimental to pregnancy, Endocrinology 148:2326, 2007.

23. Garzia E, Borgato S, Cozzi V, et al: Lack of expression of endometrial prolactin in early implantation failure: A pilot study, Hum Reprod 19:1911, 2004.

24. Miller WL, Baxter JD, Eberhardt NL: Peptide hormone genes: Structure and evolution. In Krieger DT, Brownstein MJ, Martin JB, editors: Brain Peptides, vol 21, New York, 1983, John Wiley, p 16.

25. Horseman ND, Yu-Lee L-Y: Transcriptional regulation by the helix bundle peptide hormones: GH, PRL, and hematopoietic cytokines, Endocr Rev 15:627, 1994.

26. Sinha YN: Structural variants of prolactin: Occurrence and physiological significance, Endocr Rev 16:354, 1995.

27. Lee H, Struman I, Clapp C, et al: Inhibition of urokinase activity by the antiangiogenic factor 16K prolactin: Activation of plasminogen activator inhibitor 1 expression, Endocrinology 139:3696, 1998.

28. Hilfiker-Kleiner D, Kaminski K, Podewski E, et al: A Cathepsin D-cleaved 16 kDa form of prolactin mediates postpartum cardiomyopathy, Cell 128:589, 2007.

29. Hilfiker-Kleiner D, Limbourg A, Drexler H. STAT3-mediated activation of myocardial capillary growth, Trends Cardiovasc Med 15:152, 2005.

30. Jahns B, Stein W, Hilfiker-Kleiner D, et al: Peripartum cardiomyopathy—a new treatment option by inhibition of prolactin secretion, Am J Obstet Gynecol 199:e5, 2008.

31. Hilfiker-Kleiner D, Meyer GP, Schieffer E, et al: Recovery from postpartum cardiomyopathy in two patients by blocking prolactin release with bromocriptine, J Am Coll Cardiol 50:2354, 2007.

32. Wang Y-F, Walker AM: Dephosphorylation of standard prolactin produces a more biologically active molecule: Evidence for antagonism between nonphosphorylated and phosphorylated prolactin in the stimulation of Nb2 cell proliferation, Endocrinology 133:2156, 1993.

33. Kenyon C: If birds can fly, why can't we? Homeotic genes and evolution, Cell 78:175, 1994.

34. Frawley SL: Mammosomatotropes: Current status and possible functions, Trends Endocrinol Metab 1:31, 1989.

35. Asa SL, Ezzat S: The cytogenesis and pathogenesis of pituitary adenomas, Endocr Rev 19:798, 1998.

36. Vankelecom H: Stem cells in the postnatal pituitary? Neuroendocrinology 85:110, 2007.

37. Theill LE, Castrillo J-L, Wu D, et al: Dissection of functional domains of the pituitary-specific transcription factor GHF-1, Nature 342:945, 1989.

38. He X, Treacy MN, Simmons DM, et al: Expression of a large family of POU-domain regulatory genes in mammalian brain development, Nature 340:35, 1989.

39. Ingraham HA, Chen R, Mangalam HJ, et al: A tissue-specific transcription factor containing a homeodomain specifies a pituitary phenotype, Cell 55:519, 1988.

40. Simmons DM, Voss JW, Ingraham HA, et al: Pituitary cell phenotypes involve cell-specific Pit-1 mRNA translation and synergistic interactions with other classes of transcription factors, Genes Dev 4:695, 1990.

41. Morris AE, Kloss B, McChesney RE, et al: An alternatively spliced Pit-1 isoform altered in its ability to transactivate, Nucleic Acids Res 20:1355, 1992.

42. Seyfred MA, Kladde MP, Gorski J: Transcriptional regulation by estrogen of episomal prolactin gene regulatory elements, Mol Endocrinol 3:305, 1989.

43. Cai A, Bowers RC, Moore JPJ, et al: Function of galanin in the anterior pituitary of estrogen-treated Fischer 344 rats: Autocrine and paracrine regulation of prolactin secretion, Endocrinology 139:2452, 1998.

44. Wynick D, Small CJ, Bacon A, et al: Galanin regulates prolactin release and lactotroph proliferation, Proc Natl Acad Sci U S A 95:12671, 1998.

45. Shen ES, Hardenburg JL, Meade EH, et al: Estradiol induces galanin gene expression in the pituitary of the mouse in an estrogen receptor alpha-dependent manner, Endocrinology 140:2628, 1999.

46. Schweppe RE, Frazer-Abel AA, Gutierrez-Hartmann A, et al: Functional components of fibroblast growth factor (FGF) signal transduction in pituitary cells: Identification of FGF response elements in the prolactin gene, J Biol Chem 272:30852, 1997.

47. Zhang K, Kulig E, Jin L, et al: Effects of estrogen and epidermal growth factor on prolactin and Pit-1 mRNA in GH3 cells, Proc Soc Exp Biol Med 202:193, 1993.

48. Ben-Jonathan N: Regulation of prolactin secretion. In Imura H, editor: The Pituitary Gland, 2d ed, New York, 1994, Raven Press, p 261.

49. Lea RW, Vowles DM: Vasoactive intestinal polypeptide stimulates prolactin release in vivo in the ring dove (Streptopelia risoria), Experientia 42:420, 1986.

50. Lea RW, Talbot RT, Sharp PJ: Passive immunization against chicken vasoactive intestinal polypeptide suppresses plasma prolactin and crop sac development in incubating ring doves, Horm Behav 25:283, 1991.

51. Sassin JF, Frantz AG, Kapen S, et al: The nocturnal rise of human prolactin is dependent upon sleep, J Clin Endocrinol Metab 37:436, 1973.

52. Obál F Jr, Payne L, Kacsóh B, et al: Involvement of prolactin in the REM sleep-promoting activity of systemic vasoactive intestinal peptide (VIP), Brain Res 645:143, 1994.

53. Roky R, Obal F, Valatx J-L, et al: Prolactin and rapid eye movement sleep regulation, Sleep 18:536, 1995.

54. Kelly M, Rubinstein M, Asa S, et al: Pituitary lactotroph hyperplasia and chronic hyperprolactinemia in dopamine D2 receptor-deficient mice, Neuron 19:103, 1997.

55. Pi X, Grattan DR: Expression of prolactin receptor mRNA is increased in the preoptic area of lactating rats, Endocrine 1:91, 1999.

56. Login IS, MacLeod RM: Prolactin in human and rat serum and cerebrospinal fluid, Brain Res 132(3):477, 1977.

57. Steger RW, Chandrashekar V, Zhao W, et al: Neuroendocrine and reproductive functions in male mice with targeted disruption of the prolactin gene, Endocrinology 139:3691, 1998.

58. Gregerson K, Flagg T, Anderson M, et al: Identification of the G-protein-coupled, inward rectifying potassium channel gene products in rat anterior pituitary gland, Endocrinology 142:2820, 2001.

59. Koch BD, Blalock JB, Schonbrunn A: Characterization of the cyclic AMP-independent actions of somatostatin in GH cells: I. An increase in potassium conductance is responsible for both the hyperpolarization and the decrease in intracellular free calcium produced by somatostatin, J Biol Chem 263:216, 1988.

60. Shah GV, Pedchenko V, Stanley S, et al: Calcitonin is a physiological inhibitor of prolactin secretion in ovariectomized female rats, Endocrinology 137:1814, 1996.

61. Kanyicska B, Lerant A, Freeman ME: Endothelin is an autocrine regulator of prolactin secretion, Endocrinology 139:5164, 1998.

62. Sarkar DK, Kim KH, Minami S: Transforming growth factor β-1 messenger RNA and protein expression in the pituitary gland: Its action on prolactin secretion and lactotropic growth, Mol Endocrinol 6:1825, 1992.

63. Seyfred MA, Gorski J: An interaction between the 5′ flanking distal and proximal regulatory domains of the rat prolactin gene is required for transcriptional activation by estrogens, Mol Endocrinol 4:1226, 1990.

64. Yan G-Z, Pan WT, Bancroft C: Thyrotropin-releasing hormone action on the prolactin promoter is mediated by the POU protein Pit-1, Mol Endocrinol 5:535, 1991.

65. Johnston CA, Negro-Vilar A: Role of oxytocin on prolactin secretion during proestrus and in different physiological or pharmacological paradigms, Endocrinology 122:341, 1988.

66. Bredow S, Kacsóh B, Obál F Jr, et al: Increase of prolactin mRNA in the rat hypothalamus after intracerebroventricular injection of VIP or PACAP, Brain Res 660:301, 1994.

67. López FJ, Merchenthaler I, Ching M, et al: Galanin: A hypothalamic-hypophysiotropic hormone modulating reproductive functions, Proc Natl Acad Sci U S A 88:4508, 1991.

68. Pickett CA, Gutierrez-Hartmann A: Ras mediates Src but not epidermal growth factor-receptor tyrosine kinase signaling pathways in GH4 neuroendocrine cells, Proc Natl Acad Sci U S A 91:8612, 1994.

69. Porter TE, Wiles CD, Frawley LS: Stimulation of lactotrope differentiation in vitro by fibroblast growth factor, Endocrinology 134:164, 1994.

70. Aguilera G, Hyde CL, Catt KJ: Angiotensin II receptors and prolactin release in pituitary lactotrophs, Endocrinology 111:1045, 1982.

71. Koves K, Molnar J, Kantor O, et al: New aspects of the neuroendocrine role of PACAP, Ann N Y Acad Sci 805:648, 1996.

72. El Halawani ME, Burke WH, Millam JR, et al: Regulation of prolactin and its role in gallinaceous bird reproduction, J Exp Zool 232:521, 1984.

73. Horseman ND, Buntin JD: Regulation of pigeon crop milk secretions and parental behaviors by prolactin, Annu Rev Nutr 15:213, 1995.

74. Hinuma S, Habata Y, Fujii R, et al: Prolactin-releasing peptide in the brain, Nature 393:272, 1998.

75. Samson WK, Keown C, Samson CK, et al: Prolactin-releasing peptide and its homology RFRP-1 act in hypothalamus but not in anterior pituitary gland to stimulate stress hormone secretion, Endocrine 20:59, 2003.

76. Castano JP, Kineman RD, Frawley LS: Dynamic fluctuations in the secretory activity of individual lactotropes as demonstrated by a modified sequential plaque assay, Endocrinology 135:1747, 1994.

77. Nicoll CS: Bioassay of prolactin. Analysis of the pigeon crop-sac response to local protein injection by objective and quantitative methods, Endocrinology 80:641, 1967.

78. Gout PW, Beer CT, Noble RL: Prolactin-stimulated growth of cell cultures established from malignant Nb rat lymphomas, Cancer Res 40:2433, 1980.

79. Kauppila A, Chatelain P, Kirkinen P, et al: Isolated prolactin deficiency in a woman with puerperal alactogenesis, J Clin Endocrinol Metab 64:309, 1987.

80. Falk RJ: Isolated prolactin deficiency: A case report, Fertil Steril 58:1060, 1992.

81. Douchi T, Nakae M, Yamamoto S, et al: A woman with isolated prolactin deficiency, Acta Obstet Gynecol Scand 80:368, 2001.

82. Zargar AH, Masoodi SR, Laway BA, et al: Familial puerperal alactogenesis: Possibility of a genetically transmitted isolated prolactin deficiency, Br J Obstet Gynaecol 104:629, 1997.

83. Vomachka AJ, Pratt SL, Lockefeer JA, et al: Prolactin gene-disruption arrests mammary gland development and retards T-antigen-induced tumor growth, Oncogene 19:1077, 2000.

84. Horseman ND, Zhao W, Montecino-Rodriguez E, et al: Defective mammopoiesis, but normal hematopoiesis, in mice with a targeted disruption of the prolactin gene, EMBO J 16:6926, 1997.

85. Ormandy C, Camus A, Barra J, et al: Null mutation of the prolactin receptor gene produces multiple reproductive defects in the mouse, Genes Dev 11:167, 1997.

86. Cruz-Soto ME, Scheiber MD, Gregerson KA, et al: Pituitary tumorigenesis in prolactin gene-disrupted mice, Endocrinology 143:4429, 2002.

87. Schuff KG, Hentges ST, Kelly MA, et al: Lack of prolactin receptor signaling in mice results in lactotroph proliferation and prolactinomas by dopamine-dependent and independent mechanisms, J Clin Invest 110:973, 2002.

88. Radovick S, Nations M, Du Y, et al: A mutation in the POU-homeodomain of Pit-1 responsible for combined pituitary hormone deficiency, Science 257:1115, 1992.

89. Voss JW, Rosenfeld MG: Anterior pituitary development: Short tales from dwarf mice, Cell 70:527, 1992.

90. Cosman D, Lyman SD, Idzerda RL, et al: A new cytokine receptor superfamily, Trends Biochem Sci 15:265, 1990.

91. Somers W, Ultsh M, De Vos AM, et al: The x-ray structure of a growth hormone-prolactin receptor complex, Nature 372:478, 1994.

92. Chen X, Horseman ND: Cloning, expression, and mutational analysis of the pigeon prolactin receptor, Endocrinology 135:269, 1994.

93. Schuler LA, Nagel RJ, Gao J, et al: Prolactin receptor heterogeneity in bovine fetal and maternal tissues, Endocrinology 138:3187, 1997.

94. de Vos AM, Ultsch M, Kossiakoff AA: Human growth hormone and extracellular domain of its receptor: Crystal structure of the complex, Science 255:306, 1992.

95. Gertler A, Grosclaude J, Djiane J: Interaction of lactogenic hormones with prolactin receptors, Ann N Y Acad Sci 839:177, 1998.

96. Chang W-P, Clevenger CV: Modulation of growth factor receptor function by isoform heterodimerization, Proc Natl Acad Sci U S A 93:5947, 1996.

97. Bogorad RL, Courtillot C, Mestayer C, et al: Identification of a gain-of-function mutation of the prolactin receptor in women with benign breast tumors, Proc Natl Acad Sci USA 105:14533, 2008.

98. Campbell GS, Argentsinger LS, Ihle JN, et al: Activation of JAK2 tyrosine kinase by prolactin receptors in Nb2 cells and mouse mammary gland explants, Proc Natl Acad Sci U S A 91:5232, 1994.

99. Gao J, Hughes JP, Auperin B, et al: Interaction among JANUS kinases and the prolactin (PRL) receptor in the regulation of a PRL response element, Mol Endocrinol 10:847, 1995.

100. Parganas E, Wang D, Stravopodis D, et al: Jak2 is essential for signaling through a variety of cytokine receptors, Cell 93:385, 1998.

101. Berchtold S, Volarevic S, Moriggl R, et al: Dominant negative variants of the SHP-2 tyrosine phosphatase inhibit prolactin activation of Jak2 (janus kinase 2) and induction of Stat5 (signal transducer and activator of transcription 5)-dependent transcription, Mol Endocrinol 12:556, 1998.

102. Das R, Vonderhaar BK: Prolactin as a mitogen in mammary cells, J Mammary Gland Biol Neoplasia 2:29, 1997.

103. Darnell JE Jr, Kerr IM, Stark GR: Jak-Stat pathways and transcriptional activation in response to IFNs and other extracellular signaling proteins, Science 264:1415, 1994.

104. Sidis Y, Horseman ND: Prolactin induces rapid p95/p70 tyrosine phosphorylation, and protein binding to GAS-like sites in the anx Icp^{35} and c-fos genes, Endocrinology 134:1979, 1994.

105. Wakao H, Gouilleux F, Groner B: Mammary gland factor (MGF) is a novel member of the cytokine regulated transcription factor gene family and confers the prolactin response, EMBO J 13:2182, 1994.

106. Liu X, Robinson GW, Wagner K-U, et al: Stat5a is mandatory for adult mammary gland development and lactogenesis, Genes Dev 11:179, 1997.

107. Udy GB, Towers RP, Snell RG, et al: Requirement of STAT5b for sexual dimorphism of body growth rates and liver gene expression, Proc Natl Acad Sci U S A 94:7239, 1997.

108. Teglund S, McKay C, Schuetz E, et al: Stat5a and Stat5b proteins have essential and nonessential, or redundant, roles in cytokine responses, Cell 93:841, 1998.

109. Gouilleux F, Wakao H, Mundt M, et al: Prolactin induces phosphorylation of tyr694 of Stat5 (MGF), a prerequisite for DNA binding and induction of transcription, EMBO J 13:4361, 1994.

110. Stocklin E, Wissler M, Gouilleux, et al: Functional interactions between Stat5 and the glucocorticoid receptor, Nature 383:726, 1996.

111. Helman D, Sandowski Y, Cohen Y, et al: Cytokine-inducible SH2 protein (CIS3) and Jak2 binding protein (JAB) abolish prolactin receptor-mediated Stat5 signaling, FEBS Lett 441:287, 1998.

112. Luo G, Yu-Lee L-Y: Transcriptional inhibition by Stat5, J Biol Chem 272:26841, 1997.

113. Wysolmerski JJ, Stewart AF: The physiology of parathyroid hormone-related protein: An emerging role as a developmental factor, Annu Rev Physiol 60:431, 1998.

114. Topper YJ, Freeman CS: Multiple hormone interactions in the developmental biology of the mammary gland, Physiol Rev 60:1049, 1980.

115. Kleinberg DL: Early mammary development: Growth hormone and IGF-1, J Mammary Gland Biol Neoplasia 2:49, 1997.

116. Srivastava S, Matsuda M, Hou Z, et al: Receptor activator of NF-kappaB ligand induction via Jak2 and Stat5a in mammary epithelial cells, J Biol Chem 278:46171, 2003.

117. Hovey RC, Harris J, Hadsell DL, et al: Local insulin-like growth factor-II mediates prolactin-induced mammary gland development, Mol Endocrinol 17:460, 2003.

118. Brisken C, Ayyannan A, Nguyen C, et al: IGF-2 is a mediator of prolactin-induced morphogenesis in the breast, Dev Cell 3:877, 2002.

119. Schmitt-Ney M, Happ B, Hofer P, et al: Mammary gland-specific nuclear factor activity is positively regulated by lactogenic hormones and negatively by milk stasis, Mol Endocrinol 6:1988, 1992.

120. Lyons W, Li CH, Johnson RE: Hormonal control of mammary growth and lactation, Recent Prog Horm Res 14:219, 1958.

121. Chepko G, Smith GH: Three division-competent, structurally-distinct cell populations contribute to murine mammary epithelial renewal, Tissue Cell 29:239, 1997.

122. Smith GH: Experimental mammary epithelial morphogenesis in an in vivo model: Evidence for distinct cellular progenitors of the ductal and lobular phenotype, Breast Cancer Res Treat 39:21, 1996.

123. Travers MT, Barber MC, Tonner E, et al: The role of prolactin and growth hormone in the regulation of casein gene expression and mammary cell survival: Relationships to milk synthesis and secretion, Endocrinology 137:1530, 1996.

124. Humphreys RC, Hennighausen L: Signal transducer and activator of transcription 5a influences mammary epithelial cell survival and tumorigenesis, Cell Growth Differ 10:685, 1999.

125. Capuco AV, Li M, Long E, et al: Concurrent pregnancy retards mammary involution: Effects on apoptosis and proliferation of the mammary epithelium after forced weaning of mice, Biol Reprod 66:1471, 2002.

126. Bailey JP, Nieport K, Herbst MP, et al: Prolactin and transforming growth factor-beta signaling exert opposing effects on mammary gland morphogenesis, involution, and the Akt-forkhead pathway, Mol Endocrinol 12:1171, 2004.

127. Sarkar D, Yen S: Hyperprolactinemia decreases the luteinizing hormone releasing hormone concentration in pituitary portal plasma: A possible role for β-endorphin as a mediator, Endocrinology 116:2080, 1985.

128. Cohen-Becker I, Selmanoff M, Wise P: Hyperprolactinemia alters the frequency and amplitude of pulsatile luteinizing hormone secretion in the ovariectomized rat, Neuroendocrinology 42:328, 1986.

129. Larsen J, Bhanu A, Odell W: Prolactin inhibition of pregnant mare's serum stimulated follicle development in the rat ovary, Endocr Res 16:449, 1990.

130. Tsai-Morris C, Ghosh M, Hirshfield A, et al: Inhibition of ovarian aromatase by prolactin in vivo, Biol Reprod 29:342, 1983.

131. Krasnow J, Hickey G, Richards J: Regulation of aromatase mRNA and estradiol biosynthesis in rat ovarian granulosa and luteal cells by prolactin, Mol Endocrinol 4:13, 1990.

132. Albarracin CT, Parmer TG, Duan WR, et al: Identification of a major prolactin-regulated protein as 20α-hydroxysteroid dehydrogenase: Coordinate regulation of its activity, protein content, and messenger ribonucleic acid expression, Endocrinology 134:2453, 1994.

133. Freeman ME, Smith MS, Nazian SJ, et al: Ovarian and hypothalamic control of the daily surges of prolactin secretion during pseudopregnancy, Endocrinology 94:875, 1974.

134. Voogt JL, de Greef WJ, Visser TJ, et al: In vivo release of dopamine, luteinizing hormone-releasing hormone and thyrotropin-releasing hormone in male rats bearing a prolactin-secreting tumor, Neuroendocrinol 46:110, 1987.

135. Bex FJ, Bartke A: Testicular LH binding in the hamster: Modification by photoperiod and prolactin, Endocrinology 100:1223, 1977.

136. Wennbo H, Kindblom J, Isaksson OG, et al: Transgenic mice overexpressing the prolactin gene develop dramatic enlargement of the prostate gland, Endocrinology 138:4410, 1997.

137. Mainoya JR, Bern HA, Regan JW: Influence of ovine prolactin on transport of fluid and sodium chloride by the mammalian intestine and gall bladder, J Endocrinol 63:311, 1974.

138. Ferrari SL, Rizzoli R, Bonjour JP: Parathyroid hormone-related protein production by primary cultures of mammary epithelial cells, J Cell Physiol 150:304, 1992.

139. Klibanski A, Neer RM, Beitins IZ, et al: Decreased bone density in hyperprolactinemic women, N Engl J Med 303:1511, 1980.

140. Klibanski A, Greenspan SL: Increase in bone mass after treatment of hyperprolactinemic amenorrhea, N Engl J Med 315:542, 1986.

141. Clément-Lacroix P, Ormandy C, Lepescheux L, et al: Osteoblasts are a new target for prolactin: Analysis of bone formation in prolactin receptor knockout mice, Endocrinology 140:96, 1999.

142. Freemark M, Nagano M, Edery M, et al: Prolactin receptor gene expression in the fetal rat, J Endocrinol 144:285, 1995.
143. Bridges RS: The role of lactogenic hormones in maternal behavior in female rats, Acta Paediatr Suppl 397:33, 1994.
144. Lucas BK, Ormandy CJ, Binart N, et al: Null mutation of the prolactin receptor gene produces a defect in maternal behavior, Endocrinology 139:4102, 1998.
145. Shingo T, Gregg C, Enwere E, et al: Pregnancy-stimulated neurogenesis in the adult female forebrain mediated by prolactin, Science 299:117, 2003.
146. Sobrinho LG: The psychogenic effects of prolactin, Acta Endocrinol 129:38, 1993.
147. Buntin JD: Time course and response specificity of prolactin-induced hyperphagia in ring doves, Physiol Behav 45:903, 1989.

148. Sauve D, Woodside B: The effect of central administration of prolactin on food intake in virgin female rats is dose-dependent, occurs in the absence of ovarian hormones and the latency to onset varies with feeding regimen, Brain Res 729:75, 1996.
149. Ramaswamy S, Pillai NP, Bapna JS: Analgesic effect of prolactin: Possible mechanism of action, Eur J Pharmacol 96:171, 1983.
150. Walker SE, Allen SH, McMurray RW: Prolactin and autoimmune disease, Trends Endocrinol Metab 4:147, 1993.
151. Zellweger R, Zhu X-H, Wichmann MW, et al: Prolactin administration following hemorrhagic shock improves macrophage cytokine release capacity and decreases mortality from subsequent sepsis, J Immunol 157:5748, 1996.

152. Krishnan N, Thellin O, Buckley DJ, et al: Prolactin suppresses glucocorticoid-induced apoptosis in vivo, Endocrinology 144:2102, 2003.
153. Bates RW, Riddle O, Lahr EL, et al: Aspects of splanchnomegaly associated with the action of prolactin, Am J Physiol 119:603, 1937.
154. Buckley AR, Crowe PD, Russell DR: Rapid activation of protein kinase C in isolated rat liver nuclei by prolactin, a known hepatic mitogen, Proc Natl Acad Sci U S A 85:8649, 1988.
155. Liu Y, Hyde JF, Vore M: Prolactin regulates maternal bile secretory function post partum, J Pharmacol Exp Ther 261:560, 1992.
156. Brelje TC, Sorenson RL: Role of prolactin versus growth hormone on islet B-cell proliferation in vitro: Implications for pregnancy, Endocrinology 128:45, 1991.

Chapter 3

ADRENOCORTICOTROPIC HORMONE

ADAM STEVENS and ANNE WHITE

History

Pro-Opiomelanocortin Gene
Structure of the *POMC* Gene
Expression of the *POMC* Gene
Regulation of *POMC* Gene Expression

Adrenocorticotropic Hormone and Related Peptides
Structure and Processing of POMC and Related Peptides
The Processing Pathway and Processing Enzymes
Processing in Different Tissues
Biological Activity of ACTH-Related Peptides
Factors Regulating Secretion of ACTH and Related Peptides
Mechanisms Regulating Secretion of ACTH and Related Peptides
Measurement of ACTH and Related Peptides

Adrenocorticotropic hormone (ACTH) is synthesized as part of the precursor pro-opiomelanocortin (POMC) and as such represents a challenge to endocrinologists in understanding how ACTH is cleaved from the precursor to produce the peptide that acts on the adrenal gland to stimulate the release of adrenal steroids.

This chapter focuses on ACTH in humans. The first section describes the structure, expression, and regulation of the *POMC* gene, with emphasis on the difference between POMC in the pituitary and POMC in other tissues and tumors.

In the second section, information is provided on ACTH and related peptides in the context of the structure of the precursor, how it is processed, and the biological activity of the different peptides derived from POMC. It is important to understand which peptides are present in the circulation and how differential processing of POMC produces an alternative spectrum of peptides (including precursors and fragments) in different tissues.

The hypothalamic-pituitary-adrenal (HPA) axis (Fig. 3-1) is well recognized for its role in the homeostatic mechanisms regulating the stress response. The hypothalamic secretion of corticotropin-releasing hormone (CRH) stimulates ACTH synthesis and release from the anterior pituitary, which in turn regulates the synthesis of glucocorticoids in the adrenal cortex. The impact of the host of factors and mechanisms known to regulate ACTH and related peptides is considered in the context of biological activity both at the adrenal and in other tissues.

History

The many important contributions made to the understanding of ACTH physiology make it difficult to provide a synopsis. However, the following events are some of the major milestones:

1930—Discovery by Smith that ACTH is a factor produced by the pituitary that maintains the weight of the adrenal cortex[1]
1954—Primary structure of ACTH[2]
1964—Isolation of β-lipotropic pituitary hormone (β-lipotropin)[3]
1975—Peptide with opioid activity isolated from the pituitary and named β-*endorphin*[4]
1978—Proof that POMC is the common precursor[5]
1979—Nucleotide sequence of POMC[6]
1981—Isolation and sequencing of corticotropin-releasing hormone (CRH)[7]
1992—Cloning of the ACTH receptor[8,9]
1998—Inherited mutations in *POMC* and *PC1* associated with early-onset obesity, adrenal insufficiency, and red hair pigmentation[10,11]
2005—Differential control of hypothalamic POMC transcription[12]
2006—Mechanism for glucocorticoid regulation of POMC identified[13]
2007—Identification of the differential expression of an "HPA axis" equivalent in the skin[14]

Pro-Opiomelanocortin Gene

STRUCTURE OF THE *POMC* GENE

Humans have a single *POMC* gene located on the short arm of chromosome 2 at 2p23 (the mouse and pig have two copies of the gene). The structure of the gene is well conserved and has been characterized in humans[15-17] as well as in other species.[18] The *POMC* gene consists of three exons interspersed with two large introns (Fig. 3-2). The first exon, which consists of 87 base pairs (bp), contains no coding sequence, and its RNA transcript is thought to act as a leader sequence that binds the ribosome at the start of translation. Exon 2 (152 bp) contains the initiation sequence, a signal sequence that translocates the nascent peptide into the endoplasmic reticulum, and then the N-terminal part of the coding sequence for the POMC peptide. The third exon (835 bp) encodes most of the mature protein, including ACTH,[15-17] the termination codon, and the signal for addition of the poly A tail.

POMC Transcripts

The *POMC* gene has three RNA transcripts of 1200 (T1), 800 (T2), and 1380 (T3) nucleotides, respectively (Fig. 3-3).

The Pituitary Transcript T1

T1 is the mRNA transcript found in corticotrope cells of the anterior pituitary in man and has a size of 1200 nucleotides as detected by Northern blotting.[19] In the hypothalamus, the POMC mRNA transcript seems to be identical to the pituitary transcript except for a longer poly A tail.[20]

The Upstream Transcript T3

The T3 transcript is 1380 nucleotides in size and is presumed to be under the regulation of promoter elements that lie upstream of the pituitary promoter. This transcript produces the same peptide product as T1, because the only relevant translation initiation site is in exon 1. This longer POMC mRNA transcript has been found in normal tissues (e.g., placenta[21,22]) and has also been associated with abnormal expression of POMC such as that seen in small cell lung carcinoma (SCLC).[23]

The Downstream Transcript T2

The downstream T2 transcript is an 800-nucleotide RNA transcript that has been shown in humans and rats to arise from transcription initiation at the 5′ end of exon 3.[24,25] This finding suggests that regulatory sequences may occur starting from the 3′ end of intron 2.[18] This transcript could not give rise to a mature POMC molecule and would lack a signal peptide, so its physiologic role is unclear.[26] The smaller POMC transcript is found primarily in a variety of peripheral tissues, which indicates possible differential regulation in these tissues.

Regulatory Sites for Transcription

The *POMC* promoter has a number of common elements found in other genes that may contribute to regulation of *POMC* gene transcription (Fig. 3-4). Owing to the lack of availability of a human corticotrope cell line, the mouse-equivalent cell

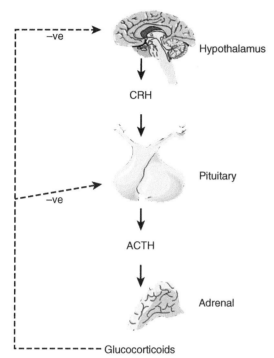

FIGURE 3-1. Schematic representation of the hypothalamic-pituitary-adrenal axis, showing sites of glucocorticoid negative feedback. *ACTH*, Adrenocorticotropic hormone; *CRH*, corticotropin-releasing hormone.

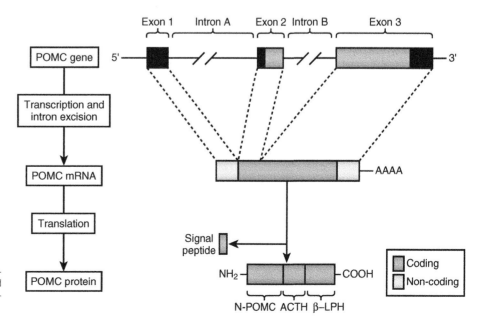

FIGURE 3-2. Genomic structure of human proopiomelanocortin (POMC) with the major spliced product and preprohormone. *ACTH*, Adrenocorticotropic hormone; *βLPH*, β-lipotropin.

line (AtT20) has been used to assess POMC transcriptional regulation along with transgenic mouse models,[27] although some studies have utilized primary human pituitary cells from surgical procedures.[28]

The T1 and T3 mRNA transcripts of POMC are initiated from a TATA box that is located close to the start of exon 1.

The correct spatial, temporal, and hormonal regulation of POMC transcription in the pituitary is conferred by two promoter regions immediately 5′ of exon 1. These regions are between −314 and −276 bp and between −67 and −27 bp in the human *POMC* gene.[27,29,30]

Hypothalamic and CNS-specific expression of POMC has been shown to require DNA control elements distal to those required for POMC expression in the pituitary. A 13 kb region immediately 5′ of the *POMC* gene has been demonstrated to control CNS and hypothalamic expression in transgenic mice.[31] A 4-kb distal region of the *POMC* gene situated −13 to −9 kb in mouse and −11 to −7 kb in human from POMC exon 1 has been shown to contain two neuronal-specific enhancer regions capable

of directing POMC expression in the arcuate nucleus of the hypothalamus.[12] These two neuronal POMC enhancer regions (nPE1 and nPE2) have been shown by deletion studies to be individually capable of driving POMC transcription in the arcuate nucleus and have also been demonstrated to be inactive in the pituitary, implying that there is a modular independence between the promoter regions used to control pituitary and hypothalamic POMC transcription.[12]

The expression of the short POMC mRNA transcript (T2) seems to be regulated by "GC box" promoter sequences located in the 3′ end of intron 2.[19]

EXPRESSION OF THE *POMC* GENE

Expression in the Pituitary

In humans, expression of POMC is most abundant in the corticotrope cells of the anterior pituitary, and in healthy subjects, these cells are the only ones that express the gene at high levels.[32,33] POMC is one of the top 10 most abundant transcripts

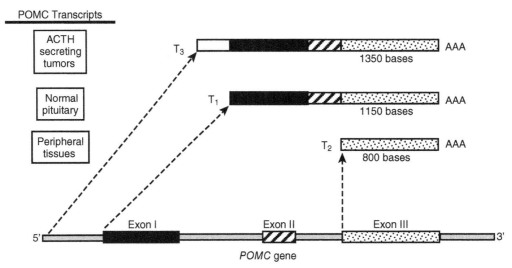

FIGURE 3-3. Tissue-specific transcriptional variants of the human pro-opiomelanocortin *(POMC)* gene. T1 has high-level expression of POMC in pituitary tissue. T2 has low-level expression in numerous extrapituitary tissues. T3 is present in some extrapituitary tumors causing the ectopic adrenocorticotropic hormone (ACTH) syndrome. *AAA,* Poly A tail.

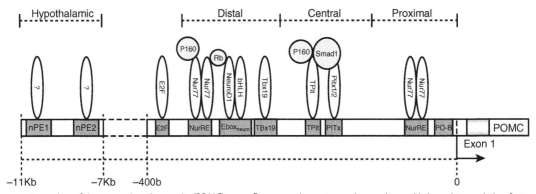

FIGURE 3-4. The promoter region of the pro-opiomelanocortin *(POMC)* gene. Response elements are shown along with bound transcription factors in association with known coregulators *(light grey).* *bHLH,* Basic-helix-loop-helix transcription factors; *E2F,* transcription factors involved in cell cycle regulation and synthesis of DNA; *Ebox,* specific DNA sequence that binds heterodimers of Neuro D1 and other bHLH proteins; *Neuro D1,* neurogenic differentiation 1 transcription factor; *nPE,* neural pro-opiomelanocortin enhancer; *Nur77,* also known as *nerve growth factor IB* (NGFIB), a member of a family of transcription factors involved in cell cycle mediation, inflammation, and apoptosis; *NurRE,* Nur factor response element; *P160,* family of coactivators; *Pitx,* a homeobox family member which is involved in organ development; *PO-B,* a transcription factor originally described as POMC specific. *Rb,* Retinoblastoma protein, a tumor suppressor protein; *Smad1,* a transcriptional modulator that mediates multiple signaling pathways; *Tbx19,* transcription factors present only in pituitary POMC-expressing cells and involved in the regulation of developmental processes; *Tpit,* transcription factors involved in regulation of development.

in the pituitary gland.[34] The main POMC mRNA expressed in the pituitary is the T1 transcript with a size of 1200 nt. POMC mRNA is also detected in the intermediate lobe of the pituitary, which is present during fetal life in humans and is found in other species such as the mouse and rat.[35-37]

Pituitary expression is conferred by the 5′ flanking region of the gene[25,27,38-40] (see Fig. 3-4), but there does not appear to be a specific element sufficient to direct high-level transcription, as for example, in the prolactin gene, where the pituitary-specific transcription factor Pit-1 binds to multiple sites to direct transcription. Rather, in the case of the *POMC* gene, there appears to be a requirement for integrity of the promoter.

The region just 5′ to the start site close to the TATA box confers basal expression and contains the binding sites for PO-B (at −27 nucleotides) and NUR 77 (−67 nucleotides). Further upstream, in the central region of the pituitary promoter, there is a response element which binds the homeobox protein Pitx1[41] and the related Pitx2.[42] During development, Pitx1/2 play an important role in corticotrope development and in the development of the anterior pituitary in general.[42-45] Close to the response element which binds Pitx1, there is a binding site for the T box factor, Tpit, which acts in synergy with Pitx1 and is required for expression of the *POMC* gene and for terminal differentiation of the pituitary corticotrope lineage.[46] Tpit functions as an activator of transcription by recruiting SRC/p160 co-activators to its cognate DNA target in the POMC promoter.[47]

Evidence for the importance of the role of Tpit comes from Tpit-deficient mice, which represent a model of isolated ACTH deficiency, and from humans with Tpit gene mutations which are associated at high frequency with early-onset isolated ACTH deficiency (IAD).[48,49] One cause of neonatal death has been identified as congenital IAD associated with mutations of the Tpit gene.[50] Different Tpit mutations have been associated with IAD, but all these mutations are likely to manifest functionally through disruption of DNA-protein and protein-protein interactions. In one case, a mutation of the Tpit gene (M86R) has been shown to inhibit the binding of other DNA-bound proteins, ultimately leading to loss of recruitment of the p160 coactivator SRC-2.[51]

Other evidence for the importance of Tpit relates to bone morphogenic proteins (BMP) 4 and 2, which are signaling molecules associated with early organogenesis and cell differentiation of the pituitary. BMP4 stimulation leads to the recruitment of activated phospho-Smad1 by the POMC promoter through "tethered" interactions with Pitx1 and Tpit, thus reducing their transcriptional activity and resulting in repression of POMC transcription.[52]

The distal region of the pituitary promoter cannot confer activity independently of the central region but does contain a binding site (Ebox$_{neuro}$) for NeuroD/1A acting as a heterodimer with other basic helix-loop-helix (bHLH) factors and synergizing with Pitx.[40,53] The Ebox$_{neuro}$ element of the distal pituitary promoter, and a nearby Nur response element (NurRE), are required to modulate expression of POMC throughout pituitary development.[54] A member of the T-box gene family, Tbx19, a pituitary development–specific transcription factor, has been shown to have a putative binding site at −310 nt, close to the Ebox$_{neuro}$ site. However, this protein may also exert POMC transcriptional effects synergistically with other pituitary-specific transcription factors.[55]

Expression in Other Tissues

POMC is also expressed, but at a much lower level, in other tissues such as the arcuate nucleus of the hypothalamus, skin, testis, ovary, placenta, duodenum, liver, kidney, adrenal medulla, lung, thymus, heart, and lymphocytes.[14,19,22,25,56-59] Extrapituitary POMC mRNA is frequently expressed as the 1200 nt T1 transcript (similar to that in the pituitary), for example in the hypothalamus, skin, and placenta. However, POMC mRNA from extracranial tissues can also have a preponderance of the shorter 800 nt T3 transcript.[58,60,61] As indicated earlier, this shorter T2 transcript could not give rise to mature POMC and would lack a signal sequence, so its physiologic role is unclear. It may be that low-level expression of longer POMC transcripts (T1 and T3) account for POMC transcription and expression even when there is high expression of the short transcript, for example as demonstrated in the testes.[20,60,62]

POMC expression and regulation in the skin is now well established.[14,63,64] Current evidence would suggest that POMC transcription in the skin is regulated by the region immediately 5′ of exon 1 in keratinocytes[64] and melanocytes.[65]

Expression in Pituitary Tumors

In corticotrope adenomas that give rise to pituitary-dependent Cushing's disease, POMC is the most highly expressed gene,[66] similar to that in the normal pituitary.[34,67] The loss of retinoblastoma tumor-suppressor protein (Rb) expression has been linked to pituitary corticotrope tumor progression.[68] It has been shown that Rb is a transcriptional activator of POMC by bridging between NeuroD and Nurr77 and potentiating interactions between Nurr77 and the p160 co-activator SRC-2.[69,70]

Expression in Nonpituitary Tumors

Tumors giving rise to the ectopic ACTH syndrome produce an mRNA transcript of 1200 bp, similar to that found in the pituitary, and approximately 20% of tumors express a larger transcript of 1400 to 1500 bp.[67] This larger transcript seems to be under the regulation of a promoter region located at −392 and −432 bp relative to the conventional start site.[21,71-73] Analysis of this domain in the human small cell lung carcinoma cell line DMS-79 showed that it binds the E2F family of *trans*-acting factors.[74]

The expression of this promoter in the ectopic ACTH syndrome suggests loss of the tight tissue-specific expression. This promoter is embedded within a CpG island which has been shown to be unmethylated in a number of tumors giving rise to the ectopic ACTH syndrome and in the POMC-expressing small cell lung carcinoma cell line, DMS-79.[75] In contrast, the CpG island was methylated in normal nonexpressing tissues.[27]

Recently it has been shown that hypomethylation of the POMC promoter in thymic carcinoid tumors correlates with POMC overexpression and the ectopic ACTH syndrome. The region of the POMC promoter that underwent change in methylation status was shown to correspond to the E2F binding region of the POMC promoter.[76]

REGULATION OF *POMC* GENE EXPRESSION
Regulation of the *POMC* Gene in the Pituitary

Numerous factors are known to regulate *POMC* gene expression in the pituitary, but perhaps the most important are CRH and glucocorticoids (Fig. 3-5). Expression of the *POMC* gene appears to be predominantly controlled at the level of gene transcription.[77]

Corticotropin-Releasing Hormone Stimulation of the POMC Gene

CRH binds transmembrane receptors on corticotrope cells and stimulates cyclic adenosine monophosphate (cAMP) production

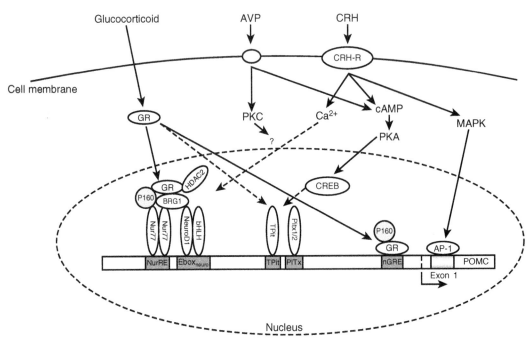

FIGURE 3-5. Intracellular signaling pathways regulating transcription of the pro-opiomelanocortin (POMC) gene. Through its receptor, corticotropin-releasing hormone (CRH) induces cyclic adenosine monophosphate (cAMP), which activates protein kinase A (PKA) and thereby phosphorylation of cAMP response element–binding protein (CREB). CRH also activates mitogen-activated protein kinase (MAPK) pathways, which ultimately induce activator protein-1 (AP-1) binding to an exon 1 response element. Arginine-vasopressin (AVP) activates cAMP and/or protein kinase C (PKC) pathways, which may also feed into this pathway. Glucocorticoids acting through the glucocorticoid receptor (GR) can repress transcription through two cooperative binding sites.

and activation of protein kinase A (PKA)[78] (see Fig. 3-5). CRH effects on POMC transcription do not require de novo protein synthesis.[79] There is no cAMP response element (CRE) in the promoter region of the POMC immediately 5' of exon 1, but two DNA elements have been identified that appear capable of conferring CRH responsiveness to the gene. One element at −171 to −160 nt upstream from the transcription start site binds a protein termed the *CRH response element–binding protein*.[80,81] The second element reported to be CRH responsive is found in the noncoding exon 1 of the rat *POMC* gene.[81,82] This element in exon 1 (+41/+47) shares close homology with a consensus activator protein-1 (AP-1) transcription factor–binding site and binds recombinant AP-1 protein and cAMP response element–binding protein (CREB) in a sequence-specific manner.[82,83]

CRH causes activation of mitogen-activated protein kinase (MAPK) and induction of the DNA-binding activity of AP-1 in the mouse pituitary corticotrope cell line, AtT20.[78,84] In addition, the POMC exon 1 element confers both phorbol ester and CRH responsiveness to a heterologous promoter.[84] Therefore, there is considerable evidence for a physiologic role of the MAPK/AP-1 cascade in mediating some actions of CRH.[81,85,86]

In AtT-20 corticotropes, CRH, and cAMP induce Nur77 expression, and POMC transcription is activated through the NurRE site by protein kinase A (PKA) and calcium-dependent and calcium-independent mechanisms.[78] The NGFI-B (Nur77) subfamily of orphan nuclear receptors (NRs), which also includes Nurr1 and NOR1, bind the NurRE as either homo- or heterodimers formed between subfamily members. Nur factors behave as endpoint effectors of the PKA signaling pathway acting through dimers and AF-1-dependent recruitment of co-activators, such as TIF2.[79]

Tpit/PitxRE also mediates CRH-induced activation of *POMC* gene expression in a calcium-dependent manner. Clearly Tpit/

PitxRE is an important element by which both CRH and Gcs regulate the *POMC* gene expression.[87]

Glucocorticoid Inhibition of the POMC Gene

Glucocorticoids are known to decrease ACTH levels, mainly as a result of inhibition of POMC transcription, as highlighted in the GR knockout mouse, where there is an increase in POMC expression in corticotropes,[88] although they also act at the level of translation[89] and antagonize actions of CRH[90] (see Fig. 3-5). Considerable evidence indicates that glucocorticoids suppress transcription of the *POMC* gene.[91-95]

Glucocorticoids enter the cell, where they bind glucocorticoid receptors complexed to heat shock proteins in the cytoplasm. This results in the translocation of the ligand-bound receptor to the nucleus, where it recruits co-regulator proteins and acts as a transcription factor, binding (usually as a dimer with another glucocorticoid receptor) to the promoter region of a gene in order to regulate gene expression. This process is modulated by the presence of tissue-specific co-regulators.[96]

In the pituitary corticotrope, the glucocorticoid receptor mediates inhibition of the *POMC* gene. In the rat *POMC* gene, there are four sites through which glucocorticoid action is mediated, although only those at −63 and between −480 and −320 are needed in vivo.[97] This latter glucocorticoid-regulated element is required to interact for the full glucocorticoid repression of pituitary POMC expression to be manifested. The −63 negative glucocorticoid-regulated element overlaps the putative COUP (chicken albumin upstream promoter) box[98] and the proximal Nur response element.[99] It has been suggested that the inhibitory effect of glucocorticoids on POMC transcription may occur by displacement of a stimulatory factor such as Nurr 77.[99,100] In the mouse corticotrope cell line, AtT20, the Nurr77-mediated actions of CRH are antagonized by glucocorticoids. The mechanism of glucocorticoid transcriptional repression through this region of the POMC promoter involves the co-repressor HDAC2 and the Swi/Snf chromatin-remodeling protein Brg1 in the modulation of the recruitment of GR to the Nur77-bound NurRE site.[13,101] The loss of nuclear expression of Brg1 or HDAC2 has been associated with 50% of glucocorticoid-resistant human and dog corticotrope adenomas.[13]

The importance of co-regulators in glucocorticoid receptor-mediated regulation of POMC transcription is demonstrated by the inhibition of pituitary POMC transcript levels in mice with a deletion of SRC-1, a glucocorticoid receptor co-activator.[102] However, this inhibition of POMC may be through SRC-1 interaction with other transcription factors that affect POMC transcription.

Stimulation of the POMC Gene by Arginine Vasopressin

A number of other hypothalamic factors act on the pituitary corticotrope to influence POMC expression; however, their modes of action are less well defined. In particular, arginine vasopressin (AVP) augments the effect of CRH and can act independently, though rather weakly, to stimulate POMC expression.[32,103-105] AVP acts on corticotropes via V1b receptors, resulting in the activation of the protein kinase C pathway and leading to a "cross-talk" interaction with the cAMP/protein kinase A pathway activated by binding of CRH to CRH1 receptors.[106]

Leukemia Inhibitory Factor Stimulation of the POMC Gene

A number of lines of evidence point to intrapituitary factors as important modulators of corticotrope function. One such factor is the proinflammatory cytokine, leukemia inhibitory factor (LIF). This factor has been shown to stimulate the POMC gene through STAT-3 at a response element that overlaps with the −166-nucleotide CRH response element, although this site does not directly bind STAT transcription factors.[85,107,108] However, a functional STAT1-3 binding site was identified in the distal region of the POMC promoter,[108] and this region has been shown to mediate LIF-CRH synergy through a mechanism involving synergy with the NurRE.[109]

Recently an interaction between LIF and glucocorticoids has been demonstrated that reduces the repressive properties of GR on POMC expression. This may occur by the loss of a co-repressor from GR tethered to Nurr77 at the NurRE.[110] Other modulators of LIF effects on POMC transcription include CCAAT/enhancer–binding protein β (C/EBPβ) and glial cell–derived neurotrophic factor (GDNF)-inducible factor (GIF).[111]

Regulation of the POMC Gene in Other Tissues

POMC expression can occur in a wide range of nonpituitary tissues, as described earlier, although in many of these extrapituitary tissues, the shorter POMC transcript predominates, leading to extremely low levels of protein.[19] However, there are several tissues where there is significant POMC expression, and subtle differences occur in regulation compared to the pituitary.

Brain

POMC is expressed mainly in the arcuate nucleus of the hypothalamus, although it is also expressed at lower levels in the hippocampus and cortex.[112,113] In the arcuate nucleus, POMC plays a major role in regulating food intake and energy balance.[114] Its importance is highlighted by children with mutations in the POMC gene who are obese.[115] POMC is regulated by leptin, insulin, and glucose to generate an anorexigenic effect[116,117] (Fig. 3-6). Fasting in rats causes a decrease in both POMC and ACTH peptides.[118]

Surprisingly, POMC expression is up-regulated by glucocorticoids in the hypothalamus. Adrenalectomized rats have a

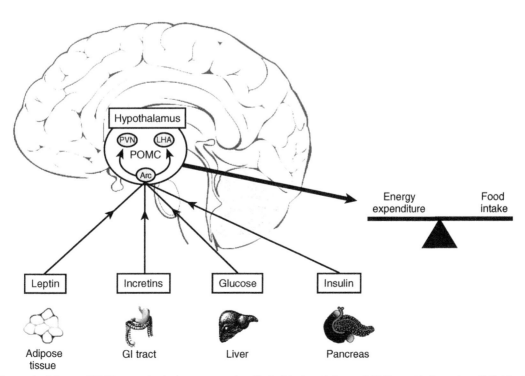

FIGURE 3-6. Factors that influence POMC expression in the arcuate nucleus (Arc) of the hypothalamus. *PVN,* Paraventricular nucleus; *LHA,* lateral hypothalamus.

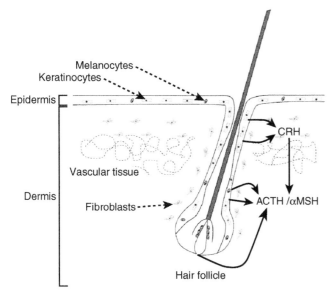

FIGURE 3-7. Components of the hypothalamic-pituitary axis present in the skin. Corticotropin-releasing hormone (CRH) released from skin and hair follicle cells can induce the secretion of adrenocorticotropic hormone (ACTH) and alpha melanocyte-stimulating hormone (αMSH) elsewhere in the skin.

marked decrease in POMC mRNA, an effect that is completely reversed by glucocorticoid treatment.[119,120]

Skin

POMC is expressed in several components of the skin, including melanocytes, keratinocytes,[121,122] and dermal microvascular endothelial cells[123] (Fig. 3-7). The expression of POMC in the skin is regulated by both glucocorticoids and CRH but also by ultraviolet radiation.

The effect of glucocorticoids on POMC expression has been shown in mouse skin, where a down-regulation has been demonstrated which is coupled to hair follicle cycling.[14,124] CRH expressed in skin cells up-regulates local POMC expression,[14,64] and this is inhibited by glucocorticoids.[125] POMC expression in the skin is increased by ultraviolet light,[65,126] which also induces CRH production in human melanocytes, with subsequent stimulation of the CRH signaling pathway resulting in POMC expression.[65] UV induction of POMC expression in mouse skin can be directly controlled by p53, and the mouse POMC promoter is stimulated by p53 in response to UV,[127] although p53 is not the main or sole regulator of POMC expression.[128]

Placenta

The placenta expresses the *POMC* gene at a relatively low level, although the large size of the tissue implies that significant amounts of POMC may be produced.[129,130] Placental POMC expression is up-regulated by CRH but does not seem to be modified by glucocorticoids.[131]

Regulation of the *POMC* Gene in Tumors

Corticotropin-Releasing Hormone Regulation of the *POMC* Gene in Tumors

In general, CRH stimulates POMC expression only in pituitary corticotrope tumors, but a few exceptions occur in ectopic tumors.[132-134] However, it is likely that the increased ACTH stimulation of glucocorticoids will result in inhibition of the *CRH*

gene. Therefore CRH may not be relevant in POMC-expressing tumors.

Glucocorticoid Regulation of the POMC *Gene in Tumors*

In pituitary corticotrope cells, expression of the *POMC* gene is repressed by glucocorticoids, and in pituitary corticotrope tumors, glucocorticoids are able to repress ACTH secretion. In contrast, in extrapituitary tumors, ACTH is characteristically resistant to glucocorticoids.[135] This concept is the basis of the high-dose dexamethasone suppression test used to distinguish pituitary from ectopic sources of ACTH in Cushing's syndrome. Most extrapituitary tumors are resistant to glucocorticoid inhibition of POMC expression, and this suggests that the mechanism of this glucocorticoid resistance is of importance.

A panel of human small cell lung carcinoma cell lines have been established as models of the ectopic ACTH syndrome.[33,136] These cell lines express the *POMC* gene, and the glucocorticoid receptor has been found to be present, although at low levels.[18,33,137] Significantly, all cell lines studied are resistant to glucocorticoid suppression. To determine whether glucocorticoid signaling was functional, a synthetic, glucocorticoid-responsive gene linked to a reporter gene was transfected into the cells. In contrast to the brisk induction of expression seen in control pituitary cells, none of the human small cell lung carcinoma cells responded to either natural or synthetic glucocorticoids.[137] Thus resistance of the *POMC* gene to glucocorticoids is part of a global resistance of these malignant cells to glucocorticoid action. Expression of high concentrations of wild-type glucocorticoid receptor in the cells was found to be sufficient to restore glucocorticoid signaling.[137] In two of the cell lines, mutations in the endogenous glucocorticoid receptor appeared to be the cause of the resistance,[136,138] and in another cell line, altered co-regulator expression and recruitment by the glucocorticoid receptor was the cause of resistance.[139]

Because glucocorticoids can inhibit proliferation in some cell types and induce differentiation in others, it is possible that evasion of glucocorticoid signaling confers a survival advantage to the malignant cells. Indeed, when high levels of a wild-type glucocorticoid receptor were expressed in one of the resistant cell lines, it led to cell death by apoptosis,[139a] this suggests that the glucocorticoid resistance does confer a survival advantage, and because it also disinhibits POMC expression and ACTH secretion, these become biomarkers of a malignant phenotype.

Adrenocorticotropic Hormone and Related Peptides

STRUCTURE AND PROCESSING OF POMC AND RELATED PEPTIDES

Many bioactive peptides are synthesized from large precursor molecules, and a number of techniques have been used to elucidate the structures of these peptides. Studies have used pulse chase analysis whereby labeled amino acids are incubated with cells to detect the labeled precursors and the peptides derived from them. Subsequently, sequence analysis and cDNA cloning have been important approaches to determine peptide structures. Discovery of the structure and biosynthesis of POMC and ACTH-related peptides and the differences between species is reviewed extensively by Eipper and Mains.[140]

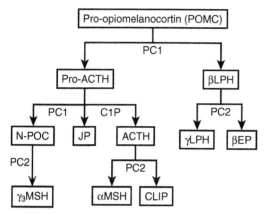

FIGURE 3-8. Processing of pro-opiomelanocortin (POMC). POMC is cleaved into pro-adrenocorticotropic hormone (pro-ACTH) and β-lipotropin (βLPH). Further processing of pro-ACTH yields ACTH, joining peptide, and N-pro-opiomelanocortin (N-POC), all of which are found in human plasma. Cleavage to smaller fragments occurs in a tissue- and species-specific manner. *Shaded boxes* represent peptides found in the human circulation. *CLIP,* Corticotropin-like intermediate lobe peptide; *EP,* endorphin; *JP,* joining peptide; *LPH,* lipotropin; *MSH,* melanocyte-stimulating hormone; *PC,* prohormone convertase.

POMC

In 1973, high-molecular-weight forms of ACTH were identified in human plasma,[141] mouse pituitary cells,[142,143] and human tumors,[144] which led to predictions of the presence of a precursors of ACTH.

Expression of the *POMC* gene leads to synthesis of the preprohormone POMC. This protein undergoes proteolytic cleavage at dibasic amino acid residues, which generates a series of small molecules, including ACTH[140] (Fig. 3-8). Processing of POMC to its constituent peptides varies in a tissue-specific fashion, in that both the nature of the processing and the degree of processing varies in different tissues. This results in different groups of peptides being secreted from different tissues, although the exact ratios of the constituent peptides and precursors are still not fully understood.

ACTH

The ACTH peptide consists of 39 amino acids, is a single polypeptide chain, and has a molecular weight of 4.5 kD[145] (see Fig. 3-8). The N-terminal 12 amino acids are highly conserved between species, thus reflecting the importance of this region for biological activity. In comparison with the human sequence, ACTH in other mammals has only one or two substitutions, which are in the region of amino acids 24 to 39. In birds, amphibians, and fish, although the N-terminal sequence is conserved, the ACTH sequence is more variable, particularly between amino acids 24 and 39. The melanocyte-stimulating hormone (MSH) sequence His-Phe-Arg-Trp is found at ACTH 6–9 and is termed α-*MSH*. Identical sequences are present in β-lipotropin (as β-MSH) and N-pro-opiomelanocortin (N-POC) (as γ-MSH). Given that these three forms of MSH bind different melanocortin receptors, it is thought that the surrounding amino acids influence their specific activity.

α-Melanocyte-Stimulating Hormone

α-MSH consists of ACTH 1–13 and is derived from ACTH 1–39 by proteolysis at the C-terminal, which is followed by C-terminal amidation and N-terminal acetylation. α-MSH is produced predominantly by melanotrope cells in the intermediate lobe of the pituitary, particularly in species such as the rat and mouse. The adult human pituitary does not have a distinct intermediate lobe, and therefore this is not a source of α-MSH in humans. In addition, α-MSH is not thought to be produced in the anterior lobe. Therefore, it is not clear whether α-MSH circulates in humans under normal circumstances.[146,147]

CLIP

Corticotropin-like intermediate lobe peptide (CLIP) consists of ACTH 18–39 and is produced during the cleavage that generates α-MSH. Because this process occurs primarily in the intermediate lobe of the pituitary, which is not present in humans, CLIP is not thought to circulate in humans under normal circumstances.

N-Pro-opiomelanocortin

Also called N-*pro-opiomelanocortin,* N-POC (see Fig. 3-8) comes from the N-terminal sequence of POMC, and in humans, it is a 76–amino acid peptide with an MSH sequence in the midregion.[148] The peptide has a tryptophan residue at the N terminus and two disulfide bridges linking cysteines 2 to 24 and 8 to 20, which are thought to be important for the sorting signal that directs POMC to the regulated pathway.[149] N-POC can also undergo N-glycosylation at Asn65 and O-glycosylation at Thr45.

γ-Melanocyte-Stimulating Hormone

$γ_1$-MSH is found at position 51 to 62 of human N-POC and has sequence homology with α-MSH. There are C-terminally extended forms of $γ_1$-MSH, which are called $γ_2$-MSH (51–63) and $γ_3$-MSH (51–76).

Joining Peptide

Joining peptide is found between N-POC and ACTH and is a 30–amino acid peptide, amidated at the C terminus. It was isolated from human pituitaries in 1981[148] and has been shown to circulate in humans in the form of homodimers.[150]

β-Lipotropin

β-Lipotropin lies at the C terminus of POMC and can be cleaved to γ-lipotropin (which contains the β-MSH sequence at its C terminus) and β-endorphin (see Fig. 3-8). In the human anterior pituitary, cleavage appears to be limited, inasmuch as the main form of this peptide in the human circulation is β-lipotropin, with very little β-endorphin.[151,152]

β-Endorphin

This 31–amino acid peptide contains the sequence for met-enkephalin as the first five amino acids at its N terminus. β-Endorphin can undergo N-acetylation, which is thought to be a tissue-specific effect, and C-terminally truncated peptides have been found, such as α-endorphin (β-endorphin 1–16), γ-endorphin (β-endorphin 1–17), and δ-endorphin (β-endorphin 1–27).

THE PROCESSING PATHWAY AND PROCESSING ENZYMES

Processing

After translation of POMC mRNA into peptide, a series of processing stages are needed for release of the constituent peptides.[112,114,130,153] The N-terminal signal sequence involved in movement of the peptide into the endoplasmic reticulum is no longer required and is removed at an early phase of posttranslational modification. Subsequently, POMC undergoes glycosyl-

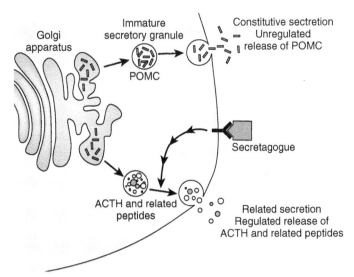

FIGURE 3-9. Pro-opiomelanocortin (POMC) processing and peptide release from cells. POMC is processed in secretory vesicles, which are released after stimulation by secretagogues.

ation and phosphorylation in the Golgi apparatus before transport to secretory vesicles, where it undergoes cleavage into its constituent peptides. The ACTH-related peptides are stored in dense core secretory granules and released from the cell on stimulation (e.g., by CRH), as in the stress response (Fig. 3-9). The prohormone, POMC, is found in the human circulation[154] and could be released from the constitutive pathway perhaps as an "overflow" mechanism.

N-Glycosylation and Phosphorylation

These events occur in the Golgi apparatus before cleavage of the peptides. γ-MSH has the sequence Asn-X-Ser, which can be glycosylated on the Asn residue, and in mouse POMC, N-glycosylation of the CLIP sequence can occur. Some evidence indicates phosphorylation of serine 31 in ACTH, although the significance of this finding is unclear.[155]

Processing Enzymes

POMC is cleaved to its constituent peptides by limited proteolysis at pairs of basic amino acids, primarily Lys-Arg and Arg-Arg. The mammalian convertases responsible for this endoproteolytic cleavage are precursor converting enzymes from the subtilisin/Kex2 serine proteases, which include furin, a protease known to cleave peptides in the constitutive pathway of secretion.[156] Prohormone convertase 1, or PC1 (also called *PC3*),[157] cleaves POMC preferentially at pairs of basic residues and produces ACTH, β-lipotropin, N-POC, and joining peptide in the anterior pituitary. Although cleavage can begin in the Golgi apparatus, it continues in secretory vesicles. PC1 can be regulated in a manner similar to POMC in that PC1 mRNA is up-regulated by CRH and decreased by glucocorticoids in mouse AtT20 cells.[158]

ACTH 1–39 can be further cleaved by PC2 to produce ACTH 1–17 and CLIP. PC2 cleaves at different pairs of basic residues to PC1 to produce the smaller peptides[159] (see Fig. 3-8). PC2 is not expressed in the human anterior pituitary but is found in the neurointermediate lobe, hypothalamus, and skin. This selective expression explains the tissue-specific presence of the MSH peptides and β-endorphin. PC2 can only cleave peptides within secretory vesicles, and therefore the MSH peptides are only produced intracellularly.

Cleavage by PC2 generates ACTH 1–17, which then has amino acids removed from the C terminus by carboxypeptidase E to produce ACTH 1–13. Subsequently, α-amidation is catalyzed by peptidylglycine α-amidating monooxygenase, an enzyme that has multiple molecular forms, and acetylation occurs by the action of specific acetyltransferases.[112] These posttranslational modifications yield α-MSH (see Fig. 3-8).

Given that POMC can be released intact from cells, then cleavage by extracellular peptidases is theoretically possible in some circumstances. This phenomenon has been recently demonstrated by the extracellular peptidases angiotensin-converting enzyme and neprilysin derived from dermal microvascular endothelial cells.[160]

PROCESSING IN DIFFERENT TISSUES

POMC processing varies depending on the species and the tissue. Although POMC is expressed primarily in the pituitary, POMC mRNA has been detected in many extrapituitary tissues.[130] However, such detection does not provide evidence that the peptides are synthesized or secreted there. POMC derived from the pituitary and placenta has been shown to be released into maternal blood.[129,154] Whether the POMC peptides produced in other extrapituitary tissues reach the circulation is debatable, and it is more likely that they act in a paracrine role.

Anterior Pituitary

In the human anterior pituitary, POMC is cleaved to give pro-ACTH, which is then cleaved to ACTH, N-POC, and joining peptide (see Fig. 3-8). Interestingly, the ACTH precursors, POMC and pro-ACTH, are found in the human circulation with ACTH, N-POC, joining peptide, and β-lipotropin.[154] That very little β-endorphin appears to be present indicates that processing of β-lipotropin is minimal (Fig. 3-10). However, reports can be confounded by the fact that in some β-endorphin assays, the antibodies also detect β-lipotropin. In the rat and sheep anterior pituitary, some ACTH is also processed to des-acetyl-α-MSH and α-MSH.[112]

Studies in the mouse pituitary tumor cell line, AtT20, suggest that cleavage is sequential, starting with the C terminus of ACTH.[140] However, the same pair of basic amino acids is found between ACTH and β-lipotropin, joining peptide and ACTH, ACTH 1–16 and ACTH 17–39, and γ-lipotropin and β-endorphin. Therefore, the adjacent amino acids and peptide folding must influence the sequential processing.

Intermediate Lobe

In the rodent intermediate lobe, POMC is found in melanotrope cells and undergoes more comprehensive processing to give the smaller fragments α-, β-, and γ-MSH, CLIP, and β-endorphin. The protease responsible for this cleavage is PC2. After endopeptidase cleavage, ACTH 1–17 is further modified by an exopeptidase that removes amino acids from the C terminus to give ACTH 1–13. Subsequently, ACTH 1–13 undergoes N-acetylation and C-terminal amidation.

Hypothalamus

POMC is produced primarily in the neurons of the hypothalamic arcuate nucleus where the peptides are central to regulation of food intake and energy balance[114] (see Fig. 3-6). POMC is also expressed in the median eminence and ventromedial border of the third ventricle and much smaller amounts in the tractus solitarius. Processing is different from the anterior pituitary, in that smaller peptides characteristic of the neurointermediate lobe are

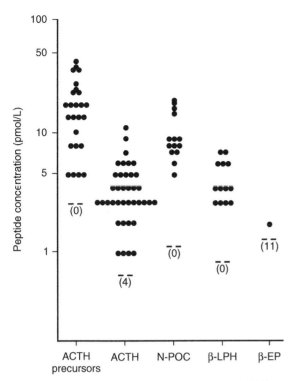

FIGURE 3-10. Concentrations of adrenocorticotropic hormone (ACTH) precursors and derived peptides in the circulation of normal subjects. *EP,* Endorphin; *LPH,* lipotropin; *N-POC,* N-pro-opiomelanocortin. (From Gibson S, Crosby SR, Stewart MF et al: Differential release of pro-opiomelanocortin-derived peptides from the human pituitary: Evidence from a panel of two-site immunoradiometric assays. J Clin Endocrinol Metab 78:835–841, 1994.)

produced.[161] However, most of the studies are limited to the rat hypothalamus. In these extracts, high-performance liquid chromatographic separation of peptides suggests that ACTH is processed to CLIP and that des-acetyl-α-MSH is detected rather than α-MSH, thus indicating that N-terminal acetylation is limited. β-Endorphin 1–31 is found in the rat hypothalamus, again suggesting more extensive processing.[114,112,162] PC1 and PC2 expression in the hypothalamus are increased by leptin and further regulated by the transcription factor Nescient Helix-Loop-Helix (Nhlh)-2, suggesting possible physiologic control of POMC peptide function at the level of peptide processing.[163]

POMC has also been detected in cerebrospinal fluid (CSF), although whether it originates from the pituitary or hypothalamus is uncertain. Evidence from changes in precursors and ACTH in rat CSF in relation to food intake and obesity suggest that they originate from the hypothalamus.[118] In human CSF, the POMC precursor peptide has been shown to occur at high concentrations and predominates over ACTH when molar ratios are compared.[164] However, several of the POMC peptides can be detected in CSF.[165,166]

Other Tissues

POMC peptides have been detected in the thyroid, pancreas, gastrointestinal tract, placenta, testis, ovary, adrenal gland, and immune system.[112] However, in comparison to the pituitary, other tissues produce only low levels of POMC peptides.

POMC peptides are also produced in the skin (see Fig. 3-7). The first peptide to be detected, α-MSH, was found, by immunostaining, to predominate in human melanocytes, but ACTH has also been detected in human keratinocytes.[167] A role for POMC peptides in hair pigmentation is also suggested by two

patients with inherited mutations in POMC that prevented synthesis of the ACTH/α-MSH region; both patients had red hair pigmentation.[11] The presence of PC1 and PC2 has been demonstrated in melanocytes and keratinocytes, along with functional POMC processing.[63,168] The possibility of extracellular peptide processing of POMC by other peptidases has been demonstrated in dermal cells.[160]

Processing of POMC in the placenta results in significant amounts of POMC secretion along with ACTH, β-LPH, α-MSH, and β-endorphin.[22,129]

Pituitary Tumors

In patients with pituitary-dependent Cushing's syndrome, the processing of precursors to ACTH appears to be relatively normal as judged by the molar ratios of these peptides in plasma.[152] However, the molar ratio of precursors to ACTH is much higher for corticotrope macroadenomas, thus suggesting that processing is impaired.[169] In pituitary corticotrope adenomas not associated with Cushing's syndrome, defective PC1 expression may result in an increase of secreted unprocessed POMC.[170]

Extrapituitary Tumors

Data on tumor extracts suggest that most extrapituitary tumors causing the ectopic ACTH syndrome do not process the prohormone efficiently. In an early study, analysis of tumor tissue from patients without clinical features of hormone excess identified a high-molecular-weight form of ACTH, and this purified material could be cleaved to mature ACTH (4.5 kD) by the action of trypsin. The ACTH immunoreactivity was found to have no biological activity and was assumed to be due to ACTH precursors.[171]

Evidence that processing is impaired in tumors from patients with the ectopic ACTH syndrome also comes from the elevated levels of ACTH precursors in plasma and the high ratio of precursors to ACTH.[152,172] Identification of ACTH precursors predominating in the circulation of patients with clinically apparent Cushing's syndrome suggests that these precursors may have some activity at the ACTH receptor or are processed at the adrenal. Most of these patients had clinically obvious small cell carcinoma of the lung. However, patients with highly differentiated, slowly growing tumors, typically bronchial carcinoids, have lower but nevertheless elevated levels of ACTH precursors.[173] CLIP has also been detected in four tumor extracts from patients with carcinoid tumors,[174] thus suggesting that some tumors may process POMC in the manner of the neurointermediate lobe. It is not yet clear whether the same tumors give rise to increased precursors and smaller fragments or whether processing varies in different tumors.

BIOLOGICAL ACTIVITY OF ACTH-RELATED PEPTIDES

ACTH and Its Receptor

The major role of ACTH is to stimulate steroidogenesis in the adrenal cortex, which results in the synthesis and release of cortisol in humans and corticosterone in rodents. In pathologic conditions, it is evident that ACTH can increase the production of adrenal androgens and aldosterone; however, under physiologic situations these pathways are regulated by other factors. Long-term overexpression of ACTH can cause adrenal cell proliferation,[175,176] although peptides from the N-terminal of POMC have also been implicated in this process. ACTH is thought to have a role in adrenal cortical development,[177,178] particularly since ACTH replacement in POMC knockout mice causes normal adrenal development.[179]

In situations with prolonged ACTH excess such as Nelson's syndrome, Addison's disease, and ectopic ACTH syndrome, skin pigmentation can occur and is thought to be due to ACTH binding through its MSH sequence to melanocortin receptors in the skin, although whether the skin pigmentation results from cleavage of ACTH to MSH peptides is unclear. ACTH receptors are also present on human mononuclear leukocytes and have been identified on other rat and mouse immune cells, which suggests that ACTH may have a role in immune function.[130]

ACTH Receptors and Signaling

The ACTH 1–39 sequence is most potent in stimulating steroidogenesis, but ACTH 1–24 is also known to have full agonist activity in certain systems. It is clear that the ACTH 1–13 sequence is involved in binding and activation, but ACTH 6–24 has been shown to have some steroidogenic activity.

ACTH binds to the melanocortin-2 receptor (MC2R),[180] which has been identified in human adrenal glands,[181,182] although in rat and ovine adrenocortical cells, there is a suggestion that low-affinity ACTH binding sites are also present. Binding of ACTH to human receptors requires calcium[181] and occurs with a K_d of approximately 2.0 nmol/L. However, ACTH at 0.01 nmol/L causes maximal steroidogenesis, and therefore only a small number of the predicted 3500 sites per cell need to be occupied to achieve this activity. ACTH 1–16 is the minimal peptide required for binding to the human MC2R and signaling; the presence of a broad binding pocket in human MC2R, utilizing both conserved and unique amino acid residues, may be the reason why α-MSH was not able to bind hMC2R.[183]

The ACTH receptor is a member of the melanocortin receptor family, which all have similar seven-membrane-spanning domains and are G-protein coupled.[182] On binding to its receptor, ACTH stimulates cAMP production,[181] and cAMP in turn stimulates a cAMP-dependent protein kinase that activates the steroidogenic pathway. Calcium is also involved in ACTH stimulation of cAMP in human adrenal cells.

Corticostatins, low-molecular-weight inhibitors of ACTH-induced steroidogenesis, are thought to act by preventing ACTH binding to its receptor, although their physiologic role is unclear.

ACTH Effects on the Adrenal

ACTH acts at a number of levels to increase cortisol production. On binding to its receptor, it stimulates lipoprotein uptake, activates hydrolysis of cholesterol, and increases transport of cholesterol to mitochondria. Importantly, ACTH also regulates cholesterol side-chain cleavage, which is the rate-limiting step in steroidogenesis and results in the production of pregnenolone. This activity takes place in the inner membrane of the mitochondria and is catalyzed by cytochrome P450 side-chain cleavage enzyme.[184]

Longer stimulation by ACTH will eventually result in downregulation of the ACTH receptor, but it is known to cause increased transcription of enzymes in the steroidogenic pathway and can result in adrenal cell proliferation.

α-Melanocyte-Stimulating Peptide

In most mammals, α-MSH is produced in the melanotrope cells of the neurointermediate lobe, but because these cells are absent from the human pituitary, it is unlikely that this peptide has a role as a secreted peptide in humans. In mice, α-MSH acting at the MC-1 receptor causes changes in coat color, and in frogs, it

affects skin pigmentation. It is also thought that locally produced α-MSH peptides stimulate melanogenesis in human skin.[167] Recently α-MSH has been shown to have immunoregulatory functions in the human hair follicle[185] as well as cytoprotective activity against UVB-induced apoptosis and DNA damage in the skin.[65,186]

α-MSH-related peptides produced in the arcuate nucleus of the hypothalamus and acting at the MC-4 receptor in the paraventricular nucleus of the hypothalamus are important in the regulation of food intake and energy balance and are the principal mediators of the effects of leptin.[161] The role of POMC peptides is evidenced by a number of inherited deletions in the POMC gene which are associated with obesity.[11,115,187] Recently, antagonists of α-MSH function have been shown to increase food intake in mice when injected peripherally, thus demonstrating the importance of α-MSH in the regulation of appetite and energy balance.[188]

The antiinflammatory and immunomodulatory properties of α-MSH have resulted in the hypothesis that α-MSH and its cognate receptors might present potential antiinflammatory treatment options.[189,190]

N-Pro-opiomelanocortin and Joining Peptide

N-POC has been reported to potentiate ACTH-induced steroidogenesis in human and rat adrenocortical cells, and it is thought that the γ3-MSH region, from mid- to C-terminal of N-POC, is responsible for this activity. It has also been shown that N-POC 1–48 and not the γ3-MSH region stimulates adrenal growth after unilateral adrenalectomy in the rat.[191] N-POC 1–28 has also been shown to decrease adrenal steroidogenesis in opposition to ACTH.[192] Since N-POC circulates intact, it has been proposed that cleavage of N-POC occurs at the adrenal gland, and a serine protease capable of cleaving N-POC has been identified in the outer adrenal cortex.[193] In addition, N-POC stimulates the release of aldosterone from human adrenal tumor cells.[194,195]

The role of joining peptide is unclear. It has been suggested that it is the adrenal androgen-stimulating hormone, but subsequently, several reports have shown that joining peptide lacks the ability to increase adrenal androgens.[196]

β-Lipotropin and β-Endorphin

β-Lipotropin was named because of its lipolytic activity, and it was suggested that the β-MSH sequence in the mid-region was responsible for this activity. Subsequently, most studies have concentrated on this peptide as a precursor of β-endorphin.

Data are conflicting regarding whether β-endorphin circulates in human plasma.[151,154] It may have a more important role when released locally in the brain because, when administered, it has opiate-like analgesic activity associated with the met-enkephalin sequence at its N terminus, and mice lacking β-endorphin exhibit absence of stress-induced analgesia.[197] β-Endorphin has also been shown to affect sexual behavior and learning. In the skin, β-endorphin modifies human hair follicle physiology via its ability to up-regulate melanogenesis, dendricity, and proliferation in melanocytes.[198]

ACTH Precursors

It has proved difficult to get a clear indication of ACTH precursor bioactivity because of problems in obtaining pure preparations of the peptides and the limitations of available bioassays. POMC itself is thought to have relatively little biological activity,[171] whereas pro-ACTH was shown to be equipotent with ACTH in a rat adrenal cell bioassay or 8% to 33% as potent in a cytochemical ACTH bioassay.[199] Nothing is currently known about the binding of POMC and pro-ACTH to the ACTH receptor (MC2-R) and the other MSH receptors (MC3-R, MC5-R).[200] However, at the MC4-R, the receptor for α-MSH in the brain, β-MSH and ACTH bind MC4-R with similar affinity to α-MSH, and POMC itself functions with low potency.[201] Also, at the MC1-R which is considered to be the receptor for α-MSH in the skin, again ACTH and α-MSH have similar affinity, and POMC can function at low potency.[63] The possible biological effect of POMC was examined in human pigment cells, where functional activity was shown but only at concentrations in excess of 10^{-7} M, considerably higher than the concentrations of POMC released from the cells (~1 × 10^{-10} M).[63] However, it is possible that POMC is degraded extracellularly to ACTH-like peptides.

Because ACTH precursors are present in the circulation at concentrations greater than those of ACTH,[154] it would be valuable to examine the agonist/antagonist activity of the precursors at the other human melanocortin receptors. In patients with hyperpigmentation related to post-adrenalectomy Cushing's disease, concentrations of both ACTH and ACTH precursors correlated with pigmentation scores.[202] The interaction of ACTH precursor peptides with the recently cloned receptor MC4-R found exclusively in the brain may also be of interest, inasmuch as concentrations of ACTH precursors in CSF are 100-fold those of ACTH (414 versus 3.2 pmol/L).[164]

Some information regarding in vivo POMC bioactivity can be gained from clinical studies. If patients with the ectopic ACTH syndrome produce ACTH precursors in preference to ACTH,[152] it must either have biological activity when present at very high levels or be cleaved to ACTH at the level of the adrenal as previously suggested.[191]

FACTORS REGULATING SECRETION OF ACTH AND RELATED PEPTIDES

Glucocorticoids

Glucocorticoids exert a classic feedback inhibitory effect on the production of CRH and ACTH (Fig. 3-11). Therefore, ACTH stimulation of cortisol release from the adrenal directly determines the concentration of cortisol feeding back to inhibit the ACTH release from the pituitary. However, there is also regeneration of cortisol from cortisone by the enzyme 11β-hydroxysteroid dehydrogenase (11β-HSD1) in tissues such as the liver and adipose,[203-205] and this will influence circulating cortisol concentrations, particularly in conditions such as obesity.

There are multiple ways in which glucocorticoids negatively regulate the activity of the HPA axis, and their interactions are not fully understood. Much is known about the molecular mechanisms whereby the glucocorticoid receptor acts as a transcription factor to activate gene transcription, but less is known about specific mechanisms of glucocorticoid inhibition of the human *POMC* gene (see section on regulation of *POMC* gene expression) or about the early effects which must involve nongenomic mechanisms. These interactions have been grouped into fast, intermediate, and slow feedback, based on the timing of the phenomena.

Fast Glucocorticoid Feedback

Fast feedback occurs over minutes and is linked to the rate of increase in glucocorticoid concentration. It was first identified in humans in 1979.[206] An acute reduction in ACTH release takes place, but fast feedback has no impact on gene expression or peptide synthesis. It appears that the targets of glucocorticoid action are hypothalamic CRH secretion and direct action on the

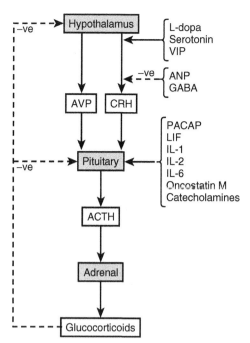

FIGURE 3-11. Factors regulating pituitary secretion of adrenocorticotropic hormone (ACTH)-related peptides. *ANP,* Atrial natriuretic peptide; *AVP,* arginine-vasopressin; *CRH,* corticotropin-releasing hormone; *GABA,* γ-aminobutyric acid; *LIF,* leukemia inhibitory factor; *PACAP,* pituitary adenylate cyclase-activating polypeptide; *VIP,* vasoactive intestinal polypeptide.

pituitary corticotrope to reduce ACTH release. Given the timeframe of the effect, this fast feedback glucocorticoid inhibition of ACTH is most likely to act on release of secretory granules. Experiments in rats, using antagonists of the glucocorticoid receptor and mineralocorticoid receptor, have shown that glucocorticoids may mediate fast feedback via the mineralocorticoid receptor.[207,208]

Intermediate Glucocorticoid Feedback

Intermediate feedback occurs over a few hours (typically maximal at 2 hours in vivo) and again appears to be due to acute inhibition of ACTH and CRH release, with no discernible effect on gene transcription or peptide synthesis. Annexin 1 is a key mediator of the inhibitory effects of glucocorticoids over this time frame, and because it is produced by the folliculo-stellate cells in the pituitary, it is probably a paracrine mediator of glucocorticoid action.[209]

Slow Glucocorticoid Feedback

The slow component is dependent on the concentration and time of exposure and occurs over days. *POMC* gene transcription and POMC peptide synthesis are reduced, but changes in CRH expression are uncertain, and glucocorticoids may also inhibit hypothalamic AVP levels. To effect inhibition of the *POMC* gene, glucocorticoids enter the cell, where they bind to the glucocorticoid receptor (GR) in the cytoplasm, which translocates to the nucleus, where it inhibits *POMC* gene transcription. A recent study in the rat, using a GR antagonist, has shown that GR modulates slow but not fast feedback of regulation of basal corticosterone secretion.[210]

Differential Glucocorticoid Regulation in Other Tissues

Glucocorticoids also act on *POMC* gene expression in the hypothalamus, where they influence food intake and energy balance. However, the evidence is controversial, since adrenalectomy (and therefore loss of glucocorticoids) has been shown to increase POMC mRNA in rat hypothalamus[211] and to decrease POMC mRNA in the hypothalamus.[119] Nevertheless, in rodents, adrenalectomy reverses many forms of obesity, suggesting removal of glucocorticoids increases POMC; alternatively, this could be explained by adrenalectomy affecting a number of other related pathways.[211a]

Corticotropin-Releasing Hormone

CRH is an important physiologic activator of ACTH. This is evidenced by mice with inactivating mutations in the *CRH* gene which die at birth with dysplastic lungs, preventable by prenatal maternal glucocorticoids.[212] Thus CRH activation of ACTH is necessary to provide sufficient glucocorticoids for lung development. Both CRH and arginine vasopressin (AVP) are considered important for activation of pituitary ACTH, but CRH is a more potent secretagogue in rat and horse, whereas AVP is thought to be more potent in sheep. In all cases, there is a marked synergism, with CRH functioning permissively, while AVP is the main dynamic signal.

CRH stimulates ACTH secretion from dispersed pituitary cells in a sustained manner, initially causing the release of preformed peptide but simultaneously stimulating peptide synthesis (see Fig. 3-9). In humans, a biphasic response to exogenous CRH reflects these two mechanisms of action.[213]

The effects of CRH on the levels of ACTH precursors in the human circulation have been examined only during petrosal sinus sampling, which is used as a diagnostic test in patients with suspected Cushing's syndrome. In this test, CRH is given intravenously, and ACTH peptides are measured in the petrosal sinuses draining the pituitary. In this situation, the increase in ACTH is much greater than the increase in precursors, which suggests that CRH is stimulating release of processed ACTH from secretory granules.[154]

Hypothalamic CRH is subject to regulation by multiple afferent signals and will in turn influence ACTH release. These signals include upregulation by catecholamines via β- and α₁-adrenoceptors, serotonin (5-HT) acting via the 5-HT1A, 5-HT2A, and 5-HT2C receptors,[214] acetylcholine acting through both muscarinic and nicotinic receptors, and the cytokines interleukin 1 (IL-1) and IL-6 possibly acting by generation of prostaglandins. In addition, CRH expression may be inhibited by glucocorticoids, catecholamines via α₂-receptors, and γ-aminobutyric acid (GABA) released by neuronal input from the hippocampus and amygdala.

Vasopressin

Vasopressin (AVP) is synthesized in the same cells of the paraventricular nucleus of the hypothalamus as CRH (see Fig. 3-11). The two peptides are released concurrently from the median eminence into the hypophysial portal system. In addition, AVP reaches portal blood from the supraoptic nucleus. AVP exerts weak, direct stimulation on ACTH release but powerfully synergizes with CRH. In vivo evidence indicates a role for AVP in stress-induced ACTH secretion.[215,216] In contrast to CRH, which acts via protein kinase A, AVP acts by stimulation of protein kinase C. AVP also increases the cAMP response to CRH in isolated pituicytes, which suggests multiple sites of interaction between the two signaling cascades.

Other Regulatory Factors

L-Dopa and serotonin both increase ACTH secretion by means of neuronal release into the paraventricular nucleus of the hypo-

thalamus.[217-219] Pituitary adenylate cyclase-activating polypeptide (PACAP) and vasoactive intestinal polypeptide (VIP) both enhance ACTH secretion, but while PACAP directly stimulates pituitary ACTH, VIP promotes release of CRH. The role of these two peptides is probably most relevant in regulating HPA responses to inflammatory and cold stressors.[220]

In contrast, GABA inhibits ACTH when released from hippocampal afferents to the hypothalamus by inhibiting release of CRH and AVP.[221] Atrial natriuretic peptide (ANP) has been shown to decrease ACTH secretion and inhibit *CRH* gene expression. In comparison, opiate receptor agonists inhibit ACTH release, probably by effects at the hypothalamic or hippocampal level, although it has been reported that met-enkephalin can directly inhibit ACTH release at the level of the corticotrope. Oxytocin inhibits CRH stimulated ACTH secretion in humans, but in rats, oxytocin stimulates ACTH, probably by binding to AVP receptors.

Cytokines and Growth Factors

Cytokines are pleiotropic polypeptides released from immune cells in response to inflammation, infection, and tissue injury.[222,223] Proinflammatory cytokines stimulate the HPA axis in vivo,[224] and while some act via CRH, several cytokines, including interleukin 2 (IL-2), interferons, and the gp130 cytokine family (IL-6, leukemia inhibitory factor [LIF], oncostatin M) act at the pituitary.

Interleukin 1

IL-1 α and β are endogenous pyrogenic proteins induced by bacterial endotoxin. The two forms bind to the same receptor, the IL-1 receptor type 1, and display identical biological activities. IL-1β is released by several cell types, including activated macrophages, monocytes, and cells within the hypothalamus, where it can stimulate its own expression.[225]

The specifics of the action of IL-1 on ACTH release are controversial. In the intact rat, infusion of human IL-1 increased circulating levels of ACTH, but IL-1 acted at the hypothalamus by stimulating CRH release.[226] However, primary cultures of rat pituitary cells responded to IL-1β by increasing secretion of ACTH,[227] showing a direct effect can occur. In another study using primary rat pituitary cultures, no effects of acute IL-1 administration on *POMC* gene transcription or ACTH peptide release were observed. Interestingly, chronic treatment of these cultures with either IL-1α or IL-1β exerted weak induction of ACTH release with no effect on POMC mRNA accumulation.[228] An explanation for these divergent results may be that IL-1 modulates the actions of other ACTH secretagogues, including catecholamines.

Interleukin 2

Expression of IL-2 mRNA and IL-2 receptor mRNA was detected in human corticotrope adenoma cells and in mouse pituitary AtT20 cells.[229]

IL-2 enhances *POMC* gene expression in the pituitary and ACTH secretion in AtT20 cells and primary rat pituitary cultures. IL-2, when administered to human subjects during cancer therapy trials, was found to increase circulating β-endorphin and ACTH levels,[230,231] thus demonstrating a role for IL-2 in activating the HPA axis in vivo.

Interleukin 6

IL-6 is synthesized and secreted by bovine pituitary folliculostellate cells, which do not express pituitary trophic hormones or their precursors in vitro.[232] In addition, cultured primary rat pituitary cells release IL-6 relatively abundantly,[233] and IL-6 is synthesized by both normal human and neoplastic anterior pituitary tissue.[234-236]

In vivo, IL-6 is a potent stimulus of the HPA axis in humans and probably acts at the hypothalamus to stimulate AVP release and subsequent ACTH induction.[237] Because IL-6 is also present in the circulation, especially during inflammatory stress, the relative importance of locally derived versus systemically available IL-6 in pituitary function remains to be determined.[238]

Leukemia Inhibitory Factor

LIF regulates differentiation and development of pituitary corticotropes during ontogenesis and is involved in the HPA response to inflammation.[239] The peptide is produced by human pituitary cells, and its receptors (LIF-Rs) are present in murine AtT20 pituicytes and human fetal corticotropes.[240] Pituitary LIF-R mRNA is induced by lipopolysaccharide (LPS) in vivo, although the changes were less pronounced than those observed for LIF mRNA.[241]

LIF acts principally on the pituitary corticotrope, potently inducing POMC gene transcription and enhancing ACTH secretion.[240,242,243] In addition, it potentiates the action of CRH to induce ACTH secretion in AtT20 cells[242] and has been shown to reverse glucocorticoid-dependent repression of POMC expression.[110]

Studies of the HPA axis in LIF knockout mice revealed a defect in activation of the axis in response to stress. Circulating ACTH levels are attenuated after fasting in the knockout animals, and chronic replacement by LIF infusion restores HPA responses to levels seen in wild-type littermates.[244] Interestingly, in mice with a double knockout of LIF and CRH, the POMC response to inflammation was robust and similar to wild-type animals. These animals had increased TNF-α, IL-1β, and IL-6, suggesting that increased central proinflammatory cytokines may compensate for the impaired HPA axis function caused by loss of CRH and LIF.[239] A study in LIF-receptor knockout mice shows a decrease in POMC expression in the fetus, highlighting the importance of LIF signaling in HPA axis development.[245]

Integrated Control of ACTH Secretion

Three tiers of control subserve the regulation of ACTH secretion (see Fig. 3-11).

Tier I

Tier 1 consists of central signals from the brain and hypothalamus and includes the hypothalamic hormones, neurotransmitters, and brain peptides. These molecules traverse the portal venous system in classic endocrine fashion to impinge on their respective distal receptors located on the corticotrope cell surface. These highly differentiated receptors transduce their signals to the cell nucleus, thus determining biosynthesis and ultimate secretion of POMC peptides. The hypothalamic hormones also determine pituitary cell mitotic activity, and clinically, pathologic oversecretion of these hormones results in pituitary hyperplasia and adenoma formation.

Tier II

The second tier of pituitary control consists of an intrapituitary network of cytokines. These molecules provide highly specific unique signals to the pituicyte or an overlapping redundancy (e.g., interleukin regulation of ACTH). Furthermore, they may often synergize with hypothalamic hormones (e.g., LIF and CRH).

The pituitary factors invariably have dual functions—regulating cell development and replication and controlling differentiated gene expression. These two functions are often subserved independently and may in fact be discordant (e.g., LIF induces POMC transcription while blocking corticotrope cell proliferation).

Tier III

The third tier of pituitary control comes from the peripheral target hormones such as glucocorticoids. Clinically, loss of negative feedback inhibition by glucocorticoid target hormones results in hypersecretion of ACTH, pituitary hyperplasia, and sometimes adenoma formation, as may be encountered in hypoadrenalism.

Differential Regulation of POMC and ACTH

The relative concentrations of POMC and ACTH in the circulation will depend not only on regulatory mechanisms influencing expression of the POMC gene but also on precursor processing and mechanisms of secretion from the corticotrope cells. Evidence from studies with the mouse corticotrope adenoma cell line AtT20 suggests that in the absence of stimulation, corticotrope cells release newly synthesized POMC.[246] Therefore, the levels of POMC and ACTH in the circulation at any given time could well vary because of the differing regulatory mechanisms.

MECHANISMS REGULATING SECRETION OF ACTH AND RELATED PEPTIDES

The many factors which regulate secretion of ACTH and related peptides are integrated into the mechanisms which underpin the regulatory processes (see Fig. 3-11). There is a marked circadian rhythm for ACTH, and underlying this is a pulsatile release process. However, it is clear that stress responses can be superimposed on these, as can the feedback regulation of cortisol, which down-regulates ACTH secretion. The details of this feedback inhibition are described in the section on glucocorticoid regulation. A number of studies describe the factors involved in the stress response and feedback regulation, but much less is known about circadian control and pulsatile secretion.

Circadian Rhythmicity

The circadian rhythm for ACTH originates from a primary "clock" which is located in the suprachiasmatic nucleus. Neuronal afferents from this nucleus feed into the paraventricular nucleus of the hypothalamus and regulate CRH expression. ACTH secretion is pulsatile, and the circadian rhythm is generated by variation in the amplitude of the pulses rather than variation in pulse frequency. Therefore, the amplitude of ACTH pulses during peak secretion is fourfold higher than during the ACTH nadir. Peak levels of ACTH, and concordantly cortisol, are reached at 6 AM, decline during the day to 4 PM, and then further decline to a nadir between 11 PM and 3 AM (Fig. 3-12). The 6 AM peak is reached after an abrupt increase in ACTH secretion. Although all the circulating POMC peptides show a diurnal variation and peak at the same time, their decline occurs at different rates, probably conferred by different circulatory half-lives and/or variation in extrapituitary processing.

Pulsatility

ACTH is secreted in a pulsatile manner which is reflected in the pulsatile release of cortisol. However, the analysis of this is very

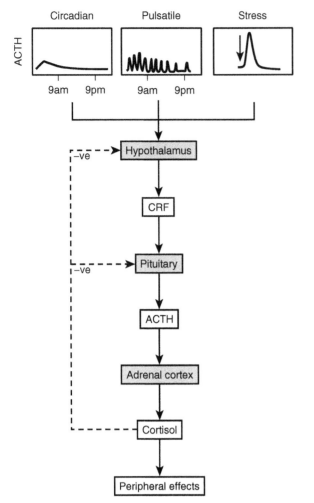

FIGURE 3-12. Mechanisms regulating pituitary secretion of adrenocorticotropic hormone (ACTH) and related peptides. *CRF,* Corticotropin-releasing factor.

much dependent on the sampling techniques. In humans, studies have shown 12 or 40 pulses per 24 hours, depending on the sampling frequency.[247,248] There are fewer pulses during the nadir of ACTH secretion, and there are more pulses, with greater peak amplitude and higher mean level, in males.[249] The pulsatility may be a mechanism for overcoming desensitization of the ACTH receptor and may reflect pulsatile release of CRH.

The Stress Response

The HPA axis is stimulated by a number of different types of stress. These include exercise, acute illness, surgical stress, hemorrhage, and hypoglycemia. Infection which activates the immune system causes release of cytokines which in turn stimulate the HPA axis. This network of interactions between the immune system and the HPA axis provides a mechanism whereby activation of the immune system is inhibited by glucocorticoid feedback on the immune cells, leading to the well-recognized immune suppression, which limits the overall response. Chronic stress, as for example in depression, also activates the HPA axis, but this persistent activation can be attributed to failures in the normal feedback regulatory loops.

In response to stress, peripheral and central signals are integrated by the pituitary to modulate adrenal glucocorticoid production. Several lines of evidence suggest a unifying hypothesis linking hypothalamic releasing factors, activation of peripheral

cytokine cascades, and intrapituitary cytokine expression with pituitary-mediated modulation of the systemic inflammatory response.[247,250]

An acute septic insult provokes a local inflammatory response, with coordinated and sequential activation of a series of proinflammatory cytokines[238,251,252] and neural and bacterial toxin signals that activate the HPA axis.[253] Initially, peripheral activation of local and distal tumor necrosis factor (TNF) expression is followed by IL-1, IL-6, and LIF.[238] A number of the proinflammatory cytokines exert most if not all their activities at the hypothalamus, notably IL-6 acting on hypothalamic AVP[237] and IL-1 and TNF acting on CRH.[226] Hypothalamic LIF mRNA is also up-regulated by lipopolysaccharide (LPS) treatment, a well-recognized model of gram-negative septic shock.[241]

Other cytokines clearly act at the pituitary, notably LIF.[242,254] The pituitary is also a site of de novo cytokine synthesis, and thus in addition to the circulating, peripherally derived cytokines, an intrapituitary network of cytokines is established in the acute phase of septic shock. IL-1β and LIF are up-regulated by LPS,[241,255] and macrophage migration inhibitory factor is acutely released from pituicytes in vitro and in vivo in response to LPS.[256] In addition, intrapituitary IL-6 is up-regulated by IL-1.[238,257]

The pituitary response to septic shock involves cytokines such as IL-6 and LIF, which limit the inflammatory response. These cytokines cause activation of the HPA axis and increased glucocorticoid production, thus limiting the extent of the inflammatory response and protecting against lethality. The increase in intrapituitary LIF stimulates POMC expression and strongly potentiates CRH action on the corticotrope.[242,244] The key role of HPA activation in limiting the lethal effects of unrestrained activation of proinflammatory cytokine cascades is underscored by the poor performance of the CRH knockout mouse exposed to endotoxin.[258] IL-1, TNF, and IL-6 have also been shown by some but not all studies to exert direct effects on pituitary ACTH secretion.[227,259,260]

A further level of action of the cytokines is to antagonize the negative feedback loop of adrenal glucocorticoids on hypothalamic CRH expression and pituitary POMC secretion.[253] The pattern of acute proinflammatory cytokines induced by septic shock opposes effective glucocorticoid signaling,[261,262] in part by activation of the NF-κB nuclear transcription factor, which inhibits glucocorticoid receptor action.[263-265]

Stress-associated disorders, such as melancholic depression, are characterized by persistent activation of the HPA axis. In this situation, there are multiple feedback loops which activate central CRH pathways, including down-regulation of the glucocorticoid receptor which prevents the normal negative feedback on the HPA axis, resulting in the vicious circle of continued activation of the HPA.[266]

MEASUREMENT OF ACTH AND RELATED PEPTIDES

ACTH and ACTH Precursors

ACTH was one of the first peptides to be measured by radioimmunoassay and presented a significant challenge because of the difficulty in generating high-affinity antisera and in labeling ACTH. The development of sensitive immunoradiometric assays for ACTH has improved the reliability of ACTH measurement.[173,267] The assays are based on a labeled monoclonal antibody that usually binds the N-terminal region of ACTH and a solid-phase antibody that recognizes a different sequence in ACTH. Because binding of both antibodies is required to generate a signal, the assay does not recognize α-MSH or CLIP. However, it is not always clear whether current ACTH assays recognize the ACTH precursors.

Recent years have seen a shift toward the measurement of ACTH by two-site immunometric assays in preference to radioimmunoassay. This change provides many benefits, including improved sensitivity, speed, reproducibility, and parallel results. The high sample throughput and wide working range of these assays make them ideal for measuring samples taken during inferior petrosal sinus sampling, a test that is fast becoming an important component in the diagnosis of pituitary tumors secreting ACTH.

However, we must recognize that in some clinical situations, the use of an assay that is highly specific for ACTH 1–39 may be insufficient or misleading. In one patient with the ectopic ACTH syndrome, shown by chromatography to be producing high-molecular-weight ACTH precursors, the ACTH concentration was very low when measured by immunoradiometric assay.[267] To ensure that patients with the ectopic ACTH syndrome are flagged by an ACTH assay, it is important that the ACTH precursors have a high degree of cross-reactivity in the ACTH assay or that a separate specific assay for ACTH precursors be available.

Detection of ACTH precursors in plasma was first demonstrated in normal subjects after stimulation with metyrapone,[268] and it was later observed after insulin-induced hypoglycemia.[269] However, complex chromatographic techniques were required to separate ACTH precursors from ACTH. Clearly, this approach cannot be used for large numbers of patient samples and would not provide a quantitative assessment of the concentrations of ACTH precursors in plasma.

Direct measurement of ACTH precursors was made possible by the development of a two-site immunoradiometric assay for the ACTH precursors POMC and pro-ACTH.[270] The assay is based on a labeled monoclonal antibody that binds within the ACTH region of POMC and a solid-phase antibody that recognizes N-POC (see Fig. 3-8). Because binding of both antibodies is required to generate a signal, the assay does not detect ACTH. With this assay, the concentrations of ACTH precursors in normal subjects were found to be 5 to 40 pmol/L, which is equivalent to or greater than the concentrations of ACTH, N-POC, β-lipotropin, and β-endorphin.[154] Measurement of ACTH precursors in patients with ectopic ACTH syndrome has indicated that the precursors are present at much higher concentrations than is ACTH.[172,173] A similar approach has been used to measure POMC in aggressive ACTH-secreting tumors.[271]

Other POMC-Derived Peptides

The development of radioimmunoassays and/or immunoradiometric assays for N-POC, γ-MSH, α-MSH, β-lipotropin, and β-endorphin has proved extremely valuable in understanding the production and action of POMC peptides. The development of specific immunometric assays that distinguish circulating levels of β-lipotropin and β-endorphin has shown that β-lipotropin is the main form in human plasma and that relatively little β-endorphin is secreted.[151] Nevertheless, questions relating to the relative molar ratios of the family of POMC peptides are still unanswered.

REFERENCES

1. Smith PE: Hypophysectomy and a replacement therapy in the rat, American Journal of Anatomy 45:205–273, 1930.
2. Bell PH: Purification and structure of beta-corticotropin, J Am Chem Soc 76:5565–5567, 1954.
3. Li CH: Lipotropin, a new active peptide from pituitary glands, Nature 201:924, 1964.
4. Li CH: Isolation, characterization and opiate activity of beta-endorphin from human pituitary glands, Biochem Biophys Res Commun 72:1542–1547, 1976.
5. Eipper BA, Mains RE: Analysis of the common precursor to corticotropin and endorphin, J Biol Chem 253:5732–5744, 1978.
6. Inoue A, Kita T, Nakamura M, et al: Nucleotide sequence of cloned cDNA for bovine corticotropin-β-lipotropin precursor, Nature 278:423–427, 1979.
7. Vale W, Spiess J, Rivier C, et al: Characterization of a 41-residue ovine hypothalamic peptide that stimulates secretion of corticotropin and beta endorphin, Science 213:1394–1397, 1981.
8. Mountjoy K, Robbins L, Mortrud M, et al: The cloning of a family of genes the encode the melanocortin receptors, Science 257:1248–1251, 1992.
9. Lefkowitz RJ, Roth J, Pricer W, et al: ACTH receptors in the adrenal: specific binding of ACTH-125I and its relation to adenyl cyclase, Proc Natl Acad Sci U S A 65:745–752, 1970.
10. Jackson RS, et al: Obesity and impaired prohormone processing associated with mutations in the human prohormone convertase 1 gene, Nat Genet 16:303–306, 1997.
11. Krude H, et al: Severe early-onset obesity, adrenal insufficiency and red hair pigmentation caused by POMC mutations in humans, Nat Genet 19:155–157, 1998.
12. de Souza FS, et al: Identification of neuronal enhancers of the proopiomelanocortin gene by transgenic mouse analysis and phylogenetic footprinting, Mol Cell Biol 25:3076–3086, 2005.
13. Bilodeau S, et al: Role of Brg1 and HDAC2 in GR *trans*-repression of the pituitary POMC gene and misexpression in Cushing disease, Genes Dev 20:2871–2886, 2006.
14. Slominski A, Wortsman J, Tuckey RC, et al: Differential expression of HPA axis homolog in the skin, Mol Cell Endocrinol 265–266:143–149, 2007.
15. Cochet M, Chang ACY, Cohen SN: Characterisation of the structural gene and putative 5′ regulatory sequences for human proopiomelanocortin, Nature 297:335–339, 1982.
16. Takahashi H, Teranishi Y, Nakanishi S, et al: Isolation and structural organisation of the human corticotropin-beta-lipotropin precursor gene, FEBS Lett 135:97–102, 1981.
17. Whitfield PL, Shire J: The human proopiomelanocortin gene: organisation sequence and interspersion with repetitive DNA, DNA 1:133–143, 1982.
18. White A, Clark AJ, Stewart MF: The synthesis of ACTH and related peptides by tumours, Bailliers Clin Endocrinol Metab 4:1–27, 1990.
19. Lacaze-Masmonteil T, De Keyzer Y, Luton JP, et al: Characterization of proopiomelanocortin transcripts in human nonpituitary tissues, Proc Natl Acad Sci USA 84:7261–7265, 1987.
20. Jeannotte L, Burbach JP, Drouin J: Unusual proopiomelanocortin ribonucleic acids in extrapituitary tissues: intronless transcripts in testes and long poly(A) tails in hypothalamus, Mol Endocrinol 1:749–757, 1987.
21. Nakai Y, Nakao K: Adrenocorticotropic hormone and related peptides in human tissue. In Black PM, et al, editors: Secretory Tumours of the Pituitary Gland, New York, 1984, Raven, pp 227–243.
22. Grigorakis SI, Anastasiou E, Dai K, et al: Three mRNA transcripts of the proopiomelanocortin gene in human placenta at term, Eur J Endocrinol 142:533–536, 2000.
23. Chang AC, Israel A, Gazdar A, et al: Initiation of proopiomelanocortin mRNA from a normally quiescent promoter in a human small cell lung cancer cell line, Gene 84:115–126, 1989.
24. Jeannotte L, Trifiro MA, Plante RK, et al: Tissue-specific activity of the pro-opiomelanocortin gene promoter, Mol Cell Biol 7:4058–4064, 1987.
25. Jingami H, Nakanishi S, Numa S: Tissue distribution of messenger RNAs coding for opioid peptide precursors and related RNA, Eur J Biochem 142:441–447, 1984.
26. Clark AJ, Lavender PM, Coates P, et al: In vitro and in vivo analysis of the processing and fate of the peptide products of the short proopiomelanocortin mRNA, Mol Endocrinol 4:1737–1743, 1990.
27. Newell-Price J: Proopiomelanocortin gene expression and DNA methylation: implications for Cushing's syndrome and beyond, J Endocrinol 177:365–372, 2003.
28. Kraus J, Buchfelder M, Hollt V: Regulatory elements of the human proopiomelanocortin gene promoter, DNA Cell Biol 12:527–536, 1993.
29. Liu B, Mortrud M, Low MJ: DNA elements with AT-rich core sequences direct pituitary cell-specific expression of the pro-opiomelanocortin gene in transgenic mice, Biochem J 312(Pt 3):827–832, 1995.
30. Liu B, Hammer GD, Rubinstein M, et al: Identification of DNA elements cooperatively activating proopiomelanocortin gene expression in the pituitary glands of transgenic mice, Mol Cell Biol 12:3978–3990, 1992.
31. Young JI, et al: Authentic cell-specific and developmentally regulated expression of pro-opiomelanocortin genomic fragments in hypothalamic and hindbrain neurons of transgenic mice, J Neurosci 18:6631–6640, 1998.
32. Lundblad JR, Roberts JL: Regulation of proopiomelanocortin gene expression in pituitary, Endocr Rev 9:135–158, 1988.
33. White A, Clark AJ: The cellular and molecular basis of the ectopic ACTH syndrome, Clin Endocrinol (Oxf) 39:131–141, 1993.
34. Nishida Y, Yoshioka M, St-Amand J: The top 10 most abundant transcripts are sufficient to characterize the organs functional specificity: evidences from the cortex, hypothalamus and pituitary gland, Gene 344:133–141, 2005.

35. Mauri A, et al: Alpha-melanocyte-stimulating hormone during human perinatal life, J Clin Endocrinol Metab 77:113–117, 1993.
36. Rosa PA, Policastro P, Herbert E: A cellular basis for the differences in regulation of synthesis and secretion of ACTH/endorphin peptides in anterior and intermediate lobes of the pituitary, J Exp Biol 89:215–237, 1980.
37. Schachter BS, Johnson LK, Baxter JD, et al: Differential regulation by glucocorticoids of proopiomelanocortin mRNA levels in the anterior and intermediate lobes of the rat pituitary, Endocrinology 110:1442–1444, 1982.
38. Roberts JL, Lundblad JR, Eberwine JH: Hormonal regulation of POMC gene expression in the pituitary, Ann N Y Acad Sci 512:275–285, 1988.
39. Hammer GD, Fairchild-Huntress V, Low MJ: Pituitary specific and hormonally regulated gene expression directed by the rat proopiomelanocortin promoter in transgenic mice, Mol Endocrinol 4:1689–1697, 1990.
40. Therrien M, Drouin, J: Cell-specific helix-loop-helix factor required for pituitary expression of the pro-opiomelanocortin gene, Mol Cell Biol 13:2342–2353, 1993.
41. Lamonerie T, et al: Ptx1, a bicoid-related homeo box transcription factor involved in transcription of the pro-opiomelanocortin gene, Genes Dev 10:1284–1295, 1996.
42. Suh H, Gage PJ, Drouin J, et al: Pitx2 is required at multiple stages of pituitary organogenesis: pituitary primordium formation and cell specification, Development 129:329–337, 2002.
43. Drouin J, Lamolet B, Lamonerie T, et al: The PTX family of homeodomain transcription factors during pituitary developments, Mol Cell Endocrinol 140:31–36, 1998.
44. Tremblay JJ, Goodyer CG, Drouin J: Transcriptional properties of Ptx1 and Ptx2 isoforms, Neuroendocrinology 71:277–286, 2000.
45. Tremblay JJ, Lanctot C, Drouin J: The pan-pituitary activator of transcription, Ptx1 (pituitary homeobox 1), acts in synergy with SF-1 and Pit1 and is an upstream regulator of the Lim-homeodomain gene Lim3/Lhx3, Mol Endocrinol 12:428–441, 1998.
46. Lamolet B, et al: A pituitary cell-restricted T box factor, Tpit, activates POMC transcription in cooperation with Pitx homeoproteins, Cell 104:849–859, 2001.
47. Maira M, et al: The T-box factor Tpit recruits SRC/p160 co-activators and mediates hormone action, J Biol Chem 278:46523–46532, 2003.
48. Pulichino AM, et al: Human and mouse TPIT gene mutations cause early onset pituitary ACTH deficiency, Genes Dev 17:711–716, 2003.
49. Metherell LA, et al: TPIT mutations are associated with early-onset, but not late-onset isolated ACTH deficiency, Eur J Endocrinol 151:463–465, 2004.
50. Vallette-Kasic S, et al: Congenital isolated adrenocorticotropin deficiency: an underestimated cause of neonatal death, explained by TPIT gene mutations, J Clin Endocrinol Metab 90:1323–1331, 2005.
51. Vallette-Kasic S, et al: The TPIT gene mutation M86R associated with isolated adrenocorticotropin deficiency interferes with protein: protein interactions, J Clin Endocrinol Metab 92:3991–3999, 2007.
52. Nudi M, Ouimette JF, Drouin J: Bone morphogenic protein (Smad)-mediated repression of proopiomelanocortin transcription by interference with Pitx/Tpit activity, Mol Endocrinol 19:1329–1342, 2005.
53. Poulin G, Turgeon B, Drouin J: NeuroD1/beta2 contributes to cell-specific transcription of the proopiomelanocortin gene, Mol Cell Biol 17:6673–6682, 1997.
54. Lavoie PL, Budry L, Balsalobre A, et al: Developmental dependence on NurRE and EboxNeuro for expression of pituitary proopiomelanocortin, Mol Endocrinol 22:1647–1657, 2008.
55. Liu J, et al: Tbx19, a tissue-selective regulator of POMC gene expression, Proc Natl Acad Sci U S A 98:8674–8679, 2001.
56. Buzzetti R, McLoughlin L, Lavender PM, et al: Expression of pro-opiomelanocortin gene and quantification of adrenocorticotropic hormone-like immunoreactivity in human normal peripheral mononuclear cells and lymphoid and myeloid malignancies, J Clin Invest 83:733–737, 1989.
57. Chen C-LC, Chang AC, Krieger DT, et al: Expression and regulation of pro-opiomelanocortin-like gene in the ovary and placenta: comparison with the testis, Endocrinology 118:2382–2389, 1986.
58. DeBold CR, Menefee JK, Nicholson WE, et al: Proopiomelanocortin gene is expressed in many normal human tissues and in tumors not associated with ectopic adrenocorticotropin syndrome, Mol Endocrinol 2:862–870, 1988.
59. Millington WR, Rosenthal DW, Unal CB, et al: Localization of pro-opiomelanocortin mRNA transcripts and peptide immunoreactivity in rat heart, Cardiovasc Res 43:107–116, 1999.
60. Gizang-Ginsberg E, Wolgemuth DJ: Localization of mRNAs in mouse testes by in situ hybridization: distribution of alpha-tubulin and developmental stage specificity of pro-opiomelanocortin transcripts, Dev Biol 111:293–305, 1985.
61. Andjelkov N, et al: Detection of mRNA transcripts of truncated opiate precursor (POMC) in human cartilage, Cell Biochem Funct 24:229–235, 2006.
62. Ivell R: The proopiomelanocortin gene is expressed as both full-length and 5′truncated transcripts in rodent Leydig cells, Reprod Fertil Dev 6:791–794, 1994.
63. Rousseau K, et al: Proopiomelanocortin (POMC), the ACTH/melanocortin precursor, is secreted by human epidermal keratinocytes and melanocytes and stimulates melanogenesis, FASEB J 21:1844–1856, 2007.
64. Slominski A, et al: Corticotropin releasing hormone and the skin, Front Biosci 11:2230–2248, 2006.
65. Zbytek B, Wortsman J, Slominski A: Characterization of a ultraviolet B-induced corticotropin-releasing hormone-proopiomelanocortin system in human melanocytes, Mol Endocrinol 20:2539–2547, 2006.
66. Morris DG, et al: Differential gene expression in pituitary adenomas by oligonucleotide array analysis, Eur J Endocrinol 153:143–151, 2005.
67. De Keyzer Y, et al: Altered proopiomelanocortin gene expression in adrenocorticotropin-producing nonpituitary tumors. Comparative studies with corticotropic adenomas and normal pituitaries, J Clin Invest 76:1892–1898, 1985.
68. Hinton DR, Hahn JA, Weiss MH, et al: Loss of Rb expression in an ACTH-secreting pituitary carcinoma, Cancer Lett 1998 Apr 24 126(2):209–214, 1998.
69. Batsche E, Moschopoulos P, Desroches J, et al: Retinoblastoma and the related pocket protein p107 act as coactivators of NeuroD1 to enhance gene transcription, J Biol Chem 280:16088–16095, 2005.
70. Batsche E, Desroches J, Bilodeau S, et al: Rb enhances p160/SRC coactivator-dependent activity of nuclear receptors and hormone responsiveness, J Biol Chem 280:19746–19756, 2005.
71. De Keyzer Y, Bertagna X, Luton JP, et al: Variable modes of proopiomelanocortin gene transcription in human tumors, Mol Endocrinol 3:215–223, 1989.
72. De Keyzer Y, et al: Pro-opiomelanocortin gene expression in human phaeochromocytomas, J Mol Endocrinol 2:175–181, 1989.
73. Texier PL, et al: Proopiomelanocortin gene expression in normal and tumoral human lung, J Clin Endocrinol Metab 73:414–420, 1991.
74. Picon A, Bertagna X, De Keyzer Y: Analysis of the human proopiomelanocortin gene promoter in a small cell lung carcinoma cell line reveals an unusual role for E2F transcription factors, Oncogene 18:2627–2633, 1999.
75. Newell-Price J, King P, Clark AJ: The CpG island promoter of the human proopiomelanocortin gene is methylated in nonexpressing normal tissue and tumors and represses expression, Mol Endocrinol 15:338–348, 2001.
76. Ye L, et al: Hypomethylation in the promoter region of POMC gene correlates with ectopic overexpression in thymic carcinoids, J Endocrinol 185:337–343, 2005.
77. Birnberg NC, Lissitsky J-C, Hinman M, et al: Glucocorticoids regulate proopiomelanocortin gene expression in vivo at the levels of transcription and secretion, Proc Natl Acad Sci USA 80:6982–6986, 1983.
78. Kovalovsky D, et al: Activation and induction of NUR77/NURR1 in corticotrophs by CRH/cAMP: involvement of calcium, protein kinase A, and MAPK pathways, Mol Endocrinol 16:1638–1651, 2002.
79. Maira M, Martens C, Batsche E, et al: Dimer-specific potentiation of NGFI-B (Nur77) transcriptional activity by the protein kinase A pathway and AF-1-dependent coactivator recruitment, Mol Cell Biol 23:763–776, 2003.
80. Boutillier AL, Sassone-Corsi P, Loeffler JP: The protooncogene c-fos is induced by corticotropin-releasing factor and stimulates proopiomelanocortin gene transcription in pituitary cells, Mol Endocrinol 5:1301–1310, 1991.
81. Jin WD, et al: Characterization of a corticotropin-releasing hormone-responsive element in the rat proopiomelanocortin gene promoter and molecular cloning of its binding protein, Mol Endocrinol 8:1377–1388, 1994.
82. Boutillier AL, Gaiddon C, Lorang D, et al: Transcriptional activation of the proopiomelanocortin gene by cyclic AMP-responsive element binding protein, Pituitary 1:33–43, 1998.
83. Autelitano DJ: Stress-induced stimulation of pituitary POMC gene expression is associated with activation of transcription factor AP-1 in hypothalamus and pituitary, Brain Res Bull 45:75–82, 1998.
84. Boutillier AL, et al: Corticotropin-releasing hormone stimulates proopiomelanocortin transcription by cFos-dependent and -independent pathways: characterization of an AP1 site in exon 1, Mol Endocrinol 9:745–755, 1995.
85. Bousquet C, Ray DW, Melmed S: A common pro-opiomelanocortin-binding element mediates leukemia inhibitory factor and corticotropin-releasing hormone transcriptional synergy, J Biol Chem 272:10551–10557, 1997.
86. Becquet D, Guillaumond F, Bosler O, et al: Long-term variations of AP-1 composition after CRH stimulation: consequence on POMC gene regulation, Mol Cell Endocrinol 175:93–100, 2001.
87. Murakami I, Takeuchi S, Kudo T, et al: Corticotropin-releasing hormone or dexamethasone regulates rat proopiomelanocortin transcription through Tpit/Pitx-responsive element in its promoter, J Endocrinol 193:279–290, 2007.
88. Reichardt HM, Schutz G: Feedback control of glucocorticoid production is established during fetal development, Mol Med 2:735–744, 1996.
89. Svec F: Interactions of glucocorticoids with the AtT-20 cell: effect on protein accumulation, Arch Biochem Biophys 240:184–190, 1985.
90. Itoi K, Jiang YQ, Iwasaki Y, et al: Regulatory mechanisms of corticotropin-releasing hormone and vasopressin gene expression in the hypothalamus, J Neuroendocrinol 16:348–355, 2004.
91. Eberwine JH, Jonassen JA, Evinger MJ, et al: Complex transcriptional regulation by glucocorticoids and corticotropin-releasing hormone of proopiomelanocortin gene expression in rat pituitary cultures, DNA 6:483–492, 1987.
92. Eberwine JH, Roberts JL: Glucocorticoid regulation of pro-opiomelanocortin gene transcription in the rat pituitary, J Biol Chem 259:2166–2170, 1984.
93. Fremeau RT, Lundblad JR, Pritchett DB, et al: Regulation of pro-opiomelanocortin gene transcription in individual cell nuclei, Science 234:1265–1269, 1986.
94. Gagner JP, Drouin J: Opposite regulation of pro-opiomelanocortin gene transcription by glucocorticoids and CRH, Mol Cell Endocrinol 40:25–32, 1985.
95. Israel A, Cohen SN: Hormonally mediated negative regulation of human pro-opiomelanocortin gene expression after transfection into mouse L-cells, Mol Cell Biol 5:2443–2453, 1985.
96. Stevens A, et al: Dissociation of steroid receptor coactivator 1 and nuclear receptor corepressor recruitment to the human glucocorticoid receptor by modification of the ligand-receptor interface: the role of tyrosine 735, Mol Endocrinol 17:845–859, 2003.
97. Riegel AT, et al: Proopiomelanocortin gene promoter elements required for constitutive and glucocorticoid-repressed transcription, Mol Endocrinol 5:1973–1982, 1991.
98. Therrien M, Drouin J: Pituitary pro-opiomelanocortin gene expression requires synergistic interactions of several regulatory elements, Mol Cell Biol 11:3492–3503, 1991.
99. Philips A, et al: Novel dimeric Nur77 signaling mechanism in endocrine and lymphoid cells, Mol Cell Biol 17:5946–5951, 1997.
100. Philips A, et al: Antagonism between Nur77 and glucocorticoid receptor for control of transcription, Mol Cell Biol 17:5952–5959, 1997.

101. Martens C, Bilodeau S, Maira M, et al: Protein-protein interactions and transcriptional antagonism between the subfamily of NGFI-B/Nur77 orphan nuclear receptors and glucocorticoid receptor, Mol Endocrinol 19:885–897, 2005.

102. Winnay JN, Xu J, O'Malley BW, et al: Steroid receptor coactivator-1-deficient mice exhibit altered hypothalamic-pituitary-adrenal axis function, Endocrinology 147:1322–1332, 2006.

103. Abou-Samra AB, Harwood JP, Manganiello VC, et al: Phorbol 12-myristate 13-acetate and vasopressin potentiate the effect of corticotropin-releasing factor on cyclic AMP production in rat anterior pituitary cells. Mechanisms of action, J Biol Chem 262:1129–1136, 1987.

104. Smoak B, Deuster P, Rabin D, et al: Corticotropin releasing hormone is not the sole factor mediating exercise induced adrenocorticotropin release in humans, J Clin Endocrinol Metab 73:302–306, 1991.

105. Watts AG: Glucocorticoid regulation of peptide genes in neuroendocrine CRH neurons: a complexity beyond negative feedback, Front Neuroendocrinol 26:109–130, 2005.

106. Carvallo P, Aguilera G: Protein kinase C mediates the effect of vasopressin in pituitary corticotrophs, Mol Endocrinol 3:1935–1943, 1989.

107. Bousquet C, Melmed S: Critical role for STAT3 in murine pituitary adrenocorticotropin hormone leukemia inhibitory factor signaling, J Biol Chem 274:10723–10730, 1999.

108. Mynard V, Guignat L, vin-Leclerc J, et al: Different mechanisms for leukemia inhibitory factor-dependent activation of two proopiomelanocortin promoter regions, Endocrinology 143:3916–3924, 2002.

109. Mynard V, et al: Synergistic signaling by corticotropin-releasing hormone and leukemia inhibitory factor bridged by phosphorylated 3′,5′-cyclic adenosine monophosphate response element binding protein at the Nur response element (NurRE)-signal transducers and activators of transcription (STAT) element of the proopiomelanocortin promoter, Mol Endocrinol 18:2997–3010, 2004.

110. Latchoumanin O, et al: Reversal of glucocorticoids-dependent proopiomelanocortin gene inhibition by leukemia inhibitory factor, Endocrinology 148:422–432, 2007.

111. Abbud RA, Kelleher R, Melmed S: Cell-specific pituitary gene expression profiles after treatment with leukemia inhibitory factor reveal novel modulators for proopiomelanocortin expression, Endocrinology 145:867–880, 2004.

112. Smith AI, Funder JW: Proopiomelanocortin processing in the pituitary, central nervous system, and peripheral tissues, Endocr Rev 9:159–179, 1988.

113. Wikberg JES, et al: New aspects on the melanocortins and their receptors, Pharmacological Research 42:393–420, 2000.

114. Pritchard LE, White A: Neuropeptide processing and its impact on melanocortin pathways, Endocrinology 148:4201–4207, 2007.

115. Krude H, Biebermann H, Gruters A: Mutations in the human proopiomelanocortin gene, Ann N Y Acad Sci 994:233–239, 2003.

116. Chaptini L, Peikin S: Neuroendocrine regulation of food intake, Curr Opin Gastroenterol 24:223–229, 2008.

117. Valassi E, Scacchi M, Cavagnini F: Neuroendocrine control of food intake, Nutr Metab Cardiovasc Dis 18:158–168, 2008.

118. Pritchard LE, et al: Proopiomelanocortin-derived peptides in rat cerebrospinal fluid and hypothalamic extracts: evidence that secretion is regulated with respect to energy balance, Endocrinology 144:760–766, 2003.

119. Wardlaw SL, McCarthy KC: Glucocorticoid regulation of hypothalamic proopiomelanocortin, Neuroendocrinol 67:51–57, 1998.

120. Pelletier G: Regulation of proopiomelanocortin gene expression in rat brain and pituitary as studied by in situ hybridization, Ann N Y Acad Sci 680:246–259, 1993.

121. Schauer E, et al: Proopiomelanocortin-derived peptides are synthesized and released by human keratinocytes, J Clin Invest 93:2258–2262, 1994.

122. Wintzen M, Yaar M, Burbach JP, et al: Proopiomelanocortin gene product regulation in keratinocytes, J Invest Dermatol 106:673–678, 1996.

123. Scholzen TE, et al: Expression of proopiomelanocortin peptides in human dermal microvascular endothelial cells: evidence for a regulation by ultraviolet light and interleukin-1, J Invest Dermatol 115:1021–1028, 2000.

124. Paus R, et al: The skin POMC system (SPS). Leads and lessons from the hair follicle, Ann N Y Acad Sci 1999 Oct 885:350–363, 1999.

125. Ito N, et al: Human hair follicles display a functional equivalent of the hypothalamic-pituitary-adrenal axis and synthesize cortisol, FASEB J 19:1332–1334, 2005.

126. Schiller M, et al: Solar-simulated ultraviolet radiation-induced upregulation of the melanocortin-1 receptor, proopiomelanocortin, and alpha-melanocyte-stimulating hormone in human epidermis in vivo, J Invest Dermatol 122:468–476, 2004.

127. Cui R, et al: Central role of p53 in the suntan response and pathologic hyperpigmentation, Cell 128:853–864, 2007.

128. Slominski A, Tobin DJ, Paus R: Does p53 regulate skin pigmentation by controlling proopiomelanocortin gene transcription? Pigment Cell Res 20:307–308, 2007.

129. Raffin-Sanson ML, et al: High precursor level in maternal blood results from the alternate mode of proopiomelanocortin processing in human placenta, Clin Endocrinol (Oxf) 50:85–94, 1999.

130. Bicknell AB: The tissue-specific processing of proopiomelanocortin, J Neuroendocrinol 20:692–699, 2008.

131. Margioris AN, Grino M, Protos P, et al: Corticotropin-releasing hormone and oxytocin stimulate the release of placental proopiomelanocortin peptides, Journal of Clinical Endocrinology Metabolism 66:922–926, 1988.

132. Kubo M, Nakagawa K, Akikawa K, et al: In vivo and in vitro ACTH response to ovine corticotropin-releasing factor in a bronchial carcinoma from a patient with ectopic ACTH syndrome, Endocrinol Jpn 32:577–581, 1985.

133. Malchoff CD, et al: Ectopic ACTH syndrome caused by a bronchial carcinoid tumor responsive to dexamethasone, metyrapone, and corticotropin-releasing factor, Am J Med 84:760–764, 1988.

134. Suda T, et al: Corticotropin-releasing hormone, proopiomelanocortin, and glucocorticoid receptor gene expression in adrenocorticotropin-producing tumors in vitro, J Clin Invest 92:2790–2795, 1993.

135. Liddle GW, et al: Clinical and laboratory studies of ectopic humoral syndromes, Recent Prog Horm Res 25:283–314, 1969.

136. Gaitan D, et al: Glucocorticoid receptor structure and function in an adrenocorticotropin-secreting small cell lung cancer, Mol Endocrinol 9:1193–1201, 1995.

137. Ray DW, Littlewood AC, Clark AJ, et al: Human small cell lung cancer cell lines expressing the proopiomelanocortin gene have aberrant glucocorticoid receptor function, J Clin Invest 93:1625–1630, 1994.

138. Ray DW: Molecular mechanisms of glucocorticoid resistance, J Endocrinol 149:1–5, 1996.

139. Waters CE, Stevens A, White A, et al: Analysis of cofactor function in a glucocorticoid-resistant small cell carcinoma cell line, J Endocrinol 183:375–383, 2004.

139a. Sommer P, Le Rouzic P, Gillingham H, et al: Glucocorticoid receptor expression exerts an anti-survival effect on human small cell lung cancer cells, Oncogene 26:1–11, 2007.

140. Eipper BA, Mains RE: Structure and biosynthesis of pro-adrenocorticotropin/endorphin and related peptides, Endocr Rev 1:1–27, 1980.

141. Yalow RS, Berson SA: Characteristics of "big ACTH" in human plasma and pituitary extracts, J Clin Endocrinol Metab 36:415–423, 1973.

142. Eipper BA, Mains RE: High molecular weight forms of adrenocorticotropic hormone in the mouse pituitary and in a mouse pituitary cell line, Biochemistry 14:3836, 1975.

143. Orth DN, et al: ACTH and MSH production by a single cloned mouse pituitary tumor cell line, Endocrinology 92:385–393, 1973.

144. Lowry PJ, Rees L, Tomlin S, et al: Chemical characterization of ectopic ACTH purified from a malignant thymic carcinoid tumour, J Clin Endocrinol Metab 43:831, 1976.

145. Schwyzer R: ACTH: a short introductory review, Ann N Y Acad Sci 297:3–26, 1977.

146. Croughs RJ, Thijssen JH, Mol JA: Absence of detectable immunoreactive alpha melanocyte stimulating hormone in plasma in various types of Cushing's disease, J Endocrinol Invest 14:197–200, 1991.

147. Kortlandt W, De Rotte AA, Arts CJM, et al: Characterization of alpha-MSH-like immunoreactivity in human plasma, Acta Endocrinological (Copenh) 113:175–180, 1986.

148. Seidah NG, Chretien M: Complete amino acid sequence of a human pituitary glycopeptide: an important maturation product of proopiomelanocortin, Proc Natl Acad Sci USA 78:4236–4240, 1981.

149. Cool DR, Fenger M, Snell CR, et al: Identification of the sorting signal motif within pro-opiomelanocortin for the regulated secretory pathway, J Biol Chem 270:8723–8729, 1995.

150. Bertagna X, Camus F, Lenne F, et al: Human joining peptide: a proopiomelanocortin product secreted as a homodimer, Mol Endocrinol 2:1108–1114, 1988.

151. Gibson S, Crosby SR, White A: Discrimination between beta-endorphin and beta-lipotropin in human plasma using two-site immunoradiometric assays, Clin Endocrinol (Oxf) 39:445–453, 1993.

152. Stewart PM, et al: ACTH precursors characterize the ectopic ACTH syndrome, Clin Endocrinol (Oxf) 40:199–204, 1994.

153. Wilson H, White A: Prohormones: their clinical relevance, Trends Endocrinol Metab 9:396–402, 1998.

154. Gibson S, et al: Differential release of proopiomelanocortin-derived peptides from the human pituitary: evidence from a panel of two-site immunoradiometric assays, J Clin Endocrinol Metab 78:835–841, 1994.

155. Mountjoy KG, Wong J: Obesity, diabetes and functions for proopiomelanocortin-derived peptides, Mol Cell Endocrinol 128:171–177, 1996.

156. Steiner DF: The proprotein convertases, Curr Opin Chem Biol 2:31–39, 1998.

157. Thomas L, Leduc R, Thorne BA, et al: Kex2-like endoproteases PC2 and PC3 accurately cleave a model prohormone in mammalian cells: evidence for a common core of neuroendocrine processing enzymes, Proc Natl Acad Sci USA 88:5297–5301, 1991.

158. Bloomquist BT, Eipper BA, Mains, RE: Prohormone-converting enzymes: regulation and evaluation of function using antisense RNA, Mol Endocrinol 5:2014–2024, 1991.

159. Benjannet S, Rondeau N, Day R, et al: PC1 and PC2 are proprotein convertases capable of cleaving proopiomelanocortin at distinct pairs of basic residues, Proc Natl Acad Sci USA 88:3564–3568, 1991.

160. Scholzen TE, Konig S, Fastrich M, et al: Terminating the stress: peripheral peptidolysis of proopiomelanocortin-derived regulatory hormones by the dermal microvascular endothelial cell extracellular peptidases neprilysin and angiotensin-converting enzyme, Endocrinology 148:2793–2805, 2007.

161. Pritchard LE, Turnbull AV, White A: Pro-opiomelanocortin processing in the hypothalamus: impact on melanocortin signalling and obesity, J Endocrinol 172:411–421, 2002.

162. Castro MG, Morrison E: Post-translational processing of proopiomelanocortin in the pituitary and in the brain, Crit Rev Neurobiol 11:35–57, 1997.

163. Nillni EA: Regulation of prohormone convertases in hypothalamic neurons: implications for prothyrotropin-releasing hormone and proopiomelanocortin, Endocrinology 148:4191–4200, 2007.

164. Tsigos C, Crosby SR, Gibson S, et al: Proopiomelanocortin is the predominant adrenocorticotropin-related peptide in human cerebrospinal fluid, J Clin Endocrinol Metab 76:620–624, 1993.

165. McLoughlin L, Lowry PJ, Ratter SJ, et al: Characterisation of the proopiocortin family of peptides in human cerebrospinal fluid, Neuroendocrinology 32:209–212, 1981.

166. Nakao K, Oki S, Tanaka I: Immunoreactive beta-endorphin and adrenocorticotropin in human cerebrospinal fluid, J Clin Invest 66:1383–1390, 1980.

167. Thody AJ, Graham A: Does alpha-MSH have a role in regulating skin pigmentation in humans? Pigment Cell Res 11:265–274, 1998.

168. Peters EM, Tobin DJ, Seidah NG, et al: Pro-opiomelanocortin-related peptides, prohormone convertases 1 and 2 and the regulatory peptide 7B2 are present in

melanosomes of human melanocytes, J Invest Dermatol 114:430–437, 2000.

169. Gibson S, et al: Impaired processing of proopiomelanocortin in corticotroph macroadenomas, J Clin Endocrinol Metab 81:497–502, 1996.

170. Tateno T, et al: Defective expression of prohormone convertase 1/3 in silent corticotroph adenoma, Endocr J 54:777–782, 2007.

171. Odell WD: Ectopic ACTH syndrome: a misnomer, Endocrinol Metab Clin North Am 20:371–379, 1991.

172. Oliver RL, Davis JR, White A: Characterisation of ACTH related peptides in ectopic Cushing's syndrome, Pituitary 6:119–126, 2003.

173. White A, Gibson S: ACTH precursors: biological significance and clinical relevance, Clin Endocrinol (Oxf) 48:251–255, 1998.

174. Vieau D, Massias JF, Girard F, et al: Corticotrophin-like intermediary lobe peptide as a marker of alternate pro-opiomelanocortin processing in ACTH-producing non-pituitary tumours, Clin Endocrinol (Oxf) 31:691–700, 1989.

175. Dallman MF, Makara GB, Roberts JL, et al: Corticotrope response to removal of releasing factors and corticosteroids in vivo, Endocrinology 117:2190–2197, 1985.

176. Dallman MF, et al: Regulation of ACTH secretion: variations on a theme of B, Recent Prog Horm Res 43:113–173, 1987.

177. Karpac J, Kern A, Hochgeschwender U: Pro-opiomelanocortin peptides and the adrenal gland, Mol Cell Endocrinol 265–266:29–33, 2007.

178. Kempna P, Fluck CE: Adrenal gland development and defects, Best Pract Res Clin Endocrinol Metab 22:77–93, 2008.

179. Coll AP, et al: The effects of proopiomelanocortin deficiency on murine adrenal development and responsiveness to adrenocorticotropin, Endocrinology 145:4721–4727, 2004.

180. Clark AJ: The melanocortin-2 receptor in normal adrenocortical function and familial adrenocorticotrophic hormone resistance. In Cone RD editor: The Melanocortin Receptors, Totowa NJ, 2000, Humana Press, pp 361–384.

181. Catalano RD, Stuve L, Ramachandran J: Characterization of corticotrophin receptors in human adrenocortical cells, J Clin Endocrinol Metab 62:300–304, 1986.

182. Cone RD, et al: The melanocortin receptors: agonists, antagonists, and the hormonal control of pigmentation, Recent Prog Horm Res 51:287–317, 1996.

183. Chen M, Aprahamian CJ, Kesterson RA, et al: Molecular identification of the human melanocortin-2 receptor responsible for ligand binding and signaling, Biochemistry 46:11389–11397, 2007.

184. Miller WL: Molecular biology of steroid hormone synthesis, Endocr Rev 9:295–318, 1988.

185. Bohm M, et al: Detection of functionally active melanocortin receptors and evidence for an immunoregulatory activity of alpha-melanocyte-stimulating hormone in human dermal papilla cells, Endocrinology 146:4635–4646, 2005.

186. Bohm M, Luger TA, Tobin DJ, et al: Melanocortin receptor ligands: new horizons for skin biology and clinical dermatology, J Invest Dermatol 126:1966–1975, 2006.

187. Challis BG, et al: A missense mutation disrupting a dibasic prohormone processing site in pro-opiomelanocortin (POMC) increases susceptibility to early-onset obesity through a novel molecular mechanism, Hum Mol Genet 11:1997–2004, 2002.

188. Sutton GM, Josephine BM, Gu X, et al: A derivative of the melanocortin receptor antagonist SHU9119 (PG932) increases food intake when administered peripherally, Peptides 29:104–111, 2008.

189. Maaser C, Kannengiesser K, Kucharzik T: Role of the melanocortin system in inflammation, Ann N Y Acad Sci 1072:123–134, 2006.

190. Lasaga M, Debeljuk L, Durand D, et al: Role of alpha-melanocyte stimulating hormone and melanocortin 4 receptor in brain inflammation, Peptides 29:1825–1835, 2008.

191. Lowry PJ, Silas L, McLean C, et al: Pro-γ-melanocyte-stimulating hormone cleavage in adrenal gland undergoing compensatory growth, Nature 306:70–73, 1983.

192. Fassnacht M, et al: N-terminal proopiomelanocortin acts as a mitogen in adrenocortical tumor cells and decreases adrenal steroidogenesis, J Clin Endocrinol Metab 88:2171–2179, 2003.

193. Bicknell AB, et al: Characterization of a serine protease that cleaves pro-gamma-melanotropin at the adrenal to stimulate growth, Cell 105:903–912, 2001.

194. Al-Dujaili EAS, Hope J, Estivariz FE, et al: Circulating human pituitary pro-γ-melanotropin enhances the adrenal response to ACTH, Nature 291:156–159, 1981.

195. Rochemont J, Hamelin J: The missing fragment of the pro-sequence of human pro-opiomelanocortin: sequence and evidence for C-terminal amidation, Biochem Biophys Res Commun 102:710–716, 1981.

196. Robinson P, et al: Isolation and characterization of three forms of joining peptide from adult human pituitaries: lack of adrenal androgen-stimulating activity, Endocrinology 129:859–867, 1991.

197. Rubinstein M, et al: Absence of opioid stress-induced analgesia in mice lacking beta-endorphin by site-directed mutagenesis, Proc Natl Acad Sci USA 93:3995–4000, 1996.

198. Kauser S, Thody AJ, Schallreuter KU, et al: Beta-endorphin as a regulator of human hair follicle melanocyte biology, J Invest Dermatol 123:184–195, 2004.

199. Ratter SJ, et al: Pro-opiocortin related peptides in human pituitary and ectopic ACTH secreting tumours, Clin Endocrinol (Oxf) 18:211–218, 1983.

200. Hruby VJ, Han G: The molecular pharmacology of alpha-melanocyte stimulating hormone. In Cone RD, editor: The melanocortin receptors, Totowa, New Jersey, 2000, Humana Press Inc, pp 255–257.

201. Pritchard LE, et al: Agouti-related protein (83–132) is a competitive antagonist at the human melanocortin-4 receptor: no evidence for differential interactions with pro-opiomelanocortin-derived ligands, J Endocrinol 180:183–191, 2004.

202. Ray DW, et al: Elevated levels of adrenocorticotropin (ACTH) precursors in post-adrenalectomy Cushing's disease and their regulation by glucocorticoids, J Clin Endocrinol Metab 80:2430–2436, 1995.

203. Morton NM, Seckl JR: 11Beta-hydroxysteroid dehydrogenase type 1 and obesity, Front Horm Res 36:146–164, 2008.

204. Tomlinson JW, Stewart PM: Modulation of glucocorticoid action and the treatment of type-2 diabetes, Best Pract Res Clin Endocrinol Metab 21:607–619, 2007.

205. Hughes KA, Webster SP, Walker BR: 11-Beta-hydroxysteroid dehydrogenase type 1 (11beta-HSD1) inhibitors in type 2 diabetes mellitus and obesity, Expert Opin Investig Drugs 17:481–496, 2008.

206. Daly JR, Reader SCJ, Alaghband-Zadeh J, et al: Observations on feedback regulation of corticotropin (ACTH) in man. In Jones MT, Gillham B, Dallman MF, Chattopadhyay S, editors: Interaction within the brain-pituitary-adrenocortical system, London, 1979, Academic, pp 181–188.

207. de Kloet ER, Vreugdenhil E, Oitzl MS, et al: Brain corticosteroid receptor balance in health and disease, Endocr Rev 19:269–301, 1998.

208. Atkinson HC, et al: Corticosteroids mediate fast feedback of the rat hypothalamic-pituitary-adrenal axis via the mineralocorticoid receptor, Am J Physiol Endocrinol Metab 294:E1011-E1022, 2008.

209. Tierney T, Christian HC, Morris JF, et al: Evidence from studies on co-cultures of TtT/GF and AtT20 cells that Annexin 1 acts as a paracrine or juxtacrine mediator of the early inhibitory effects of glucocorticoids on ACTH release, J Neuroendocrinol 15:1134–1143, 2003.

210. Spiga F, et al: Effect of the glucocorticoid receptor antagonist Org 34850 on fast and delayed feedback of corticosterone release, J Endocrinol 196:323–330, 2008.

211. Beaulieu S, Gagne B, Barden N: Glucocorticoid regulation of proopiomelanocortin messenger ribonucleic acid content of rat hypothalamus, Mol Endocrinol 2:727–731, 1988.

211a. Drazen DL, Wortman MD, Schwartz MW, et al: Adrenalectomy alters the sensitivity of the central nervous system melanocortin system, Diabetes 52(12):2928–2934, 2003.

212. Venihaki M, Carrigan A, Dikkes P, et al: Circadian rise in maternal glucocorticoid prevents pulmonary dysplasia in fetal mice with adrenal insufficiency, Proc Natl Acad Sci USA 97:7336–7341, 2000.

213. DeBold CR, et al: Effect of synthetic ovine corticotropin-releasing factor: prolonged duration of action and biphasic response of plasma adrenocorticotropin and cortisol, J Clin Endocrinol Metab 57:294–298, 1983.

214. Jorgensen H, Knigge U, Kjaer A, et al: Serotonergic stimulation of corticotropin-releasing hormone and pro-opiomelanocortin gene expression, J Neuroendocrinol 14:788–795, 2002.

215. Guillaume V, Conte-Devolx B, Magnan E: Effect of chronic active immunization with antiarginine vasopressin on pituitary-adrenal function in sheep, Endocrinology 130:3007–3014, 1992.

216. Whitnall MH: Regulation of the hypothalamic corticotropin-releasing hormone neurosecretory system, Prog Neurobiol 40:573–629, 1993.

217. Elias AN, Valenta LJ, Szekeres AV, et al: Regulatory role of gamma-aminobutyric acid in pituitary hormone secretion, Psychoneuroendocrinology 7:15–30, 1982.

218. Fish HR, Chernow B, O'Brian JT: Endocrine and neurophysiologic responses of the pituitary to insulin-induced hypoglycemia: a review, Metabolism 35:763–780, 1986.

219. Hornby PJ, Piekut DT: Opiocortin and catecholamine input to CRF-immunoreactive neurons in rat forebrain, Peptides 10:1139–1146, 1989.

220. Nussdorfer GG, Malendowicz LK: Role of VIP, PACAP, and related peptides in the regulation of the hypothalamo-pituitary-adrenal axis, Peptides 19:1443–1467, 1998.

221. Koenig JI: Pituitary gland: neuropeptides, neurotransmitters and growth factors, Toxicol Pathol 17:256–265, 1989.

222. Johnson KL, Rn CR: The hypothalamic-pituitary-adrenal axis in critical illness, AACN Clin Issues 17:39–49, 2006.

223. Ray D, Melmed S: Pituitary cytokine and growth factor expression and action, Endocr Rev 18:206–228, 1997.

224. Turnbull AV, Rivier CL: Regulation of the hypothalamic-pituitary-adrenal axis by cytokines: actions and mechanisms of action, Physiol Rev 79:1–71, 1999.

225. Skurlova M, Stofkova A, Jurcovicova J: Exogenous IL-1beta induces its own expression, but not that of IL-6 in the hypothalamus and activates HPA axis and prolactin release, Endocr Regul 40:125–128, 2006.

226. Sapolsky R, Rivier C, Yamamoto G, et al: Interleukin 1 stimulates the secretion of hypothalamic corticotropin-releasing factor, Science 238:522–524, 1987.

227. Bernton EW, Beach JE, Holaday JW, et al: Release of multiple hormones by a direct action of interleukin 1 on pituitary cells, Science 238:652–654, 1987.

228. Suda T, Tozawa F, Ushiyama T: Effects of protein kinase C related adrenocorticotrophin secretogogues and interleukin 1 on proopiomelanocortin gene expression in rat anterior pituitary cells, Endocrinology 124:1444–1449, 1989.

229. Arzt E, et al: Interleukin 2 and interleukin-receptor expression in human corticotrophic adenoma and mouse pituitary cell cultures, J Clin Invest 90:1944–1951, 1992.

230. Denicoff KD, Durkin TM, Lotze MT: The neuroendocrine effects of interleukin 2 treatment, Clin Endocrinol Metab 69:402–410, 1989.

231. Lotze MT, Frana LW, Sharrow SO, et al: In vivo administration of purified human interleukin alpha I half-life and immunologic effects of the JURKAT cell-line derived IL-2, J Immunol 134:157–166, 1985.

232. Vankelecom H, Carmeliet P, Van Damme J, et al: Production of interleukin 6 by folliculostellate cells of the anterior pituitary gland in a histiotypic cell aggregate culture system, Neuroendocrinol 49:102–106, 1989.

233. Spangelo BL, MacLeod RM, Isakson PC: Production of interleukin 6 by anterior pituitary cells in-vitro, Endocrinology 126:582, 1990.

234. Jones TH, Justice S, Price A, et al: Interleukin-6-secreting human pituitary adenomas in vitro, J Clin Endocrinol Metab 73:207–209, 1991.

235. Jones TH, et al: Production of bioactive and immunoreactive interleukin 6 (IL-6) and expression of IL-6 messenger ribonucleic acid by human pituitary adenomas, J Clin Endocrinol Metab 78:180–187, 1994.

236. Tsagarakis S, Kontogeorgos G, Giannou P: Interleukin-6, a growth promoting cytokine, is present in human pituitary adenomas: an immunocytochemical study, Clin Endocrinology 37:163–167, 1992.

237. Mastorakos G, Weber JS, Magiakou MA, et al: Hypothalamic-pituitary-adrenal axis activation and stimulation of systemic vasopressin secretion by recombinant interleukin-6 in humans: potential implications for the syndrome of inappropriate vasopressin secretion, J Clin Endocrinol Metab 79:934–939, 1994.

238. Fong Y, Moldawer LL, Marano M: Endotoxemia elicits increased circulating beta2-IFN/IL-6 in man, J Immunol 142:2321–2324, 1989.

239. Kariagina A, Romanenko D, Ren SG, et al: Hypothalamic-pituitary cytokine network, Endocrinology 145:104–112, 2004.

240. Akita S, et al: Human and murine pituitary expression of leukemia inhibitory factor: novel intrapituitary regulation of adrenocorticotropin synthesis and secretion, J Clin Invest 95:1288–1298, 1995.

241. Wang Z, Ren SG, Melmed S: Hypothalamic and pituitary leukemia inhibitory factor gene expression in vivo: a novel endotoxin-inducible neuro-endocrine interface, Endocrinology 137:2947–2953, 1996.

242. Ray DW, Ren SG, Melmed S: Leukemia inhibitory factor (LIF) stimulates proopiomelanocortin (POMC) expression in a corticotroph cell line. Role of STAT pathway, J Clin Invest 97:1852–1859, 1996.

243. Stefana B, Ray DW, Melmed S: Leukemia inhibitory factor induces differentiation of pituitary corticotroph function: an immuno-neuroendocrine phenotypic switch, Proc Natl Acad Sci USA 93:12502–12506, 1996.

244. Akita S, Malkin J, Melmed S: Disrupted murine leukemia inhibitory fact (LIF) gene attenuates adrenocorticotrophic hormone (ACTH) secretion, Endocrinology 137:3140–3143, 1996.

245. Ware CB, Kariagina A, Zonis S, et al: Leukemia inhibitory factor signaling is implicated in embryonic development of the HPA axis, FEBS Lett 579:4465–4469, 2005.

246. Kelly RB: Pathways of protein secretion in eukaryotes, Science 230:25–32, 1985.

247. Lightman SL, et al: The significance of glucocorticoid pulsatility, Eur J Pharmacol 583:255–262, 2008.

248. Gudmundsson A, Carnes M: Pulsatile adrenocorticotropic hormone: an overview, Biol Psychiatry 41:342–365, 1997.

249. Horrocks PM, et al: Patterns of ACTH and cortisol pulsatility over twenty-four hours in normal males and females, Clin Endocrinol (Oxf) 32:127–134, 1990.

250. Smith SM, Vale WW: The role of the hypothalamic-pituitary-adrenal axis in neuroendocrine responses to stress, Dialogues Clin Neurosci 8:383–395, 2006.

251. Hesse DG, Tracey KJ, Fong Y: Cytokine appearance in human endotoxemia and primate bacteremia, Surg Gynecol Obstet 166:147–153, 1988.

252. Van Deventer SJH, et al: Experimental endotoxemia in humans: analysis of cytokine release and coagulation, fibrolytic and complement pathways, Blood 76:2500–2526, 1990.

253. Chrousos GP: The hypothalamic-pituitary-adrenal axis and immune-mediated inflammation, N Engl J Med 332:1351–1362, 1995.

254. Ray DW, Stefana B, Zand O, et al: Leukaemia inhibitory factor: a potent modulator of CRH action on pituitary corticotroph cells. In Proceedings of the Annual Meeting of the Endocrine Society, San Francisco, 1996, pp 532.

255. Takao T, Culp SG, De Souza EB: Reciprocal modulation of interleukin 1 beta and interleukin-1 receptors by lipopolysaccharide (endotoxin) treatment in the mouse brain-endocrine-immune axis, Endocrinology 132:1497–1504, 1993.

256. Bernhagen J, et al: MIF is a pituitary-derived cytokine that potentiates lethal endotoxaemia, Nature 365:756–959, 1993.

257. Yamaguchi M, Matsuzaki N, Hirota K, et al: Interleukin 6 possibly induced by interleukin-1 beta in the pituitary gland stimulates the release of gonadotrophins and prolactin, Acta Endocrinology (Copenh) 122:201–20556, 1990.

258. Muglia L, Jacobson L, Dikkes P, et al: Corticotrophin-releasing hormone deficiency reveals major fetal but not adult glucocorticoid need, Nature 373:427–432, 1995.

259. Milenkovic L, Rettori V, Snyder GD, et al: Cachectin alters pituitary hormone release by a direct action in vitro, Proc Natl Acad Sci USA 86:2418–2422, 1989.

260. Spangelo BL, Judd AM, Isakson PC, et al: Interleukin 6 stimulates anterior pituitary hormone release in vitro, Endocrinology 125:575–577, 1989.

261. Almawi WY, et al: Abrogation of glucocorticoid-mediated inhibition of T-cell proliferation by the synergistic actions of IL-6 and IFN-gamma, J Immunol 146:3523–3527, 1991.

262. Kam JC, Szeffer SJ, Surs W, et al: Combination IL-2 and IL-4 reduces glucocorticoid receptor-binding affinity and T cell response to glucocorticoids, J Immunol 151:3460–3466, 1993.

263. Caldenhoven E, et al: Negative cross-talk between Re1A and the glucocorticoid receptor: a possible mechanism for the anti-inflammatory action of glucocorticoids, Mol Endocrinol 9:401–412, 1995.

264. Ray A, Prefontaine KE: Physical association and functional antagonism between the p65 subunit of transcription factor NK-kappa B and the glucocorticoid receptor, Proc Natl Acad Sci USA 91:752–756, 1994.

265. Scheinman RI, Gualberto A, Jewell CM, et al: Characterization of mechanisms involved in transrepression of NF-kappa B by activated glucocorticoid receptors, Mol Cell Biol 15:943–953, 1995.

266. Makino S, Hashimoto K, Gold PW: Multiple feedback mechanisms activating corticotropin-releasing hormone system in the brain during stress, Pharmacol Biochem Behav 73:147–158, 2002.

267. Raff H, Findling JW: A new immunoradiometric assay for corticotropin evaluated in normal subjects and patients with Cushing's syndrome, Clin Chem 35:596–600, 1989.

268. Yalow RS, Berson SA: Size heterogeneity of immunoreactive human ACTH in plasma and in extracts of pituitary glands and ACTH-producing thymoma, Biochem Biophys Res Commun 44:439–445, 1971.

269. Hale AC, Besser GM, Rees LH: Characterization of pro-opiomelanocortin-derived peptides in pituitary and ectopic adrenocorticotrophin-secreting tumours, J Endocrinol 108:49–56, 1986.

270. Crosby SR, Stewart MF, Ratcliffe JG, et al: Direct measurement of the precursors of adrenocorticotropin in human plasma by two-site immunoradiometric assay, J Clin Endocrinol Metab 67:1272–1277, 1988.

271. Raffin-Sanson ML, et al: High plasma proopiomelanocortin in aggressive adrenocorticotropin-secreting tumors, J Clin Endocrinol Metab 81:4272–4277, 1996.

Chapter 4

ENDOCRINE RHYTHMS, THE SLEEP-WAKE CYCLE, AND BIOLOGICAL CLOCKS

GEORGES COPINSCHI, FRED W. TUREK, and EVE VAN CAUTER

Major Mechanisms Controlling 24-Hour Endocrine Rhythms

A prominent feature of the endocrine system is its high degree of temporal organization. Indeed, far from obeying the concept of constancy of the internal milieu, circulating hormonal levels undergo pronounced temporal oscillations ranging from a few minutes to a year. This intricate temporal organization provides the endocrine system with remarkable flexibility. Not only can specific physiologic processes be turned on and off, depending on the presence or absence of a particular hormone, but the precise pattern of hormonal release may provide specific signaling information.

Hormonal variations in the circadian (i.e., approximately once per 24 hours) and ultradian (i.e., once per 1 to 2 hours) range are ubiquitous in endocrine systems. However, the whole spectrum of endocrine rhythms includes both higher and lower frequency ranges. Indeed, secretory oscillations with periods in the 5 to 15 minute range have been observed for a number of hormones. The menstrual cycle and seasonal rhythms belong to the so-called infradian range, corresponding to periods longer than the circadian range.

As is illustrated schematically in Figure 4-1, the temporal variability and organization of hormonal concentrations during the 24-hour cycle ultimately result from the activity of two interacting time-keeping mechanisms in the central nervous system: endogenous circadian rhythmicity and sleep-wake homeostasis, a mechanism that relates the timing and intensity of sleep to the duration of prior wakefulness. Although this dual control was first demonstrated for hormones of the hypothalamic-pituitary axis, a similar regulation appears to apply to other endocrine subsystems. In mammals, endogenous circadian rhythmicity is generated by a master circadian clock located in the paired suprachiasmatic nucleus (SCN) of the hypothalamus.[1] The SCN controls the timing of most, if not all, circadian rhythms and partially regulates the sleep-wake cycle. The sleep-wake cycle in turn regulates the timing of many rhythms that depend on the presence or absence of sleep and wakefulness. Indeed, the timing and expression of many endocrine rhythms appear to depend upon direct control from the SCN, as well as on the presence and quality of sleep, with some 24-hour endocrine rhythms influenced more by the SCN (e.g., melatonin and cortisol), and others more regulated by the sleep-wake state (e.g., growth hormone). Thus, combined inputs of the master circadian clock and the sleep-wake state[2] control the overall temporal organization of the endocrine system, as well as many other behavioral and physiologic systems, across the 24-hour cycle. The two major pathways by which circadian rhythmicity and sleep-wake homeostasis affect peripheral endocrine function are the hypothalamic-pituitary axis and the autonomous nervous system.

The first section of this chapter provides an overview of current concepts and recent advances in our understanding of circadian rhythmicity and sleep-wake regulation, and introduces the general properties, physiologic significance, and medical implications of ultradian rhythmicity. This section concludes

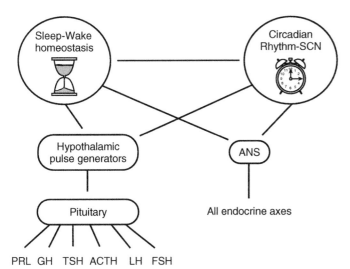

FIGURE 4-1. Schematic representation of the central mechanisms involved in the control of temporal variations in pituitary hormone secretions over the 24-hour cycle. *ACTH*, Adrenocorticotropic hormone; *ANS*, autonomous nervous system; *FSH*, follicle-stimulating hormone; *GH*, growth hormone; *LH*, luteinizing hormone; *PRL*, prolactin; *SCN*, suprachiasmatic nucleus of the hypothalamus; *TSH*, thyrotropin.

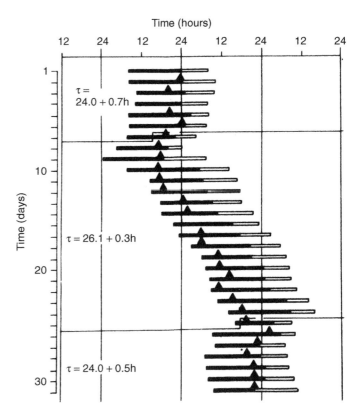

FIGURE 4-2. Circadian rhythms of wakefulness *(black bars)*, sleep *(white bars)*, and maximal rectal temperature *(triangles)* in a human subject who was exposed to external synchronizing agents for the first and last 7 days and was isolated from all time cues in an underground bunker between days 8 and 24.

with a review of the impact of age on these mechanisms. Methodologic aspects specific to the study of hormonal rhythms in human subjects are described in the second section. The third section summarizes the present state of knowledge on circadian and ultradian endocrine rhythms in health and disease for the major endocrine axes. Conditions of altered or abnormal circadian and/or sleep regulation that have implications for the temporal organization of hormonal release are presented in the last section.

Because of limitations on length and in the scope of this chapter, this review is limited to findings in adults.

CIRCADIAN RHYTHMICITY

General Characteristics

One of the most obvious characteristics of life on earth is the ability of almost all species to change their behavior on a daily or 24-hour basis. A remarkable feature of these daily or diurnal rhythms is that they are not simply a response to 24-hour changes in the physical environment imposed by the principles of celestial mechanics, but instead arise from an internal time-keeping system[1,3] that has the intrinsic capability to continuously generate rhythmic activity over a nearly 24-hour period. Thus, under laboratory conditions devoid of any external time-giving cues, it has been found that nearly all 24-hour rhythms continue to be expressed. However, under such constant conditions, the period of the rhythm rarely remains exactly 24 hours but instead is "about" 24 hours, and this is why these rhythms are referred to as *circadian,* from the Latin "circa diem," meaning "around a day." When a circadian rhythm is expressed in the absence of any 24 hour signals in the external environment, it is said to be free-running. Under free-running conditions, the endogenous period generally is close to, but is nearly never exactly, 24 hours. Strictly speaking, a diurnal rhythm should not be referred to as circadian until it has been demonstrated that such a rhythm persists under constant environmental conditions. The purpose of this distinction is to separate out those rhythms that are simply a response to 24-hour changes in the environment from those that are endogenous. However, for practical purposes, there is little reason to make a distinction between diurnal and circadian rhythms, since an endogenous timing device underlies the generation of almost all diurnal rhythms. In this chapter, we therefore extend the use of the term *circadian rhythm* to include all diurnal variations that recur regularly at a time interval of approximately 24 hours.

An immense variety of circadian rhythms have been observed in man. Human circadian rhythms have been characterized for blood constituents such as white blood cells, amino acids, and hormones, innumerable physiologic variables such as body temperature, heart rate, blood pressure, and urinary volume, and behavioral parameters such as food intake, sleep, mood, vigilance, and cognitive performance. Rhythms have also been noted in response to various challenges such as drugs and stress. Circadian rhythmicity is maintained when subjects are sleep deprived, when they are starved, or when they receive equal amounts of food at short intervals over the day. The timing of single meals, however, can have effects on the pattern of at least some variables, including hormones, and the timing, duration, and quality of sleep and wake can alter the expression of many rhythms, especially those of the endocrine system.

The endogenous nature of human circadian rhythms has been established by experiments in which subjects were isolated with no access to the natural light-dark cycle and no time cues. Such experiments were first performed in natural caves, then in underground bunkers, and finally in specially designed windowless soundproof apartments. The results of one such early experiment, conducted in an artificial underground unit in Germany, are shown in Figure 4-2.[4] The rest-activity cycle of the subject is plotted horizontally, day by day, and the times of occurrence of the daily maximum of the body temperature cycle are indicated by closed triangles. During the first 7 days of the experiment, the door of the isolation unit was left open, and the subjects knew the time of day. The average duration (t) of the rest-activity cycle and of the rhythm of body temperature was 24 hours. When, thereafter, the subject lived in complete isolation, both rhythms free-ran but with a mean period of about 26 hours. The free-running period varies from one individual to another. In humans, free-running periods of around 25 hours have been observed under conditions of prolonged temporal isolation. However, assessments of the human free-running period based on the so-called forced desynchrony protocol have provided estimations of between 24.1 and 24.2 hours.[5]

The Suprachiasmatic Nucleus: A Master Circadian Pacemaker

In mammals, the suprachiasmatic nucleus (SCN), which consists of two small, bilaterally paired nuclei in the anterior hypothalamus, each of which contains about 10,000 cells in rodents, functions as the master circadian clock. Under both free-running and entrained conditions, destruction of the SCN in a variety of species leads to abolishment or severe disruption of many endocrine, behavioral, and physiologic rhythms.[1,6] The role of the SCN as the control center for the circadian system, first suggested by lesion studies, was confirmed by studies involving transplantation of the SCN from one animal to another. Indeed, circadian rhythmicity can be restored in adult arrhythmic SCN-lesioned rodents by transplanting fetal SCN tissue into the region of the SCN.[7,8] A number of SCN rhythms, including those of neural firing, vasopressin release, glucose metabolism, and gene expression, persist in vitro.[9-12] The ability of SCN cells to generate a circadian signal does not rely on some inherent network property of many cells acting together: Single SCN cells in culture can generate circadian neural signals.[13] Neurons within the SCN appear to be organized into two groups: a core group of light responsive but nonrhythmic cells, and a shell of rhythmic cells.[14,15]

The generation and maintenance of circadian oscillations in the SCN involve a series of clock genes (including *per1, per 2, per3, cry1, cry2, tim, clock, B-mal1,* and *CKIε/δ*), often referred to as canonical, which interact in a complex feedback loop of transcription/translation.[16,17] Indeed, improved tissue culture techniques and real-time monitoring of the expression of circadian clock genes have revealed that circadian oscillations in gene expression can persist in the SCN in vitro (as well as in other tissues, see later) for many cycles.[16] It is important to note that mutations or deletions of canonical circadian clock genes have been found to profoundly affect endocrine rhythms and normal endocrine function in a variety of central and peripheral tissues.[18-20] For reviews on the molecular and genetic control of circadian rhythmicity, the reader is referred to references 16, 17, and 21.

In recent years, it has been recognized that circadian oscillations can be generated in areas of the brain other than the SCN, as well as in many peripheral tissues.[9,22] These local oscillators appear to be under the control of the SCN and of the canonical circadian clock genes in the SCN, through the synchronization or entrainment of the same circadian clock machinery at the local tissue level. The SCN controls or synchronizes these autonomous circadian clocks in non-SCN tissues directly via neural and/or endocrine signals, or indirectly via its control of behavioral rhythms such as the sleep-wake cycle and the rhythm of feeding. However, the precise mechanisms are not well understood.

Photic Entrainment of Circadian Rhythms

The fact that the endogenous circadian period is not exactly equal to 24 hours implies that changes in the physical environment must synchronize or entrain the internal clock. Otherwise, a clock with a period only a few minutes shorter or longer than 24 hours soon would be totally out of synchrony with the environmental day. Agents that are capable of entraining or synchronizing circadian rhythms are often called *zeitgebers*, a German neologism meaning "time giver."

The light-dark (LD) cycle is the primary agent that synchronizes most circadian rhythms. Thus, in the presence of a 24-hour LD cycle, the period of circadian rhythms exactly matches the period of the LD cycle. In addition to establishing period control, an entraining LD cycle establishes phase control, such that specific phases of the circadian rhythm occur at the same time in each cycle. Entrainment is restricted to cycles with periods that are close to 24 hours in duration and, in general, is not possible for LD cycles that are more than a few hours shorter or longer than the endogenous circadian period. If the period of the LD cycle is too short or too long for entrainment to occur, the circadian rhythm free-runs. This rigidity of the circadian pacemaker has been used in so-called forced desynchrony studies, where subjects are maintained on a light-dark and sleep-wake cycle with a period outside the range of entrainment, such as 20 hours or 28 hours.[5,23] As mentioned earlier, such protocols have provided estimations of the endogenous period of the human circadian system that are closer to 24 hours (i.e., averaging 24.1 hours) than those obtained in prolonged studies of temporal isolation.[5] The fact that the human endogenous circadian period probably is very close to 24 hours is consistent with the findings of a study showing that a schedule of sleep-wake and dark-light cycles with very low light intensity during wakefulness is able to maintain entrainment to the 24-hour day but not to a 23.5- or 24.6-hour day.[24]

The eyes are involved in relaying entraining information from the LD cycle to the circadian timing system in mammals via a unique pathway, separate from the visual system, and referred to as the retinohypothalamic tract.[25] At the level of the optic chiasm, retinal projections first enter the brain in the region of the SCN and surrounding hypothalamic areas.[25] Thus, the integrity of the primary visual centers of the brain and/or of the perception of light is not necessary for entrainment of circadian rhythms by the LD cycle. The independence of photic input to the circadian clock from the visual system in mammals actually is not surprising from an evolutionary point of view. In all non-mammalian vertebrates, entrainment of circadian rhythms can occur in the absence of the eyes and relies on nonretinal photoreceptors in the brain.[26] The independence of the circadian light sensing system from the visual system in mammals was suggested in early studies showing that rod-less/cone-less mice could still entrain to the light-dark cycle, even though the eyes were necessary.[27] Early in this century, several laboratories discovered almost simultaneously that a special subset of retinal ganglion cells containing melanopsin could act as photoreceptors for relaying light information to the circadian clock in the SCN.[28-31] This breakthrough not only demonstrated a new light sensing system in the retina, but also opened up new avenues of research regarding the impact of light on brain function independent of the visual system, including possible neuroendocrine effects.[32,33] The finding that visual light perception is not necessary for circadian light perception can explain why in some totally blind humans, light exposure is capable of suppressing melatonin levels, indicating that visual blindness should not be equated with circadian blindness.[34] In addition to the retinohypothalamic tract, the SCN receives retinal information indirectly from the lateral geniculate nucleus (LGN), which receives a direct projection from the retina.[25]

To examine how a zeitgeber such as light influences the circadian system, the organism is maintained in constant conditions (e.g., constant darkness) and then is exposed to the zeitgeber for a brief period (e.g., 1 hour) before it is returned to constant conditions.[35] The effects of zeitgeber exposure on a phase reference point of an overt circadian rhythm (e.g., onset of locomotor activity, minimum of body temperature) in subsequent cycles then are determined. A plot of the direction and magnitude of the phase-shift as a function of the circadian time of zeitgeber exposure is called a phase response curve (PRC).[36] In the human, light exposure during the late evening and the first half of the usual sleep period results in phase delays, but light exposure at the end of the usual sleep period and in the early morning results in phase advances. The transition from phase delays to phase advances occurs around the time of the minimum of body temperature, that is, at between 04.00 and 06.00 hours in most subjects. The magnitude of the phase-shifts is also wavelength dependent, with exposure to short-wavelength monochromatic light (shifted to the blue) resulting in much larger shifts than exposure to longer-wavelength light of equal photon density,[37] because the retinal ganglion cells that contain melanopsin are most sensitive to blue light.

Although differences in amplitude may exist, the general shape and characteristics of the PRC to light pulses are similar for all species. Based on this PRC, appropriate exposure to bright light can accelerate adaptation to shifts such as those occurring in jet lag and shift work. The amplitude of the phase-shifts depends on light intensity and duration, and on the number of consecutive exposures.[38] For example, exposure to single 3- to 7-hour light pulses can induce phase-shifts on the order of 1 to 3 hours[39-41]; repeated exposure for 2 to 3 consecutive days may cause much larger 6- to 12-hour shifts.[5,42] Intervening periods of dark/sleep exposure could play a role in enhancing the phase-shifting effects of repeated exposure to light.

Exposure to dark also can cause a phase-shift of mammalian circadian rhythms. Because under most circumstances exposure to dark is associated with changes in activity levels (i.e., increases in activity in nocturnal animals and decreases in activity and/or sleep induction in diurnal animals), it has been unclear whether the phase-shifts occurred in response to dark exposure per se, or in response to associated changes in activity levels.[43] A study in hamsters, however, has demonstrated that resetting of the rhythm of locomotor activity and concomitant downregulation of circadian clock gene expression following exposure to dark pulses could occur independently of wheel running activity.[44] In humans, abrupt 8-hour advances or 8-hour delays of the sleep-wake cycle result in immediate 2-hour phase-shifts in the same direction.[45,46] Daytime naps of 6 hours' duration in total darkness presented over a background of very dim light were found to cause delay shifts when initiated in the morning and advance shifts when initiated in the evening.[47] Naps initiated in the afternoon cause no significant phase-shifts.

Nonphotic Zeitgebers

Nonphotic cues, for example, social and/or behavioral cues, also may alter the rest-activity cycle by eliciting activity during the normal rest period or by preventing activity during the normal active period, resulting in phase-shifts in circadian rhythms of activity, as well as other behavioral, physiologic, and endocrine markers.[48-51] In nocturnal rodents, the PRC to activity-inducing stimuli is about 12 hours out of phase with the PRC to light pulses.[52]

How nonphotic information reaches the SCN still is not known, although evidence from lesion studies suggests that a distinct subdivision of the LGN, the intergeniculate leaflet (IGL), may be involved in mediating the effects of activity on the clock.[53] Furthermore, the IGL is the source of neuropeptide Y (NPY) innervation of the SCN, and the administration of NPY into the SCN area, as well as electrical stimulation of the geniculohypothalamic tract, induces phase-shifts in hamster locomotor activity rhythm that are similar to those induced by activity-inducing stimuli.[53] The LGN/IGL may be a common pathway by which information about the lighting environment and the activity-rest state reaches the circadian clock, and it may be involved in integrating information from the external and the internal environment. Both the LGN/IGL and the SCN receive a dense serotonergic projection from the midbrain raphe nuclei, and substantial evidence now indicates that these projections play a role in both photic and nonphotic regulation of the mammalian circadian clock.[54-56]

Nonphotic stimuli may affect human circadian rhythms. Exposure to a single session of 3 hours of moderate-intensity exercise during the usual nighttime period was found to result in phase-shifts of markers of circadian phase on the next day, with the direction and magnitude of the phase-shifts being dependent on the timing of exercise.[57] Similar findings were obtained with nocturnal exposure to high-intensity 1 hour exercise sessions.[58] Supporting evidence for a zeitgeber effect of exercise was obtained in a field study, which found that adaptation to night work could be facilitated by nocturnal exercise.[59] These findings were confirmed by a study demonstrating that daily exposure to nighttime exercise facilitated phase delays in circadian melatonin rhythm, even when subjects were maintained in very dim light.[60] Nocturnal exercise of low intensity also causes phase-delays in circadian rhythms in older adults, suggesting that it could be a useful treatment for the adjustment of circadian rhythmicity in older populations.[61]

Another nonphotic agent that has been shown to induce phase-shifts in human circadian rhythms is melatonin.[62] This action of melatonin is often referred to as chronobiotic. Specific neural connections are present between the SCN and the pineal gland, and diurnal variation in plasma melatonin levels is driven by the circadian clock.[63] Phase-shifts of the central circadian signal induced by changes in the LD cycle will be faithfully reflected in the synchronization of the onset of nocturnal melatonin secretion.[40,64,65] Evidence suggests that, in turn, the melatonin rhythm feeds back on the clock (where melatonin receptors have been identified) and exerts synchronizing effects.[63]

The timing of feeding, when restricted to a narrow temporal window, can affect the entrainment pattern of behavioral rhythms through what has been referred to as a food-entrainable oscillator that is independent of the SCN. Recent findings in rodents have led to a renewed interest in the role of feeding in overall circadian organization in mammals, including the following: (1) alterations in circadian clock genes can lead to obesity and other metabolic abnormalities,[2,20] (2) metabolic transcription factor and nuclear receptors involved in metabolism can alter the expression of circadian clock genes,[66,67] (3) the timing of feeding can alter rhythmicity in several peripheral circadian oscillators,[20,68] and (4) a high-fat diet can alter behavioral and molecular circadian rhythms in central and peripheral tissues involved in the regulation of energy balance.[69] Although controversy exists as to the location of an SCN-independent food entrainable oscillator,[70,71] now overwhelming evidence suggesting that the circadian and metabolic systems are linked together at molecular, cellular, and behavioral levels has fueled great interest in the possible role of circadian disorganization in obesity, diabetes, and other cardio-metabolic disorders.[20,72,73]

Sleep-Wake Regulation

General Characteristics

The sleep-wake cycle may be viewed as a 24-hour rhythm driven partially by the circadian pacemaker and partially by the homeostatic regulation of sleep pressure. Sleep itself is an ultradian rhythm in that it involves two states of distinct brain activity, each of which is generated in specific brain regions. The ultradian rhythm of normal sleep is an approximate 90-minute oscillation between non-REM (rapid eye movement) and REM stages. In healthy subjects, this pattern usually is repeated four to six times per night. REM sleep and non-REM sleep are characterized by distinct patterns of cerebral and peripheral activity.

In the normal sequence, sleep is intiated by the lighter stages of non-REM sleep (i.e., stages I and II), followed within 10 to 20 minutes by slow-wave sleep (SWS; stages III and IV). These deeper stages of sleep are maintained for nearly 60 minutes in normal young subjects but usually are much shorter (5 to 10 minutes), if present at all, in older adults. Then, lighter stages of non-REM sleep reappear, and the first REM period is initiated. As the night progresses, non-REM sleep becomes shallower, the duration of REM episodes becomes longer, and the number and duration of awakenings increase. In normal young subjects, approximately 50% of a normal night is spent in stages I and II sleep, 20% in SWS, 25% in REM, and 5% in wake. In adults over 60 years of age, SWS usually is reduced to only 5% to 10% and REM sleep to 10% to 15%, while the proportion of time awake may reach 30% of the night.

During deep non-REM sleep (SWS), the electroencephalogram (EEG) is synchronized with low-frequency, high-amplitude waveforms, referred to as slow waves or delta waves. During REM sleep, eye movements are present, muscle tone is inhibited, and the EEG resembles that of active waking. During REM sleep, cerebral glucose utilization is similar to that of waking, but it is decreased during SWS.

The all-night recording of EEG, muscle tone, and eye movements, called the polysomnogram, is scored visually over 20 or 30 second periods in stages I, II, III, IV, REM, and Wake with the use of standardized criteria.[74] This procedure allows determination of the duration of each sleep stage but does not quantify the intensity of non-REM sleep. In contrast, the quantification of EEG recordings by power spectral analysis provides useful information regarding sleep depth or sleep intensity, because spectral analysis is sensitive to the amplitude of the delta waves. Higher-amplitude delta waves reflect more intense, deeper sleep, with less sensitivity to arousal stimuli. Slow-wave activity (SWA), i.e., spectral EEG power in the low-frequency range (also called delta range; 0.5 to 4.0 Hz), is a marker of the intensity of non-REM sleep.

As detailed below, the timing, duration, and architecture of sleep are under the dual control of a homeostatic mechanism that relates sleep pressure to the duration of prior wakefulness and of central circadian rhythmicity.

Neuroanatomic Basis of Sleep Regulation

Normal waking is associated with neuronal activity in regions of the so-called ascending arousal system, which includes mono-aminergic neurons in the brain stem and posterior hypothalamus, cholinergic neurons in the brain stem and basal forebrain, and orexin (hypocretin) neurons in the lateral hypothalamus.[75,76] Initiation of sleep therefore requires the inhibition of these multiple arousal systems. In recent years, the ventrolateral preoptic area (VLPO) of the hypothalamus has been identified as involved in the inhibition of arousal. The VLPO contains sleep-active neurons that use the inhibitory neurotransmitter GABA (gamma-aminobutyric acid) and have much higher firing rates during deep sleep than during wakefulness.[77-79] Lesions of the central cell cluster of the VLPO drastically reduce SW activity. Neurons of the VLPO provide GABAergic inhibitory innervation of the major monoamine arousal systems in the brain stem. Reciprocally, inhibitory pathways result from the monoamine arousal nuclei to the VLPO.[80] The orexin neurons in the lateral hypothalamus project to all components of the ascending arousal system and stimulate the cortex.[81] REM sleep is regulated primarily by cholinergic nuclei in the pons.

Interactions Between Circadian Rhythmicity and Sleep-Wake Homeostasis

Several features of the interaction between sleep and circadian rhythmicity appear to be fairly unique to the human species. First, human sleep generally is consolidated in a single 6- to 9-hour period, whereas fragmentation of the sleep period in several bouts is the rule in most other mammals. Possibly as a result of this consolidation of the sleep period, the wake-sleep transition in man is associated with physiologic changes that usually are more marked than those observed in animals. For example, the secretion of growth hormone (GH) in normal adults is tightly associated with the beginning of the sleep period, whereas the relationship between GH secretory pulses and sleep stages is much less evident in rodents, primates, and dogs. Second, man is unique in his capacity to ignore circadian signals and to maintain wakefulness despite increased pressure to go to sleep. Finally, approximately 25% of human subjects maintained for prolonged periods in temporal isolation have shown behavioral modifications that have not been observed in laboratory animals under constant conditions. These modifications consist of a desynchronization between the sleep-wake cycle and other rhythms, such as those of body temperature and cortisol secretion, which continue to free-run with a circadian period. Under conditions of so-called internal desynchronization, the sleep-wake cycle may be lengthened suddenly to 30 hours or more, while the rhythm of body temperature continues to free-run with a circadian period.[4] Wakefulness may last longer than 30 hours. Remarkably, the subjects are not aware of these drastic changes in their way of living. Instead, most of them believe that they are living on a more or less regular 24-hour schedule. This can be explained by the observation that time perception is altered profoundly: Subjective estimations of 1 hour intervals are positively correlated with the duration of wakefulness.[82] Of particular interest is that subjects continue to have three meals per "day," irrespective of the actual number of hours they are awake.[83] The intervals between meals as well as those between wake-up and breakfast, or between dinner and bedtime, are stretched or compressed in strong proportionality to the duration of wakefulness.[84] The mechanisms that cause spontaneous internal desynchronization are not completely understood.

Detailed analyses of data obtained during temporal isolation and forced desynchrony protocols show that the timing, duration, and architecture of sleep are regulated in part by circadian rhythmicity.[23,85] Thus, the duration of sleep episodes is correlated with the phase of the circadian rhythm of body temperature and not with the duration of prior wakefulness. Short (i.e., 7 to 8 hours) sleep episodes occur in free-running conditions when the subject goes to sleep around the minimum of body temperature, whereas long (i.e., 12 to 14 hours) sleep episodes occur when sleep starts at around the maximum of body temperature. Moreover, the distribution of REM sleep is markedly modulated by circadian timing. In contrast, the hourglass-like mechanism of sleep-wake homeostasis originally was thought to be largely independent of the circadian system and to involve one or several putative neural sleep factors, which rise during waking and decay exponentially during sleep.[86] This homeostatic mechanism regulates the timing, amount, and intensity of SWS and SWA. The VLPO has been proposed as a neuroanatomic locus for the interaction of the homeostatic process and central circadian rhythmicity, as it receives dense projections from the dorsomedial hypothalamic nucleus, which itself receives direct and indirect projections from the SCN.[87] Based on human studies described later, it is thought that the SCN generates a waking signal that promotes alertness during the active period. In support of this theory, studies have shown that rodents and monkeys with SCN lesions have increased sleep duration.[88,89] Furthermore, studies in rats have described an indirect neuronal circuit from the SCN to the locus coeruleus, an area of the midbrain involved in the control of arousal.[90] A role for the SCN in promoting sleep at other circadian times is suggested by the finding of decreased sleep in a mouse with a mutation of the *Clock* gene.[91] The recent finding that the mutation or deletion of a number of circadian clock genes affects not only the timing of sleep but also many other sleep-wake traits, including traits linked to the homeostatic drive to sleep,[15,91-94] indicates that circadian and homeostatic processes underlying the regulation of the sleep-wake cycle may be linked at molecular and anatomic levels of organization.

The dual control of sleep by circadian and homeostatic mechanisms extends to the control of objective and subjective measures of sleep tendency, mood, and vigilance.[95-98] When wakefulness is extended beyond the usual 16 to 18 hours, maximum subjective sleepiness coincides with the minimum of body temperature, mood, and performance. Remarkably, despite continued sleep deprivation, subjective fatigue then decreases, and mood and performance partially recover during the daytime hours, reflecting an interaction of circadian timing with the accumulation of waking time.[96-102] Currently, it is believed that the circadian clock generates a waking signal that increases from morning to evening and is expressed maximally in the early evening hours, 1 to 2 hours before the onset of nocturnal melatonin secretion.[97] This circadian waking signal counteracts the buildup of the putative factor "S" underlying the homeostatic process, allowing the individual to maintain a high level of alertness throughout the usual waking period. Current data from human studies are compatible with the hypothesis that the SCN generates a sleep signal in the early evening hours.[103]

Circadian rhythmicity and sleep-wake homeostasis also interact to regulate hormonal secretion. These modulatory effects were long thought to be present only in hormones directly dependent on the hypothalamic-pituitary axis. However, it is now clear that modulation by circadian rhythmicity and sleep is also present in other endocrine systems, such as glucose regulation and the renin-angiotensin system.[104,105] The multiple pathways by which circadian rhythmicity, sleep-wake homeostasis, and their interaction modulate hormonal release are incompletely understood. As is illustrated in Fig. 4-1, humoral and/or neural signals originating from the hypothalamic circadian pacemaker and from brain regions involved in sleep regulation affect the pulsatile release of hypothalamic neuroendocrine factors, which stimulate or inhibit intermittent secretion of pituitary hormones. The autonomic nervous system is another pathway linking the central control of sleep-wake homeostasis and circadian rhythmicity with peripheral endocrine organs. It appears that stimulatory or inhibitory effects of sleep on endocrine release are primarily associated with SW rather than REM sleep.[106-110] Pituitary hormones that influence endocrine systems not directly controlled by hypothalamic factors probably mediate, together with the autonomous nervous system, the modulatory effects of sleep and circadian rhythmicity on these systems (e.g., counterregulatory effects of GH and cortisol on glucose regulation[105]).

To delineate the relative roles of circadian and sleep effects in the temporal organization of hormonal secretion, strategies based on the fact that circadian rhythmicity needs several days to adapt to abrupt shifts in the sleep-wake cycle have been used. Thus, by shifting sleep times by 8 to 12 hours, masking effects of sleep on circadian inputs are removed, and the effects of sleep at an abnormal circadian time are revealed. Fig. 4-3 illustrates the mean profiles of plasma cortisol, GH, prolactin, and thyrotropin (TSH) as observed in normal subjects who were studied before and during an abrupt 12-hour shift in the sleep-wake and dark-light cycles. The study period extended over a 53-hour span and included an 8-hour period of nocturnal sleep, a 28-hour period of continuous wakefulness, and a daytime period of recovery sleep. To eliminate the effects of feeding, fasting, and postural changes, subjects remained recumbent throughout the study, and the normal meal schedule was replaced by intravenous glucose infusion at a constant rate. As shown in Figure 4-3, this drastic manipulation of sleep had only modest effects on the wave shape of the cortisol profile, in sharp contrast with the immediate shift of GH and prolactin rhythms, which followed the shift in the sleep-wake cycle. As will be reviewed in subsequent sections, numerous studies have indicated that control of diurnal rhythms of corticotropic activity is primarily dependent on circadian timing, whereas sleep-wake homeostasis appears to be an important factor in control of the 24-hour profiles of GH and prolactin.[111] Nevertheless, small modulatory effects of sleep-wake homeostasis on cortisol secretion and, conversely, influences of circadian timing on somatotropic function have been clearly demonstrated.[112] The diurnal variation in TSH levels includes an evening elevation that is thought to be under circadian control and nocturnal inhibition by sleep-dependent processes that is clearly demonstrated during sleep deprivation, when a large increase in nocturnal TSH levels is apparent, as is shown in the lower panel of Fig. 4-3.[111]

Hormonal profiles thus are easily measurable reflections of central mechanisms of biologic time keeping. In clinical investigations of conditions of abnormal circadian rhythmicity such as jet lag, and in human studies of the effects of exposure to natural or artificial zeitgebers, hormonal profiles are commonly used as markers of the status of the circadian clock and of its interactions with sleep.

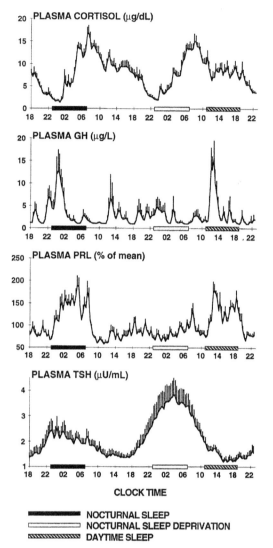

FIGURE 4-3. Mean (+standard error of the mean [SEM]) 24-hour profiles of plasma cortisol, growth hormone (GH), prolactin (PRL), and thyrotropin (TSH) in a group of eight normal young men (20 to 27 years old) studied during a 53-hour period that include 8 hours of nocturnal sleep, 28 hours of sleep deprivation, and 8 hours of daytime sleep. The black bars represent the sleep periods. The open bars represent the period of nocturnal sleep deprivation. The dashed bars represent the period of daytime sleep. Data were sampled at 20-minute intervals. (From Van Cauter E, Spiegel K: Circadian and sleep control of endocrine secretions. In Turek FW, Zee PC [eds]: Neurobiology of Sleep and Circadian Rhythms, vol 133. New York, Marcel Dekker, 1999, pp 397–426.)

ULTRADIAN RHYTHMICITY

Range of Ultradian Rhythms

The term *ultradian* is used primarily to designate rhythms with periods ranging from fractions of hours to several hours. Ultradian oscillations often are less regular and less reproducible than circadian rhythms. In most cases, they appear to represent an optimal functional status within the system where they occur rather than serving the primary function of a clock, that is, an accurate time measuring device. A wide variety of ultradian rhythms have been noted. The most prominent include pulsatile hormonal release and the alternation of REM and non-REM stages in sleep. In the human, the approximately 90-minute REM–non-REM cycle is accompanied by similar periodicity of dreaming, penile erections, sympathovagal balance, and breath-

ing. It has been suggested that this ultradian rhythm during sleep may be a reflection of a basic rest-activity cycle (BRAC), which would occur during wakefulness as well.[113] This concept has received some experimental support from a study demonstrating the existence of an ultradian rhythm of brain electrical activity in the frequency range of 13 to 35 Hz, an index of central alertness, during waking.[114] It is interesting to note that pulses of cortisol release were significantly associated with ultradian oscillations in alertness.[114]

Oscillations at frequencies higher than the hourly (i.e., circhoral) range characterizing pulsatile release have been observed for a variety of hormones and metabolic variables. In particular, rapid oscillations of insulin secretion with periods in the 10- to 15-minute range have been well characterized in humans.[115,116] Oscillations with a similar period also characterize lipolysis from omental fat, resulting in pulsatile free fatty acid release that appears driven by bursts of sympathetic drive to the adipocytes.[117]

Properties and Clinical Implications of Pulsatile Hormonal Release

In the endocrine system, ultradian variations have been observed for anterior and posterior pituitary hormones, for hormones under direct pituitary control, and for other endocrine variables such as parathyroid hormone, norepinephrine, plasma renin activity, and leptin and insulin secretion. The interval of recurrence of pulses varies from hormone to hormone and from species to species. The relative importance of pulsatile or oscillatory secretory activity versus tonic release also varies from one axis to another. For some hormones, secretory activity appears to be entirely pulsatile, with no detectable secretion between pulses. In normal men, evidence suggestive of intermittent secretion without tonic release has been obtained for luteinizing hormone (LH), follicle-stimulating hormone (FSH), GH, and adrenocorticotropic hormone (ACTH).[118-120] For some hormones, pulsatile release is superimposed on a tonic level of secretion, or secretion occurs continuously but is increased and decreased in an oscillatory fashion. Pancreatic insulin secretion is a well-established example of this type of ultradian oscillation.[121,122] Evidence for the existence of tonic secretion also has been obtained for pituitary prolactin and TSH release.[118,119]

The pulsatile nature of hormonal release implies that changes well in excess of 100% may occur within 1 hour. Therefore, it is necessary to obtain multiple samples to estimate the mean circulating level of many hormones and to determine the presence or absence of a circadian rhythm.

The physiologic significance of pulsatile hormone secretion was first proved when the essential role of the episodic nature of gonadotropin-releasing hormone (GnRH) release for normal functioning of the pituitary-ovarian axis was demonstrated.[123] Landmark studies showed that continuous infusions of exogenous GnRH in Rhesus monkeys with lesions of the arcuate nucleus, which abolished endogenous GnRH production, inhibited the secretion of LH and FSH. In contrast, the pulsatile administration of the synthetic hypothalamic hormone at a rate of one 6-minute pulse per hour restored normal LH and FSH levels.[123] Furthermore, if the rate of pulse delivery was increased to three pulses per hour, or if it was decreased to one pulse every 2 hours, serum LH and FSH levels were partially inhibited. These findings were rapidly applied to treatment for a variety of disorders of the pituitary-gonadal axis[124] and led the way to the discovery of the functional significance of pulsatility in other endocrine systems. For example, it was found that oscillatory administration of insulin with a period matching that of the normal pulsatility of endogenous insulin secretion is more effective in lowering glucose levels than is constant infusion.[125]

IMPACT OF AGING ON MECHANISMS CONTROLLING ENDOCRINE RHYTHMS

Age-related changes in endocrine, metabolic, and behavioral circadian rhythms have been reported in a variety of species, including humans.[126-128] One of the most prominent changes is a reduction in rhythm amplitude. The overall findings of a study that examined age-related differences in 24-hour endocrine rhythms in healthy subjects are shown in Fig. 4-4.[126] A marked

decrease in nocturnal release of TSH, melatonin, prolactin, GH, and melatonin was observed among older volunteers. The amplitude of the cortisol rhythm was decreased among elderly men, primarily because of an elevation of the nocturnal nadir. A retrospective analysis of polygraphic sleep recordings and concomitant profiles of plasma GH and cortisol from 149 normal healthy men, ages 16 to 83 years, showed a different rate of aging of SW sleep and REM sleep[129] (Fig. 4-5). SW sleep decreased markedly from early adulthood to midlife and was replaced by lighter sleep (stages I and II) without significant increases in sleep fragmentation or decreases in REM sleep. The transition from midlife to late life involved an increase in wake at the expense of both non-REM and REM sleep. The chronology of aging of GH secretion paralleled that of SW sleep. In contrast, the elevation in evening cortisol levels became significant only after 50 years, when sleep became more fragmented and REM sleep declined. These results were confirmed by a meta-analysis of 65 studies, which found that most of the impact of age on sleep occurs before midlife.[130] Despite the fact that older women have more subjective sleep complaints than men,[131-133] it was generally assumed that SWS and SWA are less affected by aging in women than in men.[134] However, when SWA in non-REM sleep is expressed relative to SWA in REM sleep (i.e., accounting for background SWA), SWA is actually lower in older women than in older men, consistent with the higher frequency of subjective complaints.[135]

Deficits in the maintenance and quality of nocturnal sleep in older adults are paralleled by decreased alertness, attention and memory deficits, and decreased performance during the daytime.[136] In both rodents and humans, many circadian rhythms are advanced under entrained conditions such that specific phase points of these rhythms occur earlier than in young subjects.[126,137] Both amplitude reduction and phase advance of the rhythm of body temperature have been observed in elderly subjects, and these alterations in circadian regulation were closely associated with changes in sleep-wake habits (i.e., earlier bedtimes and wake times).[127,138]

Age-related changes in the amplitude and/or the phase of circadian rhythms could be due to changes in the inner workings of the master clock, to alterations in the input pathways to the clock, or to factors downstream between the circadian clock and the system that is expressing the rhythm. Some early studies[139,140] have reported that the free-running period of various rhythms in rodents is systematically shortened with age, suggesting that the circadian clock itself is altered in advanced age. This concept has been confirmed in rats via measurement of *Per1-luc* expression in transgenic animals.[141] Age-related phase advances of a number of different behavioral and endocrine rhythms are consistent with the hypothesis that the period of the human circadian clock is shorter in the elderly. However, a study that measured the free-running period in healthy young and older adults using the forced desynchrony protocol has found no age difference.[5] Nevertheless, the very healthy older individuals who participated in this demanding protocol exhibited marked decreases in sleep consolidation and had greater difficulties sleeping at adverse circadian phases than did young subjects. These alterations and the clear advance of the propensity to awaken from sleep are thought to be related to both a reduction in the homeostatic drive to sleep and a reduction in the strength of the circadian signal.[142] In older adults, in contrast to young subjects, no significant correlation has been noted between the length of the circadian period and the phase angle of entrainment.[143]

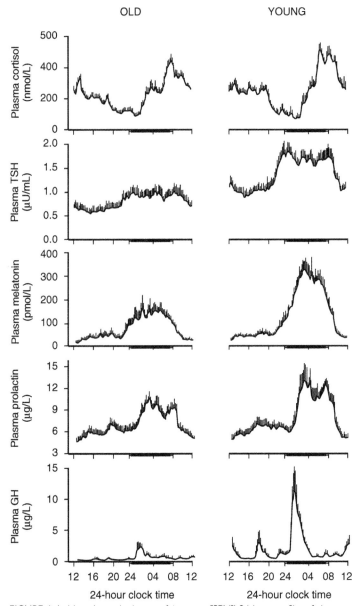

FIGURE 4-4. Mean (+standard error of the mean [SEM]) 24-hour profiles of plasma cortisol, thyrotropin (TSH), melatonin, prolactin (PRL), and growth hormone (GH) levels in eight old (67 to 84 years) and eight young (20 to 27 years) subjects. Data were sampled at 15-minute intervals. The black bars represent the mean sleep period. (From van Coevorden A, Mockel J, Laurent E, et al: Neuroendocrine rhythms and sleep in aging men. Am J Physiol 260:E651–E661, 1991.)

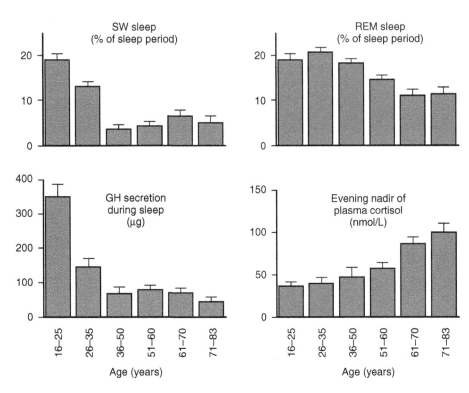

FIGURE 4-5. *Left,* Slow-wave (SW) sleep and growth hormone (GH) secretion during sleep as a function of age. Note the temporal concomitance between the decrease in SW sleep and in GH secretion. *Right,* Rapid eye movement (REM) sleep and level of evening nadir of plasma cortisol as a function of age. Note the temporal concomitance between the decrease in REM sleep and the increase in evening cortisol levels. Values shown are means (+standard error of the mean [SEM]) for each age group. Data were obtained in 149 healthy men, ages 16 to 83 years. (Data from Van Cauter E, Leproult R, Plat L: Age-related changes in slow-wave sleep and relationship with growth hormone and cortisol levels in healthy men. JAMA 284:861–868, 2000.)

Studies in rodents indicate that aging is associated with decreased responsiveness to the phase-shifting effects of both photic and nonphotic stimuli. Old hamsters show a decreased response to the phase-shifting effects of low-intensity light pulses.[144] This observation raises the possibility that in old age, signal transmission of light information to the SCN itself may be decreased, or that SCN responsiveness to photic stimulation may be lessened. Similarly, although induction of locomotor activity during a time of normal inactivity can induce pronounced phase-shifts in the circadian rhythm of locomotor activity in young animals, in old animals the response is greatly diminished or is completely abolished.[145,146] It is interesting to note that transplantation of fetal SCN tissue into the SCN region of old hamsters with an intact SCN can restore the response to the phase-shifting effects of triazolam on the activity rhythm.[147]

Behavioral changes in the elderly also may lead to changes in environmental inputs to the clock. In older adults, exposure to bright light and social cues, both potential entraining agents, is markedly diminished when compared with that seen in young adults.[148-150] Furthermore, age-related lens pigmentation decreases the transmission of blue light (i.e., the wavelength to which the circadian system is most sensitive) to the retina.[151] Absence of professional constraints, decreased mobility due to illness, and reduced socialization and outdoor activities are all hallmarks of old age. Thus, decreased exposure to environmental stimuli that entrain circadian rhythms could contribute to disruptions in circadian rhythmicity. The use of exposure to bright light and enriched social schedules to reinforce circadian rhythms in older adults and improve nighttime sleep and daytime alertness has proved beneficial in several studies.[152] In elderly insomniacs living in a nursing home with limited exposure to environmental light, supplementary light exposure during the middle of the day significantly increased nocturnal melatonin secretion without circadian phase-shifting.[153] Evidence indicates that older adults are capable of phase-shifting to the same extent as younger subjects in response to appropriately timed light exposure.[154]

The ultradian rhythmicity of pulsatile hormonal release is also affected by aging. For a number of individual hormones, including GH, insulin, LH, and ACTH, analyses of 24-hour profiles have shown increased irregularity, or disorderliness, of pulsatile release. Furthermore, the synchrony of pulsatile release between the pituitary hormone and the peripheral hormone (e.g., LH and testosterone, ACTH and cortisol) is partially disrupted in healthy older adults.[155]

Methodologic Aspects of the Study of Endocrine Rhythms

EXPERIMENTAL PROTOCOLS

Most investigations of circadian rhythms of hormonal release are based on a transversal design; that is, a group of individuals are studied for a minimum of 24 hours each, following the same experimental protocol. The demonstration of circadian rhythmicity then is based on the observation of consistently reproducible characteristics in the observed set of temporal profiles. The group of subjects should be as homogeneous as possible, not only in terms of physical parameters such as age and sex, but also in terms of living habits such as sleep-wake cycles, exercise habits, and meal schedules. Subjects who have regular social habits and describe themselves as "good sleepers" should be preferred. Shift workers and subjects who have made a transmeridian flight less than 2 months before the experiment should be excluded. Before the experiment is begun, volunteers should be asked to adhere to a standardized schedule of meals and bedtimes for several days so as to maximize interindividual synchronization. The use of continuous wrist activity recording during the prestudy period is a convenient way to monitor compliance. At least 1 night of habituation to the laboratory environment and recording procedures should be included. To avoid disruptions in sleep due to the sampling procedure, the catheter should be connected to tubing that extends to an adjoining room during the night. Because of the modulatory effects exerted by sleep stages on hormonal release, it is important to obtain polygraphic sleep recordings by using standardized methods for recording and scoring. Daytime naps should be avoided. The catheter should be inserted at least 2 hours before the first sample is collected so that observation of the effects of venipuncture stress can be avoided. To obtain valid estimations of the circadian parameters, it is necessary to sample at intervals not exceeding 1 hour.

If hormonal profiles are measured as markers of the output of the central circadian oscillator, direct effects of other factors should be minimized. Sleep-wake transitions, meals, stressful activities, and changes in physical activity all may affect hormonal levels. To eliminate these "masking" effects, experimental protocols usually referred to as constant routines have been developed to reliably derive estimates of circadian amplitude and phase from temporal patterns of peripheral hormones and other physiologic variables, such as body temperature. Constant routine conditions generally involve a regimen of continuous wakefulness, constant recumbent posture, constant illumination, and constant caloric intake either under the form of hourly identical aliquots of liquid diet or solid food, or under the form of a constant glucose infusion. Although such constant routine conditions have been used extensively in basic studies of human circadian rhythmicity, the sleep deprivation inherent to this protocol is an obvious limitation. The use of circadian markers that are not masked by sleep, meals, and other factors, such as the 24-hour profile of melatonin, has been advocated. Finally, if only circadian phase, and not amplitude, is of interest, measurements of saliva levels of melatonin during the evening provide a noninvasive way to observe the timing of the onset of nocturnal melatonin secretion, a neuroendocrine event timed by the circadian clock.

In characterizing episodic hormonal fluctuations, consideration of the total amount of blood withdrawn and of the amount of plasma needed to assay the hormones under study is obviously essential to the definition of an adequate sampling protocol. The definition of an optimal sampling protocol depends thus on the type of phenomenon under study. Sampling rates of 1 and 2 minutes will uncover high-frequency, low-amplitude episodic variations superimposed on the slower pulsatile release at intervals of 1 to 2 hours. Sampling rates of 20 and 30 minutes will detect only major pulses lasting longer than 1 hour. As compared with older studies, ultrasensitive assays now available allow detection of small-amplitude pulses at low hormonal concentrations, resulting in the finding of additional, previously undetected, secretory episodes.

PROCEDURES TO QUANTIFY CIRCADIAN VARIATIONS

Among the methods proposed for and applied to the analysis of 24-hour profiles of blood components, the oldest is the Cosinor test.[156] The major disadvantage of this test and of its derivatives is its assumption that the observed profile may be described adequately by a single sinusoidal curve. This assumption is practically never met for biological rhythms that are asymmetric in nature (e.g., the sleep-wake cycle is a 08:16 alternation, not a 12:12). Therefore, the Cosinor test generally provides unreliable estimations of rhythm parameters. Unfortunately, in recent years, the Cosinor analysis has regained popularity and has been applied indiscriminately to asymmetric profiles.

Other procedures for the detection and estimation of circadian variation have been based on periodogram calculations or on nonlinear regression procedures.[157,158] These methods provide an adequate description of asymmetric wave shapes. The times of occurrence of the maximum and the minimum of the best-fit curve often are referred to as the acrophase and the nadir, respectively. The amplitude of the rhythm may be estimated as 50% of the difference between the maximum and the minimum of the best-fit curve. With the periodogram procedure, confidence intervals for the amplitude, acrophase, and nadir may be calculated.

PROCEDURES TO QUANTIFY PULSATILE HORMONAL SECRETION

Analysis of pulsatile variations may be considered at two levels.[159] One may wish to define and characterize significant variations in peripheral levels, based on estimations of the size of the measurement error (i.e., primarily assay error). However, under certain circumstances, it is possible to mathematically derive secretory rates from the peripheral concentrations.[160-162] This procedure, often referred to as deconvolution, often reveals more pulses of secretion than does analysis of peripheral concentrations. It also more accurately defines the temporal limits of each pulse. However, deconvolution involves amplification of measurement error, with increased risk for false-positive error. Whether peripheral concentrations or secretory rates are examined, two major approaches are used to analyze the episodic fluctuations. The first and most commonly used is the time domain analysis, wherein the data are plotted against time, and pulses are detected and identified. The second is the frequency domain analysis, in which amplitude is plotted against frequency or period. The time domain analysis provides an estimation of pulse frequency, calculated as the total number of pulses detected divided by the duration of the study period. The regularity of pulsatile behavior may be quantified by examining the distribution of interpulse intervals. Alternatively, the issue of regularity of pulsatile behavior may be approached by examining the distribution of spectral power in a frequency domain analysis.[163] Finally, another analytic tool, the approximate entropy (ApEn), has been introduced to quantify the regularity of oscillatory behavior in endocrine and other physiologic time series.[164,165]

A number of computer algorithms for identification of pulses of hormonal concentration have been proposed. A detailed presentation of the operating principles of each of these procedures is beyond the scope of this chapter. Review articles[166,167] have provided comparisons of performance of several pulse detection algorithms. These comparisons have indicated that ULTRA and CLUSTER perform similarly when used with appropriate choices of parameters.[167]

Endocrine Rhythms in Health and Disease

Diurnal and/or ultradian oscillations have been observed in essentially all endocrine systems. An exhaustive review of all such observations is not possible. The following summary of findings therefore will be limited to the various hypothalamic-pituitary axes, parathyroid hormone, hydromineral hormones, glucose and insulin, and hormones involved in appetite regulation.

PITUITARY AXES

The Corticotropic Axis

Normal Rhythms of Adrenocorticotropic Hormone and Adrenal Secretions

Outputs from the SCN activate rhythmic release of corticotropin-releasing hormone (CRH) that stimulates circadian ACTH release. The 24-hour rhythm of adrenal secretion is primarily dependent on the diurnal pattern of ACTH release. In addition, neuronal signals generated by the SCN are transmitted by a multisynaptic neural pathway to the adrenal cortex.[168] The presence in the adrenal cortex of an intrinsic circadian oscillator consisting of interacting positive and negative feedback loops in circadian gene expression has been demonstrated in various animals, including monkeys,[169-171] and it has been shown that this adrenal circadian pacemaker gates the physiologic adrenal response to ACTH (i.e., defines a time window during which the adrenal most effectively responds to ACTH).[172]

The 24-hour profiles of ACTH and cortisol show an early morning maximum, declining levels throughout daytime, a quiescent period of minimal secretory activity centered around midnight, and an abrupt elevation during late sleep, resulting in an early morning maximum. Mathematical derivations of secretory rates from plasma concentrations have suggested that the 24-hour profile of plasma cortisol reflects a succession of secretory pulses of magnitude modulated by a circadian rhythm with no evidence of tonic secretion.[120,173] In normal conditions, the acrophase of the pituitary-adrenal periodicity occurs between 06.00 and 10.00 hours. With a 15-minute sampling interval, 12 to 18 significant pulses of plasma ACTH and cortisol can be detected per 24-hour span.[174] Circadian and pulsatile variations parallel to those of cortisol have been demonstrated for the plasma levels of several other adrenal steroids, in particular dehydroepiandrosterone (DHEA).[175] The temporal concomitance of 24-hour profiles of ACTH, cortisol, and DHEA is illustrated in Fig. 4-6.

The profile shown in the upper panel of Fig. 4-3 illustrates the remarkable persistence of the cortisol and, by inference, ACTH secretory rhythm when sleep is manipulated. Indeed, the overall wave shape of the profile was not markedly affected by the absence of sleep or the presence of sleep at an abnormal time of day. Thus, this rhythm is controlled primarily by the circadian pacemaker.

However, modulatory effects of sleep-wake homeostasis have been clearly demonstrated. As illustrated in Fig. 4-7, sleep onset is consistently associated with short-term inhibition of cortisol secretion, which may not be detectable when sleep is initiated in the morning (i.e., at the peak of corticotropic activity).[176-179] This inhibitory effect of sleep appears to be related to SW sleep.[109,180] Conversely, final awakenings from sleep, as well as transient awakenings that interrupt the sleep period, consistently trigger pulses of cortisol secretion (see Fig. 4-7),[120,178,180-183] and the number of nocturnal microarousals predicts morning plasma and saliva cortisol levels.[184] In an analysis of cortisol profiles during nocturnal sleep, it was observed that all transient awakenings that interrupt sleep and last at least 10 minutes were followed within the next 20 minutes by significant bursts of cortisol secretion.[183] In addition, a temporal coupling between pulses of cortisol secretion and ultradian variations in an EEG marker of alertness has been reported.[114] Total nocturnal wake time is associated with increased 24-hour plasma cortisol concentrations,[185] and chronic insomnia with reduced total sleep time is associated with higher cortisol levels across the night.[186]

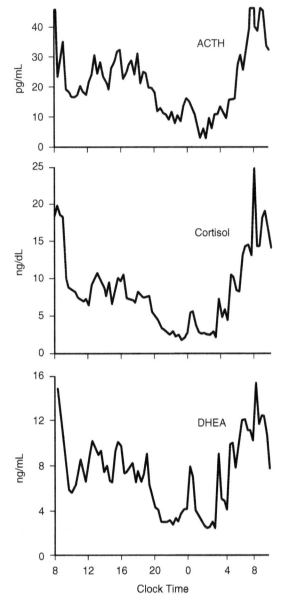

FIGURE 4-6. Twenty-four-hour profiles of plasma adrenocorticotropic hormone (ACTH), cortisol, and dehydroepiandrosterone (DHEA) levels sampled at 20-minute intervals in a healthy young man. Note the temporal concomitance of circadian and pulsatile variations of the three hormones. (Unpublished data kindly provided by Dr. K. Spiegel.)

Modulatory effects of dark-light transitions also have been noted. Cortisol secretory pulses associated with morning awakening are enhanced by increasing light intensity.[187] Moreover, the transition from darkness to dim light and from dim to bright light may stimulate cortisol secretion in subjects who are awake at bed rest.[183,188] The stimulatory effects of bright light exposure on nocturnal cortisol levels appear to be dependent on the timing of exposure.[189] When dark-light and sleep-wake transitions occur concomitantly, associated cortisol elevations are nearly two times as high as when the final awakening occurs in continuous darkness[183] (see Fig. 4-7). Thus, under usual bedtime schedules, both sleep-wake and dark-light transitions amplify the effects of circadian rhythmicity.

Studies of the 24-hour cortisol profile in the course of adaptation to shifts of the sleep-wake cycle have demonstrated that the end of the quiescent period, which coincides with the onset of the early morning rise, takes longer to adjust and appears to

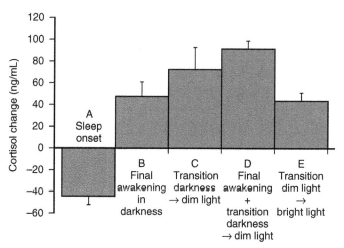

FIGURE 4-7. Mean (and standard error of the mean [SEM]) changes in plasma cortisol levels: *A,* Within 120 minutes following sleep onset at 15.00 hours (n = 32). *B,* Within 20 minutes following final spontaneous awakening in darkness (scheduled sleep period 23.00 to 07.00 hours or 15.00 to 23.00 hours; n = 10). *C,* Within 20 minutes following transition from darkness to dim light at 07.00 or 23.00 hours in subjects awake at bed rest (n = 10). *D,* Within 20 minutes following final awakening concomitant with transition from darkness to dim light at 07.00 or 23.00 hours (n = 38). *E,* Within 15 minutes following transition from dim to bright light at 05.00 hours in subjects awake at bed rest (n = 8). (Panels *A* to *D,* Data from Caufriez A, Moreno-Reyes R, Leproult R, et al: Immediate effects of an 8-h advance shift of the rest-activity cycle on 24-h profiles of cortisol. Am J Physiol 282:E1147–E1153, 2002; panel *E,* Data from Leproult R, Colecchia EF, L'Hermite-Balériaux M, et al: Transition from dim to bright light in the morning induces an immediate elevation of cortisol levels. J Clin Endocrinol Metab 86:151–157, 2001.)

be a robust marker of circadian timing. Twin studies have demonstrated that the timing of the nadir is influenced by genetic factors,[190] providing evidence for genetic control of the human circadian phase. In contrast, the timing of the morning acrophase is more labile and may be influenced by the timing of sleep offset,[182] the transition from dark to bright light,[187] and breakfast intake.[191] Finally, anticipation of the expected time of waking has been reported to be associated with a rise in levels of ACTH, but not cortisol, during the end of the sleep period.[192]

In addition to the immediate modulatory effects of sleep-wake transitions on ACTH and cortisol levels, acute total or partial (4 hours in bed) nocturnal sleep deprivation results in elevated cortisol concentrations in late afternoon and evening on the following day,[193] and the amplitude of the cortisol circadian variations is reduced by approximately 15%. Similarly, as illustrated in Fig. 4-8, recurrent partial sleep deprivation (4 hours in bed per night for 6 nights) also results in an elevation of cortisol levels in the late afternoon and evening.[194] These disturbances, which were observed in young healthy subjects, are strikingly similar to those noted in older healthy subjects with normal sleep schedules.[126,195,196] In any case, sleep loss appears to delay the return to quiescence of the hypothalamic-pituitary-adrenal axis (HPA) that normally occurs in the evening. This suggests that sleep loss, similar to aging, may slow down the rate of recovery of the HPA axis response following a challenge and therefore could facilitate the development of central and peripheral disturbances associated with glucocorticoid excess, in particular when cortisol concentrations are elevated at the time of the normal daily nadir, such as memory deficits, insulin resistance, and osteoporosis.[197-201] Conversely, decreased HPA resiliency results in HPA hyperactivity that inhibits SW sleep and promotes nocturnal awakenings, initiating a feed-forward cascade of negative events generated by both HPA and sleep disruptions.

The circadian rhythm of cortisol persists throughout adulthood and has been observed through the ninth decade.[126,196] Among young adults, 24-hour cortisol levels are slightly lower in women than in men, primarily because of lower morning maxima. With aging, evening cortisol levels increase progressively in both men and women, so that the cortisol nadir is markedly higher in healthy subjects over 70 years of age than in young adults (see Fig. 4-4). It is interesting to note that this elevation of evening cortisol levels occurs with a chronology similar to that observed for a progressive decrease in the duration of REM sleep[129] (see Fig. 4-5). As a result, older subjects have elevated 24-hour mean cortisol levels and reduced amplitude of cortisol variations. In addition, the timing of the nadir is advanced by 1 to 2 hours, indicating that aging is associated with an advance in the circadian phase.[126,196]

In pregnancy, placental CRH is secreted into the maternal circulation in a pulsatile but not in a circadian fashion, and no correlation has been noted between maternal levels of CRH and ACTH. However, ACTH and cortisol concentrations remain strongly correlated with each other over time, suggesting that diurnal variation in maternal ACTH probably is driven by another ACTH secretagogue.[202]

Alterations in Disease States

The 24-hour profile of pituitary-adrenal secretion remains largely unaltered in a wide variety of pathologic states. Disease states in which pronounced alterations of the cortisol rhythm have been observed include primarily (1) disorders involving abnormalities in binding and/or metabolism of cortisol; (2) the various forms of Cushing's syndrome; and (3) depression and posttraumatic stress disorder (PTSD).

The relative amplitude of the circadian rhythm and of the episodic fluctuations in cortisol is blunted in patients with liver disease[203] and in those with anorexia nervosa,[204] primarily because of the decreased metabolic clearance of cortisol. Pulsatile secretion of ACTH, but not cortisol, was reportedly enhanced in obese premenopausal women.[205] In hypothyroid patients, the mean level is markedly elevated and the relative amplitude of the rhythm is dampened.[206] These alterations are thought to be due to both diminished clearance and decreased efficiency of feedback control. In contrast, in hyperthyroidism, where cortisol production and peripheral metabolism are increased, episodic pulses are enhanced.[207]

A low-amplitude circadian variation may persist in pituitary-dependent Cushing's disease. Cortisol pulsatility is blunted in about 70% of patients with Cushing's disease, suggesting autonomous tonic secretion of ACTH by a pituitary tumor. However, in about 30% of these patients, the magnitude of the pulses is enhanced instead.[208] These hyperpulsatile patterns could be caused by enhanced hypothalamic release of CRH or persistent pituitary responsiveness to CRH. It also has been shown that patients with Cushing's disease secrete ACTH and cortisol jointly more asynchronously than healthy subjects.[209] The left and middle panels of Fig. 4-9 compare representative and mean 24-hour cortisol profiles in normal subjects and in patients with Cushing's disease.

In patients with primary adrenal Cushing's syndrome, increased cortisol secretion appears to result from both increased basal secretion and increased pulse frequency.[210] Although the persistence of a low-amplitude circadian cortisol variation has been claimed,[210] examination of the individual profiles does not support this notion. Nevertheless, the partial persistence of cortisol rhythmicity in the absence of ACTH could reflect the newly

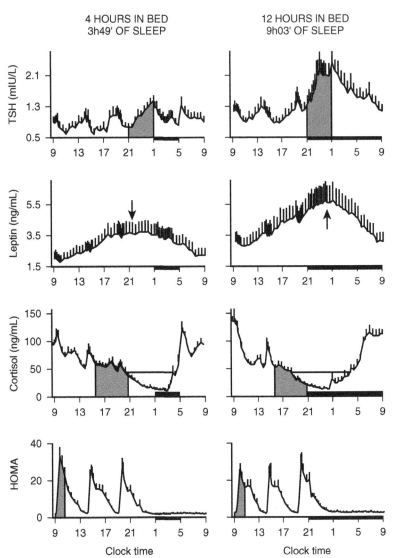

FIGURE 4-8. Impact of recurrent sleep curtailment (4 hours in bed for 6 nights) and of sleep recovery (12 hours in bed for 6 nights) on 24-hour plasma profiles of thyrotropin (TSH), leptin, and cortisol, and on homeostatic model assessment (HOMA) in healthy young men. HOMA was calculated as glucose concentration (mg/dL) × insulin concentration (μU/mL). Values shown are means ± SEM. (Adapted from Spiegel K, Leproult R, Van Cauter E: Impact of sleep debt on metabolic and endocrine function. Lancet 354:1435–1439, 1999, and from Spiegel K, Leproult R, L'Hermite-Balériaux M, et al: Leptin levels are dependent on sleep duration: relationships with sympathovagal balance, carbohydrate regulation, cortisol and thyrotropin. J Clin Endocrinol Metab 89:5762–5771, 2004.)

described neural pathway between the SCN and the adrenal cortex.[168]

The absence or even the dampening of cortisol circadian variations in Cushing's syndrome has obvious implications for clinical diagnosis, as time of day when plasma samples are obtained has to be taken into account during evaluation of the result. Differentiation between normal and pathologic levels may be greatly improved by adequate selection of the sampling time, because the overlap between normal individual values and values in patients with Cushing's syndrome is minimal during a 4-hour interval centered around midnight.

Hypercortisolism with persistent circadian rhythmicity and increased pulsatility is found in a majority of severely depressed patients.[211-213] This is illustrated in the right panels of Fig. 4-9. In these patients, who do not develop the clinical signs of Cushing's syndrome despite high circulating cortisol levels, the quiescent period of cortisol secretion is shorter and more fragmented, and it often starts later and ends earlier than in normal subjects of comparable age. These alterations could reflect the impact of sleep disturbances, as well as an advance in circadian phase. When clinical remission of the depressed state is obtained, hypercortisolism and alterations in the quiescent period disap-

pear, indicating that these disturbances are "state" rather than "trait" dependent.[214]

In PTSD, some authors have reported that plasma cortisol levels are decreased in the afternoon and/or in the evening, and that the amplitude of circadian variations is enhanced.[215-217] In fibromyalgia and in the chronic fatigue syndrome, cortisol levels have been reported to be low, normal, or elevated, depending on the study, but ACTH and cortisol pulsatility were found to be normal.[218] In a well-documented study performed in constant routine conditions, normal circadian variations of plasma cortisol levels were evidenced in women with fibromyalgia.[219]

The Somatotropic Axis

The 24 Hour Profile of Growth Hormone in Normal Subjects

Pituitary secretion of GH is stimulated by hypothalamic GH-releasing hormone (GHRH) and is inhibited by somatostatin. In addition, the acylated form of ghrelin (acyl-ghrelin), a peptide produced predominantly by the stomach, binds to the GH-secretagogue receptor and therefore is another potent endogenous stimulus of GH secretion.[220,221] In normal adult subjects, the 24-hour profile of plasma GH levels consists of stable low

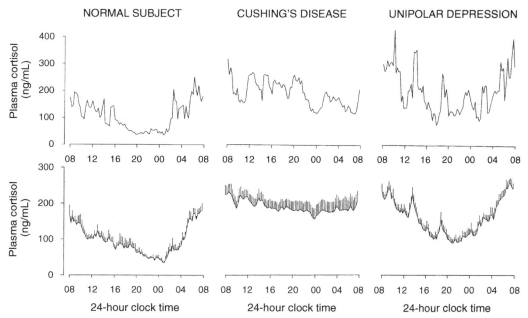

FIGURE 4-9. Twenty-four-hour profiles of plasma cortisol in normal subjects, patients with pituitary Cushing's disease, and patients with major endogenous depression of the unipolar subtype. For each condition, a representative example is shown in the top panel, and mean (+standard error of the mean [SEM]) profiles from 8 to 10 subjects are shown in the lower panel. (From Van Cauter E: Physiology and pathology of circadian rhythms. In Edwards CW, Lincoln DW [eds]: Recent Advances in Endocrinology and Metabolism. Edinburgh, Churchill Livingstone, 1989, vol 3, pp 109–134.)

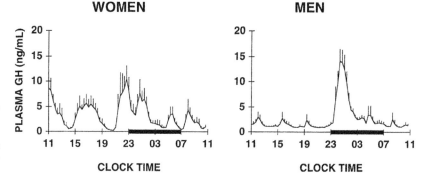

FIGURE 4-10. Mean (+standard error of the mean [SEM]) 24-hour plasma growth hormone profiles in nine men, age 18 to 30 years, and in seven women, age 21 to 33 years, during the follicular phase. The black bars represent the sleep periods. (Adapted from Van Cauter E, Plat L, Copinschi G: Interrelations between sleep and the somatotropic axis. Sleep 21:533–566, 1998.)

levels abruptly interrupted by bursts of secretion. The most reproducible pulse occurs shortly after sleep onset, in association with the first phase of SW sleep.[222] Other secretory pulses may occur in later sleep and during wakefulness, in the absence of any identifiable stimulus. Studies in young male twins have evidenced a major genetic effect on GH secretion during waking, but not during sleep.[223] In adult men, the sleep-onset GH pulse generally is the largest pulse observed over the 24-hour span. In normally cycling women, 24-hour GH levels are higher than in age-matched men, daytime pulses are more frequent, and the sleep-associated pulse, although still present in most cases, does not generally account for most of the 24-hour GH release.[224] Typical profiles of young men and women are shown in Fig. 4-10. Well-documented studies have demonstrated that in women, the amplitude of GH secretory pulses is correlated with the circulating level of estradiol.[224,225] In normally cycling young women, it also was observed that daytime GH secretion was increased during the luteal phase as compared with the follicular phase, and that this elevation correlated positively with plasma levels of progesterone but not estradiol.[226]

Sleep onset will elicit a GH secretory pulse, whether sleep is advanced, delayed, interrupted, or fragmented.[222] Thus, as illustrated in Fig. 4-3, shifts in the sleep-wake cycle are followed immediately by parallel shifts in GH rhythm.[222] In night workers, the main GH secretory episode occurs during the first half of the shifted sleep period.[227] The release of GH in early sleep is temporally and quantitatively associated with the amount of SW sleep.[228,229] Both SW sleep and GH levels are increased during the recovery night following nocturnal total sleep deprivation as compared with the baseline predeprivation night, especially during the first 4 hours of sleep.[230] Good evidence suggests that the mechanisms underlying the relationship between SW sleep and GH release involve synchronous activity of at least two different populations of hypothalamic GHRH neurons.[231] Indeed, inhibition of endogenous GHRH by administration of a specific antagonist or by immunoneutralization inhibits both sleep and GH secretion.[232] Additional evidence for the existence of a robust relationship between SW activity and GH release has been provided by studies using pharmacologic stimulation of SW sleep. Indeed, enhancement of SW sleep by oral administration of low doses of gamma-hydroxybutyrate (GHB), a natural metabolite of GABA used in treatment for narcolepsy, or of ritanserin, a selective serotonin $(5-HT)_2$ antagonist, results in simultaneous and highly correlated increases in nocturnal GH secretion.[108,233] Conversely, transient awakenings during sleep inhibit GH secretion.[234] Thus, sleep fragmentation generally will decrease nocturnal GH release.

However, although sleep is clearly the major determinant of GH secretion in man, evidence for the existence of a circadian modulation of the occurrence and amplitude of GH pulses also has been found. This may reflect decreased somatostatin inhibitory activity in the evening and during the night,[235] or it could result from the nocturnal rise in ghrelin, which occurs even in the absence of sleep.[236] Thus, the major sleep-onset associated GH pulse is caused by a surge of hypothalamic GHRH coincident with a circadian period of relative somatostatin disinhibition.[222,232] In normal-weight subjects, fasting, even for only 1 day, enhances GH secretion via an increase in pulse amplitude.[237] Presleep GH pulses, reported by some investigators in normal men,[238] may reflect the presence of a sleep debt, thus unmasking the circadian component of GH secretion.[239] A recent study provides evidence for modulation of GH secretion by endogenous acyl-ghrelin, leading to higher GH peaks before times of food intake in subjects given regular meals.[237]

After a night of total sleep deprivation, a compensatory increase in GH release is observed during the daytime, so that the overall 24-hour secretion is not altered significantly.[240] The mechanisms underlying this compensatory increase might involve decreased somatostatinergic tone and/or elevated ghrelin levels. Recurrent partial sleep restriction is associated consistently with the appearance of a presleep GH pulse.[239]

Aging is associated with dramatic decreases in circulating levels of GH (see Figs. 4-4 and 4-5).[126,224] This reduction is achieved by a decrease in amplitude, rather than in frequency, of GH pulses.[126,241,242] It also has been reported that the orderliness of GH secretion is decreased in the elderly.[243] As illustrated in Fig. 4-5, this age-related GH decrease occurs in an exponential fashion between young adulthood and midlife and follows the same chronology as the decrease in SW sleep. Despite the persistence of high levels of sex steroids, plasma concentrations and pulsatile secretion rates of GH fall in midlife to less than half the values achieved in young adulthood. Thereafter, smaller and more progressive decrements occur from midlife to old age.[129] Among the elderly, GH secretory profiles are similar in men and in women.[224] The age-related reduction of GH secretion appears to result from increased somatostatin secretion and diminished GHRH responsiveness.[244]

It is interesting to note that during pregnancy, a placental GH variant, which substitutes for pituitary GH to regulate maternal insulin-like growth factor-1 (IGF-1) levels,[245] is released in a tonic rather than a pulsatile fashion.[246]

Alterations in Disease States

Abnormalities in the 24-hour profile of plasma GH have been reported in a variety of metabolic, endocrine, neurologic, and psychiatric conditions.

An inverse relationship between adiposity and GH release has been noted, which results in marked suppression of GH levels throughout the 24-hour span in obese subjects. A normal pattern can be restored after prolonged fasting.[247] In anorexia nervosa, GH pulse amplitude and frequency are increased, and the orderliness of GH release is disrupted.[248] Nonobese juvenile or maturity-onset diabetic patients hypersecrete GH during wakefulness as well as during sleep, primarily because of an increase in the amplitude of pulses.[249] This abnormality may disappear when glycemia is strictly controlled.

In functional hypothalamic amenorrhea, 24-hour mean GH levels are normal, but the pattern of pulsatile GH release is distinctly altered, with a decrease in pulse amplitude, a 40% increase in pulse frequency, and a twofold increase in interpulse GH concentrations.[250] In lean women with the polycystic ovary syndrome (PCOS), the amplitude, but not the frequency, of GH pulses is increased as compared with body mass index (BMI)-matched normal cycling controls. In contrast, pulse amplitude is similarly reduced in obese patients with PCOS and obese controls.[251]

Diurnal and nocturnal episodes of GH secretion are more frequent and of higher amplitude in adult subjects with hyperthyroidism, who have an overall daily GH production rate fourfold greater than normal.[252] Patients with major endogenous depression often have the major nocturnal GH pulse before, rather than after, sleep onset.[253]

In Cushing's disease, an inverse relationship has been noted between the degree of cortisol hypersecretion and total GH secretion, and the frequency and the disorderliness of GH pulses are increased.[254] In acromegaly, GH is hypersecreted throughout the 24-hour span, with a highly irregular pulsatile pattern superimposed on elevated basal levels, indicating the presence of tonic secretion.[255,256] After pituitary surgery, a normal 24-hour pattern of GH release can be restored in most, but not all, patients.[255,257]

The Lactotropic Axis

The 24-Hour Profile of Prolactin in Normal Subjects

Under normal conditions, the 24-hour profile of prolactin levels exhibits minimal levels around noon, a modest increase in the afternoon, and a major nocturnal elevation starting shortly after sleep onset and culminating around midsleep at levels corresponding to an average increase of more than 200% above minimum levels (see Fig. 4-3).[258,259] Episodic pulses occur throughout the 24-hour span, but their amplitude and their frequency are higher during the night than during the day. Decreased dopaminergic inhibition of prolactin secretion during sleep is likely to be the primary mechanism underlying this nocturnal elevation. Mean prolactin levels, pulse amplitude, and pulse frequency are higher in normally cycling women than in postmenopausal women or in normal young men.[260] In normally cycling young women, it has also been observed that daytime prolactin pulsatility was enhanced during the luteal phase as compared with the follicular phase, leading to increased late afternoon and evening levels.[226] In the luteal phase, the magnitude of the evening prolactin rise correlated positively with both estradiol and progesterone levels.[226] These data indicate that endogenous estrogens and progesterone play a critical role in the differential regulation of prolactin secretion associated with sex and age. Deconvolution analysis has shown that the prolactin profile reflects both tonic and intermittent release.[119] Twin studies have revealed that genetic factors determine partially the temporal organization of prolactin secretion.[261]

Diurnal prolactin variations are regulated primarily by sleep-wake homeostasis. Sleep onset is invariably associated with an increase in prolactin secretion, irrespective of the time of the day. Thus, as illustrated in Fig. 4-3, shifts in the sleep-wake cycle are followed immediately by parallel shifts in the prolactin rhythm,[222] but the amplitude of the prolactin rise may be dampened when associated with daytime sleep as compared with nocturnal sleep.[262] Conversely, modest elevations in prolactin levels may occur during waking around the time of the usual sleep onset, particularly in women.[259] Thus, prolactin secretion appears to be modulated in part by circadian rhythmicity, and maximal secretion occurs when sleep and circadian effects are superimposed (i.e., at the usual bedtime).[258,259,263] Benzodiazepine (e.g., triazolam) and imidazopyridine (e.g., zolpidem) hypnotics taken at bedtime generally enhance the nocturnal prolactin elevation.[264,265]

A close temporal relationship has been evidenced between increased prolactin secretion and SW activity when sleep structure was characterized by power spectral analysis of the EEG.[110] Conversely, prolonged awakenings that interrupt sleep are consistently associated with decreasing prolactin concentrations.[110] Thus, SW sleep is associated with elevated prolactin secretion, and shallow and fragmented sleep generally is associated with dampening of the nocturnal prolactin rise. This is indeed observed in elderly subjects, who have a nearly 50% dampening of the nocturnal prolactin elevation (see Fig. 4-4).[126,266]

During pregnancy, serum prolactin levels rise but the 24-hour pattern of secretion is maintained, albeit at a higher level. During the postpartum period, prolactin secretory pulses follow suckling episodes, and the nocturnal rise, independent of suckling, is evident only after breastfeeding has ceased.[267]

Alterations in Disease States

Absence or blunting of the nocturnal increase in plasma prolactin has been reported in a variety of pathologic states, including uremia and breast cancer in postmenopausal women. In Cushing's disease, prolactin levels are elevated throughout the 24-hour cycle, and the relative amplitude of the nighttime rise is reduced.[268] In subjects with insulin-dependent diabetes, the circadian and sleep modulation of prolactin secretion is preserved, but overall levels are markedly diminished.[269] Obesity is associated with an increase in overall prolactin secretion, in proportion to excess visceral fat, without alteration of the diurnal variation. This enhancement is achieved by an increase in the amplitude and duration of secretory pulses.[270]

In hyperprolactinemia associated with prolactinomas, or secondary to functional pituitary stalk disconnection, the number of prolactin pulses is increased, and the regularity of the pulsatile pattern is decreased.[271,272] The nocturnal elevation in prolactin may be preserved.[271,273] Selective removal of prolactin-secreting adenomas generally results in normalization of the prolactin pattern.

Abnormal prolactin profiles have been reported in a variety of neurologic and psychiatric disorders, including narcolepsy, depression, and schizophrenia.

The Gonadotropic Axis

Normal Diurnal Profiles of Gonadotropins and Sex Steroids

Rhythms in the gonadotropic axis cover a wide range of frequencies, from episodic release in the ultradian range, to diurnal rhythmicity and menstrual cycles. These various rhythms interact to provide a coordinated temporal program that governs the development of the reproductive axis and its operation at every stage of maturation. The following description of the current state of knowledge in this area will be limited to 24-hour rhythms and their interaction with pulsatile release during adulthood.

Patterns of LH release in adult men exhibit episodic pulses with large interindividual variability.[274] LH secretory episodes mainly reflect GnRH pulsatility. A recent study indicates that LH pulsatility is inhibited by acyl-ghrelin, suggesting that the ghrelin system may play a centrally mediated inhibitory role in the gonadal axis.[275] The diurnal variation is of low amplitude or is even undetectable. During the sleep period, LH pulses appear to be temporally related to the REM–non-REM cycle.[276] FSH profiles may show some occasional pulses, with no diurnal variation.

In contrast, a marked diurnal rhythm in circulating testosterone levels is present in young normal men, with minimal levels in the late evening and maximal levels in the early morning.[175,277] In young adult men, the amplitude of the testosterone rhythm averages 25%.[175] With a 15-minute sampling interval, 17 to 18 testosterone pulses per 24-hour span can be detected.[175] Growing evidence suggests that diurnal testosterone variations are controlled primarily by the sleep-wake cycle. Experimental sleep fragmentation (schedule allowing 7 minutes of sleep every 20 minutes) results in dampening of the nocturnal testosterone rise, particularly in subjects who do not achieve REM sleep.[278] Daytime sleep, as well as nocturnal sleep, is associated with a robust rise in testosterone levels.[279] However, a progressive elevation in testosterone levels persists during nocturnal wakefulness, albeit blunted as compared with nocturnal sleep,[279] indicating the existence of a circadian component that could reflect adrenal androgen secretion. Diurnal profiles of testosterone are paralleled by inhibin B variations, with peak values in the early morning and nadirs in the late afternoon, and significant cross-correlations between inhibin B and testosterone or estradiol have been detected.[280]

A progressive decline in testosterone levels, together with an increase in sex hormone–binding globulin (SHBG) levels, is observed in normal men from 30 years of age onward, so that the decrease in bioavailable testosterone is more important than the decline in total testosterone.[281] In elderly men, the diurnal variation in testosterone is still present but may be markedly dampened.[277,282] A strong positive correlation has been evidenced between total sleep time and morning testosterone levels.[283] Pulsatile testosterone secretion is attenuated, suggesting possible partial desensitization of Leydig cells to LH.[284] Mean LH levels are increased, but the amplitude of LH pulses is decreased,[285,286] their frequency is increased,[284] and no significant diurnal pattern can be detected.[282] In contrast, pulsatile FSH secretion is increased in older men.[287] In addition, older males secrete LH and testosterone more irregularly, and jointly more asynchronously, than do younger men.[288]

In adult women, diurnal profiles of LH, FSH, estradiol, and progesterone exhibit episodic pulses throughout the 24-hour span.[289] The 24-hour variations in plasma LH are markedly modulated by the menstrual cycle.[290] Nocturnal slowing of pulsatile LH secretion is observed during the early follicular phase.[290] This nocturnal slowing is related specifically to sleep rather than to time of day, since it is also observed during daytime sleep but not during nighttime wake.[291] During periods of sleep, LH pulses were found to occur preferentially in association with brief awakenings, suggesting an inhibitory effect of sleep on pulsatile LH secretion.[291] Since night and shift work is consistently associated with shorter and more fragmented sleep, these results indicate that altered menstrual function, which frequently is observed in night and shift workers, could result directly from altered sleep patterns. Evening elevation of LH levels and LH pulse amplitude is observed in the absence of sleep, suggesting the existence of a circadian modulation of LH secretion.[291] Circulating levels of LH and FSH and LH pulse frequency increase with aging and are higher in normal women older than 40 years of age with regular menstrual cycles than in women younger than age 40.[292] Gonadotropin levels remain elevated after menopause.

Alterations in Disease States

Early studies on the 24-hour profile of plasma LH in anorexia nervosa have established the importance of an adequate temporal secretory program in the maintenance of normal reproductive function. In women with amenorrhea secondary to anorexia nervosa, the secretory pattern of LH regresses to the pubertal or prepubertal pattern, with low daytime pulsatility and increased secretion at night.[293] Secretory profiles of LH usually return to normal following weight gain and clinical remission. Short-term fasting was shown to suppress pulsatile LH secretion while enhancing its regularity in young, but not older, men.[294]

Abnormalities in the 24-hour profile of gonadotropin secretion are present in hypothalamic amenorrhea, hyperprolactinemia, and PCOS.

In most men with idiopathic hypogonadotropic hypogonadism, LH pulses are undetectable.[295] In a small number of patients, an early pubertal pattern, with enhanced pulse amplitude during the nighttime, may be observed.[295] Attenuation of pulsatile LH secretion has been reported in men, but not in women, during both hypocortisolism and hypercortisolism. The authors have speculated that this sex difference could be due to a higher level of hypothalamic opioid activity in men.[296] Poorly controlled type 1 diabetes mellitus has been found to be associated with decreased amplitude of pulsatile LH secretion.[297]

The Thyrotropic Axis

The 24-Hour Profile of Thyrotropin in Normal Subjects

In normal adult men and women, TSH levels are low and relatively stable throughout the daytime and begin to increase in the late afternoon or early evening. Maximal levels occur around the beginning of the sleep period.[298] TSH levels progressively decline during the latter part of sleep, and daytime values resume shortly after morning awakening. Onset of the nocturnal rise in TSH well before sleep onset is believed to reflect a circadian effect. This 24-hour pattern of TSH levels appears to be generated by frequency, as well as amplitude modulation, of thyrotropin-releasing hormone (TRH)-driven secretory pulses.[118] Studies involving sleep deprivation and shifts in the sleep-wake cycle have consistently indicated that sleep exerts an inhibitory influence on TSH secretion; sleep deprivation relieves this inhibition.[298,299] It is interesting to note that when sleep occurs during the daytime, TSH secretion is not suppressed significantly below normal daytime levels.[300] Profiles of plasma TSH during normal nocturnal sleep, nocturnal sleep deprivation, and daytime sleep are illustrated in the lower panel of Fig. 4-3. When depth of sleep at the habitual time is enhanced by previous sleep deprivation, inhibition of the nocturnal TSH rise is more pronounced than in basal conditions. Descending slopes of TSH concentrations during sleep are consistently associated with SW stages, and negative cross-correlations have been found between TSH fluctuations and SW activity,[107,301] suggesting that SW sleep probably is the primary determinant of the sleep-associated TSH decrease. Conversely, awakenings are frequently associated with TSH increments.[300] The timing of the TSH evening rise seems to be controlled by circadian rhythmicity and shifts in concordance with the melatonin rhythm following exposure to light or nocturnal exercise.[58] Free triiodothyronine shows a diurnal rhythm that parallels TSH variations.[302]

Under conditions of sleep deprivation, the increased amplitude of the TSH rhythm may result in a detectable increase in plasma triiodothyronine levels, paralleling the nocturnal TSH rise,[300] although negative findings also have been reported.[303] If sleep deprivation is prolonged for a second night, the nocturnal rise in TSH is markedly diminished as compared with that occurring during the first night.[303] It is likely that, following the first night of sleep deprivation, elevated thyroid hormone levels, which persist during the daytime period because of the prolonged half-life of these hormones, limit the subsequent TSH rise. A study involving 64 hours of sleep deprivation demonstrated, during the second night of sleep deprivation, a nocturnal increase in both triiodothyronine and thyroxine levels, contrasting with the decreases seen during normal sleep.[304] These data suggest that prolonged sleep loss may be associated with upregulation of the thyroid axis. Consistent findings have been reported in a study of 6 days of partial sleep loss (4 hours in bed per night) wherein the nocturnal TSH rise was strikingly decreased and overall mean TSH levels were reduced by more than 30%, probably as the result of increased levels of thyroid hormones caused by TSH elevation at the beginning of sleep curtailment (see Fig. 4-8).[194]

Because inhibitory effects of sleep on TSH secretion are time dependent, elevations in plasma TSH levels may occur in conditions of misalignment of sleep and circadian timing. This is illustrated in Fig. 4-11, which shows the mean profiles of plasma TSH observed in a group of normal young men in the course of adaptation to a simulated jet lag involving an abrupt 8-hour advance of the sleep-wake cycle and the dark period, following a 24-hour baseline period.[300] In the course of adaptation, TSH levels increased progressively because nighttime wakefulness was associated with large circadian-dependent TSH elevations, and daytime sleep failed to inhibit TSH. As a result, mean TSH levels were more than twofold higher following awakening from the second shifted period than during the same time interval after normal nocturnal sleep. This study indicates that the subjective discomfort and fatigue associated with jet lag may involve pro-

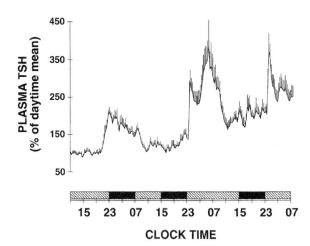

FIGURE 4-11. Mean (+standard error of the mean [SEM]) profile of plasma thyrotropin (TSH) from eight normal young men submitted to an 8-hour advance of the sleep-wake and light-dark cycles. Black bars indicate bedtime periods. (Data from Hirschfeld U, Moreno-Reyes R, Akseki E, et al: Progressive elevation of plasma thyrotropin during adaptation to simulated jet lag: effects of treatment with bright light or zolpidem. J Clin Endocrinol Metab 81:3270–3277, 1996.)

longed elevation of a hormonal concentration in the peripheral circulation.

Aging is associated with a progressive decrease in overall TSH secretion (which is achieved by a decrease in amplitude, rather than in frequency, of secretory pulses) and in circulating TSH levels, and with dampening of the amplitude of the circadian variation.[126] In subjects in the seventh and eighth decades, TSH levels are lower than in young adults throughout the 24-hour span, although the difference is more marked during sleep than during the daytime period (see Fig. 4-4). In middle-aged subjects, age-related decreases in TSH levels may be evidenced only in response to nocturnal sleep deprivation. Thus, it appears that TSH secretory capacity declines progressively with aging.

Alterations in Disease States

A decreased or absent nocturnal rise in TSH has been observed in a wide variety of nonthyroidal illnesses,[305] which suggests that hypothalamic dysregulation generally will affect the circadian TSH surge. This contrasts with the circadian variation of plasma cortisol, which persists in a wide variety of disease states. The nocturnal TSH surge is diminished or absent in various conditions of hypercortisolism,[306] as well as in hyperthyroidism and in primary and secondary hypothyroidism.[307,308] In poorly controlled diabetic states, whether insulin-dependent or non–insulin-dependent, the surge also disappears.[309] Correction of hyperglycemia is associated with a reappearance of the nocturnal elevation.[309] It is interesting to note that morning TSH values in hyperglycemic patients do not differ from those of control subjects, and the TSH response to TRH is only marginally reduced.[309] Obesity is associated with an increase in overall TSH secretion (which is achieved by an increase in amplitude, rather than in frequency, of secretory pulses) without alteration of the diurnal variation. TSH profiles tend to return toward normal levels after body weight loss induced by caloric restriction.[310]

PARATHYROID HORMONE

The 24-hour profile of circulating parathyroid hormone (PTH) levels shows a major nocturnal peak occurring at around 01.00 to 03.00 hours and morning minimal values at around 10.00 to 11.00 hours. This diurnal rhythm persists, albeit dampened, in constant routine conditions.[311] Thus, it appears to be regulated primarily by the circadian pacemaker but modulated by other factors. Although serum calcium, the major modulator of PTH secretion, also may exhibit diurnal variations, the timing of the maximum was found to be highly variable among individuals and did not have any apparent relation to PTH.[311] An early study suggested that the nocturnal rise in PTH was related to SW sleep,[312] but in more recent studies, shifts in the sleep-wake cycle did not alter the timing of the nocturnal PTH peak.[313] In contrast, this nocturnal rise was completely suppressed following a 4 day fast.[314] Diurnal profiles of circulating PTH levels are temporally related to diurnal variations in urinary calcium and phosphate and are likely to play an important role in the optimization of calcium balance.[311] The nocturnal rise in PTH has been reportedly abolished in osteoporotic women[315] and in subjects with primary hyperparathyroidism.[316]

HYDROMINERAL HORMONES

Hormones of the renin-angiotensin-aldosterone system exhibit diurnal variations with higher nocturnal levels. These diurnal variations are regulated primarily by sleep-wake homeostasis, since shifts in the sleep-wake cycle are followed immediately by parallel shifts in hormonal profiles.[104] During nocturnal and

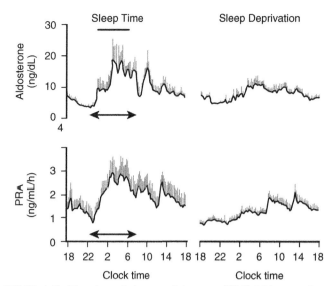

FIGURE 4-12. Mean (+standard error of the mean [SEM]) 24-hour profiles of plasma aldosterone and plasma renin activity (PRA) in eight normal young men (21 to 28 years old) during a period of normal nocturnal sleep and a period of total acute sleep deprivation. (Adapted from Charloux A, Gronfier C, Chapotot F, et al: Sleep deprivation blunts the nighttime increase in aldosterone release in humans. J Sleep Res 10:27–33, 2001.)

shifted sleep periods, a close temporal relationship has been evidenced between increases in SW activity and parallel increases in plasma renin activity (PRA) and aldosterone levels.[104,317,318] Sleep-associated PRA pulses are blunted by awakenings,[319] and nocturnal increases in PRA and aldosterone levels are dampened markedly by acute total sleep deprivation[320] (Fig. 4-12).

In conditions of abnormal sleep architecture (e.g., narcolepsy, sleeping sickness), disturbances in the REM–non-REM cycle are faithfully reflected in the PRA temporal pattern.[321] Vasopressin release is pulsatile but shows no apparent relationship to sleep stages.[321] Diurnal variations in plasma levels of atrial natriuretic peptide (ANP) have been evidenced in some, but not all, studies, and the existence of a circadian rhythm of ANP is still a matter of controversy.[322]

GLUCOSE TOLERANCE AND INSULIN SECRETION
Diurnal and Ultradian Variations in Normal Subjects

In normal man, glucose tolerance varies with the time of day. Fig. 4-13 shows circadian variations in glucose tolerance to oral glucose, identical meals, constant glucose infusion, and continuous enteral nutrition. In all four conditions, plasma glucose levels are markedly higher in the evening than in the morning.[105] Studies of fasting during nocturnal sleep have consistently observed that, despite the prolonged fasting condition, glucose levels remain stable or decrease only minimally during the night, contrasting with a clear decrease during daytime fasting. Thus, a number of mechanisms operative during nocturnal sleep are likely to maintain stable glucose levels during the overnight fast. Experimental protocols involving intravenous glucose infusion or enteral nutrition while allowing for normal nocturnal sleep have shown that glucose tolerance deteriorates further as the evening progresses, reaches a minimum around midsleep, and then improves to return to morning levels.[178,323] During the first half of sleep, SWS is the dominant sleep stage. During SWS, cerebral glucose utilization is lower than during either wake or REM sleep.[324,325] A strong correlation between SWA and regional

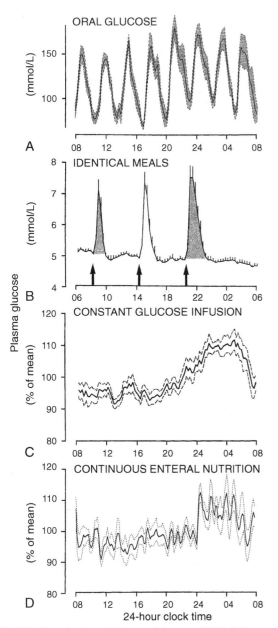

FIGURE 4-13. Mean (and standard error of the mean [SEM]) 24-hour pattern of plasma glucose changes in response to oral glucose 50 g every 3 hours, identical meals, constant glucose infusion, and continuous enteral nutrition in normal young adults. (From Van Cauter E, Polonsky KS, Scheen AJ: Roles of circadian rhythmicity and sleep in human glucose regulation. Endocr Rev 18:716–738, 1997.)

decreased β cell responsiveness are involved in reduced glucose tolerance later in the day. Under conditions of constant glucose infusion, sleep-associated rises in glucose were found to correlate with the amount of concomitant GH secreted. Thus, during the first part of the night, decreased glucose tolerance is due to decreased glucose utilization both by peripheral tissues—resulting from muscle relaxation and rapid insulin-like effects of sleep-onset GH secretion—and by the brain.[325,330] During the second part of the night, these effects subside as sleep becomes shallow and more fragmented and GH is no longer secreted. Thus, complex interactions of circadian and sleep effects, possibly mediated in part by cortisol and GH, result in a consistent pattern of changes in set point of glucose regulation over the 24-hour period. A recent study has demonstrated a continuous decline in plasma glucagon levels during nighttime sleep in healthy nondiabetic subjects.[331] Because this nocturnal decline is preserved in patients with type 1 diabetes, it has been suggested that nocturnal regulation of spontaneous glucagon release occurs independent of circulating glucose and insulin levels.[331]

Consistent with the important modulatory effects of sleep on glucose regulation, recurrent sleep loss is associated with marked alterations in parameters of glucose tolerance. In a study of sleep curtailment (4 hours in bed per night for 6 nights) performed in young healthy subjects,[194,332] the overall glucose response to breakfast was increased and subjects were more insulin resistant, as assessed by an elevation in the homeostatic model assessment (HOMA) index (see Fig. 4-8). Moreover, following an intravenous glucose tolerance test, insulin release was reduced by 30%, and glucose tolerance was found to fall in the range observed in older adults with impaired glucose tolerance. The deleterious impact of sleep restriction on glucose metabolism was subsequently confirmed in a follow-up study that used a randomized crossover design.[333] Recently, a laboratory study in young healthy adults demonstrated that reduced sleep quality, without change in sleep duration, also has a clear negative impact on glucose tolerance. Indeed, this study indicated that all-night selective suppression of SWS, without any change in total sleep time, resulted in marked decreases in insulin sensitivity without adequate compensatory increases in insulin release, leading to reduced glucose tolerance and increased diabetes risk.[334] To date, seven prospective epidemiologic studies have found an association between short and/or poor sleep and diabetes risk, even after controlling for many covariates such as BMI, shift work, hypertension, exercise, and depression (reviewed in reference 335).

Human insulin secretion is a complex oscillatory process involving rapid pulses of small amplitude that recur every 10 to 15 minutes superimposed on slower ultradian oscillations with periods in the 90- to 120-minute range.[121,336] The ultradian oscillations are tightly coupled to glucose, with a tendency for glucose pulses to lead insulin pulses by 10 minutes, and they have been shown to promote more efficient glucose utilization.[125] They are best seen in conditions in which insulin secretion is stimulated, including ingestion of a meal, continuous enteral nutrition, and constant intravenous glucose infusion.[121,323] Under these conditions, their relative amplitude is about 50% to 70% for insulin secretory pulses and 20% for plasma glucose. Their amplitude is maximal immediately after a meal, then decreases progressively. Moreover, the periodicity of the insulin secretory oscillations can be entrained to the period of an oscillatory glucose infusion,[337] thus supporting the concept that these ultradian oscillations are generated by the glucose-insulin feedback mechanism.[338] However, ultradian oscillations, but less regular and of smaller amplitude, are still present in fasting conditions. Stimula-

blood flow in the prefrontal regions was demonstrated by positron emission tomography (PET) scans of subjects who were undergoing continuous polygraphic recordings.[324,326] Brain glucose metabolism represents 30% to 50% of total body glucose utilization[327,328]; therefore, a robust link between SWS and glucose tolerance should be expected. Evidence also indicates that the diurnal variation in glucose tolerance is driven in part by the wide and highly reproducible diurnal rhythm of plasma cortisol, an important counterregulatory hormone.[105,200,329] Indeed, the diurnal variation in insulin secretion was found to be inversely related to the cortisol rhythm, with significant correlation of the magnitudes of morning to evening excursions. Rises in plasma levels of glucose and insulin following short-term elevations in plasma cortisol are more pronounced in the evening than in the morning.[200] Diminished insulin sensitivity and tory effects of sleep on insulin secretion are mediated by an increase in the amplitude of the oscillation.[323] During constant glucose infusion, REM sleep and wake episodes coincide significantly with decreasing levels of glucose and insulin, and increasing glucose levels occur during the deeper stages of non-REM sleep.[330]

Rapid 10- to 15-minute pulsations seem to have a different origin than ultradian oscillations. Indeed, they may appear independently of glucose, since they have been observed in the isolated perfused pancreas and in perifused islets.[121] Rapid insulin pulsations also have been observed in perfused human islets.[339] Administration of insulin by pulsatile infusion improves insulin-mediated glucose uptake.[340] The frequency, amplitude, and regularity of rapid insulin pulses are decreased by aging.[341] Omental lipolysis is also pulsatile and has a rapid frequency, similar to that of insulin.[342] However, the oscillation of free fatty acids appears to be driven by the central nervous system, rather than by insulin.[342]

Alterations in Disease States

In obese and diabetic subjects, diurnal and ultradian variations in glucose regulation are abnormal. In obesity, the morning versus evening difference in glucose tolerance is abolished. Obese adult subjects show no diurnal variation in glucose tolerance, no decline in insulin sensitivity in the afternoon, and only a marginally significant decline in β cell responsiveness to glucose in the latter part of the day.[343]

In patients with insulin-dependent diabetes, an increase in glucose levels and/or insulin requirements occurs during a prebreakfast period ranging from 05:00 to 09:00 hours and has been called the dawn phenomenon.[344] A role for nocturnal GH secretion in the pathogenesis of the dawn phenomenon has been demonstrated.[345,346] The observation of a dawn phenomenon in patients with non–insulin-dependent diabetes mellitus (NIDDM) under normal dietary conditions has been less consistent. However, prominent late night and early morning elevations in glucose levels and insulin secretion in both normal subjects and diabetic patients become apparent during prolonged fasting.[347]

Counterregulatory mechanisms that are already deficient in type 1 diabetes are further impaired during sleep as compared with wakefulness, as autonomic responses to hypoglycemia are reduced during sleep in diabetic patients. As a result, patients with type 1 diabetes are substantially less likely to be awakened by hypoglycemia than are nondiabetic subjects.[348] Patients with type 1 diabetes present distinct alterations in sleep architecture and nocturnal neuroendocrine release.[349] Levels of GH, epinephrine, ACTH, and cortisol are elevated, and patients have less deep SWS and more shallow stage II sleep.[349]
The rapid and ultradian oscillations of insulin secretion are perturbed in NIDDM and in impaired glucose tolerance without hyperglycemia.[121,350,351] Ultradian oscillations, which have an exaggerated amplitude in obese subjects without apparent changes in frequency or pattern of recurrence, are also more irregular and of lower amplitude in subjects with established NIDDM.[121]

HORMONES INVOLVED IN APPETITE REGULATION

Leptin

Leptin is an anorexigenic hormone, mainly released by the adipocytes, that provides information about energy status to hypothalamic regulatory centers.[352,353] As illustrated in Fig. 4-14,

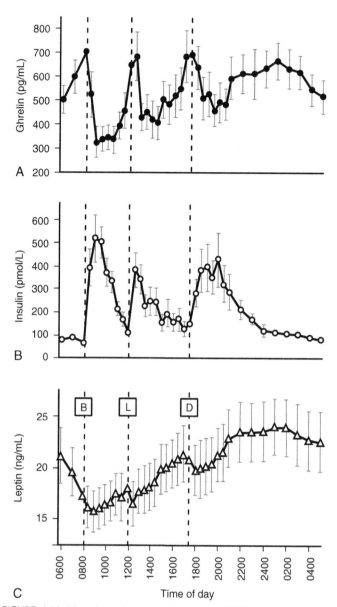

FIGURE 4-14. Mean (±standard error of the mean [SEM]) 24-hour profiles of plasma ghrelin, insulin, and leptin levels in 10 healthy subjects 29 to 64 years of age (body mass index [BMI], 22 to 30 kg/m²) receiving breakfast, lunch, and dinner at 08.00, 12.00, and 17.30 hours, respectively. (Adapted from Cummings DE, Purnell JQ, Frayo RS, et al: A preprandial rise in plasma ghrelin levels suggests a role in meal initiation in humans. Diabetes 50:1714–1719, 2001.)

plasma leptin levels in normal lean men and women show a robust diurnal rhythm, with minimal values during the daytime and a nocturnal rise with maximal values during early sleep to midsleep.[354] The amplitude of the diurnal variation averages 25% to 30% of the mean level.[355]

The timing of the daily maximum of plasma leptin levels is markedly dependent on the timing of meals, as shifts in meal timings induce immediate shifts in leptin profiles: Fasting and eating are associated with a decrease and an increase in leptin levels, respectively.[356] However, the diurnal rhythm was found to persist, albeit with a smaller amplitude, in subjects who received continuous enteral nutrition,[323] and in subjects who received identical snacks at 2-hour intervals.[357] The rhythm also persisted in subjects who were submitted to 38 or 88 consecutive hours of wakefulness.[357,358] Following an abrupt shift in the sleep period, nocturnal leptin levels rose despite the absence of sleep, and a second rise was observed following the onset of daytime recovery sleep.[323] Thus, leptin diurnal variations reflect the combined effects of the circadian pacemaker, the sleep-wake cycle, and the schedule of food intake.

Several studies have reported that human leptin levels, including those in subjects receiving continuous enteral nutrition rather than separate meals, are pulsatile.[323,355,359-361]

Leptin levels reflect cumulative energy balance, with a decline or an increase in response to underfeeding or overfeeding, respectively.[362,363] These changes have been found to be associated with reciprocal changes in hunger.[363] Circulating leptin concentrations are higher and the relative amplitude of their diurnal variation is lower in obese subjects than in normal-weight controls.[355] Marked sex differences have been reported in 24-hour mean leptin levels, which are twofold to tenfold higher in women than in men, regardless of fat mass.[355,361] In anorexia nervosa, as in amenorrheic female athletes, leptin levels are low and diurnal variations are abolished.[364,365] Aging is associated with dampening of the amplitude of the 24-hour rhythm of plasma leptin and an advance in the nocturnal acrophase.[366]

Sleep restriction (2 to 6 nights of 4-hour bedtimes) under controlled conditions of caloric intake and physical activity is associated with a 20% to 30% reduction in mean leptin levels, acrophase, and amplitude of the diurnal variation.[332,367] The magnitude of this impact of sleep restriction on leptin levels is comparable with that observed in young adults under normal sleep conditions after 3 days of dietary restriction by approximately 900 kcal per day.[363] Consistent findings have been obtained in two epidemiologic studies that found an association between short sleep and lower morning leptin levels after controlling for BMI[368] or the degree of adiposity.[369] Diurnal variations in leptin and cortisol levels form an approximate mirror image,[360,361,370,371] and in fully rested subjects, maximal leptin levels coincide with minimal cortisol levels,[332] consistent with the well-documented action of leptin on HPA activity.[353] Recurrent partial sleep deprivation results in an advance in the leptin acrophase such that high levels of leptin occur when cortisol concentrations are still elevated relative to the nocturnal nadir, possibly acting in concert to increase appetite at the end of the day.[332]

Normal 24-hour leptin levels and diurnal leptin variations were found in patients with primary adrenal failure.[371] Increased leptin levels,[372,373] caused by equal amplification of basal and pulsatile secretion,[374] with preservation of the diurnal pattern[372] have been reported in patients with Cushing's syndrome. A normal diurnal leptin pattern also has been reported in patients with GH deficiency[375] or with perinatal stalk-transection syndrome.[376]

Another secretory product of differentiated adipocytes is adiponectin, a hormone that enhances insulin sensitivity.[377,378] In normal-weight men, adiponectin levels exhibit ultradian pulsatility, as well as diurnal variation, with a significant nocturnal decline, reaching minimal values in the early morning.[379] So far, possible relations between adiponectin rhythm and sleep have not been reported. Adiponectin levels are decreased, adiponectin pulsatility is blunted, and diurnal variations are abolished in obese subjects.[380-382] In severely obese subjects, massive weight loss coupled with the reversibility of insulin resistance is associated with a restoration of adiponectin pulsatility.[382]

Ghrelin and Peptide YY

Ghrelin is an orexigenic hormone that is secreted primarily by the stomach and the duodenum.[221,383,384] Ghrelin also stimulates

GH secretion and displays ACTH- and prolactin-releasing activities.[221] One report claimed that ghrelin was found to promote SW sleep in man,[385] but others found suppressive effects on sleep in rats.[386] Ghrelin secretion is pulsatile.[381,387] Daytime profiles are regulated primarily by the schedule of food intake: Levels rise sharply before each designated mealtime and fall to trough levels within 1 hour after eating. A study examining spontaneous meal initiation in the absence of time- and food-related cues provided good evidence of a role for ghrelin in meal initiation.[388] This pattern seems to be exaggerated after the dinner meal, as ghrelin levels peak at around 01:00 hours and remain elevated until the latter part of the night, when they tend to decrease spontaneously[389-391] (see Fig. 4-14). Ghrelin levels are increased in anorexia nervosa and decreased in young obese subjects.[390,392] In obese subjects, the diurnal pattern was found to remain largely unaltered[390] or to be markedly blunted.[381] A diet-induced weight loss was associated with increased 24-hour ghrelin levels.[390]

Diurnal variations in ghrelin levels persist after 3 days of total fasting. However, the timings of acrophase and nadir are not consistent across studies.[393] Studies concur in indicating that ghrelin levels are not increased by prolonged fasting, and that women have higher levels than men.[393] Diurnal variations in ghrelin likely reflect the combined effects of the circadian pacemaker, the schedule of food intake, and possibly the sleep-wake cycle.

Acute total sleep deprivation was found to be associated with a blunted but prolonged nocturnal ghrelin elevation.[236] A 2-day sleep restriction (4 hours bedtime per night) under controlled conditions of caloric intake and physical activity was reportedly associated with a nearly 30% elevation in daytime levels (Fig. 4-15).[367] Consistent with these laboratory findings is the recent observation of a 22% increase in plasma ghrelin levels after a single night of total sleep deprivation.[394] In a large epidemiologic study, short sleep was associated with higher ghrelin levels after controlling for sex, age, and BMI.[368]

Another gut hormone that is thought to play an important role in the regulation of hunger and body weight is peptide YY (PYY), which is synthesized by gut-endocrine L cells.[395] Exogenous administration of PYY3-36 reduces food intake in obese humans and rodents. The diurnal variation of plasma PYY levels in normal adults mirrors that of ghrelin, both after meal intake and during the overnight fast.

Conditions of Altered Sleep and Circadian Rhythmicity

SLEEP CURTAILMENT

Whether voluntary or not, sleep restriction is a hallmark of modern society. "Normal" sleep duration has decreased from approximately 8.5 hours in 1960 to an average of less than 7 hours today. Many individuals voluntarily choose to curtail their sleep to the shortest amount tolerable to maximize the time available for work and leisure activities, and more than 30% of American adult men and women between the ages of 30 and 64 years report sleeping less than 6 hours per night. To meet the demands of around the clock operations, millions of shift workers sleep on average less than 6 hours per day.

Despite the fact that sleep is a major modulator of metabolic and endocrine regulation, the consensus that prevailed until recently was that sleep loss results in increased sleepiness and decreased cognitive performance but has little or no effect on

RANDOMIZED CROSS-OVER DESIGN: 2 DAYS
OF SLEEP RESTRICTION OR EXTENSION

After 2 days of 10-H bedtimes
After 2 days of 4-H bedtimes

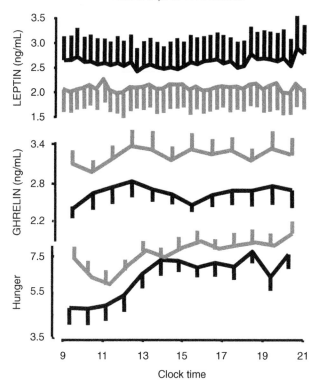

FIGURE 4-15. Mean (and standard error of the mean [SEM]) daytime profiles of plasma leptin and ghrelin and of hunger ratings in healthy young men after 2 days of 10-hour bedtimes and 2 days of 4-hour bedtimes. (Data from Spiegel K, Tasali E, Penev P, Van Cauter E: Brief communication: sleep curtailment in healthy young men is associated with decreased leptin levels, elevated ghrelin levels, and increased hunger and appetite. Ann Intern Med 141:846–850, 2004.)

peripheral function. However, as reported in previous sections, partial sleep curtailment induces potentially harmful alterations in hormonal profiles. Two to 6 nights of sleep restriction (4 hours per night) under controlled conditions of caloric intake and physical activity in healthy young men were found to result in the following:

- Elevated evening total and free cortisol concentrations,[194,332] strikingly similar to those observed in the elderly.[126,195,196] This disturbance may reflect decreased efficacy of the negative feedback regulation of the hypothalamic-pituitary-adrenal axis and could promote the development of insulin resistance and memory impairments.[200,396]
- A clinically significant impairment of carbohydrate tolerance,[194,332,333] consistent with a state of impaired glucose tolerance as observed in older adults.
- A decrease in circulating levels of leptin,[332,367] an anorexigenic hormone, and a concomitant increase in circulating levels of ghrelin,[367] an orexigenic hormone (see Fig. 4-15). Moreover, sleep curtailment was associated with an increase in hunger, and this increase in hunger was strongly correlated with the increase in the ghrelin-to-leptin ratio.[367]

These data suggest that recurrent partial sleep curtailment may increase the risk for obesity and diabetes and may accelerate the senescence of endocrine and metabolic function. An obvious limitation of these studies is that the investigation period was not extended beyond 6 days. Thus, a progressive adaptation to chronic partial sleep deprivation cannot be excluded. However, the findings from these laboratory studies are consistent with the conclusions of epidemiologic studies. Several prospective cross-sectional epidemiologic studies, which varied considerably in geographic location and subject population, were remarkably consistent in indicating that short sleep may increase the risk of developing type 2 diabetes and/or obesity (reviewed in references 335 and 397). One major limitation of all of these epidemiologic studies is that they used only subjective reporting of sleep. Laboratory and epidemiologic studies now need to be complemented by large field studies incorporating objective measures of sleep duration and interventional methods to enhance our understanding of the mechanisms linking sleep loss to endocrine and metabolic alterations. Given the morbidity and mortality associated with obesity and diabetes, the identification of novel risk factors that are potentially modifiable, such as sleep curtailment, is particularly important.

SLEEP DISORDERS

A recent laboratory study has shown that decreased sleep quality without a change in sleep duration results in a marked decrease in insulin sensitivity, without appropriate compensation of insulin release.[334] Thus, diabetes risk was markedly increased. This study suppressed SWS, thus replacing deep non-REM sleep with shallow non-REM sleep, as occurs in the course of normal aging and in a variety of sleep disorders, including obstructive sleep apnea (OSA). It is important to note that this study demonstrated that a sleep disruption can cause hormonal and metabolic alterations.

Obstructive Sleep Apnea

OSA is the most common sleep disorder, and its incidence is rising rapidly in parallel with the current epidemic of obesity. A few studies have examined pituitary hormonal release in patients with OSA before and after treatment.[398-400] Nocturnal release of the two pituitary hormones that are markedly dependent on sleep (i.e., GH and prolactin) is decreased in untreated apneic subjects. As illustrated in Fig. 4-16, treatment with continuous positive airway pressure (CPAP) results in a clear increase in the amount of GH secreted during the first few hours of sleep.[398,399] The total amount of prolactin secreted during the sleep period is not modified by CPAP treatment, but the frequency of prolactin pulses is restored to values similar to those observed in normal subjects.[400] Nocturnal LH and testosterone secretions are decreased in men with untreated OSA. These alterations are partially corrected during long-term CPAP treatment.[401]

Morning leptin levels are elevated in patients with OSA when compared with weight-matched nonapneic subjects, and CPAP treatment decreases morning leptin levels.[402-409]

Whereas obesity is a major risk for OSA, OSA is now recognized as a risk for insulin resistance, independently of BMI, as supported by a large set of nine cross-sectional studies that have assessed OSA by polysomnography (reviewed in reference 410). All but the earliest study (which also involved the smallest sample size) found an association between increased severity of OSA and alterations in glucose metabolism consistent with an increased risk for diabetes. The only prospective study that used polysomnography to assess OSA did not find an independent relationship between severity of OSA at baseline and incident diabetes, but the duration of follow-up was only 4 years. Findings from clinic-based studies are largely consistent with those of epidemiologic studies. Indeed, despite differences in sample

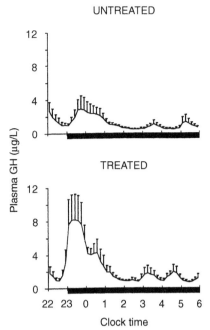

FIGURE 4-16. Mean (+standard error of the mean [SEM]) profiles of plasma growth hormone (GH) in patients with sleep apnea studied before and after treatment with continuous positive airway pressure (CPAP). (Data from Saini et al: Adapted from Van Cauter E, Spiegel K: Circadian and sleep control of endocrine secretions. In Turek FW, Zee PC [eds]: Neurobiology of Sleep and Circadian Rhythms. In Lenfant C: Lung Biology in Health and Disease, vol 133. New York, Marcel Dekker, 1999, pp 397–426.)

size, study design, measurement techniques, cut points, and control for possible confounders, most clinic-based studies (10 out of 13) were consistent in finding an independent association between OSA and abnormal glucose metabolism.[410]

Accumulating evidence suggests that metabolic abnormalities can be partially corrected by CPAP treatment, which supports the concept of a causal link between OSA and altered glucose control.[410,410a] When hyperinsulinemic euglycemic clamp evaluations were performed in nondiabetic patients with OSA, it was found that CPAP significantly improves insulin sensitivity after 2 days of treatment, and this improvement persists after nearly 3 years of treatment. In obese patients with type 2 diabetes, insulin sensitivity was improved after 3 months, but not after 2 days, of CPAP treatment. This finding suggests that the time course of improvement may be longer in obese patients who have diabetes. Two studies found that postprandial interstitial glucose levels and elevated hemoglobin A1C levels were reduced by CPAP use in type 2 diabetes. A population-based study showed reductions in fasting insulin levels and insulin resistance (estimated by HOMA) after 3 weeks of CPAP treatment in men with OSA compared with nonapneic controls followed over the same time period without CPAP. However, several studies did not show a beneficial effect of CPAP treatment on glucose metabolism.[410] Conflicting results could be due to differences in sample sizes and populations, variable durations of therapy, variable compliance, and changes in body composition during the study period.

The pathophysiologic mechanisms that lead to alterations in glucose metabolism in OSA are likely to be multiple. High sympathetic nervous system activity, intermittent hypoxia, low levels of SWS, sleep fragmentation and sleep loss, dysregulation of the hypothalamic-pituitary axis, endothelial dysfunction, and altera-

tions in cytokine and adipokine release all have been proposed as potential mechanisms for abnormal glucose metabolism in OSA.

The overall prevalence of OSA in diabetic men has been estimated at 23%, compared with 6% in a community-based sample.[411] However, preliminary analysis of cross-sectional data from a multicenter study recently revealed an exceptionally high prevalence of undiagnosed OSA in obese patients with type 2 diabetes, with more than 75% of patients having moderate to severe OSA diagnosed by polysomnography.[412] These remarkable associations raise the possibility that OSA may be a novel risk factor for type 2 diabetes and/or, conversely, that chronic hyperglycemia may promote OSA. Whether treatment for OSA may delay the development or reduce the severity of type 2 diabetes is another important question.

Other Sleep Disorders

A paucity of data is available regarding endocrine and metabolic abnormalities in sleep disorders other than OSA.

Narcolepsy is a sleep disorder that is characterized by excessive daytime sleepiness, reduced quality of nocturnal sleep with sleep-onset REM episodes, and cataleptic attacks. Narcolepsy is caused by impaired orexin (hypocretin) neurotransmission. Consistent with the role of orexin in the control of energy balance, narcoleptic patients have increased BMI and lower basal metabolism. The 24-hour rhythm of ACTH and cortisol persists in narcolepsy, suggesting that the circadian clock is not affected.[413,414] In contrast, the 24-hour profiles of hormones known to be dependent on sleep-wake homeostasis, such as GH and prolactin, are markedly disrupted, with dampened or absent nocturnal GH and prolactin release.[413,415] Leptin levels are decreased, and the nocturnal rise is abolished.[416]

Despite the high prevalence of insomnia in modern society, very little is known regarding the neuroendocrine and metabolic consequences of poor or insufficient sleep in this condition. The 24-hour profiles of ACTH and cortisol have been assessed in patients with insomnia who were monitored in a sleep laboratory for four consecutive nights. An increase in ACTH and cortisol secretion was observed in the evening and the early part of the night in patients who had objectively documented short total sleep time and poor sleep efficiency. However, patients with insomnia who had a normal sleep time did not show alterations in ACTH and cortisol profiles.[186] Certain, much less prevalent, forms of sleep disorders seem to originate from a disturbance in the circadian system. Delayed sleep phase insomnia is characterized by a chronic inability to fall asleep at a normal bedtime and to awake in the morning. Nonpharmacologic chronotherapy involving repeated scheduled exposure to bright light is the treatment of choice for this disorder.[417] In contrast, in the advanced sleep phase syndrome, the timing of the major sleep episode is advanced in relation to normal bedtime, resulting in symptoms of extreme evening sleepiness and early morning awakening. Familial forms of this syndrome may reflect an autosomal dominant mutation.[418]

Circadian Misalignment

Circadian rhythms provide synchronization with pronounced periodic fluctuations in the external environment and organize the internal milieu so that coordination and synchronization of internal processes are evident. External synchronization is of obvious importance for the survival of the species and ensures that the organism does the "right thing" at the right time of the day. Of equal importance is the fact that the circadian clock system provides internal temporal organization (i.e., internal synchrony) between the myriad of biochemical and physiologic systems in the body. The concept of internal synchrony had to be reevaluated in recent years in view of the discovery that circadian clock genes, which are part of the transcription-translation feedback loop that generates self-sustained oscillations in the central master circadian clock in the SCN, also are expressed rhythmically in other regions of the brain and in a variety of peripheral tissues, including adipocytes, hepatocytes, pancreatic β cells, cardiomyocytes, and vascular smooth muscle cells.[20,419] Under normal conditions, the central SCN pacemaker maintains synchrony between central and peripheral oscillators. In conditions of circadian misalignment, such as those that occur in jet lag and shift work, the alignment of central and peripheral oscillators is disrupted. Thus, the concept of internal desynchrony has to include *desynchrony between different centrally controlled rhythms* (e.g., cortisol vs. GH) and *desynchrony between central and peripheral rhythms*. Lack of synchrony within the internal environment may lead to chronic difficulties with serious consequences for the health and well-being of the organism. The physical and mental malaise that occurs following rapid travel across time zones (i.e., the jet lag syndrome) and the pathologies associated with long-term shift work are assumed to be due in part to alterations in the normal phase relationships between various internal rhythms. In addition, it has been speculated that alterations in internal phase relationships between rhythms underlie certain forms of affective illness.

Jet Lag

Subjects who travel rapidly across time zones are confronted with a desynchronization between their internal circadian rhythms and the periodicity of the new external environment. Upon arrival, the timings of the light-dark cycle, social schedule, and meals are abnormally matched to the phase of physiologic rhythm of the traveler. Associated with this lack of synchronization are symptoms of fatigue, subjective discomfort, sleep disturbances, reduced mental and psychomotor performance, and gastrointestinal disorders.

The rate of adaptation is generally slower for overt rhythms that are strongly dependent on the circadian system, such as those of cortisol and melatonin secretions, than for those that are markedly modulated by sleep-wake homeostasis, such as prolactin and GH secretions. As a result, during the period of adaptation, abnormal phase relationships between overt rhythms occur. Thus, the jet lag syndrome involves not only desynchronization between internal and external rhythms but also perturbation of internal temporal organization of physiologic functions. Depending on the strength of the zeitgebers, the rate of adaptation can be as low as half an hour a day or as high as 3 hours a day. The rate of adaptation is not constant: Adaptation to a large shift occurs at a faster rate during the first few days and progresses at a slower pace thereafter.[420] The rate of adaptation is also dependent on the direction of the shift, with adaptation generally occurring faster after a delay (i.e., westward) shift than after an advance (i.e., eastward) shift.[420] This eastward-westward difference in rate of adaptation is believed to be due to the fact that the endogenous circadian period of the human is slightly longer than 24 hours, and thus adjustment by delays is achieved more easily than adjustment by advances. Strong evidence suggests that reentrainment after a transmeridian flight is facilitated by exposure to bright light at appropriate circadian phases. It is widely believed that adherence to the local social and meal schedule upon arrival will accelerate adaptation to jet lag, but this has not been rigorously demonstrated. Laboratory studies suggest that physical exercise scheduled during the period corresponding to the nighttime before travel will facilitate adaptation to a delay (i.e., westward) shift.[57,421]

Shift Work

Shift work, which is—voluntarily or not—accepted by millions of workers, is a major health hazard, involving increased risks for cardiometabolic illness, gastrointestinal disorders, infertility, and insomnia.[422-424] Epidemiologic studies have indicated that shift work is a risk factor for weight gain,[425] dyslipidemia,[426,427] and insulin resistance.[427,428] The medical consequences of shift work are associated with chronic misalignment of physiologic circadian rhythms and the activity-rest cycle. In addition, shift work almost invariably results in substantial sleep loss because daytime sleep generally is shorter and more fragmented than nocturnal sleep. Shift work usually creates conditions in which some zeitgebers (e.g., an artificial light-dark cycle) and additional phase-setting factors such as the rest-activity cycle are shifted, while others (e.g., the natural light-dark cycle, the routines of family life) remain unaltered. Shift workers thus live in a situation of conflicting zeitgebers that almost never allow a complete shift of the circadian system. Indeed, several studies have shown that workers on permanent or rotating night shifts do not adapt to these schedules, even after several years.[227,429,430]

Besides its health implications, this misalignment with the circadian system has important social and economic implications, because night work is associated with substantial decrements in performance and vigilance, resulting in diminished productivity and increased accident rates. Scheduled exposure to bright light during night work and complete darkness during daytime sleep following night work can accelerate adjustment to the new schedule and improve nighttime alertness and performance; exogenous melatonin may facilitate sleep at abnormal circadian phases.[431]

REFERENCES

1. Rosenwasser AM, Turek FW: Physiology of the Mammalian Circadian System. Section 4—Chronobiology. In Kryger MH, Roth T, Dement WC, editors: Principles and Practices of Sleep Medicine, ed 4, New York, 2005, WB Saunders, pp 351–362.
2. Turek FW, Dugovic C, Laposky A: Master Circadian Clock, Master Circadian Rhythm. Section 4—Chronobiology. In Kryger MH, Roth T, Dement WC, editors: Principles and Practices of Sleep Medicine, ed 4, New York, 2005, W B Saunders; pp 318–320.
3. Turek FW: Circadian rhythms, Horm Res 49:103–113, 1998.
4. Aschoff J: Circadian rhythms: general features and endocrinological aspects. In Krieger DT, editor: Endocrine Rhythms, New York, 1979, Raven Press, pp 1–61.
5. Czeisler CA, Duffy JF, Shanahan TL, et al: Stability, precision, and near-24-hour period of the human circadian pacemaker, Science 284:2177–2181, 1999.
6. Saper CB, Scammell TE, Lu J: Hypothalamic regulation of sleep and circadian rhythms, Nature 437:1257–1263, 2005.
7. Lehman MN, Silver R, Bittman EL: Anatomy of suprachiasmatic nucleus grafts. In Klein DC, Moore RY, Reppert SM, editors: Suprachiasmatic Nucleus: The Mind's Clock, New York, 1991, Oxford University Press, pp 349–374.
8. Ralph M, Foster RG, Davis FC, et al: Transplanted suprachiasmatic nucleus determines circadian period, Science 247:975–978, 1990.
9. Abe M, Herzog ED, Yamazaki S, et al: Circadian rhythms in isolated brain regions, J Neurosci 22:350–356, 2002.
10. Earnest DJ, Sladek CD: Circadian vasopressin release from perifused rat suprachiasmatic explants in vitro: effects of acute stimulation, Brain Res 422:398–402, 1987.
11. Gillette MU: SCN electrophysiology in vitro: rhythmic activity and endogenous clock properties. In Klein DC, Moore RY, Reppert SM, editors: Suprachiasmatic Nucleus—The Mind's Clock, New York, 1991, Oxford University Press.

12. Panda S, Antoch MP, Miller BH, et al: Coordinated transcription of key pathways in the mouse by the circadian clock, Cell 109:307–320, 2002.
13. Welsh DK, Logothetis DE, Meister M, et al: Individual neurons dissociated from rat suprachiasmatic nucleus express independently phased circadian firing rhythms, Neuron 14:697–706, 1995.
14. Lee HS, Billings HJ, Lehman MN: The suprachiasmatic nucleus: a clock of multiple components, J Biol Rhythms 18:435–449, 2003.
15. Laposky A, Easton A, Dugovic C, et al: Deletion of the mammalian circadian clock gene BMAL1/Mop3 alters baseline sleep architecture and the response to sleep deprivation, Sleep 28:395–409, 2005.
16. Lowrey PL, Takahashi JS: Mammalian circadian biology: elucidating genome-wide levels of temporal organization, Annu Rev Genomics Hum Genet 5:407–441, 2004.
17. Vitaterna MH, Pinto LH, Turek FW: Molecular Genetic Basis for Mammalian Circadian Rhythms. Section 4—Chronobiology. In Kryger MH, Roth T, Dement WC, editors: Principles and Practices of Sleep Medicine, ed 4, New York, 2005, WB Saunders, pp 363–374.
18. Miller BH, Olson SL, Turek FW, et al: Circadian clock mutation disrupts estrous cyclicity and maintenance of pregnancy, Curr Biol 14:1367–1373, 2004.
19. Turek FW, Joshu C, Kohsaka A, et al: Obesity and metabolic syndrome in circadian clock mutant mice, Science 308:1043–1045, 2005.
20. Laposky AD, Bass J, Kohsaka A, et al: Sleep and circadian rhythms: key components in the regulation of energy metabolism, FEBS Lett 582:142–151, 2008.
21. Reppert SM, Weaver DR: Coordination of circadian timing in mammals, Nature 418:935–941, 2002.
22. Yoo SH, Yamazaki S, Lowrey PL, et al: PERIOD2::LUCIFERASE real-time reporting of circadian dynamics reveals persistent circadian oscillations in mouse peripheral tissues, Proc Natl Acad Sci U S A 101:5339–5346, 2004.
23. Dijk DJ, Czeisler CA: Contribution of the circadian pacemaker and the sleep homeostat to sleep propensity, sleep structure, electroencephalographic slow waves, and sleep spindle activity in humans, J Neurosci 15:3526–3538, 1995.
24. Wright KP Jr, Hughes RJ, Kronauer RE, et al: Intrinsic near-24-h pacemaker period determines limits of circadian entrainment to a weak synchronizer in humans, Proc Natl Acad Sci U S A 98:14027–14032, 2001.
25. Card JP, Moore RY: The organization of visual circuits influencing the circadian activity of suprachiasmatic nucleus. In Klein DC, Moore RY, Reppert SM, editors: Suprachiasmatic Nucleus: The Mind's Clock, New York, 1991, Oxford University Press, pp 51–76.
26. Underwood H: Circadian Organization in Nonmammalian Vertebrates. In Takahashi JS, Turek FW, Moore RY, editors: Handbook of Behavioral Neurobiology, New York, 2001, Plenum Press.
27. Foster RG, Provencio I, Hudson D, et al: Circadian photoreception in the retinally degenerate mouse (rd/rd), J Comp Physiol A 169:39–50, 1991.
28. Panda S, Sato TK, Castrucci AM, et al: Melanopsin (Opn4) requirement for normal light-induced circadian phase shifting, Science 298:2213–2216, 2002.
29. Panda S, Provencio I, Tu DC, et al: Melanopsin is required for non-image-forming photic responses in blind mice, Science 301:525–527, 2003.
30. Lupi D, Oster H, Thompson S, et al: The acute light-induction of sleep is mediated by OPN4-based photoreception, Nat Neurosci 11:1068–1073, 2008.
31. Guler AD, Ecker JL, Lall GS, et al: Melanopsin cells are the principal conduits for rod-cone input to non-image-forming vision, Nature 453:102–105, 2008.
32. Turek FW: Lighting up the brain, Journal of Biological Rhythms 14:171, 1999.
33. Foster RG: Seeing the light … in a new way, J Neuroendocrinol 16:179–180, 2004.
34. Klein T, Martens H, Dijk DJ, et al: Circadian sleep regulation in the absence of light perception: chronic non-24-hour circadian rhythm sleep disorder in a blind man with a regular 24-hour sleep-wake schedule, Sleep 16:333–343, 1993.
35. Turek FW: Pharmacological probes of the mammalian circadian clock: use of the phase response curve approach, Trends Pharmacol Sciences 8:212–217, 1987.

36. Turek FW: Pharmacological probes of the mammalian circadian clock: use of the phase response curve approach, Trends Pharmacol Sci 8:212–217, 1987.
37. Lockley SW, Brainard GC, Czeisler CA: High sensitivity of the human circadian melatonin rhythm to resetting by short wavelength light, J Clin Endocrinol Metab 88:4502–4505, 2003.
38. Boivin DB, Duffy JF, Kronauer RE, et al: Dose-response relationships for resetting of human circadian clock by light, Nature 379:540–542, 1996.
39. Minors DS, Waterhouse JM, Wirz-Justice A: A human phase-response curve to light, Neurosci Lett 13:36–40, 1991.
40. Van Cauter E, Sturis J, Byrne MM, et al: Demonstration of rapid light-induced advances and delays of the human circadian clock using hormonal phase markers, Am J Physiol 266:E953–E963, 1994.
41. Khalsa SB, Jewett ME, Cajochen C, et al: A phase response curve to single bright light pulses in human subjects, J Physiol 549:945–952, 2003.
42. Jewett M, Kronauer RE, Czeisler CA: Light-induced suppression of endogenous circadian amplitude in humans, Nature 350:59–62, 1991.
43. Van Reeth O, Turek FW: Stimulated activity mediates phase shifts in the hamster circadian clock induced by dark pulses or benzodiazepines, Nature 339:49–51, 1989.
44. Mendoza JY, Dardente H, Escobar C, et al: Dark pulse resetting of the suprachiasmatic clock in Syrian hamsters: behavioral phase-shifts and clock gene expression, Neuroscience 127:529–537, 2004.
45. Van Cauter E, Moreno-Reyes R, Akseki E, et al: Rapid phase advance of the 24-h melatonin profile in response to afternoon dark exposure, Am J Physiol 275:E48–E54, 1998.
46. Goichot B, Weibel L, Chapotot F, et al: Effect of the shift of the sleep-wake cycle on three robust endocrine markers of the circadian clock, Am J Physiol 275:E243–E248, 1998.
47. Buxton OM, L'Hermite-Baleriaux M, Turek FW, et al: Daytime naps in darkness phase shift the human circadian rhythms of melatonin and thyrotropin secretion, Am J Physiol Regul Integr Comp Physiol 278:R373–R382, 2000.
48. Mrosovsky N: Locomotor activity and non-photic influences on the circadian clock, Biol Rev 71:343–372, 1996.
49. Mrosovsky N: Phase response curves for social entrainment, J Comp Physiol A 162:35–46, 1988.
50. Turek FW: Effects of stimulated physical activity on the circadian pacemaker of vertebrates, J Biol Rhythms 4:135–148, 1989.
51. Turek FW, Smith R, Van Reeth O, et al: Disturbances of the activity rest cycle alter the circadian clock of mammals. In Inouye S, Krieger JM, editors: Endogenous sleep factors, The Hague, 1990, SPB Academic Publishing, pp 277–283.
52. Smith R, Turek FW, Takahashi JS: Two families of phase-response curves characterize the resetting of the hamster circadian clock, Am J Physiol 262:R1149–R1153, 1992.
53. Zlomanczuk P, Schwartz W: Cellular and molecular mechanisms of circadian rhythms in mammals. In Turek FW, Zee PC, editors: Regulation of sleep and circadian rhythms, New York, 1999, Marcel Dekker, pp 309–342.
54. Penev PD, Zee PC, Wallen EP, et al: Aging alters the phase-resetting properties of a serotonin agonist on hamster circadian rhythmicity, Am J Physiol 268:R293–R298, 1995.
55. Pickard GE, Rea MA: Serotonergic innervation of the hypothalamic suprachiasmatic nucleus and photic regulation of circadian rhythms, Biol Cell 89:513–523, 1997.
56. Mistleberger RE, Rusak B: Circadian rhythms in mammals: formal properties and environmental Influences. In MH Kryger MH, Roth T, Dement WC, editors: Practices of Sleep Medicine, ed 4, New York, 2005, WB Saunders, pp 363–374.
57. Van Reeth O, Sturis J, Byrne MM, et al: Nocturnal exercise phase delays circadian rhythms of melatonin and thyrotropin in normal men, Am J Physiol 266:E964–E974, 1994.
58. Buxton OM, Frank SA, L'Hermite-Baleriaux M, et al: Roles of intensity and duration of nocturnal exercise in causing phase-shifts of human circadian rhythms, Am

J Physiol (Endocrinol & Metab) 273:E536–E542, 1997.
59. Eastman CI, Hoese EK, Youngstedt SD, et al: Phase-shifting human circadian rhythms with exercise during the night shift, Physiol Behav 58:1287–1291, 1995.
60. Barger LK, Wright KP Jr, Hughes RJ, et al: Daily exercise facilitates phase delays of circadian melatonin rhythm in very dim light, Am J Physiol Regul Integr Comp Physiol 286:R1077–R1084, 2004.
61. Baehr EK, Eastman CI, Revelle W, et al: Circadian phase-shifting effects of nocturnal exercise in older compared with young adults, Am J Physiol Regul Integr Comp Physiol 284:R1542–R1550, 2003.
62. Scheer FA, Cajochen C, Turek FW, et al: Melatonin in the Regulation of Sleep and Circadian Rhythms. In Kryger MH, Roth T, Dement WC, editors: Principles and Practices of Sleep Medicine, ed 4, New York, 2005, WB Saunders, pp 395–404.
63. Turek FW, Gillette MU: Melatonin, sleep, and circadian rhythms: rationale for development of specific melatonin agonists, Sleep Med 5:523–532, 2004.
64. Rosenthal NE: Plasma melatonin as a measure of the human clock, J Clin Endocrinol Metab 73:225–226, 1991.
65. Shanahan TL, Czeisler CA: Light exposure induces equivalent phase shifts of the endogenous circadian rhythms of circulating plasma melatonin and core body temperature in men, J Clin Endocrinol Metab 73:227–235, 1991.
66. Duez H, Staels B: The nuclear receptors Rev-erbs and RORs integrate circadian rhythms and metabolism, Diab Vasc Dis Res 5:82–88, 2008.
67. Yin L, Wu N, Curtin JC, et al: Rev-erbalpha, a heme sensor that coordinates metabolic and circadian pathways, Science 318:1786–1789, 2007.
68. Stokkan KA, Yamazaki S, Tei H, et al: Entrainment of the circadian clock in the liver by feeding, Science 291:490–493, 2001.
69. Kohsaka A, Laposky AD, Ramsey KM, et al: High-fat diet disrupts behavioral and molecular circadian rhythms in mice, Cell Metab 6:414–421, 2007.
70. Fuller PM, Lu J, Saper CB: Differential rescue of light- and food-entrainable circadian rhythms, Science 320:1074–1077, 2008.
71. Landry GJ, Yamakawa GR, Webb IC, et al: The dorsomedial hypothalamic nucleus is not necessary for the expression of circadian food-anticipatory activity in rats, J Biol Rhythms 22:467–478, 2007.
72. Turek FW: Staying off the dance floor: when no rhythm is better than bad rhythm, Am J Physiol Regul Integr Comp Physiol 294:R1672–R1674, 2008.
73. Martino TA, Oudit GY, Herzenberg AM, et al: Circadian rhythm disorganization produces profound cardiovascular and renal disease in hamsters, Am J Physiol Regul Integr Comp Physiol 294:R1675–R1683, 2008.
74. Rechtschaffen A, Kales A: A manual of standardized terminology, techniques and scoring system for sleep stages of human subjects, Los Angeles, 1968, UCLA Brain Information Service/Brain Research Institute.
75. Jones BE: Modulation of cortical activation and behavioral arousal by cholinergic and orexinergic systems, Ann N Y Acad Sci 1129:26–34, 2008.
76. Szymusiak R, McGinty D: Hypothalamic regulation of sleep and arousal, Ann N Y Acad Sci 1129:275–286, 2008.
77. Sherin JE, Shiromani PJ, McCarley RW, et al: Activation of ventrolateral preoptic neurons during sleep, Science 271:216–219, 1996.
78. Gallopin T, Fort P, Eggermann E, et al: Identification of sleep-promoting neurons in vitro, Nature 404:992–995, 2000.
79. Gaus SE, Strecker RE, Tate BA, et al: Ventrolateral preoptic nucleus contains sleep-active, galaninergic neurons in multiple mammalian species, Neuroscience 115:285–294, 2002.
80. Saper CB, Chou TC, Scammell TE: The sleep switch: hypothalamic control of sleep and wakefulness, Trends Neurosci 24:726–731, 2001.
81. Sakurai T: Roles of orexin/hypocretin in regulation of sleep/wakefulness and energy homeostasis, Sleep Med Rev 9:231–241, 2005.
82. Aschoff J: On the perception of time during prolonged temporal isolation, Hum Neurobiol 4:41–52, 1985.
83. Aschoff J, von Goetz C, Wildgruber C, et al: Meal timing in humans during isolation without time cues, J Biol Rhythms 1:151–162, 1986.

84. Aschoff J: On the dilatability of subjective time, Persp Biol Med 35:276–280, 1992.

85. Czeisler CA, Weitzman ED, Moore-Ede MC, et al: Human sleep: its duration and organization depends on its circadian phase, Science 210:1264–1267, 1980.

86. Borbely AA: Processes underlying sleep regulation, Horm Res 49:114–117, 1998.

87. Chou TC, Bjorkum AA, Gaus SE, et al: Afferents to the ventrolateral preoptic nucleus, J Neurosci 22:977–990, 2002.

88. Edgar DM, Dement WC, Fuller CA: Effect of SCN lesions on sleep in squirrel monkeys: evidence for opponent processes in sleep-wake regulation, J Neurosci 13:1065–1079, 1993.

89. Mendelson WB, Bergmann BM, Tung A: Baseline and post-deprivation recovery sleep in SCN-lesioned rats, Brain Res 980:185–190, 2003.

90. Aston-Jones G, Chen S, Zhu Y, et al: A neural circuit for circadian regulation of arousal, Nat Neurosci 4:732–738, 2001.

91. Naylor E, Bergmann BM, Krauski K, et al: The circadian clock mutation alters sleep homeostasis in the mouse, J Neurosci 20:8138–8143, 2000.

92. Franken P, Thomason R, Heller HC, et al: A non-circadian role for clock-genes in sleep homeostasis: a strain comparison, BMC Neurosci 8:87, 2007.

93. Viola AU, Archer SN, James LM, et al: PER3 polymorphism predicts sleep structure and waking performance, Curr Biol 17:613–618, 2007.

94. Landolt HP: Sleep homeostasis: a role for adenosine in humans? Biochem Pharmacol 75:2070–2079, 2008.

95. Monk TH, Buysse DJ, Reynolds CF III, et al: Rhythmic versus homeostatic influences on mood, activation and performance in the elderly, J Gerontol 47:221–227, 1991.

96. Monk TH, Buysse DJ, Reynolds CF, et al: Circadian rhythms in human performance and mood under constant conditions, J Sleep Res 6:9–18, 1997.

97. Dijk DJ, Czeisler CA: Paradoxical timing of the circadian rhythm of sleep propensity serves to consolidate sleep and wakefulness in humans, Neurosci Lett 166:63–68, 1994.

98. Boivin DB, Czeisler CA, Dijk DJ, et al: Complex interaction of the sleep-wake cycle and circadian phase modulates mood in healthy subjects, Arch Gen Psychiatry 54:145–152, 1997.

99. Folkard S, Hume KI, Minors DS, et al: Independence of the circadian rhythm in alertness from the sleep-wake cycle, Nature 313:678–679, 1985.

100. Johnson MP, Duffy JF, Dijk DJ, et al: Short-term memory, alertness and performance: a reappraisal of their relationship to body temperature, J Sleep Res 1:24–29, 1992.

101. Akerstedt T, Folkard S: Validation of the S and C components of the three-process model of alertness regulation, Sleep 18:1–6, 1995.

102. Leproult R, Van Reeth O, Byrne MM, et al: Sleepiness, performance and neuroendocrine function during sleep deprivation: Effects of exposure to bright light or exercise, J Biol Rhythms 12:245–258, 1997.

103. Dijk DJ, Duffy JF: Circadian regulation of human sleep and age-related changes in its timing, consolidation and EEG characteristics, Ann Med 31:130–140, 1999.

104. Brandenberger G, Follenius M, Goichot B, et al: Twenty-four hour profiles of plasma renin activity in relation to the sleep-wake cycle, J of Hypertension 12:277–283, 1994.

105. Van Cauter E, Polonsky KS, Scheen AJ: Roles of circadian rhythmicity and sleep in human glucose regulation, Endocr Rev 18:716–738, 1997.

106. Follenius M, Brandenberger G, Simon C, et al: REM sleep in humans begins during decreased secretory activity of the anterior pituitary, Sleep 11:546–555, 1988.

107. Gronfier C, Luthringer R, Follenius M, et al: Temporal link between plasma thyrotropin levels and electroencephalographic activity in man, Neurosci Letters 200:97–100, 1995.

108. Gronfier C, Luthringer R, Follenius M, et al: A quantitative evaluation of the relationships between growth hormone secretion and delta wave electroencephalographic activity during normal sleep and after enrichment in delta waves, Sleep 19:817–824, 1996.

109. Gronfier C, Luthringer R, Follenius M, et al: Temporal relationships between pulsatile cortisol secretion and electroencephalographic activity during sleep in man, Electroencephalogr Clin Neurophysiol 103:405–408, 1997.

110. Spiegel K, Luthringer R, Follenius M, et al: Temporal relationship between prolactin secretion and slow-wave electroencephalographic activity during sleep, Sleep 18:543–548, 1995.

111. Van Cauter E, Spiegel K: Circadian and sleep control of endocrine secretions. In Turek FW, Zee PC, editors: Neurobiology of Sleep and Circadian Rhythms, New York, 1999, Marcel Dekker.

112. Van Cauter E, Copinschi G: Interactions between growth hormone secretion and sleep. In Smith RG, Thorner MO, editors: Human growth hormone secretion: basic and clinical research, Totowa, NJ, 1999, Humana Press, Inc.

113. Kleitman N: Basic rest activity cycle: 22 years later, Sleep 5:311–317, 1982.

114. Chapotot F, Gronfier C, Jouny C, et al: Cortisol secretion is related to electroencephalographic alertness in human subjects during daytime wakefulness, J Clin Endocrinol Metab 83:4263–4268, 1998.

115. Lang DA, Matthews DR, Peto J, et al: Cyclic oscillations of basal plasma glucose and insulin concentrations in human beings, N Engl J Med 301:1023–1027, 1979.

116. O'Meara NM, Sturis J, Blackman JD, et al: Analytical problems in detecting rapid insulin secretory pulses in normal humans, J Clin Endocrinol Metab 27:231–238, 1993.

117. Hucking K, Hamilton-Wessler M, Ellmerer M, et al: Burst-like control of lipolysis by the sympathetic nervous system in vivo, J Clin Invest 111:257–264, 2003.

118. Veldhuis JD, Iranmanesh A, Johnson ML, et al: Twenty-four-hour rhythms in plasma concentrations of adeno-hypophyseal hormones are generated by distinct amplitude and/or frequency modulation of underlying pituitary secretory bursts, J Clin Endocrinol Metab 71:1616–1623, 1990.

119. Veldhuis JD, Johnson ML, Lizarralde G, et al: Rhythmic and nonrhythmic modes of anterior pituitary gland secretion, Chronobiology International 9:371–379, 1992.

120. Van Cauter E, van Coevorden A, Blackman JD: Modulation of neuroendocrine release by sleep and circadian rhythmicity. In Yen S, Vale W, editors: Advances in neuroendocrine regulation of reproduction, Norwell, 1990, Serono Symposia USA, pp 113–122.

121. Polonsky KS, Sturis J, Van Cauter E: Temporal profiles and clinical significance of pulsatile insulin secretion, Horm Res 49:178–184, 1998.

122. Simon C, Brandenberger G, Saini J, et al: Slow oscillations of plasma glucose and insulin secretion rate are amplified during sleep in humans under continuous enteral nutrition, Sleep 17:333–338, 1994.

123. Knobil E, Hotchkiss J: The menstrual cycle and its neuroendocrine control. In Knobil E, Neil JD, editors: The Physiology of Reproduction, New York, 1988, Raven Press, pp 1971–1994.

124. Conn PM, Crowley WF: Gonadotropin-releasing hormone and its analogues, The New England Journal of Medicine 324:93–103, 1991.

125. Sturis J, Scheen AJ, Leproult R, et al: 24-hour glucose profiles during continuous or oscillatory insulin infusion, J Clin Invest 95:1464–1471, 1995.

126. van Coevorden A, Mockel J, Laurent E, et al: Neuroendocrine rhythms and sleep in aging men, Am J Physiol 260:E651–E661, 1991.

127. Czeisler CA, Dumont M, Duffy JF, et al: Association of sleep-wake habits in older people with changes in output of circadian pacemaker, Lancet 340:933–936, 1992.

128. Van Cauter E, Plat L, Leproult R, et al: Alterations of circadian rhythmicity and sleep in aging: endocrine consequences, Horm Res 49:147–152, 1998.

129. Van Cauter E, Leproult R, Plat L: Age-related changes in slow-wave sleep and REM sleep and relationship with growth hormone and cortisol levels in healthy men, JAMA 284:861–868, 2000.

130. Ohayon MM, Carskadon MA, Guilleminault C, et al: Meta-analysis of quantitative sleep parameters from childhood to old age in healthy individuals: developing normative sleep values across the human lifespan, Sleep 27:1255–1273, 2004.

131. Unruh ML, Newman AB, Larive B, et al: The Influence of Age on Changes in Health-Related Quality of Life over Three Years in a Cohort Undergoing Hemodialysis, J Am Geriatr Soc 56:1608–1617, 2008.

132. Vitiello MV, Larsen LH, Moe KE: Age-related sleep change: gender and estrogen effects on the subjective-objective sleep quality relationships of healthy, non-complaining older men and women, J Psychosom Res 56:503–510, 2004.

133. Groeger JA, Zijlstra FR, Dijk DJ: Sleep quantity, sleep difficulties and their perceived consequences in a representative sample of some 2000 British adults, J Sleep Res 13:359–371, 2004.

134. Mourtazaev MS, Kemp B, Zwinderman AH, et al: Age and gender affect different characteristics of slow waves in the sleep EEG, Sleep 18:557–564, 1995.

135. Latta F, Leproult R, Tasali E, et al: Sex differences in delta and alpha EEG activities in healthy older adults, Sleep 28:1525–1534, 2005.

136. Ancoli-Israel S: Sleep and aging: prevalence of disturbed sleep and treatment considerations in older adults, J Clin Psychiatry 66(Suppl 9):24–30; quiz 42–23, 2005.

137. Zee PC, Rosenberg RS, Turek FW: Effects of aging on entrainment and rate of resynchronization of the circadian locomotor activity, Am J Physiol 263:1099–1103, 1992.

138. Monk TH: Aging human circadian rhythms: conventional wisdom may not always be right, J Biol Rhythms 20:366–374, 2005.

139. Pittendrigh CS, Daan S: Circadian oscillations in rodents: a systematic increase of their frequency with age, Science 186:548–550, 1974.

140. Morin LP: Age-related changes in hamster circadian period, entrainment and rhythm splitting, J Biol Rhythms 3:237–248, 1988.

141. Yamazaki S, Straume M, Tei H, et al: Effects of aging on central and peripheral mammalian clocks, Proc Natl Acad Sci U S A 99:10801–10806, 2002.

142. Dijk DJ, Duffy JF, Riel E, et al: Ageing and the circadian and homeostatic regulation of human sleep during forced desynchrony of rest, melatonin and temperature rhythms, J Physiol 516(Pt 2):611–627, 1999.

143. Duffy JF, Czeisler CA: Age-related change in the relationship between circadian period, circadian phase, and diurnal preference in humans, Neurosci Lett 318:117–120, 2002.

144. Zhang Y, Kornhauser JM, Zee PC, et al: Effects of aging on light-induced phase-shifting of circadian behavioral rhythms, Fos expression, and Creb phosphorylation in the hamster suprachiasmatic nucleus, Neuroscience 70:951–961, 1996.

145. Van Reeth O, Zhang Y, Zee PC, et al: Aging alters feedback effects of the activity-rest cycle in the circadian clock, Am J Physiol 263:R981–R986, 1992.

146. Van Reeth O, Zhang Y, Reddy A, et al: Aging alters the entraining effects of an activity-inducing stimulus on the circadian clock, Brain Res 607:286–292, 1993.

147. Van Reeth O, Zhang Y, Zee PC, et al: Grafting fetal suprachiasmatic nuclei in the hypothalamus of old hamsters restores responsiveness of the circadian clock to a phase shifting stimulus, Brain Res 643:338–342, 1994.

148. Campbell SS, Kripke DF, Gillin JC, et al: Exposure to light in healthy elderly subjects and Alzheimer's patients, Physiol Behav 42:141–144, 1988.

149. Ehlers CL, Frank E, Kupfer DJ: Social zeitgebers and biological rhythms, Arch Gen Psychiatry 45:948–952, 1988.

150. Ancoli-Israel S, Kripke DF, Jones DW, et al: 24-hour sleep and light rhythms in nursing home patients. Sleep Res 20A:410, 1991.

151. Brainard GC, Rollag MD, Hanifin JP: Photic regulation of melatonin in humans: ocular and neural signal transduction, J Biol Rhythms 12:537–546, 1997.

152. Campbell SS, Dawson D, Anderson MW: Alleviation of sleep maintenance insomnia with timed exposure to bright light, J Am Geriatric Soc 41:829–836, 1993.

153. Mishima K, Okawa M, Shimizu T, et al: Diminished melatonin secretion in the elderly caused by insufficient environmental illumination, J Clin Endocrinol Metab 86:129–134, 2001.

154. Benloucif S, Green K, L'Hermite-Baleriaux M, et al: Responsiveness of the aging circadian clock to light, Neurobiol Aging 27:1870–1879, 2006.

155. Veldhuis JD: Mechanisms and biological significance of pulsatile hormone secretion. Symposium proceedings.

London, United Kingdom, 2–4 March 1999, Novartis Found Symp 227:1–4, 2000.
156. Halberg F, Tong YL, Johnson EA: Circadian system phase: an aspect of temporal morphology; procedures and illustrative examples. In Cellular aspects of biorhythms. Berlin, 1967, Springer-Verlag, pp 20–48.
157. Cleveland WS: Robust locally weighted regression and smoothing scatterplots, J Am Stat Assoc 74:829–836, 1979.
158. Van Cauter E. Method for characterization of 24-h temporal variation of blood constituents, Am J Physiol 237:E255–E264, 1979.
159. Van Cauter E. Computer-assisted analysis of endocrine rhythms. In Rodbard D, Forti G, editors: Computers in Endocrinology, New York, 1990, Raven Press, pp 59–70.
160. Polonsky KS, Licinio-Paixao J, Given BD, et al: Use of biosynthetic human C-peptide in the measurement of insulin secretion rates in normal volunteers and type I diabetic patients, J Clin Invest 77:98–105, 1986.
161. De Nicolao G, Rocchetti M: Stable and efficient techniques for the deconvolution of hormone time series. In Guardabasso V, Rodbard D, Forti G, editors: Computers in Endocrinology: Recent Advances, New York, 1990, Raven Press, pp 83–91.
162. Veldhuis JD, Johnson ML: A review and appraisal of deconvolution methods to evaluate in vivo neuroendocrine secretory events, J Neuroendocrinol 2:755–771, 1990.
163. Sturis J, Polonsky KS, Shapiro ET, et al: Abnormalities in the ultradian oscillations of insulin secretion and glucose levels in type 2 (non-insulin-dependent) diabetic patients, Diabetologia 35:681–689, 1992.
164. Pincus SM, Keefe DL: Quantification of hormone pulsatility via an approximate entropy algorithm, Am J Physiol 262:E741–E754, 1992.
165. Pincus SM: Orderliness of hormone release, Novartis Found Symp 227:82–96; discussion 96–104, 2000.
166. Urban RJ, Evans WS, Rogol AD, et al: Contemporary aspects of discrete peak-detection algorithms. I. The paradigm of the luteinizing hormone pulse signal in men, Endocr Rev 9:3–37, 1988.
167. Urban RJ, Kaiser DL, Van Cauter E, et al: Comparative assessment of objective pulse detection algorithms. II. Studies in men, Am J Physiol 254:E113–E119, 1988.
168. Buijs RM, Wortel J, Van Heerikhuize JJ, et al: Anatomical and functional demonstration of a multisynaptic suprachiasmatic nucleus adrenal (cortex) pathway, Eur J Neurosci 11:1535–1544, 1999.
169. Lemos DR, Downs JL, Urbanski HF: Twenty-four-hour rhythmic gene expression in the rhesus macaque adrenal gland, Mol Endocrinol 20:1164–1176, 2006.
170. Torres-Farfan C, Rocco V, Monso C, et al: Maternal melatonin effects on clock gene expression in a nonhuman primate fetus, Endocrinology 147:4618–4626, 2006.
171. Valenzuela FJ, Torres-Farfan C, Richter HG, et al: Clock gene expression in adult primate suprachiasmatic nuclei and adrenal: is the adrenal a peripheral clock responsive to melatonin? Endocrinology 149: 1454–1461, 2008.
172. Oster H, Damerow S, Kiessling S, et al: The circadian rhythm of glucocorticoids is regulated by a gating mechanism residing in the adrenal cortical clock, Cell Metab 4:163–173, 2006.
173. Veldhuis JD, Iranmanesh A, Johnson ML, et al: Amplitude, but not frequency, modulation of adrenocorticotropin secretory bursts gives rise to the nyctohemeral rhythm of the corticotropic axis in man, J Clin Endocrinol Metab 71:452–463, 1989.
174. Van Cauter E, Honinckx E: Pulsatility of Pituitary Hormones, Exp Brain Res Suppl 12:41–60, 1985.
175. Lejeune-Lenain C, Van Cauter E, Desir D, et al: Control of circadian and episodic variations of adrenal androgens secretion in man, J Endocrinol Invest 10:267–276, 1987.
176. Weitzman ED, Zimmerman JC, Czeisler CA, et al: Cortisol secretion is inhibited during sleep in normal man, J Clin Endocrinol Metab 56:352–358, 1983.
177. Born J, Muth S, Fehm HL: The significance of sleep onset and slow wave sleep for nocturnal release of growth hormone (GH) and cortisol, Psychoneuroendocrinology 13:233–243, 1988.
178. Van Cauter E, Blackman JD, Roland D, et al: Modulation of glucose regulation and insulin secretion by circadian rhythmicity and sleep, J Clin Invest 88:934–942, 1991.
179. Weibel L, Follenius M, Spiegel K, et al: Comparative effect of night and daytime sleep on the 24-hour cortisol secretory profile, Sleep 18:549–556, 1995.
180. Follenius M, Brandenberger G, Bardasept J, et al: Nocturnal cortisol release in relation to sleep structure, Sleep 15:21–27, 1992.
181. Spath-Schwalbe E, Gofferje M, Kern W, et al: Sleep disruption alters nocturnal ACTH and cortisol secretory patterns, Biol Psychiatry 29:575–584, 1991.
182. Pruessner JC, Wolf OT, Hellhammer DH, et al: Free cortisol levels after awakening: a reliable biological marker for the assessment of adrenocortical activity, Life Sci 61:2539–2549, 1997.
183. Caufriez A, Moreno-Reyes R, Leproult R, et al: Immediate effects of an 8-h advance shift of the rest-activity cycle on 24-h profiles of cortisol, Am J Physiol Endocrinol Metab 282:E1147–E1153, 2002.
184. Ekstedt M, Akerstedt T, Soderstrom M: Microarousals during sleep are associated with increased levels of lipids, cortisol, and blood pressure, Psychosom Med 66:925–931, 2004.
185. Vgontzas AN, Zoumakis M, Bixler EO, et al: Impaired nighttime sleep in healthy old versus young adults is associated with elevated plasma interleukin-6 and cortisol levels: physiologic and therapeutic implications, J Clin Endocrinol Metab 88:2087–2095, 2003.
186. Vgontzas AN, Bixler EO, Lin HM, et al: Chronic insomnia is associated with nyctohemeral activation of the hypothalamic-pituitary-adrenal axis: clinical implications, J Clin Endocrinol Metab 86:3787–3794, 2001.
187. Scheer FA, Buijs RM: Light affects morning salivary cortisol in humans, J Clin Endocrinol Metab 84:3395–3398, 1999.
188. Leproult R, Colecchia EF, L'Hermite-Baleriaux M, et al: Transition from dim to bright light in the morning induces an immediate elevation of cortisol levels, J Clin Endocrinol Metab 86:151–157, 2001.
189. Ruger M, Gordijn MC, Beersma DG, et al: Time-of-day-dependent effects of bright light exposure on human psychophysiology: comparison of daytime and nighttime exposure, Am J Physiol Regul Integr Comp Physiol 290:R1413–R1420, 2006.
190. Linkowski P, Van Onderbergen A, Kerkhofs M, et al: Twin study of the 24-h cortisol profile: evidence for genetic control of the human circadian clock, Am J Physiol 264:E173–E181, 1993.
191. Van Cauter E, Shapiro ET, Tillil H, et al: Circadian modulation of glucose and insulin responses to meals: relationship to cortisol rhythm, Am J Physiol 262:E467–E475, 1992.
192. Born J, Hansen K, Marshall L, et al: Timing the end of nocturnal sleep, Nature 397:29–30, 1999.
193. Leproult R, Copinschi G, Buxton O, et al: Sleep loss results in an elevation of cortisol levels the next evening, Sleep 20:865–870, 1997.
194. Spiegel K, Leproult R, Van Cauter E: Impact of sleep debt on metabolic and endocrine function, Lancet 354:1435–1439, 1999.
195. Sherman B, Wysham C, Pfohl B: Age-related changes in the circadian rhythm of plasma cortisol in man, J Clin Endocrinol Metab 61:439–443, 1985.
196. Van Cauter E, Leproult R, Kupfer DJ: Effects of gender and age on the levels and circadian rhythmicity of plasma cortisol, J Clin Endocrinol Metab 81:2468–2473, 1996.
197. McEwen BS, Stellar E: Stress and the individual, Arch Intern Med 153:2093–2101, 1993.
198. McEwen B: Protective and damaging effects of stress mediators, N Engl J Med 338:171–179, 1998.
199. Dallman MF, Strack AL, Akana SF, et al: Feast and famine: Critical role of glucocorticoids with insulin in daily energy flow, Frontiers in Neuroendocrinology 14:303–347, 1993.
200. Plat L, Féry F, L'Hermite-Balériaux M, et al: Metabolic effects of short-term physiological elevations of plasma cortisol are more pronounced in the evening than in the morning, J Clin Endocrinol Metab 84:3082–3092, 1999.
201. Dennison E, Hindmarsh P, Fall C, et al: Profiles of endogenous circulating cortisol and bone mineral density in healthy elderly men, J Clin Endocrinol Metab 84:3058–3063, 1999.
202. Magiakou MA, Mastorakos G, Rabin D, et al: The maternal hypothalamic-pituitary-adrenal axis in the third trimester of human pregnancy, Clin Endocrinol (Oxf) 44:419–428, 1996.
203. Rosman PM, Farag A, Benn R, et al: Modulation of pituitary-adrenal function: decreased secretory episodes and blunted circadian rhythmicity in patients with alcoholic liver disease, J Clin Endocrinol Metab 55:709–717, 1981.
204. Boyar RM, Hellman LD, Roffwarg H, et al: Cortisol secretion and metabolism in anorexia nervosa, N Engl J Med 296:190–193, 1977.
205. Kok P, Kok SW, Buijs MM, et al: Enhanced circadian ACTH release in obese premenopausal women: reversal by short-term acipimox treatment, Am J Physiol Endocrinol Metab 287:E848–E856, 2004.
206. Iranmanesh A, Lizarralde G, Johnson ML, et al: Dynamics of 24-hour endogenous cortisol secretion and clearance in primary hypothyroidism assessed before and after partial thyroid hormone replacement, J Clin Endocrinol Metab 70:155–161, 1990.
207. Gallagher TF, Hellman L, Finkelstein J, et al: Hyperthyroidism and cortisol secretion in man, J Clin Endocrinol Metab 34:919–927, 1972.
208. Van Cauter E, Refetoff S: Evidence for two subtypes of Cushing's disease based on the analysis of episodic cortisol secretion, N Engl J Med 312:1343–1344, 1985.
209. Roelfsema F, Pincus SM, Veldhuis JD: Patients with Cushing's disease secrete adrenocorticotropin and cortisol jointly more asynchronously than healthy subjects, J Clin Endocrinol Metab 83:688–692, 1998.
210. van Aken MO, Pereira AM, van Thiel SW, et al: Irregular and frequent cortisol secretory episodes with preserved diurnal rhythmicity in primary adrenal Cushing's syndrome, J Clin Endocrinol Metab 90: 1570–1577, 2005.
211. Linkowski P, Mendlewicz J, Leclercq R, et al: The 24-hour profile of adrenocorticotropin and cortisol in major depressive illness, J Clin Endocrinol Metab 61:429–438, 1985.
212. Rubin RT, Poland RE, Lesser IM, et al: Neuroendocrine aspects of primary endogenous depression: I. Cortisol secretory dynamics in patients and matched controls, Arch Gen Psychiatry 44:328–336, 1987.
213. Sachar ED: Twenty-four-hour cortisol secretory patterns in depressed and manic patients. In Gispen WH, Van Wimersma Greidanus TB, Bohus B, De Wied D, editors: Hormones, homeostasis and the brain prog in brain research, vol 42, Amsterdam, 1975, Elsevier, pp 81–91.
214. Linkowski P, Mendlewicz J, Kerkhofs M, et al: 24-hour profiles of adrenocorticotropin, cortisol, and growth hormone in major depressive illness: effect of antidepressant treatment, J Clin Endocrinol Metab 65:141–152, 1987.
215. Yehuda R, Teicher MH, Trestman RL, et al: Cortisol regulation in posttraumatic stress disorder and major depression: a chronobiological analysis, Biol Psychiatry 15:79–88, 1996.
216. Yehuda R: Hypothalamic-pituitary-adrenal alterations in PTSD: are they relevant to understanding cortisol alterations in cancer? Brain Behav Immun 17(Suppl 1):S73–S83, 2003.
217. Bremner JD, Vythilingam M, Anderson G, et al: Assessment of the hypothalamic-pituitary-adrenal axis over a 24-hour diurnal period and in response to neuroendocrine challenges in women with and without childhood sexual abuse and posttraumatic stress disorder, Biol Psychiatry 54:710–718, 2003.
218. Crofford LJ, Young EA, Engleberg NC, et al: Basal circadian and pulsatile ACTH and cortisol secretion in patients with fibromyalgia and/or chronic fatigue syndrome, Brain Behav Immun 18:314–325, 2004.
219. Klerman EB, Goldenberg DL, Brown EN, et al: Circadian rhythms of women with fibromyalgia, J Clin Endocrinol Metab 86:1034–1039, 2001.
220. Muccioli G, Tschop M, Papotti M, et al: Neuroendocrine and peripheral activities of ghrelin: implications in metabolism and obesity, Eur J Pharmacol 440:235–254, 2002.
221. van der Lely AJ, Tschop M, Heiman ML, et al: Biological, physiological, pathophysiological, and pharmacological aspects of ghrelin, Endocr Rev 25:426–457, 2004.
222. Van Cauter E, Plat L, Copinschi G: Interrelations between sleep and the somatotropic axis, Sleep 21:553–566, 1998.

223. Mendlewicz J, Linkowski P, Kerkhofs M, et al: Genetic control of 24-hour growth hormone secretion in man: a twin study, J Clin Endocrinol Metab 84:856–862, 1999.
224. Ho KY, Evans WS, Blizzard RM, et al: Effects of sex and age on the 24-hour profile of growth hormone secretion in man: importance of endogenous estradiol concentrations, J Clin Endocrinol Metab 64:51–58, 1987.
225. Shah N, Evans WS, Veldhuis JD: Actions of estrogen on pulsatile, nyctohemeral, and entropic modes of growth hormone secretion, Am J Physiol 276:R1351–R1358, 1999.
226. Caufriez A, Leproult R, L'Hermite-Balériaux M, et al: A potential role of endogenous progesterone in modulation of GH, prolactin and thyrotropin secretion during normal menstrual cycle, Clin Endocrinol (Oxf) 71: 535–542, 2009.
227. Weibel L, Spiegel K, Gronfier C, et al: Twenty-four-hour melatonin and core body temperature rhythms: their adaptation in night workers, Am J Physiol 272:R948–R954, 1997.
228. Van Cauter E, Kerkhofs M, Caufriez A, et al: A quantitative estimation of GH secretion in normal man: reproducibility and relation to sleep and time of day, J Clin Endocrinol Metab 74:1441–1450, 1992.
229. Holl RW, Hartmann ML, Veldhuis JD, et al: Thirty-second sampling of plasma growth hormone in man: correlation with sleep stages, J Clin Endocrinol Metab 72:854–861, 1991.
230. Vgontzas AN, Mastorakos G, Bixler EO, et al: Sleep deprivation effects on the activity of the hypothalamic-pituitary-adrenal and growth axes: potential clinical implications, Clin Endocrinol (Oxf) 51:205–215, 1999.
231. Obal F Jr, Krueger JM: Biochemical regulation of non-rapid-eye-movement sleep, Front Biosci 8:d520–d550, 2003.
232. Ocampo-Lim B, Guo W, DeMott Friberg R, et al: Nocturnal growth hormone (GH) secretion is eliminated by infusion of GH-releasing hormone antagonist, J Clin Endocrinol Metab 81:4396–4399, 1996.
233. Van Cauter E, Plat L, Scharf M, et al: Simultaneous stimulation of slow-wave sleep and growth hormone secretion by gamma-hydroxybutyrate in normal young men, J Clin Invest 100:745–753, 1997.
234. Van Cauter E, Caufriez A, Kerkhofs M, et al: Sleep, awakenings and insulin-like growth factor I modulate the growth hormone secretory response to growth hormone-releasing hormone, J Clin Endocrinol Metab 74:1451–1459, 1992.
235. Jaffe C, Turgeon D, DeMott Friberg R, et al: Nocturnal augmentation of growth hormone (GH) secretion is preserved during repetitive bolus administration of GH-releasing hormone: potential involvement of endogenous somatostatin—A clinical research center study, J Clin Endocrinol Metab 80:3321–3326, 1995.
236. Dzaja A, Dalal MA, Himmerich H, et al: Sleep enhances nocturnal plasma ghrelin levels in healthy subjects, Am J Physiol Endocrinol Metab 286:E963–E967, 2004.
237. Nass R, Farhy LS, Liu J, et al: Evidence for acyl-ghrelin modulation of growth hormone release in the fed state, J Clin Endocrinol Metab 93:1988–1994, 2008.
238. Steiger A, Herth T, Holsboer F: Sleep-electroencephalography and the secretion of cortisol and growth hormone in normal controls, Acta Endocrinol 116:36–42, 1987.
239. Spiegel K, Leproult R, Colecchia EF, et al: Adaptation of the 24-h growth hormone profile to a state of sleep debt, Am J Physiol Regul Integr Comp Physiol 279:R874–R883, 2000.
240. Brandenberger G, Gronfier C, Chapotot F, et al: Effect of sleep deprivation on overall 24 h growth-hormone secretion, Lancet 356:1408, 2000.
241. Vermeulen A: Nyctohemeral growth hormone profiles in young and aged men: correlation with somatomedin-C levels, J Clin Endocrinol Metab 64:884–888, 1987.
242. Veldhuis J, Liem A, South S, et al: Differential impact of age, sex steroid hormones, and obesity on basal versus pulsatile growth hormone secretion in men as assessed in an ultrasensitive chemiluminescence assay, J Clin Endocrinol Metab 80:3209–3222, 1995.
243. Veldhuis JD, Iranmanesh A, Weltman A: Elements in the pathophysiology of diminished growth hormone (GH) secretion in aging humans, Endocrine 7:41–48, 1997.
244. Martin FC, Yeo AL, Sonksen PH: Growth hormone secretion in the elderly: ageing and the somatopause, Baillieres Clin Endocrinol Metab 11:223–250, 1997.
245. Caufriez A, Frankenne F, Hennen G, et al: Regulation of maternal IGF-I by placental GH in normal and abnormal human pregnancies, Am J Physiol 265:E572–E577, 1993.
246. Eriksson L, Frankenne F, Eden S, et al: Growth hormone 24-h serum profiles during pregnancy–lack of pulsatility for the secretion of the placental variant, Br J Obstet Gynaecol 96:949–953, 1989.
247. Copinschi G, De Laet MH, Brion JP, et al: Simultaneous study of cortisol, GH and PRL circadian variations of hourly integrated concentrations in normal and obese subjects, Clin Endocrinol 9:15–26, 1978.
248. Stoving RK, Veldhuis JD, Flyvbjerg A, et al: Jointly amplified basal and pulsatile growth hormone (GH) secretion and increased process irregularity in women with anorexia nervosa: indirect evidence for disruption of feedback regulation within the GH-insulin-like growth factor I axis, J Clin Endocrinol Metab 84:2056–2063, 1999.
249. Edge JA, Dunger DB, Matthews DR, et al: Increased overnight growth hormone concentrations in diabetic compared with normal adolescents, J Clin Endocrinol Metab 71:1356–1362, 1990.
250. Laughlin GA, Dominguez CE, Yen SS: Nutritional and endocrine-metabolic aberrations in women with functional hypothalamic amenorrhea, J Clin Endocrinol Metab 83:25–32, 1998.
251. Morales AJ, Laughlin GA, Butzow T, et al: Insulin, somatotropic, and luteinizing hormone axes in lean and obese women with polycystic ovary syndrome: common and distinct features, J Clin Endocrinol Metab 81:2854–2864, 1996.
252. Iranmanesh A, Lizarralde G, Johnson ML, et al: Nature of altered growth hormone secretion in hyperthyroidism, J Clin Endocrinol Metab 72:108–115, 1991.
253. Mendlewicz J, Linkowski P, Kerkhofs M, et al: Diurnal hypersecretion of growth hormone in depression, J Clin Endocrinol Metab 60:505–512, 1985.
254. Veldman RG, Frolich M, Pincus SM, et al: Growth hormone and prolactin are secreted more irregularly in patients with Cushing's disease, Clin Endocrinol (Oxf) 52:625–632, 2000.
255. Hartman ML, Veldhuis JD, Vance ML, et al: Somatotropin pulse frequency and basal concentrations are increased in acromegaly and are reduced by successful therapy, J Clin Endocrinol Metab 70:1375–1384, 1990.
256. Hartman ML, Pincus SM, Johnson ML, et al: Enhanced basal and disorderly growth hormone secretion distinguish acromegalic from normal pulsatile growth hormone release, J Clin Invest 94:1277–1288, 1994.
257. van den Berg G, Pincus SM, Frolich M, et al: Reduced disorderliness of growth hormone release in biochemically inactive acromegaly after pituitary surgery, Eur J Endocrinol 138:164–169, 1998.
258. Spiegel K, Follenius M, Simon C, et al: Prolactin secretion and sleep, Sleep 17:20–27, 1994.
259. Waldstreicher J, Duffy JF, Brown EN, et al: Gender differences in the temporal organization of prolactin (PRL) secretion: evidence fort a sleep-independent circadian rhythm of circulating PRL levels—A Clinical Research Center study, J Clin Endocrinol Metab 81:1483–1487, 1996.
260. Katznelson L, Riskind PN, Saxe VC, et al: Prolactin pulsatile characteristics in postmenopausal women, J Clin Endocrinol Metab 83:761–764, 1998.
261. Linkowski P, Spiegel K, Kerkhofs M, et al: Genetic and environmental influences on prolactin secretion during wake and during sleep, Am J Physiol 274:E909–E919, 1998.
262. Van Cauter E, Refetoff S: Multifactorial control of the 24-hour secretory profiles of pituitary hormones, J Endocrinol Invest 8:381–391, 1985.
263. Desir D, Van Cauter E, L'Hermite M, et al: Effects of "jet lag" on hormonal patterns. III. Demonstration of an intrinsic circadian rhythmicity in plasma prolactin, J Clin Endocrinol Metab 55:849–857, 1982.
264. Copinschi G, Van Onderbergen A, L'Hermite-Balériaux M, et al: Effects of the short-acting benzodiazepine triazolam, taken at bedtime, on circadian and sleep-related hormonal profiles in normal men, Sleep 13:232–244, 1990.
265. Copinschi G, Akseki E, Moreno-Reyes R, et al: Effects of bedtime administration of zolpidem on circadian and sleep-related hormonal profiles in normal women, Sleep 18:417–424, 1995.
266. Greenspan SL, Klibanski A, Rowe JW, et al: Age alters pulsatile prolactin release: influence of dopaminergic inhibition, Am J Physiol 258:E799–E804, 1990.
267. Tay CC, Glasier AF, McNeilly AS: Twenty-four hour patterns of prolactin secretion during lactation and the relationship to suckling and the resumption of fertility in breast-feeding women, Hum Reprod 11:950–955, 1996.
268. Caufriez A, Désir D, Szyper M, et al: Prolactin secretion in Cushing's disease, J Clin Endocrinol Metab 53:843–846, 1981.
269. Iranmanesh A, Veldhuis JD, Carlsen EC, et al: Attenuated pulsatile release of prolactin in men with insulin-dependent diabetes mellitus, J Clin Endocrinol Metab 71:73–78, 1990.
270. Kok P, Roelfsema F, Frolich M, et al: Prolactin release is enhanced in proportion to excess visceral fat in obese women, J Clin Endocrinol Metab 89:4445–4449, 2004.
271. Groote Veldman R, van den Berg G, Pincus SM, et al: Increased episodic release and disorderliness of prolactin secretion in both micro- and macroprolactinomas, Eur J Endocrinol 140:192–200, 1999.
272. Veldman RG, Frolich M, Pincus SM, et al: Basal, pulsatile, entropic, and 24-hour rhythmic features of secondary hyperprolactinemia due to functional pituitary stalk disconnection mimic tumoral (primary) hyperprolactinemia, J Clin Endocrinol Metab 86:1562–1567, 2001.
273. Boyar RM, Kapen S, Finkelstein JW, et al: Hypothalamic-pituitary function in diverse hyperprolactinemic states, J Clin Invest 53:1588–1598, 1974.
274. Spratt DI, O'Dea LL, Schoenfeld D, et al: Neuroendocrine-gonadal axis in men: frequent sampling of LH, FSH and testosterone, Am J Physiol 254:E658–E666, 1988.
275. Lanfranco F, Bonelli L, Baldi M, et al: Acylated ghrelin inhibits spontaneous luteinizing hormone pulsatility and responsiveness to naloxone but not that to gonadotropin-releasing hormone in young men: evidence for a central inhibitory action of ghrelin on the gonadal axis, J Clin Endocrinol Metab 93:3633–3639, 2008.
276. Fehm HL, Clausing J, Kern W, et al: Sleep-associated augmentation and synchronization of luteinizing hormone pulses in adult men, Neuroendocrinology 54:192–195, 1991.
277. Bremner WJ, Vitiello MV, Prinz PN: Loss of circadian rhythmicity in blood testosterone levels with aging in normal men, J Clin Endocrinol Metab 56:1278–1280, 1983.
278. Luboshitzky R, Zabari Z, Shen-Orr Z, et al: Disruption of the nocturnal testosterone rhythm by sleep fragmentation in normal men, J Clin Endocrinol Metab 86:1134–1139, 2001.
279. Axelsson J, Ingre M, Akerstedt T, et al: Effects of acutely displaced sleep on testosterone, J Clin Endocrinol Metab 90:4530–4535, 2005.
280. Carlsen E, Olsson C, Petersen JH, et al: Diurnal rhythm in serum levels of inhibin B in normal men: relation to testicular steroids and gonadotropins, J Clin Endocrinol Metab 84:1664–1669, 1999.
281. Lejeune H, Dechaud H, Pugeat M: Contribution of bioavailable testosterone assay for the diagnosis of androgen deficiency in elderly men, Ann Endocrinol (Paris) 64:117–125, 2003.
282. Tenover JS, Matsumoto AM, Clifton DK, et al: Age-related alterations in the circadian rhythms of pulsatile luteinizing hormone and testosterone secretion in healthy men. J of Gerontology 43:M163–M169, 1988.
283. Penev PD: Association between sleep and morning testosterone levels in older men, Sleep 30:427–432, 2007.
284. Mulligan T, Iranmanesh A, Gheorghiu S, et al: Amplified nocturnal luteinizing hormone (LH) secretory burst frequency with selective attenuation of pulsatile (but not basal) testosterone secretion in healthy aged men: possible Leydig cell desensitization to endogenous LH signaling–a clinical research center study, J Clin Endocrinol Metab 80:3025–3031, 1995.
285. Vermeulen A, Deslypere JP, Kaufman JM: Influence of antiopioids on luteinizing hormone pulsatility in aging men, J Clin Endocrinol Metab 68:68–72, 1989.

286. Veldhuis JD, Urban RJ, Lizarralde G, et al: Attenuation of luteinizing hormone secretory burst amplitude as a proximate basis for the hypoandrogenism of healthy aging in men, J Clin Endocrinol Metab 75:52–58, 1992.
287. Veldhuis JD, Iranmanesh A, Demers LM, et al: Joint basal and pulsatile hypersecretory mechanisms drive the monotropic follicle-stimulating hormone (FSH) elevation in healthy older men: concurrent preservation of the orderliness of the FSH release process: a general clinical research center study, J Clin Endocrinol Metab 84:3506–3514, 1999.
288. Pincus SM, Mulligan T, Iranmanesh A, et al: Older males secrete luteinizing hormone and testosterone more irregularly, and jointly more asynchronously, than younger males, Proc Natl Acad Sci U S A 93:14100–14105, 1996.
289. Backstrom CT, McNeilly AS, Leask RM, et al: Pulsatile secretion of LH, FSH, prolactin, oestradiol and progesterone during the human menstrual cycle. Clin Endocrinol (Oxf) 17:29–42, 1982.
290. Filicori M, Santoro N, Merriam GR, et al: Characterization of the physiological pattern of episodic gonadotropin secretion throughout the menstrual cycle, J Clin Endocrinol Metab 62:1136–1144, 1986.
291. Hall JE, Sullivan JP, Richardson GS: Brief wake episodes modulate sleep-inhibited luteinizing hormone secretion in the early follicular phase, J Clin Endocrinol Metab 90:2050–2055, 2005.
292. Reame NE, Kelche RP, Beitins IZ, et al: Age effects of follicle-stimulating hormone and pulsatile luteinizing hormone secretion across the menstrual cycle of premenopausal women, J Clin Endocrinol Metab 81:1512–1518, 1996.
293. Turek FW, Van Cauter E: Rhythms in Reproduction. In Knobil E, Neil JD, editors: The Physiology of Reproduction, New York, 1993, Raven Press, pp 487–540.
294. Bergendahl M, Aloi JA, Iranmanesh A, et al: Fasting suppresses pulsatile luteinizing hormone (LH) secretion and enhances orderliness of LH release in young but not older men, J Clin Endocrinol Metab 83:1967–1975, 1998.
295. Spratt DI, Carr DB, Merriam GR, et al: The spectrum of abnormal patterns of gonadotropin-releasing hormone secretion in men with idiopathic hypogonadotropic hypogonadism: clinical and laboratory correlations, J Clin Endocrinol Metab 64:283–291, 1987.
296. Hangaard J, Andersen M, Grodum E, et al: Pulsatile luteinizing hormone secretion in patients with Addison's disease. Impact of glucocorticoid substitution, J Clin Endocrinol Metab 83:736–743, 1998.
297. Lopez-Alvarenga JC, Zarinan T, Olivares A, et al: Poorly controlled type I diabetes mellitus in young men selectively suppresses luteinizing hormone secretory burst mass, J Clin Endocrinol Metab 87:5507–5515, 2002.
298. Brabant G, Prank K, Ranft U, et al: Physiological regulation of circadian and pulsatile thyrotropin secretion in normal man and woman, J Clin Endocrinol Metab 70:403–409, 1990.
299. Parker DC, Rossman LG, Pekary AE, et al: Effect of 64-hour sleep deprivation on the circadian waveform of thyrotropin (TSH): further evidence of sleep-related inhibition of TSH release, J Clin Endocrinol Metab 64:157–161, 1987.
300. Hirschfeld U, Moreno-Reyes R, Akseki E, et al: Progressive elevation of plasma thyrotropin during adaptation to simulated jet lag: effects of treatment with bright light or zolpidem, J Clin Endocrinol Metab 81:3270–3277, 1996.
301. Goichot B, Brandenberger G, Saini J, et al: Nocturnal plasma thyrotropin variations are related to slow-wave sleep, J Sleep Res 1:186–190, 1992.
302. Russell W, Harrison RF, Smith N, et al: Free triiodothyronine has a distinct circadian rhythm that is delayed but parallels thyrotropin levels, J Clin Endocrinol Metab 93:2300–2306, 2008.
303. Allan JS, Czeisler CA: Persistence of the circadian thyrotropin rhythm under constant conditions and after light-induced shifts of circadian phase. Journal of Clinical Endocrinology and Metabolism 79:508–512, 1994.
304. Gary KA, Winokur A, Douglas SD, et al: Total sleep deprivation and the thyroid axis: effects of sleep and waking activity, Aviat Space Environ Med 67:513–519, 1996.
305. Romijn JA, Wiersinga WM: Decreased nocturnal surge of thyrotropin in nonthyroidal illness. J Clin Endocrinol Metabolism 70:35–42, 1990.
306. Bartalena F, Martino E, Petrini L, et al: The nocturnal serum thyrotropin surge is abolished in patients with ACTH-dependent or ACTH-independent Cushing's syndrome, J Clin Endocrinol Metab 72:1195–1199, 1991.
307. Caron PJ, Nieman LK, Rose SR, et al: Deficient nocturnal surge of thyrotropin in central hypothyroidism, J Clin Endocrinol Metab 62:960–964, 1986.
308. Samuels MH, Lillehei K, Kleinschmidt-Demasters BK, et al: Patterns of pulsatile pituitary glycoprotein secretion in central hypothyroidism and hypogonadism, J Clin Endocrinol Metab 70:391–395, 1990.
309. Bartalena L, Cossu E, Grasso L, et al: Relationship between nocturnal serum thyrotropin peak and metabolic control in diabetic patients, J Clin Endocrinol Metab 76:983–987, 1993.
310. Kok P, Roelfsema F, Langendonk JG, et al: High circulating thyrotropin levels in obese women are reduced after body weight loss induced by caloric restriction, J Clin Endocrinol Metab 90:4659–4663, 2005.
311. el-Hajj Fuleihan G, Klerman EB, Brown EN, et al: The parathyroid hormone circadian rhythm is truly endogenous—a general clinical research center study, J Clin Endocrinol Metab 82:281–286, 1997.
312. Kripke DF, Lavie P, Parker D, et al: Plasma parathyroid hormone and calcium are related to sleep stage cycles, J Clin Endocrinol Metab 47:1021–1027, 1978.
313. Logue FC, Fraser WD, O'Reilly DS, et al: Sleep shift dissociates the nocturnal peaks of parathyroid hormone (1–84), nephrogenous cyclic adenosine monophosphate, and prolactin in normal men, J Clin Endocrinol Metab 75:25–29, 1992.
314. Fraser WD, Logue FC, Christie JP, et al: Alteration of the circadian rhythm of intact parathyroid hormone following a 96-hour fast, Clin Endocrinol (Oxf) 40:523–528, 1994.
315. Fraser WD, Logue FC, Christie JP, et al: Alteration of the circadian rhythm of intact parathyroid hormone and serum phosphate in women with established postmenopausal osteoporosis, Osteoporos Int 8:121–126, 1998.
316. Lobaugh B, Neelon FA, Oyama H, et al: Circadian rhythms for calcium, inorganic phosphorus, and parathyroid hormone in primary hyperparathyroidism: functional and practical considerations, Surgery 106:1009–1016; discussion 1016–1007, 1989.
317. Luthringer R, Brandenberger G, Schaltenbrand N, et al: Slow wave electroencephalographic activity parallels renin oscillations during sleep in humans. Electroenceph and Clin Neurophysiol 95:318–322, 1995.
318. Charloux A, Gronfier C, Lonsdorfer-Wolf E, et al: Aldosterone release during the sleep-wake cycle in humans, Am J Physiol 276:E43–E49, 1999.
319. Brandenberger G, Follenius M, Simon C, et al: Nocturnal oscillations in plasma renin activity and REM—NREM sleep cycles in man: a common regulatory mechanism? Sleep 11:242–250, 1988.
320. Charloux A, Gronfier C, Chapotot F, et al: Sleep deprivation blunts the night time increase in aldosterone release in humans, J Sleep Res 10:27–33, 2001.
321. Brandenberger G, Charloux A, Grongier C, et al: Ultradian rhythms in hydromineral hormones, Horm Res 49:131–135, 1998.
322. Follenius M, Brandenberger G, Saini J: Lack of diurnal rhythm in plasma atrial natriuretic peptide, Life Sci 51:143–149, 1992.
323. Simon C, Gronfier C, Schlienger JL, et al: Circadian and ultradian variations of leptin in normal man under continuous enteral nutrition: relationship to sleep and body temperature, J Clin Endocrinol Metab 83:1893–1899, 1998.
324. Maquet P: Positron emission tomography studies of sleep and sleep disorders, J Neurol 244:S23–S28, 1997.
325. Maquet P: Functional neuroimaging of normal human sleep by positron emission tomography, J Sleep Res 9:207–231, 2000.
326. Dang-Vu TT, Desseilles M, Laureys S, et al: Cerebral correlates of delta waves during non-REM sleep revisited, Neuroimage 28:14–21, 2005.
327. DeFronzo RA: Pathogenesis of type 2 diabetes mellitus, Med Clin North Am 88:787–835, ix, 2004.
328. Magistretti PJ: Neuron-glia metabolic coupling and plasticity, J Exp Biol 209:2304–2311, 2006.
329. Plat L, Byrne MM, Sturis J, et al: Effects of morning cortisol elevation on insulin secretion and glucose regulation in humans, Am J Physiol 270:E36–E42, 1996.
330. Scheen AJ, Byrne MM, Plat L, et al: Relationships between sleep quality and glucose regulation in normal humans, Am J Physiol 271:E261–E270, 1996.
331. Jauch-Chara K, Hallschmid M, Schmid SM, et al: Plasma glucagon decreases during night-time sleep in Type 1 diabetic patients and healthy control subjects, Diabet Med 24:684–687, 2007.
332. Spiegel K, Leproult R, L'Hermite-Baleriaux M, et al: Leptin levels are dependent on sleep duration: relationships with sympathovagal balance, carbohydrate regulation, cortisol, and thyrotropin, J Clin Endocrinol Metab 89:5762–5771, 2004.
333. Spiegel K, Knutson K, Leproult R, et al: Sleep loss: a novel risk factor for insulin resistance and Type 2 diabetes, J Appl Physiol 99:2008–2019, 2005.
334. Tasali E, Leproult R, Ehrmann DA, et al: Slow-wave sleep and the risk of type 2 diabetes in humans, Proc Natl Acad Sci U S A 105:1044–1049, 2008.
335. Knutson KL, Van Cauter E: Associations between sleep loss and increased risk of obesity and diabetes, Ann N Y Acad Sci 1129:287–304, 2008.
336. Simon C, Brandenberger G: Ultradian oscillations of insulin secretion in humans, Diabetes 51(Suppl 1):S258–S261, 2002.
337. Sturis J, Van Cauter E, Blackman JD, et al: Entrainment of pulsatile insulin secretion by oscillatory glucose infusion, J Clin Invest 87:439–445, 1991.
338. Sturis J: Possible mechanisms underlying slow oscillations of human insulin secretion [PhD dissertation], Lyngby, Denmark, 1991, The Technical University of Denmark.
339. Song SH, Kjems L, Ritzel R, et al: Pulsatile insulin secretion by human pancreatic islets, J Clin Endocrinol Metab 87:213–221, 2002.
340. Porksen N, Hollingdal M, Juhl C, et al: Pulsatile insulin secretion: detection, regulation, and role in diabetes. Diabetes 51(Suppl 1):S245–S254, 2002.
341. Meneilly GS, Veldhuis JD, Elahi D: Disruption of the pulsatile and entropic modes of insulin release during an unvarying glucose stimulus in elderly individuals, J Clin Endocrinol Metab 84:1938–1943, 1999.
342. Getty L, Panteleon AE, Mittelman SD, et al: Rapid oscillations in omental lipolysis are independent of changing insulin levels in vivo, J Clin Invest 106:421–430, 2000.
343. Van Cauter E, Polonsky KS, Blackman JD, et al: Abnormal temporal patterns of glucose tolerance in obesity: relationship to sleep-related growth hormone and circadian cortisol rhythmicity, J Clin Endocrinol Metab 79:1797–1805, 1994.
344. Bolli GB, Gerich JE: The "dawn phenomenon"—a common occurrence in both non-insulin-dependent and insulin-dependent diabetes mellitus, N Engl J Med 310:746–750, 1984.
345. Campbell PJ, Bolli GB, Cryer PE, et al: Pathogenesis of the dawn phenomenon in patients with insulin-dependent diabetes mellitus, N Engl J Med 312:1473–1479, 1985.
346. Davidson MB, Harris MD, Ziel FH, et al: Suppression of sleep-induced growth hormone secretion by anticholinergic agent abolishes dawn phenomenon, Diabetes 37:166–171, 1988.
347. Shapiro ET, Polonsky KS, Copinschi G, et al: Nocturnal elevation of glucose levels during fasting in noninsulin-dependent diabetes, J Clin Endocrinol Metab 72:444–454, 1991.
348. Banarer S, Cryer PE: Sleep-related hypoglycemia-associated autonomic failure in type 1 diabetes: reduced awakening from sleep during hypoglycemia, Diabetes 52:1195–1203, 2003.
349. Jauch-Chara K, Schmid SM, Hallschmid M, et al: Altered neuroendocrine sleep architecture in patients with type 1 diabetes, Diabetes Care 31:1183–1188, 2008.
350. O'Meara NM, Sturis J, Van Cauter E, et al: Lack of control by glucose of ultradian insulin secretory oscillations in impaired glucose tolerance and in non-insulin-dependent diabetes mellitus, J Clin Invest 92:262–271, 1993.
351. Schmitz O, Juhl CB, Hollingdal M, et al: Irregular circulating insulin concentrations in type 2 diabetes mel-

litus: an inverse relationship between circulating free fatty acid and the disorderliness of an insulin time series in diabetic and healthy individuals, Metabolism 50:41–46, 2001.

352. Kershaw EE, Flier JS: Adipose tissue as an endocrine organ, J Clin Endocrinol Metab 89:2548–2556, 2004.

353. Flier JS: Obesity wars: molecular progress confronts an expanding epidemic, Cell 116:337–350, 2004.

354. Sinha MK, Ohannesian JP, Heiman ML, et al: Nocturnal rise of leptin in lean, obese and non-insulin-dependent diabetes mellitus subjects, J Clin Invest 97:1344–1347, 1996.

355. Saad MF, Riad-Gabriel MG, Khan A, et al: Diurnal and ultradian rhythmicity of plasma leptin: effects of gender and adiposity, J Clin Endocrinol Metab 83:453–459, 1998.

356. Schoeller DA, Cella LK, Sinha MK, et al: Entrainment of the diurnal rhythm of plasma leptin to meal timing, J Clin Invest 100:1882–1887, 1997.

357. Shea SA, Hilton MF, Orlova C, et al: Independent circadian and sleep/wake regulation of adipokines and glucose in humans, J Clin Endocrinol Metab 90:2537–2544, 2005.

358. Mullington JM, Chan JL, Van Dongen HP, et al: Sleep loss reduces diurnal rhythm amplitude of leptin in healthy men, J Neuroendocrinol 15:851–854, 2003.

359. Sinha MK, Sturis J, Ohannesian J, et al: Ultradian oscillations of leptin secretion in humans, Biochem Biophys Res Commun 228:733–738, 1996.

360. Licinio J, Mantzoros C, Negrao AB, et al: Human leptin levels are pulsatile and inversely related to pituitary-adrenal function, Nat Med 3:575–579, 1997.

361. Licinio J, Negrao AB, Mantzoros C, et al: Sex differences in circulating human leptin pulse amplitude: clinical implications, J Clin Endocrinol Metab 83:4140–4147, 1998.

362. Kolaczynski JW, Considine RV, Ohannesian J, et al: Responses of leptin to short-term fasting and refeeding in humans: a link with ketogenesis but not ketones themselves, Diabetes 45:1511–1515, 1996.

363. Chin-Chance C, Polonsky KS, Schoeller DA: Twenty-four-hour leptin levels respond to cumulative short-term energy imbalance and predict subsequent intake, J Clin Endocrinol Metab 85:2685–2691, 2000.

364. Laughlin GA, Yen SS: Hypoleptinemia in women athletes: absence of a diurnal rhythm with amenorrhea, J Clin Endocrinol Metab 82:318–321, 1997.

365. Balligand JL, Brichard SM, Brichard V, et al: Hypoleptinemia in patients with anorexia nervosa: loss of circadian rhythm and unresponsiveness to short-term refeeding, Eur J Endocrinol 138:415–420, 1998.

366. Franceschini R, Corsini G, Cataldi A, et al: Twenty-four-hour variation in serum leptin in the elderly, Metabolism 48:1011–1014, 1999.

367. Spiegel K, Tasali E, Penev P, et al: Brief communication: sleep curtailment in healthy young men is associated with decreased leptin levels, elevated ghrelin levels, and increased hunger and appetite, Ann Intern Med 141:846–850, 2004.

368. Taheri S, Lin L, Austin D, et al: Short sleep duration is associated with reduced leptin, elevated ghrelin, and increased body mass index, PLoS Med 1:e62, 2004.

369. Chaput JP, Despres JP, Bouchard C, et al: Short sleep duration is associated with reduced leptin levels and increased adiposity: results from the Quebec family study, Obesity (Silver Spring) 15:253–261, 2007.

370. Elimam A, Knutsson U, Bronnegard M, et al: Variations in glucocorticoid levels within the physiological range affect plasma leptin levels, Eur J Endocrinol 139:615–620, 1998.

371. Purnell JQ, Samuels MH: Levels of leptin during hydrocortisone infusions that mimic normal and reversed diurnal cortisol levels in subjects with adrenal insufficiency, J Clin Endocrinol Metab 84:3125–3128, 1999.

372. Leal-Cerro A, Considine RV, Peino R, et al: Serum immunoreactive-leptin levels are increased in patients with Cushing's syndrome, Horm Metab Res 28:711–713, 1996.

373. Masuzaki H, Ogawa Y, Hosoda K, et al: Glucocorticoid regulation of leptin synthesis and secretion in humans: elevated plasma leptin levels in Cushing's syndrome, J Clin Endocrinol Metab 82:2542–2547, 1997.

374. Veldman RG, Frolich M, Pincus SM, et al: Hyperleptinemia in women with Cushing's disease is driven by high-amplitude pulsatile, but orderly and eurhythmic, leptin secretion, Eur J Endocrinol 144:21–27, 2001.

375. Kousta E, Chrisoulidou A, Lawrence NJ, et al: The circadian rhythm of leptin is preserved in growth hormone deficient hypopituitary adults, Clin Endocrinol (Oxf) 48:685–690, 1998.

376. Pombo M, Herrera-Justiniano E, Considine RV, et al: Nocturnal rise of leptin in normal prepubertal and pubertal children and in patients with perinatal stalk-transection syndrome, J Clin Endocrinol Metab 82:2751–2754, 1997.

377. Yamauchi T, Kamon J, Waki H, et al: The fat-derived hormone adiponectin reverses insulin resistance associated with both lipoatrophy and obesity, Nat Med 7:941–946, 2001.

378. Kubota N, Terauchi Y, Yamauchi T, et al: Disruption of adiponectin causes insulin resistance and neointimal formation, J Biol Chem 277:25863–25866, 2002.

379. Gavrila A, Peng CK, Chan JL, et al: Diurnal and ultradian dynamics of serum adiponectin in healthy men: comparison with leptin, circulating soluble leptin receptor, and cortisol patterns, J Clin Endocrinol Metab 88:2838–2843, 2003.

380. Weyer C, Funahashi T, Tanaka S, et al: Hypoadiponectinemia in obesity and type 2 diabetes: close association with insulin resistance and hyperinsulinemia, J Clin Endocrinol Metab 86:1930–1935, 2001.

381. Yildiz BO, Suchard MA, Wong ML, et al: Alterations in the dynamics of circulating ghrelin, adiponectin, and leptin in human obesity, Proc Natl Acad Sci U S A 101:10434–10439, 2004.

382. Calvani M, Scarfone A, Granato L, et al: Restoration of adiponectin pulsatility in severely obese subjects after weight loss, Diabetes 53:939–947, 2004.

383. Date Y, Kojima M, Hosoda H, et al: Ghrelin, a novel growth hormone-releasing acylated peptide, is synthesized in a distinct endocrine cell type in the gastrointestinal tracts of rats and humans, Endocrinology 141:4255–4261, 2000.

384. Wren AM, Seal LJ, Cohen MA, et al: Ghrelin enhances appetite and increases food intake in humans, J Clin Endocrinol Metab 86:5992, 2001.

385. Weikel JC, Wichniak A, Ising M, et al: Ghrelin promotes slow-wave sleep in humans, Am J Physiol Endocrinol Metab 284:E407–E415, 2003.

386. Szentirmai E, Hajdu I, Obal F Jr, et al: Ghrelin-induced sleep responses in ad libitum fed and food-restricted rats, Brain Res 1088:131–140, 2006.

387. Koutkia P, Canavan B, Breu J, et al: Nocturnal ghrelin pulsatility and response to growth hormone secretagogues in healthy men, Am J Physiol Endocrinol Metab 287:E506–E512, 2004.

388. Cummings DE, Frayo RS, Marmonier C, et al: Plasma ghrelin levels and hunger scores in humans initiating meals voluntarily without time- and food-related cues, Am J Physiol Endocrinol Metab 287:E297–E304, 2004.

389. Cummings DE, Purnell JQ, Frayo RS, et al: A preprandial rise in plasma ghrelin levels suggests a role in meal initiation in humans, Diabetes 50:1714–1719, 2001.

390. Cummings DE, Weigle DS, Frayo RS, et al: Plasma ghrelin levels after diet-induced weight loss or gastric bypass surgery, N Engl J Med 346:1623–1630, 2002.

391. Teff KL, Elliott SS, Tschop M, et al: Dietary fructose reduces circulating insulin and leptin, attenuates postprandial suppression of ghrelin, and increases triglycerides in women, J Clin Endocrinol Metab 89:2963–2972, 2004.

392. Misra M, Miller KK, Kuo K, et al: Secretory dynamics of ghrelin in adolescent girls with anorexia nervosa and healthy adolescents, Am J Physiol Endocrinol Metab 289:E347–E356, 2005.

393. Espelund U, Hansen TK, Hojlund K, et al: Fasting unmasks a strong inverse association between ghrelin and cortisol in serum: studies in obese and normal-weight subjects, J Clin Endocrinol Metab 90:741–746, 2005.

394. Schmid SM, Hallschmid M, Jauch-Chara K, et al: A single night of sleep deprivation increases ghrelin levels and feelings of hunger in normal-weight healthy men, J Sleep Res 17:331–334, 2008.

395. Jayasena CN, Bloom SR: Role of gut hormones in obesity, Endocrinol Metab Clin North Am 37:769–787, 2008.

396. McEwen BS: Stress, adaptation, and disease. Allostasis and allostatic load, Ann N Y Acad Sci 840:33–44, 1998.

397. Van Cauter E, Knutson K: Sleep and the epidemic of obesity in children and adults, Eur J Endocrinol 159(suppl 1):S59–S66, 2008.

398. Cooper BG, White JES, Ashworth LA, et al: Hormonal and metabolic profiles in subjects with obstructive sleep apnea syndrome and the effects of nasal continuous positive airway pressure (CPAP) treatment, Sleep 18:172–179, 1995.

399. Saini J, Krieger J, Brandenberger G, et al: Continuous positive airway pressure treatment: effects on growth hormone, insulin and glucose profiles in obstructive sleep apnea patients, Hormone Metab Res 25:375–381, 1993.

400. Spiegel K, Follenius M, Krieger J, et al: Prolactin secretion during sleep in obstructive sleep apnea patients, J Sleep Res 4:56–62, 1995.

401. Luboshitzky R, Lavie L, Shen-Orr Z, et al: Pituitary-gonadal function in men with obstructive sleep apnea. The effect of continuous positive airways pressure treatment, Neuro Endocrinol Lett 24:463–467, 2003.

402. Ozturk L, Unal M, Tamer L, et al: The association of the severity of obstructive sleep apnea with plasma leptin levels, Arch Otolaryngol Head Neck Surg 129:538–540, 2003.

403. Patel SR, Palmer LJ, Larkin EK, et al: Relationship between obstructive sleep apnea and diurnal leptin rhythms, Sleep 27:235–239, 2004.

404. Phillips BG, Kato M, Narkiewicz K, et al: Increases in leptin levels, sympathetic drive, and weight gain in obstructive sleep apnea, Am J Physiol Heart Circ Physiol 279:H234–H237, 2000.

405. Ip MS, Lam KS, Ho C, et al: Serum leptin and vascular risk factors in obstructive sleep apnea, Chest 118:580–586, 2000.

406. Sanner BM, Kollhosser P, Buechner N, et al: Influence of treatment on leptin levels in patients with obstructive sleep apnoea, Eur Respir J 23:601–604, 2004.

407. Harsch IA, Konturek PC, Koebnick C, et al: Leptin and ghrelin levels in patients with obstructive sleep apnoea: effect of CPAP treatment, Eur Respir J 22:251–257, 2003.

408. Shimizu K, Chin K, Nakamura T, et al: Plasma leptin levels and cardiac sympathetic function in patients with obstructive sleep apnoea-hypopnoea syndrome, Thorax 57:429–434, 2002.

409. Chin K, Shimizu K, Nakamura T, et al: Changes in intra-abdominal visceral fat and serum leptin levels in patients with obstructive sleep apnea syndrome following nasal continuous positive airway pressure therapy, Circulation 100:706–712, 1999.

410. Tasali E, Mokhlesi B, Van Cauter E: Obstructive sleep apnea and type 2 diabetes: interacting epidemics, Chest 133:496–506, 2008.

410a. Schahin SP, Nechanitzky T, Dittel C, et al: Long-term improvement of insulin sensitivity during CPAP therapy in the obstructive sleep apnoea syndrome, Med Sci Monit 14:CR11121, 2008.

411. West SD, Nicoll DJ, Stradling JR: Prevalence of obstructive sleep apnoea in men with type 2 diabetes, Thorax 61:945–950, 2006.

412. Foster G, Kuna S, Sanders M, et al: Sleep Apnea In Obese Adults With Type 2 Diabetes: Baseline Results From The Sleep Ahead Study, Sleep 25:abstract 066, 2008.

413. Higuchi T, Takahashi Y, Takahashi K, et al: Twenty-four-hour secretory patterns of growth hormone, prolactin, and cortisol in narcolepsy, J Clin Endocrinol Metab 49:197–204, 1979.

414. Kok SW, Roelfsema F, Overeem S, et al: Dynamics of the pituitary-adrenal ensemble in hypocretin-deficient narcoleptic humans: blunted basal adrenocorticotropin release and evidence for normal time-keeping by the master pacemaker, J Clin Endocrinol Metab 87:5085–5091, 2002.

415. Overeem S, Kok SW, Lammers GJ, et al: Somatotropic axis in hypocretin-deficient narcoleptic humans: altered circadian distribution of GH-secretory events, Am J Physiol Endocrinol Metab 284:E641–E647, 2003.

416. Kok SW, Meinders AE, Overeem S, et al: Reduction of plasma leptin levels and loss of its circadian rhythmicity in hypocretin (orexin)-deficient narcoleptic humans, J Clin Endocrinol Metab 87:805–809, 2002.

417. Rosenthal RE, Vanderpool JRJ, Levendosky AA, et al: Phase-shifting effects of bright morning light as treatment for delayed sleep phase syndrome, Sleep 13:354–361, 1990.

418. Jones CR, Campbell SS, Zone SE, et al: Familial advanced sleep-phase syndrome: a short-period circadian rhythm variant in humans, Nat Med 5:1062–1065, 1999.

419. Young ME: The circadian clock within the heart: potential influence on myocardial gene expression, metabolism, and function, Am J Physiol Heart Circ Physiol 290:H1–H16, 2006.

420. Aschoff J, Hoffmann K, Pohl H, et al: Re-entrainment of circadian rhythms after phase-shifts of the zeitgeber, Chronobiologia 28:119–133, 1975.

421. Buxton OM, L'Hermite-Baleriaux M, Hirshfeld U, et al: Acute and delayed effects of exercise on human melatonin secretion, J Biol Rhythms 12:568–574, 1997.

422. Czeisler CA, Johnson MP, Duffy JF, et al: Exposure to bright light and darkness to treat physiologic maladaptation to night work, N Engl J Med 322:1253–1259, 1990.

423. Knutsson A, Akerstedt T, Orth-Gomer K, et al: Increased risk of ischaemic heart disease in shift workers, Lancet 2:89–92, 1986.

424. Rosa RR: Extended workshifts and excessive fatigue, J Sleep Res 4:51–56, 1995.

425. van Amelsvoort LG, Schouten EG, Kok FJ: Duration of shiftwork related to body mass index and waist to hip ratio, Int J Obes Relat Metab Disord 23:973–978, 1999.

426. Karlsson B, Knutsson A, Lindahl B: Is there an association between shift work and having a metabolic syndrome? Results from a population based study of 27,485 people, Occup Environ Med 58:747–752, 2001.

427. Nagaya T, Yoshida H, Takahashi H, et al: Markers of insulin resistance in day and shift workers aged 30–59 years, Int Arch Occup Environ Health 75:562–568, 2002.

428. Sookoian S, Gemma C, Fernandez Gianotti T, et al: Effects of rotating shift work on biomarkers of metabolic syndrome and inflammation, J Intern Med 261:285–292, 2007.

429. Roden M, Koller M, Pirich K, et al: The circadian melatonin and cortisol secretion pattern in permanent night shift workers, Am J Physiol 265:R261–R267, 1993.

430. Weibel L, Spiegel K, Follenius M, et al: Internal dissociation of the circadian markers of the cortisol rhythm in night workers, Am J Physiol 270:E608–E613, 1996.

431. Burgess HJ, Sharkey KM, Eastman CI: Bright light, dark and melatonin can promote circadian adaptation in night shift workers, Sleep Med Rev 6:407–420, 2002.

Chapter 5

HYPOTHALAMIC SYNDROMES

GLENN D. BRAUNSTEIN

Hypothalamic Disorders: Pathophysiologic Principles

Manifestations of Hypothalamic Disease
Disorders of Water Metabolism
Dysthermia
Disorders of Appetite Control and Caloric Balance
Sleep/Wake Cycle and Circadian Abnormalities
Abnormalities of Emotional Expression or Behavior
Disordered Control of Anterior Pituitary Function

Specific Hypothalamic Disorders
Prader-Willi Syndrome
Bardet-Biedl and Related Syndromes
Septo-Optic Pituitary Dysplasia
Hyperphagic Short Stature (Psychosocial Dwarfism)
Pseudocyesis
Hypothalamic Hamartoma
Suprasellar Arachnoid Cyst
Infiltrative Disorders
Hypothalamic Dysfunction after Brain Irradiation
Traumatic Brain Injury

The hypothalamus houses multiple nuclei along with afferent and efferent nerve fibers that connect the hypothalamus to the various portions of the brain and brainstem. It is divided into four regions: from anterior to posterior, the preoptic, supraoptic, tuberal, and mamillary regions; and three zones: laterally from the third ventricle, the periventricular, medial, and lateral[1-4] zones (Table 5-1, Figs. 5-1 and 5-2).

The hypothalamus is responsible for many of the body's homeostatic mechanisms, including water metabolism, temperature regulation, appetite control, the sleep/wake cycle, circadian rhythms, and control of the sympathetic and parasympathetic nervous systems. In addition, this area has activity in regard to emotional expression, behavior, and memory. Finally, the hypothalamus is essential to the neuroendocrine control of anterior pituitary function. Table 5-2 lists the various functions of the hypothalamus, the hypothalamic nuclei or hypothalamic regions that have been identified as being responsible for these functions, and the disorders that result from either destructive or stimulatory lesions in or around the nuclei or region.[1,4-25]

Hypothalamic Disorders: Pathophysiologic Principles

First, the small overall size of the hypothalamus and the close association of the nuclei and nerve tracts mean that a variety of different pathologic processes may give rise to the same signs and symptoms of neurologic and hypothalamic dysfunction.[4] The spectrum of disorders that can affect the hypothalamus is shown in Table 5-3. Tumors, infiltrative disorders, and infections, among other conditions, frequently give rise to headaches, neuro-ophthalmologic disorders, pyramidal tract or sensory nerve dysfunction, extrapyramidal cerebellar signs, and recurrent vomiting.[9,10] Other common manifestations include gonadal dysfunction (either hypogonadism or precocious puberty), diabetes insipidus, somnolence, dysthermia, and evidence of a caloric imbalance (either with hyperphagia and obesity or anorexia with emaciation).[9,10]

Second, although exceptions exist, most patients who have a systemic disorder such as Langerhans' cell histiocytosis, sarcoidosis, tuberculosis, or leukemia will exhibit manifestations of the disease outside the hypothalamus and central nervous system.

Third, a lesion may disrupt a function that is subserved by a hypothalamic nucleus distant from the lesion. Because the afferent and efferent tracts to and from the hypothalamic nuclei traverse other areas of the hypothalamus and brain distant from the nuclei, lesions that affect those tracts may result in dysfunction of several hypothalamic nuclei.

Fourth, most lesions that result in chronic hypothalamic syndromes involve more than one nucleus. As can be seen in Table 5-2, most of the hypothalamic functions are controlled by more than one nucleus, and this redundancy allows some degree of compensation should one nucleus be affected. In addition, most of the nuclei are paired, and destruction of a single nucleus may not be sufficient to result in a clinical syndrome. Thus lesions that affect the basal tuberal region of the hypothalamus (pituitary adenomas with suprasellar extension, optic gliomas, and craniopharyngiomas), are multiple (granulomatous disorders, metastatic tumors, infiltrative disease), or cause enlargement of the third ventricle (aqueductal stenosis, colloid cysts, pinealomas, germ cell tumors, midbrain gliomas) will more likely result in clinical hypothalamic dysfunction than will disorders affecting the more lateral portions of the hypothalamus.

Fifth, the rate of progression of the pathologic process affects the patient's clinical manifestations. Slowly progressive lesions

Table 5-1. Major Hypothalamic Nuclei

Region	Periventricular	Medial	Lateral
		Zone	
Preoptic	Preoptic periventricular nucleus	Medial preoptic nucleus	Lateral preoptic nucleus
	Anterior periventricular nucleus		
Supraoptic	Suprachiasmatic nucleus	Anterior hypothalamic nucleus	Lateral portion of supraoptic nucleus
	Paraventricular nucleus	Medial portion of supraoptic nucleus	
Tuberal	Arcuate (infundibular) nucleus	Dorsomedial hypothalamic nucleus	Lateral hypothalamic nucleus
		Ventromedial hypothalamic nucleus	
Mamillary	Posterior hypothalamic nucleus	Premamillary nucleus	Lateral mamillary nucleus
		Medial mamillary nucleus	Intercalatus nucleus

From Braunstein GD: The hypothalamus. In Melmed S (ed): The Pituitary, 2nd ed. Cambridge, MA: Blackwell Scientific, 2002, pp 317–348.

Table 5-2. Hypothalamic Functions, the Nuclei or Regions Involved with the Specific Functions, and the Disorders Resulting from Stimulatory or Destructive Lesions in the Regions

Function	Nuclei [n] or Region Involved [r]	Disorders
Water metabolism	Supraoptic [n]; paraventricular [n]	Diabetes insipidus
	Circumventricular organs [r]	Essential hypernatremia SIADH
Temperature regulation	Preoptic anterior hypothalamic [r]	Hyperthermia
	Posterior hypothalamus [r]	Hypothermia Poikilothermia
Appetite control	Ventromedial [n] (satiety center)	Hypothalamic obesity Cachexia
	Lateral hypothalamic [r] (feeding center)	Anorexia nervosa Diencephalic syndrome Diencephalic glycosuria
Sleep/wake cycle and circadian rhythm	Ventrolateral preoptic anterior hypothalamic [r] (sleep center)	Somnolence Reversal of sleep/wake cycle
	Posterior hypothalamic [r] including tuberomamillary [n] (arousal center)	Akinetic mutism Coma
	Suprachiasmatic [n]	
Visceral (autonomic) fraction	Posterior medial [r] (sympathetic region)	Sympathetic activation Parasympathetic activation
	Preoptic anterior hypothalamus [r] (parasympathetic region)	
Emotional expression and behavior	Ventromedial [n]	Sham rage
	Medial and posterior hypothalamus [r]	Fear or horror Apathy
	Caudal hypothalamic [r]	Hypersexual behavior
Memory	Ventromedial [n] Mamillary bodies	Short-term memory loss
Control of anterior pituitary	Arcuate [n]	Hyperfunction function
	Preoptic [n]	Hypofunction syndromes
	Suprachiasmatic [n]	
	Paraventricular [n]	
	Neovascular zone (median eminence)	

SIADH, Syndrome of inappropriate secretion of antidiuretic hormone.

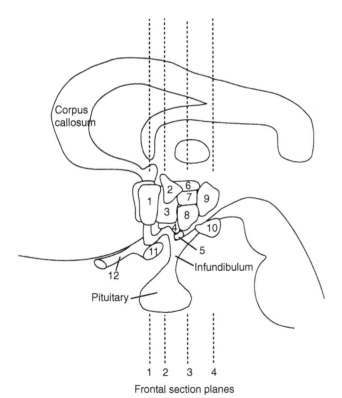

Frontal section planes

FIGURE 5-1. Schematic representation of lateral brain section demonstrating hypothalamic nuclei. *Dashed lines* represent the frontal (coronal) section planes illustrated in Figures 5-2 and 5-3. *1,* preoptic nucleus; *2,* paraventricular nucleus; *3,* anterior hypothalamic areas; *4,* supraoptic nucleus; *5,* arcuate nucleus; *6,* dorsal hypothalamic area; *7,* dorsomedial nucleus; *8,* ventromedial nucleus; *9,* posterior hypothalamic area; *10,* mamillary body; *11,* optic chiasm; *12,* optic nerve. (From Braunstein GD: The hypothalamus. In Melmed S [ed]: The Pituitary, 2nd ed. Cambridge, MA: Blackwell Scientific, 2002, pp 317–348.)

may give few or no symptoms until they achieve a large size, at which time, altered endocrine function and deterioration of cognitive ability may be present. Small, acute lesions may result in profound clinical manifestations such as alterations in consciousness, thermal dysregulation, and diabetes insipidus.

Sixth, the clinical syndrome due to involvement of a hypothalamic nucleus or tract may differ depending on whether the pathologic lesion is destructive or stimulatory. As an example, chronic, destructive lesions of the preoptic region may result in hypothermia and insomnia, whereas hyperthermia and lethargy may be seen with acute stimulatory lesions.

Finally, the clinical manifestations of the hypothalamic disease depend in part on the age of the patient. Thus prepubertal gonadotropin deficiency results in sexual infantilism, whereas in the postpubertal state, regression of secondary sexual characteristics (but not disappearance) occurs. Similarly, prepubertal growth hormone deficiency due to a hypothalamic lesion disturbing growth hormone–releasing hormone (GHRH) function results in short stature, whereas a similar lesion occurring in an adult may manifest only as adult growth hormone deficiency syndrome.

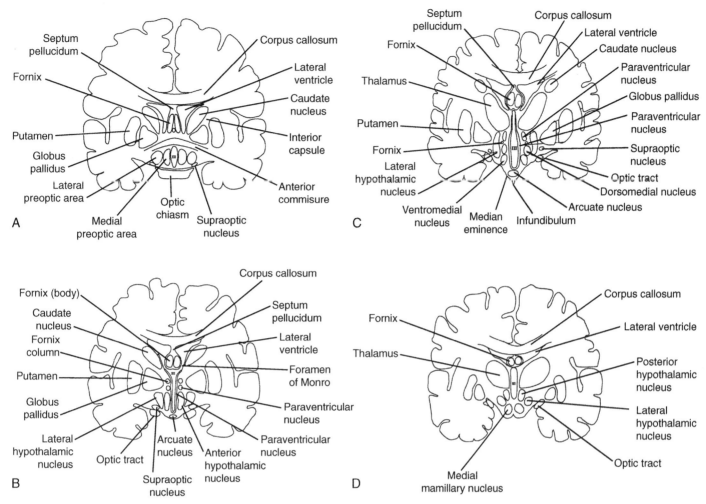

FIGURE 5-2. Frontal (coronal) sections of the hypothalamic regions. **A,** Preoptic region (frontal section plane 1 in Fig. 5-1). **B,** Supraoptic region (frontal section plane 2 in Fig. 5-1). **C,** Tuberal region (frontal section plane 3 in Fig. 5-1). **D,** Mamillary region (frontal section plane 4 in Fig. 5-1). (From Braunstein GD: The hypothalamus. In Melmed S [ed]: The Pituitary, 2nd ed. Cambridge, MA: Blackwell Scientific, 2002, pp 317–348.)

Manifestations of Hypothalamic Disease

DISORDERS OF WATER METABOLISM

Central Diabetes Insipidus

Complete or partial central diabetes insipidus results from (1) destruction of the antidiuretic hormone (ADH)-producing magnocellular neurons in the supraoptic and paraventricular nuclei or (2) interruption of the transport of ADH through their axons, which terminate in the pituitary stalk and posterior pituitary. Diabetes insipidus is relatively common in patients with chronic hypothalamic disorders, being found in approximately 35% of such patients.[9,10] It also is frequently found in patients with acute insults to the hypothalamus or pituitary stalk, as is seen in vascular accidents and neurosurgical trauma. Obesity and hypogonadism frequently are present in patients with diabetes insipidus due to tumors or infiltrative disorders (Fig. 5-3).

The majority of patients with diabetes insipidus have idiopathic or familial diabetes insipidus associated with gliosis of the supraoptic and paraventricular nuclei.[26] Approximately one third of patients with idiopathic diabetes insipidus have detectable anti-ADH–producing cell antibodies, suggesting an autoimmune cause.[27] Autosomal-recessive, X-linked-recessive, and autosomal-dominant forms of familial diabetes insipidus have been

described. In the more common autosomal-dominant form, nucleotide deletions or substitutions in the *ADH* gene on chromosome 20 have been identified.[28] The DIDMOAD syndrome (Wolfram's syndrome) represents a rare autosomal-recessive form of central diabetes insipidus (DI) associated with type 1 diabetes mellitus (DM), optic atrophy (OA), bilateral sensorineural deafness (D), and occasionally ataxia and autonomic neurogenic bladder.[29] Diabetes insipidus is a frequent manifestation of suprasellar and pineal germinomas, sarcoidosis, lymphocytic infundibuloneurohypophysitis, and the chronic disseminated form of Langerhans' cell histiocytosis.[30-37]

Adipsic or Essential Hypernatremia

Adipsic hypernatremia occurs when the osmoreceptors that are present in the anterior medial and anterior lateral preoptic regions are damaged. Affected patients have an impaired thirst mechanism, which results in insufficient fluid intake despite the hypernatremia. Although most of the affected patients have partial diabetes insipidus, their extracellular fluid volume remains normal, and they are not dehydrated. Therefore, they exhibit chronic elevations of serum sodium but normal blood pressure, pulse rate, serum creatinine, and creatinine clearance and can release ADH and concentrate their urine during fluid deprivation. When serum sodium concentrations are less than 160 mmol/L, few symptoms are

Table 5-3. Causes of Hypothalamic Dysfunction

Congenital	**Nutritional, Metabolic**
Acquired	Anorexia nervosa
Developmental malformations	Kernicterus
Anencephaly	Wernicke-Korsakoff syndrome
Porencephaly	Weight loss
Agenesis of the corpus callosum	**Degenerative**
Septo-optic dysplasia	Glial scarring
Suprasellar arachnoid cyst	Parkinson's disease
Colloid cyst of the third ventricle	**Infectious**
Hamartoma	Bacterial
Aqueductal stenosis	Meningitis
Trauma	Mycobacterial
Intraventricular hemorrhage	Tuberculosis
Genetic (familial or sporadic cases)	Spirochetal
Hypothalamic hypopituitarism	Syphilis
Familial diabetes insipidus	Viral
Prader-Willi syndrome	Encephalitis
Bardet-Biedl and associated syndromes	Jakob-Creutzfeldt disease
DIDMOAD syndrome	Kuru
Pallister-Hall syndrome	Poliomyelitis
Leptin/leptin receptor mutations	Varicella
Tumors	Cytomegalovirus infection
Primary intracranial tumors	**Vascular**
Angioma of the third ventricle	Aneurysm
Craniopharyngioma	Arteriovenous malformation
Ependymoma	Pituitary apoplexy
Ganglioneuroma	Subarachnoid hemorrhage
Germ cell tumors	**Trauma**
Glioblastoma multiforme	Birth injury
Glioma	Head injury
Hamartoma	Postneurosurgical
Hemangioma	**Functional**
Lipoma	Diencephalic epilepsy
Lymphoma	Drugs
Medulloblastoma	Hayek-Peake syndrome
Meningioma	Idiopathic syndrome of inappropriate secretion of antidiuretic hormone
Neuroblastoma	(SIADH)
Pinealomas	Kleine-Levin syndrome
Pituitary tumors	Periodic syndrome of Wolff
Plasmacytoma	Psychosocial deprivation syndrome
Sarcoma	**Other**
Metastatic tumors	Radiation
Infiltrative	Porphyria
Histiocytosis	Toluene exposure
Leukemia	
Sarcoidosis	
Immunologic	
Idiopathic diabetes insipidus	
Paraneoplastic syndrome	

Modified from Braunstein GD: The hypothalamus. In Melmed S (ed): The Pituitary, 2nd ed. Cambridge, MA: Blackwell Scientific, 2002, pp 317–348.
DIDMOAD, Diabetes insipidus, diabetes mellitus, optic atrophy, deafness.

present. However, between 160 and 180 mmol/L, patients may have fatigue, weakness, lethargy, muscle tenderness, cramps, anorexia, depression, and irritability; at 180 mmol/L, stupor and coma may be present. Close to half of these patients have hypothalamic obesity, and almost three fourths demonstrate some degree of anterior pituitary hormone deficiency.[6,9,10,13,38,39]

Essential hypernatremia has been described with a variety of lesions, including craniopharyngiomas, suprasellar germinomas, optic nerve gliomas, pineal tumors, Langerhans' cell histiocytosis, sarcoidosis, trauma, hydrocephalus, cysts, inflammatory conditions, ruptured aneurysms of the anterior communicating artery, and toluene exposure.[38-40] The Hayek-Peake syndrome is the association of essential hypernatremia with hypodipsia, obesity, lethargy, increased perspiration, central hypoventilation,

hyperprolactinemia, hypothyroidism, and hyperlipidemia without an identifiable structural hypothalamic defect.[41]

Syndrome of Inappropriate Secretion of Antidiuretic Hormone

Syndrome of inappropriate secretion of antidiuretic hormone (SIADH) is characterized by serum hyponatremia and hypo-osmolarity, with an inappropriately elevated urine osmolarity, in a patient with normal renal, adrenal, and thyroid function and no clinical evidence of intravascular or extracellular fluid volume expansion. The clinical symptoms depend on the rate of decrease of serum sodium, as well as the absolute serum sodium concentration. At serum sodium levels greater than 120 mmol/L, symptoms are generally mild and nonspecific and include anorexia,

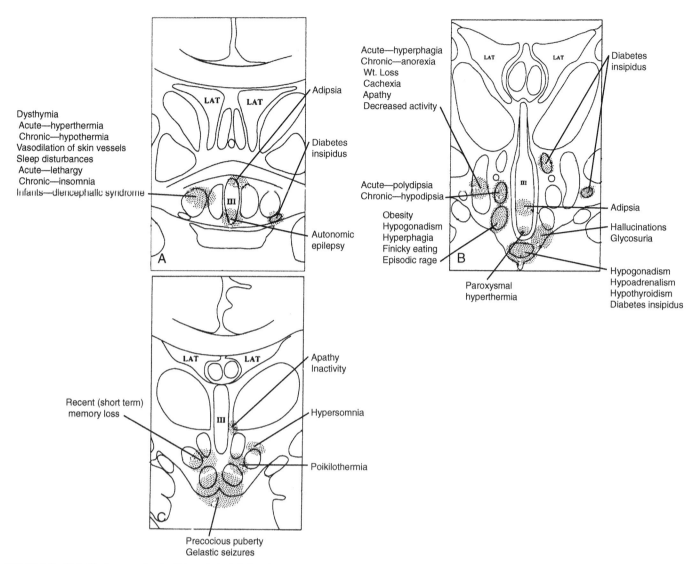

FIGURE 5-3. Clinical findings associated with hypothalamic lesions located at various anatomic sites. Clinicopathologic correlation based on multiple studies.[15-25] **A,** Corresponds to region depicted in Figure 5-2A. **B,** Corresponds to region depicted in Figure 5-2C. **C,** Corresponds to section depicted in Figure 5-2D. (From Braunstein GD: The hypothalamus. In Melmed S [ed]: The Pituitary, 2nd ed. Cambridge, MA: Blackwell Scientific, 2002, pp 317–348.)

nausea, headache, weakness, and lethargy. At less than 120 mmol/L, these symptoms are accompanied by nausea, vomiting, and mental confusion; at very low levels, by seizure and coma.[42] The syndrome is found with a variety of intracranial abnormalities, including head trauma, intracranial bleeding, meningitis, encephalitis, neurosurgery, hydrocephalus, acute intermittent porphyria, craniopharyngiomas, germinomas, and pinealomas.[6,13,30] An idiopathic form has been described in young women who exhibit menstrual irregularities, have enlarged lateral ventricles, and have SIADH cyclically. No structural defect has been described in these patients.[4]

Reset Osmostat

The osmoreceptors, located in the circumventricular organs of the lamina terminalis, may become "reset" in some patients with tuberculosis, malnutrition, quadriplegia, and psychosis. The osmoreceptors activate release of ADH at a lower serum osmolality than normal and appropriately decrease ADH release when the serum osmolality falls further.[42]

Cerebral Salt Wasting

Hyponatremia and the other manifestations of SIADH also co-occur in the syndrome of cerebral salt wasting, which is primarily seen in postoperative neurosurgical patients treated for subarachnoid bleeding, intracranial aneurysms, or following head injury. In contrast to SIADH in which patients are euvolemic or have an expansion of their effective arterial blood volume, patients with cerebral salt wasting are hypovolemic due to renal salt loss. The salt wasting and hypovolemia are felt to be the result of disruption of the normal sympathetic nervous system input into the kidneys and/or relapse of a natriuretic factor from the brain.[43]

DYSTHERMIA

Hyperthermia

The warm receptors present in the preoptic anterior hypothalamus are stimulated by an increase in the temperature of the blood. Together with signals from peripheral warm receptors that respond to an increase in external temperature, the afferent signals travel through the median forebrain bundle to the lateral portion of the posterior hypothalamus, which leads to vasodilation and sweating to dissipate heat. Conversely, stimulation of the preoptic anterior hypothalamic cold receptors through a decrease in temperature of the blood, or stimulation of the peripheral cold receptors through a decrease in ambient temperature, results in medial neurons in the posterior hypothalamus activating heat production through muscular shivering and heat conservation through vasoconstriction.[5,6]

Acute injury to the anterior hypothalamic and preoptic areas may result in a rapid temperature elevation (as high as 41°C) associated with tachycardia and unconsciousness from failure of the heat-dissipating mechanisms to function while heat production continues. Chronic hyperthermia may be secondary to lesions in the tuberoinfundibular region. In contrast to patients with elevated temperature due to the inflammation of infections, these patients generally do not experience malaise and paradoxically may have peripheral vasoconstriction.[1,5,6,9,11]

Wolff and colleagues[44] described a syndrome of hyperthermia associated with shaking chills, fever, hypertension, vomiting, and peripheral vasoconstriction that occurred cyclically at 3-week intervals, without a pathologic lesion in the hypothalamus being found. Similar paroxysms of hyperthermia have been noted in other patients without the cyclicity, and together these episodes may represent a variant of diencephalic epilepsy.[6,44,45]

Between 0.02% and 2.4% of patients receiving neuroleptic drugs develop the neuroleptic malignant syndrome (NMS), which is characterized by hyperthermia to 38°C or higher; severe extrapyramidal signs, including "lead-pipe" muscle rigidity and tremor; signs of autonomic nervous system dysfunction such as pallor, tachycardia, arrhythmias, blood pressure lability, and diaphoresis; and changes in mental status, including mutism, delirium, and coma.[46] All antipsychotic medications have been reported to cause NMS, and most evidence suggests that disruption of dopamine neurotransmission by neuroleptic-induced dopamine receptor blockade is the major pathophysiologic abnormality in susceptible individuals. Indeed, the greater the potency of the neuroleptic in regard to its dopamine D_2-receptor antagonism activity, the greater the frequency of NMS occurrence.[46] NMS is successfully treated with a variety of dopamine agonists. Injury to the preoptic medial and tuberal nuclei has been demonstrated at autopsy, as has a depletion of hypothalamic norepinephrine concentrations.[47] The syndrome generally begins within 2 weeks of initiating the neuroleptic and evolves over a 24- to 72-hour period. The most common complication is rhabdomyolysis, which may result in myoglobinuria and acute renal failure. The mortality of this syndrome is currently less than 10%, which reflects increased recognition of the disorder and initiation of prompt therapy.[46]

The serotonin syndrome is closely related to NMS and presents with the triad of altered mental status (somnolence, confusion, agitation, seizures, and coma), autonomic instability (fever, diaphoresis, tachycardia, hypo- or hyperthermia, mydriasis), and abnormal neuromuscular activity (myoclonus, rigidity, hyperreflexia). Any drug or combination of drugs which elevates the concentration of serotonin in the central nervous system can cause the syndrome. These include selective serotonin reuptake inhibitors (SSRIs), tricyclic antidepressants, monoamine oxidase inhibitors, cocaine, and amphetamines. These drugs either directly or indirectly activate thermogenesis via the hypothalamus.[46]

Hypothermia

Large, destructive lesions of the anterior or posterior hypothalamus may result in inability to generate heat through vasoconstriction and muscular shivering. This occurs in 10% to 15% of patients with a variety of hypothalamic lesions, especially neoplasms, infiltrative disorders, and infections.[9,10,13] It also has been noted in patients with Parkinson's disease and Wernicke's encephalopathy, which are associated with lesions in the posterior hypothalamus and mamillary bodies, respectively.[48,49]

Diencephalic autonomic epilepsy refers to episodic or paroxysmal hypothermia during which the body temperature decreases to 32°C or less over minutes to days, along with evidence of autonomic nervous system dysfunction, including flushing, sweating, hypotension, bradycardia, salivation, lacrimation, pupillary dilation, Cheyne-Stokes respiration, nausea, vomiting, asterixis, ataxia, and obtundation.[6,15,50-53] Electroencephalographic (EEG) abnormalities occur during the episodes. Autopsy studies have shown gliosis and loss of the arcuate nucleus and premamillary area in some patients, whereas others have been found to have tumors involving the floor and lower portion of the third ventricle.[15,50] The corpus callosum has been found to be absent in approximately half of patients with episodic hypothermia; these individuals may also exhibit diabetes insipidus, reset osmostat, growth hormone deficiency, hypogonadism, or precocious puberty (Shapiro's syndrome).[54]

Poikilothermia

When both the heat-loss and heat-conserving homeostatic mechanisms are impaired, wide fluctuations of body temperature might take place without the patient's experiencing thermal discomfort. This condition, known as *poikilothermia,* is found with both anterior and posterior hypothalamic destruction, as well as in patients with large lesions that may involve the posterior hypothalamus and rostral mesencephalon.[6,9,10] Rarely, patients with Wernicke's encephalopathy may experience poikilothermia.[6]

DISORDERS OF APPETITE CONTROL AND CALORIC BALANCE

Hypothalamic Obesity

Approximately 25% of patients with structural hypothalamic lesions exhibit hyperphagia and obesity.[9,10] Usually, the patients have lesions involving a large portion of the hypothalamus, although bilateral destruction of only the ventromedial nucleus may lead to hypothalamic obesity.[1,9,10,17,18,22,25,55] The majority of patients harbor a neoplasm, especially craniopharyngioma, with a minority having inflammatory or granulomatous processes, a history of trauma, or infiltrative disorders.[55] Common clinical findings in these patients include headaches, visual abnormalities, hypogonadism, diabetes insipidus, and somnolence. Less commonly, behavioral abnormalities, such as antisocial behavior or sham rage, and seizures may be present.[55] Hypothalamic obesity also is found with defects of the leptin and leptin receptor genes, the melanocortin 4 receptor gene, and the proopiomelanocortin gene.[56-59]

Diencephalic Syndrome of Infancy

Infants harboring a low-grade hypothalamic or optic nerve glioma, or rarely ependymomas, gangliogliomas, or dysgerminomas that destroy the ventromedial nuclei, may develop an unusual syndrome at approximately age 1 to 2 years, in which they begin to lose weight and subcutaneous fat, while maintaining an apparently good food intake and normal growth. They exhibit hyperactivity and a cheerful affect and often demonstrate nystagmus, pallor, vomiting, tremor, and optic atrophy.[60-62] Endocrine evaluation is generally normal or may show nonspecific abnormalities that include elevated growth hormone levels.[63] If the patients live beyond age 2 years, they begin to gain weight and become obese. Their euphoria and cheerful affect disappear and are replaced by rage and irritability. Somnolence and precocious puberty also may be present.[5,60-63] A similar syndrome rarely has been described in adults with tumors involving the optic chiasm or anterior hypothalamic region.[64]

Hypothalamic Cachexia in Adults

In patients with destructive lesions of the lateral hypothalamus, rapid weight loss, decreased activity, hypophagia, muscle wasting, cachexia, and death may ensue, usually due to a neoplasm.[9,10,17,18,21] Malignant multiple sclerosis also may cause the lateral hypothalamic syndrome.[17,21]

Anorexia Nervosa

Anorexia nervosa is a common disorder, usually seen in young women beginning before the age of 25 years. Although it is not associated with a structural hypothalamic defect, functional hypothalamic abnormalities are present. These patients may exercise excessively, induce vomiting, and have amenorrhea with a prepubertal pattern of gonadotropin release.[65] Elevations of basal serum growth hormone, ghrelin, and peptide YY are found, with reduction of insulin-like growth factor 1 (IGF-1) and leptin concentrations. Patients may demonstrate abnormalities in hypothalamic-pituitary-adrenal activity, with elevated plasma cortisol concentrations, decreased adrenocorticotropic hormone (ACTH) levels, and an attenuated ACTH response to corticotropin-releasing hormone (CRH). Low concentrations of thyroxine (T_4) and triiodothyronine (T_3) are found, with elevated reverse T_3 and a thyroid-stimulating hormone (TSH) response to thyrotropin-releasing hormone (TRH) that is either normal or demonstrates a delayed peak consistent with hypothalamic hypothyroidism.[66,67] Additionally, these patients may have hyperprolactinemia with galactorrhea, evidence of thermal dysregulation, and a partial diabetes insipidus.[68] The neuroendocrine and functional hypothalamic abnormalities remit when the patients regain their weight.

Diencephalic Glycosuria

Acute injuries to the tuberoinfundibular region from basal skull fractures, intracranial hemorrhage, or neurosurgical intervention around the third ventricle may lead to transient hyperglycemia and glycosuria.[1,69] Although many of the "stress hormones" with glucose contraregulatory activity are elevated in these patients, they do not appear to be responsible for the glucose abnormality.

SLEEP/WAKE CYCLE AND CIRCADIAN ABNORMALITIES

Approximately 10% of patients with hypothalamic disease will first be seen with somnolence, and this condition is found in 30% of such patients at some time during the course of their illness.[9,10] Somnolence is commonly seen in lesions involving the posterior hypothalamus, often in association with hypothermia.[1,6,70] Approximately 40% of patients with hypersomnolence also have hypothalamic obesity.[55] Most patients with these manifestations have neoplasms, especially craniopharyngiomas,

epithelial pineal tumors, and suprasellar germinomas.[31,71] Encephalitis and Wernicke's nutritional encephalopathy are other causes of hypothalamic hypersomnia.[1,5,6] As previously noted, acute hypothalamic injury may lead to a transient coma. Narcolepsy, which is characterized by sudden episodes of sleep that last minutes to hours, may in some instances have a hypothalamic cause. The syndrome has been found in patients with third ventricular tumors, with multiple sclerosis, after head injuries, and with encephalitis.[1] Deficiency of the hypothalamic orexin, hypocretin-1, have been found in the cerebrospinal fluid (CSF) of patients with narcolepsy, and a loss of hypocretin neurons occurs in the lateral hypothalamus in affected patients.[72,73]

Patients with lesions of the anterior and preoptic hypothalamic nuclei may exhibit hyperactivity and insomnia or, more commonly, alterations in the sleep/wake cycle, with daytime sleepiness and nighttime hyperactivity.[6,23,74] This is characteristically seen in patients with cystic craniopharyngiomas. Anterior tuberal lesions also may lead to alterations in the sleep/wake cycle, as well as an akinetic mutism type of syndrome in which the patient appears awake but does not respond to verbal stimuli and demonstrates little spontaneous movement.[74]

The suprachiasmatic nuclei are responsible for the maintenance of many of our circadian rhythms, and lesions involving this region will alter the sleep/wake cycle, temperature control, and cognitive function.[72,75]

ABNORMALITIES OF EMOTIONAL EXPRESSION OR BEHAVIOR

Sham rage reactions with emotional lability; marked agitation; and aggressive, destructive behavior are found in patients with lesions involving the ventromedial nuclei.[6,23,70] Activation of the sympathetic nervous system is present during the episodes. In contrast, apathy, somnolence, and hypoactivity, as well as vocal and auditory unresponsiveness and akinetic mutism, have been found in patients with destruction of the mamillary bodies or lesions in the medial posterior hypothalamus.[1,6]

Hypersexual behavior is seen in individuals with lesions involving the caudal hypothalamus.[76] The Kleine-Levin syndrome is believed to represent a functional abnormality of the hypothalamus. It generally affects adolescent boys, who have recurrent episodes of somnolence with periodic arousal that is associated with irritability, abnormal speech, forgetfulness, food gorging, and masturbation and other sexual activity. The episodes may occur at 3- to 6-month intervals and generally last 5 to 7 days. The disorder usually remits spontaneously in late adolescence or early adulthood.[77]

Gelastic or laughing seizures are a form of diencephalic epilepsy due to lesions involving the floor of the third ventricle and mamillary area, especially hamartomas of the tuber cinereum.[78] The affected child does not lose consciousness but stops his or her activity and begins to laugh or giggle or make bubbling noises, associated with a grimace from tightening of the facial muscles.[79,80] EEG abnormalities are present during the seizure.

DISORDERED CONTROL OF ANTERIOR PITUITARY FUNCTION
Hyperfunction Syndromes
Precocious Puberty

Isosexual pubertal development in girls younger than 8 years or boys younger than 9 years represents sexual precocity, which most often is due to premature activation of the hypothalamic-pituitary-gonadal axis. The majority of girls have no discernible

Table 5-4. Causes of Central Precocious Puberty

Idiopathic

Congenital Abnormalities

Hypothalamic hamartoma
Arachnoid cyst
Myelomeningocele
Aqueductal stenosis with hydrocephalus
Tuberous sclerosis
Congenital optic nerve hypoplasia
Congenital adrenal hyperplasia
McCune-Albright syndrome
Septo-optic dysplasia

Neoplasms

Optic nerve glioma
Hypothalamic glioma
Neurofibroma
Astrocytoma
Ependymoma
Infundibuloma
Pinealoma
Neuroblastoma
Germinoma
Craniopharyngioma

Inflammatory Conditions

Tuberculosis
Sarcoidosis
Meningoencephalitis

Subdural Hematoma

Primary Hypothyroidism

From Braunstein GD: The hypothalamus. In Melmed S (ed): The Pituitary, 2nd ed. Cambridge, MA: Blackwell Scientific, 2002, pp 317–348.

lesion and are therefore classified as having idiopathic central precocious puberty, whereas only 10% of boys have idiopathic precocious puberty.[81] In the latter, close to half have hypothalamic hamartomas, and a third have other benign or malignant neoplasms that are located in the posterior hypothalamus or near the mamillary bodies.[81] The spectrum of pathologic conditions that can cause central precocious puberty are listed in Table 5-4.[4,81-89] Some of these lesions may bring about early activation of the hypothalamic-pituitary-gonadal axis through increased intracranial pressure or irritation of the basal hypothalamus. Hypothalamic hamartomas involving the tuber cinereum are often associated with precocious puberty through premature activation of the normal hypothalamic gonadotropin-releasing hormone (GnRH) secretory mechanisms or through direct secretion of GnRH by the hamartoma, because GnRH has been located immunohistochemically within hamartomatous neurons.[90,91] In addition to pressure effects, germ cell tumors may result in precocious puberty through the secretion of human chorionic gonadotropin (hCG), which may stimulate the child's gonads to secrete sex steroid hormones, bringing about precocious sexual development. Finally, premature activation of the normal hypothalamic-pituitary-gonadal axis has been described in some patients who have had incomplete sexual precocity from congenital adrenal hyperplasia or polyostotic fibrous dysplasia (McCune-Albright) syndrome, in which the hypothalamus is exposed to elevated sex steroid hormone levels at an early age. Premature activation of the normal hypothalamic-pituitary-gonadal axis has also occurred in patients with primary hypothyroidism, who also may exhibit galactorrhea with elevated

prolactin levels (Van Wyk-Grumbach syndrome), in which the mechanism for the premature activation is unknown but usually ceases with correction of the hypothyroidism.[89]

Acromegaly

Acromegaly due to the ectopic secretion of GHRH is rare. In most instances, the source of the ectopic GHRH is a bronchial carcinoid, islet cell neoplasm, adrenal tumor, or lung carcinoma.[92,93] However, acromegaly has also been found in patients with hypothalamic hamartomas, gangliocytomas, gliomas, and choristomas.[92-95] Some of these tumors have been shown to contain GHRH, and they presumably secrete the releasing factor, which in turn stimulates the somatotrophs to hypersecrete growth hormone.

Cushing's Disease

Several lines of evidence suggest that Cushing's disease has a hypothalamic component to its pathophysiology.[96] First, it has been noted that the onset of the disease often follows an emotionally stressful event.[97] Because depression may be associated with pseudo-Cushing's syndrome with hypersecretion of glucocorticoids, it is conceivable that chronic corticotroph stimulation by hypothalamic CRH could lead to the development of a corticotroph adenoma and Cushing's disease and may account for the recurrence of Cushing's disease after apparently successful removal of an ACTH-secreting corticotroph adenoma.[98,99] Second, most patients with Cushing's disease, when given exogenous glucocorticoids in sufficient quantities, are able to suppress their ACTH secretion, a fact that has been known for some time and forms the basis for the high-dose portion of the dexamethasone suppression test.[96] Presumably, this phenomenon reflects an increased set point for negative feedback of glucocorticoids at the hypothalamic level. Third, some patients with Cushing's disease exhibit a reduction in ACTH and cortisol secretion and amelioration of symptoms after the administration of cyproheptadine, bromocriptine, or sodium valproate, which may work through the hypothalamus.[100-103] Nevertheless, most if not all corticotroph adenomas are of clonal origin rather than polyclonal, as would be anticipated if CRH hypersecretion were responsible for the pituitary abnormality.[104] Hypothalamic factors such as CRH may promote clonal expansion of corticotroph cells that have become intrinsically abnormal.[105] An unusual cause of pituitary-dependent Cushing's disease is the secretion of CRH by an intracranial neoplasm, as was demonstrated with an intrasellar gangliocytoma.[106]

Hyperprolactinemia

Because prolactin secretion by the lactotrophs is under hypothalamic dopamine inhibitory control, it is not surprising that patients with a variety of hypothalamic disorders may exhibit hyperprolactinemia. This is seen in 79% of patients with suprasellar germinomas, 36% of patients with craniopharyngiomas, and 14% of patients with pineal germinomas.[32] Most patients have a prolactin concentration less than 70 ng/mL, and galactorrhea is infrequently seen, probably because of the coexistence of hypogonadism.[107] Nevertheless, amenorrhea and galactorrhea may be present in women, and erectile dysfunction in men.

Idiopathic hyperprolactinemia in patients without any demonstrable structural abnormality in the pituitary or hypothalamus is presumably due to a hypothalamic dopamine deficiency. The prolactin secretory dynamics of these patients in response to various stimulatory and inhibitory agents is similar to that seen in patients with prolactin-secreting pituitary adenomas. Indeed, when followed for a long period, some patients with idiopathic hyperprolactinemia will eventually be found to have a prolactin-secreting pituitary microadenoma. Additional evidence supporting a hypothalamic cause for the pituitary adenoma is the finding of lactotroph hyperplasia in some patients who have had documented adenomas, as well as the recurrence of prolactin-secreting pituitary adenoma after successful removal of a microadenoma and an interval of normal prolactin-secretory dynamics.[108,109]

Hypofunction Syndromes

Hypothalamic Hypogonadism

Kallmann's syndrome (olfactory-genital dysplasia) is the most common form of congenital isolated gonadotropin deficiency and can occur sporadically or in a familial setting as an X-linked, autosomal-dominant, or autosomal-recessive trait with incomplete penetrance.[110] The X-linked disorder, which accounts for 10% to 15% of sporadic cases and 30% to 60% of familial cases, is due to a defect in the *KAL-1* gene whose product, anosmin-1, normally directs the migration of GnRH neurons from the olfactory placode to the hypothalamus. This results in a deficiency or absence of GnRH-secreting neurons in the hypothalamus, as well as agenesis or hypoplasia of the olfactory bulb, the latter defect being responsible for the hyposmia or anosmia seen in this syndrome. Boys are affected more commonly than girls and often exhibit cryptorchidism and microphallus at birth, reflecting the lack of fetal gonadotropins, which stimulate testosterone secretion from the fetal testes. At the time of expected puberty, there is a failure of gonadotropins to increase, of testicular enlargement, and secondary sexual characteristic development. After a single bolus injection of GnRH, little or no increase in gonadotropin levels is seen. However, if GnRH is given in a pulsatile fashion every 90 minutes, an increase in luteinizing hormone (LH) and follicle-stimulating hormone (FSH) will occur, reflecting the fact that the gonadotrophs are normal but understimulated in this syndrome. Pulsatile GnRH therapy may result in full virilization. Other components of this syndrome include color blindness, nerve deafness, cleft palate, exostosis, and renal abnormalities.[110] An autosomal-dominant form of anosmic and normosmic congenital hypogonadotropic hypogonadism is due to mutations of the fibroblast growth factor-1 receptor and accounts for 7% to 10% of patients with hypogonadotropic hypogonadism.[111] Another 5% of patients have a loss-of-function mutation of the GnRH receptor.[110]

Hypogonadotropic hypogonadism has been found with leptin and leptin-receptor gene mutations, as well as *GPR54* and *DAX1* mutations.[110] Congenital gonadotropin deficiency also is seen as a manifestation of panhypopituitarism (which may be on a hypothalamic basis), as well as with several complex hypothalamic disorders, including the Prader-Willi, Bardet-Biedl, and Laurence-Moon syndromes.

Hypogonadism is a relatively common manifestation of hypothalamic tumors and infiltrative disease, especially those that involve the floor of the third ventricle and median eminence. Obesity, diabetes insipidus, and neuro-ophthalmologic abnormalities often accompany the hypogonadism.[9,10]

Growth Hormone Deficiency

A variety of congenital structural defects involving the hypothalamus, such as anencephaly, holoprosencephaly, encephalocele, and septo-optic dysplasia, may result in growth hormone deficiency, either alone or with other anterior pituitary hormone deficiencies.[4] Monotropic growth hormone deficiency may occur sporadically or on a familial basis because of a deficient production or secretion of GHRH. Such patients will demonstrate an increase in growth hormone secretion after multiple injections of GHRH. Growth hormone deficiency also occurs as a manifestation of panhypopituitarism and is the hormone that is most frequently absent in these patients. As in patients with isolated growth hormone deficiency, those with panhypopituitarism generally have a hypothalamic basis for the abnormality, with deficiencies of multiple hypothalamic-releasing hormones.[112]

At birth, patients with congenital growth hormone deficiency have a normal length and weight but may exhibit microphallus. During the first year, growth retardation is seen, with a delay in both height and bone ages. Hypoglycemia due to loss of the glucose contraregulation effect of growth hormone may be found. During childhood, an increase in subcutaneous fat along with proportional short stature is noted. Even in the presence of normal gonadotrophs, puberty is often delayed in these patients. Treatment with growth hormone increases linear growth, reduces subcutaneous fat and glucose intolerance, and stimulates pubertal progression.[112]

Growth hormone deficiency is generally the earliest endocrine manifestation of a hypothalamic tumor or infiltrative process and results in growth retardation. Even in patients with structural hypothalamic disease who have no clinical evidence of growth retardation, provocative testing reveals a high frequency of inadequate growth hormone secretion.[110,113]

Hypothalamic Hypoadrenalism

Congenital or acquired isolated ACTH deficiency is quite rare. However, ACTH deficiency does commonly occur in association with other anterior pituitary hormone deficiencies due to craniopharyngiomas, suprasellar germinomas, and septo-optic dysplasia.[31,82,83,113-116] Clinical manifestations include nausea, vomiting, hypotension, and hypoglycemia, without the hyperpigmentation and electrolyte abnormalities from aldosterone deficiency seen in primary adrenocortical insufficiency.

Hypothalamic Hypothyroidism

Isolated TSH deficiency also is quite rare. However, TSH deficiency is found in approximately one third of the patients with craniopharyngiomas, suprasellar germinomas, and in patients with septo-optic dysplasia.[30,31,82,83,113,115] Clinically, patients may exhibit dry skin, puffiness, pallor, lethargy, bradycardia, hypothermia, and weight gain, with evidence of an atrophic thyroid gland. Serum free-T_4 levels are low, and the serum TSH may be low or slightly elevated, the latter reflecting abnormal glycosylation of the TSH molecule, which results in decreased biologic activity.[117] After an injection of TRH, a delayed and prolonged increase in TSH is seen in patients with hypothalamic hypothyroidism.[30,31,77]

Specific Hypothalamic Disorders

PRADER-WILLI SYNDROME

Prader-Willi syndrome, first described in 1956, occurs in approximately 1 in 25,000 live births.[118,119] The major clinical manifestations include infantile hypotonia; feeding problems; failure to thrive; rapid weight gain occurring between ages 1 and 6 years; a characteristic dysmorphic facial appearance with a narrow bitemporal diameter, almond-shaped eyes, palpebral fissures, down-turned mouth; developmental delay and mental retardation. Hypogonadism may be present at birth, with cryptorchidism, scrotal hypoplasia, and a small penis in boys; poor development of the labia minora and clitoris in girls; and delayed onset of puberty associated with low sex steroid hormones, low gonadotropins, and blunting of the gonadotropin response to GnRH. In addition, these patients have short stature (associated with growth hormone deficiency) and behavioral problems that appear during childhood and are characterized by temper tantrums, aggressive behavior, and obsessive-compulsiveness. One of the major characteristics of these patients is marked, indiscriminate hyperphagia and central obesity. These patients will exhibit abnormal food-seeking behavior, often eating discarded or spoiled food or pet food. Sleep disturbances and abnormalities in temperature control and heat generation also suggest a hypothalamic cause.[118-121] The only anatomic abnormality found in these patients is a decrease in the size of the paraventricular nuclei and oxytocin-producing neurons.[72]

Prader-Willi syndrome is a disorder of genetic (genomic) imprinting, in most cases due to a microdeletion of the paternally contributed chromosome 15q11-q13.[119,120] Because only the paternal genes are normally expressed in this region, a mutation of the paternal gene results in absence of expression. A minority of patients have maternal uniparental disomy (both members of the chromosome pair inherited from the same parent). An even rarer cause is a translocation involving chromosome 15.[119,120]

BARDET-BIEDL AND RELATED SYNDROMES

The Bardet-Biedl syndrome represents an autosomal-recessive disorder characterized by retinal pigmentary dystrophy (retinitis pigmentosa), mental retardation, central obesity, polydactyly, a variety of renal abnormalities, and hypogonadotropic hypogonadism.[122] Those with the Laurence-Moon syndrome also exhibit retinal pigmentary dystrophy, mental retardation, and hypogonadotropic hypogonadism. These patients also have progressive spastic paraparesis and distal muscle weakness but do not exhibit polydactyly.[123] The Biemond syndrome is another autosomal-recessive condition with mental retardation, polydactyly or brachydactyly, obesity, and hypogonadotropic hypogonadism. Retinal pigmentary dystrophy does not occur in this condition; rather, these patients have iris coloboma. The autosomal-recessive Alström syndrome is associated with atypical retinal pigmentary dystrophy, obesity, nerve deafness, diabetes mellitus, and acanthosis nigricans. Affected patients have hypogonadism due to primary gonadal failure rather than hypothalamic dysfunction.[123,124] The overlapping features of these different syndromes raise the possibility that they are due to a similar genetic abnormality.

SEPTO-OPTIC PITUITARY DYSPLASIA

The anatomic features of septo-optic pituitary dysplasia, a midline developmental abnormality, are an absence of the septum pellucidum, agenesis of the corpus callosum, unilateral or bilateral hypoplasia of the optic nerves, and absence of the supraoptic and paraventricular nuclei, with posterior pituitary hypoplasia.[82,83,114,115,125-127] The nonendocrine manifestations of this disease include visual abnormalities, mental retardation, nystagmus, seizures, and various forms of cerebral palsy.[82] Approximately two thirds of affected patients have short stature associated with growth hormone deficiency; approximately 40% have ACTH deficiency; 20% TSH deficiency; and one fourth exhibit gonadotropin deficiency. Close to one fourth of the patients exhibit diabetes insipidus, and approximately 20% have hyperprolactinemia.[82,83,114,115,125-127] This disorder is caused by recessive mutation in the homeobox gene on chromosome 3, HESX1.[128]

HYPERPHAGIC SHORT STATURE (PSYCHOSOCIAL DWARFISM)

Hyperphagic short stature, a rare syndrome which has its onset before age 2 years, occurs in some children exposed to a disturbed parent-child home environment. The clinical manifestations include short stature and delayed bone age associated with abnormal growth-hormone response to provocative tests; low body weight despite an enormous appetite that is associated with gorging, pica, food hoarding, vomiting, and production of foul-smelling stools; polydipsia; bizarre behavior; emotional or mental retardation; and a protuberant abdomen. In addition to the abnormal growth hormone responses, these patients may have an inadequate ACTH response to provocative testing, although thyroid function and urine-concentrating ability are normal. The clinical findings are reversible and disappear when the children are placed in a nurturing environment.[129,130]

PSEUDOCYESIS

An extreme example of a functional hypothalamic disorder is seen in women who develop a conversion reaction in which they think they are pregnant but in fact are not. Amenorrhea, morning nausea, breast enlargement and engorgement, and abdominal distension due to retained colonic gas are present in these women. Hyperprolactinemia is found, and some women exhibit galactorrhea.[131,132] Elevated levels of LH may account for the persistent corpus luteum activity that is seen in this syndrome.[133] When these women are informed of the diagnosis, the clinical manifestations rapidly disappear.

HYPOTHALAMIC HAMARTOMA

These benign hyperplastic malformations contain ganglion cells, myelinated nerve fibers, and glial matrix, and are generally located between the tuber cinereum and mamillary bodies.[79,134] Most patients exhibit onset of clinical symptoms before age 2 years, with the major endocrine abnormality being isosexual precocious puberty. Other common manifestations include gelastic seizures, emotional lability, hyperactivity, and neurodevelopmental delay.[78,80,89,90,134-138] During late childhood or adolescence, obesity develops in many of these patients. The precocious puberty in these patients responds to long-acting GnRH agonists that down-regulate GnRH receptors.[89] Neurosurgical removal of the hamartomas is indicated if signs of increased intracranial pressure, progressive growth, intractable seizures, or neurologic deterioration are present.[90]

The Pallister-Hall syndrome consists of hypothalamic hamartomas, panhypopituitarism, polydactyly, imperforate anus, and multiple craniofacial and limb abnormalities.[139-142] This may occur sporadically or be transmitted as an autosomal-dominant trait associated with a mutation of the GLP3 gene on chromosome 7p13.[143]

SUPRASELLAR ARACHNOID CYST

Suprasellar arachnoid cyst, an uncommon developmental anomaly of the arachnoid membrane, leads to a CSF-filled cyst that obstructs CSF flow through the foramen of Monro, leading to hydrocephalus and increased intracranial pressure. Thus headache, vomiting, lethargy, and increased head size are commonly found in these patients. The cysts also may compress the brainstem, optic nerve, and optic chiasm, leading to spasticity, ataxia, tremor, decreased visual acuity, and visual field defects. Endocrine abnormalities include growth hormone and ACTH deficiency, as well as precocious puberty.[144] Surgical decompression or percutaneous ventriculocystostomy is used to drain the cyst and reduce intracranial pressure.[145]

INFILTRATIVE DISORDERS

Sarcoidosis may involve the basal hypothalamus and floor of the third ventricle and lead to diminished visual acuity, visual field abnormalities, diabetes insipidus, thermal dysregulation, somnolence, personality changes, obesity, and hypothalamic hypopituitarism. Most patients with hypothalamic sarcoidosis also have involvement outside of the central nervous system.[34,35,37,146-147]

The chronic disseminated form of Langerhans' cell histiocytosis (Hand-Schüller-Christian disease) is classically composed of the triad of membranous bone lesions, exophthalmos, and diabetes insipidus. Growth retardation, hyperprolactinemia, hypogonadism, hypodipsia or adipsia, sleep disturbances, hyperphagia with obesity, temperature dysregulation, and behavioral abnormalities also may be found in these patients.[33,148,149]

HYPOTHALAMIC DYSFUNCTION AFTER BRAIN IRRADIATION

Both whole-brain irradiation and localized radiotherapy for brain or head or neck neoplasms are associated with delayed onset of hypothalamic dysfunction, most often manifested by progressive loss of growth hormone secretion and hyperprolactinemia. ACTH and gonadotropin deficiency are also found, as are changes in personality and abnormalities in thirst, sleep/wake cycle, and appetite regulation. Children are more susceptible to hypothalamic damage than are adults, and the incidence of hypothalamic abnormality increases with increasing radiation dose and decreasing intervals over which the radiation is administered.[150,151]

TRAUMATIC BRAIN INJURY

Posttraumatic hypopituitarism with multiple deficiencies of anterior pituitary hormones and elevation of prolactin due to damage to the hypothalamus, pituitary stalk, the hypophyseal artery or the pituitary is a relatively common occurrence following head trauma. Following the acute phase, anterior pituitary function may recover.[152,153]

REFERENCES

1. Boshes B: Syndromes of the diencephalons: The hypothalamus and the hypophysis. In Vinken PJ, Bruyn GW, editors: Localization in Clinical Neurology: Handbook of Clinical Neurology, Vol 2, Amsterdam, 1969, North-Holland, pp 432–468.
2. Kirgis HD, Locke W: Anatomy and embryology. In Locke W, Schally AV, editors: The Hypothalamus and Pituitary in Health and Disease. Springfield, IL, 1972, Charles C Thomas, pp 3–21.
3. Bruesch SR: Anatomy of the human hypothalamus. In Givens JR, Kitabchi AE, Robertson JT, editors: The Hypothalamus, St Louis, 1984, Mosby-Year Book, pp 1–16.
4. Braunstein GD: The hypothalamus. In Melmed S, editor: The Pituitary, 2nd ed, Cambridge, MA, 2002, Blackwell Scientific, pp 317–348.
5. Carmel PW: Surgical syndromes of the hypothalamus, Clin Neurosurg 27:133–159, 1980.
6. Plum F, Van Uitert R: Nonendocrine diseases and disorders of the hypothalamus. In Reichlin S, Baldessarini RJ, Martin JB, editors: The Hypothalamus. New York, 1978, Raven Press, pp 415–473.
7. Sano K, Mayanagi Y, Sekino H, et al: Results of stimulation and destruction of the posterior hypothalamus in man, J Neurosurg 33:689–707, 1970.
8. Garnica AD, Netzloff ML, Rosenbloom AL: Clinical manifestations of hypothalamic tumors, Ann Clin Lab Sci 10:474–485, 1980.
9. Bauer HG: Endocrine and other clinical manifestations of hypothalamic disease: A survey of 60 cases, with autopsies, J Clin Endocrinol Metab 14:13–31, 1954.
10. Bauer HG: Endocrine and metabolic conditions related to pathology in the hypothalamus: A review, J Nerv Ment Dis 128:323–338, 1959.
11. Thompson HJ, Tkacs NC, Saatman KE, et al: Hypothermia following traumatic brain injury: A critical evaluation, Neurobiol Dis 12:163–173, 2003.
12. Dott NM: Surgical aspects of the hypothalamus. In Le Gros Clark WE, Beattie J, Riddoch G, et al, editors: The Hypothalamus: Morphological, Functional, Clinical and Surgical Aspects, London, 1938, Oliver & Boyd, pp 131–185.
13. Frohman LA: Clinical aspects of hypothalamic disease. In Motta M, editor: The Endocrine Functions of the Brain, New York, 1980, Raven Press, pp 419–446.
14. Riddoch G: Clinical aspects of hypothalamic derangement. In Le Gros Clark WE, Beattie J, Riddoch G, et al, editors: The Hypothalamus: Morphological, Functional, Clinical and Surgical Aspects, London, 1938, Oliver & Boyd, pp 101–130.
15. McLean AJ: Autonomic epilepsy, Arch Neurol 32:189–197, 1934.

16. Rothballer AB, Dugger GS: Hypothalamic tumor: Correlation between symptomatology, regional anatomy, and neurosecretion, Neurology 5:160–177, 1955.
17. White LE, Hain RF: Anorexia in association with a destructive lesion of the hypothalamus, Arch Pathol Lab Med 68:275–281, 1959.
18. Reeves AG, Plum F: Hyperphagia, rage, and dementia accompanying a ventromedial hypothalamic neoplasm, Arch Neurol 20:616–624, 1969.
19. Fox RH, Davies TW, Marsh FP, et al: Hypothermia in a young man with an anterior hypothalamic lesion, Lancet 2:185–188, 1970.
20. Lewin K, Mattingly D, Millis RR: Anorexia nervosa associated with hypothalamic tumour, Br Med J 2:629–630, 1972.
21. Kamalian N, Keesey RE, Zurhein GM: Lateral hypothalamic demyelination and cachexia in a case of "malignant" multiple sclerosis, Neurology 25:25–30, 1975.
22. Celesia GG, Archer CR, Chung HD: Hyperphagia and obesity: Relationship to medial hypothalamic lesions, JAMA 246:151–153, 1981.
23. Haugh RM, Markesbery WR: Hypothalamic astrocytomas: Syndrome of hyperphagia, obesity, and disturbances of behavior and endocrine and autonomic function, Arch Neurol 40:560–563, 1983.
24. Schwartz WJ, Busis NA, Hedley-Whyte ET: A discrete lesion of ventral hypothalamus and optic chiasm that disturbed the daily temperature rhythm, J Neurol 233:1–4, 1986.
25. Pinkney J, Wilding J, Williams G, et al: Hypothalamic obesity in humans: what do we know and what can be done? Obes Rev 3:27–34, 2002.
26. Bergeron C, Kovacs K, Ezrin C, et al: Hereditary diabetes insipidus: An immunohistochemical study of the hypothalamus and pituitary gland, Acta Neuropathol 81:345–348, 1991.
27. Maghnie M, Ghirardello S, De Bellis A, et al: Idiopathic central diabetes insipidus in children and young adults is commonly associated with vasopressin-cell antibodies and markers of autoimmunity, Clin Endocrinol (Oxf) 65:470–478, 2006.
28. McLeod JF, Kovacs L, Gaskill MB, et al: Familial neurohypophyseal diabetes insipidus associated with a signal peptide mutation, J Clin Endocrinol Metab 77:599A–599G, 1997.
29. Minton JA, Ranibow LA, Ricketts C, et al: Wolfram syndrome, Rev Endocr Metab Disord 4:53–59, 2003.
30. Verbalis JG: Management of disorders of water metabolism in patients with pituitary tumors, Pituitary 22:119–132, 2002.

31. Buchfelder M, Fahlbusch R, Walther M, et al: Endocrine disturbances in suprasellar germinomas, Acta Endocrinol 120:337–342, 1989.
32. Jennings MT, Gelman R, Hochberg F: Intracranial germ-cell tumors: Natural history and pathogenesis, J Neurosurg 63:155–167, 1985.
33. Kaltsas GA, Powles TB, Evanson J, et al: Hypothalamo-pituitary abnormalities in adult patients with Langerhans cell histiocytosis: Clinical, endocrinological, and radiological features and response to treatment, J Clin Endocrinol Metab 85:1370–1376, 2000.
34. Delaney P: Neurologic manifestations in sarcoidosis: Review of the literature, with a report of 23 cases, Ann Intern Med 87:336–345, 1977.
35. Stuart CA, Neelon FA, Lebovitz HE: Hypothalamic insufficiency: The cause of hypopituitarism in sarcoidosis, Ann Intern Med 88:589–594, 1978.
36. Jawadi MH, Hanson TJ, Schemmel JE, et al: Hypothalamic sarcoidosis and hypopituitarism, Horm Res 12:1–9, 1980.
37. Vesely DL, Maldonado A, Levey GS: Partial hypopituitarism and possible hypothalamic involvement in sarcoidosis, Am J Med 62:425–431, 1977.
38. Ouma JR, Farrell VJR: Lymphocytic infundibulo-neurohypophysitis with hypothalamic and optic pathway involvement: Report of a case and review of the literature, Surg Neurol 57:49–54, 2002.
39. McKenna K, Thompson C: Osmoregulation in clinical disorders of thirst appreciation, Clin Endocrinol 49:139–152, 1998.
40. Teelucksingh S, Steer CR, Thompson CJ, et al: Hypothalamic syndrome and central sleep apnoea associated with toluene exposure, Q J Med 78:185–190, 1991.
41. Hayek A, Peake GT: Hypothalamic adipsia without demonstrable structural lesion, Pediatrics 70:275–278, 1982.
42. Ellison DH, Berl T: Clinical practice. The syndrome of inappropriate antidiuresis, N Engl J Med 356:2064–2072, 2007.
43. Palmer BF: Hyponatremia in patients with central nervous system disease: SIADH versus CSW, Trends Endocrinol Metab 14:182–187, 2003.
44. Wolff SM, Adler RC, Buskirk ER, et al: A syndrome of periodic hypothalamic discharge, Am J Med 36:956–967, 1964.
45. Martin JB, Reichlin S: Clinical Neuroendocrinology, Philadelphia, 1987, FA Davis, p 393.
46. Rusyniak DE, Sprague JE: Hyperthermic syndromes induced by toxins, Clin Lab Med 26:165–184, 2006.
47. Horn E, Lach B, Lapierre Y, et al: Hypothalamic pathology in the neuroleptic malignant syndrome, Am J Psychiatry 145:617–620, 1988.

48. Sandyk R, Iacono RP, Bamford CR: The hypothalamus in Parkinson disease, Ital J Neurol Sci 8:227–234, 1987.

49. Haak HR, van Hilten JJ, Roos RAC, et al: Functional hypothalamic derangement in a case of Wernicke's encephalopathy, Neth J Med 36:291–296, 1990.

50. Penfield W: Diencephalic autonomic epilepsy, Arch Neurol Psychiatry 22:358–369, 1929.

51. Fox RH, Wilkins DC, Bell JA, et al: Spontaneous periodic hypothermia: Diencephalic epilepsy, Br Med J 2:693–695, 1973.

52. Mooradian AD, Morley GK, McGeachie R, et al: Spontaneous periodic hypothermia, Neurology 34:79–82, 1984.

53. Flynn MD, Sandeman DD, Mawson DM, et al: Cyclical hypothermia: Successful treatment with ephedrine, J R Soc Med 84:752–753, 1991.

54. Kloos RT: Spontaneous periodic hypothermia, Medicine (Baltimore) 74:268–280, 1995.

55. Bray GA, Gallagher TF Jr: Manifestations of hypothalamic obesity in man: A comprehensive investigation of eight patients and a review of the literature, Medicine (Baltimore) 54:301–330, 1975.

56. Montague CT, Farooqi IS, Whitehead JP, et al: Congenital leptin deficiency is associated with severe early-onset obesity in humans, Nature 387:903–908, 1997.

57. Clement K, Vaisse C, Lahlou N, et al: A mutation in the human leptin receptor gene causes obesity and pituitary dysfunction, Nature 392:398–401, 1998.

58. Yeo GS, Farooqi IS, Aminian S, et al: A frameshift mutation in MC4R associated with dominantly inherited human obesity, Nat Genet 20:111–112, 1998.

59. Krude H, Biebermann H, Luck W, et al: Severe early-onset obesity, adrenal insufficiency and red hair pigmentation caused by POMC mutations in humans, Nat Genet 19:155–157, 1998.

60. Russell A: A diencephalic syndrome of emaciation in infancy and childhood, Arch Dis Child 26:274, 1951.

61. Burr IM, Slonim AE, Danish RK, et al: Diencephalic syndrome revisited, J Pediatr 88:439–444, 1976.

62. Poussaint TY, Barnes PD, Nichols K, et al: Diencephalic syndrome: clinical features and imaging findings, Am J Neuroradiol 18:1499–1505, 1997.

63. Fleishchman A, Brue C, Poussaint TY, et al: Diencephalic syndrome: a cause of failure to thrive and a model of partial growth hormone resistance, Pediatrics 115:e742–e748, 2005.

64. Miyoshi Y, Yunoki M, Yano A, et al: Diencephalic syndrome of emaciation in an adult associated with a third ventricle intrinsic craniopharyngioma: Case report, Neurosurgery 52:224–227, 2003.

65. Rome ES: Eating disorders, Obstet Gynecol Clin North Am 30:353–377, 2003.

66. Muñoz MT, Argente J: Anorexia nervosa in female adolescents: Endocrine and bone mineral density disturbances, Eur J Endocrinol 147:275–286, 2002.

67. Misra M, Miller KK, Tsai P, et al: Elevated peptide YY levels in adolescent girls with anorexia nervosa, J Clin Endocrinol Metab 91:1027–1033, 2006.

68. Mecklenberg RS, Loriaux DL, Thompson RH, et al: Hypothalamic dysfunction in patients with anorexia, Medicine (Baltimore) 53:147–159, 1974.

69. Clark LG: The hypothalamus in man. In Le Gros Clark WE, Beattie J, et al, editors: The Hypothalamus: Morphological, Functional, Clinical and Surgical Aspects, London, 1938, Oliver & Boyd, pp 59–68.

70. Carpenter MB, Sutin J: Human Neuroanatomy, Baltimore, 1983, Williams & Wilkins, pp 552–578.

71. Locke W, Schally AV: The Hypothalamus and Pituitary in Health and Disease, Springfield, IL, 1972, Charles C Thomas, pp 427–432.

72. Overeem S, van Vliet JA, Lammers GJ, et al: The hypothalamus in episodic brain disorders, Lancet 1:437–444, 2002.

73. Nishino S: Clinical and neurobiological aspects of narcolepsy, Sleep Med 8:373–399, 2007.

74. Martin JB, Reichlin S: Clinical Neuroendocrinology, Philadelphia, 1987, FA Davis, p 411.

75. Cohen RA, Albers HE: Disruption of human circadian and cognitive regulation following a discrete hypothalamic lesion: A case study, Neurology 41:726–729, 1991.

76. Fenzi F, Simonati A, Crosato F, et al: Clinical features of Kleine-Levin syndrome with localized encephalitis, Neuropediatrics 24:292–295, 1993.

77. Arnulf I, Seitzer JM, File J, et al: Kleine-Levin syndrome: a systemic review of 186 cases in the literature, Brain 128:2763–2776, 2005.

78. Breningstall GN: Gelastic seizures, precocious puberty, and hypothalamic hamartoma, Neurology 35:1180–1183, 1985.

79. Sharma RR: Hamartoma of the hypothalamus and tuber cinereum: A brief review of the literature, J Postgrad Med 33:1–13, 1987.

80. Harvey AS, Freeman JL: Epilepsy in hypothalamic hamartoma: clinical and EEG features, Semin Pediatr Neurol 14:60–64, 2007.

81. Shankar RR, Pescovitz OH: Precocious puberty, Adv Endocrinol Metab 6:55–89, 1995.

82. Margalith D, Jan JE, McCormick AQ, et al: Clinical spectrum of congenital optic nerve hypoplasia: Review of 51 patients, Dev Med Child Neurol 26:311–322, 1984.

83. Margalith D, Tze WJ, Jan JE: Congenital optic nerve hypoplasia with hypothalamic-pituitary dysplasia, Am J Dis Child 139:361–366, 1985.

84. Gross RE: Neoplasms producing endocrine disturbances in childhood, Am J Dis Child 59:579–628, 1940.

85. Laue L, Comite F, Hench K, et al: Precocious puberty associated with neurofibromatosis and optic gliomas, Am J Dis Child 139:1097–1100, 1985.

86. Gillett GR, Symon L: Hypothalamic glioma, Surg Neurol 28:291–300, 1987.

87. Banna M: Pathology and clinical manifestations. In Hankinson J, Banna M, editors: Pituitary and Parapituitary Tumours, London, 1976, Saunders, pp 13–58.

88. Weinberger LM, Grant FC: Precocious puberty and tumors of the hypothalamus, Arch Intern Med 67:762–792, 1941.

89. Chemaitilly W, Trivin C, Adan L, et al: Central precocious puberty: clinical and laboratory features, Clin Endocrinol (Oxf) 54:289–294, 2001.

90. Rosenfeld JV, Harvey AS, Wrennal J, et al: Transcallosal resection of hypothalamic hamartomas, with control of seizures, in children with gelastic epilepsy, Neurosurgery 48:108–118, 2001.

91. Hochman HI, Judge DM, Reichlin S: Precocious puberty and hypothalamic hamartoma, Pediatrics 67:236–244, 1981.

92. Losa M, von Werder K: Pathophysiology and clinical aspects of the ectopic GH-releasing hormone syndrome, Clin Endocrinol 47:123–135, 1997.

93. Saeger W, Puchner MJA, Ludecke DK: Combined sellar gangliocytomas and pituitary adenoma in acromegaly or Cushing's disease, Virchows Arch 425:93–99, 1994.

94. Asa SL, Bilbao JM, Kovacks K, et al: Hypothalamic neuronal hamartoma associated with pituitary growth hormone cell adenoma and acromegaly, Acta Neuropathol 52:231–234, 1980.

95. Asa SL, Scheithauer BW, Bilbao JM, et al: A case for hypothalamic acromegaly: A clinicopathological study of six patients with hypothalamic gangliocytomas producing growth hormone releasing factor, J Clin Endocrinol Metab 58:796–803, 1984.

96. Biller BMK: Pathogenesis of pituitary Cushing's syndrome: Pituitary versus hypothalamic, Endocrinol Clin North Am 23:547–554, 1994.

97. Gifford S, Gunderson JG: Cushing's disease as a psychosomatic disorder: A selective review of the clinical and experimental literature and a report of ten cases, Perspect Biol Med 13:169–221, 1970.

98. Bigos ST, Somma M, Rasio E, et al: Cushing's disease: Management by transsphenoidal pituitary microsurgery, J Clin Endocrinol Metab 50:348–354, 1980.

99. Lamberts SW, Stefanko SZ, DeLang SE, et al: Failure of clinical remission after transsphenoidal removal of a microadenoma in a patient with Cushing's disease: Multiple hyperplastic and adenomatous cell nests in surrounding pituitary tissues, J Clin Endocrinol Metab 50:793–795, 1980.

100. Krieger DT, Amorosa L, Linick F: Cyproheptadine-induced remission of Cushing's disease, N Engl J Med 293:893–896, 1975.

101. Lankford HU, Tucker HS, Blackard WG: A cyproheptadine-reversible defect in ACTH control persisting after removal of the pituitary tumor in Cushing's disease, N Engl J Med 305:1244–1248, 1981.

102. Cavagnini F, Invitti C, Polli EE: Sodium valproate in Cushing's disease, Lancet 2:162–163, 1984.

103. Lamberts SWJ, Klijn JG, deQuijada M, et al: The mechanism of the suppressive action of bromocriptine on adrenocorticotropin secretion in patients with Cushing's disease and Nelson's syndrome, J Clin Endocrinol Metab 51:307–311, 1980.

104. Biller BMK, Alexander JM, Zervas NT, et al: Clonal origins of adrenocorticotropin-secreting pituitary tissue in Cushing's disease, J Clin Endocrinol Metab 75:1303–1309, 1992.

105. Faglia G, Spada A: The role of hypothalamus in pituitary neoplasia, Clin Endocrinol 9:225–242, 1995.

106. Asa SL, Kovacs K, Tindall GT, et al: Cushing's disease associated with an intrasellar gangliocytoma producing corticotrophin-releasing factor, Ann Intern Med 101:789–793, 1984.

107. Kapcala LP, Molitch ME, Post KD, et al: Galactorrhea, oligo/amenorrhea, and hyperprolactinemia in patients with craniopharyngiomas, J Clin Endocrinol Metab 51:798–800, 1980.

108. McKeel DW Jr, Fowler M, Jacobs LS: The high prevalence of prolactin cell hyperplasia in the human adenohypophysis. In Proceedings of the Endocrine Society 60th Annual Meeting, Miami Beach, 1978, abstract 353.

109. Feigenbaum SL, Downey DE, Wilson CB, et al: Transsphenoidal pituitary resection for preoperative diagnosis of prolactin-secreting pituitary adenoma in women: Long-term follow-up, J Clin Endocrinol Metab 81:1711–1719, 1996.

110. Layman LC: Hypogonadotropic hypogonadism, Endocrinol Metab Clin North Am 36:283–296, 2007.

111. Gonzalez-Martinez D, Kim SH, Hu Y, et al: Anosmin-1 modulates fibroblast growth factor receptor 1 signaling in human gonadotropin-releasing hormone olfactory neuroblasts through a heparan sulfate-dependent mechanism, J Neurosci 24:10384–10392, 2004.

112. Dattani M, Preece M: Growth hormone deficiency and related disorders: insights into causation, diagnosis, and treatment, Lancet 363:1977–1987, 2004.

113. Fahlbusch R, Muller OA, Werder KV: Functional endocrinological disturbances in parasellar processes, Acta Neurochir 28(Suppl):456–460, 1979.

114. Arslanian SA, Rothfus WE, Foley TP Jr, et al: Hormonal, metabolic, and neuroradiologic abnormalities associated with septo-optic dysplasia, Acta Endocrinol 107:282–288, 1984.

115. Willnow S, Kiess W, Butenandt O, et al: Endocrine disorders in septo-optic dysplasia (De Morsier syndrome): Evaluation and follow up of 18 patients, Eur J Pediatr 155:179–184, 1996.

116. Korsgaard O, Lindholm J, Rasmussen P: Endocrine function in patients with suprasellar and hypothalamic tumours, Acta Endocrinol 83:1–8, 1976.

117. Beck-Peccoz P, Amr S, Menezes-Ferreira M, et al: Decreased receptor binding of biologically inactive thyrotropin in central hypothyroidism, N Engl J Med 312:1085–1090, 1985.

118. State MW, Dykens EM: Genetics of childhood disorders: XV. Prader-Willi syndrome: genes, brain, and behavior, J Am Acad Child Adolesc Psychiatry 39:797–800, 2000.

119. Cassidy SB: Prader-Willi syndrome, J Med Genet 34:917–923, 1997.

120. Hoybye C, Hilding A, Jacobsson H, et al: Metabolic profile and body composition in adults with Prader-Willi syndrome and severe obesity, J Clin Endocrinol Metab 87:3590–3597, 2002.

121. Goldstone AP: Prader-Willi syndrome: advances in genetics, pathophysiology and treatment, Trends Endocrinol Metab 15:12–20, 2004.

122. Beales PL, Elcioglu N, Woolf AS, et al: New criteria for improved diagnosis of Bardet-Biedl syndrome: Results of a population survey, J Med Genet 36:437–446, 1999.

123. Beales PL, Warner AM, Hitman GA, et al: Bardet-Biedl syndrome: A molecular and phenotypic study of 18 families, J Med Gent 34:922–928, 1997.

124. Charles SJ, Moore AT, Yates JAW, et al: Alström's syndrome: Further evidence of autosomal recessive inheritance and endocrinological dysfunction, J Med Genet 27:590–592, 1990.

125. Birkebaek NH, Patel L, Wright NB, et al: Endocrine status in patients with optic nerve hypoplasia: Relationship to midline central nervous system abnormalities and appearance of the hypothalamic-pituitary axis on

magnetic resonance imaging, J Clin Endocrinol Metab 88:5281–5286, 2003.

126. Roessmann U, Velasco ME, Small EJ, et al: Neuropathology of "septo-optic dysplasia" (de Morsier syndrome) with immunohistochemical studies of the hypothalamus and pituitary gland, J Neuropathol Exp Neurol 46:597–608, 1987.

127. Yukizane S, Kimura Y, Yamashita Y, et al: Growth hormone deficiency of hypothalamic origin in septo-optic dysplasia, Eur J Pediatr 150:30–33, 1990.

128. Polizzi A, Pavone P, Iannetti P, et al: Septo-optic dysplasia complex: a heterogeneous malformation syndrome, Pediatr Neurol 34: 66–71, 2006.

129. Skuse D, Albanese A, Stanhope R, et al: A new stress-related syndrome of growth failure and hyperphagia in children, associated with reversibility of growth-hormone insufficiency, Lancet 348:353–358, 1996.

130. Gilmour J, Skuse D, Pembrey M: Hyperphagic short stature and Prader-Willi syndrome: A comparison of behavioural phenotypes, genotypes and indices of stress, Br J Psychiatry 179:129–137, 2001.

131. Zuber T, Kelly J: Pseudocyesis, Am Fam Physician 30:131–134, 1984.

132. Bray MA, Muneyyirci-Delale A, Kofinas GD, et al: Circadian, ultradian, and episodic gonadotropin and prolactin secretion in human pseudocyesis, Acta Endocrinol 124:501–509, 1991.

133. Yen SSC, Rebar RW, Quesenberry W: Pituitary function in pseudocyesis, J Clin Endocrinol Metab 43:132–136, 1976.

134. List CF, Dowman CE, Bagchi BS, et al: Posterior hypothalamic hamartomas and gangliogliomas causing precocious puberty, Neurology 8:164–174, 1958.

135. Diebler C, Ponsot G: Hamartomas of the tuber cinereum, Neuroradiology 25:93–101, 1983.

136. Comite F, Psescovitz OH, Rieth KG: Luteinizing hormone-releasing hormone analog treatment of boys with hypothalamic hamartoma and true precocious puberty, J Clin Endocrinol Metab 59:888–892, 1984.

137. Nguyen D, Singh S, Zaatreh M, et al: Hypothalamic hamartomas: seven cases and review of the literature, Epilepsy Behav 4: 246–258, 2003.

138. Arita K, Kurisu K, Kiura Y, et al: Hypothalamic hamartoma, Neurol Med Chir (Tokyo) 45:221–231, 2005.

139. Hall JG, Pallister PD, Clarren SK, et al: Congenital hypothalamic hamartoblastoma, hypopituitarism, imperforate anus, and postaxial polydactyly: A new syndrome? Part I: Clinical, causal, and pathogenetic considerations, Am J Med Genet 7:47–74, 1980.

110. Clarren SK, Alvord EC Jr, Hall JG: Congenital hypothalamic hamartoblastoma, hypopituitarism, imperforate anus, and postaxial polydactyly: A new syndrome? Part II: Neuropathological considerations, Am J Med Genet 7:75–83, 1980.

141. Biesecker LG, Abbott M, Allen J, et al: Report from the Workshop on Pallister-Hall Syndrome and Related Phenotypes, Am J Med Genet 65:76–81, 1996.

142. Biesecker LG, Graham JM Jr: Pallister-Hall syndrome, J Med Genet 33:585–589, 1996.

143. Boudreau EA, Liow K, Frattali CM, et al: Hypothalamic hamartomas and seizures: distinct natural history of isolated and Pallister-Hall syndrome cases, Epilepsia 46:42–47, 2005.

144. Pradilla G, Jallo G: Arachnoid cysts: case series and review of the literature, Neurosurg Focus 22:E7, 2007.

145. Kirollos RW, Javadpour M, May P, et al: Endoscopic treatment of suprasellar and third ventricle-related arachnoid cysts, Childs Nerv Syst 17:713–718, 2001.

146. Bihan H, Christozova V, Dumas JL, et al: Sarcoidosis: clinical, hormonal, and magnetic resonance imaging (MRI) manifestations of hypothalamic-pituitary disease in 9 patients and review of the literature, Medicine (Baltimore) 86:259–268, 2007.

147. Porter N, Beynon HL, Randeva HS: Endocrine and reproductive manifestations of sarcoidosis, QJM 96:553–561, 2003.

148. Makras P, Alexandraki KI, Chrousos GP, et al: Endocrine manifestations in Langerhans cell histiocytosis, Trends Endocrinol Metab 18:252–257, 2007.

149. Amato MC, Elias LL, Elias J, et al: Endocrine disorders in pediatric-onset Langerhans Cell Histiocytosis, Horm Metab Res 38:746–751, 2006.

150. Rutter MM, Rose SR: Long-term endocrine sequelae of childhood cancer, Curr Opin Pediatr 19:480–487, 2007.

151. Gurney JG, Kadan-Lottick NS, Packer RJ, et al: Endocrine and cardiovascular late effects among adult survivors of childhood brain tumors: Childhood Cancer Survivor Study, Cancer 97:663–673, 2003.

152. Agha A, Thompson CJ: Anterior pituitary dysfunction following traumatic brain injury (TBI), Clin Endocrinol (Oxf) 64:481–488, 2006.

153. Schneider HJ, Kreitschmann-Andermahr I, Ghigo E, et al: Hypothalamopituitary dysfunction following traumatic brain injury and aneurysmal subarachnoid hemorrhage: a systematic review, JAMA 298:1429–1438, 2007.

Chapter 6

HYPOPITUITARISM AND GROWTH HORMONE DEFICIENCY

PAUL LEE and KEN K.Y. HO

Hypopituitarism refers to the deficiency of one or more pituitary hormones. It is seen commonly in endocrine practice and, it is important to note, is associated with increased morbidity and mortality. Clinical manifestations are influenced by the cause, severity, and rate of onset of pituitary hormone deficiency.

Adult patients with hypopituitarism receive substitutive hormone treatment for secondary glucocorticoid, sex steroid, and thyroid hormone deficiency. Until recently, growth hormone (GH) deficiency was not regarded as clinically important, as it was assumed that GH had no physiologic relevance after cessation of childhood growth. The advent of genetic engineering resulting in abundant supplies of recombinant GH has led to a major reappraisal of its physiologic role in adult life. GH continues to be produced throughout adult life and is the most abundant hormone in the adult pituitary gland. Many countries, including the United States, the United Kingdom, member countries of the European Union, and Australia, have approved the use of GH for replacement therapy in adults with GH deficiency.

Epidemiology

Limited information is available on the epidemiology of hypopituitarism. A Swedish survey estimates the prevalence of hypopituitarism to be 175 cases per million.[1] A Spanish study has reported a prevalence of hypopituitarism of 290 and 450 cases per million from two cross-sectional surveys in 1992 and 1999, respectively, and a corresponding incidence of 60 per million per year.[2] Sixty percent of the patients were GH deficient, giving a prevalence of GH deficiency of 114 to 270 cases per million and an incidence of 24 per million per year. A recent nationwide study in Denmark of GH deficiency identified an average incidence of approximately 20 million per year.[3]

Mortality

Mortality is increased in hypopituitarism. Data from six epidemiologic studies,[4-9] comprising patients aged between 46 and 52 years who were followed for 10 to 13 years, report increased mortality with standardized mortality rates (SMRs) from 1.2 to 2.2. The higher mortality arises from cardiovascular and cerebrovascular disease and appears to be greater in women[10] (Fig. 6-1).[5-8,11,12] Risk ratios for malignancies and respiratory disease varied. Comparison of these studies is difficult because of different definitions, causes, and degrees of hypopituitarism. For example, patients with craniopharyngioma and/or patients treated with radiotherapy were included in some[4,6,8,9] but not all studies.[5,7] Craniopharyngiomas carry a worse prognosis than pituitary adenomas,[13] and radiotherapy has been identified as a factor that increases mortality.[8] However, it is unclear whether it is radiotherapy or the result of more aggressive disease requiring radiotherapy that reduces survival.[8] A recent study, which included only postoperative hypopituitarism from pituitary

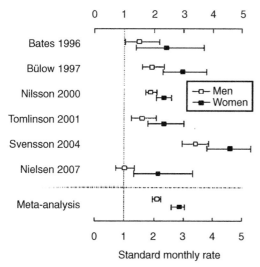

FIGURE 6-1. Standard mortality rates (SMR) and 95% confidence intervals (CI) in individual studies on patients with nonmalignant pituitary diseases not associated with excess adrenocorticotropic hormone (ACTH) or growth hormone (GH) secretion, and in the weighted meta-analysis *(bottom line)*. Results are shown for men *(open boxes)* and women *(black boxes)* separately. (From Nielsen EH, Lindholm J, Laurberg P. Excess mortality in women with pituitary disease: a meta-analysis. Clin Endocrinol 67:693–697, 2007.)

Table 6-1. Causes of Hypopituitarism

Neoplastic: Tumors involving the hypothalamic-pituitary (HP) axis
    Pituitary adenoma
    Craniopharyngioma
    Glioma (hypothalamus, third ventricle, optic nerve)
Surgery: for HP axis tumors
Radiotherapy
    HP axis tumors
    Brain tumors
    Head and neck cancer
    Acute lymphoblastic leukemia
Autoimmune
    Lymphocytic hypophysitis
Vascular
    Sheehan's syndrome
    Pituitary apoplexy
    Intrasellar carotid artery aneurysm
    Subarachnoid hemorrhage
Granulomatous disease
    Sarcoidosis
    Tuberculosis
    Histiocytosis X
    Wegener's granulomatosis
Genetic (see Table 6-2)
    Combined pituitary hormone deficiencies
    Isolated pituitary hormone deficiencies
Developmental
    Midline cerebral and cranial malformations
Traumatic
    Head injury
    Perinatal trauma
Infection
    Encephalitis
    Pituitary abscess
Iron-overload states
    Hemochromatosis
    Hemosiderosis (thalassemia)
Idiopathic

adenoma followed for a mean duration of 12.4 years, demonstrated increased mortality only in women, with an SMR of 1.97.[14]

GH deficiency has been implicated as a major contributor to excess mortality in hypopituitarism because it is the only defect not replaced in the studies of hypopituitarism. However, the contribution to overall mortality of other risk factors, such as radiotherapy and suboptimal replacement therapies for other hormone deficits, is the subject of ongoing investigation.

Causes

Major causes of hypopituitarism are shown in Table 6-1. The most common cause is a pituitary adenoma or treatment with pituitary surgery or radiotherapy.

PITUITARY AND HYPOTHALAMIC MASS LESIONS

Pituitary adenomas account for the vast majority of pituitary mass lesions, although secondary tumors do occur, from metastases to the pituitary gland from carcinomas of the breast, lung, colon, and prostate. Pituitary microadenomas are surprisingly common and are found in between 1.5% and 27% of patients at autopsy[15]; these tumors are very rarely, if at all, associated with hypopituitarism and tend to run a benign course. Macroadenomas are less common but are more frequently associated with pituitary hormone deficiencies; some 30% of patients with pituitary macroadenomas have one or more anterior pituitary hormone deficiencies. The causative mechanism of hypopituitarism is compression of the portal vessels in the pituitary stalk, secondary to the expanding tumor mass directly or to increased intrasellar pressure,[16] which explains the potential reversibility of pituitary dysfunction after surgery in some patients.

Many hypothalamic mass lesions arise from developmental abnormalities such as craniopharyngiomas, Rathke's cleft cysts, and arachnoid cysts. Craniopharyngiomas, the third most common intracranial tumor, account for most parapituitary tumors that occur. A bimodal peak in incidence occurs at 5 to 14 years and again after the age of 50. Their development origin is uncertain. They frequently have large cystic components and may be intrasellar, extrasellar, or both. Rathke's cleft cysts are cystic sellar and suprasellar lesions lined by a single epithelial layer. Arachnoid cysts present at a later age and are less common than both craniopharyngiomas and Rathke's cleft cysts.

Derangement of central endocrine regulation also occurs with other parapituitary space-occupying lesions such as chondromas, chordomas, suprasellar meningiomas, astrocytomas of the optic nerve, and primary tumors of the third ventricle.

Pituitary Surgery

The incidence and degree of hypopituitarism after surgery depend on the size of the original tumor, the degree of infiltration, and the experience of the surgeon. About 50% of patients already had evidence of GH, gonadotropin, or cortisol deficiency[17] before surgery. The patient should also be warned of a possible deterioration of postoperative pituitary function, and assessment of pituitary function should be performed promptly after surgery. However, a postoperative decline in pituitary function is not universal. After surgery, about 80% had evidence of GH or gonadotropin deficiency. In patients who received postoperative radiotherapy, evaluation after 5 years revealed that all patients were GH deficient.[17] On the other hand, surgery for pituitary adenomas may be associated with significant recovery of pituitary function. About half of the patients recover at least

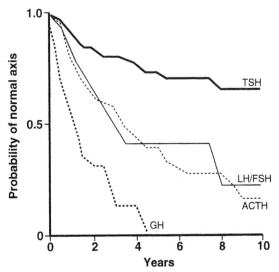

FIGURE 6-2. Life-table analysis indicating probabilities of initially normal hypothalamic-pituitary-target gland axes remaining normal after radiotherapy (3750 to 4250 cGy). Growth hormone (GH) secretion is the most sensitive of the anterior pituitary hormones to the effects of external radiotherapy, and thyroid-stimulating hormone (TSH) secretion is the most resistant. In two thirds of patients, gonadotropin deficiency develops before adrenocorticotropic hormone (ACTH) deficiency. *FSH*, Follicle-stimulating hormone; *LH*, luteinizing hormone. (From Littley MD, Shalet SM, Beardwell CG, et al: Hypopituitarism following external radiotherapy for pituitary tumors in adults. Q J Med 70:145–160, 1989.)

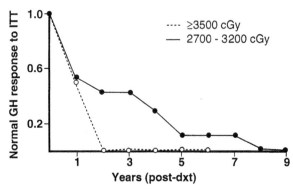

FIGURE 6-3. The incidence of growth hormone (GH) deficiency in children receiving 27 to 32 Gy or ≥35 Gy of cranial irradiation for a brain tumor in relation to time from irradiation (dxt). This illustrates that the speed at which individual pituitary hormone deficits develop is dose dependent; the higher the radiation dose, the earlier GH deficiency occurs. (Courtesy the Department of Medical Illustrations, Withington Hospital, Manchester, England.)

one pituitary insufficiency after transsphenoidal surgery. Postoperative improvement is more likely if no tumor is found on postoperative imaging, or if the tumor is not invasive.[18] The pituitary hormone most likely to recover is thyroid-stimulating hormone (TSH), followed in order by adrenocorticotropic hormone (ACTH), gonadotropins, and GH.[19] Recovery of pituitary function occurs early, within 8 weeks after surgery.[20]

Radiotherapy

Deficiency of one or more anterior pituitary hormones is almost invariable when the hypothalamic-pituitary axis lies within the fields of radiation. Hypopituitarism also develops in patients who received radiation therapy for nasopharyngeal carcinomas, parasellar tumors, and primary brain tumors, as well as in children who underwent prophylactic cranial irradiation for acute lymphoblastic leukemia or total body irradiation (TBI) for a variety of tumors and other diseases.[21]

The radiobiological impact of an irradiation schedule is dependent on the total dose, the number of fractions, and the duration and length of follow-up. Somatotrophs are the most sensitive to radiation damage, and thus, after lower radiation doses (<30 Gy), isolated GH deficiency ensues, whereas higher doses (30 to 50 Gy) increase the frequency of GH deficiency to 50% to 100% and may produce panhypopituitarism (Fig. 6-2). Radiation dose also determines the speed of onset of hormonal deficiency. The greater the dose, the earlier is the occurrence of GH deficiency, so that between 2 and 5 years after irradiation, 100% of children receiving more than 30 Gy (over a 3-week period) to the hypothalamic-pituitary axis developed subnormal GH responses to an insulin tolerance test (ITT), whereas 35% of those receiving less than 30 Gy (over a 3-week period) still showed a normal GH response[22] (Fig. 6-3). However, interpretation of the impact of radiation-induced damage to the hypothalamic-pituitary axis on GH status is complicated in the early years after irradiation. Discordant results to different

GH-provocative agents may be seen, such that up to 50% of patients classified as severely GH deficient with use of the ITT showed normal or mildly insufficient GH response during the combined GH-releasing hormone (GHRH) plus arginine stimulation test.[23,24] The discordant response to dynamic testing in patients with GH deficiency is discussed in greater detail later in the chapter, under Diagnosis in Growth Hormone Deficiency.

Paradoxically, whereas high doses of cranial irradiation may render a child gonadotropin-deficient, lesser doses of irradiation may be associated with early puberty. The mechanism for early puberty after irradiation is likely to be related to disinhibition of cortical influences on the hypothalamus.

Fractionated stereotactic conformal radiotherapy (SCRT) is a more precise technique of localized irradiation that may reduce radiation damage to normal structures in the brain. However, despite this theoretical advantage of normal-tissue sparing, hypopituitarism remains a common complication. At a median follow-up of 32 months, 22% of patients with previously normal pituitary function or partial hypopituitarism developed new hormonal deficit, and 18% developed panhypopituitarism.[25] The incidence of hypopituitarism was not different between conventional radiotherapy and SCRT,[25] and it may occur as late as 10 years after therapy, reaching as high as 66% after a median follow-up of 17 years.[26,27] Therefore, with increased survival, follow-up evaluation of patients irradiated for tumors of the brain and surrounding structures must focus equally on the possibility of tumor recurrence and on the delayed effects of therapy, including the endocrine effects. Endocrine testing should be performed on a yearly basis for at least 10 years and again at 15 years.

GENETIC CAUSES

Major advances in our understanding of the developmental biology of the pituitary in recent years have provided insights into the molecular pathology of genetic causes of hypopituitarism. During embryonic development, the pituitary gland is formed by the association of neural ectodermal cells from the ventral diencephalons with ectodermal cells from the oral cavity. The former give rise to the posterior pituitary, and the latter give rise to the anterior pituitary. The formation and differentiation of Rathke's pouch, the primordial anterior pituitary lobe structure, into the mature pituitary gland are regulated by the actions of specific transcription factors in a spatial and temporal fashion. These include KAL, HESX-1, Prop-1, and Pit-1. Mutations in genes encoding for these transcription factors result in deficiency of one or more anterior pituitary hormones.

Combined Pituitary Hormone Deficit

A cascade of pituitary transcription factors regulates the differentiation of cells of Rathke's pouch into somatotrophs, lactotrophs, thyrotrophs, gonadotrophs, and corticotrophs. Mutations in early appearing transcription factors tend to cause more extensive hormone deficiencies (Table 6-2).

Pit-1 (pituitary-specific transcription factor-1) is a pituitary-specific transcription factor that is responsible for the development of somatotrophs, lactotrophs, and thyrotrophs in mammals. Pit-1 abnormalities account for only a small minority of the total number of worldwide cases of hypopituitarism. *Pit-1* gene mutations also have been discovered in patients with idiopathic GH deficiency associated with preserved basal prolactin and TSH secretion, illustrating the variability of phenotypic presentation among these patients.

PROP1 (Prophet of Pit-1) is a novel pituitary paired-like homeodomain factor, which regulates the expression of Pit-1. Several multicenter studies of patients have reported that *PROP1* mutations are the most common genetic cause of multiple pituitary hormone deficiencies, accounting for up to 40% to 50% of cases. PROP1 abnormalities result in similar phenotypic abnormalities to *Pit-1* mutations but with associated gonadotropin deficiency. The degree of gonadotropin deficiency is variable, even among individuals within the same family with identical mutations. In individuals with a mutation of the *PROP1* gene, progressive hypopituitarism develops, with GH, TSH, and gonadotropin deficiency typically present by the end of the second decade.[28] The pituitary gland may pass through a hyperplastic phase before undergoing a phase of degeneration and late appearance of partial ACTH deficiency.

Other genetic causes of combined pituitary hormone deficiencies include mutations of *HESX1*, *LHX3/LHX4*, and *Pitx1/Pitx2*, which are transcription factors engaged in early pituitary cell development before the appearance of Pit-1 and PROP1.[29-31] For example, *HESX-1* is a homeobox gene expressed early in the ectoderm, which is the precursor of Rathke's pouch. It plays an important role in optic nerve and anterior pituitary development. *HESX-1* mutations in humans are associated with septo-optic dysplasia and GH deficiency. Other genes (e.g., *LHX3*) bind to

Pit-1 and can enhance Pit-1 activity, or synergistically activate prolactin and *TSH* genes (e.g., *Pitx1*).

Isolated Pituitary Hormone Deficiency

Isolated Growth Hormone Deficiency

Isolated GH deficiency (IGHD) can arise from mutations of the *GH* gene and of the *GH-releasing hormone (GHRH) receptor* gene.[32] The *human GH (hGH)* gene is located on chromosome 17 in a cluster of five genes: hGH-N encodes the gene for pituitary GH, hGH-V encodes the gene for placental GH, and three genes encode for human chorionic somatotropin (hCS). There are four types of Mendelian disorders of the GH gene that are due to deletion of these genes: IGHD IA and IB are both inherited in an autosomal recessive manner, resulting in absent or low GH levels. In patients with absent GH (IGHD IA), anti-GH antibodies often develop when they are treated with GH. IGHD II has an autosomal dominant mode of inheritance with variable clinical severity. IGHD III is an X-linked disorder that often is associated with hypogammaglobulinemia. Mutations of the gene encoding the GHRH receptor have been identified in a number of kindreds with severe GH deficiency in Pakistan and in Brazil.[33,34]

Isolated Gonadotropin Deficiency

Several gene mutations have been identified as causes of idiopathic hypogonadotropic hypogonadism (IHH) in humans.[35] Gonadotropin-releasing hormone (GnRH) neurons originate in the olfactory placode and migrate during embryogenesis with the olfactory nerves to the hypothalamus. The KAL protein is necessary for this process to occur. Kallmann's syndrome is characterized by the combination of IHH and anosmia or hyposmia, which usually is caused by defective GHRH secretion. It is a heterogeneous condition that manifests in an X chromosome–linked or autosomal dominant form. The X-linked form of the disorder is due to mutations in the *KAL* gene. Recently, several growth factors, including fibroblast growth factors (FGFs) and adhesion molecules, have been identified to play important regulatory roles in the development and migration of GHRH neurons. Mutation of the *FGF receptor 1 (FGFR1)* gene causes the autosomal dominant form of Kallmann's syndrome.[36] Additional clinical features associated with *KAL* mutations include bimanual synkinesia and renal agenesis; *FGFR1* mutations typically lead to cleft lip palate and dental agenesis.

Another important protein is DAX1, which is a transcription factor involved in development of pituitary gonadotrophs and the adrenal cortex. Mutations in the *DAX1* gene give rise to X-linked recessive hypogonadotropic hypogonadism and adrenal hypoplasia. Other genes implicated in IHH are *PC1* (prohormone convertase, associated with defects in prohormone processing), *OB*, and *DB* (leptin and leptin receptor, associated with obesity), whereas inactivating mutations of luteinizing hormone (LH)-β and follicle-stimulating hormone (FSH)-β genes can cause isolated deficiencies of LH and FSH, respectively.

Isolated ACTH and TSH Deficiencies

Isolated deficiencies of TSH or ACTH are very rare; however, in a number of cases, a genetic abnormality has been described or proposed. Mutations of the coding region of the *TSH-β subunit* gene[37] and the *thyrotropin-releasing hormone (TRH)-receptor* gene[38] have been found in a number of families to be the cause of hereditary isolated TSH deficiency.

Recently, a pituitary transcription factor causing isolated ACTH deficiency was identified. TBX19 (the human T-box

Table 6-2. Genetic Causes of Hypopituitarism

	Gene Defect	Hormone Deficiencies
Combined	Pit-1 (POU1F1, GHF1)	GH, TSH, PRL
	PROP-1	GH, LH/FSH, TSH, ACTH, PRL
	HESX1 (Rpx)	GH, LH/FSH, TSH, ACTH, ADH
	LHX3/LHX4	GH, LH/FSH, TSH, PRL
	PITX2	GH, PRL
Isolated	hGH	GH
	GHRH receptor gene	GH
	KAL	FSH/LH
	GnRH receptor gene	FSH/LH
	DAX1/AHC	FSH/LH
	TBX19 (Tpit)	ACTH
	TSH-β gene	TSH
	TRH receptor gene	TSH

pituitary transcription factor, analogous to Tpit in the mouse) plays an essential role in differentiation of pro-opiomelanocortin (POMC) cells in the pituitary. At least two *TBX19* gene mutations causing isolated ACTH deficiency have been described,[39,40] and this may underlie the cause of a neonatal-onset form of congenital isolated ACTH deficiency,[41] which is fatal unless diagnosed early and replaced with glucocorticoid.

Traumatic Brain Injury

Traumatic brain injury (TBI) is an under-appreciated cause of hypopituitarism. It was first reported in 1918. Meta-analysis of 19 studies, which included more than 1000 patients, demonstrated a pooled prevalence of hypopituitarism following TBI of 27.5% (1 pituitary hormone deficiency), and 7.7% of patients had multiple deficiencies. GH deficiency was the most common with a prevalence of 12.4%, followed by secondary hypogonadism (12.5%), hypoadrenalism (8.2%), and hypothyroidism (4.1%). Prevalence of diabetes insipidus is 26% in the acute phase and is decreased to 6.9% among long-term survivors.[42]

Risk factors of traumatic hypopituitarism include basal skull fracture, diffuse axonal injury, raised intracranial pressure, and prolonged stay in the intensive care unit.

TBI is common, with an overall incidence of 235 per 100,000 persons per year.[43] Traumatic hypopituitarism therefore is a major public health issue with significant clinical implications. The incidence of hypopituitarism following TBI is more than 30 patients per 100,000 population per year.[44] Patients therefore should be screened for hypopituitarism following TBI. Early (<3 months) hormonal dysfunction, including central hypothyroidism and hypogonadism, was not predictive of long-term development of hypopituitarism.[45] Assessment for GH deficiency, hypogonadism, and hypothyroidism is not necessary in the acute phase, but adrenal insufficiency should not be missed, as it can be fatal if untreated. All patients should undergo screening for hypopituitarism between 3 and 6 months after injury.

Lymphocytic Hypophysitis

Lymphocytic hypophysitis, an immune-mediated diffuse infiltration of the anterior pituitary with lymphocytes and plasma cells, occurs predominantly in women and often is first evident in pregnancy or after delivery. The classic presentation is peripartum hypopituitarism, often with a pituitary mass and visual failure. ACTH deficiency is an almost universal feature that, when undiagnosed, has proved fatal. At an early stage, the pituitary gland is enlarged and cannot be distinguished from a pituitary tumor by computed tomography (CT) or magnetic resonance imaging (MRI), whereas in later stages, the gland may atrophy, leaving an empty sella. Lymphocytic hypophysitis is more common in patients with other autoimmune endocrine diseases. Cytosolic autoantigens against the pituitary can be demonstrated in some cases but also are present in normal patients; thus the definitive diagnosis of this condition remains difficult without pituitary biopsy. Recently, identification of more specific autoantigens, such as chorionic somatomammotropin, may allow noninvasive diagnosis of hypophysitis in the future, with a sensitivity of 64% and a specificity of 86% by immunoblotting.[46] Spontaneous resolution of both the mass and the hypopituitarism has been reported, and in some cases, neurosurgical intervention has led to irreversible pituitary failure. Therefore, conservative management is appropriate in most patients. Spontaneous recovery with physiologic hydrocortisone replacement can happen,[47] and high-dose methylprednisolone pulse therapy may improve adreno-pituitary function and shrinkage of the sellar mass.[48]

Pituitary Apoplexy

Pituitary apoplexy is the abrupt destruction of pituitary tissue that results from infarction or hemorrhage into the pituitary, usually into an underlying pituitary tumor. Severe headache accompanies a variable degree of visual loss or cranial nerve palsy. Consequent pituitary hormone deficiencies may develop rapidly. In Sheehan's syndrome, pituitary infarction occurs secondary to severe postpartum hemorrhage and ensuing circulatory failure. Once common, this complication is now confined mainly to areas where obstetric services are less well developed.

Granulomatous Diseases

Granulomatous diseases, including sarcoidosis, tuberculosis, and Langerhans cell histiocytosis, can affect the hypothalamic-pituitary axis and cause hypopituitarism, including diabetes insipidus. Diabetes insipidus complicates sarcoidosis rarely (1%). This is more common, however, in Langerhans cell histiocytosis, with diabetes insipidus developing in 15% of childhood cases; it also may occur in patients first seen in adulthood.

Hypopituitarism

CLINICAL FEATURES

Presentation of hypopituitarism can be nonspecific. It is affected by degree, type, and rate of onset of the pituitary hormone deficiency. Local pressure effects or hormonal hypersecretion may complicate the clinical picture. Hypopituitarism arising from an expanding mass lesion or from irradiation produces a characteristic evolution of pituitary failure caused by an initial loss of GH secretion, followed by LH and FSH, and finally by failure of ACTH and TSH secretion.

In cases arising from loss of function caused by an expanding silent mass lesion, the onset of symptoms is insidious, typically occurring with mild headaches, lethargy, fatigue, disinterest, weight gain, low mood, and declining libido—symptoms mimicking depression. Rarely, anorexia and weight loss may arise from ACTH deficiency and may be mistaken for and lead to extensive investigations for occult malignancy. Progressive mass expansion causing increasingly severe headaches or visual symptoms from chiasmal compression usually leads to radiologic investigations that clinch the diagnosis. A high index of suspicion is required to diagnose hypopituitarism. The symptoms and signs of individual hormone deficiency are listed in Table 6-3. The features of isolated deficiencies of each axis are described below. GH deficiency is addressed separately in the section dedicated to GH deficiency in adults.

Gonadotropin Deficiency

In male patients, the clinical features of gonadotropin deficiency differ according to whether the deficiency was acquired before or after pubertal age. If acquired before pubertal age, clinical examination reveals a small penis, small testes, and eunuchoid proportions (span exceeds a height of 5 cm). Hypogonadism acquired postpubertally is associated with a reduction in testicular size, loss of facial and body hair, and thinning of the skin, leading to the characteristic finely wrinkled facial skin of the "aging youth." Other effects include a decrease in skeletal muscle mass, bone mineral density, sexual function, libido, and general well-being. Azoospermia is an almost inevitable consequence of hypogonadotropic hypogonadism. Partial LH

Table 6-3. Symptoms and Signs of Hormone Deficiencies

Hormone Deficiency	Symptoms and Signs
Growth hormone	Please refer to Table 6-6 in the section Growth Hormone Deficiency.
Gonadotropins	In men: poor libido/impotence, infertility, small soft testes, reduced facial/body hair In women: amenorrhea/oligomenorrhea dyspareunia, infertility, breast atrophy
Thyroid-stimulating hormone	Growth retardation in children; decrease in energy, constipation; sensitivity to cold, dry skin, weight gain
Adrenocorticotropic hormone	Weakness, tiredness, dizziness on standing, pallor, hypoglycemia
Prolactin	Failure of lactation
Antidiuretic hormone	Polyuria, polydipsia, nocturia, hypotension

deficiency may result in low circulating testosterone levels and gynecomastia with preserved testicular size and fertility, as intratesticular testosterone levels remain high enough to maintain spermatogenesis.

In a teenage girl, hypogonadotropic hypogonadism is associated with primary amenorrhea and absent breast development. In the adult woman, amenorrhea or oligomenorrhea, infertility, breast atrophy, vaginal dryness, and dyspareunia occur; pubic and axillary hair remains unless ACTH deficiency also is present.

Adrenocorticotropic Hormone Deficiency

ACTH deficiency is the most life-threatening component of hypopituitarism. If the onset is abrupt, as in pituitary apoplexy, the clinical picture may be dominated by profound shock in the most serious form. Patients with chronic ACTH deficiency usually present with chronic progressive symptoms of chronic fatigue, anorexia, and weight loss, sometimes mimicking anorexia nervosa or an occult malignancy. Patients on long-term glucocorticoid therapy can develop adrenal atrophy secondary to ACTH suppression.[49,50] Examination may reveal pallor of the skin, in contrast to the hyperpigmentation of Addison's disease, and in female patients particularly, loss of secondary sexual hair occurs. In severe ACTH deficiency, particularly in childhood, hypoglycemia can occur: Cortisol deficiency results in increased insulin sensitivity and a decrease in hepatic glycogen reserves. Hyponatremia, although less commonly seen than in Addison's disease because of preservation of aldosterone secretion, may be the presenting feature of ACTH deficiency, particularly in the elderly.

Thyroid-Stimulating Hormone Deficiency

Thyroid-stimulating hormone (TSH) deficiency occurs late in most pituitary disorders. Symptoms include fatigue, weakness, inability to lose weight, constipation, and cold intolerance, in keeping with the symptoms of primary hypothyroidism. However, symptoms generally are milder than in primary hypothyroidism, because some residual TSH secretion often is preserved.

Antidiuretic Hormone Deficiency

Polydipsia and polyuria with nocturia are the classic features of diabetes insipidus resulting from antidiuretic hormone (ADH) deficiency. If the patient is unable to keep up with the fluid loss, hypotension and hypovolemia ensue. The features of diabetes insipidus may be masked by the presence of ACTH deficiency, because of the consequent hypovolemia and reduced glomerular filtration rate. Only when cortisol replacement therapy is commenced may the polyuria and polydipsia of diabetes insipidus be revealed.

DIAGNOSIS AND ENDOCRINE EVALUATION
Imaging

Computerized digital imaging has revolutionized the investigation of pituitary function, as it provides unparalleled views of the anatomy of the region, readily identifying structural abnormalities. MRI is the scanning technique of choice, as it offers higher resolution than CT scanning and is able to demonstrate microadenomas as small as 3 mm in diameter. MRI also has provided insights into the morphologic abnormalities that arise from developmental defects of the pituitary gland and how morphologic abnormalities relate to dynamic tests of pituitary function, especially in GH deficiency. CT is used in situations where MRI is contraindicated, such as when arterial clips or a pacemaker is present. CT has a valuable role in defining bone anatomy in preparation for surgery.

Radiologic Phenotype of GH Deficiency

GH deficiency can be divided broadly into either genetic GH deficiency, when proven genetic mutations, such as *GH-1, GHRH-R,* and *PROP-1,* are identified, or idiopathic GH deficiency, when a genetic abnormality cannot be identified. On MRI, cases of genetic GH deficiency typically reveal a pituitary gland that is small or of normal size. The pituitary stalk is intact, and the location of the posterior lobe is normal. In contrast, idiopathic GH deficiency frequently is associated with a small pituitary gland, with evidence of stalk hypoplasia or interruption and an ectopic posterior lobe (Fig. 6-4). It has been suggested that perinatal trauma may be responsible for these abnormalities on MRI, resulting in idiopathic GH deficiency.[51,52] This is supported by the observed higher frequency of breech delivery and birth hypoxemia with idiopathic GH deficiency than in genetic cases.[53]

The stalk provides vascular communication, and its presence is significant in relation to the evaluation of diagnostic testing for GH deficiency. Maghnie and colleagues have reported that integrity of the hypothalamic-pituitary connection is necessary for GHRH-arginine to stimulate GH release, as the GH response is markedly impaired in patients with stalk agenesis.[54]

Endocrine Evaluation

The endocrine assessment of a patient with suspected hypopituitarism usually involves measurement of both baseline and stimulated hormone levels. Evaluation of baseline function involves prolactin, TSH, thyroxine (T$_4$), cortisol, LH, FSH, and testosterone in men, and estradiol in women. Baseline blood testing reliably identifies hypothyroidism, hypogonadism, and severe hypoadrenalism due to pituitary insufficiency.

Dynamic Testing

Adult Gonadotropin Deficiency. In women of postmenopausal age, gonadotropin levels are clearly low or undetectable, whereas in premenopausal women, amenorrhea (or less com-

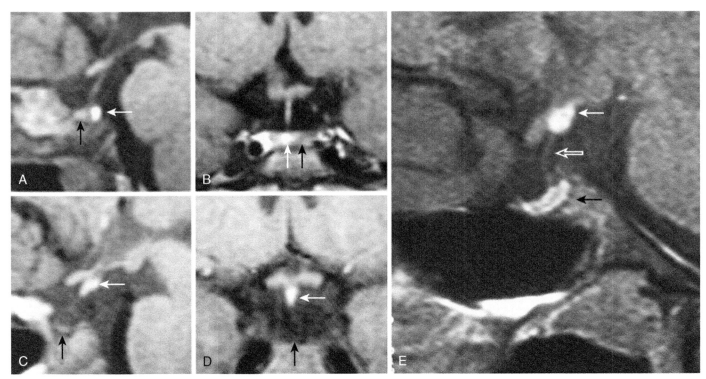

FIGURE 6-4. Magnetic resonance imaging (MRI) of congenital causes of growth hormone deficiency: Sagittal **(A)** and coronal **(B)** pituitary imaging studies of a patient with isolated growth hormone (GH) deficiency caused by *GH-1* gene deletion of 6.7 kb showing intact stalk, normal pituitary gland *(black arrow)*, and posterior lobe *(white arrow)*; sagittal **(C)** and coronal **(D)** views of a patient with idiopathic isolated GH deficiency showing stalk interruption, an ectopic posterior lobe *(white arrow)*, and pituitary gland hypoplasia *(black arrow)*. Sagittal **(E)** view of pituitary MRI of a 17-year-old patient with idiopathic GH deficiency, demonstrating a hypoplastic gland *(black arrow)*, stalk hypoplasia *(hollow white arrow)*, and an ectopic posterior pituitary gland *(white arrow)*. (From Osorio MG, Marui S, Jorge AA, Latronico AC, Lo LS, Leite CC, Estefan V, Mendonca BB, Arnhold IJ: Pituitary magnetic resonance imaging and function in patients with growth hormone deficiency with and without mutations in GHRH-R, GH-1, or PROP-1 genes. J Clin Endocrinol Metab 87:5076–5084, 2002.)

monly, oligomenorrhea), in addition to low estradiol levels and low or normal gonadotropin levels, provides sufficient evidence of the diagnosis. In adult men, a similar picture of low testosterone levels and low or inappropriately normal gonadotropin levels is seen.

Adrenocorticotropic Hormone Deficiency. A high index of clinical suspicion is most important in establishing the diagnosis. In normal people, the highest plasma cortisol levels are found between 6:00 AM and 8:00 AM, and the lowest before midnight. Plasma cortisol and ACTH concentrations are elevated during physical and emotional stress, including acute illness, trauma, surgery, infection, and starvation.

If a 9:00 AM cortisol level is less than 100 nmol/L, particularly in an unwell patient, cortisol deficiency is highly likely, whereas a baseline level greater than 500 nmol/L indicates normality; many authors suggest that dynamic assessment of the hypothalamic-pituitary-adrenal (HPA) axis is not necessary under these circumstances.[55] Unless the patient is known to have pituitary disease, a paired plasma ACTH level will help distinguish between primary and secondary glucocorticoid deficiency: In primary cortisol deficiency (Addison's disease), the ACTH level will be high, whereas in secondary glucocorticoid deficiency, the ACTH level will be low or inappropriately normal.

If cortisol deficiency is suspected in an unwell patient, baseline cortisol and ACTH samples should be taken, and replacement therapy should be commenced immediately. Provocative testing can be performed at a later date.

The insulin tolerance test (ITT) is the test of choice in those suspected of secondary adrenal failure. The ITT evaluates the response of the HPA axis to the potent stressor of hypoglycemia,

and it is generally the "gold standard" in the confirmation of secondary adrenal failure. It has the advantage of also being a test of growth hormone reserve in patients with pituitary disease.[56] Following injection of a standard dose of intravenous insulin (0.1 unit/kg),[57] cortisol concentrations are measured serially. Upon achievement of adequate hypoglycemia (<2.2 mmol/L), a peak cortisol response of between 500 and 600 nmol/L generally is accepted as adequate.[58]

The short Synacthen (tetracosactrin) test sometimes is used as a surrogate test of ACTH deficiency on the basis that the adrenal gland will respond to an exogenous bolus of synthetic ACTH when there is a normal endogenous ACTH reserve and the gland is not atrophic. Although it is a good test of adrenal reserve, it does not directly test pituitary ACTH reserve. In a patient with organic pituitary disease, a normal response to Synacthen does not exclude mild or recent ACTH deficiency.

Thyroid-Stimulating Hormone Deficiency. In secondary hypothyroidism, one might expect to find reduced concentrations of free or total T_4 in association with a serum TSH concentration below the normal range, analogous to the biochemical findings in secondary hypogonadism. Most have normal or occasionally elevated TSH levels. The mechanism behind this apparent contradiction is poorly understood, but it may be due to reduced bioactivity of TSH,[59] which suggests that TRH regulates not only the secretion of TSH but also its specific molecular and conformational features. Dynamic testing with thyrotropin-releasing hormone has little diagnostic value other than distinguishing a hypothalamic cause, which is indicated by a delayed TSH peak.

Antidiuretic Hormone Deficiency. The diagnosis of ADH deficiency first requires confirmation of polyuria, which is defined as the excretion of more than 3 L of urine per 24 hours (40 mL/kg/24 hours). Any patient with normal serum sodium and plasma osmolality who has a fluid output of <2 L/24 hours is likely to be normal and does not warrant further investigation.

Once excess urine output has been confirmed, the usual first-line investigation is an 8-hour fluid deprivation test. The test should be performed under strict observation because severe fluid and electrolyte depletion can occur. Plasma osmolality, urine volume, and osmolarity are measured hourly for 8 hours, after which a synthetic analogue of ADH (desmopressin) is given intramuscularly (IM). The urine osmolality then is remeasured. In a normal subject, ADH is secreted throughout the test, water is absorbed normally, and a subsequent elevation of urine osmolality occurs. In diabetes insipidus, the urine fails to concentrate (normal subjects achieve a urine osmolality at least twice the plasma osmolality) because of a lack of ADH; hence, plasma osmolality increases. Urine concentrates adequately only after administration of desmopressin. Sometimes in cases with long-standing polyuria, failure of urine concentration in response to desmopressin occurs not because of nephrogenic diabetes insipidus but because of a washout of interstitial solutes, including urea. This may lead to diagnostic difficulties. In cases in which the results of a water deprivation test are inconclusive, ADH measurement is helpful. A definitive diagnosis of ADH deficiency can be established by infusing hypertonic saline for 2 hours to increase plasma osmolality to more than 300 mOsm/kg, with regular 20 to 30 minute blood sampling to estimate plasma osmolality and ADH. In nephrogenic diabetes insipidus, ADH values are above the normal reference range, whereas in cranial diabetes insipidus, values are at the lower end of or below the normal reference range.

MANAGEMENT

Treatment for hypopituitarism can be separated into those therapies directed at the underlying disease process and endocrine replacement therapy (Table 6-4). Management of the underlying condition is particularly challenging for craniopharyngiomas because randomized studies are lacking and their growth pattern is often unpredictable.[60] Surgical excision in combination with external beam irradiation forms the mainstay of treatment. A recent trial demonstrated no recurrence of tumors during an average follow-up of 6.5 years in patients who received combined surgery with radiotherapy at diagnosis. Sixty percent of patients who received surgery alone had tumor recurrence.[61]

Hormone Replacement in Hypopituitarism

Endocrine replacement therapy should aim to mimic the normal hormonal milieu as far as possible, thus improving symptoms while avoiding overtreatment. GH replacement therapy is discussed separately under the section on adult GH deficiency.

Gonadotropin Deficiency

In both sexes, sex steroid replacement therapy is important for the maintenance of normal body composition, skeletal health, and sexual function, and it is the most appropriate form of replacement therapy in patients not desirous of fertility.

Estrogen Replacement. In women, this can be provided by many standard hormone replacement therapy preparations. Progesterone must be given (cyclically or continuously) in all women with an intact uterus to prevent the possible effect of unopposed estrogen on the endometrium, that is, dysfunctional bleeding or endometrial cancer. The dose of estrogen should not

Table 6-4. Endocrine Replacement Therapy for Hormone Deficiencies

Hormone Deficiency	Replacement Hormones and Typical Daily Dose Range (Oral, if Not Stated Otherwise)
Growth hormone	Please refer to Table 6-7 in the section Growth Hormone Deficiency.
Gonadotropins (female)	Estrogen: Estradiol valerate: 1-2 mg, transdermal: 25-100 µg **or** conjugated equineestrogens: 0.625-1.25 mg PLUS Progesterone (examples): Norethisterone, 0.7-1 mg, transdermal: 170-250 µg **or** Levonorgestrel, 250 µg, transdermal: 7 µg **or** Medroxyprogesterone acetate, 5 mg
Gonadotropins (male)	Testosterone: Intramuscular (as testosterone esters): 250 mg every 2-3 wk **or** Transdermal: 5-7.5 mg **or** Implant: 600-800 mg every 4-6 mo
Thyroid-stimulating hormone	Thyroxine, 75-200 µg/day
Adrenocorticotropic hormone	Glucocorticoid (preferred schedule): Hydrocortisone, 10 mg morning, 5 mg noon, 5 mg evening, to 10 mg t.i.d.
Prolactin	Nil
Antidiuretic hormone	Desmopressin (DDAVP), 300-600 µg (in divided doses); intranasal, 10-40 µg (in divided doses)

be supraphysiologic (as in the oral contraceptive pill) unless a clear indication, such as strong patient preference, exists, or a patient with partial gonadotropin deficiency still has occasional menstrual cycles, along with a desire for contraception. Although estrogen can be delivered as a tablet, patch, gel, or implant, a nonoral route is recommended because of reduction of insulin-like growth factor (IGF)-1 and fat oxidation by oral estrogen. The pathophysiology of the interaction of oral estrogen with the GH axis is discussed separately under the section on adult GH deficiency. However, an international surveillance study on 315 hypopituitary women taking estrogen replacement demonstrated significant predominance of oral versus transdermal estrogen use (86% vs. 14%). Women on oral estrogen had a significantly greater waist/hip ratio after GH treatment, with lower IGF-1 levels at the end of the study period on twice the GH dose received by women on transdermal estrogen.[62] Therefore a nonoral route is highly recommended.

Androgen Replacement. The choice of preparation of androgen replacement depends on local availability and patient preference. IM injection of testosterone can be associated with disturbing fluctuations in sexual function, energy level, and mood, mirroring the changes in testosterone concentrations. Transdermal testosterone systems, which are an alternative, are available as patch systems (nonscrotal or scrotal) or as the recently introduced testosterone gel. Both formulations are able to maintain physiologic testosterone profiles in most patients, but skin irritation, the need for scrotal shaving, and drying time after gel application are some of the potential drawbacks of both transdermal systems. Testosterone undecanoate has become available as an intramuscular injection, which achieves stable serum testosterone levels over a 10- to 14-week period. This new preparation has essentially replaced testosterone implants as replacement therapy.[63]

Androgen replacement therapy should always be monitored to ensure physiologic mean testosterone levels. Suboptimal replacement doses result in low trough levels, whereas supraphysiologic doses can promote secondary polycythemia and progression of prostate cancer; therefore, regular monitoring of hemoglobin and prostate-specific antigen is recommended.

An area of investigative concern now is the therapeutic use of testosterone in women. In postmenopausal women, particularly those who have undergone bilateral oophorectomy, evidence exists that combined estrogen and testosterone replacement improves libido and sexual function. The rationale behind such therapy is that after bilateral oophorectomy, circulating testosterone levels decrease by 50%. This reduction tends to be even greater in women with hypopituitarism, who are likely to be more severely androgen deficient from loss of adrenal androgen production. Thus symptomatic patients may benefit from androgen supplementation. Such patients demonstrate improvement in sense of well-being, libido, lean body mass, and bone mineral density with androgen supplementation with dehydroepiandrosterone[64] or low-dose testosterone.[65]

Gonadotropin and Gonadotropin-Releasing Hormone Therapy. In the hypogonadotropic hypogonadal patient, fertility can be achieved with gonadotropin therapy in both men and women. The choice of therapy lies between gonadotropin replacement and GnRH. The former is the traditional therapeutic approach; initially, LH "activity" is provided by human chorionic gonadotropin (hCG) administered subcutaneously (SC) or IM at a dose of between 1000 and 2000 IU, two to three times weekly. Spermatogenesis is unlikely within the first 3 months of therapy. Treatment with hCG alone is continued for 6 months, with regular sperm counts to monitor progress. If adequate spermatogenesis is not achieved, then FSH in the form of human menopausal gonadotropin (hMG) or a recombinant FSH is added. The dose of FSH is increased if adequate spermatogenesis is not achieved after 6 months of combination therapy. The alternative regimen in patients with idiopathic hypogonadotropic hypogonadism and Kallmann's syndrome is pulsatile GnRH therapy. GnRH is administered SC via a catheter attached to a minipump. This regimen appears to offer few advantages over gonadotropin therapy in men but may cause less gynecomastia. Both regimens may take up to 2 years to achieve adequate spermatogenesis; thus once effective, consideration should be given to storing several samples of frozen sperm for any future attempts at pregnancy.

In women with hypogonadotropic hypogonadism, pregnancy rates up to 80% are reported after therapy with pulsatile GnRH or gonadotropins. These are better than rates achieved in women undergoing ovulation induction for other pathologic conditions. Again, the choice of therapy lies between gonadotropin therapy and pulsatile GnRH, but obvious advantages accrue to GnRH therapy if the patient has enough residual gonadotroph function.

Pulsatile GnRH therapy is more likely than hMG to result in development and ovulation of a single follicle, thereby reducing the risks for ovarian hyperstimulation and multiple gestation. However, in practice, GnRH therapy may not be practicable, and in more than 50% of women with organic pituitary disease, residual gonadotroph function is not sufficient to support this method.

Adrenocorticotropic Hormone Replacement. Different forms of glucocorticoids are available for replacement, and each has its merits and disadvantages. The modern approach to glucocorticoid replacement is to mimic physiologic levels, ensuring sufficiency during times of acute illness, and to prevent over-replacement, which is associated with adverse metabolic outcomes.

Any patient identified as having ACTH deficiency should be educated about its clinical implications. It is crucial for the patient to understand the need to increase the replacement dose twofold to threefold in case of an intercurrent illness or when undergoing surgery. Patients should wear an appropriate Medic-alert bracelet or necklace and should be issued an IM hydrocortisone pack and taught how to self-administer in the event of protracted vomiting.

Hydrocortisone directly replaces the missing hormone. Cortisone acetate is metabolized to cortisol and has a slower onset of action with longer biological activity. Both prednisolone and dexamethasone have longer half-lives, thus allowing daily administration. Recent estimation of a cortisol production rate of 9 mg/m²/day demonstrated by the isotope dilution method is lower than previously shown, and the traditional cortisol replacement dose of 30 mg/day is supraphysiologic and may lead to adverse metabolic outcomes.[66,67] Generally, the lowest replacement dose tolerated by the patient is preferred (10 to 20 mg/day). Indeed higher serum concentrations of total cholesterol, low-density lipoprotein, triglycerides, and waist circumference were observed with increasing doses of glucocorticoid levels in a study comparing the metabolic phenotypes of patients with growth hormone deficiency treated with different formulations and doses of glucocorticoids. Metabolic end points were not worsened compared with ACTH-sufficient patients only in those treated with hydrocortisone-equivalent doses <20 mg/day.[68] Doses should be divided to suit individual needs.

Thyroid-Hormone Stimulating Hormone Deficiency. Secondary hypothyroidism is treated with thyroxine (T_4) replacement therapy, as is primary hypothyroidism. The normal starting dose in a young patient without evidence of cardiac disease is 1.5 mcg/kg/day. Lower starting doses are used in the elderly and in patients with evidence of ischemic heart disease. In patients with suspected hypopituitarism, thyroxine therapy should be delayed until ACTH deficiency has been excluded or treated, because the risk for worsening the features of cortisol deficiency is present. Goal of replacement is to be to restore the serum-free T_4 concentration to the normal range. Measurement of TSH is unhelpful in the monitoring of T_4 replacement therapy in secondary hypothyroidism.

Antidiuretic Hormone Deficiency. Desmopressin is the drug of choice for the treatment of ADH deficiency. It is available in a number of preparations, including oral, intranasal, parenteral, and the recently available oral form. Dosages vary as much as 10-fold between individuals, with no apparent relation to age, sex, weight, or degree of polyuria. The drug should be started at low dose and increased gradually until urine output is controlled. Overdosage carries a risk for hyponatremia, and sodium levels should be checked after therapy is commenced or changed.

Growth Hormone Deficiency in Adults

The critical role of GH in stimulating childhood growth is well recognized, and its use in treating dwarfism due to GH deficiency is an unchallenged indication worldwide. Body growth represents the result of the stimulation by GH of a complex and

Table 6-5. Causes of Growth Hormone Deficiency in 1798 Patients

	Number	%
Pituitary	991	55.1
Extrapituitary		
Cerebral*	83	4.6
Extracerebral†	233	13.0
Nontumoral		
Inflammatory	66	3.7
Trauma	40	2.2
Infiltrative	21	1.2
Other‡	20	0.7
Idiopathic	244	13.6
Total	**1798**	**100**

Data are derived from four studies (References 5-8).
*Includes gliomas, pinealomas, dysgerminomas.
†Includes craniopharyngiomas, meningiomas, epidermoid cysts, Rathke's cysts.
‡Includes developmental malformations, irradiation other than for pituitary treatment, empty sella.

Table 6-6. Syndrome of Adult Growth Hormone Deficiency

Symptoms
Increased body fat
Reduced muscle bulk
Reduced strength and physical fitness
Reduced sweating
Impaired psychological well-being
    Depressed mood
    Anxiety
    Reduced physical stamina
    Reduced vitality and energy
    Increased social isolation

Signs
Overweight
Increased adiposity, especially abdominal
Poor muscular development
Reduced exercise performance
Thin, dry skin
Depressed affect

Investigations
Peak GH response to hypoglycemia <3 µg/L (all patients)
Low IGF-1 (60% of patients)
Hyperlipidemia: high LDL cholesterol, low HDL cholesterol
Elevated fasting insulin
Reduced bone mineral density

GH, Growth hormone; *IGF*, insulin-like growth factor; *LDL*, low-density lipoprotein; *HDL*, high-density lipoprotein.

integrated series of metabolic processes that are readily demonstrable in adults, even after cessation of body growth. Growth stops at the end of puberty as a result of fusion of the growth plates in long bones. However, GH continues to be produced throughout adult life and is the most abundant hormone in the adult pituitary gland. Hormones exert their actions by binding to specific receptors on tissues. All body tissues examined to date contain receptors for GH. This observation suggests that effects of GH are widespread, and that the hormone plays a general role in maintaining the metabolic process and the integrity of many tissues.

CAUSES

The causes of adult GH deficiency from four series totaling 1798 patients are shown in Table 6-5.[69-72] Approximately 50% arise from pituitary tumors, 18% from extrapituitary tumors, and 5% from inflammatory or infiltrative lesions; up to 15% are idiopathic. Treatment for pituitary and extrapituitary tumors is the most common cause of deficiency, accounting for nearly two thirds of cases. The frequency of causes differs between patients with childhood-onset and adult-onset GH deficiency.[70] Idiopathic causes, representing the largest group in childhood disease, are likely to represent a heterogeneous collection of congenital developmental abnormalities, including mutations of *pit-1* and *PROP* genes, which cause multiple pituitary hormone deficiencies.

CLINICAL FEATURES

Adults with GH deficiency, whether dating from childhood or acquired in later adult life, have a range of metabolic, body compositional, and functional abnormalities. These patients have a recognizable clinical syndrome, associated with a characteristic history, symptoms, signs, and investigative findings (Table 6-6).

Metabolism

Hypopituitary patients in whom GH has not been replaced display biochemical abnormalities that are linked strongly to the development of vascular disease. These patients have higher concentrations of total and low-density lipoprotein (LDL) cholesterol, as well as apolipoprotein B.[73-75] Evidence is available from ultrasonographic studies of intima and media thickening

and premature atherosclerosis of large vessels.[76,77] These patients also have a higher level of plasminogen inhibitory activity and a higher concentration of fibrinogen,[78] both of which are markers of increased atherothrombotic propensity. Fibrinogen also is a risk factor for stroke and myocardial infarction. Circulating levels of proinflammatory factors linked to the development of vascular disease, such as C-reactive protein (CRP), also are increased.[79]

Body Composition

Marked abnormality of body composition is characterized by increased proportion of body fat and reduced lean mass.[80,81] These changes are a consequence of the loss of lipolytic and anabolic actions of GH. The effects of GH on body fat and muscle can be seen in Fig. 6-5, which shows striking changes in body physique in a man before and 5 years after acquisition of GH deficiency after surgery for a pituitary tumor.

These patients are more obese and display a disproportionate increase in central abdominal fat.[81] The tendency toward central fat deposition is important because visceral obesity is linked to the development of insulin resistance, diabetes, and cardiovascular disease.[82] Adults with GH deficiency have evidence of insulin resistance[83] and a higher prevalence of impaired glucose tolerance.[84]

The reduction of lean body mass in adult GH deficiency arises from the combined reduction of bone, muscle and visceral mass, and extracellular fluid volume. Bone mass at different skeletal sites is reduced in patients with childhood-onset and adult-onset GH deficiency.[85,86] The risk for fracture is increased between twofold and threefold.[87,88]

Physical Performance

Patients show significant impairment of physical performance and muscle strength.[89,90] Physical fitness, as determined by cycle ergometry, has been shown to be reduced consistently in adult GH deficiency, with rates of maximal oxygen uptake reduced on average by about 30%.[91] Exercise performance is a complex

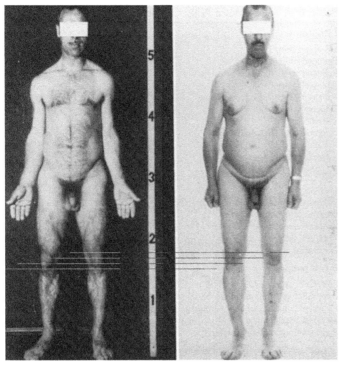

FIGURE 6-5. Body physique in a normal man before and 5 years after acquiring growth hormone deficiency as a result of pituitary surgery for a macroadenoma. Note the striking change in body composition with an accumulation of body fat, particularly in the abdomen, and marked loss of musculature. (Courtesy Professor Peter Sonksen.)

parameter that is dependent on numerous factors, including cardiorespiratory and neuromuscular muscle function. These patients have impaired cardiac function with reduced ventricular muscle mass, reduced ejection fraction, impaired ventricular filling,[92-94] and reduced lung size, all of which contribute to reduced exercise capacity. As the skin is a target tissue of GH action, another likely contributing factor to reduced exercise endurance is impairment of sweating, which arises from hypoplasia of the eccrine sweat glands. The skin of GH-deficient subjects is atrophic and dry.[73] Reduced sweating increases susceptibility to hyperthermia during exercise and may limit exercise performance.[95]

Quality of Life

Metabolic, body compositional, and functional abnormalities in adult GH deficiency are accompanied by significant impairment of psychological well-being and reduced quality of life. Fatigue, easy exhaustion, and lack of vitality are common symptoms. Early studies using generic questionnaires revealed lower self-perception of quality of life, with patients regarding themselves as having reduced health, self-control, and vitality, and experiencing increased anxiety.[96,97] A Dutch survey of social integration reported that GH-deficient adults had impaired social status.[98] These patients were on a lower professional scale, had lower income, and generally were without partners and were living at home with their parents. Recent studies based on disease-specific questionnaires evaluating life satisfaction revealed marked impairment in quality of life, regardless of country and cultural background.[99] On average, scores from GH-deficient patients were approximately half those of the normal population.[100] A recent study demonstrated significantly increased morbidity in patients with GHD, with hazard ratios approximately three times higher than in the normal population.[101]

Thus, the collective evidence indicates that adults who lack GH are not normal but suffer from metabolic abnormalities, disordered body composition, reduced physical fitness, impaired psychological well-being, and reduced quality of life.

DIAGNOSIS

Although the features of GH deficiency are recognizable, they are not particularly distinct and mimic body compositional and biochemical changes of the aging process.[102] GH secretion itself decreases progressively with aging, associated with a progressive increase in adiposity, which itself reduces GH secretion.[103,104] Thus, clinical suspicion must be confirmed by accurate biochemical diagnosis to ensure that GH-deficient patients are accurately identified and treated.

WHO TO TREAT

GH deficiency should be defined biochemically within an appropriate clinical context. Biochemical testing for GH deficiency should be considered in patients with a high probability of hypothalamic-pituitary disease who manifest clinical features of the syndrome.[105] This includes patients with a history of organic hypothalamic-pituitary dysfunction, cranial irradiation, known childhood-onset GH deficiency, and TBI. Patients with childhood-onset GH deficiency should be retested as adults before they are committed to long-term GH replacement.[105]

BIOCHEMICAL DIAGNOSIS

Three widely accepted approaches for assessing GH secretory status include measuring (1) peak GH response to a provocative test, (2) spontaneous GH secretion, and (3) serum concentrations of GH-regulated proteins such as insulin-like growth factor 1 (IGF-1) and IGF-binding protein-3 (IGFBP-3).

Provocative Test

The diagnosis of adult GH deficiency is established by provocative testing of GH secretion. Patients should be receiving adequate and stable hormone replacement for other hormonal deficits before they undergo testing.[105] Provocative tests include the insulin tolerance test (ITT); arginine, glucagon, clonidine, and growth hormone-releasing hormone (GHRH) alone or in combination with arginine or pyridostigmine are available for testing.

In 1997, the Growth Hormone Research Society recommended the ITT as the diagnostic test of choice.[106] It is superior to measuring integrated 24 hour GH concentration or IGF-1[57] (Fig. 6-6). Provided adequate hypoglycemia (<2.2 mmol/L or 40 mg/dL) is achieved, the ITT distinguishes GH deficiency from the reduced GH secretion that accompanies normal aging and obesity. The ITT should be performed in experienced endocrine units under supervision. The test is contraindicated in patients with electrocardiographic evidence or history of ischemic heart disease, and in those with seizure disorder. Given these precautions, the ITT is safe, with a risk for adverse events of less than 1 in 450.[107] Normal subjects respond to insulin-induced hypoglycemia with a peak GH concentration greater than 5 mg/L.[107,108] Severe GH deficiency is defined by a peak GH response to hypoglycemia of less than 3 mg/L. These cutoff values were defined in GH assays in which polyclonal competitive radioimmunoassays were use.[56] However, GH immunoassay results vary between different methods; therefore the cutoff value may require appropriate adjustment.

One stimulation test is sufficient for the diagnosis of adult GH deficiency. A 2007 workshop of the Growth Hormone Society has endorsed the GHRH plus arginine test, the GHRH plus GH-releasing peptide (GHRP) test, and the glucagon stimulation test as validated alternatives to the ITT.[105] The ITT evaluates the integrity of the hypothalamic-pituitary axis and has the added advantage of stimulating ACTH. Diagnostic tests employing GHRH and/or GHRP, both of which directly stimulate GH release from the pituitary gland, may miss GH deficiency due to hypothalamic disease.[109] This is exemplified by studies in those treated with cranial irradiation, in which the ITT shows the greatest sensitivity and specificity within the first 5 years after irradiation. If the peak GH level during a GHRH plus arginine test is normal in those who have received irradiation, then an ITT should also be performed. In irradiated patients and in those with inflammatory and infiltrative lesions, GH deficiency may develop many years after the initial insult. Therefore, this group should be followed over the longer term with repeat testing as clinically indicated.[24]

Biochemical Markers of GH Action

These markers include IGF-1, IGFBP-3, and the acid-labile subunit of the IGF-1-BP complex. Of the three biochemical markers, the merit of IGF-1 has been the most intensively studied. Serum IGF-1 concentrations are useful only when age-adjusted normal ranges are used. Although IGF-1 levels are reduced in adult GH deficiency, a normal concentration does not exclude the diagnosis (see Fig. 6-6). A subnormal IGF-1 level in an adult patient with coexisting pituitary hormone deficits is strongly suggestive of GH deficiency, particularly in the absence of conditions known to reduce IGF-1 levels, such as malnutrition, liver disease, poorly controlled diabetes mellitus, and hypothyroidism. The separation of IGF-1 values between GH-deficient and normal subjects is greatest in the young. As IGF-1 levels decline in normal subjects with aging, IGF-1 becomes less reliable as a biochemical marker of GH deficiency in patients older than 50 years, when the values are merged with those of normal subjects.[110] Measurement of IGFBP-3 or the acid-labile subunit does not offer any advantage over IGF-1.[111]

Which Patients Do Not Require a Stimulation Test?

In patients with organic hypothalamic-pituitary disease, the prevalence of GH deficiency is strongly linked to the number of pituitary hormone deficits, ranging from approximately 25% to 40% with no deficit to virtually 95% to 100% when more than three pituitary hormone deficiencies are present[112] (Fig. 6-7). Patients with three or more pituitary hormone deficiencies

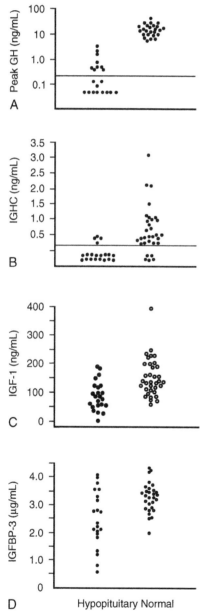

FIGURE 6-6. Comparison of peak growth hormone (GH) concentration obtained during an insulin tolerance test **(A),** integrated GH concentration (IGHC) obtained from blood withdrawal every 20 minutes for 24 hours **(B),** insulin-like growth factor (IGF)-1 **(C),** and IGF-binding protein (IGFBP)-3 concentrations **(D)** in patients with organic hypopituitarism and age- and sex-matched normal subjects. *Dotted line,* Limit of reading. (From Hoffman DM, O'Sullivan AJ, Baxter RC, Ho KKY: Diagnosis of growth hormone deficiency in adults. Lancet 343:1064–1068, 1994.)

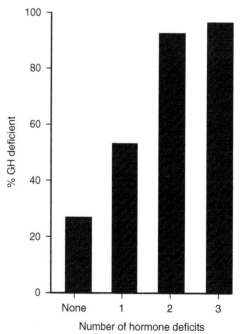

FIGURE 6-7. Relation between the number of anterior pituitary hormone deficits and the prevalence of growth hormone deficiency in 190 patients with known pituitary disease. (From Toogood AA, Beardwell C, Shalet SM: The severity of growth hormone deficiency in adults with pituitary disease is related to the degree of hypopituitarism. Clin Endocrinol 41:511–516, 1994.)

and an IGF-1 level below the reference range have a >97% chance of being GH deficient and therefore do not need a GH stimulation test.[105]

GROWTH HORMONE REPLACEMENT

The benefit effects of GH replacement in adults with hypopituitarism were first reported in 1989.[81,113] Since then, the impact of GH replacement has been studied extensively, and long-term experience of up to 10 years indicates sustained benefits.[114]

Metabolism

GH treatment induces profound effects on protein and fat metabolism, which result in significant changes in body composition. The anabolic effects arise from direct stimulation of protein synthesis and reduction of protein oxidation. GH stimulates lipolysis and fat oxidation, enhancing the utilization of fat for energy metabolism. The marked effects of GH on substrate metabolism are accompanied by significant stimulation of resting energy expenditure.[81]

In addition to exerting effects on the oxidative metabolism of fat, GH reduces a significant shift in lipoprotein metabolism to a less atherogenic profile. Most studies report a decrease in total cholesterol.[75] Less consistently reported are effects on increasing high-density lipoprotein (HDL) cholesterol and reducing levels of LDL cholesterol and apolipoprotein.[115-117] The favorable effects of improving the lipoprotein profile are more evident after treatment is provided for longer than a year.[117,118] Most studies report little effect on triglyceride levels.[75] Mechanisms that account for a less atherogenic profile include GH induction of hepatic LDL receptors and reduction in central adiposity, accompanied by an improvement in insulin sensitivity.

GH treatment reduces intima-media thickness of the carotid arteries and improves flow-mediated endothelium-dependent dilatation.[15,119] The mean intima-media thickness of the carotid vessels was significantly less after 10 years of GH treatment when compared with that of an untreated GH-deficient group.[114] The changes are not correlated to the reductions in plasma lipids. Proinflammatory factors such as CRP and interleukin (IL)-6, strongly implicated in the pathogenesis of vascular disease, decrease significantly with GH treatment.[120] It is yet to be established that improvement in these risk markers translates to a reduction in cardiovascular mortality.

Body Composition

GH replacement induces striking changes in body composition.[75,81,113,116] One of the first studies of adult replacement reported a significant reduction in body fat of 18% and a corresponding increase in lean body mass of 10% over a 6-month treatment period (Fig. 6-8). These changes in body composition occurred without a significant change in body weight. The greatest reduction in body fat occurs in abdominal and visceral fat.[121] Restoration of body composition is largely completed within the first 12 months of treatment. Significant increases in extracellular water also occur as a consequence of the antinatriuretic properties of GH, which are dose dependent and involve activation of the renin-angiotensin system, as well as a direct renal tubular effect.[122] Renal plasma flow and glomerular filtration rate are increased.

Bone remodeling is activated by GH. Markers of bone formation such as osteocalcin, alkaline phosphatase, and bone Gla protein, along with markers of resorption such as urinary hydroxyproline, are increased by GH treatment.[75] Initial studies

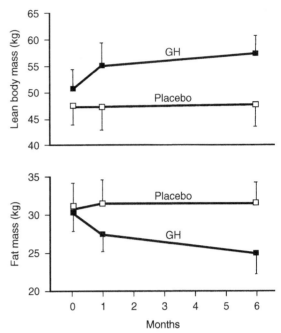

FIGURE 6-8. Body composition in growth hormone (GH)-deficient adult during treatment with GH or placebo for 6 months. **A,** Body fat. **B,** Lean body mass. (From Salomon F, Cuneo RC, Hesp R, Sonksen PH: The effects of treatment with recombinant human growth hormone on body composition and metabolism in adults with growth hormone deficiency. N Engl J Med 321:1797–1803, 1989.)

reporting changes in BMD over 6 to 12 months of treatment yielded conflicting results. However, more recent studies reporting long-term data show a progressive increase in BMD beyond 12 to 18 months of treatment[123-125] (Fig. 6-9), with a plateau reached after 3 years.[118,126] Markers of bone turnover increase over the first 12 months but return to baseline after 3 to 4 years.[127]

Physical Performance

Several studies reported that the increase in lean body and muscle mass during GH treatment is accompanied by an improvement in muscle strength. Quadriceps or hip muscle strength improves significantly after 6 months of treatment.[90,113] Muscle strength is normalized after 2 years, without further significant change at 5 years.[128,129]

Many studies reported improvement in exercise capacity and performance in parallel with an increase in maximal oxygen uptake[90,130] (Fig. 6-10). Exercise training alone significantly improves the aerobic capacity of GH-deficient adults, and this is not additive to the effects of GH treatment alone.[131]

In patients with GH deficiency, submaximal exercise performance, estimated as anaerobic threshold, increases significantly during GH treatment, suggesting that physical activities of daily living may be accomplished with less metabolic stress and subjective perception of effort.[132] Maximal workload and oxygen consumption increased progressively over a 5 year period of GH treatment.[125] In addition to increases in muscle strength, many factors may contribute to an improvement in exercise performance. These include enhanced cardiac function and improved heat dissipation through increased sweating. The data supporting a positive effect of GH on cardiac function are strong. Stroke volume, cardiac output, and diastolic function improve during GH treatment.[90,133,134]

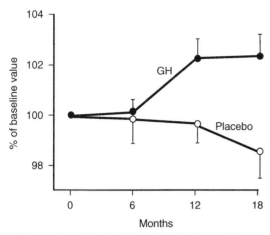

FIGURE 6-9. Bone mineral density of the lumbar spine in growth hormone (GH)-deficient adults during treatment with GH or placebo for 18 months. (From Baum HB, Biller BM, Finkelstein JS, Klibanski A: Effect of physiologic growth hormone therapy on bone density and body composition in patients with adult onset growth hormone deficiency: a randomised, placebo-controlled trial. Ann Intern Med 125:883–890, 1996.)

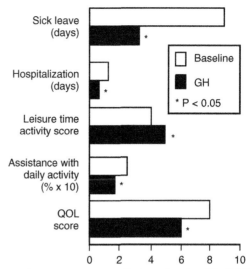

FIGURE 6-11. Changes in health care utilization and quality of life (QOL) measured at baseline and after 12 months of growth hormone replacement. The numbers of days of sick leave and hospitalization in the previous 6 months were taken as the baseline measures. QOL was assessed by a disease-specific questionnaire. (From Hernberg-Stahl E, Luger A, Abs R, et al: Healthcare consumption decreases in parallel with improvements in quality of life during GH replacement in hypopituitary adults with GH deficiency. J Clin Endocrinol Metab 86:5277–5281, 2001.)

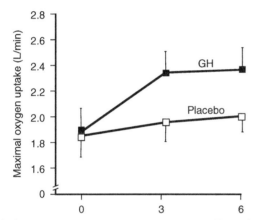

FIGURE 6-10. Maximal exercise capacity in growth hormone (GH)-deficient adults during treatment with GH or placebo for 6 months. Exercise capacity was measured as maximal oxygen uptake during incremental cycle ergometry. (From Cuneo RC, Salomon F, Wiles CM, et al: Growth hormone treatment of growth hormone deficient adults, II. Effects on exercise performance. J Appl Physiol 70:695–700, 1991.)

Quality of Life

Several double-blind, placebo-controlled studies have reported improvement in mood, energy, sleep, and vitality scores with GH treatment,[96,116,121] with continued improvement in these domains noted during the open phase. In general, GH replacement improved perceived health status and subjective well-being in the domains of health-related quality of life within 6 months. These findings were confirmed in a large randomized placebo-controlled blinded trial based on partner evaluation by questionnaire. According to the partners, patients were more alert, active, and industrious and had greater vitality and endurance during GH treatment.[135] Disease-specific tools have reported unequivocal improvement in measures of life satisfaction after GH treatment.[100] A large survey of 304 patients showed not only an improvement in quality of life, but also significant reduction in the numbers of sick leave and doctor visits during 12 months of GH therapy[136] (Fig. 6-11).

Significant differences are noted in clinical and biochemical presentation and responses to GH therapy between patients with childhood-onset and those with adult-onset GH deficiency.[70,129] Height, body weight, and lean body mass are lower in those with childhood-onset GH deficiency. The quality of life appears to be less disrupted in childhood-onset disease. During GH treatment, this group displays greater changes in body composition and greater increases in BMD and muscle strength, but lesser improvement in lipid profiles and quality-of-life measures, when compared with their adult-onset counterparts. The interesting differences at baseline and in responses to GH are likely to reflect the biological roles of GH at difference phases of life, as well as the psychological impact of GH injections given to the developing child. A patient with adult-onset disease is likely to recognize the restoration of quality of life to a level experienced before GH deficiency was acquired. In contrast, adults who received GH as a developing child have grown up with and adapted to the condition and are likely to harbor negative recollections of enforced daily injections. As GH therapy is terminated on epiphyseal closure, which occurs before somatic maturation, conventionally GH-treated children may not reach their physical and developmental potential on termination of GH treatment for dwarfism.[137] The data suggest the existence of two clinical entities, developmental and metabolic, which reflect the function of GH at different stages of life.[70]

Transition Age Patients

GH treatment of the GH-deficient child normally is terminated when final height and epiphyseal closure are reached. Strong evidence indicates that biological maturity is attained after the postpubertal period during the early years of adulthood. Muscle mass and strength continue to increase in normal subjects after puberty; this does not occur in GH-deficient subjects.[137,138] The bone mineral content of GH-treated subjects doubled that of unreplaced GH-deficient subjects after 2 years in the postpubertal period.[139]

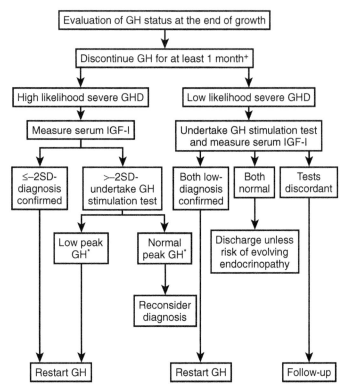

FIGURE 6-12. An approach to the reevaluation of growth hormone (GH) status for consideration of resuming GH treatment in GH deficiency diagnosed in childhood at the end of growth. *Peak GH < 5 μg/L. (Adapted from Clayton PE, Cuneo RC, Juul A, Monson JP, Shalet SM, Tauber M: European Society of Paediatric Endocrinology. Consensus statement on the management of the GH-treated adolescent in the transition to adult care. Eur J Endocrinol. 152:165–170, 2005.)

A significant proportion of patients with childhood-onset GH deficiency exhibit normal GH response when retested at the end of completion of GH treatment. The requirement for continued GH treatment should be evaluated carefully, as proposed by the European Society for Paediatric Endocrinology[140] (Fig. 6-12). GH testing is not required for those with a transcription factor mutation (e.g., Pit-1, PROP-1), those with more than three pituitary hormone deficits, and those with isolated GH deficiency associated with an identified mutation (e.g., GH-1, GHRH-R). All other patients should undergo GH testing after at least 1 month off GH treatment. Compelling reasons exist for GH-deficient children to continue GH treatment after puberty, to optimize not only physical maturation but also cardiovascular health and quality of life.

TREATMENT

Dosage

GH secretion is greater in younger individuals than in older ones, and in women than in men. It therefore is recommended that the starting dose of GH in young men and women be 0.2 and 0.3 mg/day, respectively, and in older individuals 0.1 mg/day.[105] Dose determination based on body weight is not recommended because of large interindividual variation in absorption and in sensitivity to GH, as well as the lack of evidence that a larger replacement is required for heavier individuals in adults. It is recommended that GH be administered in the evening to mimic the greater secretion of GH at night. Dose escalation should be gradual, individualized, and guided by clinical and biochemical response. Long-acting preparations

of human GH are under evaluation for long-term safety and efficacy.

A physical examination, including anthropometric measurements such as waist circumference and skin folds, and careful history, with particular attention to quality-of-life questions, are of great value in monitoring treatment; where possible, the partner's input should be sought. Serum IGF-1 is the most useful biochemical marker of GH response, the level of which should be maintained within an age-adjusted normal range. Clinical monitoring should include assessment of body composition with dual x-ray absorptiometry and lipid measurements.

Interaction

GH may influence the metabolism of many substances, including hormones and medications. GH stimulates the activity of the hepatic cytochrome P-450 system, a major pathway of the oxidative metabolism of several drugs, including anticonvulsants. It is likely that dosage adjustments may be necessary in patients commencing GH treatment. Cortisol also is metabolized by the hepatic cytochrome P-450 system. Biochemical evidence indicates that GH increases the metabolic disposition of cortisol and may increase the risk for adrenal insufficiency,[141] which has been reported in some studies.[142] Although a causal relation remains unproved, GH-deficient patients receiving GH therapy should be strongly advised to increase the dosage of glucocorticoids when unwell, as is generally recommended.

Recently, the importance of 11β-hydroxysteroid dehydrogenase type 1 (11β-HSD1) in determining tissue exposure to glucocorticoids has been recognized increasingly.[66,143] Hepatic 11β-HSD1 converts cortisone to cortisol. Its activity is inhibited by GH and therefore is increased in GHD individuals. Some studies demonstrated supraphysiologic tissue cortisol exposure in hydrocortisone-treated GHD subjects. This may explain the observation in one study of higher waist circumference and glycated hemoglobin (HbA1c) in hydrocortisone-treated GHD patients, compared with GHD patients on cortisone.[66]

GH stimulates the peripheral conversion of T_4 to triiodothyronine (T_3). This effect may be seen frequently as a decrease in circulating T_4 levels, particularly in patients taking thyroid hormone replacement for hypopituitarism.[144] If T_3 is not monitored during GH replacement, a decrease in T_4 may be misinterpreted as inadequate substitution, and this may lead to an unnecessary increase in the dosage of thyroid hormone replacement.

Sex steroids exert significant modulatory effects on GH action. Estrogen exerts significant effects on hepatic function that are dependent on the route of administration. When compared with estrogen given by the transdermal route, oral estrogen reduces IGF-1 and fat oxidation—effects that are opposite to those of GH.[145] GH-deficient women who are also hypogonadal should receive estrogen by a nonoral route during GH replacement, because oral but not transdermal estrogen attenuates the biological effects of GH.[146] Fifty percent more GH was required during oral estrogen treatment than during transdermal administration to maintain an equivalent IGF-1 level (Fig. 6-13). In contrast, androgens enhance the metabolic effects of GH. The divergent effects of estrogens and androgens on GH action provide a likely explanation for the observation that women are less responsive than men to GH[118,147] (Fig. 6-14). Over a 5-year treatment period, the average weight-adjusted dose for women was 30% higher than for men, whose IGF-1 was one standard deviation higher than that in women[118] (Fig. 6-14). Thus, women require a larger dose of GH than is required by men.

Safety

The experience from several large multicenter clinical trials indicates that GH treatment is safe and well tolerated.[116,148,149] The most common side effects arise from the antinatriuretic action of GH, which causes fluid retention (Table 6-7). These manifest as dependent edema, paresthesia, and carpal tunnel syndrome and occur with greater frequency in older patients. However, the symptoms are mild and dose related and resolve in most patients either spontaneously or with dosage reduction.[150]

Although GH antagonizes insulin action, the risk for developing hyperglycemia is very low. Only two case of reversible diabetes were reported from two European multicenter trials with a combined total of 400 patients,[148,149] whereas diabetes developed in none of 166 patients in an Australian study.[88] Insulin sensitivity did not change after 7 years of GH treatment.[151]

Because GH promotes the growth of tissues, concern has been expressed that GH therapy may increase the risk for pituitary tumor recurrence or the development of neoplasia. Analysis of the extensive pediatric experience shows no convincing evidence for a causal link between GH treatment and tumor recurrence or the development of neoplasia,[152] including leukemia.[153] In a retrospective comparison between hypopituitary adults with or without GH replacement and the normal population, an increased rate of malignancy, with colorectal cancer being the most common, was observed in hypopituitary adults without GH replacement. The rate of malignancy in patients on GH replacement was not different from that seen in the normal population.[13] In addition, overall cancer incidence rates were lower in acromegalic patients than in the general population.[154]

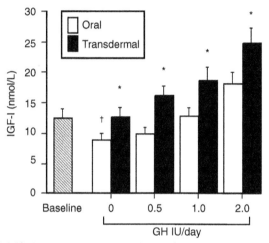

FIGURE 6-13. Mean insulin-like growth factor (IGF)-1 levels before and during incremental doses of growth hormone (GH; 0.5, 1.0, and 2.0 Units/day) during oral and transdermal estrogen therapy in eight GH-deficient adult women. *p < 0.05 oral versus transdermal. †p < 0.05 versus baseline. (From Wolthers T, Hoffman DM, Nugent AG, et al: Oral estrogen therapy impairs the metabolic effects of growth hormone [GH] in GH deficient women. Am J Physiol 281:E1191–E1196, 2001.)

Table 6-7. Treatment Guidelines for Growth Hormone (GH) Replacement in Adult GH Deficiency

Pretherapy	Adequate replacement of other hormone deficiencies
	Pituitary imaging
	Body composition
	IGF-1, BSL, lipids
Starting dose	0.2 mg/day for men and 0.3 mg/day for women
Adjustments	Small monthly increment, 0.01–0.15 mg/day
Monitor	IGF-1 (dose titration)
	BSL, lipids
	Weight, body composition, quality-of-life measures
Side effects	Edema, arthralgia, myalgia, paresthesia
Dosage considerations	Avoid weight-based regimens.
	Women require more GH than men.
	Elderly require less GH than the young.
	Requirements are greater with oral than with transdermal estrogen therapy in women.
Contraindications	Malignancy, intracranial hypertension, proliferative retinopathy

BSL, Blood sugar level; *IGF-1,* insulin-like growth factor-1.

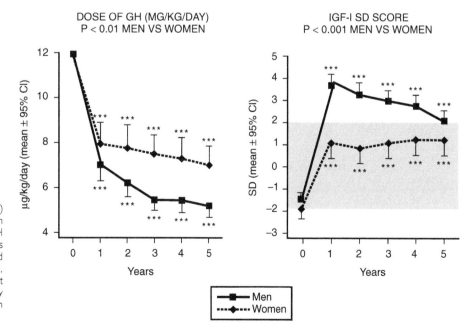

FIGURE 6-14. Growth hormone (GH) dose (μg/kg/day) and insulin-like growth factor (IGF)-1 standard deviation score in a group of 70 men and 48 women with GH deficiency treated for 5 years. The mean GH dose was lower, yet men attained higher IGF-1 responses than did women. (From Gotherstrom G, Svensson J, Koranyi J, et al: A prospective study of 5 years of GH replacement therapy in GH-deficient adults: sustained effects on body composition, bone mass and metabolic indices. J Clin Endocrinol Metab 86:4657–4665, 2001.)

These data on acromegaly provide the strongest evidence against a causal association between IGF-1 and malignancy.

Contraindications

Contraindications to GH replacement include active malignancy, benign intracranial hypertension, and proliferative retinopathy. Pregnancy is not a contraindication, although treatment should be discontinued in the second trimester, as GH is produced by the placenta.[105]

Conclusions

Hypopituitarism increases morbidity and mortality in affected patients. The extent to which GH deficiency contributes to such excess morbidity and mortality awaits confirmation from longer-term studies. Adequate and appropriate hormone replacement is mandatory in the treatment of hypopituitary patients. Based on global evidence of efficacy and safety, adults with GH deficiency should also have replacement with GH, a principle consistent with the tenet of hormone replacement for hormone deficiency in the practice of endocrinology. Because GH remains expensive, it is important that its use in adults be restricted to patients with proven GH deficiency.

The modern management of hypopituitarism and GH deficiency should also focus on their prevention. By restriction of surgery to experienced centers and replacement of conventional radiotherapy with stereotactic surgery, the incidence of long-term hypopituitarism will be significantly reduced. Furthermore, greater use of medical therapy for acromegaly with somatostatin analogues and a GH receptor antagonist should mean fewer hypopituitary patients in the future.

REFERENCES

1. Rosen T, Bengtsson BA: Epidemiology of adult onset hypopituitarism in Goteborg, Sweden during 1956–1987. Presented at the International Symposium on Growth Hormone and Growth Factors, Gothenburg, 1994, pp A3–A60 [Abstract].
2. Regal M, Paramo C, Sierra SM, et al: Prevalence and incidence of hypopituitarism in an adult Caucasian population in northwestern Spain, Clin Endocrinol (Oxf) 55:735–740, 2001.
3. Stochholm K, Gravholt CH, Laursen T, et al: Incidence of GH deficiency—a nationwide study, Eur J Endocrinol 155(July 1):61–71, 2006.
4. Rosén T, Bengtsson BA: Premature mortality due to cardiovascular disease in hypopituitarism, Lancet 336:285–288, 1990.
5. Bates AS, Van't Hoff W, Jones PJ, et al: The effect of hypopituitarism on life expectancy, J Clin Endocrinol Metab 81:1169–1172, 1996.
6. Bülow B, Hagmar L, Mikoczy Z, et al: Increased cerebrovascular mortality in patients with hypopituitarism, Clin Endocrinol (Oxf) 46:75–81, 1997.
7. Nilsson B, Gustavasson-Kadaka E, Bengtsson BA, et al: Pituitary adenomas in Sweden between 1958 and 1991: incidence, survival, and mortality, J Clin Endocrinol Metab 85:1420–1425, 2000.
8. Tomlinson JW, Holden N, Hills RK, et al: Association between premature mortality and hypopituitarism: West Midlands Prospective Hypopituitary Study Group, Lancet 357:425–431, 2001.
9. Bates AS, Bullivant B, Sheppard MC, et al: Life expectancy following surgery for pituitary tumours, Clin Endocrinol (Oxf) 50:315–319, 1999.
10. Nielsen EH, Lindholm J, Laurberg P: Excess mortality in women with pituitary disease: a meta-analysis, Clin Endocrinol (Oxf) 67(5):693–697, 2007 Nov. Epub 2007 Jul 18.
11. Svensson J, Bengtsson BA, Rosén T, et al: Malignant disease and cardiovascular morbidity in hypopituitary adults with or without growth hormone replacement therapy, J Clin Endocrinol Metab 89(7):3306–3312, 2004 Jul.
12. Nielsen EH, Lindholm J, Laurberg P, et al: Nonfunctioning pituitary adenoma: incidence, causes of death and quality of life in relation to pituitary function, Pituitary 10(1):67–73, 2007.
13. Karavitaki N, Wass JA: Craniopharyngiomas, Endocrinol Metab Clin North Am 37(1):173–193, ix–x. Review, 2008 Mar.
14. Lindholm J, Nielsen EH, Bjerre P, et al: Hypopituitarism and mortality in pituitary adenoma, Clin Endocrinol (Oxf) 65(1):51–58, 2006 Jul.
15. Molitch ME, Russell EJ: The pituitary "incidentaloma," Ann Intern Med 112:925–931, 1990.
16. Arafah BM, Prunty D, Ybarra J, et al: The dominant role of increased intrasellar pressure in the pathogenesis of hypopituitarism, hyperprolactinemia, and headaches in patients with pituitary adenomas, J Clin Endocrinol Metab 85:1789–1793, 2000.
17. Littley MD, Shalet SM, Beardwell CG, et al: Hypopituitarism following external radiotherapy for pituitary tumours in adults, Q J Med 70:145–160, 1989.
18. Webb SM, Rigla M, Wägner A, et al: Recovery of hypopituitarism after neurosurgical treatment of pituitary adenomas, J Clin Endocrinol Metab 84:3696–3700, 1999.
19. Arafah BM: Reversible hypopituitarism in patients with large nonfunctioning pituitary adenomas, J Clin Endocrinol Metab 62:1173–1179, 1986.
20. Arafah BM, Kailani SH, Nekl KE, et al: Immediate recovery of pituitary function after transsphenoidal resection of pituitary macroadenomas, J Clin Endocrinol Metab 79:348–354, 1994.
21. Littley MD, Shalet SM, Beardwell CG: Radiation and hypothalamic-pituitary function, Baillieres Clin Endocrinol Metab 4:147–175, 1990.
22. Shalet SM, Beardwell CG, Pearson D, et al: The effect of varying doses of cerebral irradiation on growth hormone production in childhood, Clin Endocrinol (Oxf) 5:287–290, 1976.
23. Darzy KH, Shalet SM: Radiation-induced growth hormone deficiency, Horm Res 59(Suppl 1):1–11, 2003.
24. Darzy KH, Aimaretti G, Wieringa G, et al: The usefulness of the combined growth hormone (GH)-releasing hormone and arginine stimulation test in the diagnosis of radiation-induced GH deficiency is dependent on the post-irradiation time interval, J Clin Endocrinol Metab 88(1):95–102, 2003 Jan.
25. Minniti G, Traish D, Ashley S, et al: Fractionated stereotactic conformal radiotherapy for secreting and non-secreting pituitary adenomas, Clin Endocrinol (Oxf) 64(5):542–548, 2006 May.
26. Hoybye C, Grenback E, Rahn T, et al: Adrenocorticotropic hormone-producing pituitary tumours: 12- to 22-year follow-up after treatment with stereotactic radiosurgery, Neurosurgery 49:284–291, 2001. And Darzy KH, Shalet SM: Hypopituitarism following radiotherapy. Pituitary. 2008 Feb 13. [Epub ahead of print.]
27. Besson A, Salemi S, Gallati S, et al: Reduced longevity in untreated patients with isolated growth hormone deficiency, J Clin Endocrinol Metab 88:3664–3667, 2003.
28. Deladoëy J, Flück C, Büyükgebiz A, et al: "Hot spot" in the PROP1 gene responsible for combined pituitary hormone deficiency, J Clin Endocrinol Metab 84:1645–1650, 1999.
29. Thomas PQ, Dattani MT, Brickman JM, et al: Heterozygous HESX1 mutations associated with isolated congenital pituitary hypoplasia and septo-optic dysplasia, Hum Mol Genet 10:39–45, 2001.
30. Netchine I, Sobrier ML, Krude H, et al: Mutations in LHX3 result in a new syndrome revealed by combined pituitary hormone deficiency, Nat Genet 25:182–186, 2000.
31. Machinis K, Pantel J, Netchine I, et al: Syndromic short stature in patients with a germline mutation in the LIM homeobox LHX4, Am J Hum Genet 69:961–968, 2001.
32. Binder G: Isolated growth hormone deficiency and the GH-1 gene: update 2002, Horm Res 58(Suppl 3):2–6, 2002.
33. Netchine I, Talon P, Dastot F, et al: Extensive phenotypic analysis of a family with growth hormone (GH) deficiency caused by a mutation in the GH-releasing hormone receptor gene, J Clin Endocrinol Metab 83:432–436, 1998.
34. Salvatori R, Hayashida CY, Aguiar-Oliveira MH, et al: Familial dwarfism due to a novel mutation of the growth hormone-releasing hormone receptor gene, J Clin Endocrinol Metab 84(3):917–923, 1999 Mar.
35. Quinton R, Duke VM, Robertson A, et al: Idiopathic gonadotrophin deficiency: genetic questions addressed through phenotypic characterization, Clin Endocrinol (Oxf) 55:163–174, 2001.
36. Falardeau J, Chung WC, Beenken A, et al: Decreased FGF8 signaling causes deficiency of gonadotropin-releasing hormone in humans and mice, J Clin Invest 118(8):2822–2831, August 1 2008.
37. Doeker BM, Pfäffle RW, Pohlenz J, et al: Congenital central hypothyroidism due to a homozygous mutation in the thyrotropin beta-subunit gene follows an autosomal recessive inheritance, J Clin Endocrinol Metab 83:1762–1765, 1998.
38. Collu R, Tang J, Castagné J, et al: A novel mechanism for isolated central hypothyroidism: inactivating mutations in the thyrotropin-releasing hormone receptor gene, J Clin Endocrinol Metab 82:1561–1565, 1997.
39. Asteria C: T-box and isolated ACTH deficiency, Eur J Endocrinol 146:463–465, 2002.
40. Tateno T, Izumiyama H, Doi M, et al: Differential gene expression in ACTH-secreting and non-functioning pituitary tumors, Eur J Endocrinol 157:717–724, 2007.
41. Vallette-Kasic S, Pulichino AM, Gueydan M, et al: A neonatal form of isolated ACTH deficiency frequently associated with Tpit gene mutations, Endocr Res 30(4):943–944, 2004 Nov.
42. Schneider HJ, Kreitschmann-Andermahr I, Ghigo E, et al: Hypothalamopituitary dysfunction following traumatic brain injury and aneurysmal subarachnoid hemorrhage: a systematic review, JAMA 298(12):1429–1438, 2007 Sep 26.
43. Tagliaferri F, Compagnone C, Korsic M, et al. A systematic review of brain injury epidemiology in Europe, Acta Neurochir (Wien) 148(3):255–268, 2006.
44. Schneider HJ, Aimaretti G, Kreitschmann-Andermahr I, et al: Hypopituitarism, Lancet 369(9571):1461–1470, 2007.
45. Klose M, Juul A, Struck J, et al: Acute and long-term pituitary insufficiency in traumatic brain injury: a prospective single-centre study, Clin Endocrinol (Oxf) 67(4):598–606, 2007 Oct.
46. Lupi I, Broman KW, Tzou SC, et al: Novel autoantigens in autoimmune hypophysitis, Clin Endocrinol (Oxf) 69(2):269–278, 2008. [Epub ahead of print.]

47. Cosman F, Post KD, Holub DA, et al: Lymphocytic hypophysitis. Report of 3 new cases and review of the literature, Medicine 68:240–256, 1989.
48. O'Dwyer DT, Smith AI, Matthew ML, et al: Identification of the 49-kDa autoantigen associated with lymphocytic hypophysitis as alpha-enolase, J Clin Endocrinol Metab 87:752, 2002.
49. Simpson ER, Waterman MR: Regulation of the synthesis of steroidogenic enzymes in adrenal cortical cells by ACTH, Annu Rev Physiol 50:427–440, 1988.
50. Cronin CC, Callaghan N, Kearney PJ, et al: Addison disease in patients treated with glucocorticoid therapy, Arch Intern Med 157:456–458, 1997.
51. Fujisawa I, Kikuchi K, Nishimura K, et al: Transection of the pituitary stalk: development of an ectopic posterior lobe assessed with MR imaging, Radiology 165:487–489, 1987.
52. Kikuchi K, Fujisawa I, Momoi T, et al: Hypothalamic-pituitary function in growth hormone-deficient patients with pituitary stalk transection, J Clin Endocrinol Metab 67:817–823, 1988.
53. Osorio MG, Marui S, Jorge AA, et al: Pituitary magnetic resonance imaging and function in patients with growth hormone deficiency with and without mutations in GHRH-R, GH-1, or PROP-1 genes, J Clin Endocrinol Metab 87(11):5076–5084, 2002 Nov.
54. Maghnie M, Salati B, Bianchi S, et al: Relationship between the morphological evaluation of the pituitary and the growth hormone (GH) response to GH-releasing hormone plus arginine in children and adults with congenital hypopituitarism, J Clin Endocrinol Metab 86(4):1574–1579, 2001 Apr.
55. Le Roux CW, Meeran K, Alaghband-Zadeh J: Is a 0900-h serum cortisol useful prior to a short Synacthen test in outpatient assessment? Ann Clin Biochem 39:148–150, 2002.
56. Hoffman DM, O'Sullivan AJ, Baxter RC, et al: Diagnosis of growth-hormone deficiency in adults, Lancet 343(8905):1064–1068, April 30 1994.
57. Trainer PJ, Besser M: The Bart's Endocrine Protocols. Livingstone, 1995, Churchhill, 4–6.
58. Nieman LK: Dynamic evaluation of adrenal hypofunction, J Endocrinol Invest 26:74–82, 2003.
59. Beck-Peccoz P, Amr S, Menezes-Ferreira MM, et al: Decreased receptor binding of biologically inactive thyrotropin in central hypothyroidism: Effect of treatment with thyrotropin-releasing hormone, N Engl J Med 312:1085–1090, 1985
60. Karavitaki N, Wass JA: Craniopharyngiomas, Endocrinol Metab Clin North Am. 37(1):173–193, ix–x, 2008 Mar.
61. Lin LL, El Naqa I, Leonard JR, et al: Long-term outcome in children treated for craniopharyngioma with and without radiotherapy. J Neurosurg Pediatrics 1(2):126–130, 2008 Feb.
62. Mah PM, Webster J, Jönsson P, et al: Estrogen replacement in women of fertile years with hypopituitarism, J Clin Endocrinol Metab 90(11):5964–5969, 2005 Nov.
63. Schubert M, Minnemann T, Hübler D, et al: Intramuscular testosterone undecanoate: pharmacokinetic aspects of a novel testosterone formulation during long-term treatment of men with hypogonadism, J Clin Endocrinol Metab 89(11):5429–5434, 2004 Nov.
64. Arlt W, Callies F, van Vlijmen JC, et al: Dehydroepiandrosterone replacement in women with adrenal insufficiency, N Engl J Med 341(14):1013–1020, 1999 Sep 30.
65. Miller KK, Biller BM, Beauregard C, et al: Effects of testosterone replacement in androgen-deficient women with hypopituitarism: a randomized, double-blind, placebo-controlled study, Clin Endocrinol Metab 91(5):1683–1690, 2006 May.
66. Filipsson H, Monson JP, Koltowska-Haggstrom M, et al: The impact of glucocorticoid replacement regimens on metabolic outcome and comorbidity in hypopituitary patients, J Clin Endocrinol Metab 91:3954–3961, 2006.
67. Lukert BP: Editorial: glucocorticoid replacement—how much is enough? J Clin Endocrinol Metab 91:793–794, 2006.
68. Filipsson H, Monson JP, Koltowska-Häggström M, et al: The impact of glucocorticoid replacement regimens on metabolic outcome and comorbidity in hypopituitary patients, J Clin Endocrinol Metab 91(10):3954–3961, 2006 Oct.

69. Rosen T, Bengtsson B-A: Premature mortality due to cardiovascular disease in hypopituitarism, Lancet 336:285–288, 1990.
70. Attanasio AF, Lamberts SWJ, Matranga AMC: Adult growth hormone deficient patients demonstrate heterogeneity between childhood-onset and adult-onset before and during human GH treatment, J Clin Endocrinol Metab 82:82–88, 1997.
71. Abs R, Verhelst J, Maiter D, et al: Cabergoline in the treatment of acromegaly: a study in 64 patients, J Clin Endocrinol Metab 83(2):374–378, 1998 Feb.
72. Christ ER, Carroll PV, Sonksen PH: The etiology of growth hormone deficiency in human adult. In Bengtsson B-A, editor: Growth Hormone, Boston, 1999, Kluwer Academic Publishers, pp 97–108.
73. Besson A, Salemi S, Gallati S, et al: Reduced longevity in untreated patients with isolated growth hormone deficiency, J Clin Endocrinol Metab 88:3664–3667, 2003.
74. De Boer H, Blok GJ, Voerman HJ, et al: Serum lipid levels in growth hormone deficient men, Metabolism 43:199–203, 1994.
75. Carroll PV, Christ ER, Bengtsson BA, et al: Growth hormone deficiency in adulthood and the effects of growth hormone replacement: a review, J Clin Endocrinol Metab 83:382–395, 1998.
76. Markussis V, Beyshah SA, Fisher C, et al: Detection of premature atherosclerosis by high resolution ultrasonography in symptom-free hypopituitary adults, Lancet 340:1188–1192, 1992.
77. Pfeiffer M, Verhovec R, Zizek B, et al: Growth hormone (GH) treatment reverses early atherosclerotic changes in GH-deficient adults, J Clin Endocrinol Metab 84:453–457, 1991.
78. Johansson JO, Landin K, Tengborn L, et al: High fibrinogen and plasminogen activator inhibitory activity in growth hormone-deficiency adults, Arterioscler Thromb 14:434–437, 1994.
79. Sesmilo G, Miller KK, Hayden D, et al: Inflammatory cardiovascular risk markers in women with hypopituitarism, J Clin Endocrinol Metab 86:5774–5781, 2001.
80. Hoffman DM, O'Sullivan AJ, Freund J, et al: Adults with growth hormone deficiency have abnormal body composition but normal energy metabolism, J Clin Endocrinol Metab 80:72–77, 1995.
81. Salomon F, Cuneo RC, Hesp R, et al: The effects of treatment with recombinant human growth hormone on body composition and metabolism in adults with growth hormone deficiency, N Engl J Med 321:1797–1803, 1989.
82. Reaven G: Banting Lecture 1988: role of insulin resistance in human disease, Diabetes 37:1595–1607, 1988.
83. Hew FL, Koschmann M, Christopher M, et al: Insulin resistance in growth hormone deficient adults: defects in glucose utilisation and glycogen synthetase activity, J Clin Endocrinol Metab 81:555–564, 1996.
84. Beshyah SA, Henderseon A, Nithayanathan R, et al: Metabolic abnormalities in growth hormone deficient adults: carbohydrate tolerance and lipid metabolism, Endocrinol Metab 1:173–180, 1994.
85. Kaufman J, Taelman P, Vermelen A, et al: Bone mineral status in growth hormone deficient males with isolated and multiple pituitary deficiencies, J Clin Endocrinol Metab 74:118–123, 1932.
86. Holmes SJ, Economou G, Whitehouse RW, et al: Reduced bone mineral densities in patients with adult onset growth hormone deficiency, J Clin Endocrinol Metab 78:669–674, 1994.
87. Wuster C, Abs R, Bengtsson BA, et al: The influence of growth hormone deficiency, growth hormone replacement therapy, and other aspects of hypopituitarism on fracture rate and bone mineral density, J Bone Miner Res 16:398–405, 2001.
88. Rosen T, Wilhelmsen L, Landin-Wilhelmsen K, et al: Increased fracture frequency in adults with hypopituitarism and growth hormone deficiency, Eur J Endocrinol 137:240–245, 1998.
89. Rutherford OM, Beshyah SA, Johnston DG: Quadriceps strength before and after growth hormone replacement in growth hormone deficient adults, Endocrinol Metab 1:44–47, 1994.
90. Cuneo RC, Salomon F, Wiles CM, et al: Growth hormone treatment of growth hormone deficient adults, I: effects on muscle mass and strength, J Appl Physiol 70:688–694, 1991

91. Cuneo RC, Salomon F, Wiles CM, et al: Growth hormone treatment of growth hormone deficient adults, II: effects on exercise performance, J Appl Physiol 70:695–700, 1991.
92. Amato G, Carella C, Fazio S, et al: Body composition, bone metabolism, and heart structure and function in growth hormone (GH) deficient adults before and after GH replacement therapy, J Clin Endocrinol Metab 77:1671–1676, 1993.
93. Merola B, Cittadini A, Coloa A, et al: Cardiac structural and functional abnormalities in adult patients with growth hormone deficiency, J Clin Endocrinol Metab 77:1658–1661, 1993.
94. Shahi M, Beshyah SA, Hackett D, et al: Myocardial dysfunction in treated adult hypopituitarism: a possible explanation for increased cardiovascular mortality, Br Heart J 67:92–96, 1992.
95. Juul A, Behrenscheer A, Tims T, et al: Impaired thermoregulation in adults with growth hormone deficiency during heat exposure and exercise, Clin Endocrinol 38:237–244, 1993.
96. McGauley GA, Cuneo RC, Salomon FC, et al: Psychological well-being before and after growth hormone treatment in adults with growth hormone deficiency, Horm Res 33(Suppl):52–54, 1990.
97. Rosen T, Wiren L, Wilhemsen L, et al: Decreased psychological well-being in adult patients with growth hormone deficiency, Clin Endocrinol 40:111–116, 1994.
98. Rikken B, Van Busschbach J, Le Cessie S, et al: Impaired social status of growth hormone deficient adults as compared to controls with short or normal stature, Clin Endocrinol 43:205–211, 1995.
99. Blum WF, Shavrikova EP, Edwards DJ, et al: Decreased quality of life in adult patients with growth hormone deficiency compared with general populations using the new, validated, self-weighted questionnaire, questions on life satisfaction hypopituitarism module, J Clin Endocrinol Metab 88:4158–4167, 2003.
100. Rosilio M, Blum WF, Edwards DJ, et al: Long-term improvement of quality of life during growth hormone (GH) replacement therapy in adults with GH deficiency, as measured by questions on life satisfaction-hypopituitarism (QLS-H), J Clin Endocrinol Metab 89:1684–1693, 2004.
101. Stochholm K, Laursen T, Green A, et al: Morbidity and GH deficiency: a nationwide study, Eur J Endocrinol 158(4):447–457, 2008 Apr.
102. Rudman D: Growth hormone, body composition and aging, J Am Geriatr Soc 33:800–807, 1985.
103. Ho KK, Evans WS, Blizzard RM, et al: Effects of sex and age on the 24 hour secretory profile of GH secretion in man: importance of endogenous estradiol concentrations, J Clin Endocrinol Metab 64:51–58, 1987.
104. Iranmanesh A, Lizarralde G, Veldhuis JD: Age and relative adiposity are specific negative determinants of the frequency and amplitude of growth hormone (GH) secretory bursts and the half-life of endogenous GH in healthy men, J Clin Endocrinol Metab 73:1081–1088, 1991.
105. Ho KK: GH Deficiency Consensus Workshop participants. Consensus guidelines for the diagnosis and treatment of adults with GH deficiency II: a statement of the GH Research Society in association with the European Society for Pediatric Endocrinology, Lawson Wilkins Society, European Society of Endocrinology, Japan Endocrine Society, and Endocrine Society of Australia, Eur J Endocrinol 157(6):695–700, 2007 Dec.
106. Growth Hormone Research Society: Consensus guidelines for the diagnosis and treatment of adults with growth hormone deficiency: summary statement of the Growth Hormone Research Society Workshop on Adult Growth Hormone Deficiency, J Clin Endocrinol Metab 83:379–381, 1998.
107. Hoffman DM, Ho KKY: Diagnosis of GH deficiency in adults. In Juul A, Jorgensen JOL, editors: Growth hormone in adults. Cambridge, 1996, Cambridge University Press, pp 168–185.
108. Ho KKY: Diagnosis of GH deficiency in adults [Editorial], Lancet 356:1125–1126, 2000.
109. Leal-Cerro A, Garcia E, Astorga R, et al: Growth hormone (GH) responses to the combined administration of GH-releasing hormone plus GH-releasing peptide 6 in adults with GH deficiency, Eur J Endocrinol 132(6):712–715, 1995 Jun.

110. Ghigo E, Aimaretti G, Gianotti L, et al: New approach to the diagnosis of growth hormone deficiency in adults, Eur J Endocrinol 134:352–356, 1996.

111. Arosio M, Garrone S, Bruzzi P, et al: Diagnostic value of the acid-labile subunit in acromegaly: evaluation in comparison with insulin-like growth factor (IGF) I, and IGF binding protein-1, 2, 3, J Clin Endocrinol Metab 86:1091–1098, 2001.

112. Toogood AA, Beardwell C, Shalet SM: The severity of growth hormone deficiency in adults with pituitary disease is related to the degree of hypopituitarism, Clin Endocrinol 41:511–516, 1994.

113. Jorgensen JOL, Theusen L, Ingemann-Hansen T, et al: Beneficial effects of growth hormone treatment in GH-deficient adults, Lancet 1:1221–1225, 1989.

114. Gibney J, Wallace JD, Spinks T, et al: The effect of 10 years of recombinant human growth hormone (GH) in adult GH-deficient patients, J Clin Endocrinol Metab 184:2596–2602, 1999.

115. Weaver JU, Monson JP, Noonan K, et al: The effect of low dose recombinant human growth hormone replacement on regional fat distribution, insulin sensitivity and cardiovascular risk factors in hypopituitary patients, J Clin Endocrinol Metab 80:153–159, 1995.

116. Cuneo RC, Judd S, Wallace JD, et al: The Australian multicentre trial of growth hormone treatment in GH-deficient adults, J Clin Endocrinol Metab 83:107–116, 1998.

117. Beshyah SA, Henderson A, Niththyananthan R, et al: The effects of short and long term growth hormone replacement in hypopituitary adults on lipid metabolism and carbohydrate tolerance, J Clin Endocrinol Metab 80:356–363, 1995.

118. Gotherstrom G, Svensson J, Koranyi J, et al: A prospective study of 5 years of GH replacement therapy in GH-deficient adults: sustained effects on body composition, bone mass and metabolic indices, J Clin Endocrinol Metab 86:4657–4665, 2001.

119. Borson-Chazot F, Serusclat A, Kalfallah Y, et al: Decrease in carotid intima-media thickness after one year growth hormone (GH) treatment in adults with GH deficiency, J Clin Endocrinol Metab 84:1329–1333, 1999.

120. Sesmilo G, Biller BM, Llevadot J, et al: Effects of growth hormone administration on inflammatory and other cardiovascular risk markers in men with growth hormone deficiency. A randomized, controlled clinical trial, Ann Intern Med 133:111–122, 2000.

121. Bengtsson B-A, Eden S, Lonn L, et al: Treatment of adults with growth hormone (GH) deficiency with recombinant human GH, J Clin Endocrinol Metab 76:309–317, 1993.

122. Hoffman DM, Crampton L, Sernia C, et al: Short term growth hormone (GH) treatment of GH deficient adults increases body sodium and extracellular water but not blood pressure, J Clin Endocrinol Metab 81:1123–1128, 1996.

123. Johannsson G, Rosen T, Bosaues I, et al: Two years of growth hormone treatment increases bone mineral content and density in hypopituitary patients with adult-onset growth hormone deficiency, J Clin Endocrinol Metab 81:2865–2873, 1996.

124. Baum HB, Biller BM, Finkelstein JS, et al: Effect of physiologic growth hormone therapy on bone density and body composition in patients with adult onset growth hormone deficiency: a randomised, placebo-controlled trial, Ann Intern Med 125:883–890, 1996.

125. Vandeweghe M, Taelman P, Kaufman J-M: Short and long term effects of growth hormone treatment on bone turnover and bone mineral content in adult growth hormone-deficient males, Clin Endocrinol 39:409–415, 1993.

126. Ter Maaten JC, Be Boer H, Kamp O, et al: Long-term effects of growth hormone (GH) replacement in men with childhood-onset GH deficiency, J Clin Endocrinol Metab 84:2373–2380, 1999.

127. Valimaki MJ, Salmela PI, Salmi J, et al: Effects of 42 months of GH treatment on bone mineral density and bone turnover in GH-deficient adults, Eur J Endocrinol 140:545–554, 1999.

128. Johannsson G, Grimby G, Sunnerhagen KS, et al: Two years of growth hormone (GH) treatment increase isometric and isokinetic muscle strength in GH-deficient adults, J Clin Endocrinol Metab 82:2877–2884, 1997.

129. Koranyi J, Svensson J, Gotherstrom G, et al: Baseline characteristics and the effects of five years of GH replacement therapy in adults with GH deficiency of childhood or adulthood onset: a comparative, prospective study, J Clin Endocrinol Metab 86:4693–4699, 2001.

130. Nass R, Huber RM, Klauss V, et al: Effect of growth hormone (hGH) replacement on physical work capacity and cardiac and pulmonary function in patients with hGH deficiency acquired in adulthood, J Clin Endocrinol Metab 80:552–557, 1995.

131. Thomas SG, Esposito JG, Ezzat S: Exercise training benefits growth hormone (GH)-deficient adults in the absence or presence of GH treatment, J Clin Endocrinol Metab 88:5734–5738, 2003.

132. Woodhouse LJ, Asa SL, Thomas SG, et al: Measures of submaximal aerobic performance evaluate and predict functional response to growth hormone (GH) treatment in GH-deficient adults, J Clin Endocrinol Metab 84:4570–4577, 1999.

133. Caidahl K, Eden S, Bengtsson BA: Cardiovascular and renal effects of growth hormone, Clin Endocrinol 40:393–400, 1994.

134. Valcavi R, Gaddi O, Zini M, et al: Cardiac performance and mass in adults with hypopituitarism: effect of one year of growth hormone treatment, J Clin Endocrinol Metab 80:659–666, 1995.

135. Burman P, Broman JE, Hetta J, et al: Quality of life in adults with growth hormone (GH) deficiency: response to treatment with recombinant GH in a placebo-controlled 21 month trial, J Clin Endocrinol Metab 80:3585–3590, 1995.

136. Hernberg-Stahl E, Luger A, Abs R, et al: Healthcare consumption decreases in parallel with improvements in quality of life during GH replacement in hypopituitary adults with GH deficiency, J Clin Endocrinol Metab 86:5277–5281, 2001.

137. Rutherford OM, Jones DA, Round JM, et al: Changes in skeletal muscle and body composition after discontinuation of growth hormone treatment in growth hormone deficient young adults, Clin Endocrinol 34:469–475, 1991.

138. Hulthen L, Bengtsson BA, Sunnerhagen KS, et al: GH is needed for the maturation of muscle mass and strength in adolescents, J Clin Endocrinol Metab 86:4765–4770, 2001.

139. Shalet SM, Shavrikova E, Cromer M, et al: Effect of growth hormone (GH) treatment on bone in postpubertal GH-deficient patients: a 2-year randomized, controlled, dose-ranging study, J Clin Endocrinol Metab 88:4124–4129, 2003.

140. Clayton PE, Cuneo RC, Juul A, et al: European Society of Paediatric Endocrinology. Consensus statement on the management of the GH-treated adolescent in the transition to adult care, Eur J Endocrinol 152(2):165–170, 2005 Feb.

141. Orme SM, McNally RI, Cartwright RA, et al: Mortality and cancer incidence in acromegaly: a retrospective cohort study, J Clin Endocrinol Metab 83:2730–2734, 1998.

142. Chan JM, Stampfer MJ, Giovannucci E, et al: Plasma insulin-like growth factor-I and prostate cancer risk: a prospective study, Science 279(5350):563–566, January 23 1998.

143. Sigurjónsdóttir HA, Koranyi J, Axelson M, et al: GH effect on enzyme activity of 11betaHSD in abdominal obesity is dependent on treatment duration, Eur J Endocrinol 154(1):69–74, 2006 Jan.

144. Jorgensen JOL, Pedersen SA, Lauberg P, et al: Effects of growth hormone therapy on thyroid function of growth hormone-deficient adults with and without concomitant thyroxine-substituted central hypothyroidism, J Clin Endocrinol Metab 69:1127–1132, 1989.

145. O'Sullivan AJ, Crampton L, Freund J, et al: Route of estrogen replacement confers divergent effects on energy metabolism and body composition in postmenopausal women, J Clin Invest 102:1035–1040, 1998.

146. Wolthers T, Hoffman DM, Nugent AG, et al: Oral estrogen therapy impairs the metabolic effects of growth hormone (GH) in GH deficient women, Am J Physiol 281:E1191–E1196, 2001.

147. Burman P, Johansson AG, Siegbahn A, et al: Growth hormone (GH)-deficient men are more responsive to GH replacement therapy than women, J Clin Endocrinol Metab 82:550–555, 1997.

148. Mardh G, Lundin K, Borg G, et al: Growth hormone replacement therapy in adult hypopituitary patients with growth hormone deficiency: combined data from 12 European placebo-controlled trials, Endocrinol Metab 1(Suppl A):43–49, 1994.

149. Chipman JJ, Attansio AF, Birkett MA, et al: The safety profile of growth hormone replacement therapy in adult based on measurement of serum markers. J Clin Endocrinol Metab 80:2069–2076, 1996.

150. De Boer H, Blok GJ, Popp-Snijders C, et al: Monitoring of growth hormone replacement therapy in adult based on measurement of serum markers, J Clin Endocrinol Metab 80:2069–2076, 1996.

151. Svensson J, Fowelin J, Landin K, et al: Effects of seven years of GH-replacement therapy on insulin sensitivity in GH-deficient adults, J Clin Endocrinol Metab 87:2121–2127, 2002.

152. Allen D: National Cooperative Growth Study Safety Symposium: safety of human growth hormone therapy, J Pediatr 128:S8–S13, 1996.

153. Nishi Y, Tanaka T, Takano K, et al: Recent status in the occurrence of leukemia in growth hormone-treated patients in Japan, J Clin Endocrinol Metab 84:1961–1965, 1999.

154. Orme SM, McNally RI, Cartwright RA, et al: Mortality and cancer incidence in acromegaly: a retrospective cohort study, J Clin Endocrinol Metab 83:2730–2734, 1998.

Chapter 7

ACROMEGALY

SHLOMO MELMED

Acromegaly is a disease of spectacular growth and metabolic disorders that has fascinated physicians for centuries. The natural history of the disorder, if left untreated, results in gross acral and facial disfigurement, musculoskeletal disability, cardiac failure, respiratory dysfunction, diabetes, and accelerated mortality.[1-3] If the disease occurs before epiphyseal closure, gigantism results.[1] After the first modern description of the disease in 1886 by Marie,[4] it was subsequently recognized that the disorder is associated with a growth hormone (GH)-secreting adenohypophyseal adenoma, resulting in both a central mass lesion and the protean peripheral effects of sustained tissue exposure to high GH levels.[1,5-7]

Pathogenesis

The pathogenetic events that underlie the etiology of pituitary acromegaly include excessive pituitary somatotroph cell proliferation and unrestrained GH hypersecretion (Fig. 7-1). GH is secreted by somatotroph cells, the largest differentiated compartment of the anterior pituitary. GH secretion is under dual hypothalamic inhibitory control: somatotropin release–inhibiting factor (SRIF) inhibits secretion, and GH-releasing hormone (GHRH) stimulates both GH synthesis and secretion.[8,9] Ghrelin, a gut-derived peptide, binds to the GHS receptor and acts primarily at the hypothalamus to induce GH. Insulin-like growth factor 1 (IGF-1), the peripheral target molecule for GH action, participates in negative GH feedback inhibition by acting both at the hypothalamus to induce SRIF and directly at the pituitary to inhibit *GH* gene transcription.[10-12] Peripheral sex and adrenal steroids also regulate GH secretion.[8,13] GH itself binds to peripheral GH receptors that elicit signaling by JAK/STAT (Janus kinase/signal transducer and activator of transcription) intracellular phosphorylation cascades.[14] GH acts directly to attenuate insulin action and induce lipolysis.[15] The growth-promoting actions of GH are indirectly mediated by IGF-1, which is synthesized in the liver, kidney, pituitary, gastrointestinal tract, muscle, and cartilage.[12,16,17] GH actions mediated by IGF-1 include protein synthesis; amino acid transportation; muscle, cartilage, and bone growth; DNA and RNA synthesis; and cell proliferation.[18,19] Local production of IGF-1 may be under autocrine and paracrine regulation,[3,20,21] acting in concert with circulating IGF-1 and GH to elicit a final tissue impact.

EXCESS GROWTH HORMONE SECRETION

Tumors may arise from clonal expansion of one or more of the anterior pituitary differentiated cell types[22,23] and thereby result in specific hormone hypersecretory syndromes. The most common cause of acromegaly is a somatotroph (GH-secreting) adenoma of the anterior pituitary, which accounts for 30% of all hormone-secreting pituitary adenomas[1] (Fig. 7-2). GH-secreting adenomas arise from differentiated cells secreting *GH* gene products[1,23,24] (Table 7-1). These cells include somatotrophs, mixed mammosomatotrophs (secreting both GH and prolactin [PRL]), or more primitive acidophilic stem cells. Regardless of their cellular origin, transformation and subsequent replication of these cells result in adenoma formation as

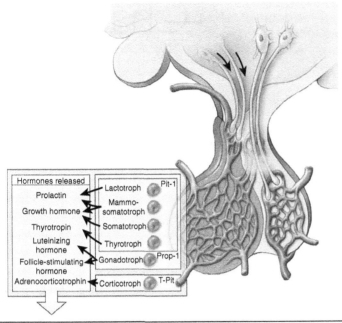

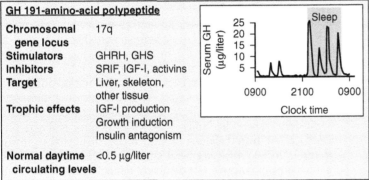

FIGURE 7-1. Synthesis and secretion of growth hormone by the anterior pituitary gland. (Modified from Melmed S: Acromegaly. New Engl J Med, 355:2558–2573, 2006.)

Table 7-1. Clinical and Pathologic Characteristics of Growth Hormone–Secreting Pituitary Tumors

Cell Type	Hormonal Products	Clinical Features	Histologic Features
Densely granulated somatotroph	GH	Slow growing	Numerous somatotrophs with large secretory granules
Sparsely granulated somatotroph	GH	Rapidly growing Often invasive	Cellular pleomorphism
Mixed cell (somatotroph/lactotrope)	GH and PRL	Variable	Densely and sparsely granulated somatotrophs and lactotrophs
Mammosomatotroph	GH and PRL	Commonly in children Gigantism Mild hyperprolactinemia	Both GH and PRL in same cell, often same secretory granule
Acidophil stem cell	PRL and GH	Rapidly growing/invasive Hyperprolactinemia dominant	Distinctive ultrastructure Giant mitochondria
Plurihormonal cell	GH (PRL) with α-GSU, FSH/LH, TSH, or ACTH	Often, secondary hormonal products are clinically silent Rarely hyperthyroidism or Cushing's disease	Variable: either monomorphous or plurimorphous
Somatotroph carcinoma	GH	Aggressive and invasive	Rigorously documented extracranial metastasis

Adapted from Melmed S: Pathogenesis of pituitary tumors. Endocrinol Metab Clin North Am 21:553–574, 1992.
ACTH, Adrenocorticotropic hormone; *GH*, growth hormone; *GSU*, α-glycoprotein subunit; *LH*, luteinizing hormone; *PRL*, prolactin; *TSH*, thyroid-stimulating hormone.

well as unrestrained GH secretion.[1] Most patients harbor densely granulated GH-cell adenomas, which are commonly encountered in older patients with indolent disease progression. Sparsely granulated GH-cell adenomas occur in younger patients with more aggressive disease onset and higher GH levels.[1,2] Mammo-

somatotroph cell tumors, or discrete mammotroph and somatotroph tumors, reflect the common stem cell origin of the somatotroph cell lineage.[2,24-26] Although acidophil stem cell adenomas secrete GH, their predominant product is PRL, thus accounting for the high incidence of hyperprolactinemic symp-

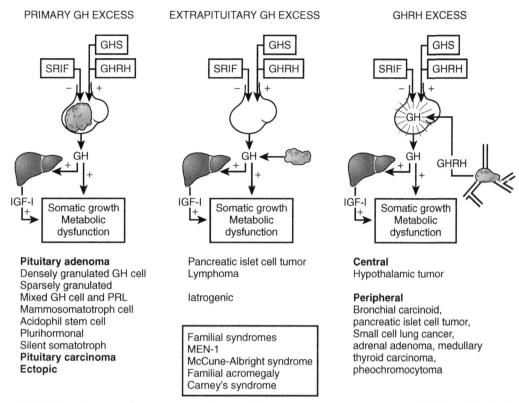

FIGURE 7-2. Pathogenesis of acromegaly. (Modified from Melmed S: Acromegaly, New Engl J Med 355:2558–2573, 2006.)

toms (galactorrhea, amenorrhea, infertility) initially seen in these patients.[27] Patients with McCune-Albright syndrome also may have acromegaly, although the presence of a discrete GH-cell adenoma has been inconsistently reported in these cases.[28] Rarely, acromegaly may occur in patients with a partially empty sella.[29] The rim of pituitary tissue surrounding the empty sella may harbor a small endocrinologically active GH-secreting adenoma not visible on magnetic resonance imaging (MRI) (i.e., <2 mm in diameter). Because embryonic pituitary tissue originates from the nasopharyngeal Rathke's pouch, ectopic pituitary adenomas may arise in remnant nasopharyngeal tissue along the line of primitive adenohypophysial migration. These adenomas may not be detected on pituitary MRI fields, and more extensive skull base imaging may be required. Very rarely, ectopic GH production by pancreatic,[30] lung,[31] ovarian,[32] or lymphocytic neoplasms may result in acromegaly.[1]

EXCESS GROWTH HORMONE–RELEASING HORMONE SECRETION

Excessive circulating levels of GHRH may overstimulate the pituitary and cause somatotroph hyperplasia, GH hypersecretion, and acromegaly.[33] Central overproduction of GHRH may occur in patients harboring hypothalamic hamartomas or gangliocytomas.[33] These rare tumors are usually diagnosed by pathologic examination of a surgically resected sellar mass causing GH hypersecretion and acromegaly.[34] Ectopic GHRH production by carcinoid tumors, although rare, accounts for most cases of acromegaly.[35] The clinical association of acromegaly with carcinoid disease had long been recognized, and the pathogenesis of ectopic GHRH production is now elucidated. Subclinical GHRH immunoreactivity has been demonstrated in about 40% of lung, abdominal, and bony carcinoid tissue specimens.

Pituitary somatotroph hyperplasia plus acromegaly associated with ectopic GHRH production has been reported in more than 100 patients, and the original isolation of GHRH was accomplished from a pancreatic carcinoid tumor.[36] Because the peripheral features of hypersomatotropism are quite similar in all forms of pituitary and nonpituitary acromegaly, diagnosis of the etiology of the disease may be clinically challenging.[1]

Acromegaloidism is a very rare syndrome characterized by acromegalic features with no discernible pituitary tumor and normal serum GH and IGF-1 concentrations. It has been presumed that this disorder is due to excess secretion of a putative, as yet unidentified, growth factor.[37]

ROLE OF THE HYPOTHALAMUS IN THE ETIOLOGY OF ACROMEGALY

Hypothalamic GHRH and SRIF selectively regulate *GH* gene expression and secretion.[8] These hypothalamic peptide hormones are expressed both within the anterior pituitary gland itself and within GH-secreting pituitary tumors.[38,39] GHRH, in addition to its hormonal regulation of GH production, induces somatotroph DNA synthesis.[40] Mice bearing an overexpressing GHRH transgene are subject to somatotroph hyperplasia and ultimately to pituitary adenomas.[41,42] In patients with carcinoid tumors and ectopic GHRH production, somatotroph hyperplasia and occasionally adenomas also may develop, which suggests that disordered endocrine or paracrine GHRH or SRIF action may be permissive for pituitary tumor growth.[43] GHRH signaling defects also have been identified in acromegaly. Constitutive activation of the GHRH receptor G-protein signaling unit facilitates ligand-independent induction of *GH* gene expression. This *gsp* mutation results in guanosine triphosphatase (GTPase) inactivation, with subsequent elevated cyclic adenosine monophosphate (cAMP) levels and GH hypersecretion.[44,45] Excessive CREB

Table 7-2. Evidence for an Intrinsic Pituitary Defect in the Pathogenesis of Acromegaly

GH-secreting adenomas are monoclonal

Absence of somatotroph hyperplasia in normal pituitary tissue surrounding pituitary adenomas

Successful surgical cure of well-circumscribed GH cell adenomas is achieved in >75% of patients

Adenoma transformation is rarely associated with generalized somatotroph hyperplasia

Unrestrained GH hypersecretion occurs independent of physiologic hypothalamic feedback control

Normalization of GH pulsatility often occurs after complete adenoma resection

Adapted from Drange MR, Melmed S: IGFs in the evaluation of acromegaly. In Rosenfeld RG, Roberts CT (eds): Contemporary endocrinology. The IGF system: molecular biology, physiology, and clinical applications. Totowa, NJ, 1999, Humana, pp 699–720.

GH, Growth hormone.

Table 7-3. Tumor-Suppressor Genes and Oncogenes Associated With GH-Cell Adenomas

	Protein	Defect	Function
Tumor-suppressor genes			
MEN1	Menin	Mutation or deletion	Nuclear; function unknown
P16INK4a	P16	Methylation	CDK4 inhibitor; loss of cell-cycle regulation
AIP	AIP	Mutation	Unclear
Oncogenes			
gsp (GNAS1)	$G_{s\alpha}$ subunit of G protein	Missense mutation at codon 201 or 227	Inactivates intrinsic GTPase; constitutive activation of adenyl cyclase
H-*ras*	Ras	Missense mutation at codon 12, 13, or 61	Constitutive activation; associated with metastases
Pttg	PTTG	Overexpression	Promotes transformation

Adapted from Drange M, Melmed S: Etiopatogenia de la acromegalia. In Webb S (ed): Libro De La Acromegalia. Barcelona, Spain, 1998, Accion Medica.

GH, Growth hormone; *GTPase*, guanosine triphosphatase; *PTTG*, pituitary tumor-transforming gene.

(cAMP response element binding protein) serine phosphorylation also may account for activation of the CREB–Pit-1 (pituitary-specific transcription factor 1) signaling unit in a subset of GH-cell adenomas.[46]

Pituitary tumor–derived paracrine GHRH or SRIF or both also may regulate tumor growth or function, although constitutively activating hormone receptor structural mutations have not been identified clinically. A truncated alternatively spliced GHRH receptor transcript has been described, but its functional significance is unclear.[47] In light of compelling evidence favoring intrinsic genetic defects occurring in GH-secreting pituitary tumors, as discussed later, it is apparent that hypothalamic influences may be permissive of tumor growth rather than being proximally involved in the initiation of somatotroph tumorigenesis.[43,48]

INTRINSIC PITUITARY LESIONS

Virtually all GH-cell adenomas arise as discrete clonal expansions of a transformed cell[22] (Table 7-2). This monoclonal origin implies that intrinsic genetic alterations account for tumorigenic initiating events and supports abundant earlier clinical observations that resection of small well-circumscribed adenomas usually results in surgical cure of GH-secreting adenomas.[24,43,49] Because adenohypophyseal tissue surrounding the pituitary adenoma is histologically normal, it is unlikely that multiple independent cellular growth events (e.g., generalized hyperplasia) precede adenoma formation. Increasing evidence points to complex molecular cascades accounting for the cellular progression, resulting in pituitary-cell transformation and, ultimately, tumor formation. Multistep development of pituitary acromegaly involves a spectrum of genetic alterations associated with dysregulation of cell proliferation, differentiation, and GH production.[43] Activation of oncogene function or inactivation of tumor-suppressor genes or both may account for these changes[43,50,51] (see Table 7-2).

CANDIDATE GENES IN THE ETIOLOGY OF ACROMEGALY

Inactivating Mutations

Several transgenic animal models have shown that disruption of tumor-suppressor genes (including *RB* [retinoblastoma] and *p27*) results in a high incidence of pituitary tumor formation in afflicted mice.[52-54] Because a variety of chromosomal loss of heterogeneity (LOH) patterns are observed in human adenomas, loss of tumor-suppressor gene activity was similarly postulated for human tumors (Table 7-3).

Several chromosomal lesions occur in pituitary tumor tissue derived from patients with sporadic nonfamilial acromegaly. LOH involving chromosomes 11q13, 13, and 9 occurs in up to 20% of sporadic[50,55,56] pituitary tumors. Despite the multiple endocrine neoplasia type 1 (*MEN1*) gene location on chromosome 11, non-*MEN1* patients with sporadic pituitary tumors and 11q LOH harbor intact coding and intronic sequences, with appropriately expressed MEN1 messenger RNA (mRNA).[56] Lesions in chromosomes 13 and 9 also are more prevalent in invasive or larger adenomas.[51] Chromosome 13q LOH occurs in proximity to the RB locus and was found in 13 aggressive pituitary tumors, whereas small circumscribed tumors exhibit intact RB alleles.[57] These results suggest the presence of putative tumor-suppressor genes located on chromosomes 11 and 13 that may be involved in controlling the propensity for pituitary tumor proliferation. Despite these heterogeneous chromosomal LOH patterns, consistent loss of tumor-suppressor gene activity has not been identified for acromegaly. Although tumor invasiveness or size correlates with an increased propensity for chromosomal LOH,[51] identification of a specific molecular lesion leading to loss of antiproliferative activity in GH-secreting tumors remains elusive[43] (see Table 7-2).

Activating Mutations

GTPase acts to inactivate stimulatory G (G_s) proteins that induce adenyl cyclase and intracellular cAMP accumulation.[58] Missense mutations replacing residue 201 (Arg → Cys or His) or 227 (Gln → Arg or Leu), termed *gsp*, result in persistently elevated ligand-independent G_s activity and constitutively elevated cAMP and GH hypersecretion.[44] *Gsp* mutations occur in a subset of GH adenomas, with a prevalence ranging from 30% to 40% in whites[58-63] to only 10% in Japanese[64] patients with acromegaly. Clinical or biochemical correlations have not been associated with *gsp* mutations.[44,65] Thus, although these mutational events suggest a compelling mechanism for explaining GH-cell hypersecretion, their clinical significance has not been apparent (see Table 7-3), because the natural course of the disease does not differ in *gsp*+ve or *gsp*–ve patients.

Rarely, *ras* mutations have been observed in highly invasive pituitary tumors or their extrapituitary metastases.[66-68] Development of true GH-cell carcinoma with documented extracranial metastases, however, is exceedingly rare[67] (see Table 7-3). A pituitary tumor-transforming gene (*PTTG*) was isolated from rat GH-secreting pituitary tumor cells[69] and is functionally homologous to yeast securin, which regulates sister chromatid separation during mitosis.[70] *PTTG* overexpression results in cell transformation in vitro and experimental pituitary tumor formation in vivo. PTTG mRNA is abundant in GH-producing tumors, with more than 10-fold increases evident in larger tumors.[71] The strong transforming potential of PTTG indicates a role in early induction of GH-cell transformation, possibly by regulating the pituitary cell cycle[70] (see Table 7-3).

Familial Syndromes

Acromegaly may occur as a component of MEN syndromes, including the Carney complex or MEN1. The Carney complex consists of myxomas, spotty skin pigmentation, and testicular, adrenal, and pituitary tumors.[72-75] About 20% of patients with this autosomal-dominant syndrome associated with chromosome 2p16 harbor GH-secreting pituitary tumors.[50,72]

The *MEN1* gene is located on chromosome 11q13, and LOH of chromosome 11q13 occurs in pancreatic, parathyroid, and pituitary tumors of patients with MEN1.[56,76] Inactivation of the MEN1 tumor-suppressor gene likely accounts for the syndrome, in accordance with Knudson's "two hit" theory whereby both inherited allelic germline mutations and a somatic deletion are required for inactivation of both specific alleles and subsequent tumor formation.[77] MEN1, an autosomal-dominant syndrome, consists of hyperplastic or adenomatous parathyroid glands, endocrine pancreas, and anterior pituitary.[76] Pituitary adenomas develop in almost half these patients, with GH-cell adenomas reported in about 10% of afflicted subjects.

Isolated familial acromegaly or gigantism not associated with MEN has rarely been reported.[50,78,79] Chromosome 11q13 LOH with no discernible MEN 1 mutation was detected in the pituitary adenomas of two brothers with gigantism.[80] Low prevalence germline mutations of the aryl hydrocarbon receptor–interacting protein (AIP, located on 11q 13.3) gene were reported as predisposing to a subset of patients with familial acromegaly and gigantism[205]; 15% of families with isolated familial acromegaly exhibit AIP mutations, and tumors are encountered earlier in subjects harboring a mutation.[206,207] AIP has also been proposed as a tumor-suppressor gene for pituitary adenomas.[209] The clinical significance of these findings to the broad population of sporadic GH-secreting tumors is at present unclear.[208]

EPIDEMIOLOGY OF ACROMEGALY

Acromegaly is a rare disease, and accurate assessment of its prevalence in the community has been difficult to ascertain. In Newcastle, England, an annual incidence of 2.8 new patients per million adult population was reported, with an approximate point prevalence of 38 cases per million adult population.[81] A higher incidence was reported in Sweden, where the average prevalence of the disease was reported to be 69 cases per million.[2,82] If these data are projected to the population of the United States, 750 to 900 new cases would be expected annually, and GH-secreting pituitary adenomas would be present but undiagnosed in another 10,000 to 20,000 persons. The mean age at diagnosis is 40 to 45 years, and its insidious onset may cause the disease to not be diagnosed until 10 to 12 years after symptom onset.[82-84] This long delay in diagnosis is often due

Table 7-4. Diagnosis of Acromegaly

Biochemical testing
GH nadir >1 ng/mL during oral glucose load
Elevated age- and gender-matched IGF-1 level
MRI
Visualization of pituitary adenoma

GH, Growth hormone; *IGF-1*, insulin-like growth factor 1; *MRI*, magnetic resonance imaging.

to the subtle and slow onset of common symptoms, including headache, joint pains, jaw malocclusion, or mild type 2 diabetes. Furthermore, this relatively long time delay allows prolonged exposure of peripheral tissues to unacceptably elevated GH and IGF-1 levels.

Diagnosis

Persistent GH hypersecretion is the hallmark of acromegaly. Excess GH stimulates hepatic production of IGF-1, which is responsible for most of the clinical manifestations of acromegaly.[85-87] The diagnosis is often delayed for up to 12 years because of slow clinical progression over many years. Heightened clinical awareness may result in earlier diagnosis.[211] Although serum GH and IGF-1 concentrations are both increased in virtually all patients with acromegaly, serum IGF-1 levels may be discordant with GH increases. When a patient is suspected to have acromegaly, biochemical testing is required to confirm the clinical diagnosis, and imaging techniques are used to localize the cause of excess GH secretion (Table 7-4).

DOCUMENTING GROWTH-HORMONE HYPERSECRETION

The diagnosis of acromegaly is confirmed by measurement of serum GH after a glucose load and by assessing levels of GH-dependent circulating molecules such as IGF-1 and IGF-binding protein 3 (IGFBP-3).[29] IGF-1 levels reflect the integrated bioeffects of GH hypersecretion, and age- and gender-matched elevated IGF-1 levels are pathognomonic of acromegaly.[88]

Measurement of the serum IGF-1 concentration is the most precise screening test for acromegaly. Unlike those of GH, serum IGF-1 concentrations do not fluctuate hourly according to food intake, exercise, or sleep, but rather reflect integrated GH secretion during the preceding day or longer. Serum IGF-1 concentrations are elevated in virtually all patients with acromegaly, thus providing excellent discrimination from subjects without acromegaly.[2,85] In normal subjects, serum IGF-1 concentrations are highest during puberty and decline gradually thereafter; values are significantly lower in adults older than 60 years than in younger subjects. Females have higher levels than do males, and pregnancy may also be associated with elevated IGF-1 levels. Thus, an inappropriately controlled "normal" IGF-1 value in an elderly male patient may in fact be truly elevated and indicative of acromegaly. Serum GH should be measured in patients with equivocal or elevated age- and sex-adjusted serum IGF-1 values.

Although all patients with acromegaly have increased GH secretion, it may be difficult to distinguish elevated random GH levels from normal. As GH levels fluctuate widely throughout the day and night, measuring random GH levels rarely provides useful information for diagnosis of the disorder.[2] Short-term fasting, exercise, stress, and sleep are associated with elevated

GH, and the availability of ultrasensitive GH assays has indicated that this pulsatile GH rhythm may occur at levels below the detectable sensitivity of previously available assays. Serum GH concentrations fluctuate widely, from less than 0.5 ng/mL (with ultrasensitive assays) during most of the day to as high as 20 or 30 ng/mL at night or after vigorous exercise. Random serum GH concentrations may be elevated in patients with uncontrolled diabetes mellitus, liver disease, and malnutrition, so dynamic tests have been proposed to confirm pituitary GH hypersecretion. The mean GH concentration obtained from 6-hourly samplings will generally provide an integrated summation of net GH secretion, and averaged pooled levels greater than 5 ng/mL are usually encountered in acromegaly.[2]

The diagnostic hallmark of excess GH hypersecretion was failure to suppress GH levels to 0.4 ng/mL or less (using a chemiluminescent immunoradiometric assay) during a 2-hour period after a 75-g oral glucose load.[29] Several factors determine the measurement of serum GH values, including age, gender, BMI, and the type of assay employed. Spontaneous GH secretion is attenuated by 50% to 70% in subjects aged 65 years or more, and IGF-1 levels also decline progressively with age.[200] GH levels also correlate inversely with BMI, and lean subjects exhibit higher GH values, as do female subjects.[201] Accordingly, criteria for the diagnosis of acromegaly requires demonstrating a mean 24-hour GH level of >2.5 µg/L, a nadir GH of >1 ng/mL after a glucose load, and/or an elevated age- and gender-watched serum IGF-1 level.[202]

When GH levels were measured by different assays in 46 patients with controlled[18] or uncontrolled[28] disease,[203] values obtained with Diagnostic Products Corporation's IMMULITE assay were ~2.3 fold higher than those determined by the Nichols assay. Using the IMMULITE assay, postglucose values of <1 µg/L were associated with disease control, while with the Nichols assay, the proposed cutoff value was 0.5 µg/L. Thus, interpretation of biochemical control should also be determined by knowledge of the specific GH assay employed, as well as the appropriateness of assay controls.[204]

Invariably, patients who fail to suppress GH after glucose exhibit elevated total IGF-1 levels, with a strong log-linear association between the 24-hour mean GH output and IGF-1 levels.[2,89] About 10% or fewer patients may have apparently "normal" GH or IGF-1 levels or both at the time of diagnosis. Repeating the assays in a reputable laboratory may often resolve an apparent clinical/biochemical discordance. Alternatively, reinterpretation of a glucose suppression test or use of a rigorous GH assay may confirm the diagnosis.

Because IGFBP-3 secretion is GH dependent, concentrations may be elevated in patients with acromegaly, thus suggesting that IGFBP-3 measurement may prove useful in diagnosis.[90] However, in contrast to the tight correlation of integrated mean 24-hour serum GH with total and free IGF-1 levels, IGFBP-3 levels do not correlate as tightly with disease activity.[91,92] Thirty-two percent of subjects with active acromegaly had normal IGFBP-3 levels, and in patients who failed to suppress GH, no consistent elevation of IGFBP-3 was observed.[91] Thus, the utility of IGFBP-3 measurements for acromegaly diagnosis or follow-up is limited.

LOCALIZING THE SOURCE OF EXCESS GROWTH HORMONE

Once a biochemical diagnosis of GH hypersecretion is confirmed, MRI of the pituitary to localize the source of hormone excess is indicated. MRI effectively delineates soft-tissue pituitary masses, and gadolinium-enhanced MRI may detect adenomas 2 mm in diameter. In about 75% of patients, the tumor is a macroadenoma (tumor diameter of ≥10 mm) and may extend to parasellar or suprasellar regions or invade the cavernous sinus. More than 90% of patients exhibit a discrete pituitary adenoma on MRI, whereas about 10% of patients may harbor a partial or even apparently total empty sella. Functional GH-secreting adenomas may arise in the remnant rim of pituitary tissue surrounding the empty sella and may not be visible on MRI. Rarely, other nonpituitary causes of acromegaly (see earlier) will require abdominal or chest imaging to localize the source of ectopic GHRH or, more rarely, GH production. Lateral skull radiographs with sellar coned-down tomography or pituitary computed tomographic scans are not usually indicated, because they expose patients to unnecessary ionizing radiation and, when compared with MRI techniques, are insensitive, especially in delineating soft-tissue changes.

Nonpituitary Acromegaly

Rare nonpituitary causes of acromegaly include a hypothalamic tumor secreting GHRH,[33,93] a nonendocrine tumor secreting GHRH,[36,94] or ectopic GH secretion by a nonendocrine tumor.[1,31,32] MRI of the head and pituitary should identify some of these tumors. If pituitary MRI findings are normal, abdominal and chest imaging should be performed, followed by catheterization studies in an attempt to demonstrate an arteriovenous GHRH gradient over the suspected tumor bed. In patients with ectopic GHRH secretion, serum GHRH and GH concentrations are both elevated, and pituitary MRI reveals a normal-sized or enlarged hyperplastic gland.[95]

An algorithm for the diagnostic evaluation of patients suspected of having acromegaly is shown in Fig. 7-3. A normal age- and gender-controlled serum IGF-1 concentration is strong evidence excluding the diagnosis of acromegaly. If the serum IGF-1 concentration is high (or equivocal), serum GH should be measured within 2 hours after oral glucose administration. If pituitary MRI fails to reveal the presence of a discrete adenoma in the presence of clear-cut biochemical evidence of hypersomatotropism, studies to identify the rarely encountered GHRH- or GH-secreting tumors should be undertaken.

CLINICAL MANIFESTATIONS

The somatotroph adenoma itself, especially if a macroadenoma, may cause local symptoms such as headache, visual-field defects (classically bitemporal hemianopia), and cranial-nerve palsies. These compressive features are not unique to acromegaly and may occur with any enlarging sellar mass. Nevertheless, the headache associated with acromegaly is uniquely debilitating and may not be exclusively caused by pressure effects.

The systemic clinical features of acromegaly occur as a consequence of the deleterious impact of elevated serum concentrations of both GH and IGF-1 on peripheral tissues (Table 7-5). The somatic impact of elevated GH includes growth stimulation of a variety of tissues, such as skin, connective tissue, cartilage, bone, and many epithelial tissues, including mucosal surfaces. The metabolic effects of excess GH include nitrogen retention, insulin antagonism, and enhanced lipolysis.[6]

The onset of acromegaly is insidious, and disease progression is usually slow. At diagnosis, about 75% of patients are shown to harbor macroadenomas (tumor diameter of ≥10 mm), and some tumors extend to the parasellar or suprasellar regions.[15] Headaches are the initial symptom in approximately 60% of patients, and 10% have visual symptoms.

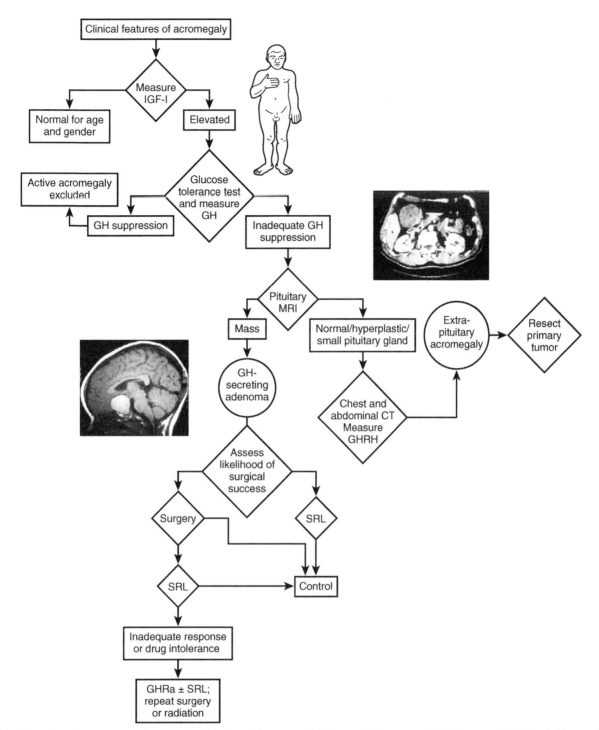

FIGURE 7-3. Diagnosis and management of acromegaly. *GH,* Growth hormone; *GHRH,* growth hormone–releasing hormone; *IGF-1,* insulin-like growth factor 1; *MRI,* magnetic resonance imaging; *OGTT,* oral glucose tolerance test; *GHRA,* GH receptor antagonist; *SRL,* somatostatin-receptor ligand. (Modified from Melmed S: Acromegaly, New Engl J Med 355:2558–2573, 2006.)

Acral Overgrowth

Acral and soft-tissue overgrowth is invariably a feature of acromegaly. Characteristic findings include an enlarged, protruding jaw (macrognathia) with associated mandibular overbite and enlarged, swollen hands and feet, resulting in increasing shoe and glove size and the need to enlarge rings. Facial features are coarse, with enlargement of the nose and frontal bones, as well as the jaw; the upper incisors are consequently spread apart.

Despite the prominence of these findings, the rate of change is so slow that few patients seek care because their appearance has changed (e.g., only 13% of 256 patients in one series[5]).

Rheumatologic Features

Musculoskeletal symptoms are leading causes of morbidity and serious functional disability in patients with acromegaly.[96,97] In several studies encompassing large series, at least half of all patients exhibited minor arthralgias, and severe, debilitating

Table 7-5. Risk of Long-Term Exposure to Elevated Growth Hormone Levels

Arthropathy
  Unrelated to age at onset or to GH levels
  Usually occurs with acromegaly of long duration
  Reversibility
    Rapid symptomatic improvement with treatment
    Irreversibility of bone and cartilage lesions
Neuropathy
  Peripheral nerves affected
    Intermittent anesthesias, paresthesias
    Sensorimotor polyneruopathy
    Impaired sensation
  Reversibility
    Onion bulbs (whorls) do not regress with lowered GH levels
Cardiovascular disease
  Cardiomyopathy
    Left ventricular diastolic function decreased
    Left ventricular mass increased; arrhythmias
    Fibrous hyperplasia of connective tissue
  Hypertension
    Exacerbates cardiomyopathic changes
  Reversibility
    May progress even with normalized GH levels
Respiratory disease
  Upper airway obstruction
    Caused by soft-tissue overgrowth and decreased pharyngeal muscle tone
  Reversibility
    Improved with reduction of GH levels
Malignancy
  Increased risk of malignancy
  Increased soft-tissue polyps
  Reversibility
    Effect of therapy on risk of malignancy unknown
Carbohydrate intolerance
  Occurs in one fourth of acromegalics, more often with family history of diabetes mellitus
  Reversibility
    Improves with reduced GH levels

From Melmed S, Dowling RH, Frohman L, et al: Acromegaly: consensus for cure, Am J Med 97:468, 1994.
GH, Growth hormone.

arthritic features ultimately developed in more than one third of patients.[97,98] The pathogenesis of joint disease in acromegaly generally begins with a noninflammatory osteoarthritic disorder and culminates in severe secondary joint and cartilage degeneration.[97] Excess GH and IGF-1 exposure leads to uneven cartilage proliferation that results in a mechanically unstable joint surface. Joint spaces then narrow as weight-bearing surfaces erode cartilage and cause excess intraarticular new fibrocartilage deposits. Subchondral cysts and osteophytes then develop in an irreversible self-perpetuating process. Severe physical deformity and functional disability result from these inexorable pathologic and mechanical stresses. Although symptomatic and functional relief of arthritic disorders is observed in most patients after reducing GH levels, structural changes are unfortunately not reversible.[98,99]

Joint arthralgias are a common initial feature of the disease, and back pain and kyphosis are common.[5] Synovial tissue and cartilage enlarge and cause hypertrophic arthropathy of the knees, ankles, hips, spine, and other joints.[97] Back pain also may occur because of osteoporosis caused either by GH excess itself or concurrent gonadal insufficiency from the enlarging pituitary tumor. Spine and hip bone density may be increased in women with acromegaly, but not if estrogen deficiency is present.[100] When excess GH secretion begins before epiphyseal fusion, linear growth increases and causes pituitary gigantism.

Skin and Soft Tissues

The skin thickens, and multiple recurrent skin tags may appear.[3,101] Hyperhidrosis at rest is common (present in 50% of patients)[2,3,5] and often malodorous. Hair growth increases, and some women have hirsutism.[2,5,102] Other manifestations of soft-tissue overgrowth include macroglossia, deepening of the voice, and paresthesias of the hands (carpal tunnel syndrome) from nerve entrapment.[2,5-7,15,98] Other patients have a symmetric sensorimotor peripheral (rarely hypertrophic) neuropathy unrelated to entrapment.[96]

Thyroid

Thyroid enlargement may be diffuse or multinodular. In a study of 37 patients with acromegaly, 92% had an enlarged thyroid gland when assessed with ultrasound; mean thyroid size was increased more than five times normal.[103] Thyroid function is, however, usually normal.

Cardiovascular

Impaired cardiovascular function in acromegaly is an important determinant of morbidity and mortality,[3,104] with exacerbated cardiovascular risk factors.[198] The deleterious direct impact of excess GH and IGF-1 on the heart, as well as the effect of hypertension, which is present in 30% of patients, contributes to the disorder.[5,105,106] Cardiac enlargement is disproportionate to the increased size of internal body organs,[107-109] and the severity of cardiomyopathy correlates significantly with the duration of exposure to hypersomatotropism.[104,108,110] Mean left ventricular mass may be significantly increased to more than 200 g, as opposed to a normal mean weight of 140 g, and end-systolic and diastolic volumes are attenuated. Concentric ventricular hypertrophy is associated with interstitial fibrosis, lymphocytic infiltration, and necrosis.[108] Resting diastolic blood pressure and left and right ventricular peak filling rates are elevated. Post-exercise systolic and diastolic blood pressure may also be elevated, and the left ventricular ejection fraction is attenuated.[111] Because physiologic doses of replacement GH also may actually improve cardiac function in patients with adult GH deficiency, a fine equilibrium may exist for the respective impacts of GH excess and GH deficiency on maintaining healthy myocardial function.[108]

Sleep Apnea

Peripheral airway obstruction caused by macroglossia, mandible deformation, mucosal hypertrophy, and inspirational laryngeal collapse has long been recognized as causing airway obstruction,[5] snoring,[3] and sleep apnea. Sleep apnea afflicts most patients with acromegaly and has been documented in up to 80% of cases.[3] Macroglossia and enlargement of the soft tissues of the pharynx and larynx lead to obstructive sleep apnea in about 50% of patients; others have central sleep apnea, possibly resulting from altered central respiratory control.[112] Sleep apnea may be an important cause of mortality in these patients. A central form of sleep apnea was recognized in acromegaly,[112-114] which appears to correlate more closely with elevated GH and IGF-1 levels and may reflect central respiratory suppression caused by the dysregulated hypothalamic-GH axis. Clearly, the strong association of sleep apnea with hypertension, coronary artery disease, and cardiac arrest also reflects the clinical phenotype of patients with acromegaly. Attenuation of GH levels, especially with octreotide, improves or abrogates sleep apnea.[112,115] Octreotide treatment is associated with improved indices for apnea, hypopnea, and oximetry.[195] After 6 months of treatment of 14 apneic acromegalic patients with octreotide, a 40% decrease in the number of apneic events per hour was seen, as well as a decrease in total apneic time from 28% to 15%. Maximum O_2 saturation rose from 76% to 84%, accompanied by a decline in daytime sleepiness, as well as improvement in central and obstructive apneic parameters.[112]

Diabetes

GH is a potent antagonist of insulin action, and glucose intolerance is encountered in up to 60% of patients. About 25% of patients may require insulin, and thus diabetes is an important systemic complication of hypersomatotropism. Diabetes is a major determinant of mortality, and only 30% of patients with diabetes at the time acromegaly is diagnosed appear to survive 20 years.[83,116]

Gonadal Function

Women with acromegaly may have amenorrhea, with or without galactorrhea,[3,15,117] and some have hot flashes and vaginal atrophy. Men may have impotence, loss of libido, decreased facial hair growth, and testicular atrophy.[3,7,117] Hypogonadism is caused either by hyperprolactinemia (present in about 30% of patients)[102,117] or by impairment of gonadotropin secretion as the expanding pituitary tumor compresses normal pituitary gonadotroph cells. Asymptomatic, reversible prostatic enlargement also is common, even in men with hypogonadism.[118,119]

Neoplasms

Acromegaly is associated with an enhanced risk for development of colonic polyps,[120-122] and prospective studies have reported premalignant adenomatous colonic polyps in up to 30% of patients, a prevalence not different from that in the general U.S. population.[122-124] In patients with acromegaly, colon length is increased, and apoptotic activity is decreased significantly.[121,209] Patients with acromegaly are more likely to have multiple adenomatous polyps, as well as polyps proximal to the splenic flexure, underscoring the need for full-length colonoscopy.[121,125] No difference in the duration or degree of acromegaly is evident in patients with or without adenomatous polyps. A multicenter retrospective study of 1362 patients with acromegaly found a lower cancer rate than in the general population (standardized incidence ratio of 0.76) but an increased colon cancer mortality rate.[126,127] The enhanced mortality correlated with persistently elevated serum GH concentrations but was not observed in patients with posttreatment serum GH levels less than 2.5 ng/mL.[128,129] Overall, a recent meta-analysis suggests a moderate doubling of colon cancer risk in acromegaly.[210] Colonoscopy is therefore recommended at diagnosis for all patients and periodically thereafter. Uncontrolled GH levels may act permissively to enhance morbidity and mortality from colon cancer. These findings underscore the requirement for tight GH control in these patients.

LABORATORY FINDINGS

Patients with acromegaly exhibit increased serum GH and IGF-1 concentrations and may have hyperglycemia, with frank diabetes occurring in 25% of patients. Some patients have hypertriglyceridemia. Hypercalciuria and hyperphosphatemia (not >5.5 mg/dL) occur in approximately 70% of patients as a result of direct stimulation of renal tubular phosphate reabsorption by IGF-1.[102]

Hyperprolactinemia occurs in about 30% of patients and is due to cosecretion of PRL and GH by the tumor or to stalk interference with hypothalamic-pituitary portal delivery of dopamine. Secretion of other pituitary hormones, especially gonadotropins, also may be decreased. Elevated plasma fibrinogen concentrations revert to normal with therapy, which suggests that effective treatment of acromegaly may prevent cardiovascular morbidity.[130]

MORTALITY

The overall mortality rate in acromegaly is about two to four times that of the general population.[126,129,131,132] Up to 50% of patients die before age 50 years, and up to 89% die before age 60 years.[2,133] In a series of 151 patients, survival was reduced an average of 10 years in comparison to age-matched controls.[83] Analyzing 18 studies of mortality outcomes in acromegaly,[126,131] there appears to be a 1.9-fold increase over expected mortality rates (range 1.16 to 3.3) for patients having undergone heterogenous treatments. Although standardized mortality outcomes have not been reported for untreated acromegaly, several mortality determinants are evident. These include the last measured GH or IGF-1 level, the prior use of radiotherapy, duration of the disease, and the presence of hypertension. Most significant predictors of survival include a postglucose GH level of <1 μg/L, a random serum GH of <2 to 2.5 μg/L, or a normal serum IGF-1 level (Fig. 7-4). Clearly attaining tight biochemical control should therefore be a goal of therapy. Aggressive management of comorbidities including hypertension, heart failure, sleep apnea, and diabetes likely also contribute to improved mortality rates[83,132,197] (Table 7-6). Several retrospective studies now indicate that survival in acromegaly may be normalized to a control age-matched rate by controlling GH levels[128,129]; in particular,

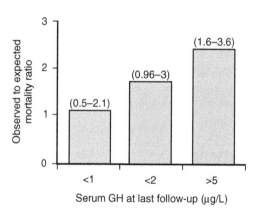

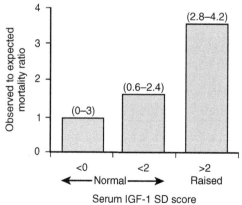

FIGURE 7-4. Growth hormone and insulin-like growth factor 1 levels as mortality determinants. (Data from Holdaway IM, Rajasoorja RC, Gamble GD: Factors influencing mortality in acromegaly, J Clin Endocrinol Metab 89:667–674, 2004.)

Table 7-6. Outcome Determinants of Acromegaly

Acromegaly Mortality

	SMR 95% CI	SMR 95% CI	Year
Wright		1.89	1970
Alexander		3.31	1980
Nabarro		1.26	1987
Bates		2.68	1993
Etxabe		3.23	1993
Abosch		1.28	1998
Orme		1.6	1998
Shimatsu		2.1	1998
Swearingen		1.16	1998
Arita		1.17	2003
Beauregard		2.14	2003
Ayuk		1.26	2004
Biermasz		1.33	2004
Holdaway		2.70	2004
Kaupinnen		1.16	2005
Trepp		1.34	2005
Total (95% CI)		**1.72**	

0.5   1   2   5

Data from Dekkers OM, Biermasz NR, Pereira AM, et al: Mortality in acromegaly: a metaanalysis, J Clin Endo Metab 93(1):61–67, 2008.

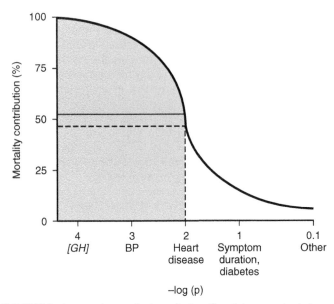

FIGURE 7-5. Acromegaly mortality determination. Growth hormone levels, hypertension, and cardiovascular disease are the most significant contributors to mortality. (Data from Melmed S: Acromegaly and cancer: not a problem? J Clin Endocrinol Metab 86:2929–2934, 2001.)

life-table analysis showed that GH levels less than 2.5 ng/mL were associated with survival rates equal to those of the general population.[126,132,134] A recent postoperative follow-up of 53 patients for a mean of 12.7 years indicated that a normal IGF-1 level and GH nadir cutoff of less than 0.25 µg/L are associated with improved blood pressure control and glucose tolerance (Fig. 7-5).[84] Thus, tight control of GH through aggressive multimodal therapy appears to reduce mortality risk to that expected for nonacromegalic subjects.[84,128,129] In particular, the role of radiotherapy in adversely skewing mortality outcomes will have to be excluded from these evaluations.[196]

Management

TREATMENT GOALS

Treatment goals for acromegaly embody principles that apply to treating hormonal hypersecretory tumors (Table 7-7). Treatment should be both safe and efficacious. GH and IGF-1 levels should be normalized, especially because elevated GH levels have been associated with mortality in these patients. Thus, tight GH control is an important therapeutic end point.[84] Tumor mass effects, especially central compression of visual tracts, should be alleviated. Importantly, the integrity of pituitary function should be preserved, and if hypopituitarism develops, patients require lifelong pituitary replacement. Clinical features of the disease that lead to the characteristic morbidity and ultimately to mortality should be ameliorated. Several treatment options are available for acromegaly. Transsphenoidal surgical resection of the adenoma; pharmacologic therapy with somatostatin analogs, dopamine agonists, and a GH-receptor antagonist; and various modes of radiation therapy are used to treat GH-secreting adenomas. The challenge of tight GH control in acromegaly can now be met with greater stringency by using single or multimodal

forms of therapy. Effective disease control should thus include sustained hormone suppression, a contained adenoma mass, improved systemic morbidity, and ultimately, normalized mortality (see Table 7-7).

SURGERY

Surgery for the treatment of GH-secreting pituitary tumors was pioneered in the early part of the century by Dr. Harvey Cushing, who demonstrated successful resection of such tumors by a transsphenoidal approach. This technique is standard, and only very rarely do large masses that extend far beyond the sella turcica require a transfrontal approach. The most important determinant of a successful surgical outcome is the experience of the surgeon. Recently, endoscopic approaches to pituitary adenoma resection have proved to be efficacious.[135,136] Surgery rapidly alleviates acromegaly symptoms, removes the tumor mass, relieves optic-tract pressure effects, and relieves headache. Tumor debulking, even if partial, also may be helpful in enhancing the effectiveness of subsequent therapy. Surgical control also is inversely correlated with initial tumor size and GH levels.[137,138] Not all patients are appropriate surgical candidates, usually because of coexisting cardiovascular and pulmonary disease, which may be a contraindication to anesthesia. If the tumor is sufficiently large or invasive and portends intraoperative damage to vital structures, the benefits of the procedure should be weighed against surgical risks.

Results of surgical resection of GH-secreting adenomas have only recently included more stringent biochemical criteria. Short-term remission (GH 5 µg/L) was achieved in 76% of 254 patients, with most of 129 patients remaining in long-term remission.[129] Although the biochemical parameter of "basal" GH less than 5 µg/L used in this study does not reflect normalization of GH hypersecretion, even with this less stringent criterion, the postsurgical mortality outcome was equivalent to that of age- and sex-matched controls, in contrast to the 2.4- to 4.8-fold

Table 7-7. Treatment Goals for Acromegaly

	Surgery	Somatostatin Receptor Ligands	GH Receptor Antagonist	Dopamine Agonist	Radiotherapy
			Acromegaly Treatment		
GH <2.5 µg/L	Macros <50% Macros >80%	~65%	Increases	<15%	60%, 10 yr
IGF-I normal	Macros <50% Macros >80%	~65%	>90%	<15%	60%, 10 yr
Onset	Rapid	Rapid	Rapid	Slow	Slow
Compliance	One-time consent	Sustained	Sustained	Good	Good
Tumor mass	Debulked or resected	No growth or shrinkage	Unknown	Unchanged	Ablated
Disadvantages					
Cost	One time	Ongoing	Ongoing	Ongoing	One time
Hypopituitarism	10%	None	Low IGF-I	None	>50%
Other	Tumor persistence or recurrence	Gallstones	Elevated liver enzymes	Nausea	Local nerve damage
	Diabetes insipidus	Nausea; diarrhea		Sinusitis	Visual and CNS disorders
	Local complications			High dose required	Cerebrovascular risk

Data from Ben-Shlomo A, Melmed S: Acromegaly, Endocrinol Metab Clin N Am 37(1):102–122, 2008.

enhanced mortality observed in patients with persistent disease (GH > 5 µg/L). Using more stringent criteria (normalized IGF-1 levels or GH suppression to ≥2 µg/L after glucose loading), more than 90% of patients with microadenomas successfully achieved control.[128,139,140] Unfortunately, most tumors encountered at diagnosis are large macroadenomas, and fewer than 50% of patients with macroadenomas are biochemically controlled.[128,138,139] In these invasive tumors, surgical resection is invariably followed by persistent GH and or IGF-1 hypersecretion. Visible residual tumor mass is often contiguous with or involves the cavernous sinus, internal carotid arteries, or suprasellar regions. Mortality risk in patients cured at surgery does not differ from that of controls, whereas in patients with persistent disease, even after adjuvant irradiation or medical therapy, mortality remains significantly increased (almost twofold). Thus, the level of GH attained postsurgically is the most important determinant of mortality outcome.[83] However, regardless of the treatment mode, normalization of GH restores mortality risk to that of age-matched population controls, and postoperative disease persistence is associated with a 3.5-fold relative mortality risk.[126,128,132] Whether or not surgical debulking improves subsequent disease control by SRIF analogs has recently been studied.[181-183] Surgical resection of at least 75% of the tumor mass enhanced the responsiveness of residual adenoma tissue to postoperative SRIF analog treatment.

Transnasal endoscopy[135,136] appears to offer a more facile tumor access and lower complication rates. Long-term outcomes are awaited to assess the efficacy of this approach.

Side Effects

The most important adverse surgical event is failure to resect invasive tumor totally and, consequently, persistent hormonal hypersecretion. Postoperative complications occur in approximately 10% of patients, and their incidence is largely dependent on the experience of the operating surgeon.[138,141] Complications include permanent diabetes insipidus, cerebrospinal fluid leaks requiring repair, meningitis, severe sinusitis, and hypopituitarism.[82,133,139-141] Perioperative morbidity and residual pituitary failure remain of concern in patients with invasive tumors, especially when operated on by less-experienced surgeons.

In summary, surgical success is based largely on skill and experience and on tumor size or invasiveness. Surgery is useful for prompt reduction of GH levels, and tumor debulking may enhance the effectiveness of medical therapy. After apparent successful resection, however, up to 8% of tumors recur within 10 years. GH levels should be measured in the immediate postoperative period; evidence of GH hypersecretion at this time portends either disease persistence or long-term recurrence. Overall, by immunoradiometric GH assay, postglucose GH values less than 1.0 µg/L are found in 50% of patients after surgery, and in 39% of patients with normalized IGF-1 levels, GH levels still fail to be suppressed.[142]

PITUITARY IRRADIATION

Techniques for pituitary radiotherapy include external radiation with either a cyclotron or a cobalt-60 source, and the radiotherapy is administered as a total dose of 4500 to 5000 rad. Higher doses are associated with a high incidence of side effects, whereas lower doses, although safer, appear to be less clinically effective. The total dose is given as 25 daily 180- to 200-rad fractions administered over a 6-week period.[143] Maximal tumor irradiation with minimal damage to nontumorous surrounding tissue has been achieved by advances in stereotactic MRI-directed tumor localization, focused-beam direction, field-size simulation, head immobilization, and isocentral rotational techniques.[144]

Proton-beam therapy also decreases GH secretion but is not widely available. Stereotactic ablation of GH-secreting adenomas by gamma knife radiosurgery is a promising new technique for which long-term results are not yet available. In 16 postsurgical patients monitored for up to 2.6 years, GH levels of less than 5 ng/mL and normalized IGF-1 concentrations were observed within 16 months of stereotactic radiosurgery.[145] However, the short follow-up precludes an assessment of complication outcome.

Tumor growth is invariably arrested after fractionated radiotherapy, but GH decline is slow, decreasing by approximately 20% per year. Within 18 years, 90% of patients have random serum GH concentrations lower than 5 ng/mL.[143] The degree and rapidity of GH attenuation are highly dependent on pretreatment GH levels.[143] However, few patients achieve the currently accepted rigorous goal of therapy, that is, a glucose-suppressed serum GH concentration less than 1 ng/mL. In one series, only 5 of 30 patients monitored for 10 or more years achieved this goal. After radiotherapy in 38 patients, 20 of whom had preradiotherapy IGF-1 data available, GH levels decreased by about 60% 3.5 years after irradiation and by about 80% 7 years after radiotherapy. However, plasma levels of IGF-1 remained almost unchanged and did not decrease to less than 80% of the initial value, even 7 years after radiotherapy. Only two patients ultimately exhibited normalized IGF levels.[146] The failure of irradiation to normalize IGF-1 levels effectively in the long term implies persistent albeit low levels of GH hypersecretion in these patients. Subsequent studies have demonstrated improved efficacy, and longer-term outcomes are awaited.[146]

Side Effects

Pituitary failure develops in 50% of patients undergoing deep x-ray therapy by 10 years and require thyroid, gonadal, or adrenal steroid replacement or a combination of these.[1,29] Rarely, optic-tract damage results in visual deficits. Ten years after radiotherapy, patients have a small but significant risk of a secondary brain malignancy, including glioma, in up to 1.7% of patients (relative risk of 16 versus expected).[147-149] Radiation also may rarely induce brain parenchymal changes[149-151] and brain dysfunction manifested as depression, decreased memory, decreased general quality of life, loss of vision, and cranial-nerve palsies.[141,152] Short-term controlled results and side-effect profiles for gamma knife radiosurgery indicate fewer local side effects, with no visual deficits reported in 30 patients for up to 4 years.[145] After maximal surgical debulking, a retrospective analysis of 83 patients who underwent single-session stereotactic radiotherapy (gamma knife), delivering high-dose radiation to the targeted mass[184] showed that 50% of patients were biochemically controlled at 5 years. The 5-year cumulative risk of hypopituitarism in this selected group was less than 5%, suggesting a lower risk of pituitary damage than that observed for fractionated radiotherapy.[185] In fact, no serious side effects were observed after 507 patient years of follow-up. In contrast, visual deficits were observed in 5.5% of patients treated for pituitary tumors with gamma knife radiation, likely reflecting high single retinal spot exposure.[186]

Thus, radiotherapy is effective in acromegaly, although its benefits are dose and time dependent, and GH reduction is delayed by 10 to 15 years. Even with the most accurate techniques, GH levels less than 2.0 ng/mL and normalization of IGF-1 levels are infrequently achieved.[146,153] Therefore, radiation therapy may be useful for patients with growing pituitary tumors whose condition is not controlled by surgery or who are resistant to medical therapy.

PHARMACOLOGIC MANAGEMENT

Somatostatin-Receptor Ligands

Octreotide is a synthetic octapeptide analog of native, naturally occurring somatostatin. This 8-amino-acid analog (molecular weight of 1019) binds selectively to the SSTR2 somatostatin-receptor subtype.[154] After subcutaneous injection, octreotide is rapidly absorbed, and peak drug concentrations (5.5 ng/mL) are achieved within 24 minutes of a 100-μg injection. The plasma distribution is about 12 minutes, and the elimination half-life is 1.5 hours, as compared with 2 minutes for natural SRIF.[154,155] The drug inhibits pituitary GH secretion, also directly suppresses hepatic IGF-1 production,[156] controls tumor growth, and relieves soft-tissue symptoms.

Octreotide inhibits GH, glucagon, and insulin release, but the analog exhibits greater selectivity in suppressing GH and glucagon than does somatostatin.[154] In normal subjects, octreotide

attenuates GH stimulation evoked by arginine,[156] exercise, and insulin-induced hypoglycemia.[157,158] The drug also may abrogate postprandial release of gastrointestinal and pancreatic peptides.[158] Because native somatostatin suppresses thyroid-stimulating hormone (TSH) secretion, it is not surprising that octreotide also blocks the TRH-induced release of TSH.[156,158,159] In acromegaly, octreotide reduces GH levels (by >50%) in more than 95% of all patients.

In the long term, about 70% of patients will have integrated GH levels suppressed to less than 5 ng/mL, and about 55% of patients have GH levels suppressed to less than 2 ng/mL. Seventy percent or more of patients will have their IGF-1 levels normalized after long-term treatment with octreotide (Fig. 7-6). Hypopituitarism does not develop during somatostatin receptor–ligand (SRL) treatment because SRIF analogs bind selectively to the somatostatin-receptor subtype that regulates GH secretion.[160] In addition to suppressing GH and IGF-1 levels, headache, fatigue, perspiration, joint pains, carpal tunnel syndrome, and paresthesias improve in most patients treated over the long term.

The starting dose of subcutaneous octreotide is 50 μg given subcutaneously in 8-hourly doses, and after 2 weeks, the dose can be increased to 100 μg 3 times daily. Thereafter, dose titrations to a maximum of 1500 μg/day may be made, depending on the nadir 2-hour postinjection GH level. The efficacy of octreotide also can be improved by increasing the dose frequency, although not necessarily increasing the total daily drug dose, or by administering the drug in a continuous-infusion minipump. Interestingly, long-term (>3 years) use of the drug is associated with enhanced sensitivity and improved biochemical control. Tachyphylaxis does not occur, and down-regulation of receptor responses does not appear to be manifested clinically.[159] About half of all patients will exhibit tumor shrinkage (30% average tumor volume change).

Responses to Long-Term Depot SRIF Analog Preparations

Long-term depot somatostatin preparations include octreotide LAR (long-acting release), and lanreotide Autogel.[155,159,161,162] Octreotide LAR incorporates octreotide into microspheres of a biodegradable poly-D,L-lactide-co-glycolide glucose polymer, whereas lanreotide Autogel is a water-soluble preparation allowing deep subcutaneous slow release. After 3-monthly injections of depot preparations, sustained concentrations are maintained.

Fig. 7-7 depicts the pharmacokinetic response to octreotide LAR in acromegaly. After a single injection of octreotide LAR, drug levels peak at about 28 days after injection and decrease slowly thereafter. GH levels decline after the injection and by day 14 are suppressed to less than 2 μg/L. GH suppression (as determined by measurement of integrated secretion over a 4-hour period) is sustained through day 49 and starts increasing thereafter. From the pharmacokinetic curve, it is apparent that a single injection administered every 30 days will allow GH levels to be persistently suppressed throughout the month. Fig. 7-8 depicts the effects of a single, monthly injection of octreotide LAR in a group of patients with acromegaly whose average GH levels were suppressed for the duration of the study (≤54 months). GH suppression appears to be sustained as long as patients receive monthly injections of octreotide LAR. About 80% of a total of 110 patients had IGF-1 levels normalized and GH suppressed to less than 2.5 ng/mL within 36 months.[155] Long-term studies indicate that >70% of patients receiving SRL therapy achieve GH levels of <2.5 μg/L and normal IGF-1 levels.[187] Several published studies include subjects preselected for prior GH

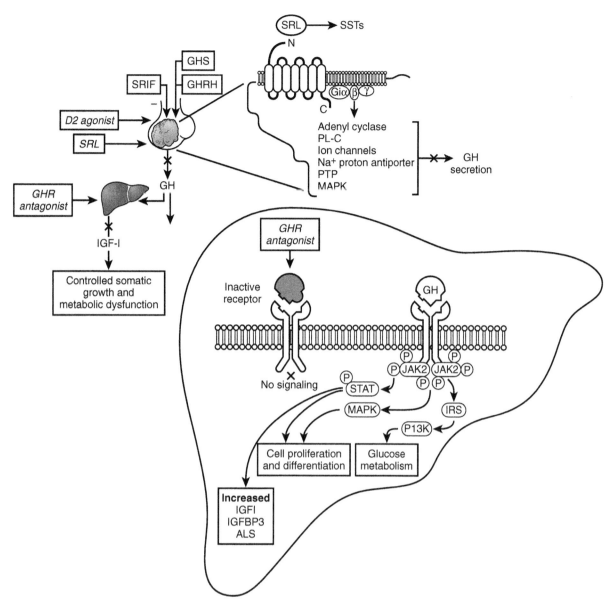

FIGURE 7-6. Acromegaly pharmacotherapy. Somatostatin-receptor ligands (SRLs) signal via G-protein coupled receptors (SST1-SST5) to suppress growth hormone (GH) secretion and action and control tumor growth. Growth hormone–receptor (GHR) antagonist blocks peripheral GH signaling to suppress insulin-like growth factor I (IGF-I). (Modified from Melmed S: Acromegaly, New Engl J Med 355:2558–2573, 2006.)

responsivity to SRLs, and a more rigorous assessment of the literature suggests an overall response rate of 40% to 50% in unselected patients.[188] SRL therapy controls tumor growth in the majority of treated patients, and continued tumor expansion while receiving these drugs has rarely been reported. A critical analysis of 15 eligible studies showed that about one third of patients receiving primary SRL therapy experience a significant reduction in pituitary tumor mass.[193,194] For those patients responding with tumor shrinkage, the dimensions of the mass decrease is ~50%. Nevertheless, several unresolved issues remain to be determined, including the effectiveness of SRL therapy in patients exhibiting optic chiasm compression, effects of SRL withdrawal on subsequent tumor mass reexpansion, and the effect of medically induced tumor shrinkage on surgical outcomes.

Clinical improvement is sustained, with little systemic or local intolerance. Thus, administration of depot SRL preparation results in persistent therapeutic serum drug concentrations and sustained suppression of both GH and IGF-1 values. The incidence of gallstones, microlithiasis, biliary sediment, or biliary sludge does not differ from that observed after subcutaneous octreotide (see following).

Side Effects

Although somatostatin-receptor ligands are relatively safe in the long term, several important adverse events are reported. Asymptomatic echogenic gallbladder lesions develop in about 25% of patients.[29] These lesions include both sludge and gallstones, which are usually diagnosed within the first 2 years of treatment, with few if any new echogenic events encountered thereafter. The prevalence of gallstones during octreotide therapy appears to vary geographically. In China, gallstones ultimately develop in most patients taking octreotide[163]; conversely, patients in southern Europe exhibit a far lower incidence. Clearly, dietary and/or other environmental factors play a role in their pathogenesis. Transient gastrointestinal symptoms, including anorexia,

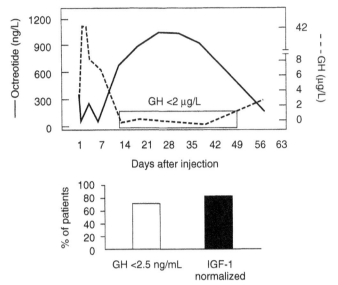

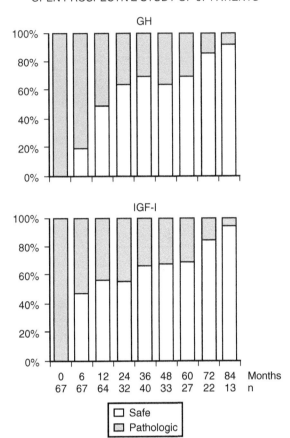

FIGURE 7-7. Pharmacokinetics of Octreotide LAR. *GH,* growth hormone; *IGF-1,* insulin-like growth factor 1; *LAR,* long-acting release.

OPEN PROSPECTIVE STUDY OF 67 PATIENTS

FIGURE 7-8. Nine years follow-up of selected patients treated with Octreotide LAR (long-acting release) shows that ~80% achieve GH and IGF-1 control. (Data from Cozzi R, Montini M, Attanasio R et al: Primary treatment of acromegaly with octreotide LAR: a long-term (up to nine years) prospective study of its efficacy in the control of disease activity and tumor shrinkage, J Clin Endocrinol Metab 91:1397–1403, 2006.)

nausea, vomiting, flatulence, and loose stools, may occur, especially during the first 2 weeks of therapy; these symptoms may be ameliorated by injecting the medication between meals or at night. Rarely, fat malabsorption and bradycardia have been reported.

In summary, long-acting somatostatin analogs are effective and safe in managing GH hypersecretion, especially in patients in whom surgical resection has failed to achieve a stringent biochemical remission. Indications for SRL therapy of acromegaly include: postoperative persistence of GH secretion from residual tumor tissue; during the latency period of GH nonresponsiveness after radiation; primary therapy of patients who decline surgery or are medically unfit for surgery or who exhibit a low probability of surgical cure. Somatostatin analogs also may be offered as primary therapy for patients who have undergone irradiation, in whom GH levels may remain unacceptably elevated.[29,164] Most patients with macroadenomas have persistent postsurgical GH hypersecretion, and the use of SRIF analogs should be weighed against radiotherapy for these patients. Long-acting injectable depot analogs administered once every 14 to 30 days provide enhanced patient convenience and compliance while retaining drug sensitivity.[84,165,166] Prior surgery appears not to alter the long-term efficacy of somatostatin analogs in attaining biochemical control. However, drug cost and patient compliance must be factored in when deciding on therapeutic options.

Further indications which have not been verified by controlled studies include the use of preoperative SRL therapy to enhance subsequent surgical results. Whether or not sustained long-term SRL therapy with or without combination with a GH receptor antagonist to tightly control GH and IGF-1 levels improves ultimate mortality outcome is not yet proven.

Dopamine Agonists

High doses of dopamine agonists have been used in the management of these patients, and bromocriptine is associated with GH normalization in fewer than 15% of patients.[167] A large meta-analysis revealed that 20% of patients will achieve GH levels less than 5 ng/mL, which is not a maximal criterion for control. Only 10% or fewer of all patients will actually have IGF-1 levels nor-

malized. However, bromocriptine does not carry with it a risk for hypopituitarism, and because it is an orally available medication, it is extremely convenient and cost effective for the patient.[168] Cabergoline, a long-acting dopamine agonist, has been used in acromegaly, but the long-term results are not compelling.[168-170]

Adverse Events

Because high doses (>20 mg/day) are required to achieve even moderate efficacy, the incidence of adverse events is far higher than usually seen when treating patients with prolactinomas. Patients receiving high doses of dopamine agonists complain of gastrointestinal symptoms, including nausea, vomiting, and abdominal cramps. Rarely, arrhythmias have been reported. Nasal stuffiness and sleep disturbances are common complaints.[167,171,172]

Growth Hormone–Receptor Antagonist

Pegvisomant, a growth hormone–receptor antagonist (GHRA), directly inhibits GH action in the periphery.[173] Unlike somatostatin and dopamine agonists that act centrally to inhibit GH secretion through somatotroph-cell somatostatin and dopamine receptors, pegvisomant interferes with the functional association of GH receptor subunits, suppressing peripheral IGF-1 generation in almost all patients with GH-secreting pituitary tumors treated for up to 36 months. Pegvisomant binds one GHR unit on site 1 but cannot bind the mutated site 2.[173] The site 2 mutation in pegvisomant involves replacement of glycine by lysine at position 120 (G120), preventing functional GHR dimerization, blocking initiation of subsequent GH signal transduction.

Daily doses of pegvisomant (10, 15, or 20 mg), given for 12 weeks, normalized IGF-1 levels in 38%, 75%, and 82% of patients with acromegaly, respectively.[174,175] A concomitant dose-dependent reduction in serum IGF-1 levels is accompanied by a dose-dependent regression of soft-tissue swelling, excessive perspiration, and fatigue, with no significant improvement in arthralgia or headache. Pegvisomant also improves insulin sensitivity and glucose tolerance in patients with acromegaly, reducing fasting serum insulin levels and fasting serum glucose levels, without observed decreased glycated hemoglobin.

Short-term (≤3 months of treatment) side effects encountered in pegvisomant-treated patients (versus placebo) included reversible injection-site reactions (11%), diarrhea, and nausea (14% versus 3%) in an 18-month study.[174] GH levels are reversibly increased approximately twofold, mirroring the IGF-1 decrease. Despite detection of anti-GH antibodies in 17% of patients, no evidence of tachyphylaxis was found. Serum cholesterol elevation also was reported.

The availability of pegvisomant allows a new approach for monitoring biochemical control of acromegaly. Pegvisomant therapy effectively normalizes IGF-1 levels in >90% of patients and also enhances insulin sensitivity in patients exhibiting glucose intolerance (Fig. 7-9). Persistent pituitary tumor growth is observed infrequently (<2% of patients), and transiently elevated (3× upper limit of normal) liver transaminase levels are observed in up to 5% of patients, with rarely reported drug-induced hepatitis.[189] Other side effects include lipohypertrophy[190] and features of hypopituitarism if IGF-1 levels are attenuated to below normal ranges.

GH levels are elevated in patients receiving pegvisomant therapy, so IGF-1 levels must be used to monitor efficacy, emphasizing the need to standardize commercial IGF-1 assays and develop age- and gender-specific reference ranges. Possible overtreatment with pegvisomant may create clinical features of GH deficiency, as pegvisomant may suppress IGF-1 levels below the lower limit of normal. It seems reasonable to titrate IGF-1 levels to midnormal ranges in these patients. Pegvisomant normalizes IGF-1 levels in somatostatin-resistant patients,[176] and promising results have been reported for combined weekly or twice-weekly pegvisomant injections and somatostatin analog cotreatment.[191,192] Pegvisomant is approved for patients who are intolerant, only partially responsive, or unresponsive to conventional treatment and effectively normalizes IGF-1 levels in patients (Fig. 7-10).

Integrated Treatment Approach to the Management of Acromegaly

PATIENTS WITH LIKELIHOOD OF GOOD SURGICAL OUTCOME

Once acromegaly is diagnosed, the likelihood of surgical cure is assessed. For small, well-circumscribed tumors, surgical excision by an experienced pituitary surgeon is the treatment of choice. Surgical cure rates are maximal for noninvasive, well-encapsulated smaller tumors. If a good surgical outcome is predicted, that is, a 60% chance or better that the disease will be controlled by tumor excision, surgery is indicated. After surgery, patients are monitored to ensure that GH responses to a glucose load are less than 1 ng/mL and that IGF-1 levels are normalized. If, however, after surgery, hormone levels are not controlled, indicative of disease persistence or recurrence, either short- or

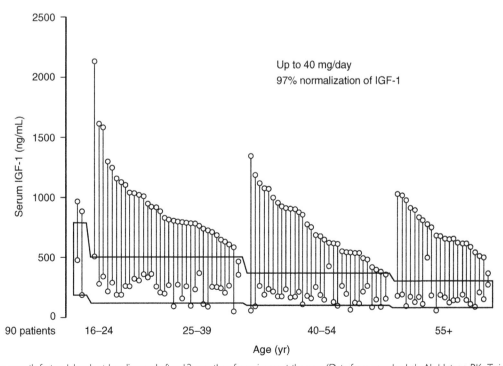

FIGURE 7-9. Insulin-like growth factor 1 levels at baseline and after 12 months of pegvisomant therapy. (Data from van der Lely AJ, Hutson RK, Trainer PJ et al: Long-term treatment of acromegaly with pegvisomant, a growth hormone–receptor antagonist, Lancet 358:1754–1759, 2001.)

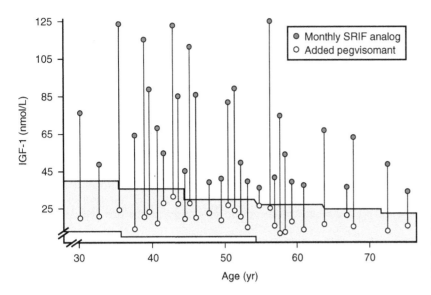

FIGURE 7-10. Combined somatostatin release–inhibiting factor (SRIF) analog and pegvisomant treatment controls insulin-like growth factor I (IGF-1) levels in patients resistant to SRIF analog monotherapy. (Data from Neggers SJ, van Aken MO, Janssen JA, et al: Long-term efficacy and safety of combined treatment of somatostatin analogs and pegvisomant in acromegaly, J Clin Endocrinol Metab 92[12]:4598–4601, 2007.)

long-acting somatostatin analogs are indicated.[29] Pegvisomant is indicated after failure of other therapy. Careful assessment of pituitary tumor size by using MRI is recommended every 6 to 12 months, depending on baseline tumor size and location. Patients should be followed up by measuring age- and gender-matched IGF-1 levels, aiming for the midnormal range levels. Pegvisomant treatment should be avoided in patients who have LFT abnormalities until further data are available, and LFTs should be evaluated monthly during the first 6 months of therapy. If the patient is still not biochemically controlled, a dopamine agonist is added, or reoperation or irradiation is considered.

PATIENTS WITH A POOR LIKELIHOOD OF SUCCESSFUL SURGICAL OUTCOME

Patients with large adenomas are likely to have a poor surgical outcome, and fewer than half of them will be biochemically controlled. Most patients in whom acromegaly is newly diagnosed have large macroadenomas, which portend a poor surgical outcome. These patients can be offered primary treatment with somatostatin analogs, as would patients in whom surgery is contraindicated or who decline surgery.[176] In 67 consecutive patients treated prospectively with octreotide LAR and followed for up to 9 years,[199] 70% exhibited GH levels <2.5 µg/L and/or normal age-matched IGF-1 levels. Interestingly, in this study over 80% of patients experienced tumor-mass shrinkage, and in 8 patients, the tumor disappeared or was reduced to an empty sella by MRI visualization. Testosterone levels and eugonadism were also restored in 64% of hypogonadal patients. Similar results were observed in an 18-year follow-up of 36 patients.[187] Use of preoperative octreotide to enhance subsequent surgical outcomes has been advocated. In a 3-month postoperative follow-up of 62 patients randomized to receive preoperative octreotide for 6 months, the drug appeared to offer improved postsurgical biochemical results for those patients harboring macroadenomas.[183] Because the drug reduces tumor bulk by approximately 50%,[161,176] subsequent surgery may therefore be facilitated. If biochemical control is not achieved, drug efficacy may be improved by dose increases and the addition of a dopamine agonist, and these patients should be offered a GHRA.[29] If

patients are resistant to medical treatment, second surgery or irradiation is indicated, depending on the size and location of the tumor remnant and the skill of the neurosurgeon.

FOLLOW-UP

Laboratory follow-up of patients includes performance of an oral glucose load and measurement of GH levels during the subsequent 2 hours. Stringent responses include GH less than 1 ng/mL, accompanied by a normalized IGF-1 level. If these goals are not achieved, medical treatment should be initiated, and if it is already being administered, efficacy may be improved by increasing medication dose frequency, adding a dopamine agonist, or starting a GHRA. Reoperation and radiation therapy are further adjuvant options. Pituitary MRI should be repeated after 6 to 12 months in patients with macroadenomas, depending on the degree of local pressure signs. In patients with tumors that have been effectively excised, serial MRI is warranted only once every 2 years after surgery. Invasive residual tumors require more frequent MRI evaluation. Although tumor mass may not invariably shrink with somatostatin analog therapy, further progressive tumor growth rarely occurs while patients are taking the medication.

GENERAL

Patients with acromegaly require management of multiple associated medical disorders. Colonoscopy should be performed at the time of diagnosis. The presence of more than three skin tags, a family history, age older than 50 years, or the presence of previous polyps requires more aggressive colonoscopic monitoring. Because cardiovascular morbidity is so high in patients with acromegaly, aggressive management of hypertension, left ventricular hypertrophy, cardiac failure, and arrhythmias should be pursued. Pulmonary function and sleep evaluation should be undertaken in all patients early in the course of the disorder, and debilitating arthritis requires aggressive rheumatologic management. Screening and therapy for insulin resistance and diabetes are important, and somatostatin analogs usually improve diabetes control dramatically. Insulin requirements may immediately decrease to 90% of pretreatment needs as GH is effectively suppressed. Headache is an extremely common symptom and usually improves with somatostatin analogs; if not, potent analgesics may be indicated. Maxillofacial disorders may require dental, maxillary, and facial cosmetic surgery. Fertility is commonly of concern to patients, and several recent reports of successful pregnancies in women treated with octreotide provide optimistic guidelines for pregnancy management.[111,177] Nevertheless, octreotide is not approved by the Food and Drug Administration for use during pregnancy. Patients with acromegaly may be depressed and have low self-esteem and other psychosocial sensitivity.[174,178] Thus, careful individual or group counseling may be indicated to assist patients with these issues. Finally, because all the available treatment modes for acromegaly are associated with therapy-specific complications, they should be carefully watched for and, if they occur, promptly treated.

The availability of long-acting depot preparations of somatostatin analogs[179] and the GHRA have changed the approach to management, inasmuch as patient compliance and medication acceptance are expected to improve markedly. Slow-release somatostatin formulations require single injections once every 2 to 4 weeks and control acromegaly in about 70% of patients; their side-effect profile appears quite similar. Availability of new formulations of SRIF receptor ligands provide promising therapeutic avenues for patients manifesting GH hypersecretory syndromes.

REFERENCES

1. Melmed S: Acromegaly, New Engl J Med 355:2558–2573, 2006.
2. Barkan AL: Acromegaly: diagnosis and therapy, Endocrinol Metab Clin North Am 18:277–310, 1989.
3. Molitch ME: Clinical manifestations of acromegaly, Endocrinol Metab Clin North Am 21:597–614, 1992.
4. Marie P: Sur deux cas d'acromegalie: hypertrophie singuliere non congenitale des extremities superieures et cephalique, Rev Med 6:297–333, 1886.
5. Nabarro JDN: Acromegaly, Clin Endocrinol (Oxf) 26:481–512, 1987.
6. Colao A, Ferone D, Marzullo P, et al: Systemic complications of acromegaly: epidemiology, pathogenesis, and management, Endocr Rev 25:102–152, 2004.
7. Jadresic A, Banks LM, Child DF, et al: The acromegaly syndrome: relation between clinical features, growth hormone values and radiological characteristics of the pituitary tumours, Q J Med 51:189–204, 1982.
8. Frohman LA, Jansson JO: Growth hormone-releasing hormone, Endocr Rev 7:223–253, 1986.
9. Thorner MO, Vance ML: Growth hormone, J Clin Invest 82:745–747, 1988.
10. Yamashita S, Melmed S: Insulin-like growth factor I regulation of growth hormone gene transcription in primary rat pituitary cells, J Clin Invest 79:449–452, 1987.
11. Berelowitz M, Szabo M, Frohman LA, et al: Somatomedin-C mediates growth hormone negative feedback by effects on both the hypothalamus and the pituitary, Science 212:1279–1281, 1981.
12. Melmed S, Yamashita S, Yamasaki H, et al: IGF-I receptor signaling: lessons from the somatotroph, Recent Prog Horm Res 51:189–215, 1996.
13. Veldhuis JD, Liem AY, South S, et al: Differential impact of age, sex steroid hormones, and obesity on basal versus pulsatile growth hormone secretion in men as assessed in an ultrasensitive chemiluminescence assay, J Clin Endocrinol Metab 80:3209–3222, 1995.
14. Carter-Su C, Schwartz J, Smit LS: Molecular mechanism of growth hormone action, Annu Rev Physiol 58:187–207, 1996.
15. Fan Y, Menon RK, Cohen P, et al: Liver-specific deletion of the growth hormone receptor reveals essential role of growth hormone signaling in hepatic lipid metabolism, J Biol Chem 284:19937–19944, 2009.
16. D'Ercole AJ, Stiles AD, Underwood LE: Tissue concentrations of somatomedin C: further evidence for multiple sites of synthesis and paracrine or autocrine mechanisms of action, Proc Natl Acad Sci U S A 81:935–939, 1984.
17. LeRoith D, Yakar S: Metabolic effects of growth hormone and insulin-like growth factor 1, Nat Clin Pract Endocrinol Metab 3:302–310, 2007.
18. Jones JI, Clemmons DR: Insulin-like growth factors and their binding proteins: biological actions, Endocr Rev 16:3–34, 1995.
19. Van Wyk JJ: The somatomedins: biological and physiologic control mechanisms. In Growth Factors, Orlando, FL, 1984, Academic Press, pp 81–125.
20. Isaksson OG, Lindahl A, Nilsson A, et al: Mechanism of the stimulatory effect of growth hormone on longitudinal bone growth, Endocr Rev 8:426–438, 1987.
21. Spencer GS, Hodgkinson SC, Bass JJ: Passive immunization against insulin-like growth factor-I does not inhibit growth hormone-stimulated growth of dwarf rats, Endocrinology 128:2103–2109, 1991.
22. Herman V, Fagin J, Gonsky R, et al: Clonal origin of pituitary adenomas, J Clin Endocrinol Metab 71:1427–1433, 1990.
23. Melmed S, Braunstein GD, Horvath E, et al: Pathophysiology of acromegaly, Endocr Rev 4:271–290, 1983.
24. Drange MR, Melmed S: Molecular pathogenesis of acromegaly, Pituitary 2:43–50, 1999.
25. Frawley LS, Boockfor FR: Mammosomatotropes: presence and functions in normal and neoplastic pituitary tissue, Endocr Rev 12:337–355, 1991.
26. Asa SL, Kovacs K, Horvath E, et al: Human fetal adenohypophysis: Electron microscopic and ultrastructural immunocytochemical analysis, Neuroendocrinology 48:423–431, 1988.
27. Horvath E, Kovacs K, Singer W, et al: Acidophil stem cell adenoma of the human pituitary: clinicopathologic analysis of 15 cases, Cancer 47:761–771, 1981.
28. Weinstein LS, Shenker A, Gejman PV, et al: Activating mutations of the stimulatory G protein in the McCune-Albright syndrome, N Engl J Med 325:1688–1695, 1991.
29. Melmed S, Colao A, Barkan A, et al: Guidelines for acromegaly management, J Clin Endocrinol Metab 94:1504–1517, 2004.
30. Melmed S, Ezrin C, Kovacs K, et al: Acromegaly due to secretion of growth hormone by an ectopic pancreatic islet-cell tumor, N Engl J Med 312:9–17, 1985.
31. Sparagana M, Phillips G, Hoffman C, et al: Ectopic growth hormone syndrome associated with lung cancer, Metabolism 20:730–736, 1971.
32. Kaganowicz A, Farkouh NH, Frantz AG, et al: Ectopic human growth hormone in ovaries and breast cancer, J Clin Endocrinol Metab 48:5–8, 1979.
33. Sano T, Asa SL, Kovacs K: Growth hormone-releasing hormone-producing tumors: clinical, biochemical, and morphological manifestations, Endocr Rev 9:357–373, 1988.
34. Asa SL, Scheithauer BW, Bilbao JM, et al: A case for hypothalamic acromegaly: a clinicopathological study of six patients with hypothalamic gangliocytomas producing growth hormone-releasing factor, J Clin Endocrinol Metab 58:796–803, 1984.
35. Oberg K, Norheim I, Wide L: Serum growth hormone in patients with carcinoid tumours: basal levels and response to glucose and thyrotrophin releasing hormone, Acta Endocrinol (Copenh) 109:13–18, 1985.
36. Thorner MO, Perryman RL, Cronin MJ, et al: Somatotroph hyperplasia: successful treatment of acromegaly by removal of a pancreatic islet tumor secreting a growth hormone-releasing factor, J Clin Invest 70:965–977, 1982.
37. Ashcraft MW, Hartzband PI, Van Herle AJ, et al: A unique growth factor in patients with acromegaloidism, J Clin Endocrinol Metab 57:272–276, 1983.
38. Levy A, Lightman SL: Growth hormone-releasing hormone transcripts in human pituitary adenomas, J Clin Endocrinol Metab 74:1474–1476, 1992.
39. Levy L, Bourdais J, Mouhieddine B, et al: Presence and characterization of the somatostatin precursor in normal human pituitaries and in growth hormone secreting adenomas, J Clin Endocrinol Metab 76:85–90, 1993.
40. Billestrup N, Swanson LW, Vale W: Growth hormone-releasing factor stimulates proliferation of somatotrophs in vitro, Proc Natl Acad Sci U S A 83:6854–6857, 1986.
41. Mayo KE, Hammer RE, Swanson LW, et al: Dramatic pituitary hyperplasia in transgenic mice expressing a human growth hormone–releasing factor gene, Mol Endocrinol 2:606–612, 1988.
42. Kovacs M, Kineman RD, Schally AV, et al: Effects of antagonists of growth hormone–releasing hormone (GHRH) on GH and insulin-like growth factor I levels in transgenic mice overexpressing the human GHRH gene, an animal model of acromegaly, Endocrinology 138:4536–4542, 1997.
43. Shimon I, Melmed S: Genetic basis of endocrine disease: pituitary tumor pathogenesis, J Clin Endocrinol Metab 82:1675–1681, 1997.
44. Spada A, Arosio M, Bochicchio D, et al: Clinical, biochemical, and morphological correlates in patients bearing growth hormone-secreting pituitary tumors with or without constitutively active adenylyl cyclase, J Clin Endocrinol Metab 71:1421–1426, 1990.
45. Vallar L, Spada A, Giannattasio G: Altered Gs and adenylate cyclase activity in human GH-secreting pituitary adenomas, Nature 330:566–568, 1987.
46. Bertherat J, Chanson P, Montminy M: The cyclic adenosine 3′,5′-monophosphate-responsive factor CREB is constitutively activated in human somatotroph adenomas, Mol Endocrinol 9:777–783, 1995.
47. Hashimoto K, Koga M, Motomura T, et al: Identification of alternatively spliced messenger ribonucleic acid encoding truncated growth hormone–releasing hormone receptor in human pituitary adenomas, J Clin Endocrinol Metab 80:2933–2939, 1995.
48. Molitch ME: Prolactinoma. In Melmed S, editor: The Pituitary, Cambridge, 1995, Blackwell, pp 443–477.
49. Melmed S, Ho K, Klibanski A, et al: Clinical review 75: recent advances in pathogenesis, diagnosis, and management of acromegaly, J Clin Endocrinol Metab 80:3395–3402, 1995.
50. Gadelha MR, Prezant TR, Une KN, et al: Loss of heterozygosity on chromosome 11q13 in two families with acromegaly/gigantism is independent of mutations of the multiple endocrine neoplasia type I gene, J Clin Endocrinol Metab 84:249–256, 1999.
51. Bates AS, Farrell WE, Bicknell EJ, et al: Allelic deletion in pituitary adenomas reflects aggressive biological activity and has potential value as a prognostic marker, J Clin Endocrinol Metab 82:818–824, 1997.
52. Fero ML, Rivkin M, Tasch M, et al: A syndrome of multiorgan hyperplasia with features of gigantism, tumorigenesis, and female sterility in p27(Kip1)-deficient mice, Cell 85:733–744, 1996.
53. Jacks T, Fazeli A, Schmitt EM, et al: Effects of an Rb mutation in the mouse, Nature 359:295–300, 1992.

54. Nakayama K, Ishida N, Shirane M, et al: Mice lacking p27(Kip1) display increased body size, multiple organ hyperplasia, retinal dysplasia, and pituitary tumors, Cell 85:707–720, 1996.

55. Herman V, Drazin NZ, Gonsky R, et al: Molecular screening of pituitary adenomas for gene mutations and rearrangements, J Clin Endocrinol Metab 77:50–55, 1993.

56. Prezant TR, Levine J, Melmed S: Molecular characterization of the MEN-1 tumor-suppressor gene in sporadic pituitary tumors, J Clin Endocrinol Metab 83:1388–1391, 1998.

57. Pei L, Melmed S, Scheithauer B, et al: Frequent loss of heterozygosity at the retinoblastoma susceptibility gene (RB) locus in aggressive pituitary tumors: evidence for a chromosome 13 tumor-suppressor gene other than RB, Cancer Res 55:1613–1616, 1995.

58. Spada A, Lania A, Ballare E: G protein abnormalities in pituitary adenomas, Mol Cell Endocrinol 142:1–14, 1998.

59. Barlier A, Gunz G, Zamora AJ, et al: Prognostic and therapeutic consequences of Gs alpha mutations in somatotroph adenomas, J Clin Endocrinol Metab 83:1604–1610, 1998.

60. Landis CA, Masters SB, Spada A, et al: GTPase inhibiting mutations activate the alpha chain of Gs and stimulate adenylyl cyclase in human pituitary tumours, Nature 340:692–696, 1989.

61. Clementi E, Malgaretti N, Meldolesi J, et al: A new constitutively activating mutation of the G_s protein alpha subunit-gsp oncogene is found in human pituitary tumours, Oncogene 5:1059–1061, 1990.

62. Lyons J, Landis CA, Harsh G, et al: Two G-protein oncogenes in human endocrine tumors, Science 249:655–659, 1990.

63. Boggild MD, Jenkinson S, Pistorello M, et al: Molecular genetic studies of sporadic pituitary tumors, J Clin Endocrinol Metab 78:387–392, 1994.

64. Hosoi E, Yokogoshi Y, Horie H, et al: Analysis of the G_s alpha gene in growth hormone-secreting pituitary adenomas by the polymerase chain reaction-direct sequencing method using paraffin-embedded tissues, Acta Endocrinol (Copenh) 129:301–306, 1993.

65. Adams EF, Brockmeier S, Friedmann E, et al: Clinical and biochemical characteristics of acromegalic patients harboring gsp-positive and gsp-negative pituitary tumors, Neurosurgery 33:198–203, 1993.

66. Cai WY, Alexander JM, Hedley-Whyte ET, et al: Ras mutations in human prolactinomas and pituitary carcinomas, J Clin Endocrinol Metab 78:89–93, 1994.

67. Pei L, Melmed S, Scheithauer B, et al: H-ras mutations in human pituitary carcinoma metastases, J Clin Endocrinol Metab 78:842–846, 1994.

68. Karga HJ, Alexander JM, Hedley-Whyte ET, et al: Ras mutations in human pituitary tumors, J Clin Endocrinol Metab 74:914–919, 1992.

69. Pei L, Melmed S: Isolation and characterization of a pituitary tumor–transforming gene (PTTG), Mol Endocrinol 11:433–441, 1997.

70. Melmed S: Mechanisms for pituitary tumorigenesis: The plastic pituitary, J Clin Invest 112:1603–1618, 2003.

71. Zhang X, Horwitz GA, Heaney AP, et al: Pituitary tumor–transforming gene (PTTG) expression in pituitary adenomas, J Clin Endocrinol Metab 84:761–767, 1999.

72. Stratakis CA, Carney JA, Lin JP, et al: Carney complex, a familial multiple neoplasia and lentiginosis syndrome: analysis of 11 kindreds and linkage to the short arm of chromosome 2, J Clin Invest 97:699–705, 1996.

73. Stratakis CA, Jenkins RB, Pras E, et al: Cytogenetic and microsatellite alterations in tumors from patients with the syndrome of myxomas, spotty skin pigmentation, and endocrine overactivity (Carney complex), J Clin Endocrinol Metab 81:3607–3614, 1996.

74. Carney JA, Hruska LS, Beauchamp GD, et al: Dominant inheritance of the complex of myxomas, spotty pigmentation, and endocrine overactivity, Mayo Clin Proc 61:165–172, 1986.

75. Carney JA, Gordon H, Carpenter PC, et al: The complex of myxomas, spotty pigmentation, and endocrine overactivity, Medicine (Baltimore) 64:270–283, 1985.

76. Teh BT, Kytola S, Farnebo F, et al: Mutation analysis of the MEN1 gene in multiple endocrine neoplasia type 1, familial acromegaly and familial isolated hyperparathyroidism, J Clin Endocrinol Metab 83:2621–2626, 1998.

77. Knudson AGJ: Mutation and cancer: statistical study of retinoblastoma, Proc Natl Acad Sci U S A 68:820–823, 1971.

78. Benlian P, Giraud S, Lahlou N, et al: Familial acromegaly: a specific clinical entity: further evidence from the genetic study of a three-generation family, Eur J Endocrinol 133:451–456, 1995.

79. Ackermann F, Krohn K, Windgassen M, et al: Acromegaly in a family without a mutation in the menin gene, Exp Clin Endocrinol Diabetes 107:93–96, 1999.

80. Gadelha MR, Rhode K, Kineman RD, et al: Author's response: isolated familial somatotropinomas: does the disease map to 11q13 or to 2p16? J Clin Endocrinol Metab 85:4921, 2000.

81. Alexander L, Appleton D, Hall R, et al: Epidemiology of acromegaly in the Newcastle region, Clin Endocrinol (Oxf) 12:71–79, 1980.

82. Bengtsson BA, Eden S, Ernest I, et al: Epidemiology and long-term survival in acromegaly, Acta Med Scand 223:327–335, 1988.

83. Holdaway IM, Rajasoorya CR, Gamble GD, et al: Long-term treatment outcome in acromegaly, Growth Horm IGF-1 Res 13:185–192, 2003.

84. Serri O, Beauregard C, Hardy J: Long-term biochemical status and disease-related morbidity in 53 postoperative patients with acromegaly, J Clin Endocrinol Metab 89:658–661, 2004.

85. Clemmons DR, Van Wyk JJ, Ridgway EC, et al: Evaluation of acromegaly by radioimmunoassay of somatomedin-C, N Engl J Med 301:1138–1142, 1979.

86. Rieu M, Kuhn JM, Bricaire H, et al: Evaluation of treated acromegalic patients with normal growth hormone levels during oral glucose load, Acta Endocrinol 107:1–8, 1984.

87. Lee PD, Durham SK, Martinez V, et al: Kinetics of insulin-like growth factor (IGF) and IGF-binding protein responses to a single dose of growth hormone, J Clin Endocrinol Metab 82:2266–2274, 1997.

88. Melmed S: Confusion in clinical laboratory GH and IGF-1 reports, Pituitary 2:171–172, 1999.

89. Barkan AL, Beitins IZ, Kelch RP: Plasma insulin-like growth factor-I/somatomedin-C in acromegaly: correlation with the degree of growth hormone hypersecretion, J Clin Endocrinol Metab 67:69–73, 1988.

90. Grinspoon S, Clemmons D, Swearingen B, et al: Serum insulin-like growth factor–binding protein-3 levels in the diagnosis of acromegaly, J Clin Endocrinol Metab 80:927–932, 1995.

91. de Herder WW, van der Lely AJ, Janssen JA, et al: IGFBP-3 is a poor parameter for assessment of clinical activity in acromegaly, Clin Endocrinol (Oxf) 43:501–505, 1995.

92. van der Lely AJ, de Herder WW, Janssen JA, et al: Acromegaly: the significance of serum total and free IGF-I and IGF-binding protein-3 in diagnosis, J Endocrinol 155(Suppl):9–16, 1997.

93. Shibasaki T, Kiyosawa Y, Masuda A, et al: Distribution of growth hormone-releasing hormone-like immunoreactivity in human tissue extracts, J Clin Endocrinol Metab 59:263–268, 1984.

94. Guillemin R, Brazeau P, Bohlen P, et al: Growth hormone–releasing factor from a human pancreatic tumor that caused acromegaly, Science 218:585–587, 1982.

95. Melmed S, Ziel FH, Braunstein GD, et al: Medical management of acromegaly due to ectopic production of growth hormone-releasing hormone by a carcinoid tumor, J Clin Endocrinol Metab 67:395–399, 1988.

96. Lieberman SA, Bjorkengren AG, Hoffman AR: Rheumatologic and skeletal changes in acromegaly, Endocrinol Metab Clin North Am 21:615–631, 1992.

97. Scarpa R, De Brasi D, Pivonello R, et al: Acromegalic axial arthropathy: a clinical case-control study, J Clin Endocrinol Metab 89:598–603, 2004.

98. Bluestone R, Bywaters EG, Hartog M, et al: Acromegalic arthropathy, Ann Rheum Dis 30:243–258, 1971.

99. Dons RF, Rosselet P, Pastakia B, et al: Arthropathy in acromegalic patients before and after treatment: a long-term follow-up study, Clin Endocrinol (Oxf) 28:515–524, 1988.

100. Lesse GP, Fraser WD, Farquharson R, et al: Gonadal status is an important determinant of bone density in acromegaly, Clin Endocrinol (Oxf) 48:59–65, 1998.

101. Melmed S: Acromegaly. In Melmed S, editor: The Pituitary, Cambridge, MA, 2002, Blackwell.

102. Wass J: Acromegaly and gigantism. In Besser GM, Thorner MO, editors: Comprehensive Clinical Endocrinology, ed 3, St. Louis, 2002, Mosby, pp 57–71.

103. Cheung NW, Boyages SC: The thyroid gland in acromegaly: An ultrasonographic study, Clin Endocrinol (Oxf) 46:545–549, 1997.

104. Pereira AM, van Thiel SW, Lindner JR, et al: Increased prevalence of regurgitant valvular heart disease in acromegaly, J Clin Encrinol Metab 89:71–75, 2004.

105. Chanson P, Megnien JL, del Pino M, et al: Decreased regional blood flow in patients with acromegaly, Clin Endocrinol (Oxf) 49:725–731, 1998.

106. Lieberman SA, Hoffman AR: Sequelae to acromegaly: reversibility with treatment of the primary disease, Horm Metab Res 22:313–318, 1990.

107. Colao A, Cuocolo A, Marzullo P, et al: Effects of 1-year treatment with octreotide on cardiac performance in patients with acromegaly, J Clin Endocrinol Metab 84:17–23, 1999.

108. Lombardi G, Colao A, Marzullo P, et al: Is growth hormone bad for your heart? Cardiovascular impact of GH deficiency and of acromegaly, J Endocrinol 155(Suppl):33–39, 1997.

109. Sacca L, Cittadini A, Fazio S: Growth hormone and the heart, Endocr Rev 15:555–573, 1994.

110. Colao A, Cuocolo A, Marzullo P, et al: Impact of patient's age and disease duration on cardiac performance in acromegaly: A radionuclide angiography study, J Clin Endocrinol Metab 84:1518–1523, 1999.

111. Colao A, Merola B, Ferone D, et al: Acromegaly, J Clin Endocrinol Metab 82:2777–2781, 1997.

112. Grunstein RR, Ho KK, Sullivan CE: Effect of octreotide, a somatostatin analog, on sleep apnea in patients with acromegaly, Ann Intern Med 121:478–483, 1994.

113. Grunstein RR, Ho KY, Sullivan CE: Sleep apnea in acromegaly, Ann Intern Med 115:527–532, 1991.

114. Grunstein RR, Ho KY, Berthon-Jones M, et al: Central sleep apnea is associated with increased ventilatory response to carbon dioxide and hypersecretion of growth hormone in patients with acromegaly, Am J Respir Crit Care Med 150:496–502, 1994.

115. Chanson P, Timsit J, Benoit O, et al: Rapid improvement in sleep apnea of acromegaly after short-term treatment with somatostatin analogue SMS 201-995 [letter], Lancet 1:1270–1271, 1986.

116. Melmed S: Unwanted effects of growth hormone excess in the adult, J Pediatr Endocrinol Metab 9:369–374, 1996.

117. Duncan E, Wass JAH: Investigation protocol: Acromegaly and its investigation, Clin Endocrinol (Oxf) 50:285–293, 1999.

118. Colao A, Marzullo P, Spiezia S, et al: Effect of growth hormone (GH) and insulin-like growth factor I on prostate diseases: an ultrasonographic and endocrine study in acromegaly, GH deficiency, and healthy subjects, J Clin Endocrinol Metab 84:1986–1991, 1999.

119. Colao A, Marzullo P, Ferone D, et al: Prostatic hyperplasia: an unknown feature of acromegaly, J Clin Endocrinol Metab 83:775–779, 1998.

120. Melmed S: Acromegaly and cancer: not a problem? J Clin Endocrinol Metab 86:2929–2934, 2001.

121. Renehan AG, Pudhupalayan B, Painter JE, et al: The prevalence and characteristics of colorectal neoplasia in acromegaly, J Clin Endocrinol Metab 85:3417–3424, 2000.

122. Jenkins PJ, Besser M: Clinical perspective: acromegaly and cancer: a problem, J Clin Endocrinol Metab 86:2935–2941, 2001.

123. Rokkas T, Pistiolas D, Sechopoulos P, et al: Risk of colorectal neoplasm in patients with acromegaly: a meta-analysis, World J Gastroenterol 14:3484–3489, 2008.

124. Leiberman DA, Weiss DG: One-time screening for colorectal cancer with combined fecal occult-blood testing and examination of the distal colon, N Engl J Med 345:555–560, 2001.

125. Jenkins PJ, Fairclough PD, Richards T, et al: Acromegaly, colonic polyps and carcinoma, Clin Endocrinol (Oxf) 47:17–22, 1997.

126. Holdaway IM, Rajasoorya RC, Gamble GD: Factors influencing mortality in acromegaly, J Clin Endocrinol Metab 89:667–674, 2004.

127. Orme SM, McNally RJ, Cartwright RA, et al: Mortality and cancer incidence in acromegaly: a retrospective cohort study: United Kingdom Acromegaly Study Group, J Clin Endocrinol Metab 83:2730–2734, 1998.

128. Swearingen B, Barker FG, Katznelson L, et al: Long-term mortality after transsphenoidal surgery and adjunctive therapy for acromegaly, J Clin Endocrinol Metab 83:3419–3426, 1998.

129. Abosch A, Tyrrell JB, Lamborn KR, et al: Transsphenoidal microsurgery for growth hormone-secreting pituitary adenomas: initial outcome and long-term results, J Clin Endocrinol Metab 83:3411–3418, 1998.

130. Landin-Wilhelmsen K, Tengborn L, Wilhelmsen L, et al: Elevated fibrinogen levels decrease following treatment of acromegaly, Clin Endocrinol (Oxf) 46:69–74, 1997.

131. Biermasz NR, Dekker FW, Pereira AM, et al: Determinants of survival in treated acromegaly in a single center: predictive value of serial insulin-like growth factor I measurements, J Clin Endocrinol Metab 89:2789–2796, 2004.

132. Ayuk J, Clayton RN, Holder G, et al: Growth hormone and pituitary radiotherapy, but not serum insulin-like growth factor-I concentrations, predict excess mortality in patients with acromegaly, J Clin Endocrinol Metab 89:1613–1617, 2004.

133. Krieger MD, Couldwell WT, Weiss MH: Assessment of long-term remission of acromegaly following surgery, J Neurosurg 98:719–724, 2003.

134. Bates AS, Van't Hoff W, Jones JM, et al: Does treatment of acromegaly affect life expectancy? Metabolism 44(Suppl 1):1–5, 1995.

135. Laws ER: Surgery for acromegaly: evolution of the techniques and outcomes, Rev Endocr Metab Disord 9:67–70, 2008.

136. Cappabianca P, Cavallo LM, Colao A, et al: Surgical complications associated with the endoscopic endonasal transsphenoidal approach for pituitary adenomas, J Neurosurg 97:293–298, 2002.

137. Biermasz NR, van Dulken H, Roelfsema F: Ten-year follow-up results of transsphenoidal microsurgery in acromegaly, J Clin Encrinol Metab 85:4596–4602, 2000.

138. Ahmed S, Elsheikh M, Stratton IM, et al: Outcome of transsphenoidal surgery for acromegaly and its relationship to surgical experience, Clin Endocrinol (Oxf) 50:561–567, 1999.

139. Kreutzer J, Vance ML, Lopes MB, et al: Surgical management of GH-secreting pituitary adenomas: an outcome study using modern remission criteria, J Clin Endocrinol Metab 86:4072–4077, 2001.

140. Shimon RL, Cohen ZR, Ram Z, et al: Transsphenoidal surgery for acromegaly: endocrinological follow-up of 98 patients, Neurosurgery 48:1239–1243, 2001.

141. Ciric I, Ragin A, Baumgartner C, et al: Complications of transsphenoidal surgery: results of a national survey, review of the literature, and personal experience, Neurosurgery 40:225–236, 1997.

142. Freda PU, Post KD, Powell JS, et al: Evaluation of disease status with sensitive measures of growth hormone secretion in 60 postoperative patients with acromegaly, J Clin Endocrinol Metab 83:3808–3816, 1998.

143. Eastman RC, Gorden P, Glatstein E, et al: Radiation therapy of acromegaly, Endocrinol Metab Clin North Am 21:693–712, 1992.

144. Laws JE, Vance ML: Radiosurgery for pituitary tumors and craniopharyngiomas, Neurosurg Clin North Am 10:327–336, 1999.

145. Attanasio R, Epaminonda P, Motti E, et al: Gamma-knife radiosurgery in acromegaly: a 4-year follow-up study, J Clin Endocrinol Metab 88:3105–3112, 2003.

146. Barkan AL, Halasz I, Dornfeld KJ, et al: Pituitary irradiation is ineffective in normalizing plasma insulin-like growth factor I in patients with acromegaly, J Clin Endocrinol Metab 82:3187–3191, 1997.

147. Tsang RW, Laperriere NJ, Simpson WJ, et al: Glioma arising after radiation therapy for pituitary adenoma: A report of four patients and estimation of risk [published erratum appears in Cancer 73:492, 1994], Cancer 72:2227–2233, 1993.

148. Ahmed M, Kanaan I, Rifai A, et al: An unusual treatment-related complication in a patient with growth hormone–secreting pituitary tumor, J Clin Endocrinol Metab 82:2816–2820, 1997.

149. Brada M, Ford D, Ashley S, et al: Risk of second brain tumour after conservative surgery and radiotherapy for pituitary adenoma, Br Med J 304:1343–1346, 1992.

150. Al-Mefty O, Kersh JE, Routh A, et al: The long-term side effects of radiation therapy for benign brain tumors in adults, J Neurosurg 73:502–512, 1990.

151. Alexander MJ, DeSalles AA, Tomiyasu U: Multiple radiation-induced intracranial lesions after treatment for pituitary adenoma: Case report, J Neurosurg 88:111–115, 1998.

152. Crossen JR, Garwood D, Glatstein E, et al: Neurobehavioral sequelae of cranial irradiation in adults: a review of radiation-induced encephalopathy, J Clin Oncol 12:627–642, 1994.

153. Jaffe CA: Reevaluation of conventional pituitary irradiation in the therapy of acromegaly, Pituitary 2:55–62, 1999.

154. Lamberts SWJ, van der Lely AJ, de Herder WW, et al: Octreotide, N Engl J Med 334:246–254, 1996.

155. Cozzi R, Attanasio R, Montini M, et al: Four-year treatment with octreotide long-acting repeatable in 110 acromegalic patients: predictive value of short-term results? J Clin Endocrinol Metab 88:3090–3098, 2003.

156. Murray RD, Kim K, Ren S-G, et al: Central and peripheral actions of somatostatin on the growth hormone-insulin-like growth factor-I axis, J Clin Invest 114:349–356, 2004.

157. Lightman SL, Fox P, Dunne MJ: The effect of SMS 201-995, a long-acting somatostatin analogue, on anterior pituitary function in healthy male volunteers, Scand J Gastroenterol Suppl 119:84–95, 1986.

158. Battershill PE, Clissold SP: Octreotide: a review of its pharmacodynamic and pharmacokinetic properties, and therapeutic potential in conditions associated with excessive peptide secretion, Drugs 38:658–702, 1989.

159. Gillis JC, Noble S, Goa KL: Octreotide long-acting release (LAR): a review of its pharmacological properties and therapeutic use in the management of acromegaly, Drugs 53:618–699, 1997.

160. Shimon I, Yan X, Taylor JE, et al: Somatostatin receptor (SSTR) subtype-selective analogues differentially suppress in vitro growth hormone and prolactin in human pituitary adenomas: novel potential therapy for functional pituitary tumors, J Clin Invest 100:2386–2392, 1997.

161. Colao A, Ferone D, Marzullo P, et al: Long-term effects of depot long-acting somatostatin analog octreotide on hormone levels and tumor mass in acromegaly, J Clin Endocrinol Metab 86:2779–2786, 2001.

162. Attanasio R, Baldelli R, Pivonello R, et al: Lanreotide 60 mg, a new long-acting formulation: effectiveness in the chronic treatment of acromegaly, J Clin Endocrinol Metab 88:5258–5265, 2003.

163. Shi YF, Zhu XF, Harris AG, et al: Prospective study of the long-term effects of somatostatin analog (octreotide) on gallbladder function and gallstone formation in Chinese acromegalic patients, J Clin Endocrinol Metab 76:32–37, 1993.

164. Ayuk J, Stewart SE, Stewart PM, et al: Long-term safety and efficacy of depot long-acting somatostatin analogs for the treatment of acromegaly, J Clin Endocrinol Metab 87:4142–4146, 2002.

165. Newman CB, Melmed S, Snyder PJ, et al: Safety and efficacy of long-term octreotide therapy of acromegaly: results of a multicenter trial in 103 patients: A clinical research center study, J Clin Endocrinol Metab 80:2768–2775, 1995.

166. Caron P, Cogne M, Gusthiot-Joudet B, et al: Intramuscular injections of slow-release lanreotide (BIM 23014) in acromegalic patients previously treated with continuous subcutaneous infusion of octreotide (SMS 201-995), Eur J Endocrinol 132:320–325, 1995.

167. Jaffe CA, Barkan AL: Treatment of acromegaly with dopamine agonists, Endocrinol Metab Clin North Am 21:713–735, 1992.

168. Jackson SN, Fowler J, Howlett TA: Cabergoline treatment of acromegaly: a preliminary dose finding study, Clin Endocrinol (Oxf) 46:745–749, 1997.

169. Abs R, Verhelst J, Maiter D, et al: Cabergoline in the treatment of acromegaly: a study in 64 patients, J Clin Endocrinol Metab 83:374–378, 1998.

170. Muratori M, Arosio M, Gambino G, et al: Use of cabergoline in the long-term treatment of hyperprolactinemic and acromegalic patients, J Endocrinol Invest 20:537–546, 1997.

171. Colao A, Ferone D, Marzullo P, et al: Effect of different dopaminergic agents in the treatment of acromegaly, J Clin Endocrinol Metab 82:518–523, 1997.

172. Vance ML, Evans WS, Thorner MO: Drugs five years later: bromocriptine, Ann Intern Med 100:78–91, 1984.

173. Kopchick JJ, Parkinson C, Stevens EC, et al: Growth hormone receptor antagonists: discovery, development and use in patients with acromegaly, Endocr Rev 23:623–646, 2002.

174. van der Lely AJ, Hutson RK, Trainer PJ, et al: Long-term treatment of acromegaly with pegvisomant, a growth hormone receptor antagonist, Lancet 358:1754–1759, 2001.

175. Trainer PJ, Drake WM, Katznelson L, et al: Treatment of acromegaly with the growth hormone–receptor antagonist pegvisomant, N Engl J Med 342:1171–1177, 2000.

176. Bonert VH, Zib K, Scarlett JA, et al: Growth hormone receptor antagonist therapy in acromegalic patients resistant to somatostatin analogs, J Clin Endocrinol Metab 85:2958–2961, 2000.

177. Herman-Bonert V, Seliverstov M, Melmed S: Pregnancy in acromegaly: successful therapeutic outcome, J Clin Endocrinol Metab 83:727–731, 1998.

178. Furman K, Ezzat S: Psychological features of acromegaly, Psychother Psychosom 67:147–153, 1998.

179. van der Hoek J, de Herder WW, Feelders RA, et al: A single-dose comparison of the acute effects between the new somatostatin analog SOM230 and octreotide in acromegalic patients, J Clin Endocrinol Metab 89:638–645, 2004.

180. Bevan JS, Atkin SL, Atkinson AB, et al: Primary medical therapy for acromegaly: an open, prospective, multicenter study of the effects of subcutaneous and intramuscular slow-release octreotide on growth hormone, insulin-like growth factor I, and tumor size, J Clin Endocrinol Metab 87:4554–4563, 2002.

181. Colao A, Attanasio R, Pivonello R, et al: Partial surgical removal of growth hormone-secreting pituitary tumors enhances the response to somatostatin analogs in acromegaly, J Clin Endocrinol Metab 91:85–92, 2006.

182. Petrossians P, Borges-Martins L, Espinoza C, et al: Gross total resection or debulking of pituitary adenomas improves hormonal control of acromegaly by somatostatin analogs, Eur J Endocrinol 152:61–66, 2005.

183. Carlsen SM, Lund-Johansen M, Schreiner T, et al: Preoperative octreotide treatment in newly diagnosed acromegalic patients with macroadenomas increases cure short-term postoperative rates: a prospective, randomized trial, J Clin Endocrinol Metab 93:2984–2990, 2008.

184. Losa M, Gioia L, Picozzi P, et al: The role of stereotactic radiotherapy in patients with growth hormone-secreting pituitary adenoma, J Clin Endocrinol Metab 93:2546–2552, 2008.

185. Jenkins PJ, Bates P, Carson MN, et al: Conventional pituitary irradiation is effective in lowering serum growth hormone and insulin-like growth factor I in patients with acromegaly, J Clin Endocrinol Metab 91:1239–1245, 2006.

186. Jagannathan J, Sheehan JP, Pouratian N, et al: Gamma Knife surgery for Cushing's disease, J Neurosurg 106:980–987, 2007.

187. Maiza JC, Vezzosi D, Matta M, et al: Long-term (up to 18 years) effects on GH/IGF-1 hypersecretion and tumour size of primary somatostatin analogue (SSTa) therapy in patients with GH-secreting pituitary adenoma responsive to SSTa, Clin Endocrinol (Oxf) 67:282–289, 2007.

188. Mercado M, Borges F, Bouterfa H, et al: A prospective, multicentre study to investigate the efficacy, safety and tolerability of octreotide LAR (long-acting repeatable octreotide) in the primary therapy of patients with acromegaly, Clin Endocrinol (Oxf) 66:859–868, 2007.

189. Schreiber I, Buchfelder M, Droste M, et al: Treatment of acromegaly with the GH receptor antagonist pegvisomant in clinical practice: safety and efficacy evaluation from the German Pegvisomant Observational Study, Eur J Endocrinol 156:75–82, 2007.

190. Bonert VS, Kennedy L, Petersenn S, et al: Lipodystrophy in patients with acromegaly receiving pegvisomant, J Clin Endocrinol Metab 93:3515–3518, 2008.

191. Feenstra J, de Herder WW, ten Have SM, et al: Combined therapy with somatostatin analogues and weekly pegvisomant in active acromegaly, Lancet 365:1644–1646, 2005.

192. Jorgensen JO, Feldt-Rasmussen U, Frystyk J, et al: Cotreatment of acromegaly with a somatostatin analog and a growth hormone receptor antagonist, J Clin Endocrinol Metab 90:5627–5631, 2005.

193. Melmed S, Sternberg R, Cook D, et al: A critical analysis of pituitary tumor shrinkage during primary medical therapy in acromegaly, J Clin Endocrinol Metab 90:4405–4410, 2005.

194. Bevan JS: Clinical review: the antitumoral effects of somatostatin analog therapy in acromegaly, J Clin Endocrinol Metab 90:1856–1863, 2005.

195. Herrmann BL, Wessendorf TE, Ajaj W, et al: Effects of octreotide on sleep apnoea and tongue volume (magnetic resonance imaging) in patients with acromegaly, Eur J Endocrinol 151:309–315, 2004.

196. Ayuk J, Clayton RN, Holder G, et al: Growth hormone and pituitary radiotherapy, but not serum insulin-like growth factor I concentrations, predict excess mortality in patients with acromegaly, J Clin Endocrinol Metab 89:1613–1617, 2004.

197. Kauppinen-Makelin R, Sane T, Reunanen A, et al: A nationwide survey of mortality in acromegaly, J Clin Endocrinol Metab 90:4081–4086, 2005.

198. Ronchi CL, Varca V, Beck-Peccoz P, et al: Comparison between six-year therapy with long-acting somatostatin analogs and successful surgery in acromegaly: effects on cardiovascular risk factors, J Clin Endocrinol Metab 91:121–128, 2006.

199. Cozzi R, Montini M, Attanasio R, et al: Primary treatment of acromegaly with octreotide LAR: a long-term (up to nine years) prospective study of its efficacy in the control of disease activity and tumor shrinkage, J Clin Endocrinol Metab 91:1397–1403, 2006.

200. Lamberts SW, van den Beld AW, van der Lely AJ: The endocrinology of aging, Science 278:419–424, 1997.

201. Colao A, Amato G, Pedroncelli AM, et al: Gender- and age-related differences in the endocrine parameters of acromegaly, J Endocrinol Invest 25:532–538, 2002.

202. Giustina A, Barkan A, Casanueva FF, et al: Criteria for cure of acromegaly: a consensus statement, J Clin Endocrinol Metab 85:526–552, 2000.

203. Arafat AM, Mohlig M, Weickert MO, et al: Growth hormone response during oral glucose tolerance test: the impact of assay method on the estimation of reference values in patients with acromegaly and in healthy controls, and the role of gender, age, and body mass index, J Clin Endocrinol Metab 93:1254–1262, 2008.

204. Colao A, Lombardi G: Should we still use glucose-suppressed growth hormone levels for the evaluation of acromegaly? J Clin Endocrinol Metab 93:1181–1182, 2008.

205. Vierimaa O, Georgitsi M, Lehtonen R, et al: Pituitary adenoma predisposition caused by germline mutations in the AIP gene, Science 312:1228–1230, 2006.

206. Daly AF, Vanbellinghen JF, Khoo SK, et al: Aryl hydrocarbon receptor-interacting protein gene mutations in familial isolated pituitary adenomas: analysis in 73 families, J Clin Endocrinol Metab 92:1891–1896, 2007.

207. Georgitsi M, Raitila A, Karhu A, et al: Molecular diagnosis of pituitary adenoma predisposition caused by aryl hydrocarbon receptor-interacting protein gene mutations, Proc Natl Acad Sci U S A 104:4101–4105, 2007.

208. Melmed S: Update in pituitary disease, J Clin Endocrinol Metab 93:331–338, 2008.

209. Bogazzi F, Russo D, Locci MT, et al: Apoptosis is reduced in the colonic mucosa of patients with acromegaly, Clin Endocrinol (Oxf) 63:683–688, 2005.

210. Renehan AG, O'Connell J, O'Halloran D, et al: Acromegaly and colorectal cancer: a comprehensive review of epidemiology, biological mechanisms, and clinical implications, Horm Metab Res 35:712–725, 2003.

211. Beauregard C, Utz AL, et al: Growth hormone decreases visceral fat and improves cardiovascular risk markers in women with hypopituitarism: a randomized, placebo-controlled study, J Clin Endocrinol Metab 93(6):2063–2071, 2008.

Chapter 8

CUSHING'S SYNDROME

DAMIAN G. MORRIS, ASHLEY GROSSMAN, and LYNNETTE K. NIEMAN

Harvey Cushing[1,2] was the first to codify the symptom complex of obesity, diabetes, hirsutism, and adrenal hyperplasia, and to postulate that the basophilic adenomas found at autopsy in six of eight patients caused the disease that now bears his name. Shortly thereafter, Walters and colleagues[3] identified the etiologic contribution of adrenal tumors and the therapeutic role of adrenalectomy. Over the ensuing century, our understanding of the pathogenesis of Cushing's syndrome has expanded to include ectopic production of adrenocorticotropic hormone (ACTH)[4] and corticotropin-releasing hormone (CRH),[5] and recognition of bilateral adrenal stimulation by factors other than ACTH.[6-9] Because florid Cushing's syndrome is ultimately fatal, early diagnosis and treatment have always been important. A plethora of tests have been developed over the years to improve the diagnostic yield. Similarly, the treatment options for Cushing's syndrome have increased to include medical agents that decrease the secretion or block the activity of circulating cortisol and surgical resection of eutopic and ectopic ACTH-producing

tumors. Despite all these advances, Cushing's syndrome continues to tax endocrinologists and is likely to continue to do so. This chapter reviews the manifestations, causes, approaches to diagnosis, and treatments for this complicated and multifaceted syndrome.

DEFINITION

Cushing's syndrome is a symptom complex that reflects chronic excessive tissue exposure to glucocorticoids. The diagnosis cannot be made unless both clinical features and biochemical abnormalities are present.

ETIOLOGY AND PATHOPHYSIOLOGY

Cushing's Syndrome

The causes of Cushing's syndrome can be divided into those that are ACTH dependent and those that are ACTH independent (Table 8-1). The ACTH-dependent forms are characterized by excessive ACTH production from a corticotroph adenoma (known as pituitary-dependent Cushing's syndrome or Cushing's disease), from an ectopic tumoral source (ectopic ACTH syndrome), or (rarely) from normal corticotrophs under the influence of excessive CRH production (ectopic CRH secretion). ACTH stimulates all three layers of the adrenal cortex to grow and secrete steroids. When excessive, this results in histologic hyperplasia and increased adrenal weight. Micronodules and macronodules (>1 cm) may be seen. Circulating glucocorticoids are increased, often in association with some increase in adrenal androgens.

ACTH-independent forms, apart from exogenous administration of glucocorticoids, represent adrenal activation by mechanisms other than trophic ACTH support. This enlarging group includes unilateral disease (adenoma and carcinoma), bilateral disease (primary pigmented nodular adrenal disease, McCune-Albright syndrome, and macronodular adrenal disease related to aberrations of the cyclic AMP signaling pathway, or caused by ectopic expression of G protein–coupled receptors), and hyperfunction of adrenal rest tissue.

Adrenal adenomas, composed of zona fasciculata cells, generally produce only glucocorticoids, in contrast to activation of the entire adrenal cortex as seen in other causes of Cushing's syndrome. ACTH levels are suppressed by hypercortisolism and the nonadenomatous tissue atrophies because of lack of this trophic factor. As a result, androgenic signs, such as pustular acne and hirsutism, are relatively uncommon, and dehydroepiandrosterone sulfate levels are typically low. By contrast, case reports have described patients with macronodular adrenal disease with secretion of mineralocorticoids, estrones, or androgens, in addition to cortisol.

Cushing's Disease

Cushing's disease is almost always caused by a solitary (probably monoclonal) corticotroph adenoma.[10] Although nodular corticotroph hyperplasia without evidence of a CRH-producing neoplasm does occur, it represents 2% or less of large surgical series,[11,12] and some doubt its existence. Most tumors are intrasellar microadenomas (<1 cm in diameter), although macroadenomas account for approximately 5% to 10% of tumors, and extrasellar extension or invasion may occur. The cause of Cushing's disease remains unknown, despite much work on the molecular characterization of these tumors. Traditionally, whether the development of pituitary adenomas is due to abnormal hypothalamic hormonal stimulation or feedback regulation or an intrinsic pituitary defect has been the subject of debate, although most data support a primary pituitary abnormality or a series of abnormalities. More recently, a model has been proposed that encompasses both theories. Here, tumors can arise either as a clonal expansion from a primary intrinsic pituitary defect or as excessive hormonal stimulation/abnormal feedback leading to hyperplasia, which in turn predisposes the cells to mutate, with subsequent clonal expansion.[13] Analysis of the primary corticotroph stimulatory and negative feedback pathways has not revealed a common defect.[14,15] Similarly, the common oncogenes and tumor suppressor genes implicated in other cancers do not seem to be commonly involved in the pathogenesis of corticotropinomas. Studies of knockout mice and analysis of human pituitary tumor samples have implicated

the cyclin-dependent kinase inhibitor p27 (Kip1) in corticotroph tumorigenesis. Overall, reduced p27 protein levels in corticotropinomas and a high phosphorylated p27/p27 ratio suggest increased inactivation of this negative cell-cycle regulator, although the cause of this change remains to be elucidated.[16] Cytogenetic studies have revealed a surprising number of gross chromosomal changes in benign pituitary adenomas, and although the number of corticotroph tumors studied has been small, gain of chromosome 6p and loss of chromosomes 2, 15q, and 22 seem to be the most common abnormalities.[17-19] Perhaps improvement in molecular biologic techniques, particularly microarray analysis, will lead to the implication of new genes in the pathogenesis of these tumors that then will require further study.[20]

Ectopic Adrenocorticotropic Hormone Syndrome

The syndrome of ectopic hormone secretion was first codified by Liddle and colleagues, who defined it as "any hormone produced by a neoplasm which is derived from tissue not normally engaged in the production of the hormone in question."[4] ACTH and other pro-opiomelanocortin (POMC) products were subsequently identified in many noncorticotroph tumors, although not all were associated with increased circulating levels or the development of Cushing's syndrome.[4,21]

Although small cell lung cancer is probably the most common cause of ectopic ACTH syndrome, it is not the most common seen in larger series of generally less obvious tumors investigated at endocrine centers, as discussed later (Table 8-2). An intrathoracic neoplasm (carcinoma of the lung or carcinoid of the bronchus or thymus) accounts for approximately 60% of ectopic ACTH secretion, followed by pancreatic tumors (islet cell or carcinoid), pheochromocytoma (≈5% to 10%), and medullary carcinoma of the thyroid (<5%).

The mechanism whereby the POMC gene becomes derepressed in noncorticotroph tumors is not understood. One hypothesis is that these cells are derived from a common multipotential progenitor cell capable of producing peptide hormones, such that ACTH production is a reversion to a less differentiated state.[22] The speculation that many ACTH-producing tumors are derived from neural crest amine precursor uptake and decarboxylation (APUD) cells may support this view,[23] although this embryological hypothesis is not supported by the most recent data. However, because endodermally derived tumors also produce ACTH, the acquisition of APUD characteristics may be but one manifestation of dedifferentiation and may not represent the cause of ectopic ACTH production.

Although the mechanism of gene derepression is not understood, the regulation of POMC production and processing has

Table 8-1. Causes of Cushing's Syndrome

ACTH-dependent
  Pituitary-dependent Cushing's syndrome (Cushing's disease)
  Ectopic ACTH syndrome
  Ectopic CRH secretion
  Exogenous ACTH administration
ACTH-independent
  Adrenal adenoma
  Adrenal carcinoma
  Primary pigmented nodular adrenal disease (PPNAD), sporadic or
    associated with the Carney complex
AIMAH
AIMAH secondary to abnormal hormone receptor expression/signaling
McCune-Albright syndrome
Exogenous glucocorticoid administration

ACTH, Adrenocorticotropic hormone; *AIMAH*, ACTH-independent bilateral macronodular adrenal hyperplasia; *CRH*, corticotropin-releasing hormone.

Table 8-2. Percentage Incidence of Tumor Types Causing Ectopic Adrenocorticotropic Hormone Syndrome in Four Large Series from 1969 to 2003

Tumor Type	Liddle et al., 1969[4] (N = 104)	Jex et al., 1985[428] (N = 21)	Torpy et al., 2002[429] (N = 58)	Morris and Grossman, 2003[430] (N = 32)
Lung carcinoma	50	20	2	19
Bronchial carcinoid	5	28	40	41
Thymic carcinoid	10	8	10	3
Pancreatic tumor	10	20	7	12
Pheochromocytoma, paraganglioma, neuroblastoma	5	12	5	3
Medullary thyroid carcinoma	2		3	9
Miscellaneous*	17	8	2	12

*Other tumors reported to uncommonly secrete adrenocorticotropic hormone include appendix, breast, cloacogenic carcinoma of the anal canal, colon, esophagus, gallbladder, gastric carcinoid, kidney, melanoma, mesothelioma, myeloblastic leukemia, ovary, prostate, salivary glands, and testes.

been investigated. POMC, corticotropin-like intermediate lobe protein, and larger forms of ACTH ("big" or pro-ACTH) that are not usually secreted may circulate, and the intracellular ratio of the POMC products may be abnormal.[24,25] Investigation of cell lines of small cell carcinoma of the lung that synthesize POMC and pro-ACTH showed that only ACTH precursors were secreted, suggesting that processing to ACTH is defective.[26] The pattern of POMC mRNA species in ACTH-producing tumors has been characterized. A 1200 bp transcript similar to that of a corticotroph adenoma,[27] a shorter than normal 800 bp mRNA lacking a signal sequence for secretion,[27,28] and a larger 1400 to 1500 bp POMC transcript have been identified. The larger species appears to originate upstream of the usual pituitary promoter, with preservation of the normal translation start site.[29,30] It is possible that the promoters that initiate this transcription are not regulated by glucocorticoids, and this may explain in part the lack of responsiveness to glucocorticoid suppression noted clinically in these patients. In vitro investigation of human small cell cancer cell lines and pancreatic islet cell tumors with normal glucocorticoid receptor binding has found, for the most part, no regulation of POMC, tyrosine aminotransferase, or the glucocorticoid receptor mRNA at doses of hydrocortisone that would normally suppress pituitary production.[31-33] However, clinical observation of suppression of ACTH production by some bronchial carcinoids during glucocorticoid administration suggests retention of a functional glucocorticoid response element that regulates POMC production, at least in some ectopic tumors.[34]

Ectopic Corticotropin-Releasing Hormone Secretion

Tumor secretion of CRH with or without ACTH secretion is a rare cause of Cushing's syndrome. Although many tumors immunostain for CRH, its secretion is less common, and most patients do not develop cushingoid features.[35] Thus, the diagnosis primarily rests on the demonstration of elevated plasma CRH levels (requiring an assay that is not readily available). The literature includes fewer than 20 patients who fit this criterion. Tumors may have negative immunostaining for ACTH, but this may be related to reduced storage and rapid secretion. In cases such as these, a CRH and ACTH gradient across the tumor bed can be suggestive that, in fact, the tumor secretes both peptides.[36] Tumors include bronchial and thymic carcinoids, small cell lung cancer, medullary thyroid carcinoma, pheochromocytoma, gangliocytoma, prostate carcinoma, and ganglioneuroblastoma.[37,38] The biochemical responses to diagnostic tests can be similar to those seen in ectopic ACTH secretion or in pituitary ACTH-dependent disease.[38] It is important to note that many, if not all, ectopic secretors of CRH causing Cushing's syndrome are also ectopic ACTH secretors.

Primary Adrenal Disease

The primary adrenal forms of Cushing's syndrome do not share a common cause. Although the cause of adrenocortical neoplasia is not known, some events important in the development of adrenal cancer have been identified. Paternal isodisomy at 11p15.5 with overexpression of insulin-like growth factor-2 (IGF-2) and reduced expression of CDKN1C (a G1 cyclin-dependent kinase inhibitor) and H19 (a putative growth suppressor) seems to be a key event. Mutations of p53 may be involved in a small subset of carcinomas, and mutations of β-catenin may be an early event. Other genes important in pathogenesis remain to be elucidated, although potential loci have been identified at chromosomes 17p, 1p, 2p16, and 11q13 for tumor suppressor genes, and at chromosomes 4, 5, and 12 for

oncogenes.[39] Adenomas and carcinomas tend to be monoclonal, although the nodular hyperplasias are often polyclonal.[40] Adrenal adenomas are encapsulated benign tumors, usually less than 40 g in weight. Adrenal carcinomas usually are encapsulated, generally weigh more than 100 g, and may lack classic histologic features of malignancy, although nuclear pleomorphism, necrosis, mitotic figures, and vascular or lymphatic invasion suggest the diagnosis.[41] The adjacent adrenal tissue is atrophic in both conditions.

Primary pigmented nodular adrenal disease (PPNAD), also known as micronodular adrenal disease, is a rare form of Cushing's syndrome characterized histologically by small to normal-size glands (combined weight <12 g) with cortical micronodules (average 2 to 3 mm) that may be dark or black in color. The intervening cortex is usually atrophic.[42] Most cases of PPNAD occur as part of the Carney complex in association with a variety of other abnormalities, including myxomatous masses of the heart, skin, or breast; blue nevi or lentigines; and other endocrine disorders (sexual precocity; Sertoli cell, Leydig cell, or adrenal rest tumors; acromegaly). The Carney complex is inherited as an autosomal dominant condition, and Cushing's syndrome occurs in approximately 30% of cases. The tumor suppressor gene PRKAR1A, coding for the type 1A regulatory subunit of protein kinase A, has been shown to be mutated in approximately one half of patients with Carney complex. Mutations in this gene and also the phosphodiesterase 11A (PDE11A) gene have been shown to be associated with an isolated distinct form of PPNAD.[43]

Cushing's syndrome resulting from bilateral nodular adrenal disease is an uncommon feature of the McCune-Albright syndrome,[44] which is characterized by fibrous dysplasia of bone, café-au-lait skin pigmentation, and endocrine dysfunction (usually precocious puberty). In this disease, an activating mutation at codon 201 of the α subunit of the G protein that stimulates cyclic adenosine monophosphate formation occurs in a mosaic pattern in early embryogenesis.[45] If this affects some adrenal cells, constitutive activation of adenylate cyclase and the steroidogenic cascade leads to nodule formation and glucocorticoid excess. The internodular adrenal cortex, where the mutation is not present, becomes atrophic.[46]

A missense mutation of the ACTH receptor, resulting in its constitutive activation and ACTH-independent Cushing's syndrome, also has been reported.[47]

ACTH-independent bilateral macronodular adrenal hyperplasia (AIMAH) is a rare form (<1%) of Cushing's syndrome that involves large or even huge adrenal glands, usually with definite nodules on imaging. Most cases are sporadic, but a few familial cases have been reported.[48] Although the cause remains unclear in most cases, some nodules express increased numbers of receptors normally found on the adrenal gland, or ectopic receptors for circulating ligands that then can stimulate cortisol production. Perhaps the best known example of this phenomenon is food-dependent Cushing's syndrome. The normal postprandial increase in gastric inhibitory peptide (GIP) appeared to cause Cushing's syndrome in two middle-aged women with bilateral multinodular adrenal enlargement, mildly elevated urinary free cortisol (UFC) values, and undetectable plasma ACTH values. Fasting morning serum cortisol values were low or normal. Cortisol values increased dramatically after meals and after in vivo or in vitro exposure to GIP.[7,8] In one patient, curative bilateral adrenalectomy revealed multinodular adrenal glands weighing 20 and 35 g.[8] In the other, treatment with octreotide ameliorated the syndrome.[7] Ectopic expression of GIP receptors was found in these patients. Aberrant expression of vasopressin, β-adrenergic luteinizing hormone/human chorionic gonadotropin, serotonin, angiotensin, leptin, glucagon, interleukin (IL)-1, and thyroid-stimulating hormone (TSH) has been described as functionally linked to cortisol production.[49] However, it is possible that this apparent ectopic induction of receptors on the adrenal is a response to the adrenal hyperplasia rather than its cause.

Adrenal rest tissue in the liver, in the adrenal beds, or in association with the gonads may rarely cause Cushing's syndrome, usually in the setting of ACTH-dependent disease after adrenalectomy.[50-53] Ectopic cortisol production by an ovarian carcinoma has been reported.[54]

PSEUDO-CUSHING'S STATES

A pseudo-Cushing's state may be defined as one in which some or all of the clinical features that resemble true Cushing's syndrome, and some evidence of hypercortisolism, are present but disappear after resolution of the underlying condition.[55] The pathophysiology of these states has not been established. One hypothesis is that these stressful conditions increase the activity of the CRH neuron, resulting in excessive ACTH secretion, adrenal hyperplasia, and increased cortisol production.[56] The model predicts only intermittent and modest hypercortisolism because of appropriate corticotroph reduction in ACTH secretion in response to negative feedback by cortisol (Fig. 8-1). This construct presumes also that hypertrophied adrenal glands produce excessive glucocorticoids in response to normal ACTH levels, an assumption that is supported by the blunted ACTH, but not cortisol, response to exogenous CRH in anorexia nervosa,[57] depression,[58] and obligate athleticism.[59]

EPIDEMIOLOGY

Iatrogenic causes account for most cases of Cushing's syndrome because of the common therapeutic use of high-dose glucocorticoids. Large series have reported the distribution of endogenous cases as follows: Cushing's disease (68%), adrenal adenomas (8% to 19%), adrenal carcinoma (6% to 7%), ectopic ACTH syndrome (6% to 15%), and nodular adrenal hyperplasia (2%).[55,60] However, a paucity of information is available on the true incidence of these causes. Perhaps the best data come from a population-based study covering the whole of Denmark (population of 5.3 million), which used stringent methods of data collection, aided by the small number of centers treating the disorder.[61] The incidences of Cushing's disease, adrenal adenoma, and adrenal carcinoma were 1.2 per million per year, 0.6 per million per year, and 0.2 per million per year, respectively. The reported incidence of ectopic ACTH syndrome was extremely low (0.1 per million per year). This is probably due (as the authors concede) to the fact that many cases were never recognized, but may be explained in part by a group of patients with ACTH-dependent Cushing's syndrome (0.5 per million per year) with presumed but unproven pituitary disease. Some of these may well have had ectopic ACTH syndrome. The incidence of ectopic ACTH syndrome most certainly is underestimated in the endocrine literature because most cases reaching endocrinologists are those caused by occult tumors as opposed to those caused by overt malignancy. However, given that Cushing's syndrome will be present in 3% to 12% of cases of small cell lung cancer,[62,63] and that the recent incidence of small cell lung cancer in Europe is approximately 120 per million per year in men and 40 per million per year in women,[64] this is by far the most common cause. Other epidemiologic studies have looked at just the incidence of Cushing's disease and have found rates between 0.7 per million per year in northern Italy[65] and 2.4 per million per year in northern Spain.[66]

Gender and age distribution varies with the cause of Cushing's syndrome. Adrenal adenomas and Cushing's disease present much more commonly in women than in men, and adrenal carcinoma is approximately 1.5 times as common as in men.[55,60] Nodular adrenal hyperplasia has an approximately equal gender ratio.

Ectopic ACTH syndrome is the only cause of the syndrome that is more common in men (other than Cushing's disease in prepubertal children), although this may change as more women are developing small cell lung cancer. Lung cancer is more common after age 40, and this accounts for the increased mean age of patients with ectopic ACTH syndrome compared with Cushing's disease, which occurs between 25 and 40 years of age.[67] The other major cause of ectopic ACTH secretion, intrathoracic carcinoids, has a peak incidence around 40 years and only a slightly increased male-to-female ratio.[68] The age distribu-

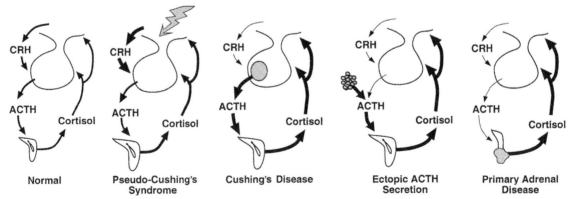

FIGURE 8-1. Physiology of the hypothalamic-pituitary-adrenal axis in normal individuals and hypercortisolemic states. Corticotropin-releasing hormone (CRH) secretion from the hypothalamus normally stimulates adrenocorticotropic hormone (ACTH) secretion from the pituitary gland. This in turn results in increased cortisol production from the adrenal glands. The system is modulated by negative feedback inhibition by cortisol of both CRH and ACTH secretion. In pseudo-Cushing's syndrome, the CRH neuron is activated by central input *(large shaded arrow)*, resulting in increased CRH output that eventuates in hypercortisolism. Increased cortisol production restrains corticotroph activation but does not completely reverse the activation of the CRH neuron, so that mild to moderate hypercortisolism may persist. In Cushing's disease, a corticotroph adenoma secretes ACTH in excess and is inhibited only partially by rising cortisol levels. In this setting and that of ectopic ACTH secretion and primary adrenal disease, the CRH neuron is suppressed by hypercortisolism. In ectopic ACTH secretion, excessive secretion of ACTH from a nonpituitary tumor is not inhibited by glucocorticoid feedback. In this setting and that of autonomous production of cortisol by the adrenal gland, ACTH secretion by normal corticotrophs is suppressed by hypercortisolism.

tion of adrenal cancer is bimodal, with peaks in childhood and adolescence and late in life, although adrenal adenoma occurs most often around 35 years of age.

CLINICAL FEATURES

Excessive cortisol production has widespread systemic effects[67,69-72] (Table 8-3). Although the full-blown cushingoid phenotype is unmistakable, the clinical diagnosis may be equivocal for patients with few of the typical characteristics (Fig. 8-2). Some nonspecific features consistent with the diagnosis of Cushing's syndrome, such as obesity, hypertension, and menstrual irregularity, are common in the general population and may provoke unwarranted and costly screening tests for patients not likely to be affected.

One useful strategy when the diagnosis of Cushing's syndrome is considered, is to look for evidence of progressive physical changes by examination of serial photographs, especially of individuals photographed at annual events such as holidays, birthdays, or school milestones (Fig. 8-3). Another approach relies on identification of signs and symptoms that correctly classify patients suspected of having the disorder. Truncal obesity, ecchymoses, plethora, proximal muscle weakness, and osteopenia are useful discriminant indices for Cushing's syndrome, with osteoporosis, ecchymoses, and muscle weakness being the most reliable.[69,73,74]

Increased deposition of fat, one of the earliest signs, occurs in almost all patients and is reported as increasing weight or difficulty in maintaining weight. The distribution of fat is altered in both men and women, with increased amounts in the visceral compartments[75] and subcutaneous sites on the face and neck. Increased intra-abdominal fat results in the truncal obesity described by Cushing in approximately 50% of patients. Increased fat in the face (moon facies), the supraclavicular or temporal fossae, and the dorsocervical area ("buffalo hump") is uncommon in normal people.

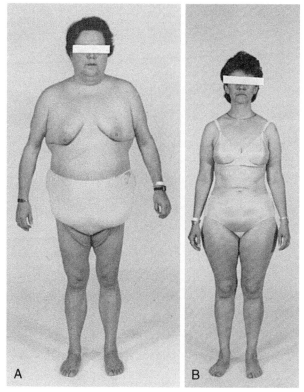

FIGURE 8-2. Body habitus of two patients with proven Cushing's syndrome. Features typical of the syndrome—central obesity, round face, and supraclavicular fat pads—are present in the patient in **A,** but not in the patient in **B,** illustrating that the diagnosis is not always apparent from the initial physical examination.

Table 8-3. Percentage Frequency of Clinical Signs and Symptoms of Cushing's Syndrome as Described in Six Large Studies from 1952 to 2003

Signs and Symptoms (Men/Women)	Plotz et al., 1952[67] (N = 33)	Sprague et al., 1956[72] (N = 100)	Soffer et al., 1961[71] (N = 50)	Urbanic and George, 1981[70] (N = 31)	Ross & Linch, 1982[69] (N = 70)	Giraldi et al., 2003[125] (N = 280)
Obesity or weight gain	97	84	86	79	97	85/86
Hypertension	84	90	88	77	74	68/67
Weakness/muscle atrophy	83		58	90	56	64/46
Plethora	89	81	78		94	89/81
Round face	89	92	92		88	
Striae	60	64	50	51	56	72/51
Thin skin				84		
Ecchymoses	60	62	68	77	62	21/32
Hirsutism	73	74	84	64	81	
Acne	82	64		35	21	19/28
Female balding			51		13	
Dorsocervical fat pad		67	34		54	51/54
Edema	60		66	48	50	
Menstrual changes	86	35	72	69	84	
Decreased libido	86		100/33	55	100/47	
Headache	58					
Backache	83			39	43	
Psychiatric disturbance	67		40	48	62	26/34
Recurrent infection		14		25		
Poor wound healing/severe infection	42					
Abdominal pain					21	
Renal calculi					15	21/6
Osteoporosis/fracture	83		56	48	50	47/32
Abnormal glucose tolerance	94		84	39	50	43/45

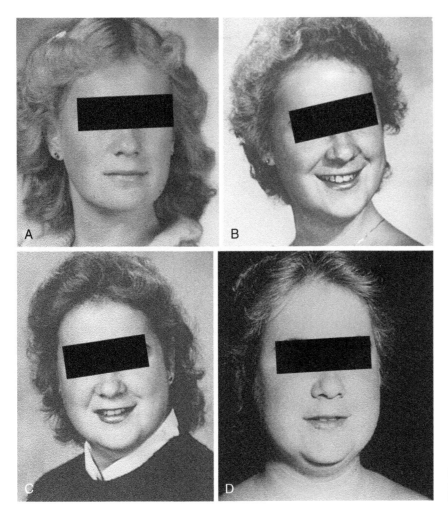

FIGURE 8-3. Progression of cushingoid features as shown in photographs taken at 1-year intervals (**A** through **D,** progress from earliest to latest).

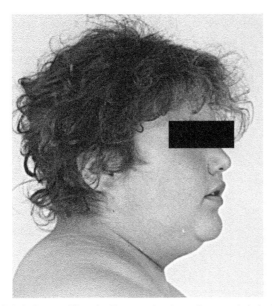

FIGURE 8-4. Fat may fill or, in this case, rise above the supraclavicular fossa of patients with Cushing's syndrome.

When extreme, the supraclavicular fat may present as a "collar" rising above the clavicles (Fig. 8-4); filling of the temporal fossae may prevent eyeglass frames from seating properly. Abnormal fat deposition may occur in the epidural space. Spinal epidural lipomatosis causing neurologic deficit, a rare complication of long-term exogenous steroid use, has been reported in a few patients with endogenous Cushing's syndrome.[76,77] Lumbosacral findings were seen in both men and women, whereas thoracic obstruction was restricted to men. The condition can be diagnosed by magnetic resonance imaging (MRI).[78]

Loss of subcutaneous tissue results in a variety of skin abnormalities that are unusual in the general population and suggest hypercortisolism. Ecchymoses, often after minimal trauma, and cutaneous atrophy, seen as a fine "cigarette paper" wrinkling or tenting over the dorsum of the hand and elbows, are typical. Cutaneous atrophy is influenced by gender and age, with men and the young having greater skin thickness. Two maxims follow: First, it is useful to compare the patient's skin with that of a near age- and gender-matched healthy person; and second, skin thickness is relatively preserved in cushingoid women with increased androgen production or preservation of ovarian function (Fig. 8-5).

Facial plethora, especially over the cheeks, also reflects loss of subcutaneous tissue. Although plethora is more obvious in pale Caucasian individuals, it may be present and should be sought in darker-skinned persons. Because erythema may be induced in normal persons by ultraviolet radiation from lamps or sunlight, wind, or medications (including topical drying agents, glucocorticoids, and antipsoriatic treatments), exposure to these agents should be ascertained before plethora is ascribed to endogenous hypercortisolism. A demarcation line, representing collar, sleeve, or shoulder straps, may differentiate exogenous from endogenous causes. Flushing caused by other conditions (e.g., mastocytosis, thyrotoxicosis, vasomotor instability or estrogen insufficiency in women, carcinoid syndrome) also should be considered.

Purple striae more than 1 cm in diameter are virtually pathognomonic for Cushing's syndrome (Fig. 8-6). Although the silvery, healed striae that are typical postpartum are not caused by active Cushing's syndrome, other pink, less pigmented, and thinner striae may be seen. Although most common over the abdomen, striae occur also over the hips, buttocks, thighs, breasts, and upper arms. The tear in the subcutaneous tissue may be best appreciated by indirect (side) lighting, which throws the striae into relief, or by light stroking of the skin. The violaceous hue is not dependent on ACTH-dependent pigmentation and may be seen in Cushing's syndrome in association with primary adrenal causes.

Proximal muscle weakness with preservation of distal strength is a hallmark of Cushing's syndrome. Histologically, this is reflected in profound atrophy of fibers without necrosis.[79-81] Weakness is best assessed historically by questions related to the use of these muscles: Is there difficulty or weakness in climbing

stairs, getting up from a chair or bed without using hand propulsion, or performing activities using the shoulders (e.g., brushing hair, reaching objects in overhead cabinets, changing ceiling light bulbs)? Formal muscle testing is useful. Assess the strength of the hip flexors by asking the patient to get out of a chair without using his or her arms. If this can be done, the patient is asked to rise from a squat. Inability to perform either task, in the absence of hip or lower extremity arthropathy or other myopathic processes, is suggestive of Cushing's syndrome. Leg extension while seated is a quantifiable test of proximal muscle strength. The number of seconds for which this position is held can be used to judge deterioration or progress after treatment.

Osteopenia is common. A history of fractures, typically of the feet, ribs, or vertebrae, may be one of the only signs of Cushing's syndrome, especially in men.[70,71,82] Avascular necrosis of bone, a rare complication of endogenous hypercortisolism, is more common in iatrogenic hypercortisolism.[83,84] It usually occurs in the hips, but we have also seen it in the knees.

Vellous hypertrichosis of the forehead or upper cheeks distinguishes Cushing's syndrome from the more common causes of hirsutism and may be appreciated only by careful visual and tactile inspection (Fig. 8-7). Excessive terminal hair on the face and body, and acne—pustular, reflecting increased androgens, or papular, reflecting pure glucocorticoid excess—may be present.[85] Severe hirsutism and virilization are uncommon and suggest adrenal carcinoma.

Most patients experience emotional and cognitive changes (including increased fatigue, irritability, crying, and restlessness, depressed mood, decreased libido, insomnia, anxiety, impaired memory, concentration, and verbal communication) and changes in appetite. These changes correlate with the degree of hypercortisolism.[86] Irritability, characterized as a decreased threshold for uncontrollable verbal outbursts, may be one of the earliest symptoms. Global impairment in neuropsychological function correlates well with the performance of seven serial subtractions and recall of the names of three cities—bedside tests that can be used by the clinician to quantify this symptom complex.[87]

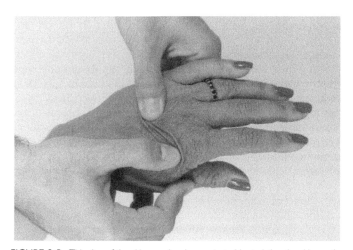

FIGURE 8-5. Thinning of the skin may be demonstrated by twisting the skin on the dorsum of the hand.

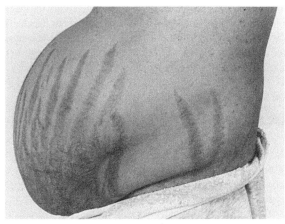

FIGURE 8-6. Typical abdominal striae of a patient with hypercortisolism. These are greater than 1 cm in width and are violaceous.

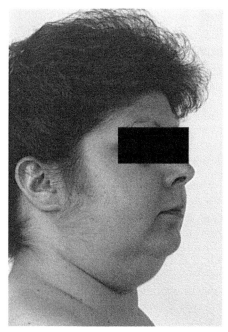

FIGURE 8-7. Vellous hirsutism, especially on the cheeks, is often present in women with Cushing's syndrome.

Approximately 80% of patients meet strict criteria for a major affective disorder—50% with unipolar depression and 30% with bipolar illness.[88,89] Although the quality of the depressed mood ranges from suicide attempts to sadness, the time course is characteristically intermittent, rarely lasting longer than 3 days, in contrast to the constant dysphoria reported by depressed patients without Cushing's syndrome.[86] A minority of patients are manic. The improvement in neuropsychiatric findings after treatment of Cushing's syndrome, coupled with similar features in patients treated with exogenous steroids, and the association of hypercortisolism with poor cognitive performance in depressed patients suggest glucocorticoid excess as a cause.[90,91]

Hypertension is present in approximately 80% of patients, and although hypertension is also common in the general population, its presence in patients younger than 40 years of age, especially if difficult to control, may alert one to the syndrome. Hypertension usually resolves with treatment of the Cushing's syndrome but may persist, possibly as the result of microvessel remodeling and/or underlying essential hypertension.[92]

The association of hypercortisolism and fungal infections of the skin, such as mucocutaneous candidiasis and pityriasis versicolor, with poor wound healing is a common feature. Wound dehiscence occurs less often but is an important consideration in patients who are treated surgically without medical pretreatment.

Patients with marked hypercortisolism (plasma cortisol >43 µg/dL [1200 nmol/L], UFC >2000 µg/day [5520 nmol/day]) are at risk for two potentially catastrophic events: perforation of the viscera and severe infection, either bacterial or opportunistic, such as *Pneumocystis carinii*, aspergillosis, nocardiosis, cryptococcosis, histoplasmosis, and *Candida*.[93-95] Classic clinical signs, such as loss of bowel sounds and fever, may be absent in peritonitis, and the typical leukocytosis of hypercortisolism may not increase further. Thus, the threshold of suspicion for opportunistic infection and a surgical abdomen must be low in patients with severe hypercortisolism.

Libido is decreased uniformly in men and to a lesser extent (44%) in women,[70] in whom *increased* libido may indicate excess androgen production by an adrenocortical carcinoma. Menstrual irregularities, amenorrhea, and infertility are common and may be the presenting complaints.[96] Impotence is common.

PATHOLOGY

The cardinal laboratory findings in endogenous Cushing's syndrome reflect overproduction of glucocorticoids. Although morning plasma cortisol values may be normal, an increased nighttime nadir blunts or obliterates the normal diurnal rhythm.[97-99] This increase in mean 24-hour plasma values is reflected in increased levels of free, or unbound, cortisol in urine[100] and saliva.[101] The capacity of corticosteroid-binding globulin for cortisol is exceeded at a serum cortisol value of approximately 20 µg/dL (≈600 nmol/L). At this point, the excretion of free cortisol increases dramatically in direct proportion to the increased unbound circulating cortisol values.

Hypokalemic metabolic alkalosis usually is observed when daily urine cortisol excretion is greater than 1500 µg (4100 nmol), and thus mainly in cases of ectopic ACTH syndrome.[102] This probably represents a mineralocorticoid action of cortisol at the renal tubule due to saturation of the enzyme 11β-hydroxysteroid dehydrogenase type 2, which inactivates cortisol to cortisone.[103] However, although a common feature of ectopic ACTH secretion, it also may occur in approximately 10% of patients with Cushing's disease. Serum albumin is inversely correlated with

cortisol levels, but this is of clinical significance only at very high cortisol levels, and it reverses with treatment for Cushing's syndrome.[104] Drastic reductions in serum albumin should alert the physician to the possibility of concomitant pathology such as infection. Circulating elevated glucocorticoids increase clotting factors, including factor VIII, fibrinogen, and von Willebrand factor, and reduce fibrinolytic activity, resulting in a fourfold risk of thrombotic events.[105-107] Lipid abnormalities show increases in very–low density lipoprotein, low-density lipoprotein, high-density lipoprotein, and consequently total cholesterol and triglycerides. These changes probably are caused by a direct cortisol effect of increased hepatic synthesis of very low–density lipoprotein without altered clearance.[108,109]

Cushing's syndrome is characterized by insulin resistance and hyperinsulinemia, with frank diabetes mellitus occurring in 30% to 40% of patients, and glucose intolerance in a further 20% to 30%.[110,111] A recent study has suggested that as many as 2% of overweight, poorly controlled patients with diabetes may have occult Cushing's syndrome if fully investigated.[112] In the absence of clinical suspicion, the yield is probably lower.[113]

Patients with Cushing's disease show accelerated cardiovascular disease, including increased carotid artery intima-media thickness and atherosclerotic plaques on Doppler ultrasonography.[114] This increased risk is maintained even as long as 5 years after cure of the hypercortisolemia is attained.[115] It also is likely that glucocorticoids have a direct pathogenic effect on the myocardium.

Hypercortisolism suppresses the thyroidal, gonadal, and growth hormone axes. Thyrotropin-releasing hormone and thyroid-stimulating hormone release is disturbed, and particularly the nocturnal surge of thyroid-stimulating hormone is lost, resulting in reduced total thyroxine, total triiodothyronine, and free triiodothyronine levels compared with controls.[116] Others have found no differences in free thyroxine or free triiodothyronine levels but have shown a significantly increased prevalence of autoimmune thyroid disease in patients treated for Cushing's syndrome.[117,118] In both men and women, low levels of luteinizing hormone, follicle-stimulating hormone, and gonadal steroids consistent with hypogonadotropic hypogonadism are common and correlate with the degree of hypercortisolemia.[119,120] In addition, the coexistence of polycystic ovarian syndrome in Cushing's syndrome may be more common than was previously thought.[96] Hypercortisolemia causes reduced growth hormone (GH) secretion during sleep and blunted GH response to stimulation tests.[121]

The prevalence of osteoporosis as assessed by dual-energy x-ray absorptiometry is approximately 50% in adult Cushing's syndrome.[122] It appears more common in adrenal Cushing's syndrome than in Cushing's disease, and this may relate to the protective effect of increased adrenal androgens in the latter.[123]

The accentuated visceral fat distribution characteristic of Cushing's syndrome can be marked when visualized by computed tomography (CT),[75] and the liver frequently (20%) is steatotic on imaging.[124]

CLINICAL SPECTRUM

The typical patient with Cushing's disease presents at midlife complaining of the gradual development of symptoms, although males tend to present at an earlier age and with more severe clinical consequences.[125] Hypokalemia, virilization, and extremely high cortisol excretion (>10-fold normal) are distinctly uncommon and should alert the physician to an alternative cause. The clinical presentation of pituitary corticotroph macroadenomas, apart from visual field changes caused by suprasellar expansion, is not unique. By contrast, invasive pituitary adenomas present at a slightly younger age; cavernous sinus and dural involvement may result in cranial neuropathies and facial neuralgia.[126,127] Only a few case reports attest to cerebrospinal or extracranial metastasis of ACTH-producing pituitary tumors.[128]

Nelson's syndrome is characterized by the development of hyperpigmentation and high ACTH levels after bilateral adrenalectomy for Cushing's disease. Tumor growth after adrenalectomy has been attributed to the relative resistance of these tumors to physiologic glucocorticoid suppression.

An abrupt onset of severe Cushing's syndrome should prompt an evaluation for ectopic ACTH secretion. This variant of ectopic ACTH secretion classically presents as a paraneoplastic syndrome in the context of a known malignancy. The features were captured in the initial formulation of Liddle[4]: weight loss, hypokalemia, weakness, and diabetes. However, Cushing's syndrome caused by less obvious ectopic ACTH secretion often presents in the more classic way with weight gain and striae and can be difficult to differentiate clinically from Cushing's disease. It is patients with this syndrome who most often present a diagnostic dilemma. They tend to have UFC excretion in the range seen in pituitary disease and may not show hypokalemia, hyperpigmentation, or the other findings typical of severe classical ectopic ACTH secretion.

Adrenocortical carcinomas are inefficient producers of cortisol and tend to evince Cushing's syndrome when the tumor is large (>6 cm), if at all. Abdominal pain or a palpable mass suggests this cause. Feminization in a man or virilization and increased libido in a woman, indicating involvement of the zona reticularis, suggest adrenal cancer or macronodular adrenal disease, which is rarer. The typical patient with PPNAD is a child or young adult who may present with an intermittent course or a family history of associated signs: Lentigines may be the initial clue to this cause. By contrast, patients with the massive macronodular variant of ACTH-independent Cushing's syndrome tend to be older than 40 years.

DIAGNOSIS AND DIFFERENTIAL DIAGNOSIS

The diagnosis of Cushing's syndrome rests on the demonstration of both physical and biochemical features of glucocorticoid excess. Thus, the diagnosis is unequivocal in a typical patient, with many of the physical features discussed earlier in the setting of UFC levels more than fourfold above normal.[129] However, many of the signs of hypercortisolism, such as obesity, hypertension, glucose intolerance, mood changes, menstrual irregularity, and hirsutism, are common in the general population. Similarly, mild glucocorticoid excess is seen in affective disorders,[130] strenuous exercise,[59] alcoholism and alcohol withdrawal states,[131] renal failure,[132] and hypoglycemia. Diagnostic strategies for distinguishing between these pseudo-Cushing's states and true Cushing's syndrome are discussed later.

Glucocorticoid resistance is characterized by an abnormal glucocorticoid receptor number or binding, which causes compensatory increases in ACTH and excessive glucocorticoid production to maintain normal glucocorticoid-mediated effects at the target tissues. The diagnosis should be considered in the hypokalemic, hypertensive, hypercortisolemic patient without typical glucocorticoid-mediated signs of Cushing's syndrome.[133]

ESTABLISHING THE DIAGNOSIS OF CUSHING'S SYNDROME

When a careful history and physical examination reveal clinical features that could be consistent with the syndrome, exogenous

Table 8-4. Evaluation of Suspected Cushing's Syndrome

History

Increased weight
Growth retardation in children
Weakness
Easy bruising
Stretch marks
Poor wound healing
Fractures
Change in libido
Impotence/irregular or no menses
Emotional, cognitive, mood changes (fatigue, irritability, anxiety, insomnia, depression, impaired memory and concentration)

Examination

Fat distribution (centripetal obesity; rounded face; dorsocervical, supraclavicular, temporal fat pads)
Hypertension
Proximal muscle weakness and atrophy
Thin skin and ecchymoses
Purple striae
Hirsutism
Acne
Facial plethora
Edema
Impaired serial 7s/recall of three cities

Laboratory Findings

Abnormal glucose tolerance/frank diabetes mellitus, hypokalemia

First-Line Screening Tests

Elevated 24-hour urinary free cortisol (three collections)
Lack of suppression to low-dose dexamethasone (LDDST)
Elevated late-night salivary cortisol

Additional Screening Tests (if required)

Cortisol circadian rhythm
Combined dexamethasone-CRH test
Insulin tolerance test
Loperamide test

CRH, Corticotropin-releasing hormone; *LDDST,* low-dose dexamethasone suppression test.

glucocorticoid use must be excluded (Table 8-4). In addition to inquiring about the use of oral, rectal, inhaled, injected, or topical glucocorticoid administration, it is important to evaluate the use of "tonics," herbs, and skin bleaching creams, which may contain glucocorticoids. In the absence of exogenous glucocorticoids, biochemical confirmation of the diagnosis of Cushing's syndrome is needed. It is important to remember that the urgency for diagnosis and treatment of Cushing's syndrome is greatest when the symptoms are severe. In milder cases, the patient may be best served by waiting until the diagnosis is clear. Periodic reevaluation with urine screening tests and documentation of body habitus with photographs may reveal progression.

Initial Screening Tests

Hypercortisolemia, demonstrated by loss of the normal circadian rhythm of cortisol secretion, and disturbed feedback of the hypothalamic-pituitary-adrenal (HPA) axis are the cardinal biochemical features of Cushing's syndrome. Tests to confirm the diagnosis are based on these principles. To screen for Cushing's syndrome, tests of high sensitivity should be used initially to avoid missing milder cases. All of these screening tests may miss identification of mild cases of hypercortisolemia, and multiple samples or a combination of tests may be needed. A recent guideline suggests that two abnormal first-line test results should be required for the diagnosis of Cushing's syndrome.[134]

Urinary Free Cortisol

Under normal conditions, 10% of plasma cortisol is free or unbound and physiologically active. Unbound cortisol is filtered by the kidney, with most being reabsorbed in the tubules and the remainder excreted unchanged. Thus, 24-hour UFC collection produces an integrated measure of serum cortisol, smoothing out variations in cortisol during the day. UFC determinations first became clinically available in 1968[135] and have superseded the historical measurement of urinary metabolites of glucocorticoids and androgens (17-hydroxycorticosteroids [17-OHCS], 17-ketosteroids, and 17-ketogenic steroids).

The major drawback of the test is the potential for overcollection or undercollection of the 24-hour specimen, and written instructions must be given to the patient. In addition, creatinine excretion in the collection can be measured to assess completeness and should equal approximately 1 g per 24 hours in a 70 kg patient (variations depend on muscle mass). This value should not vary by more than 10% between collections in the same individual.[136] It cannot be used to correct for incomplete collection, however, because rates of cortisol and creatinine excretion are not parallel over the 24-hour period. Various groups have tried to overcome the collection issue by proposing shorter collection periods, usually at night, when the loss of circadian rhythm differs most from normal controls,[137,138] but this approach has not been widely accepted. High-performance liquid chromatography and tandem mass spectrometry are now used to measure UFC, which overcomes the previous problem of cross-reactivity of some exogenous glucocorticoids and other structurally similar steroids with conventional radioimmunoassay.[139] Occasionally, substances such as carbamazepine, digoxin, and fenofibrate can coelute with cortisol during high-performance liquid chromatography, causing falsely elevated results.[140,141]

If the previous caveats have been satisfied, the UFC measurement can be interpreted. In large series, measurement of an elevated UFC above the normal range has a high sensitivity for the diagnosis of Cushing's syndrome (≈95% to 100%).[100,142] However, it should be noted that in the latter study, 11% of 146 patients with proven Cushing's syndrome had at least one of four UFC collections within the normal range, which confirms the need for multiple collections. Values greater than fourfold normal are rare except in Cushing's syndrome. Values between this and down to the upper limit of normal are compatible with Cushing's syndrome or pseudo-Cushing's states, so that one must exclude the latter diagnosis. In summary, UFC measurements have a high sensitivity if collected correctly, and several completely normal collections make the diagnosis of Cushing's syndrome very unlikely. However, when biochemical evidence of Cushing's syndrome is not obtained in the setting of clinical features that suggest the diagnosis, repeated measurement of urine cortisol may demonstrate cyclicity or progression. The specificity is somewhat lower, thus patients with marginally elevated levels require further investigation.[55]

Late-Night Salivary Cortisol

Salivary cortisol measurement offers an excellent reflection of the plasma free cortisol concentration in health and disease because it circumvents the changes in total cortisol due to corticosteroid-binding globulin alterations.[143,144] Salivary cortisol is stable for some days at room temperature, and the simple noninvasive collection procedure means that it can be performed conveniently at home and delivered via mail. Thus, it offers a number of attractive advantages over blood collection, particularly in

children. Analysis is performed using a modification of the plasma cortisol radioimmunoassay, enzyme-linked immunosorbent assay, or liquid chromatography/tandem mass spectrometry, and commercial kits are internationally available for this.[145] The diagnostic value cutoff varies between studies (0.13 µg/dL [3.6 nmol/L] to 0.55 µg/dL [15.2 nmol/L]) because of different assays and comparison groups studied.[146-153] Normal values also differ between adult and pediatric populations, and this may be affected by other comorbidities such as diabetes and hypertension.[154] However, from these studies, the sensitivity and specificity of this test appear to be relatively consistent at different centers, ranging from 92% to 100%, and from 93% to 100% respectively. It does not appear to make a difference if sampling is done at bedtime (≈23.00 hr) or at midnight, although it should be determined that the patient has a normal sleep pattern. Positive or negative results should be confirmed by repeat sampling. In summary, therefore, although late-night salivary cortisol appears to be a useful and convenient additional screening test for Cushing's syndrome, particularly in the outpatient setting, local normal ranges should be validated based on the assay used and the population studied.

Low-Dose Dexamethasone Suppression Tests

In normal individuals, administration of the potent synthetic glucocorticoid dexamethasone results in suppression of the HPA axis, whereas patients with Cushing's syndrome are resistant, at least partially, to this negative feedback. The original low-dose dexamethasone test (LDDST), as described by Liddle in 1960, measured urinary 17-OHCS before and during 48 hours of 0.5 mg dexamethasone every 6 hours, and an excretion of greater than 4 mg/day on the second day of dexamethasone treatment was considered to indicate Cushing's syndrome.[155] Dexamethasone does not cross-react with modern cortisol immunoassays, and the simpler measurement of a single plasma cortisol post dexamethasone has been validated in various series and gives the test a sensitivity of between 97% and 100% for the diagnosis of Cushing's syndrome.[156-159] The simpler overnight LDDST was proposed by Nugent and colleagues in 1965; this measured a 9:00 A.M. plasma cortisol after a single dose of 1 mg dexamethasone taken at midnight.[160] Since then, various other doses, between 0.5 and 2 mg, have been proposed for the overnight test, and various diagnostic cutoffs have been applied.[161-163] There appears to be no difference in discrimination between single doses of 1, 1.5, and 2 mg.[164] Higher doses significantly decrease the sensitivity of the test.[165] In a comprehensive review of the LDDST, both the original 2 day test and the 1 mg overnight protocol appear to have comparably high sensitivities (98% to 100%), provided a conservative postdexamethasone serum cortisol cutoff of 1.8 µg/dL (50 nmol/L) is applied. However, the specificity of the overnight test (88%) is lower compared with the 2 day test, particularly if serum cortisol is measured at both 24 and 48 hours (97% to 100%), with potential misclassification of patients with pseudo-Cushing's states and acute or chronic illnesses. Many endocrinologists use the overnight test because of its greater simplicity and lower cost, although some centers still advocate the 48-hour test because of its high sensitivity and specificity, and the information it can provide in the differential diagnosis of ACTH-dependent Cushing's syndrome (see later).[159] Written instructions should be given to the patient if the latter is to be performed on an outpatient basis. Salivary rather than serum cortisol has been evaluated as the end point for the LDDST. This offers potential benefit in terms of convenience but requires further evaluation.[149,166]

Table 8-5. Spurious Causes of Abnormal Dexamethasone Suppression Test Results

False Positive

Increased metabolism: barbiturates, phenytoin, carbamazepine, primidone, rifampicin, aminoglutethimide
Increased cortisol-binding globulin: pregnancy, oral estrogens, tamoxifen
Malabsorption
Pseudo-Cushing's states

False Negative

Reduced metabolism: high-dose benzodiazepines, indomethacin, liver disease

Factors such as variable absorption and increased or decreased dexamethasone metabolism due to other compounds (Table 8-5) can influence any oral dexamethasone test.[167] Therefore, a history of symptoms of malabsorption and a careful drug history should be taken before the test is used in a patient. Measurement of plasma dexamethasone is available in some centers and can be useful in patients of concern. One solution to overcome demonstrated malabsorption is to use one of the published intravenous dexamethasone suppression tests, recognizing that criteria for response have not been standardized.[168,169] Pregnancy and other causes of increased or decreased corticosteroid-binding globulin (such as exogenous estrogens and the nephrotic syndrome) also should be excluded because these are likely to result in false-positive and false-negative tests.[170]

Second-Line Tests

The Dexamethasone-CRH Test

In 1993, a combined dexamethasone-CRH (Dex-CRH) test was introduced for the difficult scenario of the differentiation of pseudo-Cushing's states from true Cushing's syndrome in patients with only mild hypercortisolemia and equivocal physical findings.[171] Dexamethasone 0.5 mg every 6 hours was given for eight doses, ending 2 hours before administration of ovine CRH (1 µg/kg intravenously) to 58 adults with UFC less than 360 µg/day (<1000 nmol/day). Subsequent evaluation proved that 39 had Cushing's syndrome and 19 had a pseudo-Cushing's state. The plasma cortisol value 15 minutes after CRH was less than 1.4 µg/dL (38 nmol/L) in all patients with pseudo-Cushing's states and was greater in all patients with Cushing's syndrome. A prospective follow-up study by the same group in 98 patients continued to show that the test had an impressive sensitivity and specificity of 99% and 96%, respectively.[172] However, results from a number of other smaller studies have challenged the diagnostic utility of this test over the standard LDDST.[173-175] Overall, in these reports, the specificity of the LDDST in 92 patients without Cushing's syndrome was 79%, versus 70% for the Dex-CRH. Test sensitivity in 59 patients with Cushing's syndrome was 96% for LDDST, versus 98% for the Dex-CRH group. It perhaps is not surprising that the diagnostic utility of the Dex-CRH has altered with additional studies at a greater number of centers. This might be the case for a number of reasons, including variable dexamethasone metabolism in individuals, different definitions of patients with pseudo-Cushing's, different protocols and assays, and variable diagnostic thresholds.[176] Of note, the original cortisol criteria performed poorly at these other centers, and this may have happened because many cortisol assays do not reliably measure levels <1.8 µg/dL (50 nmol/L). It does highlight that as a clinician one must be confident in the assay that is to be used for a particular test, and diagnostic criteria should be chosen that are appropriate for that assay. The Dex-CRH test remains a test that should be considered in patients with equivocal results.

Plasma Cortisol Circadian Rhythm

The normal diurnal rhythm of plasma cortisol is blunted or absent in Cushing's syndrome, with normal or increased morning values and an increase in the nighttime nadir. Although less convenient than salivary cortisol, midnight plasma cortisol levels may be useful to obtain in patients admitted for investigation. Samples are best obtained around midnight, through an indwelling line for awake patients or by direct venipuncture within 5 to 10 minutes of waking of sleeping patients. In one study, 20 normal sleeping subjects had values less than 1.8 µg/dL (50 nmol/L), whereas all 150 patients with Cushing's syndrome had midnight plasma cortisol concentrations greater than this.[158] The suggested cutoff criterion in awake patients is higher, 7.5 to 8.3 µg/dL (207 to 229 nmol/L) and less discriminatory (sensitivity 92% to 94%, and specificity 96% to 100%).[177,178] This difference probably reflects a different comparison group—patients suspected to have Cushing's but in whom it was excluded. Patients with severe medical illness, depression, and mania may have cortisol values one to three times normal.[130,164] Therefore, a sleeping midnight cortisol value less than 1.8 µg/dL (50 nmol/L) effectively excludes active Cushing's syndrome, but higher values, unless very high, are less specific for Cushing's syndrome.

Other Second-Line Tests

The insulin tolerance test has been used to distinguish Cushing's syndrome from pseudo-Cushing's states. Serum cortisol values increase in normal people after acute hypoglycemia, presumably because of central stimulation of CRH and vasopressin. The sustained hypercortisolism of Cushing's syndrome suppresses CRH and vasopressin secretion and so blunts this response. The CRH/vasopressin neurons are presumed to be overactive in pseudo-Cushing's states, particularly those that are depression associated, so a normal response to hypoglycemia (<40 mg/dL; <2.2 nmol/L) usually is maintained. Unfortunately, approximately 18% of patients with Cushing's syndrome, especially those with minimal hypercortisolism, show a normal response to adequate hypoglycemia.[164] Additionally, criteria for interpretation of results have not been established. If used, a dose of insulin of 0.3 U/kg should be used to overcome insulin resistance in these patients.[130]

The opiate agonist loperamide (16 mg orally) has been shown to inhibit CRH and thus ACTH and cortisol levels in most normal individuals, but not in patients with Cushing's syndrome. This test has not been used widely but has been evaluated in one center, revealing a sensitivity of 100% and a specificity of 95%.[179,180] However, it is unclear as to how well this test may exclude pseudo-Cushing's states because a significant proportion of patients with depression also fail to suppress the HPA axis.[181] It does not appear to be affected by drugs that affect the metabolism of dexamethasone and could potentially be useful in assessing patients on such treatment.[180]

DIFFERENTIAL DIAGNOSIS OF CUSHING'S SYNDROME

Once the diagnosis of Cushing's syndrome is made, its cause must be determined. The strategy for the differential diagnosis of Cushing's syndrome (Fig. 8-8) begins with measurement of

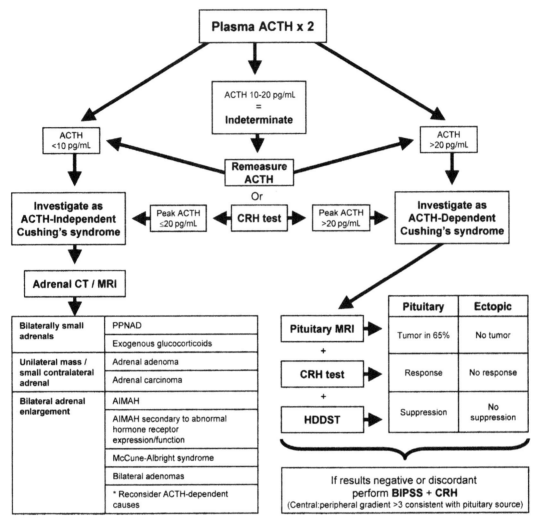

FIGURE 8-8. Suggested strategy for the differential diagnosis of Cushing's syndrome. *ACTH,* Adrenocorticotropic hormone; *AIMAH,* ACTH-independent bilateral macronodular adrenal hyperplasia; *BIPSS,* bilateral inferior petrosal sinus sampling; *CRH,* corticotropin-releasing hormone; *CT,* computed tomography; *HDDST,* high-dose dexamethasone suppression test; *MRI,* magnetic resonance imaging; *PPNAD,* primary pigmented nodular adrenal disease.

plasma ACTH to distinguish between ACTH-dependent and ACTH-independent causes. Modern two-site immunoradiometric assays are more sensitive than the older radioimmunoassays and therefore provide the best discrimination. Only assays that can reliably detect values to below 10 ng/L should be used, and appropriate collection and processing of the sample are essential, because ACTH is susceptible to degradation by peptidases; therefore the sample must be kept in an ice water bath and centrifuged, aliquoted, and frozen within a few hours to avoid a spuriously low result. Repeated measurements are usually necessary because patients with ACTH-dependent Cushing's disease have been shown to have on occasion ACTH levels less than 10 ng/L (2 pmol/L) on conventional radioimmunoassay,[182] but consistent ACTH measurements of less than 10 ng/L (2 pmol/L) at 9:00 AM with concomitant hypercortisolemia essentially confirm ACTH-independent Cushing's syndrome. When the basal ACTH level is indeterminate (10 to 20 g/L [2 to 4 pmol/L]), the response to CRH may be useful in this setting. Patients with primary adrenal disease rarely show maximal ACTH values greater than 20 ng/L (4 pmol/L), although patients with Cushing's disease usually exceed this value.

Investigating Adrenocorticotropic Hormone–Independent Cushing's Syndrome

Radiologic tests are the mainstay in differentiating between the various types of ACTH-independent Cushing's syndrome. High-resolution CT scanning of the adrenal glands has excellent diagnostic accuracy for masses greater than 1 cm and allows evaluation of the contralateral gland.[183] MRI may be useful for the differential diagnosis of adrenal masses; the T_2-weighted signal is progressively brighter in normal tissue, adenoma, carcinoma, and finally pheochromocytoma.[184] With this approach, adrenal tumors appear as a unilateral mass with an atrophic or less commonly a normal-size contralateral gland.[185] If the lesion is greater than 5 cm in diameter, it should be considered to be malignant until proven otherwise, and imaging characteristics should not be relied upon. Very rarely, bilateral adenomas may be present.[186] The adrenal glands in PPNAD appear normal or slightly lumpy from multiple small nodules but generally are not enlarged.[187] AIMAH is characterized by bilaterally huge (>5 cm) nodular or hyperplastic glands.[188] Exogenous administration of glucocorticoids results in adrenal atrophy; very small glands may provide a clue as to this entity.

The CT appearance of the adrenals in AIMAH may be similar to that of ACTH-dependent forms of Cushing's syndrome, in which adrenal enlargement is present in 70% of cases.[189] However, in our experience, the adrenal glands in Cushing's disease are smaller and usually are symmetrically enlarged with an occasional nodule, as opposed to large or huge glands with definite nodules in AIMAH. In addition, the two can usually be differentiated by the ACTH level, although some patients with the macronodular subset of Cushing's disease can develop a degree of adrenal autonomy that can cause biochemical confusion.[190] Occasionally, confusion also may arise with apparent unilateral adrenal lesions, when the biochemistry is consistent with an ACTH-dependent cause; we generally would rely on the biochemistry in this situation and would examine the contralateral gland to see whether it is hyperplastic.

Differentiating Between Adrenocorticotropic Hormone–Dependent Causes of Cushing's Syndrome

Although some patients with ectopic ACTH secretion, usually those with overt tumors, have extremely elevated values of plasma ACTH (>100 ng/L [>20 pmol/L]), complete overlap is seen between values in occult ectopic ACTH secretion and in Cushing's disease.[191] Therefore, ACTH values alone cannot differentiate reliably the ACTH-dependent forms of Cushing's syndrome.

The ACTH-dependent forms of Cushing's syndrome present the greatest diagnostic challenge. Cushing's disease accounts for by far the majority of cases of ACTH-dependent Cushing's syndrome—overall approximately 80% to 90% in most series. This percentage is gender dependent and is higher in women than in men,[192] although in prepubertal childhood, an anomalous 80% male preponderance is noted. Therefore, even before one starts further investigation, the pretest probability that the patient has Cushing's disease is very high, and any investigation must improve on this. The specificity of any test should be as close to 100% as possible for the diagnosis of Cushing's disease, to avoid inappropriate pituitary surgery in patients with ectopic ACTH production. A variety of functional tests of the HPA axis have been developed to take advantage of the differences in pathophysiology between ACTH-dependent causes of Cushing's syndrome. Some of these investigations have evolved, and others have fallen by the wayside.

Bilateral Inferior Petrosal Sinus Sampling

Bilateral inferior petrosal sinus sampling (BIPSS) is the best test for distinguishing ACTH-dependent forms of Cushing's syndrome, as long as the patient has active hypercortisolemia, which should be confirmed at the time of the procedure.[193,194] The test exploits the normal venous drainage of each half of the pituitary gland via the cavernous sinus into the corresponding petrosal sinus. Each petrosal sinus is catheterized separately via a femoral approach, and blood for measurement of ACTH is obtained simultaneously from each sinus and a peripheral vein at two timepoints before and at 3 to 5 minutes and possibly also 10 minutes after the administration of ovine or human CRH (Ferring) (1 µg/kg or 100 µg intravenously)[195] (Fig. 8-9). Where CRH is unavailable for whatever reason, recent data suggest that 10 µg desmopessin may be a suitable alternative.

ACTH concentrations are greater in the central samples in Cushing's disease and increase after CRH administration, reflecting ACTH secretion by the corticotroph adenoma. In contrast, ACTH values in the central and peripheral specimens are similar in ectopic ACTH secretion and do not increase after CRH. A ratio

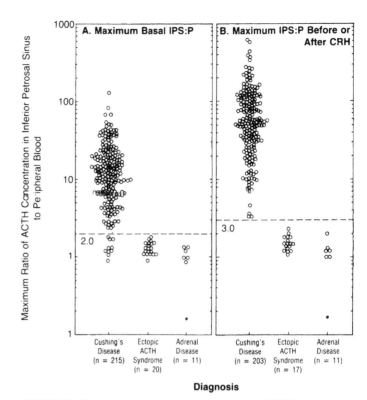

FIGURE 8-9. Maximal ratio of adrenocorticotropic hormone (ACTH) concentration in the inferior petrosal sinus to peripheral blood in patients with confirmed Cushing's disease, ectopic ACTH syndrome, or adrenal disease before corticotropin-releasing hormone (CRH) **(A)** or at any time before or after CRH administration **(B)**. A ratio of 3.0 had 100% sensitivity and specificity. (Data from Oldfield EH, Doppman JL, Nieman LK, et al: Petrosal sinus sampling with and without corticotropin-releasing hormone for the differential diagnosis of Cushing's syndrome. N Engl J Med 325:897–905, 1991.)

of central (i.e., petrosal) to peripheral ACTH values is calculated. In earlier series, pre-CRH ratios greater than 2 or post-CRH ratios greater than 3 were 100% specific for Cushing's disease,[196,197] but a small number of false positives have been reported in later series.[198,199] The sensitivity of the test is improved after CRH; however, false negatives still occur in about 6% of patients with Cushing's disease. False positives in ectopic ACTH are extremely rare.

It should be remembered that the technique is highly specialized, and allied with this are a number of important points. First, both petrosal sinuses must be cannulated adequately and catheter placement confirmed before and after sampling.[200] Second, the radiologist must confirm the venous anatomy because anomalous venous drainage can give false-negative results. Preliminary data have suggested that simultaneous measurement of prolactin can be used as an index of pituitary venous drainage, and prolactin should be measured when results indicate a noncentral source of ACTH.[201] Third, the procedure carries a small risk of complications. Transient ear discomfort or pain can occur, as can local groin hematomas. More serious transient and permanent neurologic sequelae, including brain stem infarction, have been reported, although these are rare (<1%), and most have been related to the particular type of catheter used[202,203]; if any early warning signs of such events are observed, the procedure should be halted immediately. Patients should be given heparin during sampling to prevent thrombotic events.[129] CRH itself generally is tolerated well, although patients may experience brief facial flushing and a metallic taste in the mouth. One case of CRH induced pituitary apoplexy in a patient with Cushing's disease has been reported.[204]

Another potential advantage of BIPSS involves lateralizing microadenomas within the pituitary using the inferior petrosal sinus ACTH gradient, with a basal or post-CRH intersinus ratio of at least 1.4 being the criterion used for lateralization in all large studies.[196,197,205,206] In these studies, the diagnostic accuracy of localization as assessed by operative outcome varied between 59% and 83%. This is improved if venous drainage is assessed to be symmetric.[207] Some discrepancy has been noted between studies as to whether CRH improves the predictive value of the test.[208] If a reversal of lateralization is seen pre- and post-CRH, the test cannot be relied upon.[209] Sampling of the internal jugular veins is a simpler procedure but is not as sensitive as BIPSS.[210] However, it may be a useful technique in less experienced centers, with the caveat that patients with negative results then are referred for BIPSS.[211] In our opinion, sampling from the cavernous sinus itself offers no great advantage.

High-Dose Dexamethasone Suppression Test

The original high-dose dexamethasone suppression test (HDDST) was described in the same paper as the 48-hour LDDST; 2 mg dexamethasone is used in place of 0.5 mg, with a 50% reduction in urinary 17-OHCS shown to differentiate 96% of patients with Cushing's disease rather than adrenal tumors.[155] The role of the HDDST in the differential diagnosis of ACTH-dependent Cushing's syndrome is based on the same premise, that is, that most pituitary corticotroph tumors retain some responsiveness (albeit reduced) to negative glucocorticoid feedback on ACTH secretion, whereas ectopic ACTH-secreting tumors, like adrenal tumors, typically do not. Measurement of UFC or plasma/serum cortisol has superseded that of urinary 17-OHCS, and an overnight test has been advocated, with a single dose of 8 mg dexamethasone given at 11:00 PM, and with the criterion of a 50% reduction in plasma cortisol levels on the morning after administration.[212] Despite evidence that only about 80% of patients with Cushing's disease will show suppression of plasma cortisol to less than 50% of the basal value, and large numbers of patients with ectopic Cushing's syndrome have false-positive results (≈30%),[60,213] the HDDST is still used widely. Some data suggest that that suppression to HDDST can be inferred by a greater than 30% suppression of serum cortisol to the 2 day LDDST (Fig. 8-10); therefore, in centers that use this form of the LDDST, the HDDST may not confer any extra information.[159] It should not be forgotten that patients are receiving large doses of glucocorticoids, in addition to their high endogenous cortisol production, and one should be alert for the precipitation of psychosis and/or worsening of glycemic control or other complications.

Corticotropin-Releasing Hormone Stimulation Test

The use of CRH stimulation for the differential diagnosis of ACTH-dependent Cushing's syndrome is based on two assumptions: (1) that corticotropinomas retain responsivity to CRH, whereas noncorticotroph tumors lack CRH receptors and cannot respond to the agent; and (2) that hypercortisolism has been sufficient to inhibit the normal corticotroph response. Indeed, most patients with Cushing's disease respond to CRH, either 1 μg/kg or 100 μg intravenous synthetic ovine or human sequence CRH, with increases in plasma ACTH or cortisol, and patients with ectopic ACTH secretion typically do not.[214-216] Human sequence CRH has qualitatively similar properties to ovine CRH, although it is shorter acting with a slightly smaller increase in plasma cortisol and ACTH in normal and obese

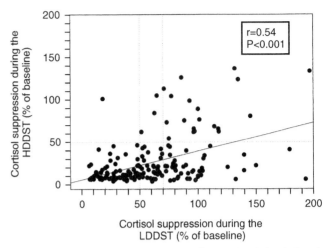

FIGURE 8-10. Correlation between the degree of suppression during the low-dose dexamethasone suppression test (LDDST) and during the high-dose dexamethasone suppression test (HDDST) in 185 patients with Cushing's disease. (Reproduced with permission from Isidori AM, Kaltsas GA, Mohammed S, et al: Discriminatory value of the low-dose dexamethasone suppression test in establishing the diagnosis and differential diagnosis of Cushing's syndrome. J Clin Endocrinol Metab 88:5299–5306, 2003. Copyright © 2003, The Endocrine Society.)

patients and in those with Cushing's disease[217]; this may be related to the more rapid clearance of the human sequence by endogenous CRH-binding protein.[218] Availability differs worldwide, with ovine CRH predominant in North America but human CRH elsewhere.

Because different centers have used differing protocols, including different types of CRH and different sampling timepoints, little consensus has been reached on a universal criterion for interpreting the test. However, where the test has been validated in experienced centers, the diagnostic utility appears similar. For instance, in the largest published series of the use of ovine CRH in ACTH-dependent Cushing's syndrome, an increase in ACTH of at least 35% from a mean basal (5 minutes and 1 minute) to a mean of 15 and 30 minutes after ovine CRH in 100 patients with Cushing's disease and in 16 patients with ectopic ACTH syndrome (Fig. 8-11) gave the test a sensitivity of 93% for diagnosing Cushing's disease and 100% specificity. The best cortisol criterion was an increase of at least 20% at a mean of 30 and 45 minutes, revealing a sensitivity of 91% and a specificity of 88%.[219] Similarly, in the largest series involving use of the human CRH test in 101 patients with Cushing's disease and in 14 with ectopic ACTH syndrome, the best criterion used to differentiate Cushing's disease from ectopic ACTH syndrome was an increase in cortisol of at least 14% from a mean basal (15 and 0 minutes) to a mean of 15 and 30 minutes, yielding a sensitivity of 85% and a specificity of 100% (Fig. 8-12). In contrast, the best ACTH response was a maximal increase of at least 105%, indicating 70% sensitivity and 100% specificity.[192] The CRH test is a useful discriminator between causes of ACTH-dependent Cushing's syndrome; however, which cutoff to use must be evaluated at individual centers, and caution should be exercised because undoubtedly there will be patients with ectopic ACTH syndrome who respond outside these cutoffs. However, an increase in cortisol outside the normal range can differentiate Cushing's disease from normality, albeit in only approximately 50% of cases, and, as noted previously, the measurement of plasma ACTH in the test can help to discriminate ACTH-dependent from ACTH-independent causes of Cushing's syn-

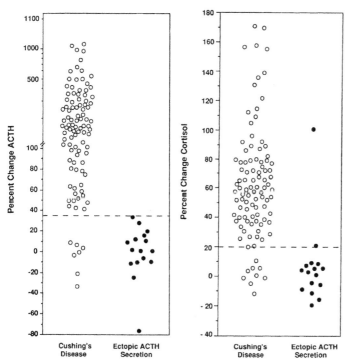

FIGURE 8-11. Response of adrenocorticotropic hormone (ACTH) and cortisol to ovine corticotropin-releasing hormone in patients with Cushing's disease and ectopic ACTH secretion. ACTH responses are expressed as the percentage of change in mean concentration 15 and 30 minutes after ovine corticotropin-releasing hormone from the mean basal value 1 and 5 minutes before the injection. The *dashed line* indicates a response of 35%, representing a diagnostic criterion with 100% specificity and 93% sensitivity. Cortisol responses are expressed as percentage of change in mean cortisol concentration 30 and 45 minutes after ovine corticotropin-releasing hormone from the mean basal value 1 and 5 minutes before the injection. The *dashed line* indicates a response of 20%, representing a diagnostic criterion with 88% specificity and 91% sensitivity. (Data from Nieman LK, Oldfield EH, Wesley R, et al: A simplified morning ovine corticotropin-releasing hormone stimulation test for the differential diagnosis of ACTH-dependent Cushing syndrome. J Clin Endocrinol Metab 77:1308–1312, 1993.)

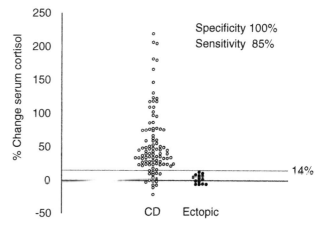

FIGURE 8-12. Percentage change in serum cortisol from a mean basal at 15 and 0 minutes to a mean value calculated from the levels at 15 and 30 minutes after the administration of human corticotropin-releasing hormone (100 mg intravenously) in 100 patients with Cushing's disease (CD) and 14 patients with ectopic adrenocorticotropic hormone syndrome. (Reproduced with permission from Newll-Price J, Morris DG, Drake WM, et al: Optimal response criteria for the human CRH test in the differential diagnosis of ACTH-dependent Cushing's syndrome. J Clin Endocrinol Metab 87:1640–1645, 2002.)

drome when basal levels of ACTH are equivocal. We therefore believe that this test plays a useful role in the investigation of patients with Cushing's syndrome.

Other Stimulation Tests

Vasopressin and desmopressin (a synthetic long-acting vasopressin analogue without V1-mediated pressor effects) are thought to stimulate ACTH release in Cushing's disease through the corticotroph-specific V3 (or V1b) receptor. Hexarelin (a growth hormone secretagogue) also stimulates ACTH release to a sevenfold greater extent than human CRH; although the mechanism has not been entirely elucidated, this probably occurs through stimulation of vasopressin release in normal subjects,[220] and through stimulation of aberrant growth hormone secretagogue receptors in patients with corticotroph tumors.[221] These peptides all have been used in a similar manner to CRH, to try to improve the differentiation of ACTH-dependent Cushing's syndrome, but they generally have proved inferior or of no advantage.[222-225] However, desmopressin may be useful in centers where CRH is unavailable. A combined desmopressin (10 μg) and human CRH (100 μg) test initially looked extremely promising.[226] However, a later study of this combined test in 26 patients with Cushing's disease and 5 patients with ectopic ACTH syndrome showed significant overlap in responses.[227] The disappointing discriminatory outcome of these stimulants is undoubtedly due to the

expression of both vasopressin and growth hormone secretagogue receptors by some ectopic ACTH-secreting tumors.[129,228]

Measurement of marker peptides, such as calcitonin, gastrin, 5-hydroxyindoleacetic acid, serotonin, and catecholamines or their metabolites, may help to identify a neuroendocrine tumor.

Combined Test Strategies

Because none of the noninvasive tests have 100% diagnostic accuracy, a number of investigators have evaluated the utility of combined test strategies. The CRH and the HDDST have been paired in this way, and combined, they have a diagnostic accuracy greater than that of either test alone, yielding 98% to 100% sensitivity and 88% to 100% specificity.[229-231] Similar high accuracy has been obtained by combining the results of the LDDST and the CRH test.[159]

Imaging of the Adrenocorticotropin Hormone Source

Pituitary MRI imaging before and after gadolinium enhancement should be performed in all patients with ACTH-dependent Cushing's syndrome via T_1-weighted spin echo and/or spoiled gradient recalled acquisition (SPGR) techniques. These will identify an adenoma in up to 80% of patients with Cushing's disease,[60,232,233] and in approximately 10% of normal individuals.[234] Most adenomas (95%) exhibit a hypointense signal with no postgadolinium enhancement, and the remaining 5% show an isointense signal post gadolinium enhancement.[235] CT imaging typically shows a hypodense lesion that fails to enhance post contrast but is less sensitive than MRI in detecting small (<5 mm) adenomas and is not recommended for this reason.[60,236]

Imaging is the most helpful way to identify the source of ectopic ACTH production. Given the likely sites of tumors, CT and/or MRI of the neck, chest, and abdomen should be obtained. The most common source is a bronchial carcinoid tumor, but small (<1 cm) lesions often can prove difficult to locate. Fine-cut high-resolution CT scanning with both supine and prone images can help differentiate between tumors and vascular shadows.[55] MRI can identify chest lesions that are not evident on CT scanning and that characteristically show a high signal on T_2-weighted and short-inversion time inversion recovery (STIR) images.[237]

Additionally, pheochromocytomas are bright on T_2-weighted MRI. CT-guided aspiration of masses for measurement of ACTH may provide useful functional information.[238]

Because most ectopic ACTH-secreting tumors are of neuroendocrine origin and therefore may express somatostatin receptor subtypes, radiolabeled somatostatin analogue (^{111}In-pentetreotide) scintigraphy may be useful to show functionality of identified tumors, and sporadic reports have indicated that it identifies lesions not apparent on conventional imaging.[239-241] However, in most patients, including a recent series of 35 patients with ectopic ACTH secretion, ^{111}In-pentetreotide scintigraphy was not able to detect tumors when the MRI or CT scan was negative, and significant numbers of false-positive scans resulted.[242] Thus, CT and MRI represent the best initial screening examinations, but scintigraphy may be a useful adjunctive imaging modality to help confirm abnormalities seen on CT or MRI. 18-Flurodeoxyglucose positron emission tomography (PET) generally does not offer any advantage over conventional CT or MRI unless the tumors are metabolically active,[243] which is not usually the case.[244] However, ^{67}Ga-octreotate PET scintigraphy may show advantages over ^{111}In-pentetreotide scintigraphy.[245]

Strategy for Diagnosis and Differential Diagnosis of Cushing's Syndrome

After an international workshop in 2002, a consensus statement was published for the diagnosis and differential diagnosis of Cushing's syndrome.[129] Most of its recommendations are still valid. We would advocate that three 24-hour UFC, late-night salivary cortisols and/or the LDDST should be used as first-line screening tests. (This approach also was advocated in a recent guidelines statement issued by the Endocrine Society.[134]) False-positive results will be common, and second-line tests should be used as necessary for confirmation. Once the diagnosis of Cushing's syndrome is unequivocal, ACTH levels, the CRH test, and a dexamethasone suppression test, together with appropriate imaging, are the most useful noninvasive investigations to determine the cause. Bilateral inferior petrosal sinus sampling is recommended in cases of ACTH-dependent Cushing's syndrome in which the clinical, biochemical, or radiologic results are discordant or equivocal, although others would recommend its use in almost all cases of ACTH-dependent Cushing's syndrome.

TREATMENT

Optimal treatment for Cushing's syndrome renders the patient eucortisolemic with minimal morbidity and mortality. With the advent of synthetic glucocorticoid therapy, adrenalectomy became the treatment of choice because it conferred rapid and, in most cases, permanent resolution of Cushing's syndrome.[246] Improvements in neurosurgical techniques and appreciation of the sources of ectopic ACTH secretion have changed the therapeutic approach to Cushing's syndrome, so that surgery now is directed toward resection of abnormal tissue, whether ACTH or cortisol producing. In patients with only mild hypercortisolemia and subclinical disease, the benefits of surgical treatment have not been proved.[247] The optimal surgical approach cannot be realized if the patient is unable to safely undergo surgery, or if the tumor is occult or metastatic. Other second-line therapies that are less specific and that may have greater morbidity must be chosen in these settings. In 2007, an international meeting of endocrinologists outlined a consensus statement on the treatment of ACTH-dependent Cushing's syndrome.[248]

SURGERY

Preoperative Evaluation and Treatment

Some centers use routine preoperative medical adrenal blockade to attain a period of eucortisolemia for 4 to 6 weeks before surgery. The aim is to allow reversal of some of the metabolic and catabolic effects of the hypercortisolemia that may inhibit wound healing and cause other complications in the perioperative period. The disadvantage of this strategy is that the normal corticotrope may be disinhibited by the time of surgery, so that expected hypocortisolism after successful tumor resection does not occur, and this index of remission is not reliable. This rationale is only empirical, and a randomized trial undertaken to see whether this approach improves outcome would be welcomed.[249]

Because Cushing's syndrome is a prothrombotic state, anticoagulant prophylaxis should be considered perioperatively.[250] The lipid abnormalities, hypertension, and diabetes common in Cushing's syndrome predispose these patients to atherosclerotic cardiac disease and should be treated by conventional approaches.

Transsphenoidal Resection of Corticotropinoma

Transsphenoidal resection is regarded as the treatment of choice in Cushing's disease.[248] The procedure usually is performed via a gingival approach, as originally devised by Kanavel and Halsted and later popularized by Cushing.[251] The development of the operating microscope led to the introduction of transsphenoidal resection of pituitary microadenomas by Hardy in 1968. Additional advances have been made over the past decade with the use of rigid endoscopes and more recently flexible endoscopes. The goal of surgery is a selective adenomectomy and thus preservation of as much normal pituitary tissue as possible; the procedure should be performed by a neurosurgeon who is experienced in transsphenoidal surgery. Most large series report immediate remission rates of approximately 70% to 90%,[252-259] with lower rates noted for macroadenomas.[254,260] These reports use variable remission criteria that include normal postoperative cortisol levels, normal UFC levels, and/or a normal response to an LDDST, associated with clinical resolution of the disease. Data are insufficient regarding whether endoscopic surgery offers any benefit.[261] However, a recent report suggests that resection achieved through a technique that enucleates microadenomas via their pseudocapsule may improve remission rates to 98%.[262]

Long-term recurrence rates are as high as 20% by 10 years after surgery. Thus, in reality, transsphenoidal surgery achieves long-term cure even in the best of hands in only approximately 60% to 80% of adult patients, and therefore is somewhat disappointing; the data emphasize the need for long-term endocrinologic follow-up of these patients.[263] Favorable indicators of long-term remission are patients older than 25 years, a microadenoma detected by MRI, lack of invasion of the dura or cavernous sinus, histologic confirmation of an ACTH-secreting tumor, low postoperative cortisol levels, and long-lasting adrenal insufficiency.[248] If a tumor cannot be identified at surgery, hemihypophysectomy on the side of the gland with an ACTH gradient on petrosal sinus sampling is usually the best way to proceed, and in some series, this yields better results than those attained by selective microadenomectomy.[256,264]

The mortality associated with transsphenoidal surgery is approximately 1% to 2%.[11,258] Transient diabetes insipidus is probably the most common complication, being reported in as many as 28% of patients.[264] Other perioperative complications, including cerebrospinal fluid leak, meningitis, and profuse bleeding, occur in less than 10% of patients. Permanent complications such as persistent diabetes insipidus and injury to the optic nerve or nerves of the cavernous sinus (causing ptosis or diplopia) occur much less frequently.[11,258] However, hypopituitarism, particularly growth hormone deficiency, is common (53% to 59%), with other anterior hormone deficits occurring in approximately 35% to 45% of patients.[264,265] Such complications are more common after resection of larger tumors or with the presence of larger amounts of normal pituitary tissue (or stalk), or after repeat surgery.

Postoperative Evaluation and Management

Patients typically receive supraphysiologic doses of glucocorticoids to cover transsphenoidal surgery at initial daily doses of as high as 400 mg hydrocortisone (4 mg dexamethasone), tapering off within 1 to 3 days. Morning (9:00 AM) serum cortisol measurements then are obtained for 3 days, starting 24 hours after the last glucocorticoid administration, during which time the patient should be observed for development of signs of adrenal insufficiency. This approach allows prompt classification of likely cure, normocortisolemia, or persistent hypercortisolism. Where close perioperative supervision is possible, such glucocorticoid "cover" may be omitted, permitting a very early postoperative assessment of cure. What defines apparent cure or remission after transsphenoidal surgery is still debated. Postoperative hypocortisolemia (<1.8 μg/dL [50 nmol/L] at 9:00 AM) is probably the best indicator of the likelihood of long-term remission. However, detectable cortisol levels of <5 μg/dL (140 nmol/L) are also compatible with sustained remission.[266,267] Higher postoperative cortisol levels are more likely to be associated with failed surgery; however, cortisol levels sometimes may decline gradually over 4 to 6 weeks, reflecting gradual infarction of remnant tumor or some degree of adrenal semiautonomy. Persistent cortisol levels >5 μg/dL (140 nmol/L) 6 weeks after surgery require further investigation.

Dynamic tests have been used to predict long-term remission. The cortisol and ACTH response to CRH in the early postoperative period may provide a useful index of the risk for recurrence of Cushing's disease, the rationale being that responsiveness may indicate residual tumor.[60,268] A study of postoperative responses to CRH in 221 patients suggested that a cortisol response greater than 5 μg/dL (138 nmol/L) at 60 minutes had a positive predictive value of 42% and a negative predictive value of 94% for recurrence of disease.[269] Because patients with partial recovery of the axis would be expected to have a normal response, regardless of the risk for recurrence, the CRH test cannot be interpreted and should not be used in this setting. Some evidence suggests that persistence of the ACTH response to desmopressin postoperatively probably is linked to a higher rate of relapse.[270,271]

Patients who are hypocortisolemic should be started on glucocorticoid replacement, and 15 to 30 mg hydrocortisone (12 to 15 mg/m²) in two to three divided doses is the preferred choice. The first dose (usually half to two thirds of the total dose) should be taken before getting out of bed, and the last dose should be taken no later than 6:00 PM, because later administration of glucocorticoids may result in disordered sleep. In this situation, the lowest possible dose of hydrocortisone should be used to avoid long-term suppression of the HPA axis. All patients receiving long-term glucocorticoid replacement therapy should be instructed that they are "dependent" on taking glucocorticoids as prescribed, and that failure to take or absorb the medication will lead to adrenal crisis and possibly death. They should be prescribed a 100 mg hydrocortisone (or other high-dose

glucocorticoid) intramuscular injection pack for emergency use. They also should obtain a medical information bracelet or necklace that identifies this requirement (Medic Alert Foundation). Education should stress the effects of glucocorticoid withdrawal[272]; the need for compliance with the daily dose of glucocorticoid; the need to double the oral dose for nausea, diarrhea, and fever; and the need for parenteral administration and medical evaluation during emesis, trauma, or severe medical stress.

The patient should be told to expect desquamation of the skin and flu-like symptoms (malaise, joint aching, anorexia, and nausea) during the postoperative months, and that these are signs that indicate remission; some of these symptoms have been related to high levels of circulating interleukin-6.[273] Most patients tolerate these symptoms of glucocorticoid withdrawal much better if they are forewarned and alerted to their positive nature. Physicians should not increase the glucocorticoid dose in the absence of intercurrent illness based on these symptoms alone but should seek signs of adrenal insufficiency, such as vomiting, electrolyte abnormalities, and postural hypotension.[274] The affective and cognitive changes associated with Cushing's syndrome are particularly slow to resolve and may not normalize. Evidence of persisting physical and emotional dysfunction has been found, even after prolonged duration of cure.[275] Postoperatively, assessment for deficiencies of other pituitary hormones should be sought, and the appropriate replacement regimen initiated as necessary.

Diuresis is common after transsphenoidal surgery and may result from intraoperative or glucocorticoid-induced fluid overload or may be due to diabetes insipidus. For these reasons, assessment of paired serum and urine osmolality and the serum sodium concentration is essential. It is advisable to withhold specific therapy unless the serum osmolality is greater than 295 mOsm/kg, the serum sodium is greater than 145 mmol/L, and the urine output is greater than 200 mL/hr, with an inappropriately low urine osmolality. Desmopressin (DDAVP, Ferring) 1 μg given subcutaneously, will provide adequate vasopressin replacement for 12 hours or longer. Hyponatremia may occur in as many as 20% of patients within 10 days of surgery. This may be due to injudicious fluid replacement or inappropriate antidiuretic hormone secretion, as is frequently seen after extensive gland exploration, and fluid intake should be restricted.[276] A small minority of patients proceed to (apparently) permanent diabetes insipidus, requiring long-term treatment with a vasopressin analogue. A dose and schedule of administration should be chosen to provide unbroken sleep but allowing a period of "breakthrough" urination each day. This goal is often achieved when 10 to 20 μg desmopressin is given intranasally (or an equivalent oral dose) in the evening.

Some glucocorticoid-induced abnormalities, including hypokalemia, hypertension, and glucose intolerance, may be normalized during the postoperative period, so that preoperative treatments for these need to reassessed. Some evidence indicates that deficits in bone mass may be partially reversed after treatment of hypercortisolemia.[277,278] Bisphosphonate treatment may induce a more rapid improvement in bone mineral density[279] and should be considered (along with calcium and vitamin D supplements) in patients with osteoporosis.

Persistent hypercortisolemia after transsphenoidal exploration should prompt reevaluation of the diagnosis of Cushing's disease, especially if previous diagnostic test results were indeterminate or conflicting, or if no tumor was found on pathologic examination. Petrosal sinus sampling after transsphenoidal surgery can confirm a pituitary source of ACTH, but the rate of correct lateralization decreases, probably because of alterations in venous anatomy caused by the previous surgery; therefore, the procedure cannot be used routinely to direct a second operative search or decision for hemihypophysectomy.

Treatment options for patients with persistent Cushing's disease include repeat surgery, radiation therapy, and adrenalectomy. If immediate surgical remission is not achieved at the first exploration, early repeat transsphenoidal surgery may be worthwhile in a significant proportion of patients, at the expense of increased likelihood of hypopituitarism.[280,281] The likelihood of remission after repeat surgery is greatest when some or all of the following outcome parameters are present: The diagnosis is correct, as evidenced by previous curative surgery with pathologic confirmation of an ACTH-staining adenoma; the initial exposure or resection was incomplete; or residual tumor is seen on MRI scan without evidence of cavernous sinus invasion. Repeat sellar exploration is less likely to be helpful in patients with empty sella syndrome or very little pituitary tissue on MRI scans. Patients with cavernous sinus or dural invasion identified at the initial procedure are not candidates for repeat surgery to treat hypercortisolism and should receive radiation therapy.

Recovery of the HPA axis can be monitored by measurement of 9:00 AM serum cortisol after omission of hydrocortisone replacement. Because recovery after transsphenoidal surgery rarely occurs before 3 to 6 months and is common at 1 year, initial testing at 6 to 9 months is cost-effective.[282] If the cortisol is undetectable on 2 consecutive days, then recovery of the axis has not occurred, and glucocorticoid replacement can be restarted. If the cortisol is measurable, adequate reserve of the HPA axis can be assessed with the insulin tolerance test,[283] with a peak cortisol value of >18 μg/dL (500 nmol/L), indicating adequate reserve on modern assays.[284] Many centers use the cortisol response to 250 μg synthetic (1-24) ACTH as an alternative means of assessing HPA reserve,[285,286] but some controversy regarding its reliability in this situation has been ongoing.[287,288] If it is used instead of the insulin tolerance test, a 30 minute cortisol of 22 μg/dL (600 nmol/L) is probably more reliable than the traditional cutoff of 18 μg/dL (500 nmol).[284] Glucocorticoid replacement can be discontinued abruptly if the cortisol response is shown to be normal.

Where recovery of the HPA axis is only partial on dynamic testing, but the 9:00 AM cortisol levels are above the lower limit of the normal range (7 μg/dL [200 nmol/L]), it is reasonable to reduce the hydrocortisone unless symptoms of adrenal insufficiency occur. Patients must continue to be aware of the continuing need for additional glucocorticoids at times of stress or illness and should be given a supply of oral hydrocortisone and an intramuscular injection pack. For patients with detectable but low 9:00 AM cortisol levels, the hydrocortisone replacement dose should be adjusted down if weight loss has occurred, and a slightly lower dose may be given. Some centers assess adequate replacement of thrice daily hydrocortisone dosing by measuring serum cortisol at various points throughout the day, ensuring that levels are always sufficient (>1.8 μg/dL; 50 nmol/L) before each dose; this may mean that peak levels after each dose appear to be unphysiologic, but there is a tradeoff between mirroring a normal physiologic rhythm as far as possible and the inconvenience of multiple dosing.

Two late but unrelated conundrums may arise: the questions of recurrence and permanent lack of recovery of the axis. Patients who articulate that Cushing's syndrome has returned are often correct, even before physical and biochemical evidence is unequivocal. Assessment is warranted in a patient with these complaints or with recurrent physical signs characteristic of the hypercortisolemic phase. If this is to be done on an outpatient basis, UFC can be measured initially on dexamethasone 0.5 mg/ day, if not yet weaned from glucocorticoids. Measurement of late-night salivary cortisol after omission of the afternoon dose of hydrocortisone also may be useful. However, ideally, assessment of a cortisol circadian rhythm can be done on an inpatient basis after the hydrocortisone has been stopped completely. If the UFC result is increased, evaluation of hypercortisolism should proceed. If recurrent Cushing's disease is diagnosed, the therapeutic options are the same as for persistent disease. It should be remembered when investigating recurrence that longstanding ACTH stimulation by a pituitary adenoma causing macronodular adrenal hyperplasia subsequently may involve autonomous cortisol production.[289]

If the UFC result is subnormal or low, the patient should be questioned about the actual dose of glucocorticoid that has been taken. Often, patients take additional hydrocortisone, either because they discover that this decreases the symptoms of glucocorticoid withdrawal, or because they have increased the dose "for stress," often without following strict guidelines. These patients have a suppressed axis and a very slow regression of cushingoid features because of exogenous hypercortisolism. They require education and support along with reduction in the daily dose of hydrocortisone to recommended levels. The patient who has a subnormal cortisol response to ACTH 2 years after transsphenoidal surgery (in the absence of overreplacement) may proceed to life-long ACTH deficiency.

Adrenalectomy

Resection of the affected adrenal gland(s) is the treatment of choice only for non–ACTH-dependent hypercortisolism of adrenal origin, or when a specific surgical approach to ACTH-dependent causes is not feasible. In adrenal adenomas, the cure rate is 100% when performed by experienced adrenal surgeons.[290] Surgery is the mainstay of treatment for adrenal cancer; more aggressive surgical approaches probably account for the increase in life span reported in this disease.[85,291] This approach may require multiple operations to resect primary lesions, local recurrences, and hepatic, thoracic, and, occasionally, intracranial metastases. Adjuvant medical treatment with mitotane and other chemotherapeutic agents is discussed later.

The mortality and morbidity of traditional open adrenalectomy via an anterior or posterior incision range from 1% to 20% in various series, probably reflecting differences in the severity of Cushing's syndrome and the presence of associated conditions, such as cardiovascular disease.[184,246] Apart from resection of suspected carcinoma, these approaches have been supplanted by laparoscopic resection, which has low mortality and morbidity when done by an experienced surgeon.[292] Glands as large as 7.5 cm may be removed through this approach.[293] Serum cortisol levels become undetectable after successful adrenalectomy. Early failure to achieve hypocortisolism usually is related to incomplete resection of the gland(s). Recurrence, especially in the ACTH-dependent forms of Cushing's syndrome, may be related to regrowth of adrenal cells in the surgical bed, or to growth of adrenal rest tissue.

Bilateral adrenalectomy as a second line of treatment for Cushing's disease has the advantage of providing rapid resolution of hypercortisolism and has no risk of hypopituitarism, in contrast to radiation therapy. Adrenalectomy may be chosen over radiation therapy by young patients who desire fertility, who have concerns about radiation-induced hypopituitarism and loss of reproductive function. Its disadvantages include perioperative morbidity and mortality and the life-long requirement of glucocorticoid and mineralocorticoid replacement therapy. In addition, patients with Cushing's disease have a risk for developing Nelson's syndrome, which may occur more frequently if adrenalectomy is performed at a younger age, and if a pituitary adenoma is confirmed at previous pituitary surgery.[259,294] Regular pituitary MRI and monitoring of ACTH levels are mandatory in these patients.[295] Prophylactic pituitary radiotherapy appears to reduce the risk for developing Nelson's syndrome from 50% to 25%,[296] but no consensus has been reached on this topic.

In the postoperative period after bilateral adrenalectomy, the hydrocortisone dose is maintained at approximately twice the replacement dose, and saline 0.9% is given intravenously until the patient can take oral medications. This provides sodium and sufficient mineralocorticoid activity until fludrocortisone 100 μg/day can be given by mouth. Serum cortisol measurement done to confirm adequacy of resection is assessed while the patient receives dexamethasone 0.5 mg/day and fludrocortisone. The patient then is switched back to hydrocortisone and fludrocortisone and must be advised regarding adrenal insufficiency, as previously discussed. The dose of fludrocortisone is adjusted according to the patient's blood pressure, exposure to heat, and salt intake; the usual dose is 100 μg/day but ranges from 50 to 400 μg. A normal plasma renin activity measurement provides evidence of adequate mineralocorticoid replacement and can be used to gauge therapy.

After unilateral adrenalectomy, the components of the HPA axis gradually recover after surgical cure of Cushing's syndrome. The time to recovery may be as short as 3 months and as long as 2 years.[268,282] The duration of recovery may be shorter in patients with mild hypercortisolism and in those with recurrence, and longer after resection of an adrenal adenoma.

Surgery for Ectopic Adrenocorticotropic Hormone Syndrome

If an ectopic ACTH-secreting tumor is localized and amenable to surgical excision, such as in a lobectomy for a bronchial carcinoid tumor, the chance for cure of Cushing's syndrome is high. However, if significant metastatic disease is present, surgery is unlikely to be of benefit. If the source of ACTH cannot be localized, or if metastatic disease precludes surgery, alternative treatment for hypercortisolism must be chosen. For the patient with occult disease, medical therapy allows interval tumor surveillance with the goal of eventual tumor resection. Because some tumors remain occult for as long as 20 years, this may not prove practical for all patients, and adrenalectomy is appropriate when the patient cannot tolerate the cost, medical side effects, or psychological effects of long-term medical therapy and monitoring. Long-term medical therapy also may be the treatment of choice for the patient with widely disseminated disease who is not a good surgical candidate for adrenalectomy. Bilateral adrenalectomy is the treatment of choice for any patient requiring rapid correction of hypercortisolism or when hypercortisolism cannot be controlled with medical therapy, when previously effective medical therapy must be discontinued because of significant medical side effects or intolerance, or when a severely hypercortisolemic patient is unable to take oral medications or etomidate.

RADIOTHERAPY

Pituitary

The role of radiation therapy to the pituitary gland in Cushing's disease is usually adjunctive in those who have failed transsphenoidal surgery, but it is also a good primary option for patients who cannot undergo surgery, and for those having a bilateral adrenalectomy for whom the risk for Nelson's syndrome is deemed great.

Conventional Radiotherapy

Conventional pituitary radiotherapy is delivered at a total dose of 4500 to 5000 cGy (rad) in 25 fractional doses over 35 days through a three-field (opposed lateral fields and vertex field) technique. Nowadays, this usually is based on stereotactic conformal field planning to optimize the tumor dose and to minimize radiation to other areas. This approach ensures that the daily dose to neural tissue does not exceed 180 cGy and avoids the complications of optic neuritis and cortical necrosis associated with larger total and fractional doses.[297] The latent onset of action of radiotherapy means that adjunctive medical therapy usually is instituted before or at the time of treatment. The therapeutic response is assessed at least with annual monitoring, with weaning of medical treatment if possible. When conventional radiotherapy is used as primary treatment for Cushing's disease, remission is achieved in only 40% to 60% of adult patients.[259,298-300] The response is even worse if a lower dose of radiation (2000 cGy) is used.[301] More usually, conventional radiotherapy is used in the setting of failure to cure after transsphenoidal surgery. In this regard, it performs rather better, with reported remission rates as high as 83%.[299,302] After conventional radiotherapy is given, remission usually starts by 9 months after treatment, and most patients are in remission within 2 years, although this can take much longer.[303]

Hypopituitarism is the most common side effect of pituitary radiotherapy, with growth hormone deficiency occurring in 36% to 68% of treated adults.[265,302] Gonadotropin and thyroid-stimulating hormone deficiency is seen less commonly. The risk for optic neuropathy is low and probably is less than 1% as long as low-dose fractions are used[304] (200 cGy). Similarly, the occurrence of brain necrosis is exceedingly rare.[305] The issue of secondary tumors remains contentious; although meningiomas and gliomas have been reported after pituitary radiotherapy, it is not clear whether the incidence is significantly greater than the background risk for developing such tumors in patients who already have one intracranial tumor and have undergone careful surveilllance.[304]

Stereotactic Radiosurgery

In stereotactic radiosurgery, concentrated beams of high doses of radiation are aimed precisely at the mapped discrete lesion, delivering very high doses to the tumor and relatively low doses to normal surrounding tissue. A number of techniques can be used to do this: using narrow beams from multiple gamma cobalt sources (gamma knife), using heavy charged particles (proton or helium beams), or using a single beam from a linear accelerator that is arced around the target (X-knife, SMART, Linac). The advent of high-resolution MRI for mapping has facilitated this therapy. Usually, only a single therapy dose is required, and this is biologically more effective than delivery of the same dose in fractions.[306] This technique also may be used to deliver radiation to the entire pituitary gland when a specific target is not known after surgery or MRI examination.

Probably the technique most widely used currently for Cushing's syndrome is the gamma knife. As adjunctive therapy after failed transsphenoidal surgery, it probably is no better than conventional radiotherapy.[307] Radiosurgery of the pituitary gland using proton beams has similar efficacy.[308] Linear accelerator radiotherapy for Cushing's disease is less well described, but success has been reported in small numbers of patients.[309]

As with conventional radiotherapy, the main side effect is hypopituitarism, and although the perceived risk of damage to adjacent structures such as the optic chiasm is less, additional studies and longer follow-up are needed. Some centers use it mainly for salvage of difficult recurrent tumors, for example, in the cavernous sinus or in Nelson's syndrome, whereas others have suggested it as an alternative to conventional radiotherapy in adenomas smaller than 30 mm with a minimal distance from the optic chiasm of 2 to 3 mm.[305]

Interstitial Radiotherapy

Two centers have used interstitial irradiation (yttrium-90 or gold-198 implants) as primary therapy for Cushing's disease.[310,311] Remission rates in these cohorts were high (75% to 77%), although some required a second implant. The principal side effect was hypopituitarism.

Other Tumors

No significant evidence suggests that radiotherapy improves overall survival in adrenocortical carcinoma, although sporadic reports indicate that it may be helpful adjuvant treatment to radical surgery in selected cases.[312,313] Local radiotherapy after surgical resection of an ectopic ACTH-secreting source may be beneficial, particularly in nonmetastatic thoracic carcinoid tumors.[314,315]

MEDICAL TREATMENT

Medical treatments for hypercortisolism have two broad mechanisms of action. One class of agents reduces cortisol levels through inhibition of adrenal steroidogenesis or cortisol action by antagonism at the level of the receptor. These compounds may be used in treatment for all forms of Cushing's syndrome. The second class of compounds, which generally are much less effective, modulate ACTH release and are restricted to treatment for ACTH-dependent Cushing's syndrome, principally Cushing's disease. The major current role of medical therapy is in the preoperative control of hypercortisolemia or as adjunctive treatment after failed surgical management, while other therapies such as radiotherapy are instituted.

Agents Inhibiting Steroidogenesis

The oral inhibitors of adrenal steroidogenesis are the most commonly used medical agents as treatment for Cushing's syndrome; of these, metyrapone, ketoconazole, and mitotane are the most effective. Aminoglutethimide[316] is no longer available, and trilostane[317] is now rarely used. Etomidate is the only available agent that can be given parenterally. We usually would recommend partial inhibition of cortisol production (adjusted adrenal blockade) with frequent monitoring to identify a dosing regimen that maintains eucortisolism while avoiding adrenal insufficiency or excess. However, in some patients, particularly those with variable cortisol production, it can be difficult to achieve this. In these cases, full adrenal blockade with glucocorticoid replacement to avoid symptoms of adrenal insufficiency (a block-and-replace regimen) may be advocated. In all forms of treatment, patients and their physicians must be alert to the signs and symptoms of adrenal insufficiency.

Metyrapone

Metyrapone acts primarily to inhibit the enzyme 11β-hydroxylase,[318] and the subsequent elevation of 11-deoxycortisol can be monitored in the serum of patients treated with metyrapone. The decrease in cortisol is rapid, with trough levels at 2 hours post dose, and a test dose of 750 mg with hourly cortisol estimation for 4 hours can be used to predict response: A rapid and sustained decrease in cortisol to less than approximately 7 µg/dL (≈200 nmol/L), as is often seen with ectopic ACTH and adrenal tumors, suggests that a smaller dose of metyrapone may be appropriate, whereas a decrease 10 to 12 µg/dL (≈300 nmol/L), as often is seen in Cushing's disease, would indicate a higher dose requirement.[319] Therapy is started at 0.75 to 1.5 g/day in three to four divided doses daily. The usual requirement is approximately 2 g/day, although higher doses (as high as 6 g/day) may be needed in ectopic ACTH syndrome.[319] Metyrapone is useful in treating patients with Cushing's syndrome from adrenal tumors, ectopic ACTH syndrome, and Cushing's disease.[319,320] The principal side effects are hirsutism and acne (as predicted by the increase in adrenal androgens), dizziness, and gastrointestinal upset. The androgenic effects can be particularly problematic and may preclude its use in some younger female patients. Hypokalemia, edema, and hypertension due to increased mineralocorticoids are infrequent[319] but may require cessation of therapy. Our experience would suggest that the only major problems are associated with the increase in adrenal androgens; careful monitoring of treatment to avoid hypoadrenalism and education of the patient are required. Although not previously reported, we have seen a case of hemolysis in a patient with glucose-6-phosphate dehydrogenase deficiency.

Ketoconazole and Other Antifungals

Ketoconazole is an imidazole derivative whose primary indication is as an oral antifungal agent. However, reports of gynecomastia in some ketoconazole-treated patients led to the realization that it is an inhibitor of cytochrome P-450 enzymes, including side-chain cleavage, C17,20-lyase, 11β-hydroxylase, and 17β-hydroxylase.[321,322] It has also been reported to have a direct effect on ectopic ACTH secretion from a thymic carcinoid tumor.[323] Treatment for Cushing's syndrome usually is started at a dose of 200 mg twice daily, and its onset of action is slower than metyrapone. It has been used successfully to lower cortisol levels in patients with Cushing's syndrome of various causes, including adrenal carcinoma, ectopic ACTH syndrome, and invasive ACTH-producing pituitary carcinoma, with doses between 200 and 1200 mg/day required in as many as four divided daily doses.[324-326] The principal side effect of ketoconazole is hepatotoxicity. Reversible elevation of hepatic serum transaminases occurs in approximately 5% to 10% of patients and need not result in discontinuation of the agent if levels remain below twofold to threefold the upper normal range. The incidence of serious hepatic injury is approximately 1 in 15,000 patients,[327] and it can be fatal or may require liver transplantation.[328,329] The hepatotoxicity appears to be idiosyncratic and has been reported within 7 days of the start of treatment in a patient with Cushing's syndrome.[330] Other adverse reactions of ketoconazole include skin rashes and gastrointestinal upset, but these occur in less than 15%,[324] and one must always be wary of causing adrenal insufficiency.[331] Because of its C17-20 lyase inhibition and consequent antiandrogenic properties, ketoconazole is particularly useful in female patients in whom hirsutism, which may be worsened with metyrapone, is an issue. Conversely, gynecomastia and reduced libido in male patients may be unacceptable and may require alternative agents. One further advantage of ketoconazole is its inhibition of cholesterol synthesis, particularly low-density lipoprotein cholesterol.[332] We have found it to be particularly useful in combination with low doses of metyrapone. Fluconazole, another oral imidazole, is less well studied but has been shown to be effective, and it provides the advantage of less toxicity.[333]

Mitotane

Mitotane, or o,p'DDD, is derived from the family of insecticides that includes DDT. It inhibits adrenal steroidogenesis catalyzed by cholesterol desmolase,[334] 11- and 18-hydroxylase, and 3β-hydroxysteroid dehydrogenase.[335] It also has marked direct cytotoxic effects on the zona fasciculata and the zona reticulosa, which led to its original use in high doses (5 to 20 g/day) as treatment for inoperable adrenocortical carcinoma.[336,337] In this condition, it now is used more commonly as adjunctive treatment to surgery, and it does appear to prolong recurrence-free survival with lower doses of between 1 and 5 g/day.[338,339] At such doses, it may take a longer time to reach therapeutic levels, and where possible, monitoring of serum levels should be undertaken. It is suggested that target levels should be between 15 and 20 µg/mL.[338,340] Combined treatment of mitotane with standard chemotherapeutic agents such as cisplatin, etoposide, and doxorubicin has been used in a number of small studies in advanced adrenal carcinoma with variable benefit.[341-343]

In Cushing's disease, mitotane alone in high doses (4 to 12 g/day) can achieve remission in as many as 83% of patients, but more commonly, it is used in lower doses (0.5 to 4 g/day), sometimes in combination with radiation therapy, with clinical and biochemical remission achieved in approximately 80%.[344,345] At these doses, the onset of effect can take approximately 6 to 8 weeks, and additional adjunctive medical treatment may be needed in this interim. Similarly, the agent has a long half-life (18 to 159 days), due in part to its lipophilic properties, and it effects can last for weeks or months after discontinuation of therapy. Mitotane, alone or in combination with metyrapone or aminoglutethimide, also has proved useful as treatment for hypercortisolism associated with ectopic secretion of ACTH.[346]

The utility of mitotane is limited by its gastrointestinal and neurologic toxicity. Nausea and anorexia are common at doses as high as 4 g/day and are ubiquitous at more than 4 g/day.[347] These side effects may be avoided by beginning at a dose of 0.5 to 1.0 g/day and increasing gradually, by 0.5 to 1.0 g every 1 to 4 weeks. Doses should be taken with meals or at bedtime with food. If significant adverse effects do occur, the drug should be discontinued for 3 to 5 days and then restarted at a lower dose.[345] At higher doses and serum levels >20 µg/mL,[340] neurologic side effects are common and include drowsiness, gait disturbances, dizziness or vertigo, confusion, and problems with language. Other adverse effects at any dose include fatigue (perhaps due to decreased cortisol levels), gynecomastia, skin rash, hypouricemia, elevated liver enzymes, and abnormal platelet function.[337,348,349] The hypercholesterolemia, which is common even at low doses, can be reversed with 3-hydroxy-3-methylglutaryl coenzyme A reductase inhibitors such as simvastatin.[350] Mitotane is relatively contraindicated in women desiring fertility within 2 to 5 years. It may induce spontaneous abortion and may act as a teratogen, effects that may persist for a number of years after discontinuation because of deposition in fat.[351] Mitotane increases hormone-binding proteins (cortisol-binding globulin, sex hormone binding–globulin[352] and thyroxine-binding globulin). Therefore, total serum cortisol cannot be relied on to monitor therapy, and UFC should be used instead. The value of serum-free or salivary cortisol remains to be determined. In addition, mitotane increases the metabolic clearance of exogenously administered steroids,[353] and replacement doses of glucocorticoid must be increased by approximately one third.

Etomidate

Etomidate, an imidazole-derived anesthetic agent, was reported in 1983 to have adrenolytic effects.[354] Compared with the other imidazole derivative ketoconazole, etomidate more potently inhibits adrenocortical 11β-hydroxylase and shows similar inhibition of 17-hydroxylase, but it has less of an effect on C17-20 lyase.[355] At higher concentrations, it also appears to have an effect on cholesterol side-chain cleavage.[356] Short-term etomidate infusions can reduce severe hypercortisolemia in patients with Cushing's syndrome of various causes at doses as high as 0.3 mg/kg/hr,[357] although such high doses tend to be sedative.[358] Most case reports of long-term therapy therefore have described the use of lower nonhypnotic total doses of between 1.2 and 8.3 mg/hr to good effect.[359-362] It may be more difficult to normalize cortisol levels in patients with Cushing's disease, which probably reflects increased ACTH drive from the pituitary, as opposed to relatively fixed production from an ectopic source.[360] Clearly, etomidate is an effective adrenolytic agent that acts rapidly but is limited in its use by the fact that it has to be given parenterally. However, in this situation, it may be lifesaving. It is important to recognize that the etomidate preparations available in Europe are dissolved in an alcohol-based vehicle, although the currently available preparation in the United States uses propylene glycol, which may have potential side effects such as nephrotoxicity.[361]

Glucocorticoid Receptor Antagonists

Mifepristone (RU 486), the antiprogesterone antagonist that is marketed as an abortifacient, is also a competitive antagonist of glucocorticoid and androgen receptors. The major drawback is the lack of biochemical markers to monitor overtreatment, and its long half-life and minimal agonist activity leave the patient open to hypoadrenalism.[363]

Agents That Modulate ACTH Release

A number of agents, including the serotonin antagonists cyproheptadine[364] and ritanserin,[365] the dopamine agonists bromocriptine[366] and cabergoline,[367] and sodium valproate,[368] have been examined in Cushing's disease. The precise mechanism of action of many of these agents is incompletely understood, although most seem to reduce ACTH secretion through an effect on the hypothalamic-pituitary axis. Their efficacy in Cushing's disease seems to be variable between individual patients; therefore, we do not recommend their routine use. However, more recent data on the use of cabergoline suggest that this drug may be more effective than was previously realized.

Somatostatin Analogues

Long-acting somatostatin analogues such as octreotide and lanreotide are used widely in the therapy of various neuroendocrine tumors, and somatostatin receptors have been demonstrated on corticotroph adenomas, in addition to ectopic sources of ACTH.[369] Octreotide appears to inhibit ACTH release in Nelson's syndrome but rarely in patients with Cushing's disease, and this has been postulated to be due to somatostatin receptor down-regulation from the circulating hypercortisolemia.[370] In ectopic ACTH-secreting tumors, octreotide has produced a prolonged (>3 months) reduction in ACTH and hypercortisolemia in approximately 70% of published cases, but this high rate of response may be due to selective reporting. Preoperative assessment with pentetreotide scintigraphy may help predict which tumors might respond to treatment. Octreotide treatment produces a temporary response in GIP-dependent Cushing's syndrome but is unhelpful in other causes of ACTH-independent Cushing's syndrome.[371] So far, little experience has been reported with use of the sustained-release preparations in treating Cushing's syndrome. Much interest surrounds somatostatin analogues with a broader spectrum of activity for somatostatin receptor subtypes. Such an agent, pasireotide (SOM230; Novartis, Basel, Switzerland), has been shown in vitro to reduce human corticotroph proliferation and ACTH secretion,[372] and early results in vivo are encouraging.[373,374] Additional clinical studies are ongoing.

Thiazolidinediones

Rosiglitazone, a peroxisome-proliferator–activated receptor-γ (PPAR-γ) agonist, at suprapharmacologic doses has been shown in vitro and in animal models to suppress ACTH secretion and corticotroph tumor size.[375] However, a number of clinical trials of the thiazolidinediones rosiglitazone and pioglitazone in patients with Cushing's syndrome have generally been disappointing, with only short-term benefit seen in occasional patients even at high doses.[376-380]

Potential Novel Medical Agents

In the rare cases of Cushing's syndrome due to AIMAH and aberrant receptor expression, specific receptor antagonists have proved useful at least in the short term, and further investigation is needed.[381] Retinoic acid has been found to inhibit ACTH secretion and cell proliferation both in vitro in ACTH-producing tumor cell lines and cultured human corticotroph adenomas and in vivo in nude mice[382] and dogs.[383] The potential antisecretory and antiproliferative activities of this agent in Cushing's syndrome have not to our knowledge been investigated further in man.

Special Clinical Scenarios

CYCLIC CUSHING'S SYNDROME

Most patients with Cushing's syndrome demonstrate consistently elevated glucocorticoid values. A small subset show significant variability in glucocorticoid secretion, alternating normal and elevated values on a regular or irregular basis.[384] The few cases of spontaneous remission of Cushing's syndrome, including Cushing's first patient, may fit into this category.[2,385,386] The clinical course of patients with this type of intermittent, cyclic, or periodic Cushing's syndrome may be invariant, usually with mild signs and cushingoid symptoms, or it may parallel the biochemical abnormalities, with exacerbation of cushingoid features that parallel increased glucocorticoid production. The etiologic distribution is altered; in a recent review, Cushing's disease, ectopic ACTH secretion, and primary adrenal causes accounted for 54%, 26%, and 11%, respectively, of 65 cases, with the remainder being unclassified.[387]

Patients with periodic Cushing's syndrome often show conflicting or "inappropriate" responses to standard diagnostic tests, particularly dexamethasone suppression.[388] Discrepant urine tests have been reported in these patients, with elevated 17-OHCS and normal UFC excretion.[389] If studied during a quiescent period, patients with nonpituitary disease may be misclassified as having Cushing's disease, and those with "normal" responses to the LDDST may be incorrectly diagnosed as not having Cushing's syndrome.[390] Dynamic testing should be performed only during a sustained period of hypercortisolism, as documented by failure to suppress on an LDDST, concurrent increased evening salivary or plasma cortisol, and/or elevated UFC excretion.

IATROGENIC AND FACTITIOUS CUSHING'S SYNDROME

Appropriate therapeutic but supraphysiologic doses of glucocorticoids given for a medical condition cause most cases of iatrogenic Cushing's syndrome, which usually is an expected, unavoidable adverse effect of therapy. Exogenous hypercortisolism may result also when a prescribed dose of glucocorticoid is increased inappropriately by the patient. Although most common with oral agents, Cushing's syndrome may result from glucocorticoids administered to the nasal or rectal mucosa, the tracheobronchial tree, or the skin.[391-393] The use of all prescription drugs, over-the-counter medications, and herbal remedies,[394] including nasal drops, inhalants, and topical agents, should be assessed in all cushingoid patients. Agents not given for their glucocorticoid activity, such as fludrocortisone acetate and megestrol,[395] also may produce cushingoid features on occasion. Agents sold for cosmetic skin whitening may contain potent glucocorticoids.

Factitious Cushing's syndrome, which may be a form of Münchausen's syndrome, is rare. The typical suppression of plasma ACTH and dehydroepiandrosterone sulfate may lead to a mistaken diagnosis of primary adrenal disease.[396] Plasma and urine cortisol values vary, depending on the route, schedule, and type of glucocorticoid ingested. For example, intravenous injection of hydrocortisone may suppress ACTH values and increase UFC levels without increasing single random plasma cortisol values.[397] If basal urine or plasma cortisol values are low, it may be useful to screen the urine for synthetic glucocorticoids.[396]

Treatment for exogenous Cushing's syndrome consists of discontinuing glucocorticoid ingestion. If this is possible, a weaning schedule should be followed until a replacement dose of hydrocortisone is reached, at which point the patient may be weaned very gradually, as discussed earlier for postoperative treatment. If the degree of suppression of the axis cannot be estimated from the medication and dose received, the response to synthetic ACTH can be used as a rough gauge of adrenal suppression.

For the patient in whom glucocorticoids cannot be discontinued, a change in dose or schedule may ameliorate symptoms of Cushing's syndrome. Patients who require supraphysiologic glucocorticoid therapy should undergo measurement of bone density and should be counseled to maintain adequate calcium and vitamin D intake, to exercise, and to receive bisphosphonate therapy when appropriate.

CHRONIC RENAL FAILURE

Cushing's syndrome has been described in the setting of chronic renal failure only rarely.[398-400] Plasma levels of cortisol are normal in chronic renal failure when assessed with radioimmunoassays using an organic extraction procedure,[401,402] but they may be increased if other assay techniques are used.[403] ACTH levels are increased.[401] Glomerular filtration rates of less than 30 mL/min result in decreased cortisol excretion, and the UFC may be normal despite excessive cortisol production.[404] ACTH and cortisol responses to ovine CRH may be suppressed in patients with renal failure, except for those undergoing continuous ambulatory peritoneal dialysis.[402] The metabolism of dexamethasone is normal in chronic renal failure, but oral absorption can be altered in some patients, which may necessitate measurement of plasma dexamethasone levels.[405,406] The reduced degree of suppression of cortisol by dexamethasone suggests a prolonged half-life of cortisol. Normal suppression of the overnight 1 mg LDDST is uncommon, and the 2 day LDDST does better in this regard.[132,406,407] The cortisol response to insulin-induced hypoglycemia is normal or absent.[405,408]

PEDIATRIC CUSHING'S SYNDROME

The most common presentation of Cushing's syndrome in children is growth retardation, often with a decrease in height percentile over time as the weight percentile increases.[409-411] However, hypercortisolemic patients with virilizing adrenal tumors may show growth acceleration; thus, the absence of growth failure does not exclude the diagnosis of Cushing's syndrome.[412] Other virilizing signs such as acne and hirsutism are seen in approximately 50% of patients regardless of etiology.[411] Hypertension and striae are seen in approximately 50% of cases.[413] Muscle weakness may be less common in the pediatric patient.[70] This may reflect the effect of exercise rather than age because older patients who follow an exercise program tend to maintain strength. In addition to the spectrum of psychiatric and cognitive changes seen in adults, which can affect school performance, children may show "compulsive diligence" and actually do well academically.[409] Depression is less common in children than in adults. Headache and fatigue are common.[411] Cushing's disease accounts for between 75% and 80% of Cushing's syndrome in children and adolescents, but before the age of 10 years, ACTH-independent causes of Cushing's syndrome are more common. Cushing's disease has a male predominance in prepubertal children. Two primary adrenal causes of Cushing's syndrome, McCune-Albright syndrome and PPNAD, are typically diseases of childhood or young adulthood. Signs of virilization or feminization in the very young (<4 years) suggest adrenal carcinoma. Ectopic secretion of ACTH occurs rarely in the pediatric population and usually is due to bronchial or thymic carcinoids.[414]

As mentioned previously, late-night salivary cortisol measurement has particular logistical benefits in children. Study of its utility in the pediatric population has been limited, and diagnostic criteria are not clear, although a cutoff of 0.27 μg/dL (7.5 nmol/L) has been suggested if the sample is taken around midnight.[166,415] Serum cortisol measurement in inpatients has high sensitivity.[416] In children, UFC should be corrected for body surface area (×1.72 m²).[417] The standard 2 day LDDST adult protocol can be used in children weighing 40 kg or more, otherwise the dexamethasone dose is adjusted to 30 μg/kg/day.[410] As in adults, there is good correlation between cortisol suppression on the LDDST and on the HDDST for the differential diagnosis; thus the latter is not necessary.[418] Although it can be argued that the ectopic ACTH syndrome is so rare in children that the CRH test or BIPSS is not necessary, they do add reassurance in those with a negative pituitary MRI, which is the case in more than 50% of cases. In addition, BIPSS has arguably better

accuracy in lateralization of the pituitary tumor.[414] MRI is at least as useful as CT in the evaluation of adrenal causes.[419]

Adrenalectomy, either unilateral or bilateral depending on the cause, is first-line therapy in ACTH-independent Cushing's syndrome. Transsphenoidal surgery is the treatment of choice in children with Cushing's disease, with similar rates of remission as in adults in expert hands.[420] Conventional radiotherapy used in the setting of failure to cure after transsphenoidal surgery performs even better than in adults with reported remission rates as high as 100%, with cure occurring within 12 months.[421] Following pituitary surgery, plus or minus radiotherapy, the incidence of growth hormone deficiency is high, but prompt diagnosis and treatment with human growth hormone ensure acceptable growth acceleration and catch-up growth, although an abnormal body composition often persists.[422] Similarly, normalization of reduced bone mineral density can be achieved.[423]

CUSHING'S SYNDROME IN PREGNANCY

The pregnant woman with possible Cushing's syndrome presents a diagnostic challenge to the physician because of the physical and biochemical changes that are common to both conditions, including weight gain, fatigue, striae, hypertension, and glucose intolerance. The investigative screening process has to be based on the recognition of physiologic changes in pregnancy.[424] Total serum cortisol levels increase in pregnancy, beginning in the first trimester and peaking at 6 months, with a decrease only after delivery, probably reflecting increased induction of hepatic corticosteroid-binding globulin production by estrogen. UFC excretion is normal in the first trimester and then rises up to threefold by term. Thus, only UFC values greater than threefold normal are diagnostic in the last two trimesters. Suppression to dexamethasone is blunted, but not because of reduced bioavailability of dexamethasone. The cortisol diurnal rhythm is maintained in pregnancy but with a higher nadir, and appropriate diagnostic cutoffs in pregnancy have yet to be established. Adrenal adenomas are frequently the cause of Cushing's syndrome in pregnancy (40% to 50%), but it is interesting to note that ACTH levels may not be suppressed in these patients, possibly because of placental CRH stimulation of the pituitary corticotrophs or placental ACTH secretion. The HDDST may be useful in distinguishing these patients from those with Cushing's disease. The CRH test also has been used to identify patients with Cushing's disease, and no evidence of harm has been found in animal studies and in the small number of pregnant patients studied with this drug. MRI without gadolinium enhancement is considered safe in the third trimester, and its use in combination with the noninvasive tests discussed earlier should resolve most diagnostic issues. IPSS with appropriate additional radiation protection for the fetus should be reserved only for cases in which diagnostic uncertainty remains.

Although Cushing's syndrome is rare in pregnancy, maternal hypercortisolism is associated with poor outcomes, both maternal and fetal. Definitive surgical treatment for adrenal or pituitary disease is recommended to achieve eucortisolemia, although adverse fetal outcomes may persist: The second trimester is probably the safest time for operative intervention. Medical treatment carries potential risk for the fetus and should be considered only as second-line therapy when the benefit outweighs the risk, and then generally only as an interim measure. Metyrapone is probably the adrenolytic agent of choice, although its association with preeclampsia has been reported. Ketoconazole has been utilized successfully in a small number of patients but is teratogenic in animals and therefore should be used cautiously.[425]

Prognosis

The life expectancy of patients with nonmalignant causes of Cushing's syndrome, at one time a uniformly fatal illness, has improved dramatically with effective surgical and medical treatments and the availability of antibiotics, antihypertensive agents, and glucocorticoids. In a 1952 review, Plotz[67] reported a 5-year mortality rate of 50% in actively hypercortisolemic patients, with 46% caused by bacterial infection and 40% due to cardiovascular complications (cardiac failure, cardiovascular accidents, or renal insufficiency). In 1961, the mortality rate was similar, but the causes had changed: Two thirds were due to postoperative adrenal crisis before cortisone was available or from metastatic adrenal cancer. Cardiovascular events related to hypertension (stroke, heart failure, renal failure, myocardial infarction) led to death in approximately 20%; infectious causes decreased to approximately 15%.[71] Ten years later, in 1971, 30% of patients with benign causes of Cushing's syndrome died within 5 years of diagnosis, most from cardiovascular disease or infection, despite decreased postoperative mortality.[426] In 1979, a lower incidence of death (6%) was noted within 2 to 10 years of radiation therapy, mitotane, or combination treatment for Cushing's disease.[344] This improvement may reflect earlier detection of Cushing's syndrome and better treatment for hypercortisolism and associated medical complications, such as hypertension, or lower perioperative mortality. Three studies on long-term survival in Cushing's disease treated in the era of transsphenoidal surgery have been completed; two were epidemiologic studies from northern Spain[66] and Denmark,[61] and the third was a series from a single neurosurgical center where all patients had undergone transsphenoidal surgery.[255] Investigators report varying standardized mortality ratios of 3.8, 1.7, and 0.98, respectively. The discrepancy in findings between the three series is not completely clear, but it is difficult to make absolute comparisons, not least because the study by Swearingen and colleagues undoubtedly is affected by selection bias. However, the latter two studies do appear to show that after curative transsphenoidal surgery, long-term mortality is not significantly different from that in the general population. This is perhaps surprising because increased cardiovascular risk markers and evidence of atherosclerotic disease persist when measured 5 years after remission of Cushing's disease.[115] The outcome of pediatric Cushing's disease is excellent if treated at centers with appropriate experience.[413]

Cushing's syndrome results in significant impairment in quality of life. Unfortunately, in the long term, this is improved only partially with treatment.[275,427]

The prognosis of the potentially malignant causes of Cushing's syndrome is variable. Adrenal cancer, as reviewed earlier, has an extremely poor prognosis. Tumors that produce ACTH ectopically tend to have a poor prognosis, particularly when compared with tumors from the same tissue that do not produce ACTH. Small cell lung cancer, islet cell tumors, and thymic carcinoids[428] illustrate this phenomenon. As many as 82% of patients with small cell lung cancer and Cushing's syndrome die within 2 weeks from the start of chemotherapy.[63] Among the causes of ectopic ACTH syndrome, pheochromocytoma and bronchial carcinoid appear to offer the best prognosis after tumor resection, but this is not universal.

REFERENCES

1. Cushing HW: The pituitary body and its disorders, Philadelphia, 1912, JB Lippincott.
2. Cushing HW: The basophil adenomas of the pituitary body and their clinical manifestations (pituitary basophilism), Bulletin of the Johns Hopkins Hospital 1:137–195, 1932.
3. Walters W, Wilder RM, Kepler EJ: The suprarenal cortical syndrome with presentation of ten cases, Ann Surg 100:670–688, 1934.
4. Liddle GW, Nicholson WE, Island DP, et al: Clinical and laboratory studies of ectopic humoral syndromes, Recent Prog Horm Res 25:283–314, 1969.
5. Howlett TA, Rees LH, Besser GM: Cushing's syndrome, Clin Endocrinol Metab 14:911–945, 1985.
6. Bertagna X: New causes of Cushing's syndrome, N Engl J Med 327:1024–1025, 1992.
7. Reznik Y, Allali-Zerah V, Chayvialle JA, et al: Food-dependent Cushing's syndrome mediated by aberrant adrenal sensitivity to gastric inhibitory polypeptide, N Engl J Med 327:981–986, 1992.
8. Lacroix A, Bolte E, Tremblay J, et al: Gastric inhibitory polypeptide-dependent cortisol hypersecretion—a new cause of Cushing's syndrome, N Engl J Med 327:974–980, 1992.
9. Malchoff CD, Orth DN, Abboud C, et al: Ectopic ACTH syndrome caused by a bronchial carcinoid tumor responsive to dexamethasone, metyrapone, and corticotropin-releasing factor, Am J Med 84:760–764, 1988.
10. Biller BM, Alexander JM, Zervas NT, et al: Clonal origins of adrenocorticotropin-secreting pituitary tissue in Cushing's disease, J Clin Endocrinol Metab 75:1303–1309, 1992.
11. Mampalam TJ, Tyrrell JB, Wilson CB: Transsphenoidal microsurgery for Cushing disease. A report of 216 cases, Ann Intern Med 109:487–493, 1988.
12. Young WF Jr, Scheithauer BW, Gharib H, et al: Cushing's syndrome due to primary multinodular corticotrope hyperplasia, Mayo Clin Proc 63:256–262, 1988.
13. Asa SL, Ezzat S: The cytogenesis and pathogenesis of pituitary adenomas, Endocr Rev 19:798–827, 1998.
14. Dahia PL, Grossman AB: The molecular pathogenesis of corticotroph tumors, Endocr Rev 20:136–155, 1999.
15. Rabbitt EH, Ayuk J, Boelaert K, et al: Abnormal expression of 11 beta-hydroxysteroid dehydrogenase type 2 in human pituitary adenomas: a prereceptor determinant of pituitary cell proliferation, Oncogene 22:1663–1667, 2003.
16. Korbonits M, Chahal HS, Kaltsas G, et al: Expression of phosphorylated p27(Kip1) protein and Jun activation domain-binding protein 1 in human pituitary tumors, J Clin Endocrinol Metab 87:2635–2643, 2002.
17. Trautmann K, Thakker RV, Ellison DW, et al: Chromosomal aberrations in sporadic pituitary tumors, Int J Cancer 91:809–814, 2001.
18. Metzger AK, Mohapatra G, Minn YA, et al: Multiple genetic aberrations including evidence of chromosome 11q13 rearrangement detected in pituitary adenomas by comparative genomic hybridization, J Neurosurg 90:306–314, 1999.
19. Fan X, Paetau A, Aalto Y, et al: Gain of chromosome 3 and loss of 13q are frequent alterations in pituitary adenomas, Cancer Genet Cytogenet 128:97–103, 2001.
20. Evans CO, Young AN, Brown MR, et al: Novel patterns of gene expression in pituitary adenomas identified by complementary deoxyribonucleic acid microarrays and quantitative reverse transcription-polymerase chain reaction, J Clin Endocrinol Metab 86:3097–3107, 2001.
21. Imura H: Ectopic hormone syndromes, Clin Endocrinol Metab 9:235–260, 1980.
22. de Bustros A, Baylin SB: Hormone production by tumours: biological and clinical aspects, Clin Endocrinol Metab 14:221–256, 1985.
23. Pearse AG: Common cytochemical and ultrastructural characteristics of cells producing polypeptide hormones (the APUD series) and their relevance to thyroid and ultimobranchial C cells and calcitonin, Proc R Soc Lond B Biol Sci 170:71–80, 1968.
24. Pullan PT, Clement-Jones V, Corder R, et al: ACTH LPH and related peptides in the ectopic ACTH syndrome, Clin Endocrinol (Oxf) 13:437–445, 1980.
25. Rees LH, Bloomfield GA, Gilkes JJ, et al: ACTH as a tumor marker, Ann N Y Acad Sci 297:603–620, 1977.
26. Stewart MF, Crosby SR, Gibson S, et al: Small cell lung cancer cell lines secrete predominantly ACTH precursor peptides not ACTH, Br J Cancer 60:20–24, 1989.
27. White A, Clark AJ, Stewart MF: The synthesis of ACTH and related peptides by tumours, Baillieres Clin Endocrinol Metab 4:1–27, 1990.
28. DeBold CR, Menefee JK, Nicholson WE, et al: Proopiomelanocortin gene is expressed in many normal human tissues and in tumors not associated with ectopic adrenocorticotropin syndrome, Mol Endocrinol 2:862–870, 1988.
29. de Keyzer Y, Bertagna X, Luton JP, et al: Variable modes of proopiomelanocortin gene transcription in human tumors, Mol Endocrinol 3:215–223, 1989.
30. Clark AJ, Lavender PM, Besser GM, et al: Pro-opiomelanocortin mRNA size heterogeneity in ACTH-dependent Cushing's syndrome, J Mol Endocrinol 2:3–9, 1989.
31. Clark AJ, Stewart MF, Lavender PM, et al: Defective glucocorticoid regulation of proopiomelanocortin gene expression and peptide secretion in a small cell lung cancer cell line, J Clin Endocrinol Metab 70:485–490, 1990.
32. Roth KA, Newell DC, Dorin RI, et al: Aberrant production and regulation of proopiomelanocortin-derived peptides in ectopic Cushing's syndrome, Horm Metab Res 20:225–229, 1988.
33. Melmed S, Yamashita S, Kovacs K, et al: Cushing's syndrome due to ectopic proopiomelanocortin gene expression by islet cell carcinoma of the pancreas, Cancer 59:772–778, 1987.

34. Limper AH, Carpenter PC, Scheithauer B, et al: The Cushing syndrome induced by bronchial carcinoid tumors, Ann Intern Med 117:209–214, 1992.
35. Asa SL, Kovacs K, Vale W, et al: Immunohistologic localization of corticotrophin-releasing hormone in human tumors, Am J Clin Pathol 87:327–333, 1987.
36. Jessop DS, Cunnah D, Millar JG, et al: A phaeochromocytoma presenting with Cushing's syndrome associated with increased concentrations of circulating corticotrophin-releasing factor, J Endocrinol 113:133–138, 1987.
37. Zangeneh F, Young WF Jr, Lloyd RV, et al: Cushing's syndrome due to ectopic production of corticotropin-releasing hormone in an infant with ganglioneuroblastoma, Endocr Pract 9:394–399, 2003.
38. Wajchenberg BL, Mendonca BB, Liberman B, et al: Ectopic adrenocorticotropic hormone syndrome, Endocr Rev 15:752–787, 1994.
39. Sidhu S, Gicquel C, Bambach CP, et al: Clinical and molecular aspects of adrenocortical tumourigenesis, ANZ J Surg 73:727–738, 2003.
40. Beuschlein F, Reincke M, Karl M, et al: Clonal composition of human adrenocortical neoplasms, Cancer Res 54:4927–4932, 1994.
41. Weiss LM, Medeiros LJ, Vickery AL Jr: Pathologic features of prognostic significance in adrenocortical carcinoma, Am J Surg Pathol 13:202–206, 1989.
42. Travis WD, Tsokos M, Doppman JL, et al: Primary pigmented nodular adrenocortical disease. A light and electron microscopic study of eight cases, Am J Surg Pathol 13:921–930, 1989.
43. Stratakis CA, Boikos SA: Genetics of adrenal tumors associated with Cushing's syndrome: a new classification for bilateral adrenocortical hyperplasias, Nat Clin Pract Endocrinol Metab 3:748–757, 2007.
44. Kirk JM, Brain CE, Carson DJ, et al: Cushing's syndrome caused by nodular adrenal hyperplasia in children with McCune-Albright syndrome, J Pediatr 134:789–792, 1999.
45. Weinstein LS, Shenker A, Gejman PV, et al: Activating mutations of the stimulatory G protein in the McCune-Albright syndrome, N Engl J Med 325:1688–1695, 1991.
46. Boston BA, Mandel S, LaFranchi S, et al: Activating mutation in the stimulatory guanine nucleotide-binding protein in an infant with Cushing's syndrome and nodular adrenal hyperplasia, J Clin Endocrinol Metab 79:890–893, 1994.
47. Swords FM, Baig A, Malchoff DM, et al: Impaired desensitization of a mutant adrenocorticotropin receptor associated with apparent constitutive activity, Mol Endocrinol 16:2746–2753, 2002.
48. Findlay JC, Sheeler LR, Engeland WC, et al: Familial adrenocorticotropin-independent Cushing's syndrome with bilateral macronodular adrenal hyperplasia, J Clin Endocrinol Metab 76:189–191, 1993.
49. Christopoulos S, Bourdeau I, Lacroix A: Aberrant expression of hormone receptors in adrenal Cushing's syndrome, Pituitary 7:225–235, 2004.
50. Maschler I, Rosenmann E, Ehrenfeld EN: Ectopic functioning adrenocortico-myelolipoma in longstanding Nelson's syndrome, Clin Endocrinol (Oxf) 10:493–497, 1979.
51. Lalau JD, Vieau D, Tenenbaum F, et al: A case of pseudo-Nelson's syndrome: cure of ACTH hypersecretion by removal of a bronchial carcinoid tumor responsible for Cushing's syndrome, J Endocrinol Invest 13:531–537, 1990.
52. Adeyemi SD, Grange AO, Giwa-Osagie OF, et al: Adrenal rest tumour of the ovary associated with isosexual precocious pseudopuberty and cushingoid features, Eur J Pediatr 145:236–238, 1986.
53. Contreras P, Altieri E, Liberman C, et al: Adrenal rest tumor of the liver causing Cushing's syndrome: treatment with ketoconazole preceding an apparent surgical cure, J Clin Endocrinol Metab 60:21–28, 1985.
54. Marieb NJ, Spangler S, Kashgarian M, et al: Cushing's syndrome secondary to ectopic cortisol production by an ovarian carcinoma, J Clin Endocrinol Metab 57:737–740, 1983.
55. Newell-Price J, Trainer P, Besser M, et al: The diagnosis and differential diagnosis of Cushing's syndrome and pseudo-Cushing's states, Endocr Rev 19:647–672, 1998.
56. Chrousos GP, Schuermeyer TH, Doppman J, et al: NIH conference. Clinical applications of corticotropin-releasing factor, Ann Intern Med 102:344–358, 1985.
57. Gold PW, Gwirtsman H, Avgerinos PC, et al: Abnormal hypothalamic-pituitary-adrenal function in anorexia nervosa. Pathophysiologic mechanisms in underweight and weight-corrected patients, N Engl J Med 314:1335–1342, 1986.
58. Gold PW, Loriaux DL, Roy A, et al: Responses to corticotropin-releasing hormone in the hypercortisolism of depression and Cushing's disease. Pathophysiologic and diagnostic implications, N Engl J Med 314:1329–1335, 1986.
59. Luger A, Deuster PA, Kyle SB, et al: Acute hypothalamic-pituitary-adrenal responses to the stress of treadmill exercise. Physiologic adaptations to physical training, N Engl J Med 316:1309–1315, 1987.
60. Invitti C, Giraldi FP, de Martin M, et al: Diagnosis and management of Cushing's syndrome: results of an Italian multicentre study. Study Group of the Italian Society of Endocrinology on the Pathophysiology of the Hypothalamic-Pituitary-Adrenal Axis, J Clin Endocrinol Metab 84:440–448, 1999.
61. Lindholm J, Juul S, Jorgensen JO, et al: Incidence and late prognosis of Cushing's syndrome: a population-based study, J Clin Endocrinol Metab 86:117–123, 2001.
62. Abeloff MD, Trump DL, Baylin SB: Ectopic adrenocorticotrophic (ACTH) syndrome and small cell carcinoma of the lung-assessment of clinical implications in patients on combination chemotherapy, Cancer 48:1082–1087, 1981.
63. Dimopoulos MA, Fernandez JF, Samaan NA, et al: Paraneoplastic Cushing's syndrome as an adverse prognostic factor in patients who die early with small cell lung cancer, Cancer 69:66–71, 1992.
64. Janssen-Heijnen ML, Coebergh JW: The changing epidemiology of lung cancer in Europe, Lung Cancer 41:245–258, 2003.
65. Ambrosi B, Faglia G: Epidemiology of pituitary tumours. In Faglia G, Beck-Peccoz P, Ambrosi B, Travaglini P, Spada A, editors: Pituitary adenomas: New trends in basic and clinical research, Amsterdam, 1991, Excerpta Medica.
66. Etxabe J, Vazquez JA: Morbidity and mortality in Cushing's disease: an epidemiological approach, Clin Endocrinol (Oxf) 40:479–484, 1994.
67. Plotz CM, Knowlton AI, Ragan C: The natural history of Cushing's syndrome, Am J Med 13:597–614, 1952.
68. Leinung MC, Young WF Jr, Whitaker MD, et al: Diagnosis of corticotropin-producing bronchial carcinoid tumors causing Cushing's syndrome, Mayo Clin Proc 65:1314–1321, 1990.
69. Ross EJ, Linch DC: Cushing's syndrome—killing disease: discriminatory value of signs and symptoms aiding early diagnosis, Lancet 2:646–649, 1982.
70. Urbanic RC, George JM: Cushing's disease—18 years' experience, Medicine (Baltimore) 60:14–24, 1981.
71. Soffer LJ, Iannaccone A, Gabrilove JL: Cushing's syndrome *1: A study of fifty patients, The American Journal of Medicine 30:129–146, 1961.
72. Sprague RG, Randall RV, Salassa RM: Cushing's syndrome: review of 100 cases, Arch Intern Med 98:389–398, 1956.
73. Nugent CA, Warner HR, Dunn JT, et al: PROBABILITY THEORY IN THE DIAGNOSIS OF CUSHING'S SYNDROME, J Clin Endocrinol Metab 24:621–627, 1964.
74. Pecori GF, Pivonello R, Ambrogio AG, et al: The dexamethasone-suppressed corticotropin-releasing hormone stimulation test and the desmopressin test to distinguish Cushing's syndrome from pseudo-Cushing's states, Clin Endocrinol (Oxf) 66:251–257, 2007.
75. Rockall AG, Sohaib SA, Evans D, et al: Computed tomography assessment of fat distribution in male and female patients with Cushing's syndrome, Eur J Endocrinol 149:561–567, 2003.
76. Roy-Camille R, Mazel C, Husson JL, et al: Symptomatic spinal epidural lipomatosis induced by a long-term steroid treatment. Review of the literature and report of two additional cases, Spine 16:1365–1371, 1991.
77. Noel P, Pepersack T, Vanbinst A, et al: Spinal epidural lipomatosis in Cushing's syndrome secondary to an adrenal tumor, Neurology 42:1250–1251, 1992.
78. Healy ME, Hesselink JR, Ostrup RC, et al: Demonstration by magnetic resonance of symptomatic spinal epidural lipomatosis, Neurosurgery 21:414–415, 1987.
79. Pleasure DE, Walsh GO, Engel WK: Atrophy of skeletal muscle in patients with Cushing's syndrome, Arch Neurol 22:118–125, 1970.
80. Muller R, Kugelberg E: Myopathy in Cushing's syndrome, J Neurol Neurosurg Psychiatry 22:314–319, 1959.
81. Afifi AK, Bergman RA, Harvey JC: Steroid myopathy. Clinical, histologic and cytologic observations, Johns Hopkins Med J 123:158–173, 1968.
82. Vertebral compression fractures with accelerated bone turnover in a patient with Cushing's disease, Am J Med 68:932–940, 1980.
83. Kingsley GH, Hickling P: Polyarthropathy associated with Cushing's disease, Br Med J (Clin Res Ed) 292:1363, 1986.
84. Phillips KA, Nance EP Jr, Rodriguez RM, et al: Avascular necrosis of bone: a manifestation of Cushing's disease, South Med J 79:825–829, 1986.
85. Bertagna C, Orth DN: Clinical and laboratory findings and results of therapy in 58 patients with adrenocortical tumors admitted to a single medical center (1951 to 1978), Am J Med 71:855–875, 1981.
86. Starkman MN, Schteingart DE: Neuropsychiatric manifestations of patients with Cushing's syndrome. Relationship to cortisol and adrenocorticotropic hormone levels, Arch Intern Med 141:215–219, 1981.
87. Starkman MN, Schteingart DE, Schork MA: Correlation of bedside cognitive and neuropsychological tests in patients with Cushing's syndrome, Psychosomatics 27:508–511, 1986.
88. Haskett RF: Diagnostic categorization of psychiatric disturbance in Cushing's syndrome, Am J Psychiatry 142:911–916, 1985.
89. Hudson JI, Hudson MS, Griffing GT, et al: Phenomenology and family history of affective disorder in Cushing's disease, Am J Psychiatry 144:951–953, 1987.
90. Rubinow DR, Post RM, Savard R, et al: Cortisol hypersecretion and cognitive impairment in depression, Arch Gen Psychiatry 41:279–283, 1984.
91. Kathol RG: Etiologic implications of corticosteroid changes in affective disorder, Psychiatr Med 3:135–162, 1985.
92. Fallo F, Sonino N, Barzon L, et al: Effect of surgical treatment on hypertension in Cushing's syndrome, Am J Hypertens 9:77–80, 1996.
93. Bakker RC, Gallas PR, Romijn JA, et al: Cushing's syndrome complicated by multiple opportunistic infections, J Endocrinol Invest 21:329–333, 1998.
94. Graham BS, Tucker WS Jr: Opportunistic infections in endogenous Cushing's syndrome, Ann Intern Med 101:334–338, 1984.
95. Sarlis NJ, Chanock SJ, Nieman LK: Cortisolemic indices predict severe infections in Cushing syndrome due to ectopic production of adrenocorticotropin, J Clin Endocrinol Metab 85:42–47, 2000.
96. Kaltsas GA, Korbonits M, Isidori AM, et al: How common are polycystic ovaries and the polycystic ovarian syndrome in women with Cushing's syndrome? Clin Endocrinol (Oxf) 53:493–500, 2000.
97. Halbreich U, Zumoff B, Kream J, et al: The mean 1300–1600 h plasma cortisol concentration as a diagnostic test for hypercortisolism, J Clin Endocrinol Metab 54:1262–1264, 1982.
98. Liu JH, Kazer RR, Rasmussen DD: Characterization of the twenty-four hour secretion patterns of adrenocorticotropin and cortisol in normal women and patients with Cushing's disease, J Clin Endocrinol Metab 64:1027–1035, 1987.
99. Refetoff S, Van Cauter E, Fang VS, et al: The effect of dexamethasone on the 24-hour profiles of adrenocorticotropin and cortisol in Cushing's syndrome, J Clin Endocrinol Metab 60:527–535, 1985.
100. Mengden T, Hubmann P, Muller J, et al: Urinary free cortisol versus 17-hydroxycorticosteroids: a comparative study of their diagnostic value in Cushing's syndrome, Clin Investig 70:545–548, 1992.
101. Evans PJ, Peters JR, Dyas J, et al: Salivary cortisol levels in true and apparent hypercortisolism, Clin Endocrinol (Oxf) 20:709–715, 1984.
102. Christy NP, Laragh JH: Pathogenesis of hypokalemic alkalosis in Cushing's syndrome, Nord Hyg Tidskr 265:1083–1088, 1961.
103. Stewart PM, Krozowski ZS: 11 beta-Hydroxysteroid dehydrogenase, Vitam Horm 57:249–324, 1999.
104. Putignano P, Kaltsas GA, Korbonits M, et al: Alterations in serum protein levels in patients with Cushing's

syndrome before and after successful treatment, J Clin Endocrinol Metab 85:3309–3312, 2000.

105. Ambrosi B, Sartorio A, Pizzocaro A, et al: Evaluation of haemostatic and fibrinolytic markers in patients with Cushing's syndrome and in patients with adrenal incidentaloma, Exp Clin Endocrinol Diabetes 108:294–298, 2000.

106. Casonato A, Pontara E, Boscaro M, et al: Abnormalities of von Willebrand factor are also part of the prothrombotic state of Cushing's syndrome, Blood Coagul Fibrinolysis 10:145–151, 1999.

107. Patrassi GM, Dal Bo ZR, Boscaro M, et al: Further studies on the hypercoagulable state of patients with Cushing's syndrome, Thromb Haemost 54:518–520, 1985.

108. Taskinen MR, Nikkila EA, Pelkonen R, et al: Plasma lipoproteins, lipolytic enzymes, and very low density lipoprotein triglyceride turnover in Cushing's syndrome, J Clin Endocrinol Metab 57:619–626, 1983.

109. Friedman TC, Mastorakos G, Newman TD, et al: Carbohydrate and lipid metabolism in endogenous hypercortisolism: shared features with metabolic syndrome X and NIDDM, Endocr J 43:645–655, 1996.

110. Biering H, Knappe G, Gerl H, et al: [Prevalence of diabetes in acromegaly and Cushing syndrome], Acta Med Austriaca 27:27–31, 2000.

111. Krassowski J, Godziejewska M, Kurta J, et al: [Glucose tolerance in adrenocortical hyperfunction. Analysis of 100 cases], Pol Arch Med Wewn 92:70–75, 1994.

112. Catargi B, Rigalleau V, Poussin A, et al: Occult Cushing's syndrome in type-2 diabetes, J Clin Endocrinol Metab 88:5808–5813, 2003.

113. Newsome S, Chen K, Hoang J, et al: Cushing's syndrome in a clinic population with diabetes, Intern Med J 38:178–182, 2008.

114. Faggiano A, Pivonello R, Spiezia S, et al: Cardiovascular risk factors and common carotid artery caliber and stiffness in patients with Cushing's disease during active disease and 1 year after disease remission, J Clin Endocrinol Metab 88:2527–2533, 2003.

115. Colao A, Pivonello R, Spiezia S, et al: Persistence of increased cardiovascular risk in patients with Cushing's disease after five years of successful cure, J Clin Endocrinol Metab 84:2664–2672, 1999.

116. Bartalena L, Martino E, Petrini L, et al: The nocturnal serum thyrotropin surge is abolished in patients with adrenocorticotropin (ACTH)-dependent or ACTH-independent Cushing's syndrome, J Clin Endocrinol Metab 72:1195–1199, 1991.

117. Colao A, Pivonello R, Faggiano A, et al: Increased prevalence of thyroid autoimmunity in patients successfully treated for Cushing's disease, Clin Endocrinol (Oxf) 53:13–19, 2000.

118. Niepomniszcze H, Pitoia F, Katz SB, et al: Primary thyroid disorders in endogenous Cushing's syndrome, Eur J Endocrinol 147:305–311, 2002.

119. Luton JP, Thieblot P, Valcke JC, et al: Reversible gonadotropin deficiency in male Cushing's disease, J Clin Endocrinol Metab 45:488–495, 1977.

120. Lado-Abeal J, Rodriguez-Arnao J, Newell-Price JD, et al: Menstrual abnormalities in women with Cushing's disease are correlated with hypercortisolemia rather than raised circulating androgen levels, J Clin Endocrinol Metab 83:3083–3088, 1998.

121. Giustina A, Bossoni S, Bussi AR, et al: Effect of galanin on the growth hormone (GH) response to GH-releasing hormone in patients with Cushing's disease, Endocr Res 19:47–56, 1993.

122. Kaltsas G, Manetti L, Grossman AB: Osteoporosis in Cushing's syndrome, Front Horm Res 30:60–72, 2002.

123. Ohmori N, Nomura K, Ohmori K, et al: Osteoporosis is more prevalent in adrenal than in pituitary Cushing's syndrome, Endocr J 50:1–7, 2003.

124. Rockall AG, Sohaib SA, Evans D, et al: Hepatic steatosis in Cushing's syndrome: a radiological assessment using computed tomography, Eur J Endocrinol 149:543–548, 2003.

125. Giraldi FP, Moro M, Cavagnini F: Gender-related differences in the presentation and course of Cushing's disease, J Clin Endocrinol Metab 88:1554–1558, 2003.

126. King AB: The diagnosis of carcinoma of the pituitary gland, Bull Johns Hopkins Hosp 89:339–353, 1951.

127. Martins AN, Hayes GJ, Kempe LG: INVASIVE PITUITARY ADENOMAS, J Neurosurg 22:268–276, 1965.

128. Della CS, Corsello SM, Satta MA, et al: Intracranial and spinal dissemination of an ACTH secreting pituitary neoplasia. Case report and review of the literature, Ann Endocrinol (Paris) 58:503–509, 1997.

129. Arnaldi G, Angeli A, Atkinson AB, et al: Diagnosis and complications of Cushing's syndrome: a consensus statement, J Clin Endocrinol Metab 88:5593–5602, 2003.

130. Besser GM, Edwards CRW: Cushing's Syndrome, Clin Endocrinol Metab 1:451–490, 1972.

131. Lamberts SW, Klijn JG, de Jong FH, et al: Hormone secretion in alcohol-induced pseudo-Cushing's syndrome. Differential diagnosis with Cushing disease, JAMA 242:1640–1643, 1979.

132. Wallace EZ, Rosman P, Toshav N, et al: Pituitary-adrenocortical function in chronic renal failure: studies of episodic secretion of cortisol and dexamethasone suppressibility, J Clin Endocrinol Metab 50:46–51, 1980.

133. Werner S, Thoren M, Gustafsson JA, et al: Glucocorticoid receptor abnormalities in fibroblasts from patients with idiopathic resistance to dexamethasone diagnosed when evaluated for adrenocortical disorders, J Clin Endocrinol Metab 75:1005–1009, 1992.

134. Nieman LK, Biller BM, Findling JW, et al: The diagnosis of Cushing's syndrome: an Endocrine Society Clinical Practice Guideline, J Clin Endocrinol Metab 93:1526–1540, 2008.

135. Murphy BE: Clinical evaluation of urinary cortisol determinations by competitive protein-binding radioassay, J Clin Endocrinol Metab 28:343–348, 1968.

136. Orth DN: Cushing's syndrome, N Engl J Med 332:791–803, 1995.

137. Contreras LN, Hane S, Tyrrell JB: Urinary cortisol in the assessment of pituitary-adrenal function: utility of 24-hour and spot determinations, J Clin Endocrinol Metab 62:965–969, 1986.

138. Laudat MH, Billaud L, Thomopoulos P, et al: Evening urinary free corticoids: a screening test in Cushing's syndrome and incidentally discovered adrenal tumours, Acta Endocrinol (Copenh) 119:459–464, 1988.

139. Lin CL, Wu TJ, Machacek DA, et al: Urinary free cortisol and cortisone determined by high performance liquid chromatography in the diagnosis of Cushing's syndrome, J Clin Endocrinol Metab 82:151–155, 1997.

140. Turpeinen U, Markkanen H, Valimaki M, et al: Determination of urinary free cortisol by HPLC, Clin Chem 43:1386–1391, 1997.

141. Meikle AW, Findling J, Kushnir MM, et al: Pseudo-Cushing Syndrome Caused by Fenofibrate Interference with Urinary Cortisol Assayed by High-Performance Liquid Chromatography, J Clin Endocrinol Metab 88:3521–3524, 2003.

142. Nieman LK, Cutler GB Jr: The sensitivity of the urine free cortisol measurement as a screening test for Cushing's syndrome, Program of the 72nd Annual Meeting of The Endocrine Society, Atlanta GA (Abstract P-822) 1990.

143. Laudat MH, Cerdas S, Fournier C, et al: Salivary cortisol measurement: a practical approach to assess pituitary-adrenal function, J Clin Endocrinol Metab 66:343–348, 1988.

144. Putignano P, Dubini A, Toja P, et al: Salivary cortisol measurement in normal-weight, obese and anorexic women: comparison with plasma cortisol, Eur J Endocrinol 145:165–171, 2001.

145. Raff H, Homar PJ, Skoner DP: New enzyme immunoassay for salivary cortisol, Clin Chem 49:203–204, 2003.

146. Papanicolaou DA, Mullen N, Kyrou I, et al: Nighttime salivary cortisol: a useful test for the diagnosis of Cushing's syndrome, J Clin Endocrinol Metab 87:4515–4521, 2002.

147. Putignano P, Toja P, Dubini A, et al: Midnight salivary cortisol versus urinary free and midnight serum cortisol as screening tests for Cushing's syndrome, J Clin Endocrinol Metab 88:4153–4157, 2003.

148. Raff H, Raff JL, Findling JW: Late-night salivary cortisol as a screening test for Cushing's syndrome, J Clin Endocrinol Metab 83:2681–2686, 1998.

149. Castro M, Elias PC, Quidute AR, et al: Out-patient screening for Cushing's syndrome: the sensitivity of the combination of circadian rhythm and overnight dexamethasone suppression salivary cortisol tests, J Clin Endocrinol Metab 84:878–882, 1999.

150. Viardot A, Huber P, Puder JJ, et al: Reproducibility of nighttime salivary cortisol and its use in the diagnosis of hypercortisolism compared with urinary free cortisol

and overnight dexamethasone suppression test, J Clin Endocrinol Metab 90:5730–5736, 2005.

151. Trilck M, Flitsch J, Ludecke DK, et al: Salivary cortisol measurement–a reliable method for the diagnosis of Cushing's syndrome, Exp Clin Endocrinol Diabetes 113:225–230, 2005.

152. Yaneva M, Mosnier-Pudar H, Dugue MA, et al: Midnight salivary cortisol for the initial diagnosis of Cushing's syndrome of various causes, J Clin Endocrinol Metab 89:3345–3351, 2004.

153. Baid SK, Sinaii N, Wade M, et al: Radioimmunoassay and tandem mass spectrometry measurement of bedtime salivary cortisol levels: a comparison of assays to establish hypercortisolism, J Clin Endocrinol Metab 92:3102–3107, 2007.

154. Liu H, Bravata DM, Cabaccan J, et al: Elevated late-night salivary cortisol levels in elderly male type 2 diabetic veterans, Clin Endocrinol (Oxf) 63:642–649, 2005.

155. Liddle GW: Tests of pituitary-adrenal suppressibility in the diagnosis of Cushing's syndrome, J Clin Endocrinol Metab 20:1539–1560, 1960.

156. Kennedy L, Atkinson AB, Johnston H, et al: Serum cortisol concentrations during low dose dexamethasone suppression test to screen for Cushing's syndrome, Br Med J (Clin Res Ed) 289:1188–1191, 1984.

157. Hankin ME, Theile HM, Steinbeck AW: An evaluation of laboratory tests for the detection and differential diagnosis of Cushing's syndrome, Clin Endocrinol (Oxf) 6:185–196, 1977.

158. Newell-Price J, Trainer P, Perry L, et al: A single sleeping midnight cortisol has 100% sensitivity for the diagnosis of Cushing's syndrome, Clin Endocrinol (Oxf) 43:545–550, 1995.

159. Isidori AM, Kaltsas GA, Mohammed S, et al: Discriminatory value of the low-dose dexamethasone suppression test in establishing the diagnosis and differential diagnosis of Cushing's syndrome, J Clin Endocrinol Metab 88:5299–5306, 2003.

160. Nugent CA, Nichols T, Tyler FH: Diagnosis of Cushing's syndrome—single dose dexamethasone suppression test, Arch Intern Med 172–176, 1965.

161. Shimizu N, Yoshida H: Studies on the "low dose" suppressible Cushing's disease, Endocrinol Jpn 23:479–484, 1976.

162. McHardy-Young S, Harris PW, Lessof MH, et al: Single dose dexamethasone suppression test for Cushing's Syndrome, Br Med J 2:740–744, 1967.

163. Seidensticker JF, Folk RL, Wieland RG, et al: Screening test for Cushing's syndrome with plasma 11-hydroxycorticosteroids, JAMA 202:87–90, 1967.

164. Crapo L: Cushing's syndrome: a review of diagnostic tests, Metabolism 28:955–977, 1979.

165. Odagiri E, Demura R, Demura H, et al: The changes in plasma cortisol and urinary free cortisol by an overnight dexamethasone suppression test in patients with Cushing's disease, Endocrinol Jpn 35:795–802, 1988.

166. Martinelli CE Jr, Sader SL, Oliveira EB, et al: Salivary cortisol for screening of Cushing's syndrome in children, Clin Endocrinol (Oxf) 51:67–71, 1999.

167. Putignano P, Kaltsas GA, Satta MA, et al: The effects of anti-convulsant drugs on adrenal function, Horm Metab Res 30:389–397, 1998.

168. Abou Samra AB, Dechaud H, Estour B, et al: Beta-lipotropin and cortisol responses to an intravenous infusion dexamethasone suppression test in Cushing's syndrome and obesity, J Clin Endocrinol Metab 61:116–119, 1985.

169. Atkinson AB, McAteer EJ, Hadden DR, et al: A weight-related intravenous dexamethasone suppression test distinguishes obese controls from patients with Cushing's syndrome, Acta Endocrinol (Copenh) 120:753–759, 1989.

170. Klose M, Lange M, Rasmussen AK, et al: Factors influencing the adrenocorticotropin test: role of contemporary cortisol assays, body composition, and oral contraceptive agents, J Clin Endocrinol Metab 92:1326–1333, 2007.

171. Yanovski JA, Cutler GB Jr, Chrousos GP, et al: Corticotropin-releasing hormone stimulation following low-dose dexamethasone administration. A new test to distinguish Cushing's syndrome from pseudo-Cushing's states, JAMA 269:2232–2238, 1993.

172. Yanovski JA, Cutler GB Jr, Chrousos GP, et al: Prospective evaluation of the dexamethasone-suppressed corticotrophin-releasing hormone test in the differential

diagnosis of Cushing's syndrome and pseudo-Cushing's states, Program of the 77th Annual Meeting of the Endocrine Society, Washington DC p 99 (abstract):1995.
173. Martin NM, Dhillo WS, Banerjee A, et al: Comparison of the dexamethasone-suppressed corticotropin-releasing hormone test and low-dose dexamethasone suppression test in the diagnosis of Cushing's syndrome, J Clin Endocrinol Metab 91:2582–2586, 2006.
174. Gatta B, Cortet C, Martinie M, et al: Reevaluation of the dex-CRH test for the differential diagnosis between Cushing's disease and pseudo-Cushing's syndrome. Program of the 88th Annual Meeting of The Endocrine Society, Boston, MA, 2006, P2–734 2006.
175. Erickson D, Natt N, Nippoldt T, et al: Dexamethasone-suppressed corticotropin-releasing hormone stimulation test for diagnosis of mild hypercortisolism, J Clin Endocrinol Metab 92:2972–2976, 2007.
176. Nieman L: Editorial: The dexamethasone-suppressed corticotropin-releasing hormone test for the diagnosis of Cushing's syndrome: what have we learned in 14 years? J Clin Endocrinol Metab 92:2876–2878, 2007.
177. Papanicolaou DA, Yanovski JA, Cutler GB Jr, et al: A single midnight serum cortisol measurement distinguishes Cushing's syndrome from pseudo-Cushing states, J Clin Endocrinol Metab 83:1163–1167, 1998.
178. Reimondo G, Allasino B, Bovio S, et al: Evaluation of the effectiveness of midnight serum cortisol in the diagnostic procedures for Cushing's syndrome, Eur J Endocrinol 153:803–809, 2005.
179. Ambrosi B, Bochicchio D, Ferrario R, et al: Effects of the opiate agonist loperamide on pituitary-adrenal function in patients with suspected hypercortisolism, J Endocrinol Invest 12:31–35, 1989.
180. Ambrosi B, Bochicchio D, Colombo P, et al: Loperamide to diagnose Cushing's syndrome, JAMA 270:2301–2302, 1993.
181. Bernini GP, Argenio GF, Cerri F, et al: Comparison between the suppressive effects of dexamethasone and loperamide on cortisol and ACTH secretion in some pathological conditions, J Endocrinol Invest 17:799–804, 1994.
182. Lytras N, Grossman A, Perry L, et al: Corticotrophin releasing factor: responses in normal subjects and patients with disorders of the hypothalamus and pituitary, Clin Endocrinol (Oxf) 20:71–84, 1984.
183. Fig LM, Gross MD, Shapiro B, et al: Adrenal localization in the adrenocorticotropic hormone-independent Cushing syndrome, Ann Intern Med 109:547–553, 1988.
184. Perry RR, Nieman LK, Cutler GB Jr, et al: Primary adrenal causes of Cushing's syndrome. Diagnosis and surgical management, Ann Surg 210:59–68, 1989.
185. Doppman JL, Miller DL, Dwyer AJ, et al: Macronodular adrenal hyperplasia in Cushing disease, Radiology 166:347–352, 1988.
186. Mimou N, Sakato S, Nakabayashi H, et al: Cushing's syndrome associated with bilateral adrenal adenomas, Acta Endocrinol (Copenh) 108:245–254, 1985.
187. Doppman JL, Travis WD, Nieman L, et al: Cushing syndrome due to primary pigmented nodular adrenocortical disease: findings at CT and MR imaging, Radiology 172:415–420, 1989.
188. Doppman JL, Nieman LK, Travis WD, et al: CT and MR imaging of massive macronodular adrenocortical disease: a rare cause of autonomous primary adrenal hypercortisolism, J Comput Assist Tomogr 15:773–779, 1991.
189. Sohaib SA, Hanson JA, Newell-Price JD, et al: CT appearance of the adrenal glands in adrenocorticotrophic hormone-dependent Cushing's syndrome, AJR Am J Roentgenol 172:997–1002, 1999.
190. Aron DC, Findling JW, Fitzgerald PA, et al: Pituitary ACTH dependency of nodular adrenal hyperplasia in Cushing's syndrome. Report of two cases and review of the literature, Am J Med 71:302–306, 1981.
191. Howlett TA, Drury PL, Perry L, et al: Diagnosis and management of ACTH-dependent Cushing's syndrome: comparison of the features in ectopic and pituitary ACTH production, Clin Endocrinol (Oxf) 24:699–713, 1986.
192. Newell-Price J, Morris DG, Drake WM, et al: Optimal response criteria for the human CRH test in the differential diagnosis of ACTH-dependent Cushing's syndrome, J Clin Endocrinol Metab 87:1640–1645, 2002.
193. Yamamoto Y, Davis DH, Nippoldt TB, et al: False-positive inferior petrosal sinus sampling in the diagnosis of Cushing's disease. Report of two cases, J Neurosurg 83:1087–1091, 1995.
194. Yanovski JA, Cutler GB Jr, Doppman JL, et al: The limited ability of inferior petrosal sinus sampling with corticotropin-releasing hormone to distinguish Cushing's disease from pseudo-Cushing states or normal physiology, J Clin Endocrinol Metab 77:503–509, 1993.
195. Miller DL, Doppman JL: Petrosal sinus sampling: technique and rationale, Radiology 178:37–47, 1991.
196. Oldfield EH, Doppman JL, Nieman LK, et al: Petrosal sinus sampling with and without corticotropin-releasing hormone for the differential diagnosis of Cushing's syndrome, N Engl J Med 325:897–905, 1991.
197. Kaltsas GA, Giannulis MG, Newell-Price JD, et al: A critical analysis of the value of simultaneous inferior petrosal sinus sampling in Cushing's disease and the occult ectopic adrenocorticotropin syndrome, J Clin Endocrinol Metab 84:487–492, 1999.
198. Colao A, Faggiano A, Pivonello R, et al: Inferior petrosal sinus sampling in the differential diagnosis of Cushing's syndrome: results of an Italian multicenter study, Eur J Endocrinol 144:499–507, 2001.
199. Swearingen B, Katznelson L, Miller K, et al: Diagnostic errors after inferior petrosal sinus sampling, J Clin Endocrinol Metab 89:3752–3763, 2004.
200. McCance DR, McIlrath E, McNeill A, et al: Bilateral inferior petrosal sinus sampling as a routine procedure in ACTH-dependent Cushing's syndrome, Clin Endocrinol (Oxf) 30:157–166, 1989.
201. Findling JW, Kehoe ME, Raff H: Identification of patients with Cushing's disease with negative pituitary adrenocorticotropin gradients during inferior petrosal sinus sampling: prolactin as an index of pituitary venous effluent, J Clin Endocrinol Metab 89:6005–6009, 2004.
202. Miller DL: Neurologic complications of petrosal sinus sampling, Radiology 183:878, 1992.
203. Lefournier V, Gatta B, Martinie M, et al: One transient neurological complication (sixth nerve palsy) in 166 consecutive inferior petrosal sinus samplings for the etiological diagnosis of Cushing's syndrome, J Clin Endocrinol Metab 84:3401–3402, 1999.
204. Rotman-Pikielny P, Patronas N, Papanicolaou DA: Pituitary apoplexy induced by corticotrophin-releasing hormone in a patient with Cushing's disease, Clin Endocrinol (Oxf) 58:545–549, 2003.
205. Tabarin A, Greselle JF, San Galli F, et al: Usefulness of the corticotropin-releasing hormone test during bilateral inferior petrosal sinus sampling for the diagnosis of Cushing's disease, J Clin Endocrinol Metab 73:53–59, 1991.
206. Landolt AM, Schubiger O, Maurer R, et al: The value of inferior petrosal sinus sampling in diagnosis and treatment of Cushing's disease, Clin Endocrinol (Oxf) 40:485–492, 1994.
207. Lefournier V, Martinie M, Vasdev A, et al: Accuracy of bilateral inferior petrosal or cavernous sinuses sampling in predicting the lateralization of Cushing's disease pituitary microadenoma: influence of catheter position and anatomy of venous drainage, J Clin Endocrinol Metab 88:196–203, 2003.
208. Morris DG, Grossman AB: Dynamic tests in the diagnosis and differential diagnosis of Cushing's syndrome, J Endocrinol Invest 26:64–73, 2003.
209. Miller DL, Doppman JL, Nieman LK, et al: Petrosal sinus sampling: discordant lateralization of ACTH-secreting pituitary microadenomas before and after stimulation with corticotropin-releasing hormone, Radiology 176:429–431, 1990.
210. Erickson D, Huston J, III, Young WF Jr, et al: Internal jugular vein sampling in adrenocorticotropic hormone-dependent Cushing's syndrome: a comparison with inferior petrosal sinus sampling, Clin Endocrinol (Oxf) 60:413–419, 2004.
211. Ilias I, Chang R, Pacak K, et al: Jugular venous sampling: an alternative to petrosal sinus sampling for the diagnostic evaluation of adrenocorticotropic hormone-dependent Cushing's syndrome, J Clin Endocrinol Metab 89:3795–3800, 2004.
212. Tyrrell JB, Findling JW, Aron DC, et al: An overnight high-dose dexamethasone suppression test for rapid differential diagnosis of Cushing's syndrome, Ann Intern Med 104:180–186, 1986.
213. Aron DC, Raff H, Findling JW: Effectiveness versus efficacy: the limited value in clinical practice of high dose dexamethasone suppression testing in the differential diagnosis of adrenocorticotropin-dependent Cushing's syndrome, J Clin Endocrinol Metab 82:1780–1785, 1997.
214. Kaye TB, Crapo L: The Cushing syndrome: an update on diagnostic tests, Ann Intern Med 112:434–444, 1990.
215. Giraldi FP, Invitti C, Cavagnini F: The corticotropin-releasing hormone test in the diagnosis of ACTH-dependent Cushing's syndrome: a reappraisal, Clin Endocrinol (Oxf) 54:601–607, 2001.
216. Ilias I, Torpy DJ, Pacak K, et al: Cushing's syndrome due to ectopic corticotropin secretion: twenty years' experience at the National Institutes of Health, J Clin Endocrinol Metab 90:4955–4962, 2005.
217. Trainer PJ, Faria M, Newell-Price J, et al: A comparison of the effects of human and ovine corticotropin-releasing hormone on the pituitary-adrenal axis, J Clin Endocrinol Metab 80:412–417, 1995.
218. Trainer PJ, Woods RJ, Korbonits M, et al: The pathophysiology of circulating corticotropin-releasing hormone-binding protein levels in the human, J Clin Endocrinol Metab 83:1611–1614, 1998.
219. Nieman LK, Oldfield EH, Wesley R, et al: A simplified morning ovine corticotropin-releasing hormone stimulation test for the differential diagnosis of adrenocorticotropin-dependent Cushing's syndrome, J Clin Endocrinol Metab 77:1308–1312, 1993.
220. Korbonits M, Kaltsas G, Perry LA, et al: The growth hormone secretagogue hexarelin stimulates the hypothalamo-pituitary-adrenal axis via arginine vasopressin, J Clin Endocrinol Metab 84:2489–2495, 1999.
221. Korbonits M, Bustin SA, Kojima M, et al: The expression of the growth hormone secretagogue receptor ligand ghrelin in normal and abnormal human pituitary and other neuroendocrine tumors, J Clin Endocrinol Metab 86:881–887, 2001.
222. Tabarin A, San Galli F, Dezou S, et al: The corticotropin-releasing factor test in the differential diagnosis of Cushing's syndrome: a comparison with the lysine-vasopressin test, Acta Endocrinol (Copenh) 123:331–338, 1990.
223. Malerbi DA, Mendonca BB, Liberman B, et al: The desmopressin stimulation test in the differential diagnosis of Cushing's syndrome, Clin Endocrinol (Oxf) 38:463–472, 1993.
224. Ghigo E, Arvat E, Ramunni J, et al: Adrenocorticotropin- and cortisol-releasing effect of hexarelin, a synthetic growth hormone-releasing peptide, in normal subjects and patients with Cushing's syndrome, J Clin Endocrinol Metab 82:2439–2444, 1997.
225. Castinetti F, Morange I, Dufour H, et al: Desmopressin test during petrosal sinus sampling: a valuable tool to discriminate pituitary or ectopic ACTH-dependent Cushing's syndrome, Eur J Endocrinol 157:271–277, 2007.
226. Newell-Price J, Perry L, Medbak S, et al: A combined test using desmopressin and corticotropin-releasing hormone in the differential diagnosis of Cushing's syndrome, J Clin Endocrinol Metab 82:176–181, 1997.
227. Tsagarakis S, Tsigos C, Vasiliou V, et al: The desmopressin and combined CRH-desmopressin tests in the differential diagnosis of ACTH-dependent Cushing's syndrome: constraints imposed by the expression of V2 vasopressin receptors in tumors with ectopic ACTH secretion, J Clin Endocrinol Metab 87:1646–1653, 2002.
228. Korbonits M, Jacobs RA, Aylwin SJB, et al: Expression of the Growth Hormone Secretagogue Receptor in Pituitary Adenomas and Other Neuroendocrine Tumors, J Clin Endocrinol Metab 83:3624–3630, 1998.
229. Nieman LK, Chrousos GP, Oldfield EH, et al: The ovine corticotropin-releasing hormone stimulation test and the dexamethasone suppression test in the differential diagnosis of Cushing's syndrome, Ann Intern Med 105:862–867, 1986.
230. Hermus AR, Pieters GF, Pesman GJ, et al: The corticotropin-releasing-hormone test versus the high-dose dexamethasone test in the differential diagnosis of Cushing's syndrome, Lancet 2:540–544, 1986.
231. Grossman AB, Howlett TA, Perry L, et al: CRF in the differential diagnosis of Cushing's syndrome: a comparison with the dexamethasone suppression test, Clin Endocrinol (Oxf) 29:167–178, 1988.

232. Doppman JL, Frank JA, Dwyer AJ, et al: Gadolinium DTPA enhanced MR imaging of ACTH-secreting microadenomas of the pituitary gland, J Comput Assist Tomogr 12:728–735, 1988.
233. Patronas N, Bulakbasi N, Stratakis CA, et al: Spoiled gradient recalled acquisition in the steady state technique is superior to conventional postcontrast spin echo technique for magnetic resonance imaging detection of adrenocorticotropin-secreting pituitary tumors, J Clin Endocrinol Metab 88:1565–1569, 2003.
234. Hall WA, Luciano MG, Doppman JL, et al: Pituitary magnetic resonance imaging in normal human volunteers: occult adenomas in the general population, Ann Intern Med 120:817–820, 1994.
235. Findling JW, Doppman JL: Biochemical and radiologic diagnosis of Cushing's syndrome, Endocrinol Metab Clin North Am 23:511–537, 1994.
236. Escourolle H, Abecassis JP, Bertagna X, et al: Comparison of computerized tomography and magnetic resonance imaging for the examination of the pituitary gland in patients with Cushing's disease, Clin Endocrinol (Oxf) 39:307–313, 1993.
237. Doppman JL, Pass HI, Nieman LK, et al: Detection of ACTH-producing bronchial carcinoid tumors: MR imaging vs CT, AJR Am J Roentgenol 156:39–43, 1991.
238. Doppman JL, Nieman L, Miller DL, et al: Ectopic adrenocorticotropic hormone syndrome: localization studies in 28 patients, Radiology 172:115–124, 1989.
239. de Herder WW, Lamberts SW: Octapeptide somatostatin-analogue therapy of Cushing's syndrome, Postgrad Med J 75:65–66, 1999.
240. Tabarin A, Valli N, Chanson P, et al: Usefulness of somatostatin receptor scintigraphy in patients with occult ectopic adrenocorticotropin syndrome, J Clin Endocrinol Metab 84:1193–1202, 1999.
241. Tsagarakis S, Christoforaki M, Giannopoulou H, et al: A reappraisal of the utility of somatostatin receptor scintigraphy in patients with ectopic adrenocorticotropin Cushing's syndrome, J Clin Endocrinol Metab 88:4754–4758, 2003.
242. Torpy DJ, Chen CC, Mullen N, et al: Lack of utility of (111)In-pentetreotide scintigraphy in localizing ectopic ACTH producing tumors: follow-up of 18 patients, J Clin Endocrinol Metab 84:1186–1192, 1999.
243. Kumar J, Spring M, Carroll PV, et al: 18Fluorodeoxyglucose positron emission tomography in the localization of ectopic ACTH-secreting neuroendocrine tumours, Clin Endocrinol (Oxf) 64:371–374, 2006.
244. Pacak K, Ilias I, Chen CC, et al: The role of [(18)F]fluorodeoxyglucose positron emission tomography and [(111)In]-diethylenetriaminepentaacetate-D-Phe-pentetreotide scintigraphy in the localization of ectopic adrenocorticotropin-secreting tumors causing Cushing's syndrome, J Clin Endocrinol Metab 89:2214–2221, 2004.
245. Sarkar R, Thompson NW, McLeod MK: The role of adrenalectomy in Cushing's syndrome, Surgery 108:1079–1084, 1990.
246. Terzolo M, Reimondo G, Bovio S, et al: Subclinical Cushing's syndrome, Pituitary 7:217–223, 2004.
247. Biller BM, Grossman AB, Stewart PM, et al: Treatment of Adrenocorticotropin-Dependent Cushing's Syndrome: A Consensus Statement, J Clin Endocrinol Metab 93:2454–2462, 2008.
248. Lamberts SW, van der Lely AJ, de Herder WW: Transsphenoidal selective adenomectomy is the treatment of choice in patients with Cushing's disease. Considerations concerning preoperative medical treatment and the long-term follow-up, J Clin Endocrinol Metab 80:3111–3113, 1995.
249. Boscaro M, Sonino N, Scarda A, et al: Anticoagulant prophylaxis markedly reduces thromboembolic complications in Cushing's syndrome, J Clin Endocrinol Metab 87:3662–3666, 2002.
250. Welbourn RB: The evolution of transsphenoidal pituitary microsurgery, Surgery 100:1185–1190, 1986.
251. Fahlbusch R, Buchfelder M, Muller OA: Transsphenoidal surgery for Cushing's disease, J R Soc Med 79:262–269, 1986.
252. Knappe UJ, Ludecke DK: Persistent and recurrent hypercortisolism after transsphenoidal surgery for Cushing's disease, Acta Neurochir Suppl 65:31–34, 1996.
253. Stevenaert A, Perrin G, Martin D, et al: [Cushing's disease and corticotrophic adenoma: results of pituitary microsurgery], Neurochirurgie 48:234–265, 2002.
254. Swearingen B, Biller BM, Barker FG, et al: Long-term mortality after transsphenoidal surgery for Cushing disease, Ann Intern Med 130:821–824, 1999.
255. Hammer GD, Tyrrell JB, Lamborn KR, et al: Transsphenoidal microsurgery for Cushing's disease: initial outcome and long-term results, J Clin Endocrinol Metab 89:6348–6357, 2004.
256. Hofmann BM, Fahlbusch R: Treatment of Cushing's disease: a retrospective clinical study of the latest 100 cases, Front Horm Res 34:158–184, 2006.
257. Bochicchio D, Losa M, Buchfelder M: Factors influencing the immediate and late outcome of Cushing's disease treated by transsphenoidal surgery: a retrospective study by the European Cushing's Disease Survey Group, J Clin Endocrinol Metab 80:3114–3120, 1995.
258. Sonino N, Zielezny M, Fava GA, et al: Risk factors and long-term outcome in pituitary-dependent Cushing's disease, J Clin Endocrinol Metab 81:2647–2652, 1996.
259. Blevins LS Jr, Christy JH, Khajavi M, et al: Outcomes of therapy for Cushing's disease due to adrenocorticotropin-secreting pituitary macroadenomas, J Clin Endocrinol Metab 83:63–67, 1998.
260. Netea-Maier RT, van Lindert EJ, den Heijer M, et al: Transsphenoidal pituitary surgery via the endoscopic technique: results in 35 consecutive patients with Cushing's disease, Eur J Endocrinol 154:675–684, 2006.
261. Oldfield EH, Vortmeyer AO: Development of a histological pseudocapsule and its use as a surgical capsule in the excision of pituitary tumors, J Neurosurg 104:7–19, 2006.
262. Atkinson AB, Kennedy A, Wiggam MI, et al: Long-term remission rates after pituitary surgery for Cushing's disease: the need for long-term surveillance, Clin Endocrinol (Oxf) 63:549–559, 2005.
263. Rees DA, Hanna FW, Davies JS, et al: Long-term follow-up results of transsphenoidal surgery for Cushing's disease in a single centre using strict criteria for remission, Clin Endocrinol (Oxf) 56:541–551, 2002.
264. Hughes NR, Lissett CA, Shalet SM: Growth hormone status following treatment for Cushing's syndrome, Clin Endocrinol (Oxf) 51:61–66, 1999.
265. Pereira AM, van Aken MO, van Dulken H, et al: Long-term predictive value of postsurgical cortisol concentrations for cure and risk of recurrence in Cushing's disease, J Clin Endocrinol Metab 88:5858–5864, 2003.
266. Esposito F, Dusick JR, Cohan P, et al: Clinical review: Early morning cortisol levels as a predictor of remission after transsphenoidal surgery for Cushing's disease, J Clin Endocrinol Metab 91:7–13, 2006.
267. Avgerinos PC, Chrousos GP, Nieman LK, et al: The corticotropin-releasing hormone test in the postoperative evaluation of patients with Cushing's syndrome, J Clin Endocrinol Metab 65:906–913, 1987.
268. Nieman LK, Gumowski J, DeVroom H, et al: Prediction of long-term remission of Cushing's disease after successful transsphenoidal resection of ACTH-secreting tumor. Presented at the 80th Annual Meeting of the Endocrine Society P345: New Orleans, LA, 1998.
269. Colombo P, Dall'Asta C, Barbetta L, et al: Usefulness of the desmopressin test in the postoperative evaluation of patients with Cushing's disease, Eur J Endocrinol 143:227–234, 2000.
270. Losa M, Mortini P, Dylgjeri S, et al: Desmopressin stimulation test before and after pituitary surgery in patients with Cushing's disease, Clin Endocrinol (Oxf) 55:61–68, 2001.
271. Byyny RL: Withdrawal from glucocorticoid therapy, N Engl J Med 295:30–32, 1976.
272. Papanicolaou DA, Tsigos C, Oldfield EH, et al: Acute glucocorticoid deficiency is associated with plasma elevations of interleukin-6: does the latter participate in the symptomatology of the steroid withdrawal syndrome and adrenal insufficiency? J Clin Endocrinol Metab 81:2303–2306, 1996.
273. Leshin M: Acute adrenal insufficiency: recognition, management, and prevention, Urol Clin North Am 9:229–235, 1982.
274. Lindsay JR, Nansel T, Baid S, et al: Long-term impaired quality of life in Cushing's syndrome despite initial improvement after surgical remission, J Clin Endocrinol Metab 91:447–453, 2006.
275. Olson BR, Rubino D, Gumowski J, et al: Isolated hyponatremia after transsphenoidal pituitary surgery, J Clin Endocrinol Metab 80:85–91, 1995.
276. Manning PJ, Evans MC, Reid IR: Normal bone mineral density following cure of Cushing's syndrome, Clin Endocrinol (Oxf) 36:229–234, 1992.
277. Di Somma C, Pivonello R, Loche S, et al: Effect of 2 years of cortisol normalization on the impaired bone mass and turnover in adolescent and adult patients with Cushing's disease: a prospective study, Clin Endocrinol (Oxf) 58:302–308, 2003.
278. Di Somma C, Colao A, Pivonello R, et al: Effectiveness of chronic treatment with alendronate in the osteoporosis of Cushing's disease, Clin Endocrinol (Oxf) 48:655–662, 1998.
279. Ram Z, Nieman LK, Cutler GB Jr, et al: Early repeat surgery for persistent Cushing's disease, J Neurosurg 80:37–45, 1994.
280. Locatelli M, Vance ML, Laws ER: Clinical review: the strategy of immediate reoperation for transsphenoidal surgery for Cushing's disease, J Clin Endocrinol Metab 90:5478–5482, 2005.
281. Doherty GM, Nieman LK, Cutler GB Jr, et al: Time to recovery of the hypothalamic-pituitary-adrenal axis after curative resection of adrenal tumors in patients with Cushing's syndrome, Surgery 108:1085–1090, 1990.
282. Plumpton FS, Besser GM: The adrenocortical response to surgery and insulin-induced hypoglycemia in corticosteroid-treated and normal subjects, Br J Surg 55:857, 1968.
283. Bangar V, Clayton RN: How reliable is the short synacthen test for the investigation of the hypothalamic-pituitary-adrenal axis? Eur J Endocrinol 139:580–583, 1998.
284. Kehlet H, Lindholm J, Bjerre P: Value of the 30 min ACTH-test in assessing hypothalamic-pituitary-adrenocortical function after pituitary surgery in Cushing's disease, Clin Endocrinol (Oxf) 20:349–353, 1984.
285. Stewart PM, Corrie J, Seckl JR, et al: A rational approach for assessing the hypothalamo-pituitary-adrenal axis, Lancet 1:1208–1210, 1988.
286. Orme SM, Peacey SR, Barth JH, et al: Comparison of tests of stress-released cortisol secretion in pituitary disease, Clin Endocrinol (Oxf) 45:135–140, 1996.
287. Ammari F, Issa BG, Millward E, Scanion MF: A comparison between short ACTH and insulin stress tests for assessing hypothalamo-pituitary-adrenal function, Clin Endocrinol (Oxf) 44:473–476, 1996.
288. Timmers HJ, van Ginneken EM, Wesseling P, et al: A patient with recurrent hypercortisolism after removal of an ACTH-secreting pituitary adenoma due to an adrenal macronodule, J Endocrinol Invest 29:934–939, 2006.
289. Valimaki M, Pelkonen R, Porkka L, et al: Long-term results of adrenal surgery in patients with Cushing's syndrome due to adrenocortical adenoma, Clin Endocrinol (Oxf) 20:229–236, 1984.
290. Bellantone R, Ferrante A, Boscherini M, et al: Role of reoperation in recurrence of adrenal cortical carcinoma: results from 188 cases collected in the Italian National Registry for Adrenal Cortical Carcinoma, Surgery 122:1212–1218, 1997.
291. McCallum RW, Connell JM: Laparoscopic adrenalectomy, Clin Endocrinol (Oxf) 55:435–436, 2001.
292. Wells SA, Merke DP, Cutler GB Jr, et al: Therapeutic controversy: The role of laparoscopic surgery in adrenal disease, J Clin Endocrinol Metab 83:3041–3049, 1998.
293. Kemink L, Pieters G, Hermus A, et al: Patient's age is a simple predictive factor for the development of Nelson's syndrome after total adrenalectomy for Cushing's disease, J Clin Endocrinol Metab 79:887–889, 1994.
294. Assie G, Bahurel H, Coste J, et al: Corticotroph tumor progression after adrenalectomy in Cushing's Disease: A reappraisal of Nelson's Syndrome, J Clin Endocrinol Metab 92:172–179, 2007.
295. Jenkins PJ, Trainer PJ, Plowman PN, et al: The long-term outcome after adrenalectomy and prophylactic pituitary radiotherapy in adrenocorticotropin-dependent Cushing's syndrome, J Clin Endocrinol Metab 80:165–171, 1995.
296. Sheline GE, Wara WM, Smith V: Therapeutic irradiation and brain injury, Int J Radiat Oncol Biol Phys 6:1215–1228, 1980.
297. Orth DN, Liddle GW: Results of treatment in 108 patients with Cushing's syndrome, N Engl J Med 285:243–247, 1971.

298. Howlett TA, Plowman PN, Wass JA, et al: Megavoltage pituitary irradiation in the management of Cushing's disease and Nelson's syndrome: long-term follow-up, Clin Endocrinol (Oxf) 31:309–323, 1989.

299. Murayama M, Yasuda K, Minamori Y, et al: Long term follow-up of Cushing's disease treated with reserpine and pituitary irradiation, J Clin Endocrinol Metab 75:935–942, 1992.

300. Littley MD, Shalet SM, Beardwell CG, et al: Long-term follow-up of low-dose external pituitary irradiation for Cushing's disease, Clin Endocrinol (Oxf) 33:445–455, 1990.

301. Estrada J, Boronat M, Mielgo M, et al: The long-term outcome of pituitary irradiation after unsuccessful transsphenoidal surgery in Cushing's disease, N Engl J Med 336:172–177, 1997.

302. Mahmoud-Ahmed AS, Suh JH: Radiation therapy for Cushing's disease: a review, Pituitary 5:175–180, 2002.

303. Plowman PN: Pituitary adenoma radiotherapy—when, who and how? Clin Endocrinol (Oxf) 51:265–271, 1999.

304. Becker G, Kocher M, Kortmann RD, et al: Radiation therapy in the multimodal treatment approach of pituitary adenoma, Strahlenther Onkol 178:173–186, 2002.

305. Marks LB: Conventional fractionated radiation therapy vs. radiosurgery for selected benign intracranial lesions (arteriovenous malformations, pituitary adenomas, and acoustic neuromas), J Neurooncol 17:223–230, 1993.

306. Jagannathan J, Sheehan JP, Pouratian N, et al: Gamma Knife surgery for Cushing's disease, J Neurosurg 106:980–987, 2007.

307. Petit JH, Biller BM, Yock TI, et al: Proton stereotactic radiotherapy for persistent adrenocorticotropin-producing adenomas, J Clin Endocrinol Metab 93:393–399, 2008.

308. Swords FM, Allan CA, Plowman PN, et al: Stereotactic Radiosurgery XVI: A Treatment for Previously Irradiated Pituitary Adenomas, J Clin Endocrinol Metab 88:5334–5340, 2003.

309. Sandler LM, Richards NT, Carr DH, et al: Long term follow-up of patients with Cushing's disease treated by interstitial irradiation, J Clin Endocrinol Metab 65:441–447, 1987.

310. Molinatti GM, Limone P, Porta M: Treatment of Cushing's disease by interstitial pituitary irradiation: short- and long-term follow-up, Panminerva Med 37:1–7, 1995.

311. Magee BJ, Gattamaneni HR, Pearson D: Adrenal cortical carcinoma: survival after radiotherapy, Clin Radiol 38:587–588, 1987.

312. de Castro F, Isa W, Aguera L, et al: [Primary adrenal carcinoma], Actas Urol Esp 17:30–34, 1993.

313. He J, Zhou J, Lu Z: Radiotherapy of ectopic ACTH syndrome due to thoracic carcinoids, Chin Med J (Engl) 108:338–341, 1995.

314. Andres R, Mayordomo JI, Cajal S, et al: Paraneoplastic Cushing's syndrome associated to locally advanced thymic carcinoid tumor, Tumori 88:65–67, 2002.

315. Misbin RI, Canary J, Willard D: Aminoglutethimide in the treatment of Cushing's syndrome, J Clin Pharmacol 16:645–651, 1976.

316. Semple CG, Beastall GH, Gray CE, et al: Trilostane in the management of Cushing's syndrome, Acta Endocrinol (Copenh) 102:107–110, 1983.

317. Carballeira A, Fishman LM, Jacobi JD: Dual sites of inhibition by metyrapone of human adrenal steroidogenesis: correlation of in vivo and in vitro studies, J Clin Endocrinol Metab 42:687–695, 1976.

318. Verhelst JA, Trainer PJ, Howlett TA, et al: Short and long-term responses to metyrapone in the medical management of 91 patients with Cushing's syndrome, Clin Endocrinol (Oxf) 35:169–178, 1991.

319. Jeffcoate WJ, Rees LH, Tomlin S, et al: Metyrapone in long-term management of Cushing's disease, Br Med J 2:215–217, 1977.

320. Feldman D: Ketoconazole and other imidazole derivatives as inhibitors of steroidogenesis, Endocr Rev 7:409–420, 1986.

321. Engelhardt D, Weber MM, Miksch T, et al: The influence of ketoconazole on human adrenal steroidogenesis: incubation studies with tissue slices, Clin Endocrinol (Oxf) 35:163–168, 1991.

322. Steen RE, Kapelrud H, Haug E, et al: In vivo and in vitro inhibition by ketoconazole of ACTH secretion from a human thymic carcinoid tumour, Acta Endocrinol (Copenh) 125:331–334, 1991.

323. Sonino N, Boscaro M, Paoletta A, et al: Ketoconazole treatment in Cushing's syndrome: experience in 34 patients, Clin Endocrinol (Oxf) 35:347–352, 1991.

324. Tabarin A, Navarranne A, Guerin J, et al: Use of ketoconazole in the treatment of Cushing's disease and ectopic ACTH syndrome, Clin Endocrinol (Oxf) 34:63–69, 1991.

325. Ahmed M, Kanaan I, Alarifi A, et al: ACTH-producing pituitary cancer: experience at the King Faisal Specialist Hospital & Research Centre, Pituitary 3:105–112, 2000.

326. Lewis JH, Zimmerman HJ, Benson GD, et al: Hepatic injury associated with ketoconazole therapy. Analysis of 33 cases, Gastroenterology 86:503–513, 1984.

327. Duarte PA, Chow CC, Simmons F, et al: Fatal hepatitis associated with ketoconazole therapy, Arch Intern Med 144:1069–1070, 1984.

328. Knight TE, Shikuma CY, Knight J: Ketoconazole-induced fulminant hepatitis necessitating liver transplantation, J Am Acad Dermatol 25:398–400, 1991.

329. McCance DR, Ritchie CM, Sheridan B, et al: Acute hypoadrenalism and hepatotoxicity after treatment with ketoconazole, Lancet 1:573, 1987.

330. Tucker WS Jr, Snell BB, Island DP, et al: Reversible adrenal insufficiency induced by ketoconazole, JAMA 253:2413–2414, 1985.

331. Miettinen TA: Cholesterol metabolism during ketoconazole treatment in man, J Lipid Res 29:43–51, 1988.

332. Riedl M, Maier C, Zettinig G, et al: Long term control of hypercortisolism with fluconazole: case report and in vitro studies, Eur J Endocrinol 154:519–524, 2006.

333. Hart MM, Swackhamer ES, Straw JA: Studies on the site of action of o,p'-DDD in the dog adrenal cortex. II, Steroids 17:575–586, 1971.

334. Ojima M, Saitoh M, Itoh N, et al: [The effects of o,p'-DDD on adrenal steroidogenesis and hepatic steroid metabolism], Nippon Naibunpi Gakkai Zasshi 61:168–178, 1985.

335. Bergenstal DM, Hertz R, Lipsett MB, et al: Chemotherapy of adrenocortical cancer with O,p'DDD, Ann Intern Med 53:672–682, 1960.

336. Gutierrez ML, Crooke ST: Mitotane (o,p'-DDD), Cancer Treat Rev 7:49–55, 1980.

337. Kasperlik-Zaluska AA: Clinical results of the use of mitotane for adrenocortical carcinoma, Braz J Med Biol Res 33:1191–1196, 2000.

338. Terzolo M, Angeli A, Fassnacht M, et al: Adjuvant mitotane treatment for adrenocortical carcinoma, N Engl J Med 356:2372–2380, 2007.

339. van Slooten H, Moolenaar AJ, van Seters AP, et al: The treatment of adrenocortical carcinoma with o,p'-DDD: prognostic implications of serum level monitoring, Eur J Cancer Clin Oncol 20:47–53, 1984.

340. Bukowski RM, Wolfe M, Levine HS, et al: Phase II trial of mitotane and cisplatin in patients with adrenal carcinoma: a Southwest Oncology Group study, J Clin Oncol 11:161–165, 1993.

341. Berruti A, Terzolo M, Pia A, et al: Mitotane associated with etoposide, doxorubicin, and cisplatin in the treatment of advanced adrenocortical carcinoma. Italian Group for the Study of Adrenal Cancer, Cancer 83:2194–2200, 1998.

342. Williamson SK, Lew D, Miller GJ, et al: Phase II evaluation of cisplatin and etoposide followed by mitotane at disease progression in patients with locally advanced or metastatic adrenocortical carcinoma: a Southwest Oncology Group Study, Cancer 88:1159–1165, 2000.

343. Luton JP, Mahoudeau JA, Bouchard P, et al: Treatment of Cushing's disease by O,p'DDD. Survey of 62 cases, N Engl J Med 300:459–464, 1979.

344. Schteingart DE, Tsao HS, Taylor CI, et al: Sustained remission of Cushing's disease with mitotane and pituitary irradiation, Ann Intern Med 92:613–619, 1980.

345. Carey RM, Orth DN, Hartmann WH: Malignant melanoma with ectopic production of adrenocorticotropic hormone. Palliative treatment with inhibitors of adrenal steroid biosynthesis, J Clin Endocrinol Metab 36:482–487, 1973.

346. Hutter AM Jr, Kayhoe DE: Adrenal cortical carcinoma. Results of treatment with o,p'DDD in 138 patients, Am J Med 41:581–592, 1966.

347. Luton JP, Cerdas S, Billaud L, et al: Clinical features of adrenocortical carcinoma, prognostic factors, and the effect of mitotane therapy, N Engl J Med 322:1195–1201, 1990.

348. Haak HR, Caekebeke-Peerlinck KM, van Seters AP, et al: Prolonged bleeding time due to mitotane therapy, Eur J Cancer 27:638–641, 1991.

349. Maher VM, Trainer PJ, Scoppola A, et al: Possible mechanism and treatment of o,p'DDD-induced hypercholesterolaemia, Q J Med 84:671–679, 1992.

350. Leiba S, Weinstein R, Shindel B, et al: The protracted effect of o,p'-DDD in Cushing's disease and its impact on adrenal morphogenesis of young human embryo, Ann Endocrinol (Paris) 50:49–53, 1989.

351. van Seters AP, Moolenaar AJ: Mitotane increases the blood levels of hormone-binding proteins, Acta Endocrinol (Copenh) 124:526–533, 1991.

352. Hague RV, May W, Cullen DR: Hepatic microsomal enzyme induction and adrenal crisis due to o,p'DDD therapy for metastatic adrenocortical carcinoma, Clin Endocrinol (Oxf) 31:51–57, 1989.

353. Ledingham IM, Watt I: Influence of sedation on mortality in critically ill multiple trauma patients, Lancet 1:1270, 1983.

354. Weber MM, Lang J, Abedinpour F, et al: Different inhibitory effect of etomidate and ketoconazole on the human adrenal steroid biosynthesis, Clin Investig 71:933–938, 1993.

355. Lamberts SW, Bons EG, Bruining HA, et al: Differential effects of the imidazole derivatives etomidate, ketoconazole and miconazole and of metyrapone on the secretion of cortisol and its precursors by human adrenocortical cells, J Pharmacol Exp Ther 240:259–264, 1987.

356. Schulte HM, Benker G, Reinwein D, et al: Infusion of low dose etomidate: correction of hypercortisolemia in patients with Cushing's syndrome and dose-response relationship in normal subjects, J Clin Endocrinol Metab 70:1426–1430, 1990.

357. Allolio B, Schulte HM, Kaulen D, et al: Nonhypnotic low-dose etomidate for rapid correction of hypercortisolaemia in Cushing's syndrome, Klin Wochenschr 66:361–364, 1988.

358. Herrmann BL, Mitchell A, Saller B, et al: [Transsphenoidal hypophysectomy of a patient with an ACTH-producing pituitary adenoma and an "empty sella" after pretreatment with etomidate], Dtsch Med Wochenschr 126:232–234, 2001.

359. Drake WM, Perry LA, Hinds CJ, et al: Emergency and prolonged use of intravenous etomidate to control hypercortisolemia in a patient with Cushing's syndrome and peritonitis, J Clin Endocrinol Metab 83:3542–3544, 1998.

360. Krakoff J, Koch CA, Calis KA, et al: Use of a parenteral propylene glycol-containing etomidate preparation for the long-term management of ectopic Cushing's syndrome, J Clin Endocrinol Metab 86:4104–4108, 2001.

361. Greening JE, Brain CE, Perry LA, et al: Efficient short-term control of hypercortisolaemia by low-dose etomidate in severe paediatric Cushing's disease, Horm Res 64:140–143, 2005.

362. Sartor O, Cutler GB Jr: Mifepristone: treatment of Cushing's syndrome, Clin Obstet Gynecol 39:506–510, 1996.

363. Waveren Hogervorst CO, Koppeschaar HP, Zelissen PM, et al: Cortisol secretory patterns in Cushing's disease and response to cyproheptadine treatment, J Clin Endocrinol Metab 81:652–655, 1996.

364. Sonino N, Fava GA, Fallo F, et al: Effect of the serotonin antagonists ritanserin and ketanserin in Cushing's disease, Pituitary 3:55–59, 2000.

365. Mercado-Asis LB, Yasuda K, Murayama M, et al: Beneficial effects of high daily dose bromocriptine treatment in Cushing's disease, Endocrinol Jpn 39:385–395, 1992.

366. Pivonello R, Ferone D, de Herder WW, et al: Dopamine receptor expression and function in corticotroph pituitary tumors, J Clin Endocrinol Metab 89:2452–2462, 2004.

367. Colao A, Pivonello R, Tripodi FS, et al: Failure of long-term therapy with sodium valproate in Cushing's disease, J Endocrinol Invest 20:387–392, 1997.

368. Greenman Y, Melmed S: Heterogeneous expression of two somatostatin receptor subtypes in pituitary tumors, J Clin Endocrinol Metab 78:398–403, 1994.

369. Lamberts SW, de Herder WW, Krenning EP, et al: A role of (labeled) somatostatin analogs in the differential diagnosis and treatment of Cushing's syndrome, J Clin Endocrinol Metab 78:17–19, 1994.

370. de Herder WW, Lamberts SW: Is there a role for somatostatin and its analogs in Cushing's syndrome? Metabolism 45:83–85, 1996.

371. Batista DL, Zhang X, Gejman R, et al: The effects of SOM230 on cell proliferation and adrenocorticotropin secretion in human corticotroph pituitary adenomas, J Clin Endocrinol Metab 91:4482–4488, 2006.

372. Boscaro M, Atkinson AB, Bertherat J, et al: SOM230 Cushing's disease study group. Early data on the efficacy and safety of the novel multi-ligand somatostatin analog SOM230 in patients with Cushing's disease. 87th Annual Meeting of The Endocrine Society, San Diego, CA, June 4–7, 2005, P2-672 2005.

373. Boscaro M, Glusman JE, Ludlam W, et al: Treatment of pituitary dependent Cushing's disease with the multi-receptor ligand somatostatin analog pasireotide (SOM230): A multicenter, phase II trial, J Clin Endocrinol Metab 94:115–122, 2009.

374. Heaney AP, Fernando M, Yong WH, et al: Functional PPAR-gamma receptor is a novel therapeutic target for ACTH-secreting pituitary adenomas, Nat Med 8:1281–1287, 2002.

375. Suri D, Weiss RE: Effect of pioglitazone on adrenocorticotropic hormone and cortisol secretion in Cushing's disease, J Clin Endocrinol Metab 90:1340–1346, 2005.

376. Ambrosi B, Dall'Asta C, Cannavo S, et al: Effects of chronic administration of PPAR-gamma ligand rosiglitazone in Cushing's disease, Eur J Endocrinol 151:173–178, 2004.

377. Pecori GF, Scaroni C, Arvat E, et al: Effect of protracted treatment with rosiglitazone, a PPARgamma agonist, in patients with Cushing's disease, Clin Endocrinol (Oxf) 64:219–224, 2006.

378. Morcos M, Fohr B, Tafel J, et al: Long-term treatment of central Cushing's syndrome with rosiglitazone, Exp Clin Endocrinol Diabetes 115:292–297, 2007.

379. Munir A, Song F, Ince P, et al: Ineffectiveness of rosiglitazone therapy in Nelson's syndrome, J Clin Endocrinol Metab 92:1758–1763, 2007.

380. Sonino N, Boscaro M, Fallo F: Pharmacologic management of Cushing syndrome: new targets for therapy, Treat Endocrinol 4:87–94, 2005.

381. Paez-Pereda M, Kovalovsky D, Hopfner U, et al: Retinoic acid prevents experimental Cushing syndrome, J Clin Invest 108:1123–1131, 2001.

382. Castillo V, Giacomini D, Paez-Pereda M, et al: Retinoic acid as a novel medical therapy for Cushing's disease in dogs, Endocrinology 147:4438–4444, 2006.

383. Shapiro MS, Shenkman L: Variable hormonogenesis in Cushing's syndrome, Q J Med 79:351–363, 1991.

384. Kammer H, Barter M: Spontaneous remission of Cushing's disease. A case report and review of the literature, Am J Med 67:519–523, 1979.

385. Hayslett JP, Cohn GL: Spontaneous remission of Cushing's disease. Report of a case, N Engl J Med 276:968–970, 1967.

386. Meinardi JR, Wolffenbuttel BH, Dullaart RP: Cyclic Cushing's syndrome: a clinical challenge, Eur J Endocrinol 157:245–254, 2007.

387. Brown RD, Van Loon GR, Orth DN, et al: Cushing's disease with periodic hormonogenesis: one explanation for paradoxical response to dexamethasone, J Clin Endocrinol Metab 36:445–451, 1973.

388. Vagnucci AH, Evans E: Cushing's disease with intermittent hypercortisolism, Am J Med 80:83–88, 1986.

389. Kreze A, Veleminsky J, Spirova E: A follow-up of the "low dose suppressible" hypercortisolism, Endocrinol Exp 17:119–123, 1983.

390. Tsuruoka S, Sugimoto K, Fujimura A: Drug-induced Cushing syndrome in a patient with ulcerative colitis after betamethasone enema: evaluation of plasma drug concentration, Ther Drug Monit 20:387–389, 1998.

391. Findlay CA, Macdonald JF, Wallace AM, et al: Childhood Cushing's syndrome induced by betamethasone nose drops, and repeat prescriptions, BMJ 317:739–740, 1998.

392. Quddusi S, Browne P, Toivola B, et al: Cushing syndrome due to surreptitious glucocorticoid administration, Arch Intern Med 158:294–296, 1998.

393. McConkey B: Adrenal corticosteroids in Chinese herbal remedies, QJM 96:81–82, 2003.

394. Mann M, Koller E, Murgo A, et al: Glucocorticoidlike activity of megestrol. A summary of Food and Drug Administration experience and a review of the literature, Arch Intern Med 157:1651–1656, 1997.

395. Cizza G, Nieman LK, Doppman JL, et al: Factitious Cushing syndrome, J Clin Endocrinol Metab 81:3573–3577, 1996.

396. O'Hare JP, Vale JA, Wood S, et al: Factitious Cushing's syndrome, Acta Endocrinol (Copenh) 111:165–167, 1986.

397. Sharp NA, Devlin JT, Rimmer JM: Renal failure obfuscates the diagnosis of Cushing's disease, JAMA 256:2564–2565, 1986.

398. Otokida K, Fujiwara T, Oriso S, et al: Cortisol and its metabolites in the plasma and urine in Cushing's syndrome with chronic renal failure (CRF), compared to Cushing's syndrome without CRF, Nippon Jinzo Gakkai Shi 31:651–656, 1989.

399. Jain S, Sakhuja V, Bhansali A, et al: Corticotropin-dependent Cushing's syndrome in a patient with chronic renal failure–a rare association, Ren Fail 15:563–566, 1993.

400. Luger A, Lang I, Kovarik J, et al: Abnormalities in the hypothalamic-pituitary-adrenocortical axis in patients with chronic renal failure, Am J Kidney Dis 9:51–54, 1987.

401. Siamopoulos KC, Dardamanis M, Kyriaki D, et al: Pituitary adrenal responsiveness to corticotropin-releasing hormone in chronic uremic patients, Perit Dial Int 10:153–156, 1990.

402. Nolan GE, Smith JB, Chavre VJ, et al: Spurious overestimation of plasma cortisol in patients with chronic renal failure, J Clin Endocrinol Metab 52:1242–1245, 1981.

403. Sederberg-Olsen P, Binder C, Kehlet H: Urinary excretion of free cortisol in impaired renal function, Acta Endocrinol (Copenh) 78:86–90, 1975.

404. Ramirez G, Gomez-Sanchez C, Meikle WA, et al: Evaluation of the hypothalamic hypophyseal adrenal axis in patients receiving long-term hemodialysis, Arch Intern Med 142:1448–1452, 1982.

405. Workman RJ, Vaughn WK, Stone WJ: Dexamethasone suppression testing in chronic renal failure: pharmacokinetics of dexamethasone and demonstration of a normal hypothalamic-pituitary-adrenal axis, J Clin Endocrinol Metab 63:741–746, 1986.

406. Rosman PM, Farag A, Peckham R, et al: Pituitary-adrenocortical function in chronic renal failure: blunted suppression and early escape of plasma cortisol levels after intravenous dexamethasone, J Clin Endocrinol Metab 54:528–533, 1982.

407. Rodger RS, Dewar JH, Turner SJ, et al: Anterior pituitary dysfunction in patients with chronic renal failure treated by hemodialysis or continuous ambulatory peritoneal dialysis, Nephron 43:169–172, 1986.

408. Streeten DH, Faas FH, Elders MJ, et al: Hypercortisolism in childhood: shortcomings of conventional diagnostic criteria, Pediatrics 56:797–803, 1975.

409. Magiakou MA, Mastorakos G, Oldfield EH, et al: Cushing's syndrome in children and adolescents. Presentation, diagnosis, and therapy, N Engl J Med 331:629–636, 1994.

410. Weber A, Trainer PJ, Grossman AB, et al: Investigation, management and therapeutic outcome in 12 cases of childhood and adolescent Cushing's syndrome, Clin Endocrinol (Oxf) 43:19–28, 1995.

411. Lee PD, Winter RJ, Green OC: Virilizing adrenocortical tumors in childhood: eight cases and a review of the literature, Pediatrics 76:437–444, 1985.

412. Savage MO, Lienhardt A, Lebrethon MC, et al: Cushing's disease in childhood: presentation, investigation, treatment and long-term outcome, Horm Res 55(Suppl 1):24–30, 2001.

413. Storr HL, Chan LF, Grossman AB, et al: Paediatric Cushing's syndrome: epidemiology, investigation and therapeutic advances, Trends Endocrinol Metab 18:167–174, 2007.

414. Gafni RI, Papanicolaou DA, Nieman LK: Nighttime salivary cortisol measurement as a simple, noninvasive, outpatient screening test for Cushing's syndrome in children and adolescents, J Pediatr 137:30–35, 2000.

415. Batista DL, Riar J, Keil M, et al: Diagnostic tests for children who are referred for the investigation of Cushing syndrome, Pediatrics 120:e575–e586, 2007.

416. Carpenter PC: Diagnostic evaluation of Cushing's syndrome, Endocrinol Metab Clin North Am 17:445–472, 1988.

417. Dias R, Storr HL, Perry LA, et al: The discriminatory value of the low-dose dexamethasone suppression test in the investigation of paediatric Cushing's syndrome, Horm Res 65:159–162, 2006.

418. Hanson JA, Weber A, Reznek RH, et al: Magnetic resonance imaging of adrenocortical adenomas in childhood: correlation with computed tomography and ultrasound, Pediatr Radiol 26:794–799, 1996.

419. Storr HL, Afshar F, Matson M, et al: Factors influencing cure by transsphenoidal selective adenomectomy in paediatric Cushing's disease, Eur J Endocrinol 152:825–833, 2005.

420. Storr HL, Plowman PN, Carroll PV, et al: Clinical and endocrine responses to pituitary radiotherapy in pediatric Cushing's disease: an effective second-line treatment, J Clin Endocrinol Metab 88:34–37, 2003.

421. Davies JH, Storr HL, Davies K, et al: Final adult height and body mass index after cure of paediatric Cushing's disease, Clin Endocrinol (Oxf) 62:466–472, 2005.

422. Scommegna S, Greening JP, Storr HL, et al: Bone mineral density at diagnosis and following successful treatment of pediatric Cushing's disease, J Endocrinol Invest 28:231–235, 2005.

423. Lindsay JR, Nieman LK: The hypothalamic-pituitary-adrenal axis in pregnancy: challenges in disease detection and treatment, Endocr Rev 26:775–799, 2005.

424. Lindsay JR, Jonklaas J, Oldfield EH, et al: Cushing's syndrome during pregnancy: personal experience and review of the literature, J Clin Endocrinol Metab 90:3077–3083, 2005.

425. Welbourn RB, Montgomery DA, Kennedy TL: The natural history of treated Cushing's syndrome, Br J Surg 58:1–16, 1971.

426. Heald AH, Ghosh S, Bray S, et al: Long-term negative impact on quality of life in patients with successfully treated Cushing's disease, Clin Endocrinol (Oxf) 61:458–465, 2004.

427. Wick MR, Rosai J: Neuroendocrine neoplasms of the thymus, Pathol Res Pract 183:188–199, 1988.

428. Jex RK, van Heerden JA, Carpenter PC, et al: Ectopic ACTH syndrome, Diagnostic and therapeutic aspects, Am J Surg 149:276–282, 1985.

429. Torpy DJ, Mullen N, Ilias I, et al: Association of hypertension and hypokalemia with Cushing's syndrome caused by ectopic ACTH secretion: a series of 58 cases, Ann N Y Acad Sci 970:134–144, 2002.

430. Morris DG, Grossman AB: Cushing's syndrome—The diagnosis and differential diagnosis. In Gaillard RC, editor: The ACTH Axis: Pathogenesis, Diagnosis and Treatment, Hingham, 2003, Kluwer, p. 270.

Chapter 9

CLINICALLY NONFUNCTIONING SELLAR MASSES

PETER J. SNYDER and SHLOMO MELMED

Many types of lesions present as a mass within or near the sella turcica (Table 9-1). The majority of sellar masses are pituitary adenomas, even those that are not obviously associated with clinical syndromes. The majority of these clinically nonfunctioning pituitary adenomas are gonadotroph adenomas, but some are relatively silent lactotroph, somatotroph, corticotroph, and thyrotroph adenomas. Determining whether a sellar mass is a pituitary adenoma or other type of sellar mass is important; and if it is a pituitary adenoma, the type of adenoma is significant, because that distinction will determine optimal treatment.

Natural History of a Pituitary or Parasellar Mass

Prior to the advent of sensitive pituitary imaging techniques, a wide spectrum of clinical sequelae were evident from the effects of an enlarging mass arising from within the pituitary or its adjacent structures (Table 9-2). Although it is today relatively uncommon for such a mass to be invasive at the time of diagnosis, the relative subtlety of clinical features may delay the anatomic imaging of such a mass.

Most pituitary and hypothalamic masses are benign neoplasms, with the very rare occurrence of a true primary malignancy with proved distant metastases. Nevertheless, these benign lesions may be aggressively invasive locally into contiguous structures, resulting in clinical features that depend on the anatomic location of the impinging mass. Hemorrhage and infarction, which may often be coincidental, may occur in these masses, especially during pregnancy, when the normal pituitary and its surrounding soft tissue structures are edematous and swollen. Diabetes mellitus and hypertension have also been associated with pituitary infarction. Hemorrhage and infarction of the pituitary and hypothalamus are true endocrine emergencies. Acute pituitary failure may lead to hypoglycemia, hypothermia, hypotension, apoplexy, and death.

Clearly, many pituitary masses undergo silent infarction as evidenced by histologic proof of old infarct tissue in patients with otherwise normal pituitary function. Large infarcts may lead to development of a partial or totally empty pituitary sella. Most of these patients exhibit normal pituitary reserve, implying that the surrounding rim of pituitary tissue is fully functional. Large cysts associated with the hypothalamic-pituitary unit will also give the radiologic appearance of an empty sella. Rarely, functional pituitary adenomas may arise within the remnant pituitary tissue, and these tumors, although their presence is indicated by classical endocrine hyperactivity, may not be visible by sensitive magnetic resonance imaging (MRI) (i.e., <2 mm in diameter). Acute or chronic infection with abscess formation may be an extremely rare occurrence in the pituitary or hypothalamic mass. Many of these mass lesions present with clinically evident hormonal derangements caused by hormone hypersecretion or, more commonly, by failure of pituitary trophic hormone reserve.

Pituitary hormone hyposecretion may be due to the direct pressure effects of the expanding mass on the anterior pituitary

Table 9-1. Types of Sellar Masses

Pituitary hyperplasia
    Lactotroph hyperplasia of pregnancy
    Thyrotroph hyperplasia due to primary hypothyroidism
    Gonadotroph hyperplasia due to primary hypogonadism
Benign tumors
    Pituitary adenomas (somatotroph, lactotroph, corticotroph, gonadotroph, thyrotroph)
    Craniopharyngioma
    Meningioma
    Pituicytoma
Malignant tumors
    Germ cell tumor (ectopic pinealoma)
    Chordoma
    Lymphoma
    Metastatic diseases
    Pituitary carcinomas
Cysts (Rathke's cleft, arachnoid, dermoid, epidermoid)
Lymphocytic hypophysitis
Infiltrative and granulomatous diseases (sarcoidosis, Langerhans cell histiocytosis, tuberculoma)
Abscess
Vascular abnormalities (aneurysm, arteriovenous fistula)

Table 9-2. Local Neurologic Effects of a Pituitary or Hypothalamic Mass

Impacted Structure	Clinical Effect
Optic tract	Loss of red perception, bitemporal hemianopsia, superior or bitemporal field defect, scotoma, blindness
Hypothalamus	Temperature dysregulation, appetite disorders, obesity, thirst disorders, diabetes insipidus, sleep disorders, behavioral dysfunction, autonomic nervous system dysfunction
Cavernous sinus	Ptosis, diplopia, ophthalmoplegia, facial numbness
Temporal lobe	Uncinate seizures
Frontal lobe	Personality disorder, anosmia
Central	Headache, hydrocephalus, psychosis, dementia, laughing seizures

Table 9-3. Spectrum of Functionality of Pituitary Adenomas

Term	Description
Clinically obvious	Typical physical features of excessive hormonal hypersecretion
Clinically subtle	Subtle physical features of excessive hormonal hypersecretion
Clinically silent	Elevated serum concentration of pituitary hormone but not even subtle clinical manifestations
Silent	Type of adenoma identifiable only by immunostaining; normal serum concentration of hormone normally secreted by that cell type

Types of Sellar Masses

PITUITARY ADENOMAS

Any pituitary adenoma type may first be recognized as a sellar mass, even those that usually cause recognizable clinical syndromes, such as corticotroph, somatotroph, and lactotroph adenomas. In some situations, the clinical syndrome (e.g., Cushing's syndrome or acromegaly) is present but not recognized; in other situations, the clinical syndrome is relatively subtle or nonexistent. The latter have been referred to as "silent" adenomas.[1-3] It is probably more accurate, however, to regard the clinical presentations of these adenomas as a spectrum from clinically obvious (e.g., frank acromegaly), to clinically subtle (e.g., slight increase in ring size but still overall normal appearance), to clinically silent (e.g., no clinical manifestations but a high IGF-1),[4,5] to silent (e.g., normal IGF-1 but immunostaining of excised tissue for growth hormone) (Table 9-3).

The most common pituitary adenoma that presents as a sellar mass is a gonadotroph adenoma. They comprise 40% to 50% of all macroadenomas and approximately 80% of clinically nonfunctioning adenomas. They are often not recognized as of gonadotroph cell origin, as they secrete inefficiently, and what they do secrete—intact gonadotropins and their subunits—often do not produce a recognizable clinical syndrome. Consequently, these adenomas are often not recognized until they become so large that they cause neurologic symptoms. Occasionally, however, they do cause recognizable clinical syndromes, as described later under "Clinical Features," and more often they are recognized by finding abnormal serum concentrations of gonadotropins and their subunits.

PITUITARY HYPERPLASIA

Hyperplasia of anterior pituitary cells can result from several causes and results in generalized enlargement of the pituitary. During pregnancy, lactotroph hyperplasia occurs as the result of estrogen stimulation. When a target gland fails, the resulting lack of feedback inhibition on the corresponding pituitary trophic hormone-secreting cells results in hyperplasia. For example, thyrotroph hyperplasia occurs as a consequence of longstanding and untreated primary hypothyroidism, and gonadotroph hyperplasia occurs as a consequence of longstanding and untreated primary hypogonadism.[6-9] When a neuroendocrine tumor secretes growth hormone–releasing hormone excessively, the result is somatotroph hyperplasia.[10]

LYMPHOCYTIC HYPOPHYSITIS

Lymphocytic infiltration of the pituitary usually occurs in late pregnancy or postpartum but can also be seen in women who are not pregnant and infrequently in men.[11] It is characterized

hormone-secreting cells. Alternatively, parasellar pressure effects may directly attenuate synthesis or secretion of hypothalamic hormones, with resultant pituitary failure. In contrast, a not uncommon association of hypothalamic masses is overproduction of a specific hypothalamic hormone with resultant hyperfunctioning of a specific hypothalamic-pituitary–target hormone axis.

The important diagnostic dilemma facing the clinician is to effectively distinguish an adenoma arising from the anterior pituitary gland from other parasellar masses. The compelling reason for this diagnosis is the fact that the management and prognosis of true anterior pituitary neoplasms differ so markedly from those of other nonpituitary masses. Most masses arising from within the sella are benign, hormonally functional or nonfunctional adenomas with comparatively good prognosis after appropriate therapy. Their invasiveness is relatively limited, and only rarely will local vital structures be compromised. In contrast, parasellar masses arising from structures contiguous with the pituitary are often malignant or invasive and usually portend a less favorable prognosis.

by headaches whose intensity is out of proportion to the size of the lesion and by hypopituitarism, in which adrenal insufficiency is unusually prominent.

BENIGN TUMORS, NONPITUITARY
Rathke's Cleft and Other Cysts

During early embryogenesis, the anterior and intermediate lobes of the pituitary gland arise from Rathke's pouch. If the pouch fails to obliterate, cystic remnants remain at the interface between the anterior and posterior pituitary lobes. These small cysts (<5 mm) are found in about 20% of pituitary glands at autopsy.[12] Occasionally a pituitary adenoma may also contain small cleft cysts.[13] The imaging of these cysts on MRI reveals hyperdense or hypodense masses on either TI or T2 images. CT scan reveals the presence of homogenous hypodense areas that may allow differentiation from pituitary adenomas.[14] Other sellar cysts include arachnoid, epidermoid, and dermoid cysts. Although these lesions develop mainly in the cerebellopontine angle, they may also occur in the suprasellar region. Clinical features of compression include internal hydrocephalus, visual disturbances, and rarely growth hormone or ACTH deficiency, hyperprolactinemia, and diabetes insipidus.[15-17] Rarely, a squamous cell carcinoma may develop in the cyst.[18]

Craniopharyngiomas

Craniopharyngiomas[19] are solid or mixed solid-cystic tumors that arise from remnants of Rathke's pouch, either intrasellar or suprasellar. About half present clinically during childhood and adolescence, but some do not present until age 70 or 80 years. The major presenting symptoms are growth retardation in children and abnormal vision in adults. Anterior pituitary hormonal deficiencies and diabetes insipidus are also common. MRI often reveals a heterogeneous signal, and CT scan often shows calcifications. When cut, they often ooze a viscous fluid described as looking like "crankcase oil." Histologically, they show their epithelial origin, either an adamantinomatous or papillary pattern.

The endocrine manifestations of craniopharyngioma usually result from partial or complete pituitary hormonal deficiencies. Growth hormone deficiency, with resultant short stature in childhood, diabetes insipidus, and other anterior pituitary hormonal deficiencies are common. Compression of the pituitary stalk or damage to the dopaminergic neurons in the hypothalamus result in hyperprolactinemia, which sometimes leads to misdiagnosis of a craniopharyngioma as a lactotroph adenoma. Although imaging may not easily distinguish the two lesions,[20] a highly asymmetrical mass (especially with preferential posterior or dorsal extension) that does not shrink in response to dopamine agonist treatment should arouse suspicion of craniopharyngioma. A decrease in serum prolactin in response to dopamine agonist treatment, however, does not distinguish between the two. Thus craniopharyngioma may mimic a lactotroph adenoma in imaging, presence of hyperprolactinemia, and response of hyperprolactinemia to dopamine agonist treatment.

The treatment of these lesions is radical surgery, radiotherapy, or a combination of these modalities.[21,22] In selected centers, stereotactic irradiation of the mass has been performed with some success. Nevertheless, regardless of which form of therapy is chosen, the ablation of the mass invariably results in anterior and/or posterior pituitary hormone deficits. Postoperative recurrence may occur in about a fifth of patients who undergo radical surgical excision,[23] while no appreciable difference is noted in the outcome in those who undergo a subtotal surgical excision

followed by radiotherapy. The presence of pure papillary squamous cellular elements may portend a higher surgical recurrence rate.[24] The long-term effects of childhood irradiation for these tumors are considered elsewhere.

Meningiomas

These are usually benign and arise from the meninges anywhere within the head. About 20% arise near the sella,[25] causing visual impairment and hormonal deficiencies. By MRI, meningiomas typically emit a low signal on T1-weighted images and a high signal on T2-weighted images and exhibit intense enhancement after gadolinium.

Pituicytomas

Pituicytomas are rare, benign tumors that arise from pituicytes,[26] which are glial cells of the posterior pituitary. They have no hormonal secretory function and can be diagnosed only histologically by the characteristic histologic pattern of elongated cells in bundles and immunostaining for cell adhesion molecules.

MALIGNANT TUMORS

Some malignant tumors arise within or near the sella, and others metastasize there. Malignancies that arise in the parasellar region include germ cell tumors, sarcomas, chordomas, and lymphomas. Pituitary carcinomas also arise within the sella but are exceedingly rare.

Germ Cell Tumors (Ectopic Pinealomas)

Suprasellar germ cell tumors[27] usually occur through the third decade of life and are histologically and biologically similar to germ cell tumors in other anatomic locations, such as germinomas, teratomas, embryonal carcinomas, and choriocarcinomas. They may present with headache, nausea, vomiting, and lethargy (from increased intracranial pressure in patients with pineal lesions), diplopia, hypopituitarism or diabetes insipidus (with suprasellar tumors), and paralysis of upward conjugate gaze. If the tumor is in the pineal, imaging will show a mass in the third ventricle; if the tumor is in the infundibulum, it will be thickened.[28] Serum concentrations of human chorionic gonadotropin beta (β-hCG), and/or alpha fetoprotein (AFP) may be increased. Although these lesions are highly malignant and metastasize readily, they are also highly radiosensitive.

Chordomas

Chordomas are slowly growing malignancies that arise from notochord remnants. Chordomas that arise in the clivus, the bone that is the base of the sella turcica, may present with headaches, visual impairment, and anterior pituitary hormonal deficiencies. MRI often shows a heterogeneous sellar mass associated with osteolytic bony erosion and calcification that may or may not be distinct from the normal pituitary. Histologically, they exhibit markers for epithelial cells, including cytokeratin and vimentin. After surgical excision, local invasion and recurrence commonly occur; mean patient survival is about 5 years. Rarely, chordomas become sarcomatous, sometimes after single fraction gamma- or proton-beam radiation,[29,30] and then they are more aggressive.

Primary Lymphoma

Primary central nervous system (CNS) lymphoma sometimes involves the pituitary and hypothalamus. A review of 13 patients with pituitary involvement noted neurologic symptoms, including headaches and visual and oculomotor impairment, and/or deficiencies of anterior pituitary hormones and vasopressin.[31] MRI shows a sellar mass with variable extrasellar extension.

Metastatic Disease

Metastases to the hypothalamus and pituitary gland occur most commonly with breast cancer in women and lung cancer in men but are encountered with other cancers.[32,33] Symptoms include diabetes insipidus, anterior pituitary dysfunction, visual field defects, retro-orbital pain, and ophthalmoplegia.[32,34] Reflecting that these are patients with metastatic disease, survival is not long; in 36 patients in one series, average survival was 6 months.[33] Up to one quarter of patients with metastatic breast cancer have pituitary metastases. Interestingly, symptomatic pituitary metastases may be the presenting sign of previously undiscovered malignancy and even of malignancy of unknown origin. Although anterior pituitary failure is rare, an isolated metastatic deposit in the pituitary stalk without involvement of the anterior lobe may also present with pituitary failure. Metastases to the posterior pituitary lobe are far more common. About 15% of patients with diabetes insipidus harbor metastases from extrapituitary sources. Unfortunately, imaging of the pituitary mass does not distinguish these deposits from a pituitary adenoma unless extensive bony erosion is present. In fact, metastatic pituitary lesions may masquerade as a pituitary adenoma. In several instances, the diagnosis of pituitary metastasis will be made only by histologic study of the specimen removed at transsphenoidal surgery.

Pituitary Carcinoma

Carcinoma arising from anterior pituitary cells is quite rare. When it does occur, the malignancy can arise from any anterior pituitary cell type. Lactotroph,[35] somatotroph, corticotroph,[35] thyrotroph,[36] and gonadotroph[37] carcinomas have been reported. Diagnosis is made by finding a distant extracranial metastasis.

Infiltrative and Granulomatous Diseases

Infiltrative diseases, such as sarcoidosis and Langerhans cell histiocytosis, may cause a sellar mass and often cause widening of the pituitary stalk. Tuberculomas of the sellar region may occur as part of systemic infection or may be isolated to this region. Because these lesions primarily affect the hypothalamus and infundibulum, diabetes insipidus is common, whereas anterior pituitary hormone deficiencies are less frequently encountered. Infiltrative sarcoidosis of the hypothalamic-pituitary unit occurs in most patients with central nervous system sarcoid involvement.[38] Typically these patients present with varying degrees of anterior pituitary failure with or without diabetes insipidus.

Abscess

Pituitary abscesses, which are rare, can occur in a normal or diseased pituitary gland. In immunocompromised subjects, they may be caused by fungi (*Aspergillus*, *Nocardia*, or *Candida albicans*) or *Pneumocystis carinii*. In a series of 24 patients, 16 presented with symptoms and physical findings consistent with a pituitary mass, while only 8 had features suggestive of infection, such as fever, leukocytosis, meningismus.[39] MRI is usually unable to distinguish between pituitary abscess and pituitary adenoma, so most patients are diagnosed at the time of surgical exploration.

Vascular Abnormalities

Aneurysms and arteriovenous fistulas can arise in this region and present as sellar masses. Because they arise from the cavernous sinus, they are more likely than other sellar lesions to cause cranial nerve palsies, eye pain, and headaches. They can usually be recognized by MRI, but a highly vascular meningioma may be confused with an aneurysm.

Etiology of Pituitary Adenomas

All pituitary adenomas appear to be true neoplasms, arising from a somatic mutation of a single progenitor cell that divides repetitively. The evidence for this view comes from studies that show that virtually all pituitary adenomas are monoclonal, that is, arise from a somatic mutation of a single cell. In one study of five women whose pituitary macroadenomas expressed some combination of FSHβ, LHβ, and α subunit and whose peripheral leukocytes were heterozygous for HPRT, the adenomas had predominantly one allele or the other, but not both[40] (Fig. 9-1). This study suggests that gonadotroph adenomas arise from a somatic mutation of a single progenitor cell that then proliferates. Other studies present similar evidence that other types of pituitary adenomas are also clonal.[41]

Specific mutations have been identified in association with hereditary pituitary adenomas in multiple endocrine neoplasia type I (MEN 1), Carney complex, and familial isolated acromegaly associated with mutations of aryl hydrocarbon receptor interacting protein (AIP). In MEN 1,[42] a mutation of the *MEN1* gene results in decreased expression of the tumor suppressor gene menin and development of adenomas of the pituitary, parathyroids, and pancreas. All pituitary adenoma types can occur in MEN 1, most commonly lactotroph and somatotroph adenomas, and rarely including gonadotroph adenomas[37,43] and those identified only as clinically nonfunctioning.[44-46] In the Carney complex, about half the patients have germ line inactivating mutations in the regulatory subunit type I of the c-AMP-dependent protein kinase A gene (*PRKARIA*).[47] The resulting phenotype consists of somatotroph adenomas, myxomas of the heart, skin, and breast, spotty skin pigmentation (multiple skin lentigines and blue nevi), schwannomas, ovarian cysts, and adrenal, testicular, and thyroid tumors. Mutations of AIP have been found in familial acromegaly in Finland[48] but infrequently in familial acromegaly in other countries.

About 40% of somatotroph adenomas are associated with mutations of the gene encoding the alpha subunit of the G

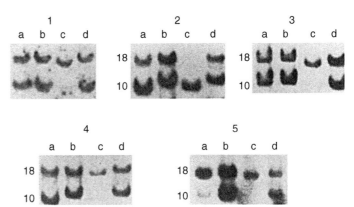

FIGURE 9-1. Demonstration of clonality of pituitary adenomas. Southern blots from extracts of gonadotroph adenomas (*c lanes*) and peripheral leukocytes (*d lanes*) of five women who were heterozygous for the HPRT gene. The peripheral leukocytes from all five women expressed both alleles of the HPRT gene, but the adenomas expressed only one allele or the other. (From Alexander JM, Biller BMK, Bikkal H, Zervas NT, Arnold A, Klibanski A: Clinically nonfunctioning pituitary tumors are monoclonal in origin. J Clin Invest 86:336–340, 1990.)

stimulatory protein ($G_{s\alpha}$), and as a consequence, constitutively activating adenylyl cyclase and increasing cAMP, which is mitogenic to somatotroph cells, thereby resulting in somatotroph adenomas.[49] Mutations that cause other pituitary adenomas, including gonadotroph adenomas, are not known. Investigators have searched for other mutations that might be causally related to development of other pituitary adenomas, but none of these has been clearly associated with the pathogenesis of any pituitary adenoma. Three genes have been identified that might be related to the pathogenesis of pituitary adenomas. One is the pituitary tumor transforming gene *(PTTG)*, which was cloned from GH4 cells, a rat pituitary tumor cell line.[50] It is overexpressed in the majority of human pituitary adenomas of all cell types compared with nonadenomatous pituitary tissue.[51] Another is a truncated form of the fibroblast growth factor receptor 4, which has been identified in all types of human pituitary adenomas. A third is the MEG3 tumor suppressor gene, expression of which is selectively lost in nonfunctioning adenomas by hypermethylation.[52]

External hormonal stimulation from the hypothalamus is unlikely to be a primary cause of gonadotroph adenomas but might have a secondary effect on adenoma growth and probably has an effect on adenoma secretion, since administration of the GnRH antagonist Nal-Glu GnRH to patients who have gonadotroph adenomas and supranormal serum FSH concentrations lowers FSH levels to normal.[53]

Clinical Features

NEUROLOGIC FEATURES

Clinically nonfunctioning sellar masses, by definition, do not cause florid syndromes of hormonal excess and as a result often grow unrecognized until they become so large as to cause neurologic symptoms, including abnormalities of vision and oculomotor function (see Table 9-2).

Visual Abnormalities

A mass within or near the sella that stretches the optic chiasm or nerves sufficiently may result in visual impairment. Masses that arise below the optic chiasm, such as pituitary adenomas, may extend superiorly to elevate and then stretch the chiasm sufficiently to cause visual field abnormalities, initially of the upper, outer quadrants (bilateral superior quadrantopsia) and then of the outer halves (bilateral hemianopsia), before much later affecting central vision and visual acuity. Masses that arise above the chiasm may first cause asymmetric impairment of inferior visual fields. They may be reversible once the masses have been partially or completely excised.

Oculomotor Abnormalities

Masses that arise within the sella and extend into a cavernous sinus may affect one or more of the oculomotor nerves on that side, resulting in diplopia, impaired extraoculomotor movements, and/or ptosis. A dramatic example of this phenomenon is the sudden development of these findings following pituitary apoplexy, the sudden occurrence of bleeding into the pituitary or into a preexisting adenoma.

Other

Other neurologic manifestations of sellar masses are headaches, cerebrospinal fluid leakage and meningitis, and hydrocephalus. Any kind of sellar mass can cause a headache; those that grow more rapidly are more likely to do so. CSF rhinorrhea is uncommon. When it does occur, it is the result of an aggressive pituitary adenoma that extends inferiorly and erodes the cribriform plate, allowing the leakage of CSF, which in turn predisposes to retrograde infection and meningitis. Hydrocephalus is also uncommon. When it occurs it is often the result of a suprasellar lesion that obstructs the fourth ventricle.

ENDOCRINOLOGIC FEATURES

Hormonal Excess—Gonadotroph Adenomas

Serum Concentrations of Gonadotropins and Their Subunits

Although gonadotroph adenomas are typically clinically nonfunctioning, because they secrete inefficiently and because their secretory products—intact gonadotropins and their subunits—usually do not cause a clinical syndrome, they often can be identified by their basal and stimulated secretory products (Table 9-4). Gonadotroph adenomas often basally secrete sufficient intact FSH to result in a supranormal serum FSH concentration. In a series of 38 men who had clinically nonfunctioning pituitary adenomas, 10 had supranormal serum FSH concentrations.[54] The degree of FSH elevation may range from minimal to 10 times the upper limit of normal. Intact FSH secreted by gonadotroph adenomas appears to be normal or nearly normal in size,[55] charge,[56] and biological activity in vitro.[57] In contrast, gonadotroph adenomas uncommonly produce supranormal serum concentrations of intact LH, but when they do, the serum testosterone concentration is elevated.[58-60] About 15% of men who have gonadotroph adenomas have supranormal basal serum concentrations of gonadotropin subunits α, FSHβ, or LHβ.[54] Administration of synthetic TRH to patients who have gonadotroph adenomas often produces an increase in the serum concentrations of intact gonadotropins and their subunits, especially of the LHβ subunit.[54,61]

Clinical Syndromes

Gonadotroph adenomas sometimes result in recognizable clinical syndromes (Table 9-5). One syndrome that is being recognized with increasing frequency is ovarian hyperstimulation when a gonadotroph adenoma secretes intact FSH.[62-66] Continu-

Table 9-4. Hormonal Criteria for the Diagnosis of Gonadotroph Adenomas

Men	Women
Supranormal Basal Serum Concentrations of	
FSH	FSH but not LH
α LHβ, or FSHβ subunits	Any subunit relative to intact FSH and intact LH
LH and testosterone	FSH and estradiol
Supranormal Response to TRH of	
FSH	FSH
LH	LH
LHβ (most common)	LHβ (most common)

Table 9-5. Clinical Syndromes Associated With Gonadotroph Adenomas

Ovarian hyperstimulation
Pituitary apoplexy following GnRH or GnRH analog administration
   Acute GnRH administration
   GnRH analog treatment for prostate carcinoma
Large testicular size
Premature puberty in a prepubertal boy

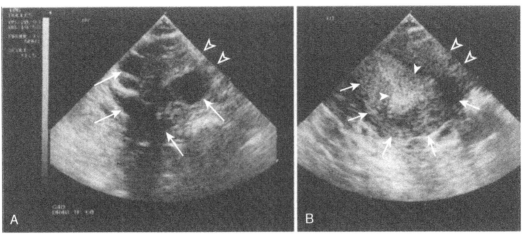

FIGURE 9-2. Ultrasound of ovaries **(A)** and uterus **(B)** in a 39-year-old woman who had a gonadotroph adenoma secreting FSH and causing ovarian hyperstimulation. In **A,** the *closed arrows* indicate large ovarian cysts. In **B,** the *thin arrows* indicate the uterus, and the *wide arrows* indicate the thickened endometrium. The distance between the *open arrows* is 1 cm. (From Djerassi A, Coutifaris C, West VA, Asa SL, Kapoor SC, Pavlou SN, Snyder PJ: Gonadotroph adenoma in a premenopausal woman secreting follicle-stimulating hormone and causing ovarian hyperstimulation. J Clin Endocrinol Metab 80:591–594, 1995.)

ous secretion of FSH by the adenoma, in contrast to cyclical secretion by normal gonadotroph cells, results in very large ovaries, oligomenorrhea, and multiple large cysts and widened endometrial stripe, all detected by pelvic ultrasound (Fig. 9-2). This clinical picture can be mistaken for polycystic ovarian syndrome, but administration of a superactive GnRH analog to a patient with the gonadotroph adenoma results in increased, rather than decreased, FSH secretion and ovarian size and function.[67] Typically in these patients, the serum FSH concentration is elevated and the LH concentration is suppressed, and the concentrations of α subunit and estradiol are elevated. The estradiol concentration is often higher than 500 pg/mL and sometimes as high as 2000 pg/mL. Excision of the gonadotroph adenoma can lead to restoration of normal gonadotropin secretion and ovarian function, and pregnancy can occur.[67,68]

Other clinical presentations of gonadotroph adenomas are less common. One is pituitary apoplexy following GnRH or GnRH analog administration to patients with a gonadotroph adenoma. Recent reports describe discovery of previously unrecognized gonadotroph adenomas when GnRH superactive analogs were administered to treat prostate cancer.[69-71] Enlargement of a gonadotroph adenoma, without apoplexy, was also reported when a superactive GnRH analog was administered for prostate cancer.[72] Another presentation is large testicular size in a hypogonadal man. Yet another presentation is premature puberty in a boy whose gonadotroph adenoma secretes intact LH.[73,74]

Hormonal Excess—Other Pituitary Adenomas

Although corticotroph, somatotroph, and lactotroph adenomas often secrete efficiently and therefore usually result in classic clinical syndromes, a minority of these adenomas secrete inefficiently and do not cause a classic clinical syndrome and therefore present as a clinically silent sellar mass. In some of these, subtle features of the syndrome can be detected, and in others no clinical features can be detected, but the serum concentration of the pituitary or target gland hormone is elevated. The latter are termed *clinically silent adenomas.*[4,5]

Hormonal Deficiencies

The large size of many sellar masses commonly causes hormonal hyposecretion due to compression of the pituitary, stalk, or hypothalamus, but these deficiencies often do not compel the patient to seek medical attention. The deficiency most likely to lead a patient to seek medical attention is that of vasopressin, due to damage to the hypothalamus or infundibulum, resulting in diabetes insipidus. Patients who have deficiencies of anterior pituitary hormones, when questioned, however, often do report symptoms. Even in the absence of symptoms, testing for hypocortisolism, hypothyroidism, and hypogonadism may detect deficiencies.

Diagnosis

Establishing the diagnosis of a clinically nonfunctioning sellar mass usually proceeds from recognizing that a patient's visual abnormality or other neurologic symptom could be caused by a sellar lesion, to confirming the presence of the lesion by an imaging procedure, to characterizing the lesion by its hormonal features. Alternatively, the sellar mass may have been found incidentally ("incidentaloma") when an MRI was performed because of symptoms unrelated to the mass, in which case the next step is to attempt to characterize the lesion by its hormonal features.

UTILITY OF DIAGNOSING A CLINICALLY NONFUNCTIONING SELLAR MASS

Identifying the specific type of sellar mass is desirable in distinguishing a pituitary from a nonpituitary lesion and in providing a marker by which to monitor the treatment response. Distinguishing the lesion as of pituitary rather than nonpituitary origin is of value because it influences treatment. If surgery is indicated, for example, a pituitary lesion is almost always approached transsphenoidally, no matter how large, because it is situated below the diaphragm sella, but a meningioma should be approached transcranially if it arises above the diaphragm sella. If the lesion is a somatotroph adenoma, identified by an elevated serum concentration of IGF-1, medical treatment may be an option. Finding a tumor marker such as an elevated IGF-1, characteristic of a somatotroph adenoma, or an elevated serum FSH, characteristic of a gonadotroph adenoma, not only identifies the lesion as of somatotroph or gonadotroph origin but also provides a means

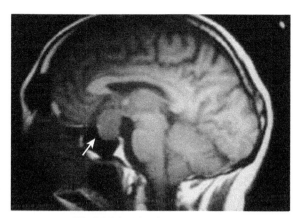

FIGURE 9-3. MRI of large sellar mass.

by which to follow the response to treatment. For example, when the serum FSH concentration is elevated prior to surgery, the decrease after surgery correlates with reduction in adenoma mass seen by imaging.[75]

IMAGING OF THE SELLAR REGION

Magnetic resonance imaging is currently the best imaging technique for the sellar region. If MRI shows a lesion that is clearly above the sella and distant from the pituitary, it is safe to say it is not a pituitary lesion, but for a lesion within the sella, with or without extrasellar extension, MRI does not distinguish a pituitary adenoma from other sellar lesions or one kind of pituitary adenoma from another (Fig. 9-3). Some MRI features suggest a greater likelihood of one type of lesion than another, but none is pathognomonic. For example, a sellar mass with a thin rim of tissue that emits a strong signal after gadolinium administration and a core that emits little signal suggests a cystic lesion, such as a Rathke's cleft cyst, but a largely cystic pituitary adenoma cannot be excluded. Another example is a sellar mass that is somewhat irregular in shape and emits a heterogeneous signal, which is typical of a craniopharyngioma, but a pituitary adenoma can also present similarly. A converse example is an invasive lesion of the clivus, which is typical of a chordoma, but some pituitary adenomas extend primarily into the clivus and therefore can be mistaken for a chordoma. Because of the limitations of imaging in distinguishing types of sellar lesions, endocrinologic testing is invariably necessary.

ENDOCRINOLOGIC TESTS

Sellar mass lesions should be evaluated by measurement of serum concentrations of pituitary hormones and related target gland hormones to determine if the lesion is of pituitary or nonpituitary origin, and if pituitary, the cell of origin. A prolactin concentration above 100 ng/mL, and especially above 200 ng/mL, suggests a lactotroph adenoma[76]; an elevated IGF-1 concentration suggests a somatotroph adenoma even if the patient does not exhibit features of acromegaly; an elevated 24-hour urine cortisol suggests a corticotroph adenoma even if the patient does not exhibit features of hypercortisolemia; and an elevated serum T_4 associated with a TSH value that is not suppressed suggests a thyrotroph adenoma.

Suspicion that the lesion is a gonadotroph adenoma depends on the absence of findings suggestive of another adenoma type, as well as the presence of specific combinations of intact gonadotropins and their subunits (see Table 9-4). The combinations differ somewhat in men and women. In a man who has a

pituitary macroadenoma, elevated basal serum concentrations of intact gonadotropins and/or their subunits alone or in combination with responses of any of these to TRH is strong evidence that the adenoma is of gonadotroph origin. An elevated basal FSH concentration is common. In a woman of postmenopausal age, elevated basal serum concentrations of intact FSH or gonadotropin subunits are usually of little diagnostic value, because either the adenoma or the nonadenomatous postmenopausal gonadotroph cells could be the source. However, a gonadotroph adenoma is likely if intact FSH is markedly elevated but LH is not at all elevated, or if one of the gonadotropin subunits is distinctly elevated but intact FSH and LH are not elevated.[61] More commonly, however, the diagnosis depends on finding an LHβ subunit response to TRH. In a woman of premenopausal age, ovarian hyperstimulation, including elevated serum estradiol concentration, as discussed earlier, elevated FSH out of proportion to LH levels, or elevated basal α subunit concentration all point to the gonadotroph nature of the sellar mass.

Gonadotroph adenomas can usually be readily distinguished from pituitary enlargement due to gonadotroph hyperplasia that results from longstanding primary hypogonadism. The pituitary enlargement seen with primary hypogonadism is not as prominent as that observed with gonadotroph adenomas at the time of presentation. In primary hypogonadism, LH as well as FSH is elevated, and neither intact gonadotropins nor their subunits respond to TRH.[77]

HISTOLOGIC EVALUATION

Even when the identity of a sellar mass cannot be determined in vivo, pathologic examination of excised tissue can usually make this identification. Pituitary adenomas have a characteristic appearance that differs from that of the normal pituitary and of other sellar masses. By light microscopy, pituitary adenoma cells do not exhibit the normal pituitary glandular pattern but are arranged in cords or sheets,[78,79] sometimes interspersed with varying amounts of fibrous tissue. In an adenoma, cells are usually homogenously similar in size, but cell size varies considerably among adenomas. Immunostaining for pituitary hormones (GH, ACTH, prolactin, FSHβ, LHβ and TSHβ, and α) usually identifies the adenoma type.

APPROACH TO THE PATIENT WITH A SELLAR MASS

The clinical approach to the patient harboring a pituitary mass is compounded by the observation that the incidence of incidental silent pituitary microadenomas discovered at autopsy is between 10% and 20%. Pituitary cysts, hemorrhages, and infarctions are also not uncommonly discovered at autopsy. With the widespread sensitive imaging techniques, asymptomatic pituitary lesions are being identified with increasing frequency.[80] Pituitary abnormalities compatible with the diagnosis of pituitary microadenomas are detectable in about 10% of the normal adult population. Considering the differential diagnosis of the intrasellar mass discussed previously, and recognizing that most observed lesions represent pituitary adenomas, several issues should be considered in the management of these masses. Of particular concern is whether the mass is hormonally functional, and whether local mass effects are apparent at the time of diagnosis or develop in the future.[80]

Evaluation of pituitary mass function is important, as the onset of symptoms and signs related to disordered hormone secretion are often insidious and may remain unnoticed for years. Clinical evaluation for changes compatible with ACTH, GH, or

PRL hypersecretion or hyposecretion may reveal long-term serious systematic complications, and each may require distinct therapeutic approaches.[81] In the absence of clinical features of a humoral hypersecretory syndrome, recommendations for cost-effective laboratory screening are debatable. The incidence of hormone-secreting tumors in asymptomatic subjects with incidental pituitary masses is low, and low-grade asymptomatic hormone hypersecretion (e.g., for PRL or α subunits) carries questionable long-term risk.

In the absence of evidence for hormone oversecretion, the presence of (or potential for) local compressive effects must be considered. The risk for macroadenoma enlargement towards a compressive macroadenoma is low, so that a decision to operate may be confidently postponed. For hypothalamic or parasellar masses of uncertain origin, a histologic tissue examination may be the only direct approach to yielding an accurate diagnosis. Although distinguishing MRI or CT features may be helpful in the differential diagnosis of the nonpituitary sellar mass, the final diagnosis usually remains elusive until pathologic confirmation is obtained. The benefits of pituitary surgery must also be weighed carefully against the potential side effects,[82] although endoscopic approaches may now facilitate safer access to sellar tissue for histologic diagnosis or resection.[83] If surgery is not indicated, subsequent imaging studies can determine the lesion's slow growth rate, if any. In the absence of tumor growth, the interval between scans may be prolonged, and surgery should not be recommended in these asymptomatic cases. When an incidentally asymptomatic macroadenoma is diagnosed, visual field and pituitary function should be comprehensively evaluated. If these are found to be normal, imaging should be repeated. Progressive enlargement or impingement of vital structures will indicate the need for surgical intervention.

Treatment

Because clinically nonfunctioning sellar masses are often not detected until they become so large that they cause significant visual impairment, treatment usually must be directed at reducing the size of the mass and restoring visual defects as soon as possible. Transsphenoidal and/or endoscopic surgery is the only treatment that meets this criterion. Pituitary adenomas and some other sellar masses are sensitive to radiation, which may be used to prevent regrowth if substantial adenoma tissue remains after surgery. Several pharmacologic treatments have been tried, but none reduces the size of clinically nonfunctioning adenomas reliably. Observation alone is a satisfactory approach in the absence of neurologic symptoms.

SURGERY

Surgical Approaches

Transsphenoidal surgery using the operating microscope replaced transcranial surgery in the 1970s as the preferred treatment for sellar masses thought to be below the diaphragm sella, because that approach allowed excision of more tissue with fewer serious complications. In the past decade, an increasing number of neurosurgeons have been using endoscopic surgery[84-86] instead of or in addition to the operating microscope, and now several series report experience with more than 100 patients who have undergone a procedure involving endoscopy. Some surgeons employ the endoscope exclusively.[87-89] Others use transsphenoidal surgery with the operative microscope for primary resection and

then use an endoscope for assistance in extending surgery within and beyond the sella.[90] Other techniques for guiding surgery are intraoperative MRI, to determine the extent of sellar mass remaining after initial debulking,[91] and intraoperative Doppler to allow operating near and within the cavernous sinuses without damaging the internal carotid arteries.[92] Neurosurgeons are using these and other techniques to extend the reach of surgery in and around the sella to include the cavernous sinuses and suprasellar regions. Some neurosurgeons are now operating on suprasellar lesions, such as craniopharyngiomas, via a transsphenoidal approach.[93-95]

Efficacy of Surgery

Efficacy of surgery for a sellar mass can be judged by the amount of the mass excised, reduction in serum concentrations of secretory products that were elevated before surgery, improvement in vision, and restoration of normal pituitary function. In one series of 230 patients whose visual fields were abnormal before transsphenoidal surgery, the fields improved in 73%, remained the same in 23%, and worsened in 4%.[96] In another series of 113 pituitary adenomas that extended beyond the sella, 81% of those with visual field defects before transsphenoidal surgery experienced improvement in fields after surgery, 19% remained the same, and none worsened.[97] In patients with gonadotroph adenomas who had elevated serum FSH concentrations before transsphenoidal surgery, improvement in vision was paralleled by a decrease in FSH hypersecretion.[75] Few reports of endoscopic surgery describe the degree of mass removal or change in postoperative vision.

Complications of Surgery

Serious complications of transsphenoidal and endoscopic surgery are uncommon when the procedures are performed by surgeons who have great experience with these procedures but are greater when the adenoma is very large and the surgeon has performed fewer procedures. In a survey in which neurosurgeons were asked to report their own experience with transsphenoidal surgery (Table 9-6), serious complications reported by the 958 respondents included some that were serious, including carotid artery injury (1.1%), central nervous system injury (1.3%), loss

Table 9-6. Relationship of a Neurosurgeon's Experience in Performing Transsphenoidal Surgery to the Rate of Complications

| Complication | % of Operations Resulting in Complications | | |
| | Number of Previous Transsphenoidal Surgeries | | |
	<20	20-500	>500
Carotid artery injury	1.4	0.6	0.4
Central nervous system injury	1.6	0.9	0.6
Hemorrhage into tumor bed	2.8	4.0	0.8
Loss of vision	2.4	0.8	0.5
Cerebrospinal fluid leak	4.2	2.8	0.5
Meningitis	1.9	0.8	0.5
Nasal septum perforation	7.6	4.6	3.3
Anterior pituitary insufficiency	20.6	14.9	7.2
Diabetes insipidus	19.0	NA	7.6
Death	1.2	0.6	0.2

Adapted from Ciric I, Ragin A, Baumgartner C, Pierce D: Complications of transsphenoidal surgery: results of a national survey, review of the literature, and personal experience. Neurosurg 40:225–237, 1997.
Data were collected from participating surgeons by questionnaire.

of vision (1.8%), ophthalmoplegia (1.4%), hemorrhage or swelling of the residual tumor (2.9%), cerebrospinal fluid leak (3.9%), meningitis (1.5%), and death (0.9%).[82] The chances of anterior pituitary insufficiencies (19.4%) and diabetes insipidus (17.8%) were higher. The incidence of each complication was higher among neurosurgeons who were less experienced. Among neurosurgeons who reported performing fewer than 200 transsphenoidal procedures, 1.2% of procedures resulted in death, but among neurosurgeons who reported performing more than 500 procedures, only 0.2% resulted in death. Although these results are based on retrospective self-reporting via questionnaire, they provide a broader assessment of complications of transsphenoidal surgery than that provided by individual pituitary surgeons,[97,98] whose complication rates are closer to those of the most experienced group above.[82]

An even broader assessment is provided by a study using the Nationwide Inpatient Sample, 1996-2000, of 5497 operations at 538 hospitals by 825 surgeons, which also demonstrated that surgeons who performed more transsphenoidal operations had fewer complications than those who performed fewer.[99] Odds ratio for one or more complications of surgery or perioperative care was 0.76 for a fivefold larger case load per surgeon (95% confidence interval 0.65 to 0.89; P = 0.005). The lowest quartile of surgeons in this survey performed only one transsphenoidal procedure a year and the highest only eight or more per year, illustrating dramatically that this survey represented a much broader sampling than that of the primarily pituitary neurosurgeons above.

Complication rates are also greater in patients who have had prior pituitary surgery than in those who never had, and even greater in those whose prior surgery was via craniotomy than in those whose prior surgery was transsphenoidal.[100] The types of complications that occur after endoscopic surgery are similar to those that occur after transsphenoidal surgery,[87-89] but no reports directly compare the two approaches.

Evaluation of the Results of Surgery

The results of surgery should initially be evaluated 4 to 6 weeks afterwards by measurement of hormones or subunits that had been elevated before surgery and by assessment of the functions of the nonadenomatous anterior pituitary and vasopressin secretion. Neuroophthalmologic function should likewise be reevaluated. Residual tissue should be evaluated by MRI, generally about 6 months after surgery, to allow time for blood and edema from surgery to resolve.

RADIATION

Techniques of Radiation

Radiation therapy has been used to treat pituitary adenomas, including clinically nonfunctioning adenomas, for decades. The technique that had been used for much of this period employed a supervoltage source to deliver a total of 45 to 50 Gy in daily 2-Gy doses via three external portals. Much of our information about the long-term effects of radiation on the adenomas and surrounding tissues is based on patients treated by this technique. This technique has now been supplanted by techniques in which the radiation is delivered stereotactically to attempt to minimize the amount of radiation to which the brain is exposed. Current techniques employ radiation from one of several sources: protons from a cyclotron, high-energy x-rays from a linear accelerator, or gamma radiation from a ^{60}Co source (Table 9-7). Radiation from a linear accelerator and cyclotron can be

Table 9-7. Types of Pituitary Radiation

Radiation Source	Type of Radiation	Availability of	
		Fractionated Doses	Single Dose
Linear Accelerator	X-radiation	Yes	Yes
^{60}Cobalt	Gamma radiation	No	Yes
Cyclotron	Protons	Yes	Yes

administered either as a single dose or multiple fractions over the course of several weeks. Single-dose techniques are often referred to, inappropriately, as "radiosurgery." All of the techniques use computer-generated models based on magnetic resonance imaging, so that the radiation conforms to boundaries of the lesion.

Efficacy of Radiation

Studies of pre-stereotactic radiation administered following surgery for a pituitary macroadenoma generally showed efficacy in preventing regrowth of the adenoma.[101-103] In one study of men who had radiation therapy following surgery for clinically nonfunctioning pituitary macroadenomas, only 7% of the 63 patients who received radiation following surgery developed new visual impairment requiring additional treatment during the subsequent 15 years, but 66% of the 63 who did not receive radiation developed new visual impairment.[103]

Several series have been reported in recent years describing the efficacy of stereotactic methods of radiation on preventing recurrence of pituitary adenomas and other sellar tumors. In series of patients treated with fractionated radiotherapy using a linear accelerator[104,105] or proton beam[106] and observed for a median of 40 months or more, adenoma size was reduced or stable in 90% to 100%. In a review of 25 studies involving 1621 patients, of whom 452 had clinically nonfunctioning pituitary adenomas and who were treated with single-dose radiation from a linear accelerator, gamma source, or proton beam, adenoma size was controlled in about 90% during a follow-up that was more than 40 months in half.[107] In a report from a single center at which 100 clinically nonfunctioning adenomas were treated with single-dose radiation from a gamma source and followed for a median of 45 months, adenoma volume decreased or remained stable in 92% of patients.[108]

Complications of Radiation

The long-term side effects after pre-stereotactic radiation include hypopituitarism and neurologic deficits. Hypopituitarism, in several studies, began about a year or more after radiation, and by 10 years afterwards, about 50% of patients had a deficiency of ACTH, TSH, or LH.[109-111] Neurologic side effects occurred less commonly. Blindness due to optic neuritis,[112] brain tumors, and cerebrovascular accidents attributed to accelerated local atherosclerosis were reported as case reports and in some series,[113,114] but other series have reported no neurologic sequelae.[115] Although decreased cognitive function has been reported anecdotally after radiation, one systematic study did not confirm this effect.[116]

Although current radiotherapy techniques offer the theoretical advantage of targeting the tumor by stereotactic means, pituitary deficiencies and neurologic complications also occur with these techniques. In the series of 100 patients with clinically nonfunctioning adenomas treated with single-dose gamma radiation and followed for a median of 45 months, 20% developed new hypopituitarism.[108] In the review of 35 studies involving 1621 patients, optic neuropathy occurred in about 1%, other cranial neuropathies in 1.3%, and parenchymal brain damage in about 0.8%.[107]

Management of Patients After Radiation

Hormonal evaluation, both for excessive secretion of whichever hormones and their subunits were secreted excessively by the adenoma prior to treatment and for deficient secretion by the nonadenomatous pituitary, should be performed 6 and 12 months after radiation and once a year thereafter. Evaluation of size by MRI should be performed 1 year after radiation; if the mass is smaller, less frequently thereafter. Neuroophthalmologic evaluation should be repeated after radiation if it was abnormal before.

PHARMACOLOGIC TREATMENT

If a clinically silent pituitary adenoma is found to be associated with an elevated serum concentration of prolactin or growth hormone, pharmacologic treatments typically used for those adenomas can be used, depending on the clinical circumstances.

Several drugs have been administered in attempts to treat gonadotroph adenomas, but none has been found that reduces their size consistently and substantially. Although dopamine does not decrease gonadotropin secretion to an appreciable degree in normal subjects, bromocriptine has been reported to reduce the secretion of intact gonadotropins and α subunit in a few patients, and even to improve vision in one, but not to reduce adenoma size.[117] CV 205-504 has been reported to reduce secretion and adenoma size in occasional patients.[118] Cabergoline has been reported to reduce α subunit concentration in a single patient with a gonadotroph adenoma[119] and to decrease adenoma volume by 10% to 18% in 7 of 13 other patients with gonadotroph adenomas.[120]

The somatostatin analog, octreotide, has been used to treat gonadotroph adenomas, because gonadotroph adenomas express somatostatin receptors and because of the demonstration that somatostatin itself may decrease secretion by gonadotroph adenomas in vitro. Although there have been occasional reports of dramatic decreases in size of gonadotroph adenomas associated with octreotide administration[121,122] and some improvement in vision, the majority of patients have little if any improvement in adenoma size or vision.[121-123] In a report of ten patients with clinically nonfunctioning adenomas, a combination of cabergoline and octreotide decreased adenoma size by 30% only in the six with evidence of secretory activity of FSH, LH, or their subunits.[124]

Several agonist analogs of GnRH have been administered to patients with gonadotroph adenomas, based on the rationale that chronic administration of these agonists causes down-regulation of GnRH receptors on, and decreased secretion of FSH and LH from, normal gonadotroph cells. Administration of GnRH agonist analogs to patients with gonadotroph adenomas, however, generally produces either an agonist effect or no effect on secretion and no effect on adenoma size.[125,126] Administration for 1 week of the GnRH antagonist, Nal-Glu GnRH, to men with gonadotroph adenomas reduced their elevated FSH concentrations to normal.[53] However, when Nal-Glu administration was continued for 6 months, although FSH remained suppressed, adenoma size did not decrease.[127]

OBSERVATION

Observation alone is a reasonable course even for patients who have sellar masses extending outside of the sella and elevating the optic chiasm, as long as the mass is not associated with neurologic symptoms, especially for patients whose surgical risk is high or who prefer not to have surgery until necessary. In a series of 40 patients with clinically nonfunctioning sellar masses, 24 "macro" and 16 "micro," who were followed for a mean of 42 months, the 48-month probability of enlargement was 19% for the micro lesions and 44% for the macros.[128] New or worse visual field defects were observed in 67% of the macro lesions that increased in size.

REFERENCES

1. Horvath E, Kovacs K, Killinger DW, et al: Silent corticotropic adenomas of the human pituitary gland. A histologic study, immunocytologic, and ultrastructural study, Am J Pathol 98:617–638, 1980.
2. Jouanneau E, Ducluzeau PH, Tilikete C, et al: Should silent corticotroph-cell adenoma be classified as a nonfunctional pituitary adenoma? Neurochirurgie 47:128–132, 2001.
3. Klibanski A, Zervas NT, Kovacs K, et al: Clinically silent hypersecretion of growth hormone in patients with pituitary tumors, J Neurosurg 66:806–811, 1987.
4. Sakharova AA, Dimaraki EV, Chandler WF, et al: Clinically silent somatotropinomas may be biochemically active, J Clin Endocrinol Metab 90:2117–2121, 2005.
5. Yamada S, Sano T, Stefaneanu L, et al: Endocrine and morphological study of a clinically silent somatotroph adenoma of the human pituitary, J Clin Endocrinol Metab 76:352–356, 1993.
6. Groff TR, Shulkin BL, Utiger RD, et al: Amenorrhea-galactorrhea, hyperprolactinemia, and suprasellar pituitary enlargement as presenting features of primary hypothyroidism. Obstet Gynecol 63:86S, 1984.
7. Samaan NA, Stephans AV, Danziger J, et al: Reactive pituitary abnormalities in patients with Klinefelter's and Turner's syndromes, Arch Intern Med 139:198–201, 1979.
8. Scheithauer BW, Kovacs K, Horvath E, et al: The pituitary in Turner syndrome, Endocr Pathol 16:195–200, 2005.

9. Scheithauer BW, Moschopulos M, Kovacs K, et al: The pituitary in Klinefelter syndrome, Endocr Pathol 16:133–138, 2005.
10. Thorner MO, Perryman RL, Cronin MJ, et al: Somatotroph hyperplasia, successful treatment of acromegaly by removal of a pancreatic islet tumor secreting a growth hormone-releasing factor, J Clin Invest 70(5):965–977, 1982.
11. Thodou E, Asa SL, Kontogeorgos G, et al: Lymphocytic hypophysitis: clinicopathologic findings, J Clin Endocrinol Metab 80:2302–2311, 1995.
12. el-Mahdy W, Powell M: Transsphenoidal management of 28 symptomatic Rathke's cleft cysts, with special reference to visual and hormonal recovery, Neurosurgery 42:7–16; discussion 16–17, 1998.
13. Nishio S, Mizuno J, Barrow DL, et al: Pituitary tumors composed of adenohypophysial adenoma and Rathke's cleft cyst elements: a clinicopathological study, Neurosurgery 21:371–377, 1987.
14. Mukherjee JJ, Islam N, Kaltsas G, et al: Clinical, radiological and pathological features of patients with Rathke's cleft cysts: tumors that may recur, J Clin Endocrinol Metab 82:2357–2362, 1997.
15. Baskin DS, Wilson CB: Transsphenoidal treatment of non-neoplastic intrasellar cysts. A report of 38 cases, J Neurosurg 60:8–13, 1984.
16. Yamakawa K, Shitara N, Genka S, et al: Clinical course and surgical prognosis of 33 cases of intracranial epidermoid tumors, Neurosurgery 24:568–573, 1989.

17. Lewis AJ, Cooper PW, Kassel EE, et al: Squamous cell carcinoma arising in a suprasellar epidermoid cyst. Case report, J Neurosurg 59:538–541, 1983.
18. Schlachter LB, Tindall GT, Pearl GS: Granular cell tumor of the pituitary gland associated with diabetes insipidus, Neurosurgery 6:418–421, 1980.
19. Karavitaki N, Cudlip S, Adams CB, et al: Craniopharyngiomas, Endocr Rev 27:371–397, 2006.
20. Pigeau I, Sigal R, Halimi P, et al: MRI features of craniopharyngiomas at 1.5 Tesla. A series of 13 cases, J Neuroradiol 15:276–287, 1988.
21. Yasargil MG, Curcic M, Kis M, et al: Total removal of craniopharyngiomas. Approaches and long-term results in 144 patients, J Neurosurg 73:3–11, 1990.
22. Wen BC, Hussey DH, Staples J, et al: A comparison of the roles of surgery and radiation therapy in the management of craniopharyngiomas, Int J Radiat Oncol Biol Phys 16:17–24, 1989.
23. Adamson TE, Wiestler OD, Kleihues P, et al: Correlation of clinical and pathological features in surgically treated craniopharyngiomas, J Neurosurg 73:12–17, 1990.
24. Honegger J, Buchfelder M, Fahlbusch R: Surgical treatment of craniopharyngiomas: endocrinological results, J Neurosurg 90:251–257, 1999.
25. Ciric I, Rosenblatt S: Suprasellar meningiomas, Neurosurgery 49:1372–1377, 2001.
26. Figarella-Branger D, Dufour H, Fernandez C, et al: Pituicytomas, a mis-diagnosed benign tumor of the

neurohypophysis: report of three cases, Acta Neuropathol 104:313–319, 2002.

27. Marsden HB, Birch JM, Swindell R: Germ cell tumours of childhood: a review of 137 cases, J Clin Pathol 34:879–883, 1981.

28. Leger J, Velasquez A, Garel C, et al: Thickened pituitary stalk on magnetic resonance imaging in children with central diabetes insipidus, J Clin Endocrinol Metab 84:1954–1960, 1999.

29. Hara T, Kawahara N, Tsuboi K, et al: Sarcomatous transformation of clival chordoma after charged-particle radiotherapy. Report of two cases, J Neurosurg 105:136–141, 2006.

30. Tsuboi Y, Hayashi N, Kurimoto M, et al: Malignant transformation of clival chordoma after gamma knife surgery—case report, Neurol Med Chir (Tokyo) 47:479–482, 2007.

31. Giustina A, Gola M, Doga M, et al: Clinical review 136: primary lymphoma of the pituitary: an emerging clinical entity, J Clin Endocrinol Metab 86:4567–4575, 2001.

32. Morita A, Meyer FB, Laws ER Jr: Symptomatic pituitary metastases, J Neurosurg 89:69–73, 1998.

33. Schubiger O, Haller D: Metastases to the pituitary-hypothalamic axis, Neuroradiology 34:131–134, 1992.

34. Fassett DR, Couldwell WT: Metastases to the pituitary gland, Neurosurg Focus 16:E8, 2004.

35. Pernicone PJ, Scheithauer BW, Sebo TJ, et al: Pituitary carcinoma. A clinicopathologic study of 15 cases, Cancer 79:804–812, 1996.

36. Mixson AJ, Friedman TC, Katz DA, et al: Thyrotropin-secreting pituitary carcinoma, J Clin Endocrinol Metab 76:529–533, 1993.

37. Benito M, Asa SL, Livolsi VA, et al: Gonadotroph tumor associated with multiple endocrine neoplasia type 1, J Clin Endocrinol Metab 90:570–574, 2005.

38. Cannavo S, Romano C, Buffa R, et al: Granulomatous sarcoidotic lesion of hypothalamic-pituitary region associated with Rathke's cleft cyst, J Endocrinol Invest 20:77–81, 1997.

39. Vates GE, Berger MS, Wilson CB: Diagnosis and management of pituitary abscess: a review of twenty-four cases, J Neurosurg 95:233–241, 2001.

40. Alexander JM, Biller BMK, Bikkal H, et al: Clinically nonfunctioning pituitary tumors are monoclonal in origin, J Clin Invest 86:336–340, 1990.

41. Melmed S: Mechanisms for pituitary tumorigenesis: the plastic pituitary, J Clin Invest 112(11):1603–1618, 2003.

42. Chandrasekhapappa SC, Guru SC, Manickam P, et al: Positional cloning of the gene for multiple endocrine neoplasia-type 1, Science 276:404–407, 1997.

43. Sztal-Mazer S, Topliss DJ, Simpson RW, et al: Gonadotroph adenoma in multiple endocrine neoplasia type 1, Endocr Pract 14:592–594, 2008.

44. Bassett JH, Forbes SA, Pannett AA, et al: Characterization of mutations in patients with multiple endocrine neoplasia type 1, Am J Hum Genet 62:232–244, 1998.

45. Cebrian A, Ruiz-Llorente S, Cascon A, et al: Mutational and gross deletion study of the MEN1 gene and correlation with clinical features in Spanish patients, J Med Genet 40:e72, 2003.

46. Verges B, Boureille F, Goudet P, et al: Pituitary disease in MEN type 1 (MEN1): data from the France-Belgium MEN1 multicenter study, J Clin Endocrinol Metab 87:457–465, 2002.

47. Carney JA, Gordon H, Carpenter PC, et al: The complex of myxomas, spotty pigmentation, and endocrine overactivity, Medicine 64:270–283, 1985.

48. Vierimaa O, Georgitsi M, Lehtonen R, et al: Pituitary adenoma predisposition caused by germline mutations in the AIP gene, Science 312:1228–1230, 2006.

49. Spada A, Arosio M, Bochicchio D, et al: Clinical, biochemical, and morphological correlates in patients bearing growth hormone–secreting pituitary tumors with or without constitutively active adenylyl cyclase, J Clin Endocrinol Metab 71:1421–1426, 1990.

50. Pei L, Melmed S: Isolation and characterization of a pituitary tumor transforming gene (PTTG), Mol Endocrinol 11:433–441, 1997.

51. Zhang X, Horwitz GA, Heaney AP, et al: Pituitary tumor transforming gene (PTTG) expression in pituitary adenomas, J Clin Endocrinol Metab 84:761–767, 1999.

52. Gejman R, Batista DL, Zhong Y, et al: Selective loss of MEG3 expression and intergenic differentially methylated region hypermethylation in the MEG3/DLK1 locus in human clinically nonfunctioning pituitary adenomas, J Clin Endocrinol Metab 93:4119–4125, 2008.

53. Daneshdoost L, Pavlou S, Molitch ME: Inhibition of follicle-stimulating hormone secretion from gonadotroph adenomas by repetitive administration of a gonadotropin-releasing hormone antagonist, J Clin Endocrinol Metab 71:92–97, 1990.

54. Daneshdoost L, Gennarelli TA, Bashey HM, et al: Identification of gonadotroph adenomas in men with clinically nonfunctioning adenomas by the LHβ subunit response to TRH, J Clin Endocrinol Metab 77:1352–1355, 1993.

55. Snyder PJ, Bashey HM, Kim SU, et al: Secretion of uncombined subunits of luteinizing hormone by gonadotroph cell adenomas, J Clin Endocrinol Metab 59:1169–1175, 1984.

56. Chappel SC, Bashey HM, Snyder PJ: Similar isoelectric profiles of FSH from gonadotroph cell adenomas and non-adenomatous pituitaries, Acta Endocrinol 113:311–316, 1986.

57. Galway AB, Hsueh JW, Daneshdoost L, et al: Gonadotroph adenomas in men produce biologically active follicle-stimulating hormone, J Clin Endocrinol Metab 71:907–912, 1990.

58. Snyder PJ, Sterling FH: Hypersecretion of LH and FSH by a pituitary adenoma, J Clin Endocrinol Metab 42:544–550, 1976.

59. Peterson RD, Kourides IA, Horwith M, et al: Luteinizing hormone and α-subunit-secreting pituitary tumor: positive feedback of estrogen, J Clin Endocrinol Metab 51:692–698, 1981.

60. Klibanski A, Deutsch PJ, Jameson JL, et al: Luteinizing hormone-secreting pituitary tumor: biosynthetic characterization and clinical studies, J Clin Endocrinol Metab 64:536–542, 1987.

61. Daneshdoost L, Gennarelli TA, Bashey HM, et al: Recognition of gonadotroph adenomas in women, N Engl J Med 324:589–594, 1991.

62. Djerassi A, Coutifaris C, West VA, et al: Gonadotroph adenoma in a premenopausal woman secreting follicle-stimulating hormone and causing ovarian hyperstimulation, J Clin Endocrinol Metab 80:591–594., 1995.

63. Christin-Maitre S, Rongieres-Bertrand C, Kottler ML, et al: A spontaneous and severe hyperstimulation of the ovaries revealing a gonadotroph adenoma, J Clin Endocrinol Metab 83:3450–3453, 1998.

64. Mor E, Rodi IA, Bayrak A, et al: Diagnosis of pituitary gonadotroph adenomas in reproductive-aged women, Fertil Steril 84:757, 2005.

65. Valimaki MJ, Tiitinen A, Alfthan H, et al: Ovarian hyperstimulation caused by gonadotroph adenoma secreting follicle-stimulating hormone in 28-year-old woman, J Clin Endocrinol Metab 84:4204–4208, 1999.

66. Cooper O, Geller JL, Melmed S: Ovarian hyperstimulation syndrome caused by an FSH-secreting pituitary adenoma, Nat Clin Pract Endocrinol Metab 4:234–238, 2008.

67. Castelbaum AJ, Bigdeli H, Post KD, et al: Exacerbation of ovarian hyperstimulation by leuprolide reveals a gonadotroph adenoma, Fertil Steril 78:1311–1313, 2002.

68. Sugita T, Seki K, Nagai Y, et al: Successful pregnancy and delivery after removal of gonadotrope adenoma secreting follicle-stimulating hormone in a 29-year-old amenorrheic woman, Gynecol Obstet Invest 59:138–143, 2005.

69. Chanson P, Schaison G: Pituitary apoplexy caused by GnRH-agonist treatment revealing gonadotroph adenoma, J Clin Endocrinol Metab 80:2267–2268, 1995.

70. Reznik Y, Chapon F, Lahlou N, et al: Pituitary apoplexy of a gonadotroph adenoma following gonadotrophin releasing hormone agonist therapy for prostatic cancer, J Endocrinol Invest 20:566–568, 1997.

71. Davis A, Goel S, Picolos M, et al: Pituitary apoplexy after leuprolide, Pituitary 9:263–265, 2006.

72. Massoud W, Paparel P, Lopez JG, et al: Discovery of a pituitary adenoma following treatment with a gonadotropin-releasing hormone agonist in a patient with prostate cancer, Int J Urol 13:87–88, 2006.

73. Ambrosi B, Bassti M, Ferrario R, et al: Precocious puberty in a boy with a PRL, LH- and FSH-secreting pituitary tumour: hormonal and immunocytochemical studies, Acta Endocrinol 122:569–576, 1990.

74. Faggiano M, Criscuolo T, Perrone I, et al: Sexual precocity in a boy due to hypersecretion of LH and prolactin by a pituitary adenoma, Acta Endocrinol 102:167–172, 1983.

75. Harris RI, Schatz NJ, Gennarelli T, et al: Follicle-stimulating hormone-secreting pituitary adenomas: correlation of reduction of adenoma size with reduction of hormone hypersecretion after transsphenoidal surgery, J Clin Endocrinol Metab 56:1288–1293, 1983.

76. Karavitaki N, Thanabalasingham G, Shore HC, et al: Do the limits of serum prolactin in disconnection hyperprolactinaemia need re-definition? A study of 226 patients with histologically verified non-functioning pituitary macroadenoma, Clin Endocrinol (Oxf) 65:524–529, 2006.

77. Snyder PJ, Muzyka R, Johnson J, et al: Thyrotropin-releasing hormone provokes abnormal follicle-stimulating hormone (FSH) and luteinizing hormone responses in men who have pituitary adenomas and FSH hypersecretion, J Clin Endocrinol Metab 51:744–748, 1980.

78. Trouillas J, Girod C, Sassolas G, et al: The human gonadotropic adenoma pathologic diagnosis and hormonal correlations in 26 tumors, Semin Diagn Pathol 3:42–57, 1986.

79. Horvath E, Kovacs K: Gonadotroph adenomas of the human related sex-related fine-structural dichotomy, Am J Pathol 117:429–440, 1984.

80. Greenman Y, Melmed S: Diagnosis and management of nonfunctioning pituitary tumors, Annu Rev Med 47:95–106, 1996.

81. Shimon I, Melmed S: Management of pituitary tumors, Ann Intern Med 129:472–483, 1998.

82. Ciric I, Ragin A, Baumgartner C, et al: Complications of transsphenoidal surgery: results of a national survey, review of the literature, and personal experience, Neurosurg 40:225–237, 1997.

83. Jho HD, Carrau RL: Endoscopic endonasal transsphenoidal surgery: experience with 50 patients, J Neurosurg 87:44–51, 1997.

84. Cappabianca P, Cavallo LM, Colao A, et al: Endoscopic endonasal transsphenoidal approach: outcome analysis of 100 consecutive procedures, Minim Invasive Neurosurg 45:193–200, 2002.

85. Jho HD: Endoscopic transsphenoidal surgery, J Neurooncol 54:187–195, 2001.

86. Kawamata T, Iseki H, Ishizaki R, et al: Minimally invasive endoscope-assisted endonasal trans-sphenoidal microsurgery for pituitary tumors: experience with 215 cases comparing with sublabial trans-sphenoidal approach, Neurol Res 24:259–265, 2002.

87. Dehdashti AR, Ganna A, Karabatsou K, et al: Pure endoscopic endonasal approach for pituitary adenomas: early surgical results in 200 patients and comparison with previous microsurgical series, Neurosurgery 62:1006–1015; discussion 1015–1007, 2008.

88. Senior BA, Ebert CS, Bednarski KK, et al: Minimally invasive pituitary surgery, Laryngoscope 118:1842–1855, 2008.

89. Frank G, Pasquini E, Farneti G, et al: The endoscopic versus the traditional approach in pituitary surgery, Neuroendocrinology 83:240–248, 2006.

90. Fatemi N, Dusick JR, de Paiva Neto MA, et al: The endonasal microscopic approach for pituitary adenomas and other parasellar tumors: a 10-year experience, Neurosurgery 63:244–256; discussion 256, 2008.

91. Nimsky C, von Keller B, Ganslandt O, et al: Intraoperative high-field magnetic resonance imaging in transsphenoidal surgery of hormonally inactive pituitary macroadenomas, Neurosurgery 59:105–114; discussion 105–114, 2006.

92. Dusick JR, Esposito F, Malkasian D, et al: Avoidance of carotid artery injuries in transsphenoidal surgery with the Doppler probe and micro-hook blades, Neurosurgery 60:322–328; discussion 328–329, 2007.

93. Gardner PA, Prevedello DM, Kassam AB, et al: The evolution of the endonasal approach for craniopharyngiomas, J Neurosurg 108:1043–1047, 2008.

94. Laufer I, Anand VK, Schwartz TH: Endoscopic, endonasal extended transsphenoidal, transplanum transtuberculum approach for resection of suprasellar lesions, J Neurosurg 106:400–406, 2007.

95. de Divitiis E, Cappabianca P, Cavallo LM, et al: Extended endoscopic transsphenoidal approach for extrasellar craniopharyngiomas, Neurosurgery 61:219–227; discussion 228, 2007.

96. Trautmann JC, Laws ER: Visual status after transsphenoidal surgery at the Mayo Clinic, 1971–1982, Am J Ophthalmol 96:200–208, 1983.

97. Black PM, Zervas NT, Candia GL: Incidence and management of complications of transsphenoidal operations for pituitary adenomas, Neurosurg 20:920–924, 1987.

98. Wilson CB: A decade of pituitary microsurgery, JNeurosurg 61:814–833, 1984.

99. Barker FG 2nd, Klibanski A, Swearingen B: Transsphenoidal surgery for pituitary tumors in the United States, 1996–2000: mortality, morbidity, and the effects of hospital and surgeon volume, J Clin Endocrinol Metab 88:4709–4719, 2003.

100. Laws ER Jr, Fode NC, Redmond MJ: Transsphenoidal surgery following unsuccessful prior therapy, J Neurosurg 63:823–829, 1985.

101. Zaugg M, Adamman O, Pescia R, et al: External irradiation of macroinvasive pituitary adenomas with telecobalt: a retrospective study with long-term follow-up in patients irradiated with doses mostly of between 40–45 Gy, Int J Radiat Oncol Biol Phys 32:671–680, 1995.

102. McCord MW, Buatti JM, Fennel EM, et al: Radiotherapy for pituitary adenoma: long-term outcome and sequelae, Int J Radiat Oncol Biol Phys 39:437–444, 1997.

103. Gittoes NJL, Bates AS, Tse W, et al: Radiotherapy for non-functioning pituitary adenomas, Clin Endocrinol 48:331–337, 1998.

104. Colin P, Jovenin N, Delemer B, et al: Treatment of pituitary adenomas by fractionated stereotactic radiotherapy: a prospective study of 110 patients, Int J Radiat Oncol Biol Phys 62:333–341, 2005.

105. Mackley HB, Reddy CA, Lee SY, et al: Intensity-modulated radiotherapy for pituitary adenomas: the preliminary report of the Cleveland Clinic experience, Int J Radiat Oncol Biol Phys 67:232–239, 2007.

106. Ronson BB, Schulte RW, Han KP, et al: Fractionated proton beam irradiation of pituitary adenomas, Int J Radiat Oncol Biol Phys 64:425–434, 2006.

107. Sheehan JP, Niranjan A, Sheehan JM, et al: Stereotactic radiosurgery for pituitary adenomas: an intermediate review of its safety, efficacy, and role in the neurosurgical treatment armamentarium, J Neurosurg 102:678–691, 2005.

108. Mingione V, Yen CP, Vance ML, et al: Gamma surgery in the treatment of nonsecretory pituitary macroadenoma, J Neurosurg 104:876–883, 2006.

109. Snyder PJ, Fowble B, Schatz NJ, et al: Hypopituitarism following radiation therapy of pituitary adenomas, Am J Med 81:457–462, 1986.

110. Littley MD, Shalet SM, Beardwell CG, et al: Hypopituitarism following external radiotherapy for pituitary tumours in adults, Q J Med 145:160, 1970.

111. Nelson P, Goodman M, Flickenger J, et al: Endocrine function in patients with large pituitary tumors treated with operative decompression and radiation therapy, Neurosurg 24:398–400, 1989.

112. Millar JL, Spry NA, Lamb DS, et al: Blindness in patients after external beam irradiation for pituitary adenoma: two cases occurring after small daily fractional doses, Clin Oncol 3:291–294, 1991.

113. Brada M, Ford D, Ashley S, et al: Risk of second brain tumour after conservative surgery and radiotherapy for pituitary adenoma, Brit Med J 304:1343–1346, 1993.

114. Fisher BJ, Gaspar LE, Noone B: Radiation therapy of pituitary adenoma: delayed sequelae, Radiology 187:843–846, 1993.

115. Dowsett RJ, Fowble B, Sergott RC, et al: Results of radiotherapy in the treatment of acromegaly: lack of ophthalmologic complications, Int J Radiat Oncol Biol Phys 19:453–459, 1990.

116. van Beek AP, van den Bergh AC, van den Berg LM, et al: Radiotherapy is not associated with reduced quality of life and cognitive function in patients treated for nonfunctioning pituitary adenoma, Int J Radiat Oncol Biol Phys 68:986–991, 2007.

117. Stewart PM, Kane KF, Stewart SE, et al: Depot long-acting somatostatin analog (Sandostatin-LAR) is an effective treatment for acromegaly, J Clin Endocrinol Metab 80:3267–3272, 1995.

118. Connor SE, Penney CC: MRI in the differential diagnosis of a sellar mass, Clin Radiol 58:20–31, 2003.

119. Giusti M, Bocca L, Florio T, et al: Cabergoline modulation of alpha-subunits and FSH secretion in a gonadotroph adenoma, J Endocrinol Invest 23:463–466, 2000.

120. Lohmann T, Trantakis C, Biesold M, et al: Minor tumour shrinkage in nonfunctioning pituitary adenomas by long-term treatment with the dopamine agonist cabergoline, Pituitary 4:173–178, 2001.

121. Warnet A, Harris AG, Renard E, et al: A prospective multicenter trial of octreotide in 24 patients with visual defects caused by nonfunctioning and gonadotropin-secreting pituitary adenomas. French Multicenter Octreotide Study Group, Neurosurgery 41:786–795; discussion 796–797, 1997.

122. Sy RAG, Bernstein R, Chynn KY, et al: Reduction in size of a thyrotropin- and gonadotropin-secreting pituitary adenoma treated with octreotide acetate (somatostatin analog), J Clin Endocrinol Metab 74:690–694, 1992.

123. Katznelson L, Oppenheim DS, Coughlin F, et al: Chronic somatostatin analog administration in patients with alpha subunit-secreting pituitary adenomas, J Clin Endocrinol Metab 75:1318–1325, 1992.

124. Andersen M, Bjerre P, Schroder HD, et al: In vivo secretory potential and the effect of combination therapy with octreotide and cabergoline in patients with clinically non-functioning pituitary adenomas. Clin Endocrinol (Oxf) 54:23–30, 2001.

125. Roman SH, Goldstein M, Kourides IA, et al: The luteinizing hormone-releasing hormone (LHRH) agonist d-TRT[6]-PRO[9]-NEt LHRH increased rather than lowered LH and alpha subunit levels in a patient with an LH-secreting pituitary tumor, J Clin Endocrinol Metab 58:313–319, 1984.

126. Klibanski A, Jameson JL, Biller BMK, et al: Gonadotropin and alpha subunit responses to chronic gonadotropin-releasing hormone analog administration in patients with glycoprotein hormone-secreting pituitary tumors, J Clin Endocrinol Metab 68:81–86, 1989.

127. McGrath GA, Goncalves RJ, Udupa JK, et al: New technique for quantitation of pituitary adenoma size: use in evaluating treatment of gonadotroph adenomas with gonadotropin-releasing hormone antagonist, J Clin Endocrinol Metab 76:1363–1368, 1993.

128. Karavitaki N, Collison K, Halliday J, et al: What is the natural history of nonoperated nonfunctioning pituitary adenomas? Clin Endocrinol (Oxf) 67:938–943, 2007.

Chapter 10

TSH-PRODUCING ADENOMAS

PAOLO BECK-PECCOZ and LUCA PERSANI

Pituitary thyrotropin-producing adenomas (TSH-omas) are rare tumors that cause hyperthyroidism by chronically stimulating an intrinsically normal thyroid gland.[1-4] The first case of hyperthyroidism related to TSH-oma (central hyperthyroidism) was reported in 1960 when serum TSH levels were measured with a bioassay.[5] In 1970, Hamilton and coworkers[6] documented the first case of TSH-oma that was indisputably proved by radioimmunoassay techniques. Since then, about 350 patients have been reported in the literature. Although early reports describe these tumors as invasive macroadenomas that cause high morbidity and, in general, are difficult to be removed surgically, some cases now are cured more easily owing to earlier diagnosis. In fact, with the advent of ultrasensitive immunometric assays for TSH measurement, which are performed routinely in association with direct measurement of circulating free thyroid hormones (free thyroxine [FT$_4$] and free triiodothyronine [FT$_3$]), it is expected that patients with TSH-oma at the stage of microadenoma will be recognized with increasing frequency, thus permitting an improved clinical outcome.

Classically, TSH-omas, together with resistance to thyroid hormone,[7-9] were defined as syndromes of "inappropriate secretion of TSH," based on the common hormonal profile character-

ized by high levels of FT$_4$ and FT$_3$ in the presence of measurable TSH concentrations—a finding that contrasted with that observed in primary hyperthyroidism in which TSH is always undetectable. Nonetheless, the term *central hyperthyroidism* seems to be more pertinent for these disorders. However, clinically and biochemically, euthyroid patients with pituitary adenomas that secrete TSH molecules, possibly with reduced bioactivity, have been described but not clearly documented.[10,11] Moreover, pituitary hyperplasia and, in rare instances, true adenoma[12-14] related to long-standing primary hypothyroidism are well-known clinical conditions.[4] In most of these so-called feedback tumors, resolution of the pituitary lesion and normalization of TSH levels occur after levothyroxine (LT4) replacement therapy, thus bringing into question the actual functional autonomy of such tumors.

The clinical importance of these rare entities is based on the diagnostic and therapeutic challenges they present. Failure to recognize these different disorders may result in dramatic consequences, such as improper thyroid ablation in patients with central hyperthyroidism or unnecessary pituitary surgery in patients with resistance to thyroid hormone. In contrast, early diagnosis and correct treatment of pituitary tumors prevent the occurrence of complications (visual defects by compression of the optic chiasm, headache, hypopituitarism) and should improve the rate of cure.

Epidemiology

TSH-producing adenoma is a rare disorder, accounting for about 0.5% to 2% of all pituitary adenomas in both clinical and surgical or pathologic series.[1,15-17] The prevalence in the general population is 1 to 2 cases per million. Indeed, the number of reported cases of TSH-omas has tripled in the decade from 1989 to 1999 (Fig. 10-1). This increased number of recorded cases results from the introduction of ultrasensitive immunometric assays for TSH as a first-line test for the evaluation of thyroid function. On the basis of the finding of measurable serum TSH levels in the presence of elevated thyroid hormone concentrations, many patients who previously were thought to have Graves' disease can be diagnosed correctly as having a TSH-secreting pituitary adenoma or, alternatively, resistance to thyroid hormone. Moreover, increased awareness by the endocrinologist and general practitioner regarding the existence of central hyperthyroidism has contributed greatly to the disclosure of a higher number of patients with such a rare disorder.

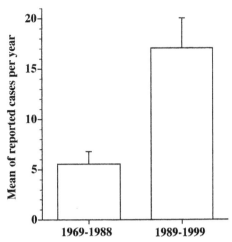

FIGURE 10-1. The significant increase in reported cases of pituitary thyrotropin (TSH)-producing adenoma in the decade from 1989 to 1999, when ultrasensitive TSH assay and direct methods for free thyroid hormone measurement became available as first-line tests of thyroid function.

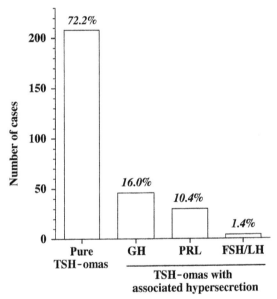

FIGURE 10-2. Classification of pituitary thyrotropin (TSH)-producing adenomas based on hormone secretion into circulation.

Pathology and Etiopathogenesis

The thyrotroph is the cell type of origin in TSH-omas. These tumors are nearly always benign; at present, transformation of a TSH-oma into a carcinoma with multiple metastases has been reported in only two patients.[18,19] Most of them (72%) secrete TSH alone, although this often is accompanied by unbalanced hypersecretion of the α subunit. About one fourth of TSH-omas are mixed adenomas, characterized by concomitant hypersecretion of other anterior pituitary hormones, mainly growth hormone (GH), prolactin (PRL), or both, which are known to share with TSH the common transcription factor Pit-1. Indeed, hypersecretion of TSH and GH is the most frequent association (16%), followed by hypersecretion of TSH and PRL (10.4%) and occasionally TSH and gonadotropins (1.4%) (Fig. 10-2). No association with adrenocorticotropic hormone (ACTH) hypersecretion has been documented to date. Two ectopic TSH-producing adenomas have been documented in the pharyngeal hypophysis.[20,21]

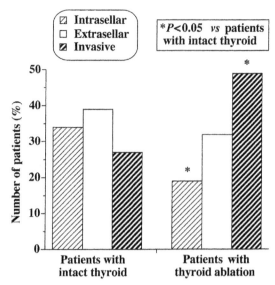

FIGURE 10-3. Effects of previous thyroid ablation on the size of pituitary thyrotropin (TSH)-producing adenomas. *Intrasellar* refers to both microadenomas and intrasellar macroadenomas, *extrasellar* to macroadenomas with suprasellar extension, and *invasive* to invasive macroadenomas. Data were calculated from 253 reported patients (163 with intact thyroid and 90 with thyroid ablation). Statistical analysis was carried out by Fisher's exact test.

At morphologic and histopathologic analysis, most TSH-omas are macroadenomas (87%), frequently with fibrous consistency, even in the absence of prior surgery or radiotherapy, and high local invasiveness.[22] However, previous thyroid ablation by surgery or radioiodine has deleterious effects on the size and invasiveness of the tumor (Fig. 10-3).[4] In fact, invasive macroadenomas were found in 49% of patients who had undergone thyroid ablation versus 27% in those who were untreated, whereas the figure was reversed in patients with microadenomas (diameter <1 cm) or intrasellar macroadenomas. Therefore, previous thyroid ablation may induce an aggressive transformation of the tumor, as is observed in Nelson's syndrome after adrenalectomy for Cushing's disease.

Light microscopy shows that adenoma cells are chromophobic, although they occasionally stain with basic or acid dyes. Ultrastructurally, adenomatous cells frequently appear monomorphous, even if they hypersecrete TSH, α subunit, and other pituitary tropins.[23-26] Cells with abnormal morphologic features or mitoses,[27] which may be misinterpreted as pituitary malignancy or metastases from distant carcinomas, are present in poorly differentiated adenomas that are characterized by the presence of fusiform cells with sparse and small secretory granules (80 to 200 nm). Indeed, there are no clear criteria of malignancy for TSH-omas except for the presence of metastases. It is worth noting that the first carcinoma reported in the literature exhibited a progressive malignant transformation accompanied by a decline in TSH and α subunit secretion.[18]

Immunostaining studies show the presence of TSH-β, either free or combined with the α subunit. In very few cases, a negative TSH-β immunostaining has been reported, possibly due to the extremely fast secretion rate of newly synthesized TSH molecules.[4,34] With the use of double immunostaining, the existence of mixed TSH-α subunit adenomas composed of one cell type secreting α subunit alone and another cosecreting α subunit and TSH has been documented.[28] In addition to α subunit, TSH frequently colocalizes with other pituitary hormones in the same tumoral cell[29] or even in the same secretory granule.[24,28,30,31] Nonetheless, positive immunohistochemistry panels for one or more pituitary hormones do not necessarily correlate with hypersecretion in vivo.[32] Indeed, positive immunostaining for ACTH and gonadotropins without evidence of in vivo hypersecretion has been reported.[33-37]

TSH-omas have been shown to be monoclonal in origin,[38] and several studies have screened a substantial number of adenomas for proto-oncogene activation[32,33,39-41] or loss of antioncogenes,[40,42] yielding negative results.[4] A highly variable expression of thyrotropin-releasing hormone (TRH) and dopamine receptors was documented in several adenomas,[43-45] whereas functional somatostatin receptors were detected constantly in TSH-omas,[46-48] thus providing the rationale for their medical treatment with somatostatin analogues. Indeed, loss of heterozygosity at the locus of the somatostatin receptor type 5 gene appears to be associated with resistance to somatostatin analogues and a more aggressive phenotype.[49]

Recently, somatic mutations[50] and aberrant alternative splicing[51] of thyroid hormone receptor β have been reported, along with dysregulation of iodothyronine deiodinase enzyme expression and function.[52,53] These findings at least in part may explain the defects in negative regulation of TSH secretion by thyroid hormones in some tumors.

Clinical Features

Patients with TSH-oma present with the signs and symptoms of either hyperthyroidism or the mass effect of an expanding intracranial tumor (Table 10-1). TSH-omas may occur at any age (range, 11 to 84 years), although most patients are in the third to sixth decade of life. Unlike the female predominance seen with other common thyroid disorders, TSH-omas occur with equal frequency in males and females. Goiter and clinical thyrotoxicosis are the most common presenting symptoms. Most patients presented with a long history of thyroid dysfunction, often mistakenly diagnosed as Graves' disease, and one third had inappropriate thyroidectomy, radioiodine thyroid ablation, or both. Thus, patients with TSH-omas may present to the specialist with hyperthyroidism that has been refractory to previous therapeutic attempts. In general, clinical features of hyperthyroidism are milder than expected on the basis of circulating thyroid hormone

Table 10-1. Clinical Characteristics of Patients With Pituitary Thyrotropin (TSH-oma) (Data from reports published until December 2007)

	Patients With TSH-oma % (n/total)*
Age, years	40.9 ± 14.5 (312)†
Sex, female	55 (180/325)
Previous thyroid ablation	33 (95/290)
Severe thyrotoxicosis	29 (60/204)
Goiter	93 (219/235)
Thyroid nodule(s)	72 (46/64)
Macroadenomas	87 (227/261)
Visual field defect	40 (61/154)
Headache	20 (23/117)
Menstrual disorders‡	33 (27/81)

*n/total refers to the number of patients for whom the information was available.
†Mean ± SD (n).
‡Data include women with or without associated prolactin (PRL) hypersecretion.

levels. Moreover, individual patients with untreated TSH-oma were reported to be clinically euthyroid.[10,54-56] This emphasizes the importance of systematic measurement of TSH and FT_4 in all patients with pituitary tumor, to disclose those with central hyperthyroidism or central hypothyroidism. In some acromegalic patients, signs or symptoms of hyperthyroidism are missed, as they are overshadowed by those of acromegaly.[24,57] Severe thyrotoxic features, such as atrial fibrillation, cardiac failure, and episodes of periodic paralysis,[58-60] are observed in about one fourth of cases.

The presence of a goiter is the rule (93%), even in patients who have undergone previous partial thyroidectomy. Because the thyroid is intrinsically normal in this disorder, it may regrow even after near total resection as a consequence of TSH hyperstimulation. Occurrence of multinodular goiter has been reported in several patients,[61] and differentiated thyroid carcinoma has been reported in other patients.[62-65] Progression toward functional autonomy seems to be infrequent.[66,67] In contrast to Graves' disease, the occurrence of circulating antithyroid autoantibodies is similar to that found in the general population. Unilateral exophthalmos due to orbital invasion by pituitary tumor was reported in three patients with TSH-omas, whereas Graves'-associated bilateral ophthalmopathy was reported in five patients.[4]

Most patients bearing a TSH-producing macroadenoma seek medical attention with signs and symptoms of an expanding intracranial tumor. Indeed, as a consequence of tumor suprasellar extension or invasiveness, signs and symptoms of tumor mass prevail over those of thyroid hyperfunction in many patients. Visual field defects are present in 40% of patients and headache in one fifth. Moreover, partial hypopituitarism is common, and loss of gonadal function is present in about one third of patients.[22,68] Galactorrhea was recorded in almost all patients with mixed TSH- and PRL-secreting tumors.[69,70]

Finally, TSH-omas may occur in families with multiple endocrine neoplasia type I[71-73] and in McCune-Albright syndrome.[74]

Biochemical Findings

TSH AND THYROID HORMONE LEVELS

High concentrations of thyroid hormones in the presence of detectable TSH levels typically are present in patients with hyperthyroidism due to a TSH-oma or with resistance to thyroid hormone. In the case of replacement therapy for prior thyroidectomy or thyroid ablation, it is crucial to assess patients in steady state, as TSH levels need 4 to 6 weeks to adjust to a change in LT4 dose. Thus, the diagnosis of TSH-producing adenoma may be difficult to establish in any patient who has had a dramatic change in thyroid hormone replacement therapy resulting from physician instruction or poor compliance. Conversely, the finding of elevated TSH levels in patients who have undergone thyroid ablation and have been overtreated with LT4 should be regarded as a possible sign of previously undiagnosed TSH-oma.[75]

Various abnormalities in the pituitary-thyroid axis, as well as laboratory artifacts, may cause a biochemical profile similar to that of central hyperthyroidism. These different conditions are more common than are TSH-omas and resistance to thyroid hormone and should be excluded before an extensive clinical assessment of the possible presence of central hyperthyroidism is conducted. Familial or drug- or estrogen-induced increases in circulating thyroxine-binding globulin (TBG) or variants of

Table 10-2. Circulating Factors That May Interfere With the Measurement of Pituitary Thyrotropin (TSH) or Total and Free Thyroid Hormones Giving Overestimation of the Actual Serum Levels of These Hormones and Thus Simulating the Presence of a TSH-Producing Adenoma

Heterophilic antibodies directed against mouse γ-globulins, leading to interference with monoclonal antibodies used in the immunometric assay*
Anti-TSH autoantibodies or antibodies cross-reacting with TSH†
Anti-iodothyronine autoantibodies (anti-T4 and/or anti-T3)‡
Abnormal forms of albumin or transthyretin (e.g., familial dysalbuminemic hyperthyroxinemia)‡

*This interference is commonly prevented by the addition of a few microliters of mouse serum to the assay buffer.
†Overestimation of TSH is very rare in the presence of such antibodies. This interference cannot be prevented, but it can be documented by performing dilution and recovery tests in the immunoassay.
‡To prevent misdiagnosis, measure free T4 and free T3 by direct "two-step" methods.[76,77]

Table 10-3. Biochemical Data of Patients With Pituitary Thyrotropin (TSH-oma) (Data from reports published until December 2007)

Parameter	Patients With Intact Thyroid (n)	Patients With Thyroid Ablation (n)	P
TSH mU/L*	9.2 ± 1.4 (145)	57.8 ± 10.2 (81)	<.0002
α-subunit, µg/L*	18.1 ± 5.9 (68)	15.3 ± 2.9 (47)	NS
α-subunit/TSH m.r.*†	42.4 ± 14.9 (68)	3.7 ± 0.7 (47)	<.03
TT4, nmol/L*	244 ± 20 (31)	177 ± 10 (45)	<.002
FT4, pmol/L*	45.3 ± 2.8 (78)	29.7 ± 2.9 (31)	<.0006
TT3, nmol/L*	5.2 ± 0.7 (27)	4.1 ± 0.3 (42)	NS
FT3, pmol/L*	14.6 ± 0.9 (59)	9.7 ± 0.9 (24)	<.0005
Normal TSH levels‡	37% (67/180)	11% (9/78)	<.0005
High α-subunit levels‡	63% (65/104)	73% (35/48)	NS
High α-subunit/TSH m.r.‡	84% (91/108)	77% (37/48)	NS
High SHBG levels‡	88% (23/26)	67% (6/9)	NS
Abnormal TSH response to TRH test‡§	83% (125/150)	83% (58/70)	NS
Abnormal TSH response to T3 suppression test‡¶	100% (47/47)	100% (33/33)	NS

FT3, Free triiodothyronine; FT4, free thyroxine; NS, not significant; SHBG, sex hormone–binding globulin; m.r., molar ratio; T3, triiodothyronine; TRH, thyrotropin-releasing hormone; TT3, total triiodothyronine; TT4, total thyroxine.
*Mean ± standard error (SE) (n).
†To calculate the α subunit/TSH molar ratio, divide α subunit (µg/L) by TSH (mU/L) and multiply by 10, provided that TSH IRP 80/558 is used in the immunometric assay.
‡% (n/total).
§Net TSH increment <4.0 mU/L.
¶Lack of complete TSH inhibition after 8 to 10 days of LT3 administration (80 to 100 µg/day).

albumin or transthyretin have led to increases in the levels of total serum thyroid hormone, particularly T4, thus producing a biochemical profile that may be confused with that of TSH-omas. Therefore, measurement of free thyroid hormones is mandatory in these conditions and should be performed by means of direct "two-step" methods (i.e., techniques by which contact between serum proteins and tracer can be avoided at the time of assay).[76,77] Indeed, normal levels of total T4 were recorded in several patients with TSH-oma, and only the measurement of FT4 allowed the right diagnosis of central hyperthyroidism. Furthermore, inhibition of T4 to T3 conversion induced by iodine-containing drugs or nonthyroidal illness may cause hyperthyroxinemia and nonsuppressed TSH that are, however, associated with normal or low-normal T3. In clinically ambiguous situations, the differential diagnosis rests on recognition of the underlying disorder, as well as on documentation of normalization of thyroid function test results at a later stage or after recovery of drug withdrawal.

Several laboratory artifacts may cause falsely high serum levels of TSH or thyroid hormones (Table 10-2). The more common factors that interfere with TSH measurement are heterophilic antibodies directed against mouse gamma globulins[78] or anti-TSH antibodies. However, preventing formation of the "sandwich" anti-TSH antibodies usually leads to an underestimation of the actual levels of TSH and rarely to an overestimation. The presence of anti-T4 or anti-T3 autoantibodies or both may cause FT4, FT3, or both to be overestimated, particularly when "one-step" analog methods are employed.[77] Finally, because patients with a TSH-oma may have T3 toxicosis, as in other forms of hyperthyroidism, there is a need to measure T3, in particular, free T3, when T4 levels are normal.

In TSH-omas, extremely variable levels of serum TSH and thyroid hormones have been reported (Table 10-3). It is interesting to note that in patients who were treated previously with thyroid ablation, TSH levels were dramatically higher than in untreated patients, although free thyroid hormone levels were still in the hyperthyroid range and the reduction of total thyroid hormone levels was minimal. The conserved sensitivity of tumoral thyrotroph cells to even small reductions in circulating free thyroid hormone levels is confirmed by the rapidly increased rate of TSH secretion during antithyroid drug administration.[57]

Although patients with TSH-oma have TSH-dependent hyperstimulation of the thyroid gland, any significant correlation between immunoreactive TSH and free thyroid hormone levels is lacking, even though only untreated patients are taken into account. Moreover, in one third of these patients, high levels of free thyroid hormones are associated with immunoreactive TSH levels within the normal range. Variations in the biologic activity of secreted TSH molecules most likely account for these findings.[79] The first demonstration that circulating TSH in patients with TSH-oma may possess an enhanced bioactivity was made in one patient with a mixed GH-TSH–secreting pituitary adenoma in whom a ratio between biologic and immunologic activities of TSH significantly higher than that of controls was documented.[24] Other studies indicate that the circulating TSH biologic/immunologic activity ratio may be normal, reduced, or increased in patients with TSH-oma,[22,79,80] probably because of altered glycosylation of circulating TSH molecules. In fact, both intrapituitary and circulating TSH exist as multiple isoforms characterized by heterogeneity of oligosaccharide chains, which has a great impact on hormone biologic properties, such as biologic activity and metabolic clearance rate. Tumoral transformation may be accompanied by variable alterations in posttranslational processing within thyrotrophs, leading to the secretion of TSH molecules with peculiar glycosylation and biologic properties.[79,81,82]

GLYCOPROTEIN HORMONE α SUBUNIT

TSH-omas commonly secrete excessive quantities of the free α subunit, resulting in high levels of circulating free α subunit in two thirds of patients (see Table 10-3). This is another expression of the altered synthetic process within tumoral thyrotropes and represents a helpful diagnostic clue to the presence of a TSH-oma. Secretion of the α subunit in these tumors is in excess not only of the TSH-β subunit, but also of the intact TSH molecule. This generally results in a molar ratio of α subunit to TSH that is higher than 1. Although previous studies have suggested that a ratio greater than 1.0 is indicative of the presence of TSH-producing adenoma,[83] similar values have been observed in normal controls, particularly in postmenopausal women, indicating the need for appropriate control groups matched for TSH and gonadotropin levels.[4,61,84] It is interesting to note that microadenomas that frequently have α subunit levels within the normal range may show a high α subunit/TSH molar ratio. Furthermore, it has been suggested that extremely high levels of free α subunit might portend future malignant behavior, and that a spontaneous and marked decrease in both TSH and α subunit might indicate that the tumor is becoming less differentiated and might correlate with invasive and metastatic behavior.[18]

PARAMETERS EVALUATING PERIPHERAL THYROID HORMONE ACTION

Measurements of several parameters of peripheral thyroid hormone action both in vivo (basal metabolic rate, cardiac systolic time intervals, Achilles' reflex time) and in vitro (sex hormone–binding globulin [SHBG], cholesterol, angiotensin-converting enzyme, osteocalcin, blood red cell sodium content, carboxyterminal cross-linked telopeptide of type I collagen [ICTP], and so on)[85] may help in quantifying the degree of peripheral hyperthyroidism, particularly in patients with mild clinical signs and symptoms[34,57,61,86-89] (see Table 10-3). In particular, evaluations of SHBG and ICTP may help to differentiate hyperthyroid patients with TSH-oma, in whom these parameters are elevated, from those with resistance to thyroid hormone, in whom they are in the range of those of euthyroid subjects.

Dynamic Testing

Several stimulatory and inhibitory tests have been employed to evaluate TSH secretory dynamics in patients with TSH-oma. None of these tests is of clear-cut diagnostic value, and the combination of some of them may enhance their accuracy in disclosing the pituitary adenoma. Among the stimulatory tests, TRH-induced TSH secretion is absent or blunted in 83% of patients (see Table 10-3). Although the α subunit response to the preceding stimulatory agents usually has paralleled that of TSH, discrepancy between α subunit and TSH response to TRH has been recorded in some cases. Such a discrepancy may be due to the presence of mixed adenomas, composed of distinct cell types that possess different receptor expression.[24,28] Most TSH-omas are unable to increase TSH secretion after administration of dopamine antagonists such as domperidone or sulpiride. Long-term treatment with antithyroid drugs induces an increase in serum TSH levels in most patients because of both the high sensitivity of adenomatous cells to the reduction of circulating levels of FT_4 and FT_3[57] and recovered TSH secretion by normal thyrotrophs surrounding the adenoma in response to the activated feedback mechanism.[4,90] In keeping with this are the observations of significantly higher TSH levels in patients who have undergone thyroid ablation, as well as the more active proliferation of tumoral cells in treated patients.

Among inhibitory tests, complete inhibition of both basal and TRH-stimulated TSH secretion after a T_3 suppression test (Werner test: 80 to 100 µg/day of LT3 for 8 to 10 days) has never been recorded in a patient with a TSH-oma (see Table 10-3), although a slight TSH reduction may occur in a minority of patients. In patients who have undergone previous thyroid ablation, this test is the most sensitive and specific in documenting the possible presence of a TSH-oma. However, high doses of LT3 are contraindicated in elderly patients and in those with coronary heart disease. Dopamine (1 to 4 µg/kg body weight/min intravenously) or dopamine agonists, such as bromocriptine (2.5 mg orally), generally are ineffective in inhibiting TSH secretion, whereas native somatostatin or its analogues reduce TSH levels in most cases and may be predictive of the efficacy of long-term treatment in the majority of patients.[61,91,92] We have demonstrated recently that long-term administration of long-acting somatostatin analogues in patients with central hyperthyroidism caused a marked decrease in both FT_4 and FT_3 circulating levels in all patients but one with TSH-omas, whereas patients with thyroid hormone resistance did not respond at all. Thus, administration of these analogues for at least 2 to 3 months can be useful in distinguishing the two forms of central hyperthyroidism.[93]

Imaging Studies and Localization

In considering the diagnosis of a TSH-oma, full imaging studies, particularly high-resolution computed tomography (CT) or nuclear magnetic resonance imaging (MRI), are necessary. Various degrees of suprasellar extension or sphenoidal sinus invasion are present in two thirds of cases. It is curious that in two patients, pituitary stones have been described.[94]

Microadenomas now are reported with increasing frequency, accounting for about 13% of all recorded cases. In contrast to other secreting pituitary tumors,[95] no correlation between serum TSH levels and tumor size was found in untreated patients with TSH-oma. Pituitary scintigraphy with radiolabeled Tyr[3]-substituted octreotide has been shown to successfully image TSH-omas.[96] Moreover, in vivo evidence for both somatostatin and dopamine D_2 receptors was obtained with the use of single-photon emission tomography with ^{111}In-pentetreotide and ^{123}I-iodobenzamide.[92,97] The presence of these receptors correlates with the sensitivity of the tumor to long-term medical treatment. ^{111}In-pentetreotide scintigraphy also may be useful in localizing possible ectopic TSH-producing adenomas. Finally, bilateral petrosal sinus sampling has been used in difficult cases, allowing the identification and lateralization of a microadenoma not seen on radiographic scans.[98] However, one should expect a certain number of false lateralizations, as already has been observed for ACTH-secreting pituitary tumors.

Differential Diagnosis

The presence of detectable TSH levels in a hyperthyroid patient rules out primary hyperthyroidism, whereas in patients receiving levothyroxine replacement for primary hypothyroidism, poor compliance is by far the most common cause of apparent inappropriate secretion of TSH, with TSH still too high for the levels of thyroid hormones. This underscores the importance of studying patients in steady state. The first step in the case of hyperthyroxinemia and detectable TSH is to measure free thyroid hormone levels and repeat TSH by ultrasensitive assays. The finding of normal TSH, FT_4, and FT_3 levels suggests euthyroid hyperthyroxinemia, whereas high FT_4 and FT_3 concentrations and suppressed TSH definitively indicate the presence of primary hyperthyroidism due to Graves' disease and other forms of thyrotoxicosis. If FT_4 and FT_3 concentrations are elevated in the presence of measurable TSH levels, it is important to exclude methodologic interference. When the existence of central hyperthyroidism is eventually confirmed, several diagnostic steps have to be carried out to differentiate a TSH-oma from resistance to thyroid hormone (RTH). This is particularly true for the variant of RTH with predominant pituitary resistance with clear clinical signs and symptoms of hyperthyroidism.[7-9] Indeed, alterations of pituitary content on CT or MRI, as well as the possible presence of neurologic signs and symptoms (visual defects, headache), or clinical features of concomitant hypersecretion of other pituitary hormones (acromegaly, galactorrhea, amenorrhea) definitely point to the presence of a TSH-oma. Nevertheless, the differential diagnosis may be difficult when the pituitary adenoma is undetectable by CT or MRI or in the case of confusing (empty sella) or incidental pituitary lesions.[99,100] No significant differences in age, sex, previous thyroid ablation, TSH levels, or free thyroid hormone concentrations occur between patients with TSH-oma and those with RTH (Table 10-4). However, in contrast to RTH patients, familial cases of TSH-oma have never been documented. The finding of measurable TSH levels and high concentrations of FT_4 and FT_3 in one relative definitely points to the diagnosis of RTH. Serum TSH levels within the normal range are found more frequently in RTH, whereas elevated α subunit concentrations or a high α subunit/TSH molar ratio typically is present in patients with TSH-omas. Moreover, absent or impaired TSH responses to TRH administration and to the T_3 suppression test favor the presence of a TSH-oma. Circulating SHBG levels are in the hyperthyroid range in patients with TSH-oma, the only patients with low SHBG being those with concomitant hypersecretion of GH, which potently inhibits SHBG secretion. The few patients with RTH and high SHBG levels were those who were treated with estrogens or those who showed profound hypogonadism.[88] Other parameters that may be useful in the differential diagnosis are markers of bone turnover, such as ICTP (altered in TSH-omas, normal in RTH) or total cholesterol (rarely high in TSH-omas).[9,89] In difficult cases, particularly after thyroidectomy, genetic investigations into thyroid hormone receptor-β_1

mutations may be the only diagnostic test. Finally, an apparent association between TSH-oma and resistance to thyroid hormone has been reported in a few patients.[86,101] Although genetic studies and familial investigations were not carried out in the Japanese patient, the occurrence of TSH-omas in patients with RTH is theoretically possible and therefore should be considered carefully.

Treatment and Outcome

PITUITARY SURGERY AND RADIATION THERAPY

The primary goal in the treatment of TSH-omas is to remove the pituitary tumor and restore euthyroidism. Therefore, the first therapeutic approach to TSH-producing adenomas should be to surgically remove or debulk the tumor by transsphenoidal or subfrontal adenomectomy, the choice of route depending on the tumor volume and its suprasellar extension.[1,16,102,103] This may be particularly difficult because of the marked fibrosis of these tumors and local invasion involving the cavernous sinus, internal carotid artery, or optic chiasm. To restore euthyroidism before surgery, antithyroid drugs or octreotide along with propranolol can be administered. If surgery is contraindicated or declined, pituitary radiotherapy (no less than 45 Gy fractionated at 2 Gy/day or 10 to 25 Gy in a single dose if a stereotactic gamma unit is available) and subsequent somatostatin analogue administration should be considered.

Surgery alone or combined with radiotherapy induces normalization of thyroid hormone levels and apparent complete removal of tumor mass in about one third of patients, whereas normalization of thyroid hormones without complete removal of the adenoma occurs in an another third of patients (Table 10-5). Collectively, about two thirds of TSH-omas are brought under control with surgery, irradiation, or both. In the remaining patients, the large size and the invasiveness of the tumor prevent successful removal of the tumor. Elevation of α subunit or cosecretion of other pituitary hormones does not seem to be an unfavorable prognostic factor. Postsurgical deaths were reported in five cases. Partial or complete hypopituitarism may be the result of surgery. Evaluation of other pituitary functions, particularly ACTH secretion, should be undertaken carefully soon after surgery and should be performed again every year, especially in patients who are treated by radiotherapy. In addition, in the case of surgical cure, postoperative TSH is undetectable and may remain low for many weeks or months, causing central hypothy-

Table 10-4. Differential Diagnosis Between TSH-Producing Adenomas (TSH-omas) and Resistance to Thyroid Hormones (RTH)

Parameter	TSH-omas	RTH	P
Sex (F/M ratio)	1.4	1.3	NS
TSH, mU/L*	2.8 ± 0.6	2.0 ± 0.3	NS
FT_4, pmol/L*	42.0 ± 4.5	28.5 ± 2.7	NS
FT_3, pmol/L*	14.2 ± 1.5	11.9 ± 1.0	NS
SHBG, nmol/L*	117 ± 18	60 ± 4	<.0001
Familial cases	0%	84%	<.0001
Lesions at CT scan or MRI	98%	6%	<.0001
High α subunit levels	63%	3%	<.0001
High α subunit/TSH m.r.	84%	3%	<.0001
Abnormal TSH response to TRH test†	83%	5%	<.0001
Abnormal TSH response to T_3 suppression test‡	100%	100%§	NS

CT, Computed tomography; FT_3, free triiodothyronine; FT_4, free thyroxine; m.r., molar ratio; MRI, magnetic resonance imaging; NS, not significant; SHBG, sex hormone–binding globulin; T_3, triiodothyronine; TRH, thyrotropin-releasing hormone; TSH, pituitary thyrotropin.

*Only patients with intact thyroid were taken into account. Data were obtained from patients followed at our institution (18 TSH-omas and 68 RTH) and are expressed as mean ± standard error (SE) (n).
†Net TSH increment <4.0 mU/L.
‡Werner's test (80 to 100 μg T3 for 8 to 10 days). Quantitatively normal responses to T_3 (i.e., complete inhibition of both basal and TRH-stimulated TSH levels) have never been recorded in either group of patients.
§Although abnormal in quantitative terms, TSH response to T_3 suppression test is qualitatively normal in most RTH patients.[7-9]

Table 10-5. Results of Pituitary Surgery Alone, Surgery Plus Irradiation (Rx), and Injection of Somatostatin Analogues in the Treatment of TSH-Producing Adenomas

	Surgery (n = 125)	Surgery + Rx (n = 57)	Somatostatin Analogues (n = 84)
Reduction of Tumor Mass			
Complete	33%	29%	0%
Partial	35%	40%	51%
Absent	32%	31%	49%
Resolution of Clinical Symptoms			
Yes	58%	62%	94%
No	42%	38%	6%

roidism. The time necessary for the recovery of normal thyrotrophs is variable, and permanent central hypothyroidism occasionally may occur as the result of damage to the normal thyrotroph by the tumor or during surgery. Thus, temporary or permanent LT4 replacement therapy may be necessary. In a few cases, total thyroidectomy was performed after pituitary surgery failed because patients were at risk for thyroid storm.

MEDICAL TREATMENT

In terms of pharmacologic therapy for TSH-omas, antithyroid drugs must not be used because they may cause worsening of goiter size or more rapid growth and invasiveness of the pituitary adenoma, and their use is recommended only as preparation of the patient for neurosurgery. For alleviating the symptoms of hyperthyroidism, β-blockers such as propranolol may be used. Glucocorticoids are effective in reducing TSH secretion, but they induce deleterious side effects in long-term treatment. Dopamine agonists, particularly bromocriptine, have been employed in some TSH-omas with variable results, with the positive effects observed in some patients with mixed TSH- and PRL-secreting adenoma diminishing over time.[104,105] Currently, medical treatment for TSH-oma rests on somatostatin analogues (SSa) such as octreotide[47,91-93,106-108] or the slow-release formulation of lanreotide.[109,110] Both SSa lead to a reduction in TSH and α subunit secretion in almost all cases, with restoration of the euthyroid state in most (see Table 10-5). Moreover, modifications of the TSH glycoisomer distribution pattern during SSa treatment have been documented in one patient,[111] suggesting that restoration of euthyroidism in some patients who show no reduction in immunoreactive levels of TSH during SSa therapy may be due to a reduction in the bioactivity of secreted molecules.[91,112] During SSa therapy, tumor shrinkage occurs in about half of patients (see Table 10-5), and vision improvement is seen in 75%.

Tachyphylaxis occurred in about one fifth of patients and responded to increasing SSa doses, whereas long-term studies demonstrated true escape from the inhibitory effects in few cases. In only 5% of cases was true resistance to SSa treatment documented. Octreotide treatment was effective in restoring euthyroidism in one pregnant woman with central hyperthyroidism and had no side effects on fetal development and thyroid function.[113,114] Patients taking octreotide have to be monitored carefully because untoward side effects, such as cholelithiasis and carbohydrate intolerance, may arise. The dose administered should be tailored for each patient, depending on therapeutic response and tolerance (including gastrointestinal side effects). The marked SSa-induced suppression of TSH secretion and consequent biochemical hypothyroidism seen in some patients may require LT4 substitution. Whether somatostatin analogue treatment may be an alternative to surgery and irradiation in patients with TSH-oma remains to be established. However, the slow-release preparation of somatostatin, lanreotide-SR, and octreotide-LAR may represent useful tools for long-term treatment of such a rare pituitary adenoma.

Criteria of Cure and Follow-Up

Evidence has accumulated about the criteria of cure and follow-up for patients undergoing operation or irradiation for TSH-omas.[4,57,61] In untreated hyperthyroid patients, it is reasonable to assume that cured patients have clinical and biochemical reversal of thyroid hyperfunction. However, normal free thyroid hormone concentrations or indices of peripheral thyroid hormone action in the euthyroid range may be associated with partial removal or destruction of tumoral cells, since transient clinical remission and euthyroidism are observed frequently.[57,61] As it occurs for other pituitary tumors, disappearance of neurologic signs and symptoms only partially reflects the radicality of tumor removal, in that it may occur even in the presence of an incomplete debulking of the tumor. Pituitary imaging performed after surgery has low predictivity because of the high frequency of false-negative imaging results. The criteria for normalization of circulating TSH are not applicable to previously thyroidectomized patients or to those with normal basal values of TSH. In our experience, undetectable TSH levels 1 week after surgery are likely to indicate complete adenomectomy, provided that the patient was hyperthyroid and presurgical treatments were stopped at least 10 days before surgery.[48] Similarly, although normalization of α subunit or the α subunit/TSH molar ratio in general is a good index for the evaluation of therapy efficacy, both parameters are normal in a remarkable number of patients with TSH-oma. The most sensitive and specific test used to document complete removal of the adenoma remains the T_3 suppression test (in the absence of clinical contraindication). In fact, regardless of the restoration of euthyroidism, only patients in whom T_3 administration completely inhibits basal and TRH-stimulated TSH secretion appear to be truly cured (Fig. 10-4).

Data on the recurrence rate of TSH-oma in patients who are judged to be cured after surgery or radiotherapy are still lacking. However, recurrence of the adenoma does not appear to be frequent, at least in the first years after successful surgery. In general, the patient should be evaluated clinically and biochemically two or three times the first year postoperatively and then every year. Pituitary imaging should be performed every 2 or 3 years but should be performed promptly whenever an increase in TSH and thyroid hormone levels or clinical symptoms occur. In the case of persistent macroadenoma, a close visual field follow-up is required, as visual function is threatened.

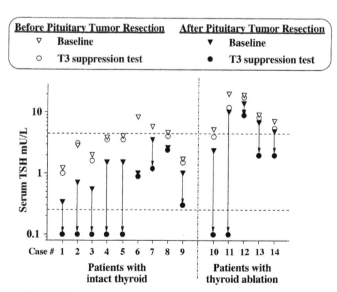

FIGURE 10-4. Results of T_3 suppression test carried out before and after pituitary surgery in patients with pituitary thyrotropin (TSH)-producing adenoma. *Horizontal dashed lines* indicate the normal range of serum TSH. Note the lack of TSH suppression in all patients before neurosurgery. Complete suppression of serum TSH levels (i.e., complete removal of the adenoma) was seen in about half of patients after neurosurgery, independent of previous thyroid ablation.

Conclusions

Central hyperthyroidism due to TSH-secreting pituitary adenomas is a rare cause of thyrotoxicosis. The diagnosis is now facilitated by the recent introduction of ultrasensitive TSH immunoassays, as well as direct free thyroid hormone measurements, which are not obscured by abnormal serum transport proteins. Increased awareness and early recognition of these tumors will prevent inappropriate treatment, such as thyroid ablation or long-term antithyroid drug administration, which undoubtedly increases TSH secretion, tumor size, and invasiveness. Although no single diagnostic test is pathognomonic in establishing the diagnosis, elevation of α subunit levels and serum SHBG concentrations and the frequently absent or impaired TSH responses to TRH and T_3 suppression tests are the most useful markers to distinguish patients with TSH-oma from those with thyroid hormone resistance. Furthermore, high-resolution CT and MRI may help in detecting tumors as small as 3 mm in diameter. Surgery still remains the first therapeutic approach to the disease, followed by radiotherapy in the case of failure. The finding of measurable TSH levels after a simple T_3 suppression test definitely indicates that removal of the tumor cells was incomplete, thus requiring closer follow-up of the patient or additional therapies, or both. If needed, treatment with somatostatin analogues is worthwhile, allowing restoration of euthyroidism in more than 90% of patients and even tumor shrinkage in half of cases.

Acknowledgment

The authors thank Professor Anna Spada for critical reading of the manuscript.

REFERENCES

1. Clarke MJ, Erickson D, Castro R, et al: Thyroid-stimulating hormone pituitary adenomas, J Neurosurg 109:17, 2008.
2. Samuels MH, Ridgway EC: Glycoprotein-secreting pituitary adenomas, Baillieres Clin Endocrinol 9:337, 1995.
3. Greenman Y, Melmed S: Thyrotropin-secreting pituitary tumors. In Melmed S, editor: The Pituitary, Boston, 1995, Blackwell Science, p 546.
4. Beck-Peccoz P, Brucker-Davis F, Persani L, et al: Thyrotropin-secreting pituitary tumors, Endocr Rev 17:610, 1996.
5. Jailer JW, Holub DA: Remission of Graves' disease following radiotherapy of a pituitary neoplasm, Am J Med 28:497, 1960.
6. Hamilton C, Adams LC, Maloof F: Hyperthyroidism due to thyrotropin-producing pituitary chromophobe adenoma, N Engl J Med 283:1077, 1970.
7. Refetoff S, Weiss RE, Usala SJ: The syndromes of resistance to thyroid hormone, Endocr Rev 14:348, 1993.
8. Beck-Peccoz P, Asteria C, Mannavola D: Resistance to thyroid hormone. In Braverman LE (ed): Contemporary Endocrinology: Diseases of the Thyroid, Totowa, NJ, 1997, Humana Press, p 199.
9. Gurnell M, Beck-Peccoz P, Chatterjee VKK: Resistance to thyroid hormone.
10. Felix I, Asa SL, Kovacs K, et al: Recurrent plurihormonal bimorphous pituitary adenoma producing growth hormone, thyrotropin, and prolactin, Arch Pathol Lab Med 118:66, 1994.
11. Bertholon-Gregoire M, Trouillas J, Guigard MP, et al: Mono and plurihormonal thyrotropic pituitary adenomas: Pathological, hormonal and clinical studies in twelve patients, Eur J Endocrinol 140:519, 1999.
12. Katz MS, Gregerman RI, Horvath E, et al: Thyrotroph cell adenoma of the human pituitary gland associated with primary hypothyroidism: Clinical and morphological features, Acta Endocrinol 95:41, 1980.
13. Ghannam NN, Hammami MM, Muttair Z, et al: Primary hypothyroidism-associated TSH-secreting pituitary adenoma/hyperplasia presenting as a bleeding nasal mass and extremely elevated TSH level, J Endocrinol Invest 22:419, 1999.
14. Losa M, Mortini P, Minelli R, et al: Coexistence of TSH-secreting pituitary adenoma and autoimmune hypothyroidism, J Endocrinol Invest 29:555, 2006.
15. Kienitz T, Quinkler M, Strasburger C, et al: Long-term management in five cases of TSH-secreting pituitary adenomas: a single center study and review of the literature, Eur J Endocrinol 157:39, 2007.
16. Socin HV, Chanson P, Delemer B, et al: The changing spectrum of TSH-secreting pituitary adenomas: Diagnosis and management in 43 patients, Eur J Endocrinol 148:433, 2003.
17. Mindermann T, Wilson CB: Thyrotropin-producing pituitary adenomas, J Neurosurg 79:521, 1993.
18. Mixson AJ, Friedman TC, David AK, et al: Thyrotropin-secreting pituitary carcinoma, J Clin Endocrinol Metab 76:529, 1993.
19. Brown RL, Muzzafar T, Wollman R, et al: A pituitary carcinoma secreting TSH and prolactin: a non-secreting adenoma gone awry, Eur J Endocrinol 154:639, 2006.
20. Cooper DS, Wenig BM: Hyperthyroidism caused by an ectopic TSH-secreting pituitary tumor, Thyroid 6:337, 1996.
21. Pasquini E, Faustini-Fustini M, Sciarretta V, et al: Ectopic TSH-secreting pituitary adenoma of the vomerosphenoidal junction, Eur J Endocrinol 148:253, 2003.
22. Gesundheit N, Petrick P, Nissim M, et al: Thyrotropin-secreting pituitary adenomas: Clinical and biochemical heterogeneity, Ann Intern Med 111:827, 1989.
23. Teramoto A, Sanno N, Tahara S, et al: Pathological study of thyrotropin-secreting pituitary adenoma: plurihormonality and medical treatment, Acta Neuropathol 108–147, 2004.
24. Beck-Peccoz P, Piscitelli G, Amr S, et al: Endocrine, biochemical, and morphological studies of a pituitary adenoma secreting growth hormone, thyrotropin (TSH), and α-subunit: Evidence for secretion of TSH with increased bioactivity, J Clin Endocrinol Metab 62:704, 1986.
25. Ozawa Y, Kameya T, Kasuga A, et al: A functional thyrotropin- and growth hormone-secreting pituitary adenoma with ultrastructurally monomorphic feature: A case study, Endocr J 45:211, 1998.
26. Ikeda H, Ogawa Y, Yoshimoto T: Ultrastructural characteristics of TSH-producing adenomas with special reference to its close similarity to BFA-treated pituitary adenoma cells, Pituitary 1:221, 1999.
27. Trouillas J, Girod C, Loras B, et al: The TSH secretion in the human pituitary adenomas, Pathol Res Pract 183:596, 1988.
28. Terzolo M, Orlandi F, Bassetti M, et al: Hyperthyroidism due to a pituitary adenoma composed of two different cell types, one secreting alpha-subunit alone and another cosecreting alpha-subunit and thyrotropin, J Clin Endocrinol Metab 72:415, 1991.
29. Jaquet P, Hassoun J, Delori P, et al: A human pituitary adenoma secreting thyrotropin and prolactin: Immunohistochemical, biochemical and cell culture study, J Clin Endocrinol Metab 59:817, 1984.
30. Kuzuya N, Inoue K, Ishibashi M, et al: Endocrine and immunohistochemical studies on thyrotropin (TSH)-secreting pituitary adenomas: Responses of TSH, alpha-subunit and growth hormone to hypothalamic releasing hormones and their distribution in adenoma cells, J Clin Endocrinol Metab 71:1103, 1990.
31. Malarkey WB, Kovacs K, O'Dorisio T: Response of GH- and TSH-secreting pituitary adenoma to a somatostatin analogue (SMS 201–995): Evidence that GH and TSH coexist in the same cell and secretory granules, Neuroendocrinology 49:267, 1989.
32. Sanno N, Teramoto A, Matsuno A, et al: Clinical and immunohistochemical studies on TSH-secreting pituitary adenoma: Its multihormonality and expression of Pit-1, Modern Pathol 7:893, 1994.
33. Dong Q, Brucker-Davis F, Weintraub BD, et al: Screening of candidate oncogenes in human thyrotroph tumors: Absence of activating mutations of the $G\alpha_q$, $G\alpha_{11}$, $G\alpha_s$, or thyrotropin-releasing hormone receptor genes, J Clin Endocrinol Metab 81:1134, 1996.
34. Lind P, Langsteger W, Koltringer P, et al: Transient prealbumin-associated hyperthyroxinemia in a TSH-producing pituitary adenoma, Nuklearmedizin 29:40, 1990.
35. Waldhausl W, Brautsch-Marrain P, Nowotony P, et al: Secondary hyperthyroidism due to thyrotropin hypersecretion: Study of pituitary tumor morphology and thyrotropin chemistry and release, J Clin Endocrinol Metab 49:879, 1979.
36. Stanley JM, Najjar SS: Hyperthyroidism secondary to a TSH-secreting pituitary adenoma in a 15-year-old-male, Clin Pediatr 30:109, 1991.
37. Patrick AW, Atkin SL, MacKenzie J, et al: Hyperthyroidism secondary to a pituitary adenoma secreting TSH, FSH, alpha-subunit and GH, Clin Endocrinol (Oxf) 40:275, 1994.
38. Ma W, Ikeda H, Watabe N, et al: A plurihormonal TSH-producing pituitary tumor of monoclonal origin in a patient with hypothyroidism, Horm Res 59:257, 2003.
39. Pellegrini I, Barlier A, Gunz G, et al: Pit-1 gene expression in the human pituitary and pituitary adenomas, J Clin Endocrinol Metab 79:189, 1994.
40. Boggild MD, Jenkinson S, Pistorello M, et al: Molecular genetics studies of sporadic pituitary tumors, J Clin Endocrinol Metab 78:387, 1994.
41. Bamberger CM, Fehn M, Bamberger AM, et al: Reduced expression levels of the cell-cycle inhibitor p27Kip1 in human pituitary adenomas, Eur J Endocrinol 140:250, 1999.
42. Sumi T, Stefaneanu L, Kovacs K, et al: Immunohistochemical study of p53 protein in human and animal pituitary tumors, Endocr Pathol 4:95, 1993.
43. Chanson P, Li JY, LeDafniet M, et al: Absence of receptors for thyrotropin (TSH)-releasing hormone in human TSH-secreting pituitary adenomas associated with hyperthyroidism, J Clin Endocrinol Metab 66:447, 1988.
44. LeDafniet M, Brandi A-M, Kujas M, et al: Thyrotropin-releasing hormone (TRH) binding sites and thyrotropin response to TRH are regulated by thyroid hormones in human thyrotropic adenomas, Eur J Endocrinol 130:559, 1994.
45. Kim K, Arai K, Sanno N, et al: The expression of thyrotrophin-releasing hormone receptor 1 messenger ribonucleic acid in human pituitary adenomas, Clin Endocrinol (Oxf) 54:309, 2001.
46. Takano K, Ajima M, Teramoto A, et al: Mechanism of action of somatostatin on human TSH-secreting adenoma cells, Am J Physiol 268:E558, 1995.
47. Bertherat J, Brue T, Enjalbert A, et al: Somatostatin receptors on thyrotropin-secreting pituitary adenomas: Comparison with the inhibitory effects of octreotide upon in vivo and in vitro hormonal secretions, J Clin Endocrinol Metab 75:540, 1992.
48. Horiguchi K, Yamada M, Umezawa R, et al: Somatostatin receptor subtypes mRNA in TSH-secreting pituitary

adenomas: a case showing a dramatic reduction in tumor size during short octreotide treatment, Endocr J 54:371, 2007.
49. Filopanti M, Ballarè E, Lania AG, et al: Loss of heterozygosity at the SS receptor type 5 locus in human GH- and TSH-secreting pituitary adenomas, J Endocrinol Invest 27:937, 2004.
50. Ando S, Sarlis NJ, Oldfield EH, Yen PM: Somatic mutation of TRbeta can cause a defect in negative regulation of TSH in a TSH-secreting pituitary tumor, J Clin Endocrinol Metab 86:5572, 2001.
51. Ando S, Sarlis NJ, Krishnan J, et al: Aberrant alternative splicing of thyroid hormone receptor in a TSH-secreting pituitary tumor is a mechanism for hormone resistance, Mol Endocrinol 15:1529, 2001.
52. Tannahill LA, Visser TJ, McCabe CJ, et al: Dysregulation of iodothyronine deiodinase enzyme expression and function in human pituitary tumours, Clin Endocrinol (Oxf) 56:735, 2002.
53. Baur A, Buchfelder M, Kohrle J: Expression of 5′-deiodinase enzymes in normal pituitaries and in various human pituitary adenomas, Eur J Endocrinol 147:263, 2002.
54. Yamakita N, Ikeda T, Murai T, et al: Thyrotropin-producing pituitary adenoma discovered as a pituitary incidentaloma, Intern Med 34:1055, 1995.
55. Koide Y, Kugai N, Kimura S, et al: A case of pituitary adenoma with possible simultaneous secretion of thyrotropin and follicle-stimulating hormone, J Clin Endocrinol Metab 54:397, 1982.
56. Scanlon MF, Howells S, Peters JR, et al: Hyperprolactinaemia, amenorrhoea and galactorrhoea due a pituitary thyrotroph adenoma, Clin Endocrinol 23:35, 1985.
57. Losa M, Giovanelli M, Persani L, et al: Criteria of cure and follow-up of central hyperthyroidism due to thyrotropin-secreting pituitary adenomas, J Clin Endocrinol Metab 81:3084, 1996.
58. Kiso Y, Yoshida K, Kaise K, et al: A case of thyrotropin (TSH)-secreting tumor complicated by periodic paralysis, Jpn J Med 29:399, 1990.
59. Alings AM, Fliers E, de Herder WW, et al: A thyrotropin-secreting pituitary adenoma as a cause of thyrotoxic periodic paralysis, J Endocrinol Invest 21:703, 1998.
60. Hsu FS, Tsai WS, Chau T, et al: Thyrotropin-secreting pituitary adenoma presenting as hypokalemic periodic paralysis, Am J Med Sci 325:48, 2003.
61. Brucker-Davis F, Oldfield EH, Skarulis MC, et al: Thyrotropin-secreting pituitary tumors: Diagnostic criteria, thyroid hormone sensitivity, and treatment outcome in 25 patients followed at the National Institutes of Health, J Clin Endocrinol Metab 84:476, 1999.
62. Calle-Pascual AL, Yuste E, Martin P, et al: Association of a thyrotropin-secreting pituitary adenoma and a thyroid follicular carcinoma, J Endocrinol Invest 14:499, 1991.
63. Gasparoni P, Rubello D, Persani L, et al: Unusual association between a thyrotropin-secreting pituitary adenoma and a papillary thyroid carcinoma, Thyroid 8:181, 1998.
64. Kishida M, Otsuka F, Kataoka H, et al: Hyperthyroidism in a patient with TSH-producing pituitary adenoma coexisting with thyroid papillary adenocarcinoma, Endocr J 47:731, 2000.
65. Ohta S, Nishizawa S, Oki Y, et al: Coexistence of thyrotropin-producing pituitary adenoma with papillary adenocarcinoma of the thyroid: A case report and surgical strategy, Pituitary 4:271, 2001
66. Beckers A, Abs R, Mahler C, et al: Thyrotropin-secreting pituitary adenomas: Report of seven cases, J Clin Endocrinol Metab 72:477, 1991.
67. Abs R, Stevenaert A, Beckers A: Autonomously functioning thyroid nodules in a patient with a thyrotropin-secreting pituitary adenoma: Possible cause-effect relationship, Eur J Endocrinol 131:355, 1994.
68. Sy ARG, Bernstein R, Chynn KI, et al: Reduction in size of a thyrotropin- and gonadotropin-secreting pituitary adenoma treated with octreotide acetate (somatostatin analogue), J Clin Endocrinol Metab 74:690, 1992.
69. Horn K, Erhardt F, Fahlbusch R, et al: Recurrent goiter, hyperthyroidism, galactorrhoea and amenorrhoea due to a thyrotropin and prolactin-producing pituitary tumor, J Clin Endocrinol Metab 43:137, 1976.
70. Adriaanse R, Brabant G, Endert E, et al: Pulsatile thyrotropin and prolactin secretion in a patient with a mixed thyrotropin- and prolactin-secreting pituitary adenoma, Eur J Endocrinol 130:113, 1994.
71. Burgess JR, Shepherd JJ, Greenaway TM: Thyrotropinomas in multiple endocrine neoplasia type 1 (MEN-1), Aust N Z J Med 24:740, 1994.
72. Wynne AG, Gharib H, Scheithauer BW, et al: Hyperthyroidism due to inappropriate secretion of thyrotropin in 10 patients, Am J Med 92:15, 1992.
73. Taylor TJ, Donlon SS, Bale AE, et al: Treatment of a thyrotropinoma with octreotide-LAR in a patient with multiple endocrine neoplasia-1, Thyroid 10:1001, 2000
74. Gessl A, Freissmuth M, Czech T, et al: Growth hormone-prolactin-thyrotropin-secreting pituitary adenoma in atypical McCune-Albright syndrome with functionally normal Gsα protein, J Clin Endocrinol Metab 79:1128, 1994.
75. Langlois M-F, Lamarche JB, Bellabarba D: Long-standing goiter and hypothyroidism: An unusual presentation of a TSH-secreting adenoma, Thyroid 6:329, 1996.
76. Ekins R: Measurement of free hormones in blood, Endocr Rev 11:5, 1990.
77. Beck-Peccoz P, Piscitelli G, Cattaneo MG, et al: Evaluation of free thyroxine methods in the presence of iodothyronine binding autoantibodies, J Clin Endocrinol Metab 58:736, 1984.
78. Zweig MH, Csako G, Spero M: Escape from blockade of interfering heterophile antibodies in a two-site immunoradiometric assay for thyrotropin, Clin Chem 34:2589, 1988.
79. Beck-Peccoz P, Persani L: Variable biological activity of thyroid-stimulating hormone, Eur J Endocrinol 131:331, 1994.
80. Bevan JS, Burke CW, Esiri MM, et al: Studies of two thyrotropin-secreting pituitary adenomas: Evidence for dopamine receptor deficiency, Clin Endocrinol 31:59, 1989.
81. Magner JA, Kane J: Binding of thyrotropin to lentil lectin is unchanged by thyrotropin-releasing hormone administration in three patients with thyrotropin-producing pituitary adenomas, Endocr Res 8:163, 1992.
82. Magner JA, Klibanski A, Fein H, et al: Ricin and lentil lectin affinity chromatography reveals oligosaccharide heterogeneity of thyrotropin secreted by 12 human pituitary tumors, Metabolism 41:1009, 1992.
83. Kourides IA, Ridgway EC, Weintraub BD, et al: Thyrotropin-induced hyperthyroidism: Use of alpha and beta subunit levels to identify patients with primary tumors, J Clin Endocrinol Metab 45:534, 1977.
84. Beck-Peccoz P, Persani L, Faglia G: Glycoprotein hormone α-subunit in pituitary adenomas, Trends Endocrinol Metab 3:41, 1992.
85. Franklyn J, Shephard M: Evaluation of thyroid function in health and disease. In DeGroot LJ (Ed): Thyroid disease, http://www.thyroidmanager.org, 2008
86. Watanabe K, Kameya T, Yamauchi A, et al: Thyrotropin-producing adenoma associated with pituitary resistance to thyroid hormone, J Clin Endocrinol Metab 76:1025, 1993.
87. Azarnivar A, Chopra IJ: Tension pneumoencephalus after transsphenoidal resection of a thyrotropin (TSH)-secreting pituitary adenoma, Endocrinologist 5:308, 1995.
88. Beck-Peccoz P, Roncoroni R, Mariotti S, et al: Sex hormone-binding globulin measurement in patients with inappropriate secretion of thyrotropin (IST): Evidence against selective pituitary thyroid hormone resistance in nonneoplastic IST, J Clin Endocrinol Metab 71:19, 1990.
89. Persani L, Preziati D, Matthews CH, et al: Serum levels of carboxyterminal cross-linked telopeptide of type I collagen (ICTP) in the differential diagnosis of the syndromes of inappropriate secretion of TSH, Clin Endocrinol 47:207, 1997.
90. Rubello D, Busnardo B, Girelli ME, et al: Severe hyperthyroidism due to neoplastic TSH hypersecretion in an old man, J Endocrinol Invest 12:571, 1989.
91. Chanson P, Weintraub BD, Harris AG: Octreotide therapy for thyroid stimulating hormone-secreting pituitary adenomas: A follow-up of 52 patients, Ann Intern Med 119:236, 1993.
92. Losa M, Magnani P, Mortini P, et al: Indium-111 pentetreotide single-photon emission tomography in patients with TSH-secreting pituitary adenomas: Correlation with the effect of a single administration of octreotide on serum TSH levels, Eur J Nucl Med 24:728, 1997.
93. Mannavola D, Persani L, Vannucchi G, et al: Different responses to chronic somatostatin analogues in patients with central hyperthyroidism, Clin Endocrinol (Oxf) 62:176, 2005.
94. Webster J, Peters JR, John R, et al: Pituitary stone: Two cases of densely calcified thyrotropin-secreting pituitary adenomas, Clin Endocrinol 40:137, 1994.
95. Nabarro JDN: Acromegaly, Clin Endocrinol (Oxf) 26:481, 1987.
96. Lamberts SWJ, Krenning EP, Reubi J-C: The role of somatostatin and its analogs in the diagnosis and treatment of tumors, Endocr Rev 12:450, 1991.
97. Verhoeff NPLG, Bemelman FJ, Wiersinga WM, et al: Imaging of dopamine D2 and somatostatin receptors in vivo using single-photon emission tomography in a patient with a TSH/PRL-producing pituitary macroadenoma, Eur J Nucl Med 20:555, 1993.
98. Frank SJ, Gesundheit N, Doppman JL, et al: Preoperative lateralization of pituitary microadenomas by petrosal sinus sampling: Utility in two patients with non-ACTH-secreting tumors, Am J Med 87:679, 1989.
99. Mariotti S, Anelli S, Bartalena L, et al: Familial hyperthyroidism due to nonneoplastic inappropriate TSH secretion associated with sellar abnormalities [Abstract], J Endocrinol Invest 10(Suppl 1):20, 1987.
100. Hall WA, Luciano MG, Doppman JL, et al: Pituitary magnetic resonance imaging in normal human volunteers: Occult adenomas in the general population, Ann Intern Med 120:817, 1994.
101. Safer JD, Colan SD, Fraser LM, et al: A pituitary tumor in a patient with thyroid hormone resistance: A diagnostic dilemma, Thyroid 11:281, 2001.
102. McCutcheon IE, Weintraub BD, Oldfield EH: Surgical treatment of thyrotropin-secreting pituitary adenomas, J Neurosurg 73:674, 1990.
103. Losa M, Mortini P, Franzin A, et al: Surgical management of thyrotropin-secreting pituitary adenomas, Pituitary 2:127, 1999.
104. Mouton F, Faivre-Defrance F, Cortet-Rudelli C, et al: TSH secreting adenoma improved with cabergoline, Ann Endocrinol (Paris) 69:244, 2008.
105. Zuniga S, Mendoza V, Espinoza IF, et al: A plurihormonal TSH-secreting pituitary microadenoma: Report of a case with an atypical clinical presentation and transient response to bromocriptine therapy, Endocr Pathol 8:81, 1997.
106. Comi R, Gesundheit N, Murray L, et al: Response of thyrotropin-secreting pituitary adenomas to a long-acting somatostatin analogue, N Engl J Med 317:12, 1987.
107. Gourgiotis L, Skarulis MC, Brucker-Davis F, et al: Effectiveness of long-acting octreotide in suppressing hormonogenesis and tumor growth in thyrotropin-secreting pituitary adenomas: report of two cases, Pituitary 4:135, 2001.
108. Caron P, Arlot S, Bauters C, et al: Efficacy of the long-acting octreotide formulation (octreotide-LAR) in patients with thyrotropin-secreting pituitary adenomas, J Clin Endocrinol Metab 86:2849, 2001.
109. Gancel A, Vuillermet P, Legrand A, et al: Effects of a slow-release formulation of the new somatostatin analogue lanreotide in TSH-secreting pituitary adenomas, Clin Endocrinol 40:421, 1994.
110. Kuhn JM, Arlot S, Lefebvre H, et al: Evaluation of the treatment of thyrotropin-secreting pituitary adenomas with a slow release formulation of the somatostatin analog lanreotide, J Clin Endocrinol Metab 85:1487, 2000.
111. Francis TB, Smallridge RC, Kane J, et al: Octreotide changes serum thyrotropin (TSH) glycoisomer distribution as assessed by lectin chromatography in a TSH macroadenoma patient, J Clin Endocrinol Metab 77:183, 1993.
112. Hill S, Falko J, Wilson C, et al: Thyrotropin-producing pituitary adenomas, J Neurosurg 57:515, 1982.
113. Caron P, Gerbaud C, Pradayrol L, et al: Successful pregnancy in an infertile woman with a thyrotropin-secreting macroadenoma treated with somatostatin analog (octreotide), J Clin Endocrinol Metab 81:1164, 1996.
114. Blackhurst G, Strachan MW, Collie D, et al: The treatment of a thyrotropin-secreting pituitary macroadenoma with octreotide in twin pregnancy, Clin Endocrinol (Oxf) 57:401, 2002.

Chapter 11

DISORDERS OF PROLACTIN SECRETION AND PROLACTINOMAS

MARCELLO D. BRONSTEIN

Nongestational/puerperal prolactin (PRL) hypersecretion is the most prevalent hypothalamic-pituitary dysfunction, and its main cause is PRL-secreting pituitary adenomas (prolactinomas). Prolactinomas are the most common pituitary tumors, with an estimated prevalence of 500 cases/1 million inhabitants.[1] These tumors are classified either as microadenomas (diameter <10 mm) or macroadenomas (>10 mm) and can be enclosed, expansive, or invasive.[2] Prolactinomas are more common in women, especially microprolactinomas; macroprolactinomas have roughly the same prevalence in both genders. PRL-secreting pituitary carcinomas are exceedingly rare.[3] Because hyperprolactinemia usually is associated with menstrual disturbances, anovulation, and sexual impairment in both genders, and pro-

lactinomas have a greater incidence in people in their 20s and 30s, these tumors are an important cause of infertility. To make the correct diagnosis of prolactinoma, other causes of hyperprolactinemia—physiologic, drug-induced, or pathologic—must be ruled out. It also is important to be aware of laboratory and imaging pitfalls that can mislead the diagnosis and treatment.[4] This chapter addresses the causes, clinical findings, diagnosis, and therapeutic options for prolactinomas and other causes of hyperprolactinemia.

History

"If a woman is neither pregnant nor has given birth, and produces milk, her menstruation has stopped." This sentence, attributed to Hippocrates (*Aphorisms*, Section 5, #39), shows that the association between menstrual disturbances and inappropriate milk secretion has been known since ancient times. It was only in the 20th century, however, that such disturbances were associated with hypersecretion of a pituitary hormone. In 1928, Striker and Grueter[5] identified a pituitary factor that was able to induce milk secretion in rabbits. Early in the 18th century, Hunter discovered that "pigeon's milk," a substance secreted by male and female parents to feed the young pigeon, is secreted by the crop, and according to Hunter, "the crop behaves like the udder of mammalian females regarding uterine gestation." In 1933, Riddle and colleagues[6] identified the stimulatory effect of a pituitary hormone on pigeons' crop growth and differentiation, which also controlled milk secretion in mammals, and called it *prolactin*. The pigeon's crop model later was used for the PRL bioassay. Coincidentally, the association of amenorrhea, infertility, and galactorrhea were described better around the 1930s.

Afterward, this clinical picture was characterized in three different contexts: (1) postpartum without sellar enlargement (Chiari-Frommel syndrome)[7]; (2) nonpuerperal period, also without sellar augmentation (Ahumada-Argonz-del Castillo syndrome)[8]; and (3) associated with a pituitary tumor (Forbes-Albright syndrome).[9] The existence of a human PRL, distinct from the growth hormone (GH), remained controversial, however, until the development of a specific radioimmunoassay for PRL in the early 1970s,[10] when it was shown that all the above-mentioned syndromes were linked to elevated serum PRL levels. The development of pituitary microsurgery and, later on, of high-resolution imaging techniques showed that most of the cases with normal sella on plain x-rays, described as nontumoral, were small pituitary tumors (microadenomas). When PRL-secreting pituitary adenomas (prolactinomas) were proved to be the main cause of pathologic hyperprolactinemia, linked or not to a previous pregnancy, the division borne by the three eponymic amenorrhea-galactorrhea syndromes became obsolete. There are many other causes of hyperprolactinemia that must be differentiated from prolactinomas so that a correct therapeutic approach can be instituted.

Epidemiology

Hyperprolactinemia is the most prevalent hypothalamic-pituitary dysfunction, with prolactinomas being the main cause. These tumors represent roughly 25% of surgically removed pituitary adenomas and nearly 50% of adenohypophyseal tumors in autopsy series.[11] This apparent discrepancy may be due to the excellent results of medical treatment of prolactinomas with dopaminergic agonists. Their prevalence is estimated at 500 cases/1 million inhabitants, with an incidence of 27 cases/1 million/year.[1] Microprolactinomas (diameter <10 mm) represent about 60% of PRL-secreting adenomas and are more common in women than in men (20:1), whereas macroadenomas have roughly the same prevalence on both genders.[12] There are no sex-related differences in autopsy series. Prolactinomas occur in all ages, with the diagnosis made predominantly in the 20s and 30s in both sexes.[12] They are the most frequent pituitary adenomas encountered in childhood and adolescence.[12] Prolactinomas represent the minority of pituitary tumors diagnosed after age 70, however. Prolactinomas are the most prevalent pituitary adenoma in the multiple endocrine neoplasia type 1 (MEN1) syndrome.[12] Isolated familial prolactinomas (not related to MEN1) have been described.[13] PRL-secreting pituitary carcinomas are exceedingly rare, with about 50 documented cases in the literature.[3]

Pathogenesis

Similar to other pituitary adenomas, prolactinomas are monoclonal in origin.[14] To date, the exact mechanisms leading to the development of lactotroph adenomas are not well established. Among the candidates are the pituitary tumor transforming gene (PTTG)[15] and the heparin-binding secretory transforming gene (HST),[16] both of which induce angiogenesis through fibroblast growth factors (FGF-2 and FGF-4). Estrogens seem to play a pivotal role in these mechanisms, because estrogen-modulator drugs (e.g., tamoxifen and raloxifene) and the antiestrogen ICI-182780 inhibit PTTG expression in prolactinomas in vitro and their growth in vivo (Fig. 11-1).[17] Reduction in the expression of the cytokine leukemia inhibitory factor[18] and nerve growth factor[19] and the overexpression of bone morphogenetic protein 4[20] and the high-mobility group A2 gene (HMGA2)[21] are among other events that potentially might be involved in prolactinoma tumorigenesis.

Studies on the microvascular density of prolactinomas show conflicting results: One study by electronic microscopy did not disclose differences between vascular density of the normal pituitary and microprolactinomas, but macroprolactinomas exhibited a much lower degree of vascularization. A more recent study using immunohistochemistry with antibodies for different

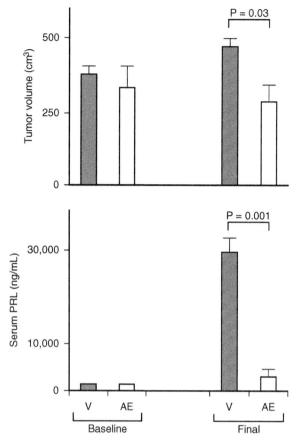

FIGURE 11-1. Selective antiestrogen treatment inhibits pituitary tumor growth in vivo. Pretreatment (baseline) and posttreatment tumor volumes and serum prolactin (PRL) levels after mini osmotic pumps infusion of vehicle or antiestrogen ICI-182780 (0.5 μg/day) was infused in 20 female Wistar-Furth rats harboring subcutaneous pituitary tumors. All animals developed tumors. Each bar represents mean ± SEM for 10 animals per group. *P = 0.03; **P < 0.001. (From Heaney AP, Fernando M, Melmed S: Functional role of estrogen in pituitary tumor pathogenesis. J Clin Invest 109:277–283, 2002.)

endothelial markers observed that microprolactinomas are less vascular than macroprolactinomas. Additionally, microvascular density was related to tumor invasiveness and malignancy.[22]

The decrease of dopaminergic inhibition seems to play a role, at least a permissive one, in prolactinoma development. Lesions in the tuberoinfundibular dopaminergic neurons in female rats bearing prolactinomas were described.[23] Several studies have shown the development of prolactinomas in mice with D2 receptor knockout, with this phenotype being more severe and presenting a faster evolution in females and in animals treated with estrogens.[24,25] To date, no "natural" mutations were found in the D2 receptor gene.[26] PRLr(–/–) mice exhibited more intense hyperprolactinemia and larger tumors than did age-matched Drd2(–/–) mice, and there were cumulative effects in compound homozygous mutant male mice. This fact suggests that PRL inhibits lactotrophs not only by the activation of hypothalamic dopamine neurons, but also directly within the pituitary in a dopamine-independent fashion.

Prolactinomas associated with MEN1 present inactivating mutations characterized by loss of heterozygosity in locus 11q13 and mutations in the menin-codifying gene. They tend to be larger and more aggressive than their sporadic counterparts.[12] Sporadic prolactinomas may exhibit loss of heterozygosity but without mutations in the menin gene detected to date, suggesting the presence of a tumor suppressor gene located within chromosome 11q13 yet distinct from MEN1.[27] The recently described inactivating mutations of the gene encoding aryl hydrocarbon receptor–interacting protein (AIP) on chromosome 11q13.3 are frequently found in isolated familial pituitary adenomas (mainly somatotropinomas but also prolactinomas)[28] but rarely in sporadic pituitary tumors.[29] Finally, mutations in the proto-oncogene *ras* and in the tumor suppressor gene *TP53* can be linked to the development of the rare PRL-secreting carcinomas.[3]

Pathology

The terms *microadenoma* and *macroadenoma*, coined by Hardy,[30] represent pituitary adenomas measuring less or more than 1 cm, respectively. Microprolactinomas are found mainly in young women, usually located in the lateral portions of the pituitary. They are generally enclosed within a pseudocapsule but also can be invasive.[31] Macroprolactinomas also can be enclosed but usually expand to the optic chiasmal region or invade local structures such as the cavernous sinus or the sellar floor and sphenoid sinus.[31] Histologically, there are no differences between microprolactinomas and macroprolactinomas, which are usually "chromophobic" on hematoxylin-eosin staining. For this reason, many pituitary adenomas previously classified as "functionless" before the development of a radioimmunoassay for PRL were prolactinomas. This fact is explained by the use of electronic microscopy, which characterized most prolactinomas as sparsely granulated: oval and slightly irregular nuclei, complex rough endoplasmic reticulum, large Golgi complexes, and sparse spherical or pleomorphic secretory granules, measuring 130 to 500 nm (Fig. 11-2).[32] The hallmark of these tumors is the so-called misplaced exocytosis, the extrusion of secretory granules along the lateral cell border. This phenomenon diagnoses PRL secretion either by normal or by neoplastic lactotrophs. The rare, densely granulated lactotroph adenoma is strongly acidophilic with strong, diffuse immunostaining for PRL in the cytoplasm. The rough endoplasmic reticulum is less prominent, and the secretory granules are bigger (500 to 700 nm) and more numerous than in its sparsely granulated counterpart.[32]

Electron microscopy usually is not required for prolactinoma diagnosis since the immunohistochemical assessment of PRL production became routinely available. This technique directly characterizes PRL-secreting adenomas, ruling out "functionless" macroadenomas associated with hyperprolactinemia due to hypothalamus-pituitary disconnection, the so-called pseudoprolactinomas.[33] A study of 120 unselected necropsies showed that 27% of them harbored pituitary microadenomas without clinical expression, 40% of which immunostained for PRL.[11] These data indicate that there could be clinically and hormonally non–PRL-secreting pituitary adenomas that are immunohistochemically positive for this hormone. The significance of this finding for the natural history of prolactinomas is unknown.

ACIDOPHIL STEM CELL ADENOMA

Exceptionally hyperprolactinemic patients might exhibit mild or no clinical features of acromegaly associated with biochemical evidence of slight serum GH elevation. This situation is due to the presence of the rare and aggressive acidophil stem cell pituitary adenoma.[34] The acidophilia is attributable to mitochondrial accumulation called *oncocytic change*. Immunohistochemical analysis is positive for PRL, and occasionally there is a scant positivity for GH. The definitive diagnosis requires electron

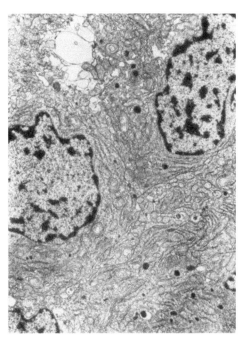

FIGURE 11-2. Electronic microscopy of a sparsely granulated prolactinoma, showing sparse secretory granules, well-developed rough endoplasmic reticulum, and prominent Golgi complexes.

microscopy, which depicts enlarged mitochondria. Scattered cells containing juxtanuclear fibrous bodies are similar to cells of sparsely granulated somatotroph adenomas. Misplaced exocytosis is present. The secretory granules are sparse and small, measuring 150 to 200 nm.

NONTUMORAL LESIONS ASSOCIATED WITH HYPERPROLACTINEMIA

Many nontumoral conditions can be mistaken for prolactinomas. Thyrotroph hyperplasia is associated with primary hypothyroidism due to loss of feedback (Fig. 11-3).[35] The correct diagnosis is important because this condition regresses with thyroid hormone replacement.[35] Idiopathic lactotroph hyperplasia is a rare cause of hyperprolactinemia that mistakenly can be taken for an expanding macroprolactinoma. The pituitary mass shape can help in the differential diagnosis. Inflammatory lesions such as lymphocytic hypophysitis (occurring mainly during pregnancy and puerperium) and sarcoidosis can be misdiagnosed as lactotroph adenoma.[36,37]

PITUITARY PROLACTIN-SECRETING CARCINOMAS

Pituitary PRL-secreting carcinomas are exceedingly rare tumors that exhibit morphologic features indistinguishable from those of PRL-secreting adenomas. In addition to local invasiveness, distant intracranial and extracranial metastases in the nervous system and visceral metastases are the clues for the diagnosis of malignancy. Regarding intracranial lesions, sometimes it is difficult to distinguish between contiguity of an invasive prolactinoma and true metastasis from a PRL-secreting carcinoma.[3]

Differential Diagnosis of Hyperprolactinemia

The main causes of hyperprolactinemia are listed in Table 11-1.

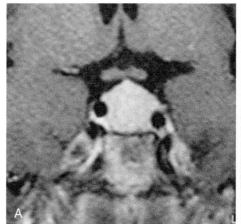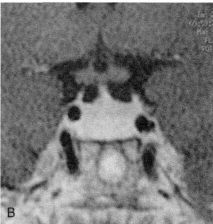

FIGURE 11-3. Magnetic resonance imaging (gadolinium-enhanced T1-weighted coronal views) of a 41-year-old woman with primary hypothyroidism before **(A)** and after 1 month on levothyroxine replacement therapy **(B).** (From Bronstein MD: Problems in the differential diagnosis of the hyperprolactinemic patient. Clinical Endocrinology Update 2003, syllabus pp 241–247; with permission of the Endocrine Society.)

Table 11-1. Causes of Hyperprolactinemia

PHYSIOLOGIC
Pregnancy and puerperium
Neonatal period
Physical activity
"Stress"

DRUG-INDUCED
Dopamine receptor blockers
   Sulpiride
   Chlorpromazine
   Haloperidol
   Risperidone
   Metoclopramide
   Domperidone
Serotonin reuptake inhibitors
Cimetidine
Tricyclic antidepressants
Verapamil
Methyldopa
Protease inhibitors

PATHOLOGIC
Pituitary disease
   Prolactinomas
   Acromegaly
   Cushing's disease
   Nelson's syndrome
   Lymphocytic hypophysitis
   "Empty sella" syndrome
Hypothalamic disease and hypothalamus/pituitary disconnection
   Tumors
      Nonfunctioning pituitary adenomas
      Meningiomas
      Dysgerminomas
      Craniopharyngiomas
   Inflammatory/granulomatous
      Sarcoidosis
      Histiocytosis
   Stalk section
   Vascular
   Actinic
Neurogenic
   Chest wall lesions
   Spinal cord lesions
Miscellaneous
   Primary hypothyroidism
   Adrenal insufficiency
   Uremia
   Cirrhosis
   Paraneoplastic
   Idiopathic

PHYSIOLOGIC HYPERPROLACTINEMIA

Throughout pregnancy, the size of a normal pituitary increases up to 136%, according to magnetic resonance imaging (MRI) studies.[38] This extensive growth is due to estrogen-induced hypertrophy and hyperplasia of lactotrophs, leading to progressive increase in PRL production and its hypersecretion during pregnancy.[39] Placental estrogen production stimulates lactotroph mitosis, PRL mRNA levels, and PRL synthesis, leading to a stepwise increase in serum PRL levels, achieving mean levels of 200 ng/mL at the end of pregnancy and up to 450 ng/mL in some cases. Serum PRL levels decline quickly after delivery but are maintained slightly increased in nursing women several months, especially after breastfeeding. At birth, newborn serum PRL concentrations are elevated nearly 10-fold, probably as a result of the stimulatory effect of maternal estrogen levels.[40]

Because exercise and nonspecific stress are physiologic causes of hyperprolactinemia, there is a concern that the stress-induced PRL increase could lead to hormone elevation during venipuncture, and a period of rest before blood withdrawal is still recommended in many laboratories. A report by Vieira and coworkers,[41] which included a large population, provided evidence that rest before blood collection may be needed in only a few patients.

PHARMACOLOGIC HYPERPROLACTINEMIA

Among medications that increase serum PRL, dopamine receptor blockers are the most potent. Neuroleptics (e.g., sulpiride, haloperidol, chlorpromazine, risperidone) and antiemetic drugs (e.g., metoclopramide, domperidone) can elevate serum PRL to levels that usually are detected with prolactinomas.[42] Serotoninergic and antihistaminergic drugs are less potent than antidopaminergic medications. The calcium channel blocker verapamil elevates serum PRL levels probably by decreasing central dopamine generation, possibly through N-type calcium channels.[43] It was shown that protease inhibitors used for treatment of acquired immunodeficiency syndrome can cause hyperprolactinemia, but the mechanism is unknown.[44] A detailed inquiry about drug use is mandatory for all hyperprolactinemic patients.

PATHOLOGIC HYPERPROLACTINEMIA

Hyperprolactinemia is present in about 40% of acromegalic patients as a result of GH/PRL co-secretion by the same or by different tumor cells or secondary to hypothalamus-pituitary disconnection.[45] Because of the characteristic features of acromegaly, the differential diagnosis is usually not a problem. As already mentioned, in patients harboring the rare acidophil stem cell pituitary adenoma, serum GH is usually low compared with PRL levels, however, and acromegalic features are usually absent or minimally expressed.[34] In some cases, PRL resistance to dopamine agonists can be a clue for the differential diagnosis with prolactinomas.

Hyperprolactinemia secondary to impaired hypothalamic/tuberoinfundibular dopamine secretion or to stalk or even intrapituitary disconnection can be caused by tumors, inflammatory diseases, or trauma. In these cases, PRL is produced by normal lactotrophs and rarely exceeds 150 μg/L. The differential diagnosis of macroprolactinomas is mainly with clinically nonfunctioning pituitary adenomas (pseudoprolactinomas) and, to a lesser extent, with craniopharyngiomas.[46] Other tumoral lesions, such as meningiomas and chordomas, and nontumoral conditions, such as "empty sella" syndrome and even intrasellar aneurysms, can be associated with hyperprolactinemia, however (Fig. 11-4).[47] The differential diagnosis between macroprolactinomas and pseudoprolactinomas is crucial regarding their primary treatment—medical for macroprolactinomas and surgical for pseudoprolactinomas. Patients with nonfunctioning tumors treated with dopamine agonists were considered as having resistant macroprolactinomas, owing to the absence of tumor shrinkage even with the (obvious) PRL decrease to very low or undetectable levels (Fig. 11-5).[48] A clue to differentiate pseudoprolactinomas from true prolactinomas is the dramatic early PRL decrease with bromocriptine doses of 1.25 mg/day.

Primary hypothyroidism can be associated with hyperprolactinemia, presumably due to high thyrotropin-releasing hormone levels that stimulate PRL release and presumably reduce prolactin metabolic clearance. Thyrotroph hyperplasia may occur, leading to pituitary enlargement mimicking a pituitary adenoma (see Fig. 11-3).[35] Cushing's disease and adrenal insufficiency can

be associated with hyperprolactinemia, which also can be present in Nelson's syndrome.[49,50] Polycystic ovary syndrome also may be associated with hyperprolactinemia.[51] Menstrual disturbances are prevalent in patients with polycystic ovary syndrome and in patients with prolactinomas, and sometimes the distinction between the two conditions may be difficult. The presence of mild hyperprolactinemia, negative pituitary imaging, high luteinizing hormone/follicle stimulating–hormone ratio, and clinical features suggestive of polycystic ovary syndrome can help in the differential diagnosis.

Uremia can be associated with hyperprolactinemia, mainly in patients with end-stage renal disease.[52] The mechanism probably is related to reduced PRL clearance and to a presumably reduced dopaminergic tonus. Serum PRL elevation is mild but can be considerably increased in uremic patients taking drugs with a dopamine receptor–blocking effect. Hyperprolactinemia is present in up to 20% of patients with liver cirrhosis, probably due to an unbalanced estrogen-to-androgen ratio and to an altered dopaminergic tonus.[53] Nipple manipulation and chest-wall lesions, such as herpes zoster and surgical scars, may increase serum PRL via stimulation of neuron pathways going through the spinal cord.[54] In contrast to paraneoplastic adrenocorticotropic hormone (ACTH) secretion, ectopic production of PRL has rarely been described.[55] Finally, when all the above-mentioned causes are ruled out, hyperprolactinemia is considered idiopathic or functional. It is likely, however, that most patients with this condition harbor small microprolactinomas that went undetected with less-sensitive imaging tools used in the past, such as hypocycloidal polytomography and computed tomography (CT) and even with MRI. If there is no radiologic evidence of a prolactinoma at initial diagnosis of hyperprolactinemia, however, an identifiable adenoma is unlikely to develop in the long-term follow-up.[56] Nevertheless, a recent study by De Bellis et al.[57]

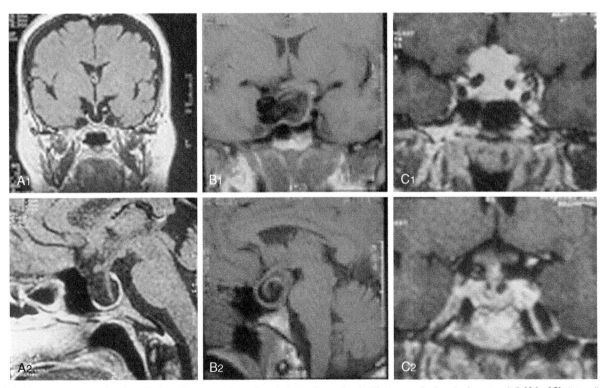

FIGURE 11-4. Magnetic resonance imaging of lesions (*1*, coronal views; *2*, sagittal views) associated with hyperprolactinemia: "empty sella" **(A1, A2)**, intrasellar aneurysm **(B1, B2)**, and meningioma **(C1, C2)**.

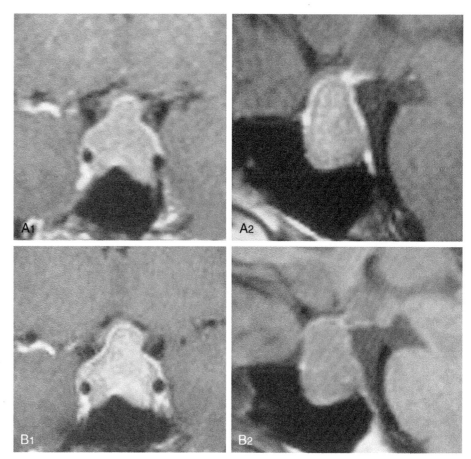

FIGURE 11-5. Magnetic resonance imaging of a 41-year-old woman with a nonfunctioning pituitary adenoma and serum prolactin level of 51 ng/mL before (**A1,** coronal view; **A2,** sagittal view) and during the 12th month of cabergoline "treatment" (**B1,** coronal view; **B2,** sagittal view). No tumor shrinkage was observed, despite serum prolactin decrease to 1.2 ng/mL. (From Bronstein MD: Problems in the differential diagnosis of the hyperprolactinemic patient. Clinical Endocrinology Update 2003, syllabus pp 241–247; with permission of the Endocrine Society.)

points out the presence of anti-pituitary antibodies in 25.7% of patients with idiopathic hyperprolactinemia versus 0% in those with microprolactinoma, suggesting an autoimmune etiology for a subset of cases of idiopathic hyperprolactinemia.

Diagnosis of Prolactinomas

CLINICAL FEATURES

Hyperprolactinemia and its impact on the gonadotropic axis is the hallmark of microprolactinomas and macroprolactinomas and their clinical manifestations. Macroprolactinomas also may cause neurologic and visual disturbances and impairment of other pituitary functions owing to the tumor-mass effect (Table 11-2).[58] Loss of visual fields and impairment of visual acuity are the main ophthalmologic manifestations. Headache is the most common neurologic presentation; it is attributed to dural stretch or cavernous sinus invasion and less frequently as part of the clinical symptoms of pituitary apoplexy.[59] There are a few reports of special types of headache, such as the SUNCT (short-lasting unilateral neuralgiform headache attacks with conjunctival injection and tearing) syndrome secondary to prolactinomas, but the role of hyperprolactinemia as causative agent is obscure.[60] Other rare presentations of invasive macroprolactinomas are hydrocephalus,[61] neuropsychiatric manifestations, and otoneurologic manifestations.[62,63]

Women generally present with a correlation between the degree of serum PRL elevation and gonadal impairment, ranging

Table 11-2. Clinical Manifestations of Prolactinomas

RELATED TO HYPERPROLACTINEMIA
Gonadal impairment
    Menstrual disturbances
    Infertility
    Sexual dysfunction
    Osteoporosis
Galactorrhea

RELATED TO TUMOR MASS EFFECT
Visual disturbances
    Visual field defects
    Reduced visual acuity
    Disturbances of ocular motility
Headache
Rare manifestations
    Trigeminal neuralgia
    Hydrocephalus
    Otoneurologic
    Neuropsychiatric
Impairment of other pituitary functions

from a short luteal phase to amenorrhea (Fig. 11-6). Most PRL-secreting pituitary adenomas are associated with amenorrhea, because hyperprolactinemia due to prolactinomas usually shows serum PRL levels greater than 100 ng/mL. Because hyperprolactinemia is present in about 20% of women with amenorrhea,[64] most patients with such menstrual disturbance and high serum PRL levels may harbor a prolactinoma. Because microprolactinomas can be associated with serum PRL levels between 40 and

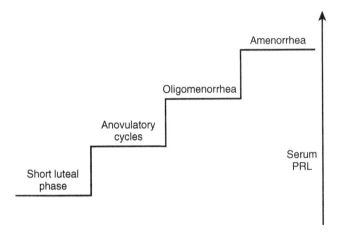

FIGURE 11-6. Serum prolactin (PRL) elevation and gonadal impairment.

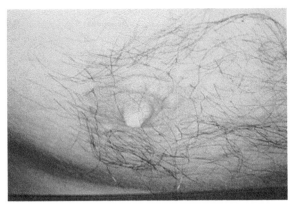

FIGURE 11-7. Galactorrhea in a man harboring a macroprolactinoma.

100 ng/mL, and because PRL biological activity does not always correspond to routine laboratory assay levels,[65] some women with prolactinomas may exhibit milder forms of gonadotropic impairment such as anovulatory cycles and oligomenorrhea.[66] In addition to menstrual disturbances, hyperprolactinemic women complain of loss of libido, vaginal dryness, dyspareunia, and psychological distress.[67] Similar to other disorders associated with hypogonadism, osteoporosis is a frequent finding in women with hyperprolactinemia/prolactinomas, mainly in prolactinomas with long-standing hypogonadism. The relative risk of developing osteoporosis in premenopausal women with prolactinomas can be 4.5%.[68] Although a direct effect of PRL on bone has been considered, there is evidence that hyperprolactinemia is not a risk factor in itself for the development of osteoporosis, with the associated hypoestrogenism being the major determinant.[69]

Galactorrhea is a frequent finding in women with hyperprolactinemia, but it can be absent, mainly in patients with macroprolactinomas associated with severe hypogonadism. Breast examination, if not adequate, also may fail to disclose mild galactorrhea. These facts may explain the discrepancy among series, which show a prevalence of galactorrhea ranging from 30% to 84%.[64,70] Galactorrhea also may occur in normoprolactinemic women. A study including 235 patients with galactorrhea associated with diverse conditions showed that serum PRL was normal in 86% of women with idiopathic galactorrhea without amenorrhea.[71] The mechanism is unknown, being attributed to different causes such as mammary hypersensitivity to PRL or "occult" transient hyperprolactinemia.

Hyperprolactinemia in men is predominantly associated with macroprolactinomas. The main clinical manifestations are hypogonadism, which is usually severe, along with loss of libido and reduced body hair growth, visual impairment, and headache.[72] Only 22.5% of 80 patients with macroprolactinomas in our series sought medical assistance due to sexual complaints, whereas most patients requested appointments because of visual or neurologic disturbances. During the interview, 85% of the patients admitted, however, that loss of libido was of utmost importance.[73] In patients with microprolactinomas ($n = 12$), sexual dysfunction was the main complaint in 67% of the cases, but that number increased to 92% after the interview.[73] Testosterone replacement without serum PRL normalization seldom restores libido, an observation that points to a direct effect of PRL on sexual behavior, as previously suggested by animal models.[74] Galactorrhea is far less frequent in men than in women

with prolactinomas.[75] It was disclosed in 15% and 25% of our patients with macroprolactinomas and microprolactinomas.[73] When present in men harboring pituitary tumors, however, it strongly suggests the presence of a prolactinoma (Fig. 11-7).[75] Osteoporosis also is present in hyperprolactinemic men.[76]

Although the prevalence of prolactinomas in both genders is higher in the 20s and 30s, prolactinomas can occur in elderly and in younger individuals. Data on 44 young patients (12 males and 32 females, aged 16.3 ± 1.9 years at diagnosis) with pituitary adenomas showed a predominance of macroadenomas (61%) over microadenomas (39%). Of those, prolactinomas were the most prevalent (68% of cases).[77] Other series on prolactinomas diagnosed in childhood or adolescence showed that the prevalence of macroadenomas was also higher (15 versus 11 cases)[78] or similar (24 versus 23 cases) compared with microadenomas.[79] The predominance of larger tumors in children and adolescents points to molecular mechanisms influencing proliferation rather than the time course of the disease influencing the progression of prolactinoma size and invasiveness.

LABORATORY EVALUATION

Basal serum PRL evaluation usually confirms the clinical suspicion of a prolactinoma. Serum PRL usually ranges from 50 to 300 ng/mL in the presence of microprolactinomas and from 200 to 5000 ng/mL in the presence of macroprolactinomas (normal values range from 2 to 15 ng/mL). Values of 30 ng/mL have been associated with microprolactinomas, however, and values of 35,000 ng/mL have been found in patients harboring large and invasive macroprolactinomas. Stimulation tests with thyrotropin-releasing hormone and metoclopramide or suppression tests using levodopa, previously popular mainly for the differential diagnosis of microprolactinomas and so-called idiopathic hyperprolactinemia, give nonspecific results and have been largely abandoned.[80]

Hyperprolactinemia secondary to hypothalamus-pituitary disconnection rarely exceeds 150 ng/mL, and lesions that mimic macroprolactinomas, especially nonfunctioning pituitary adenomas, generally exhibit serum PRL less than this value (pseudoprolactinomas).[46] A laboratory artifact may lead to an erroneous differential diagnosis between macroprolactinomas and pseudoprolactinomas, however. When serum PRL is evaluated by two-site immunometric assays, large amounts of antigen—PRL in this case—saturate capture and signal antibodies, impairing their binding and causing serum PRL to be underestimated (the so-called high-dose hook effect). Patients bearing macroprolactinomas with extremely high serum PRL levels (generally >10,000 ng/

mL, depending on the assay measuring range) may present with falsely lower levels, within the 30 to 150 ng/mL range, causing the patient to be misdiagnosed as harboring a nonfunctioning pituitary adenoma. To avoid unnecessary surgeries (treatment of choice for nonfunctioning tumors), PRL assays with serum dilution or using two-step incubation are recommended in patients with macroadenomas who may harbor a prolactinoma.[81]

If such assays are not readily available, clinical clues pointing to prolactinomas are patient age younger than 50 years, presence of galactorrhea in male patients, and tumor shrinkage under dopamine agonist drugs, as shown by fast visual improvement in cases with chiasmal compression or rapid tumor reduction evidenced by MRI.[75]

Another laboratory pitfall concerns the presence of high serum PRL levels in subjects with few or no symptoms related to PRL excess. Human PRL in circulation manifests as marked size heterogeneity, with three forms (23 kD, 50 kD, and 150 to 170 kD) that are indistinguishable by routine assays.[82] The 23-kD form (little PRL) is the most common form, but serum PRL can be elevated secondary to the presence of 150- to 170-kD aggregates with low biological activity (big-big PRL), leading to *macroprolactinemia*, a term coined by Jackson and colleagues[83] in the 1980s. Less frequently, the 50-kD form (big PRL) can be the prevalent circulating form.[84,85] The presence of molecular aggregates with low biological activity, such as big-big PRL, should be suspected when high serum PRL levels are detected in patients without or with scarce signs and symptoms related to hyperprolactinemia.[4,86] Precipitation with polyethylene glycol is an excellent screening method.[87] The predominant molecular form recovered (i.e., assayed after the precipitation) is the highly biologically active little PRL. The gel filtration chromatography confirms the presence of big-big PRL (Fig. 11-8), but being a costly and time-consuming method, it is performed for practical clinical purposes only when polyethylene glycol precipitation results are inconclusive. Macroprolactinemia is a common finding, occurring in 8% to 42% of all cases of hyperprolactinemia.[4] The pathogenesis of macroprolactinemia is still unknown. It could be in part a complex of monomeric PRL with immunoglobulin G[89]; anti-PRL autoantibodies were identified in patients with idiopathic hyperprolactinemia.[89]

Big-big PRL biological activity is still controversial in the literature. Studies in vitro with rat Nb2 cell bioassays show either the presence or the absence of biological activity.[4] To explain the dissociation of presence of activity in vitro but not in vivo, we can speculate that because of its large molecular weight, macroprolactin does not cross the capillary barrier, and it is unable to reach target cells. Additionally, the PRL receptor forms of rat cells are different from those of humans, so a bioassay using cells harboring human PRL receptors which addresses the biological activity of macroprolactin should be of interest. As a matter of fact, a study by Glezer et al.[90] showed that sera of individuals with macroprolactinemia presented lower biological activity in a bioassay using a mouse cell transfected with the long form of human PRL receptor as compared to the rat Nb2 bioassay (Fig. 11-9). Moreover, in a recent publication, Hattori et al.[89] claim that the level of bioactivity of macroprolactin in the Nb2 bioassay is present due to the dissociation of monomeric PRL from the autoantibodies, as a result of the longer incubation and more dilute assay conditions. Despite these controversies in the literature concerning the biological activity of PRL aggregates, most patients with macroprolactinemia do not manifest clinical features related to hyperprolactinemia and do not need any treatment. To avoid unnecessary medical or surgical procedures,

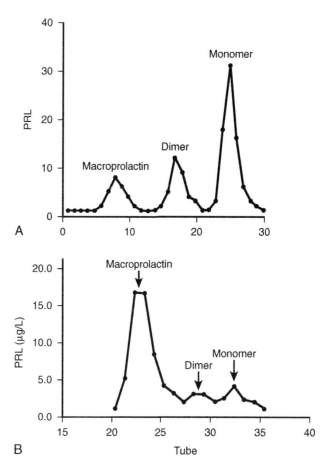

FIGURE 11-8. Gel filtration chromatography of a patient with symptomatic prolactinoma **(A)** and of an asymptomatic woman with macroprolactinemia **(B)**. *PRL,* Prolactin.

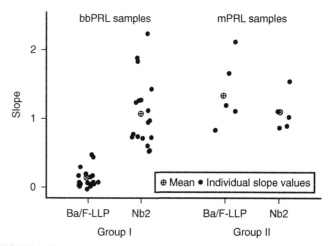

FIGURE 11-9. Individual slopes of bioactivity/immunoactivity (BA/IA) of macroprolactinemic individuals (group I) and hyperprolactinemic patients without macroprolactinemia (group II). The mean slope obtained in Ba/F-LLP assay for group I was significantly lower, compared to that obtained in the Nb2 assay for the same group. On the contrary, no significant differences between the mean slopes of both assays were found in group II. (From Glezer et al: Human macroprolactin displays low biological activity via its homologous receptor in a new sensitive bioassay. J Clin Endocrinol Metab 91:1048–1055, 2006.)

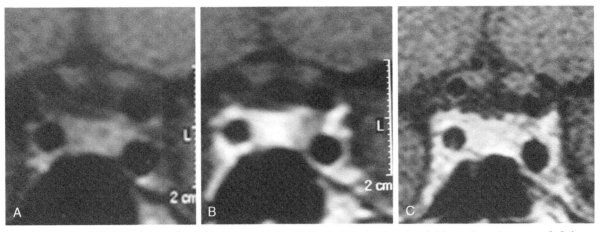

FIGURE 11-10. Magnetic resonance imaging (coronal views) of a microprolactinoma disclosed only during dynamic gadolinium-enhanced sequence. **A,** Before contrast injection. **B,** Lack of contrast enhancement on the left side of the pituitary gland suggestive of microadenoma. **C,** Whole gland contrasted.

macroprolactin screening is mandatory when clinical features and serum PRL assay results are conflicting.

Assessment of other pituitary functions is mandatory, mainly in the presence of macroprolactinomas. Insulin-like growth factor 1 must be followed either to verify GH deficiency or to disclose the rare cases of prolactinomas that progress with PRL/GH co-secretion.[91] Gonadotropin assessment may explain cases with persistent amenorrhea or sexual impairment despite PRL normalization. Although less frequently affected, thyrotropic and adrenocorticotropic axes also must be evaluated. Thyrotropin assessment also may disclose primary hypothyroidism as the cause of hyperprolactinemia.[35] Because restoration of pituitary function may occur after adenoma removal by surgery or tumor shrinkage attained by medical therapy,[92,93] these assessments have to be repeated after such procedures to avoid unnecessary hormone replacement.

IMAGING

MRI is currently the gold-standard imaging method for diagnosis and treatment follow-up of micro- and macroprolactinomas, although CT scan still have a place for sellar region assessment. MRI is superior to CT for tumor boundary delineation, especially regarding its associations with the optic chiasm and cavernous sinus (Fig. 11-10). Additionally, tumor consistency, presence of hemorrhage, and presence of cystic lesions are better shown by MRI, especially comparing T1-weighted and T2-weighted images. CT has the advantage of showing bone erosion and calcifications and may help surgical planning.[94] Although MRI is currently the most sensitive imaging method for microprolactinomas, tumors measuring less than 2 mm may remain undetected by this technique. This fact is well known for the usually tiny ACTH-secreting adenomas leading to Cushing's disease, with about 50% of them not identified by MRI.[95] It is probable that many of the so-called idiopathic hyperprolactinemic patients harbor a small microprolactinoma. Procedures such as dynamic imaging with gadolinium enhancement (Fig. 11-11) and spoiled gradient recalled acquisition technique (SPGR)[96] may contribute to improve MRI sensitivity for such tiny adenomas.

MRI can disclose the so-called pituitary incidentaloma, a term coined by Reincke in 1990 to describe incidentally discovered pituitary masses by imaging performed to evaluate conditions not linked to pituitary disease, including head trauma and sinusitis. Controversies exist in the literature concerning the definition

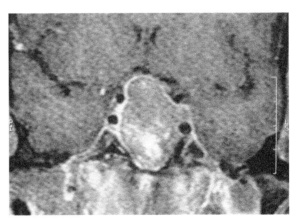

FIGURE 11-11. Magnetic resonance imaging (gadolinium-enhanced coronal view) showing optic chiasm compression and left cavernous sinus invasion by a macroadenoma.

of pituitary incidentalomas.[97] Molitch[98] included patients who presented with symptomatic pituitary disease and who were diagnosed only when a sellar mass was incidentally disclosed. In our opinion, the term *incidentaloma* should be reserved for cases with no endocrine or mass effects of a pituitary adenoma.[4] Incidental imaging findings of pituitary adenomas, mainly microadenomas, are present in up to 27% of autopsy findings in the general population.[11] Other imaging pitfalls include normal anatomic variations such as asymmetric sphenoid septum with bulging of the sellar floor or displacement of the pituitary stalk,[99] artifacts such as clips and prostheses, and global pituitary enlargement—either physiologic, as shown in puberty or even in young adults[100] and pregnancy,[101] or pathologic, as seen in primary hypothyroidism[35] and mental depression.[102]

Regarding the functional evaluation of prolactinomas by imaging, in-vivo imaging by single-photon emission computed tomography using radiolabeled high-affinity benzamine derivatives to D2 receptors, such as iodine 123–methoxybenzamide or iodine 123–epidepride, could serve as a response predictor to dopamine agonist treatment.[103,104] Positron emission tomography using 18-fluorodeoxyglucose, carbon 11–methionine, or dopamine D2 receptor ligands also has been used for in-vivo assessment of the metabolic rate and D2 receptor density of

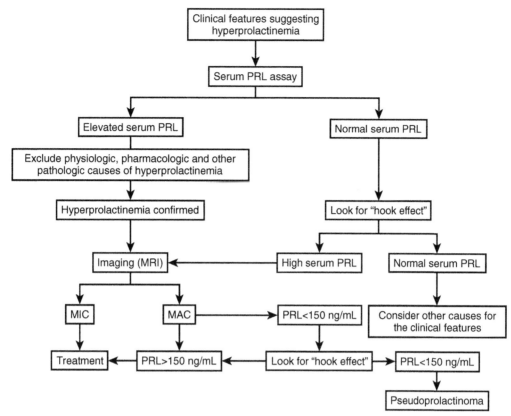

FIGURE 11-12. Flow diagram for the diagnostic evaluation of hyperprolactinemia. *MAC,* Macroadenoma; *MIC,* microadenoma; *PRL,* prolactin.

macroprolactinomas and other pituitary tumors.[105] These methods are expensive and time consuming, however, and are better reserved for the study of tumors without a hormone marker, such as clinically nonfunctioning pituitary adenomas. Regarding prolactinomas, such techniques currently should be reserved for investigational purposes or for special cases, such as searching for metastases in the rare malignant prolactinomas.[106] Fig. 11-12 is a flow diagram for the diagnostic evaluation of hyperprolactinemia.

Treatment

The therapy of hyperprolactinemia/prolactinomas aims at reverting the symptoms dependent on hormone hypersecretion and the neurologic and visual manifestations due to tumor-mass effect. The ideal treatment must spare or even improve other pituitary dysfunctions, if present. Good tolerance and low recurrence rates also are therapeutic goals.

Treatment of secondary hyperprolactinemia is intended to treat or remove the cause of the disorder. Levothyroxine usually corrects hyperprolactinemia associated with primary hypothyroidism. The surgical removal of a nonfunctioning pituitary adenoma with mass effect and withdrawal of drugs such as sulpiride and haloperidol, when possible, bring serum PRL down to normal levels.

As far as prolactinoma treatment is concerned, the 1970s brought almost concomitantly two powerful therapeutic advances: the improvement of pituitary microsurgery[2] and the development of ergot derivatives with potent dopaminergic agonistic activity.[107] Additionally, radiation therapy, including more recent stereotactic techniques, has a place, albeit restricted, in

Table 11-3. Treatment of Prolactinomas

MEDICAL
Dopamine agonist drugs
Sexual steroid replacement (for selective microprolactinomas)

SURGICAL
Transsphenoidal approach
    Sublabial
    Endonasal (with or without endoscope)

RADIOTHERAPY
Conventional
Stereotactic
    Cobalt-60 or linear acceleration (LINAC)
    Single shot ("radiosurgery") or multiple shots
Proton beam

prolactinoma treatment (Table 11-3). Therapeutic strategy must consider several aspects, such as the patient's clinical presentation, the differences between microadenomas and macroadenomas concerning their natural history, the desire for pregnancy, and the patient's treatment preference, if applicable.

SURGICAL THERAPY

Pituitary surgery by the transsphenoidal approach was used at the beginning of the 20th century and was reintroduced in the early 1960s and greatly improved when the surgical microscope was introduced.[2,108] More recently, endonasal endoscopic surgery has become available. Compared to the classic transsphenoidal approach, endoscopic pituitary surgery seems to reduce the time of hospitalization, but improvement of surgical results remains to be demonstrated.[109,110] These developments made the selective removal of the pituitary adenoma possible, sparing the normal gland, along with low complication and mortality rates, mainly for surgeons with more than 500 operations.[111] Besides serum PRL normalization, this surgical modality aims at reducing or eliminating the mass effect of expanding macroadenomas, often leading to the resolution of neurologic and visual manifestations. The transcranial surgical approach is reserved solely for tumors with a predominance of extrasellar location expanding out of the midline.[112]

The surgical success in normalizing serum PRL levels depends on the experience and ability of the surgeon and on the tumor size and invasiveness. Preoperative serum PRL levels, usually associated with tumor dimension and location, were found to be paramount in predicting surgical remission, being the only predictive factor in multivariate analysis in some reports.[113,114] Consequently, the best results were achieved in microprolactinomas with a preoperative serum PRL less than or equal to 100 ng/mL. A study on the initial outcome of 219 women with prolactinomas operated on by transsphenoidal microsurgery showed a remission rate of 92% of cases with preoperative PRL less than or equal to 100 ng/mL and 91% with intrasellar microadenomas, but only 59% in women with microadenomas with cavernous sinus extension, leading to an overall remission rate of 82% for microadenomas. Of the women with macroprolactinomas, 88% with intrasellar adenomas, 86% with moderate suprasellar extension, and 80% with focal sphenoid sinus invasion achieved remission. Surgical remission in patients with diffuse sphenoid sinus invasion, cavernous sinus invasion, and major suprasellar extension was poor, however, ranging from 0% to 44%.[113] In another large series of 120 patients with prolactinomas (93 women and 27 men) who underwent pituitary surgery by the transsphenoidal route, PRL normalization occurred in 78% of patients with microadenomas, in 87.5% of patients with intrasellar macroadenomas, and in 27% of patients with extrasellar macroadenomas.[114]

A compilation of 50 published series showed that postsurgical serum PRL normalization was achieved in 73.7% of 2137 microprolactinomas and 33.9% of 2226 macroprolactinomas.[115] Comparison among the series is difficult, however, because many authors do not mention preoperative serum PRL levels, the tumor size, and degree of invasiveness. The grade of clinical improvement in cured patients is high, mainly in smaller tumors. Menses and fertility restoration is high, and pregnancy rates ranged from 75% to 90% in different series. Some patients can achieve menstrual regulation and even become pregnant without full PRL normalization.[114,116] Sexual improvement in men is less likely to occur, probably owing to irreversible gonadotropic damage caused by the higher frequency of extrasellar and invasive prolactinomas compared with women. Nonetheless, pituitary function generally is preserved in intrasellar adenomas and is restored by the removal of suprasellar adenomas causing hypothalamus-pituitary disconnection.[114] In addition, neurologic and visual amelioration often is achieved after pituitary surgery.

Many patients bearing prolactinomas have undergone treatment with dopamine agonist drugs before surgery. The effect of previous medical therapy on surgical outcome is still a matter of debate. Some reports point to poorer results compared with nontreated patients[117,118]; others do not show significant differences.[113,114] There is also evidence, however, of improvement of surgical results in the medically pretreated group.[119,120] Because the issue of dopamine agonist–induced fibrosis remains unresolved, it is unclear whether the negative outcome was caused directly by the drug or whether it was biased by a tendency to treat medically large and invasive tumors, which present with the poorest surgical results.

An important caveat of surgical treatment is prolactinoma recurrence. This issue was raised in the early 1980s when an article from the Montreal group reported recurrence rates in surgically "cured" patients to be 50% for microprolactinomas and 80% for macroprolactinomas.[121] Subsequently, several reports on this issue were published but with less impressive figures. A literature compilation reported recurrence rates of 18.2% of 809 microprolactinomas and 22.8% of 465 macroprolactinomas.[115] In our series, the recurrence of hyperprolactinemia in surgically cured patients was 27% for microprolactinomas and 17% for macroprolactinomas.[116] Median time to recurrence varied among the different surgical series, from 1 to 7 years. Concerning recurrence predictors, many studies pointed to higher postoperative serum PRL levels in patients who recurred compared with patients without recurrence,[113,121,122] whereas others did not find serum PRL levels to be a predictor of late outcome.[123] Another marker of recurrence is the absence of PRL response to dynamic tests, especially to thyrotropin-releasing hormone.[114,123] These findings raise the question whether, in prolactinomas, serum PRL increase after surgical normalization represents true recurrence or important but incomplete tumor removal.

Although the occurrence of relapses contributes to the decrease of long-term surgical cure rate of prolactinomas, many patients with recurrent hyperprolactinemia remain asymptomatic and have no evidence of tumor regrowth.[113,124] Relapse can be transient. From a cohort of 44 patients with surgically cured microprolactinomas, 8 (18.2%) experienced recurrence and were followed up. Only two of the eight patients experienced permanent relapse.[125] Additional therapy is reserved only for patients with symptomatic recurrence.

Surgical treatment for prolactinomas is indicated for cases with persistent intolerance or hormonal or tumor resistance to dopamine agonists (see later); pituitary apoplexy[126]; tumor growth during medical therapy[127]; cerebrospinal fluid (CSF) leakage due to dopamine agonist–induced tumor shrinkage of invasive macroprolactinomas[128,129]; and (rarely) visual loss on medical therapy, secondary to optic chiasm herniation resulting from tumor retraction.[130] Additionally, surgery is an excellent alternative for patients harboring microprolactinomas, especially patients with serum PRL less than or equal to 100 ng/mL, with poor compliance to medical therapy.[113,131]

MEDICAL THERAPY

The knowledge that dopamine is a powerful inhibitor of PRL secretion has yielded insights regarding use of dopamine agonists in hyperprolactinemia treatment.

Bromocriptine

At the end of the 1960s, an ergot derivative, 2-bromo-α-ergocryptine (bromocriptine) was developed, and shortly thereafter its use in clinical trials was initiated.[107,132] Bromocriptine binds and stimulates the seven-membrane–spanning dopamine D2 receptors in normal and in adenomatous lactotrope cells, inducing activation of the G_i receptor (negatively coupled to adenylate cyclase) and, consequently, leading to postreceptor events that ultimately cause the inhibition of PRL synthesis and secretion.[133] Although many other dopamine agonist drugs were developed thereafter, bromocriptine is still the one that presents the largest and longest worldwide experience (Table 11-4).

Pharmacokinetic studies with bromocriptine show that after a single oral dose of 2.5 mg, serum levels peak, and maximal

CHAPTER 11 — DISORDERS OF PROLACTIN SECRETION AND PROLACTINOMAS   **e199**

Table 11-4. Main Dopamine Agonist Drugs

Drug	Usual Dose
Bromocriptine	2.5-10 mg/day
Pergolide	0.025-0.5 mg/day
Quinagolide*	0.075-0.6 mg/day
Cabergoline	0.5-2 mg/wk

*Not approved in the United States.

suppressive action occurs between 1 and 3 hours. The drug has a relatively short mean elimination half-life (about 6.2 hours) and generally is administered twice a day.[134] Owing to a considerable interindividual variability in the PRL-lowering effects of a given dose of bromocriptine, however, some patients need to take the drug three times a day and others just once a day, mainly when higher doses are required or normoprolactinemia already has been achieved.[135]

Bromocriptine treatment results in serum PRL normalization and clinical improvement in most patients with hyperprolactinemia/prolactinomas. A compilation of 13 series from the literature, encompassing 286 women treated with bromocriptine, showed PRL normalization and return of menses from 64% to 100% and 57% to 100% of cases.[134] Our data showed evidence of normoprolactinemia in 55% of patients with microprolactinoma treated primarily or postsurgically with bromocriptine (mean dose 3.8 mg/day), with menses return in 98% of the patients. Of women without PRL normalization, 81% also recovered menses, making unnecessary the increase of bromocriptine dose, optimizing drug tolerance and reducing costs.[116] Although less frequent, microprolactinoma in men also can be treated successfully with dopamine agonists. Of 12 patients predominantly treated with bromocriptine, 83% achieved normal PRL level and clinical improvement.[135] Eleven men with microprolactinoma have been treated by us, with serum PRL and serum testosterone normalization in 73% and 86% of them.[73]

Because macroprolactinomas often present with mass effect, they were first surgically treated and, if not cured, then treated with bromocriptine. The observation by Corenblum and colleagues[136] in the mid-1970s that bromocriptine use reduces tumor size in addition to its PRL-lowering effect, consequently relieving neurologic and visual complaints, also allowed primary treatment for macroprolactinomas. In a prospective multicenter trial, normal PRL levels were achieved in 18 of 27 patients (67%) followed up for at least 12 months while receiving variable doses of bromocriptine.[137] All patients exhibited some degree of tumor shrinkage: 9, less than 25%; 5, between 25% and 50%; and 13, greater than 50% tumor size reduction. Another study with macroprolactinomas with extrasellar extension showed serum PRL normalization in all of the 10 men and 17 of 19 women, with mean bromocriptine doses of 13 mg/day and 8 mg/day. Tumor size was reduced by more than 50% in 18 of 29 patients (62%) with a secondary empty sella in 5 cases and by less than 50% in 11 patients. Visual field improved in most of the patients who initially presented with such abnormalities.[138] Patients with giant prolactinomas (diameter >4 cm) also achieved disease control with primary bromocriptine therapy.[139] In our series, serum PRL was normalized in 60% of women with macroprolactinomas (mean bromocriptine dose 7 mg/day); 72% of these women had menses recovery. Menses also were restored in 44% of patients who remained hyperprolactinemic.[116] The lower rate of menses normalization compared with women harboring microprolactinomas is probably due to the higher prevalence of

gonadotropic impairment in the macroprolactinoma group. Regarding macroprolactinoma in men, serum PRL and testosterone levels normalized in 67% and 85% of 66 patients bearing macroprolactinomas, showing that in men also, the gonadotropic axis may normalize even when PRL is not fully normalized.[73] Other series show different figures, with PRL returning to normal levels in 83% of patients but with testosterone normalization in only 62% of them, probably reflecting different degrees of gonadotropic impairment. We obtained 80% of tumor reduction in primarily treated macroprolactinoma patients.

The mechanism of prolactinoma shrinkage by dopamine agonists is not yet fully understood. Some reports in the early 1980s suggested that tumor reduction was due to lactotrope cell size reduction.[140] Bromocriptine decreases mRNA and PRL synthesis within days and cell multiplication (antiproliferative and proapoptotic mechanisms have been suggested) and tumor growth.[141] These events are evidenced quickly microscopically by a decrease in the number of PRL secretory granules, involution of the rough endoplasmic reticulum and Golgi apparatus, and decrease of cytoplasmic volume. With longer periods of treatment (e.g., 6 months), there is evidence of cell vacuolization and fragmentation with collagen deposition.[142] These early and late morphologic changes of the tumor lactotropes may explain the rapid regrowth of macroprolactinomas when bromocriptine is discontinued after a short period of therapy,[143] whereas often no tumor expansion is observed when the drug is withdrawn after being used for a longer period.[144] Serum PRL levels may be suppressed in some patients without tumor shrinkage, although the converse does not occur.

The degree of macroprolactinoma reduction by bromocriptine and its time course have been carefully analyzed.[145] Data on 271 patients included from prospective series on primary therapy of true macroprolactinomas showed that 79% of patients presented with more than 25% shrinkage and that 89% of them had shrunk to some degree. Pretreatment serum PRL concentration and gender difference did not predict the degree of tumor reduction. Of 102 prolactinomas large enough to produce chiasmal compression, 85% showed tumor shrinkage of more than 25%. Another compilation, including eight series from the literature totaling 112 patients with macroprolactinomas,[146] showed that 40.2% had a greater than 50% reduction in tumor size; in 28.6%, the reduction was 25% to 50%; in 12.5%, the reduction was less than 25%; and 18.7% had no evidence of tumor size reduction (Table 11-5). The time course of macroprolactinoma shrinkage is highly variable. Some patients experience a dramatic improvement of visual acuity 12 hours after bromocriptine has been introduced, with tumor shrinkage being documented within 1 week. In others, significant tumor reduction is observed only 1 year after medical therapy has been started. In the U.S. multicenter study cited previously,[137] 19 patients had tumor shrinkage in 6 weeks, but in 8 others, the reduction was not observed until the 6-month imaging reassessment was performed. General data from most series show that rapid shrinkage occurs during the first 6 months in most cases, with slower reduction thereafter, and additional decreases in tumor size observed after 1 year for several years in some cases. Visual improvement generally parallels and often precedes tumor shrinkage unless the optic tract has been chronically and severely damaged. Fig. 11-13 illustrates an unusual case of long-term macroprolactinoma shrinkage, showing that minor tumor reduction, even when not depicted by imaging, is sufficient for visual field improvement. In such situations, the clinical amelioration signified that the primary medical therapy was effective even without clear tumor shrinkage, and pituitary surgery could be postponed or, as it was in this case, needless.

Macroprolactinoma reexpansion during successful medical therapy, albeit uncommon, may occur and can lead to visual impairment or headache recurrence.[127] Another rare situation is visual deterioration despite initial improvement, in parallel with tumor shrinkage during medical treatment, provoked by chiasm herniation, which may result from traction on the optic chiasm that is pulled down into the now partially empty sella. The two above-mentioned situations generally require surgical intervention, although drug reduction or discontinuation may repair the chiasm herniation.[130] In addition, pituitary surgery often is needed for a third rare situation, CSF leakage, occurring in macroprolactinomas invading the sphenoid sinus in cases treated with dopamine agonists (Fig. 11-14). In such cases, the tumor shrinkage behaves as the cork removed from a wine bottle, opening a pathway for CSF flow. CSF leakage, which brings a risk for meningitis, often occurs shortly after the beginning of medical therapy[129] but may manifest several months later.[128]

Besides its effect on visual and neurologic symptoms, bromocriptine-induced shrinkage of macroprolactinomas can recover other impaired anterior pituitary functions as a result of the restoration of hypothalamus-pituitary connection, which has been compromised by the tumor-mass effect.[92,93] To avoid the maintenance of unnecessary hormonal replacement, pituitary function must be reassessed in patients with macroprolactinoma and previous hypopituitarism successfully treated by dopamine agonists.

Despite the effectiveness of medical therapy for prolactinomas, one of the drawbacks is the need for long-term therapy. Treatment with bromocriptine and other dopamine agonists generally is considered as "symptomatic" because bromocriptine

discontinuation leads to recurrence of hyperprolactinemia in most patients and, as previously mentioned, to tumor regrowth, at least after short-term use. Concerning long-term therapy with bromocriptine, a retrospective study from our group showed that 25.8% of 62 patients with microprolactinomas and 15.9% of 69 patients with macroprolactinomas treated with bromocriptine for a median time of 47 months continued to be normoprolactinemic after a median time of 44 months of drug withdrawal.[147] There were no statistically significant differences regarding age, gender, bromocriptine initial dose and length of use, tumor size, pregnancy during treatment, and previous pituitary surgery or radiotherapy among patients who continued to be normoprolactinemic and patients who did not. Other reports from the

Male, 30 y

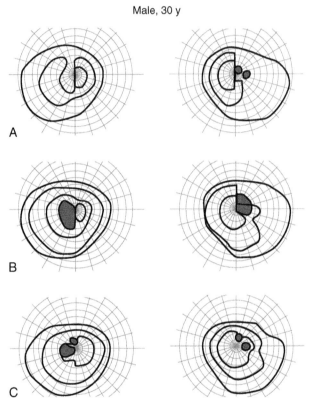

A

B

C

FIGURE 11-13. Visual fields (Goldman perimetry) of a 30-year-old man harboring a macroprolactinoma. Impaired visual fields before treatment (A) showed amelioration 3 days after the beginning of bromocriptine treatment (B) and were almost normalized after 28 days (C) of drug therapy.

Table 11-5. Comparison of Efficacy of Dopamine Agonists in Effecting Tumor Size Reduction

Dopamine Agonist	No. Cases	Tumor Size Reduction (%)			
		>50	25-50	<25	No Change
Bromocriptine	112	40.2	28.6	12.5	18.7
Pergolide	61	75.4	9.8	8.2	6.5
Quinagolide*	105	48.1	20.2	17.3	14.4*
Cabergoline	320	28.4	28.4	14.8	28.4

Data from Molitch ME: Medical management of prolactin-secreting pituitary adenomas. Pituitary 5:55–65, 2002.
*Not approved in the United States.

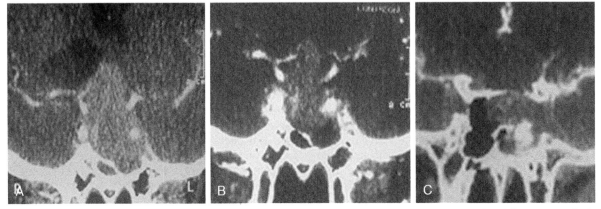

FIGURE 11-14. Computed tomography (coronal views) of a man harboring a macroprolactinoma invading the sphenoid sinus before (A) and 6 days after bromocriptine treatment, showing shrinkage mainly of the sphenoid sinus mass (B), with cerebrospinal fluid leakage confirmed by metrizamide injection (C).

Table 11-6. Overview of Studies on Normoprolactinemia After Bromocriptine (BRC) Withdrawal

Author	Year	No.	Normal Prolactin After BRC Withdrawal (%)	Mean Period of BRC Use (mo)	Period Without BRC (mo)
Zarate et al.	1983	16	37.5	24	24 (mean)
Johnston et al.	1984	15	6.6	44	1.25-3.5
Rasmussen et al.	1987	75	44	24	≥6
Wang et al.	1987	24	21	24	12-48
Winkelmann et al.	1988	40	18.4	48	5-25
Van't Verlaat et al.	1991	12	8.3	58.8	12 (mean)
Passos et al.	2002	131	20.6	47	44 (mean)
Biswas et al.	2005	22 (micro)	50	31	1-7

Data from Passos VQ, Souza JJS, Musolino NRC et al: Long-term follow-up of prolactinomas: Normoprolactinemia after bromocriptine withdrawal. J Clin Endocrinol Metab 87:3578–3582, 2002.

literature point to a percentage of patients who remained normoprolactinemic after bromocriptine interruption ranging from 6.6% to 44%.[147] Biswas et al.[148] recently reported that 50% of 22 patients with microprolactinomas on bromocriptine therapy for a mean period of 3.1 years persisted normoprolactinemic for more than 1 year after drug withdrawal (Table 11-6). The question regarding why long-term findings differ from short-term findings may be answered by the formerly described microscopic alterations of the lactotrope during bromocriptine administration, suggesting a cytostatic effect related to short-term therapy and a cytocidal effect related to long-term treatment, which could explain the maintenance of normoprolactinemia after drug withdrawal.[149]

Another factor that may influence remission of prolactinomas is their natural history. A study including 25 women with untreated hyperprolactinemia (18 microadenomas, 7 macroadenomas) for a mean period of 11.3 years (mean initial PRL levels 225 ng/mL) showed that 7 of 22 patients with amenorrhea resumed menses spontaneously. Galactorrhea resolved completely in 8 of 19 patients. Only one patient had a slight progression of sellar abnormality. At the reevaluation, mean PRL levels had decreased to 155 ng/mL.[150] Another report was concerned with 30 women with hyperprolactinemia (18 with normal pituitary imaging or empty sella) without treatment, followed for an average time of 5.2 years. Of the women, 35% showed improvement in clinical symptoms. Six of 30 women had increased PRL levels, 14 showed no changes, and 10 had a decrease with PRL normalization in 6.[151] A study of 41 patients with "idiopathic" hyperprolactinemia followed for 1 year found that 83% of patients had unchanged PRL levels or even showed a decrease, and 34% showed normalization of PRL levels.[56]

During a mean period of 31 months, 38 patients with microprolactinomas were followed without treatment. Nearly 55% of patients had normalization of PRL levels, and there was no evidence of tumor growth.[152] Finally, there is evidence that women with hyperprolactinemia who experience menopause have a significant chance of normalizing their PRL levels, pointing to estrogen influence.[153] These data on untreated patients indicate that natural history has an important role in the outcome of prolactinomas and PRL normalization. The mechanisms involved are yet to be clarified, however. Although bromocriptine use has been associated with pituitary apoplexy,[154] the evolution of one of our patients who became normoprolactinemic, shown in Fig. 11-15, which shows a bright T1-weighted image without contrast on MRI highly indicative of hemorrhage before medical treatment, suggested that subclinical pituitary apoplexy may play a role in the natural history of prolactinomas and PRL normalization.

Whatever the mechanisms involved, there is a subset of patients with prolactinomas treated with bromocriptine who maintain normoprolactinemia after drug withdrawal without any predictive factor. We suggest that a gradual drug-dose reduction should be attempted, along with PRL level monitoring in patients under dopamine-agonist use who show normalization of PRL levels. To avoid unnecessary treatment, drug withdrawal can be attempted in this group of patients, with periodic reassessments.

Among the problems associated with medical treatment of prolactinomas, drug side effects are the most prevalent. Bromocriptine is generally well tolerated with doses between 2.5 and 20 mg/day. The most frequent side effects are nausea, vomiting, and orthostatic hypotension and, to a lesser extent, nasal congestion, headache, constipation, and psychotic events, such as auditory hallucinations, delusional ideas, and mood changes. The drug should be given carefully to psychiatric patients.[155] There are isolated reports of leukopenia, hepatitis, headaches, and cardiac arrhythmias. Higher doses (20 to 140 mg daily), used for patients with Parkinson's disease, may lead to pleural effusions, thickening and parenchymal lung changes, and retroperitoneal fibrosis.[156]

Bromocriptine side effects can be minimized by starting therapy at 1.25 mg at bedtime after food intake and progressively increasing it to include 1.25 mg a day after breakfast and at bedtime, according to individual tolerance, until the therapeutic dose is achieved. When normoprolactinemia is obtained, the dose can be reduced in many cases.[157] A subset of patients remain intolerant, however, even when all such recommendations are followed. Our data show persistent intolerance to bromocriptine in 24% and 12% of women harboring microprolactinomas and macroprolactinomas and in 5% of men with macroprolactinomas. Intolerance to bromocriptine may be overcome in some cases with a slow-releasing oral formulation (bromocriptine SRO), which also can be used as a once-a-day formulation.[158] We did not find better tolerance of this extended oral form, however, compared with the regular formulation. A single long-lasting injectable form (bromocriptine LA), with 50 mg of the drug, peaking after 2 hours and lasting for 28 days, which was developed for lactation inhibition, was efficacious for prolactinoma treatment, mainly in patients with intracranial hypertension and vomiting.[159] Thereafter, an injectable repeatable form was developed (bromocriptine-LAR), with good local and systemic tolerance even in patients who were previously intolerant to the oral formulation.[63,160] The injectable forms of bromocriptine are not commercially available, however. Additionally, the use of bromocriptine by the intravaginal route offered better tolerance for some patients, probably as a result of a slower drug absorption, but the absence of a local upper gastrointestinal effect of oral bromocriptine cannot be excluded.[161] The administration is bothersome, however, and there are local side effects, such as vaginal irritation. With the development of better-tolerated new oral

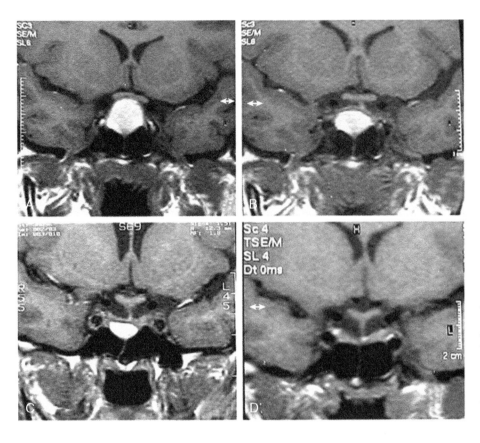

FIGURE 11-15. Magnetic resonance imaging (T1-weighted coronal views without gadolinium enhancement) of a 14-year-old girl harboring a macroadenoma. **A,** Before treatment (prolactin, 108 ng/mL). **B,** 2 months on bromocriptine (2.5 mg/day). **C,** 8 months on bromocriptine (5 mg/day) (prolactin, 18 ng/mL). **D,** 16 months after bromocriptine withdrawal (prolactin, 13 ng/mL). (From Passos VQ, Souza JJ, Musolino NR et al: Long-term follow-up of prolactinomas: normoprolactinemia after bromocriptine withdrawal. J Clin Endocrinol Metab 87:3578–3582.)

drugs, the intravaginal administration of bromocriptine for prolactinoma treatment is now seldom employed.

An even more vexing problem in the medical treatment of prolactinomas is their partial or complete lack of responsiveness to bromocriptine. The definition of bromocriptine resistance is arbitrary, with the failure of the drug in normalizing serum PRL levels or in reducing the tumor size using a dose equal to or greater than 15 mg/day for at least 3 months being the most currently accepted. According to this principle, about 10% of prolactinomas are resistant to bromocriptine.[162] This criterion has limitations regarding clinical practice, however. Patients who are intolerant to bromocriptine would not attain the dose established as limit, and although they are different conceptually, bromocriptine intolerance and resistance overlap. Patients harboring expanding tumors with visual impairment should not wait for 3 months without an improvement. As previously mentioned, clinical amelioration and tumor reduction may be achieved even if serum PRL is still above the normal range.[116] Pragmatically, *bromocriptine resistance* can be defined as the failure to obtain adequate clinical results in patients using the highest tolerable drug dose.

Mechanisms implicated for bromocriptine resistance of prolactinomas have not yet been fully elucidated. Studies in vivo and in vitro using radiolabeled dopamine antagonists as markers[103,163] or assessing D2 receptor expression by RT-PCR[164] show that dopamine D2 receptor density is reduced in resistant prolactinomas compared with tumors that are responsive to bromocriptine. When the D2 receptor density in lactotrope cell membranes is extremely low, the dopamine agonist drug paradoxically may lead to tumor growth.[163] The paucity of dopamine D2 receptors seems to be the main mechanism of bromocriptine resistance in prolactinomas. Additionally, postreceptor events have been described, including decreased ratio between the short and long isoforms of the dopamine D2 receptor, derived from alternative splicing.[165] No mutations in the dopamine D2 receptor that could be ascribed to bromocriptine resistance have been described to date.[26]

Regarding dopamine agonist resistance and tumor invasiveness, Delgrange et al.[166] recently showed that parasellar extension of macroprolactinomas, assessed on the basis of strict MRI criteria, may predict a negative response to DA. Additionally, some prolactinomas that are initially responsive to bromocriptine become resistant during therapy.[167] In such situations, especially in aggressive tumors, the diagnosis of the rare PRL-secreting carcinoma must be considered.[3]

Several other dopamine agonist drugs have been employed for the treatment of hyperprolactinemia/prolactinomas (see Table 11-3). Many show therapeutic efficacy, but three of them in particular merit detailed description, aiming mainly at overcoming intolerance and resistance to bromocriptine.

Pergolide

Pergolide is an ergot derivative, with an estimated potency 100 times that of bromocriptine, that has been approved by the U.S. Food and Drug Administration only for Parkinson's disease therapy. Considerable data concerning prolactinoma treatment have been collected, however. The drug can be given once daily in a dose ranging from 0.025 to 0.5 mg. When pergolide is compared with bromocriptine, some studies point to similar efficacy and tolerance of both drugs,[168,169] whereas others favor pergolide.[170,171] Regarding tumor reduction, a compilation of 61 patients with macroprolactinoma shows 75.4% of cases with more than 50% shrinkage and 9.8% of patients with adenoma reduction between 25% and 50% (see Table 11-5).[146] Heart valvulopathy occurring in patients taking pergolide for Parkinson's disease have been reported (see cabergoline).

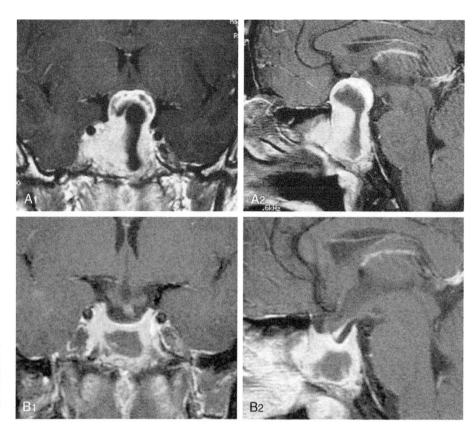

FIGURE II-I6. Magnetic resonance imaging (TI-weighted with gadolinium enhancement) of a man bearing a large macroprolactinoma. **AI** (coronal view) and **A2** (sagittal view), before treatment. **BI** (coronal view) and **B2** (sagittal view), after I month of cabergoline treatment, showing significant tumor shrinkage that was paralleled by visual improvement.

Quinagolide (CV 205-502)

Quinagolide is a non-ergot dopamine agonist drug that has specific affinity to the dopamine D2 receptor. Its efficacy in normalizing serum PRL levels is similar to that of bromocriptine, ranging from 45% to 100%, with most studies with macroprolactinomas showing PRL normalization between 58% and 75%, paralleled by clinical improvement.[172-176] Quinagolide is administered once a day in doses ranging from 0.075 mg to 0.6 mg. Some studies point to better tolerance compared with bromocriptine.[175,176] Additionally, there is evidence that about 50% of patients with bromocriptine-resistant prolactinomas attained normoprolactinemia when switched to quinagolide.[177,178] Such tumors were partially responsive to bromocriptine, however, with the further decrease attributed to better patient tolerance and a higher affinity to the already reduced but still present dopamine D2 receptors. Prolactinoma patients who are severely resistant to bromocriptine are not expected to respond to quinagolide either. Tumor size reduction evaluated in 105 patients showed more than 50% shrinkage and reduction between 25% and 50% in 48.1% and 20.2% of cases (see Table 11-5).[146] Quinagolide is commercially available only in Europe.

Cabergoline

Cabergoline is a synthetic ergoline that shows high specificity and affinity for the dopamine D2 receptor. It is a potent and long-acting inhibitor of PRL secretion, with an elimination half-life ranging between 63 and 109 hours.[179] PRL-lowering effects occur rapidly within 3 hours and were evident after a single-dose administration at the end of follow up (21 days) in puerperal women and at 14 days in patients with hyperprolactinemia. This pharmacologic profile allows cabergoline to be administrated once or twice a week in most patients, usually at a weekly dose

of 0.5 to 2 mg. In our experience, normoprolactinemia was maintained in some patients taking one tablet (0.5 mg) of cabergoline every 10 days and even every 2 weeks. Many studies have shown the efficacy of cabergoline in normalizing serum PRL levels and reducing tumor size, with consequent improvement of clinical and visual manifestations (Fig. 11-16). In 127 hyperprolactinemic patients (71 microprolactinomas, 19 macroprolactinomas, 37 idiopathic), cabergoline was administered at a dose between 0.25 and 3.5 mg/wk, given once or twice weekly in 114 patients and three times weekly or daily in 13 cases. Serum PRL levels were normalized in 114 patients (90%). Of 56 women with amenorrhea, 52 resumed menses; 17 women became pregnant, and sexual potency was restored in the three men. A total of 48 mild to moderate adverse events were reported by 29 patients (23%).[180]

In a study comprising 37 new patients, cabergoline normalized PRL levels in 88% of 26 microprolactinomas and in 100% of 11 macroprolactinomas. Regular menses were restored in 7 of 10 macroprolactinomas and in all oligomenorrheic patients with microadenoma; serum testosterone levels normalized in 2 of 3 hypogonadal men. Side effects developed in only three cases.[181] Another study with cabergoline (0.5 to 3 mg/wk) administered once per week was conducted in 15 patients (8 women) with macroprolactinomas. Normal PRL levels were attained in 73% of cases. Gonadal function was restored in all hypogonadal men and in 75% of premenopausal women with amenorrhea. Side effects were minimal.[182] A study addressing long-term cabergoline treatment in men showed that after 24 months of therapy, PRL levels normalized in 31 patients with macroprolactinoma (75.6%) and in eight with microprolactinoma (80%). Galactorrhea disappeared in all patients, and sperm volume and count normalized in all patients who normalized testosterone levels, whereas motility normalized in more than 80%.[183]

Table 11-7. Treatment of Hyperprolactinemia: Comparison Between Bromocriptine (BRC) and Cabergoline (CAB) Efficacy and Tolerability

Author (n)	Treatment Characteristics	BRC	CAB
Webster et al. 1994[185] (n = 459)	Prolactin normalization	58%	83%
	Ovulatory cycles	52%	72%
	Side effects	78%	68%
	Withdrawal	12%	3%
	Prevailing dose	2.5 mg 2×/day	0.5 mg 2×/wk
Sabuncu et al. 2001[188] (n = 34)	Prolactin normalization	59%	82%
	Side effects	53%	12%
Pascal-Vigneron et al. 1995[186] (n = 120)	Prolactin normalization	48%	93%
	Ovulatory cycles	48%	72%
	Side effects	65%	53%
	Digestive side effects	86%	37%

Many studies pointed to better efficacy and tolerance of cabergoline compared with bromocriptine (Table 11-7).[184-188] In a recent Brazilian multicenter study, data collected from 388 patients (320 women and 68 men) bearing prolactinomas (220 microadenomas and 68 macroadenomas) showed that cabergoline was significantly more effective than BCR in inducing normoprolactinemia (81.9% vs 67.1%), without any difference according to the gender.[184] In a large, multicenter European comparative study encompassing 459 women with hyperprolactinemic amenorrhea, 0.5 to 1 mg of cabergoline twice weekly was more effective than 2.5 to 5 mg of bromocriptine twice daily in the treatment of hyperprolactinemic amenorrhea, restoring ovulatory cycles in 72% of women and normalizing plasma PRL levels in 83%, compared with 52% and 59% for bromocriptine. Adverse effects were recorded in 68% of women taking cabergoline and 78% of women taking bromocriptine, but only 3% discontinued cabergoline, whereas 12% stopped taking bromocriptine because of drug intolerance.[185] Regarding cabergoline effect on macroprolactinoma size, in a compilation of 12 series including 320 patients, 28.4% had a greater than 50% tumor shrinkage, 28.4% had a reduction between 25% and 50%, and 43% had less than 25% or no reduction at all (see Table 11-5).[146] Because many of these patients had been previously intolerant or resistant to other dopamine agonists, the poorer cabergoline results for macroprolactinoma shrinkage compared with other drugs may have been biased. This bias can be illustrated by a study showing that the prevalence of macroprolactinoma shrinkage greater than 80% after cabergoline treatment was higher in naive patients (92.3%) than in patients who were previously intolerant (42.1%), resistant (30.3%), or responsive (38.4%) to bromocriptine or quinagolide.[189] As far as dopamine-agonist resistance in prolactinomas is concerned, some studies indicate that cabergoline normalized serum PRL levels in patients who were resistant to bromocriptine and even to quinagolide. In two series dealing with bromocriptine-treated prolactinomas without full PRL normalization, normoprolactinemia was achieved in 70% and 85% of patients when they were switched to cabergoline.[187,190] As previously pointed out (see section on quinagolide), such tumors did respond partially to bromocriptine, however, and the additional decrease brought up by cabergoline is probably related to its better tolerability and higher affinity to the reduced but still present dopamine D2 receptors. Consequently, severely resistant prolactinomas are not expected to respond to any dopamine agonist drug and have to be treated by a different means.

Some studies pointed out maintenance of normoprolactinemia in 23% of patients after cabergoline withdrawal for 12 months, on average.[180,181] A long-term prospective study including 200 hyperprolactinemic patients showed that after 2 to 5 years after cabergoline withdrawal, normoprolactinemia still persisted in 76% of patients with "nontumoral" hyperprolactinemia, in 70% of patients with microprolactinomas, and in 65% of patients with macroprolactinomas.[191] These results suggest that cabergoline compares favorably with bromocriptine also in terms of maintenance of normal PRL levels after drug withdrawal.[147] Nevertheless, a recent study dealing only with microprolactinomas did not show difference in remission rates between subjects treated with cabergoline and bromocriptine.[148]

Recently, two studies pointed to a high prevalence of cardiac valve dysfunction, compared to the general population, in patients treated for Parkinson's disease with cabergoline and also with pergolide but not with other dopamine agonist drugs.[192,193] The supposed mechanism is related to a serotoninergic effect presented by the drugs in addition to dopaminergic agonism. The risk of valvular regurgitation appears to be greatest in patients who have received at least 3 mg of cabergoline a day. Although this dose is much higher than that used for prolactinomas, the cumulative dose derived from the potential long-term use of cabergoline by patients harboring prolactinomas brought concerns about harmful cardiac valve effects of this drug also in this disease.

Three recently published studies addressing this issue did not show increased prevalence of clinically relevant valvular heart disease in patients with hyperprolactinemia/prolactinomas on long-term treatment with cabergoline.[194-196] However, additional findings of uncertain clinical relevance, like a higher prevalence of mild regurgitation of the tricuspid valve and of calcifications of the aortic valve, did occur in one study.[196] There was no relation between the cumulative dose of cabergoline and the presence of mild, moderate, or severe valve regurgitation.[196] Therefore, until more data are available that focus on the safety of cabergoline on the heart during long-term treatment of macroprolactinomas, it is prudent to recommend that all patients starting on this dopamine agonist receive cardiac echography and periodic reassessment during therapy.

Medical therapy seems to be the first option for prolactinoma therapy, being more effective than surgery, especially for macroprolactinomas.[197] To date, cabergoline seems to be the first-choice drug for prolactinoma treatment in view of its remarkable tolerance, capacity to normalize serum PRL levels, reduce tumor size, and induce high rates of normoprolactinemia persistence after drug withdrawal.

RADIOTHERAPY

The efficacy of conventional radiation therapy for prolactinomas is lower than medical or surgical treatment. Our results of 19 patients submitted to radiotherapy after medical/surgical failure showed that only 3 (16%) achieved serum PRL normalization 5, 6, and 15 years after the procedure.[116] A study with 63 patients treated with radiation after noncurative surgery showed that only 30% had normal PRL levels by 10 years.[198] A compilation from the literature shows serum PRL normalization in less than one third of patients 5 to 15 years after conventional radiotherapy, with hypopituitarism occurring in 5.5% to 93.3% of cases.[199] This prevalence is probably greater because many series have underestimated GH deficiency in adults. Other complications associated with conventional radiotherapy include optic nerve lesions, neurologic dysfunctions, cerebrovascular disease, and the development of other intracranial tumors.

There are emerging data on gamma-knife radiosurgery for prolactinomas. In one retrospective investigation, the authors examined the results of gamma-knife radiosurgery for tumor remnants after unsuccessful open surgery and medical treatment in 20 patients with prolactinomas. Serum PRL levels decreased into the normal range in five cases (25%). Patients treated with dopamine agonists during gamma-knife radiosurgery did significantly less well compared with the untreated group, suggesting a "radioprotective" effect of the drug.[200] This event is also suggested by a recent study[201] showing serum PRL normalization in 26% of 23 patients in an average time of 24.5 months, with new pituitary hormone deficiencies in 28% of patients and cranial nerve palsy in two cases (7%). Best results were achieved in patients with tumor volume less than 3.0 cm³ and who are not receiving dopamine agonist at the time of treatment. Another study including 128 patients estimated the efficacy of gamma-knife radiosurgery as the primary therapy for prolactinomas. The mean follow-up time was 33.2 months (range, 6 to 72 months). Tumor control was observed in all but two patients who underwent surgery 18 and 36 months after gamma-knife radiosurgery. Clinical cure was achieved in 67 cases (52%). Nine infertile women became pregnant 2 to 13 months after irradiation, and all gave birth to normal infants. There was no visual deterioration related to gamma-knife radiosurgery. This study points to better results in terms of PRL normalization but does not mention the impact of treatment on pituitary function, besides mentioning five women who experienced "premature menopause."[202] More data and follow-up time are required to assess the superiority of gamma-knife radiosurgery compared with conventional radiotherapy. To date, in the author's opinion, radiation therapy for prolactinomas is reserved for cases with medical and surgical failures, especially for invasive tumors.

THERAPEUTIC PERSPECTIVES

As a result of the efficacy of medical and surgical therapies, most patients with prolactinomas can be controlled adequately. A subset of patients resistant to dopamine agonists, especially patients harboring invasive macroadenomas, who are not expected to be surgically cured, pose an important therapeutic problem. Radiotherapy use is generally limited, efficacious only in the long term, and usually leads to hypopituitarism.

Many studies did not find tumor enlargement in patients with "idiopathic" hyperprolactinemia or microprolactinomas, before or after menopause.[153,203] When pregnancy is not a concern, and galactorrhea is not disturbing, sexual steroid replacement can be considered for those patients, who must be followed carefully. Additionally, testosterone may be given to men harboring resistant microprolactinomas and even partially resistant macroprolactinomas, with monitoring of PRL levels and with imaging. The introduction of an aromatase-inhibitor drug may be considered if there is evidence of tumor growth or serum PRL increase.[204]

Prolactinomas usually do not respond to somatostatin.[205] It has been shown, however, that a selective analogue of the somatostatin receptor subtype 5 (SSTR5) inhibited PRL secretion in human prolactinoma cell culture.[206] Nevertheless, another in-vitro study did not show better response of this selective analogue compared with quinagolide.[207] A recent publication by Fusco et al.[208] pointed to an efficacy comparable to cabergoline of a selective analogue of SSTR5, BIM-23206, and the chimeric somatostatin/dopamine D2 receptor ligant, BIM-23A760, in responsive prolactinomas but not in resistant ones. Also the "universal" somatostatin ligand SOM230 (pasireotide) was ineffective in cabergoline-resistant adenomas.[208] In summary, although the SSTRs are expressed in prolactinomas, the somatostatinergic ligands do not appear to be highly effective in suppressing PRL in tumors resistant to dopamine agonists.

Studies show that the human PTTG induces angiogenesis via basic fibroblast growth factor induction[209] and that estrogen is involved in paracrine regulation of pituitary tumorigenesis by PTTG. Selective estrogen receptor modulators, such as tamoxifen and raloxifene, and inhibitors, such as ICI 182780, abolished estrogen-induced pituitary PTTG expression in vivo, suppressed serum PRL concentrations by 88%, and attenuated PRL-secreting pituitary tumor growth by 41% in rats. Antiestrogen treatment of primary human pituitary tumor cultures reduced PTTG expression approximately 65%.[17] These findings may indicate a role for selective antiestrogens in prolactinoma treatment, including resistant ones.

The development of PRL receptor antagonists could also represent an option for medical treatment of resistant macroprolactinomas without mass effect, because they should be able to block the actions of PRL, if not its production.[210] One therapeutic approach would be the association of dopamine agonists and PRL receptor–antagonist drugs in cases of macroprolactinomas exhibiting tumor shrinkage but not PRL normalization when on dopamine agonist monotherapy.

The alkylating agent temozolomide has been experimentally used in many tumors. Its product of hydrolyzation, 5-(3-methyltriazen-1-yl) imidazole-4-carboxamide, is thought to exert a cytotoxic effect by DNA alkylation. Temozolomide can be given orally and is currently approved in the United States for the treatment of patients with refractory anaplastic astrocytoma and for the treatment of newly diagnosed patients with glioblastoma multiforme, as an adjunct to radiotherapy. Three case reports recently published describe patients with invasive prolactinoma or PRL-secreting carcinoma resistant to conventional therapy who responded to this drug[211-213] (Fig. 11-17). More data is needed to assess the efficacy and tolerability of this promising drug in a larger cohort of aggressive, resistant prolactinomas.

Finally, there is evidence that nerve growth factor expression is reduced in resistant prolactinomas and that this growth factor restores p53 function in pituitary cell lines.[214] Nerve growth factor administration to athymic mice with transplanted human bromocriptine-resistant prolactinomas results in the expression of dopamine D2 receptors in the tumor and restores sensitivity to subsequent treatment with bromocriptine. This could be a promising therapy for patients who are refractory to dopamine-agonist treatment.[215]

PROLACTINOMAS AND PREGNANCY

The development of efficacious medical and surgical therapies for prolactinomas has made pregnancy possible for women bearing such tumors. Gestational risks due to the possibility of tumor growth during pregnancy, mainly in women with macroadenomas, raise a concern, however. The management of pregnancy in patients with prolactinomas submitted to different therapies is brought into focus here.

Regarding microprolactinomas, a study including 91 pregnancies mostly induced by bromocriptine, without previous surgery or radiotherapy, indicated symptomatic tumor growth in 5.5% of cases.[216] In a compilation of pregnancies in 246 women with microprolactinomas treated with bromocriptine only, tumor growth symptoms were reported in 1.6% of patients, although an asymptomatic increase of the tumor was shown in 4.5% of the cases. None of the patients needed surgical intervention during pregnancy.[217] We followed 71 term pregnancies, and the results were similar.[218,219] Of the 22 patients with previous surgery, none presented symptoms of tumor growth; of the 41 pregnant patients who underwent treatment with bromocriptine alone, only 1 (2.4%) presented with headaches in the third month of pregnancy, which regressed with drug reintroduction. Seven patients got pregnant without treatment and did not develop any complications. There was an asymptomatic increase of the tumor in one case with previous surgery and in two cases with bromocriptine alone, as assessed by scanning postpartum. Because of the low risk of tumor growth during pregnancy in patients with microprolactinomas, there is no need to perform periodic imaging or ophthalmologic examinations. These assessments should be reserved for cases with clinical complaints suggesting tumor growth, such as headache or visual field changes.

The risk of complications during pregnancy is much greater with macroprolactinomas. One study revealed symptomatic tumor growth in 41.3% of 56 pregnancies occurring in 46 patients who were medically treated only, compared with 7.1% of 70 pregnancies that occurred in 67 women who previously had been submitted to surgery or radiotherapy.[216] A review from the literature pointed to symptoms related to tumor growth in 15.5% of 45 patients with macroprolactinomas treated with

bromocriptine only. The incidence of complications was only 4.3% in the 46 patients who underwent surgery or radiotherapy before pregnancy. Additionally, asymptomatic tumor growth was seen in 8.9% of the patients without prior surgery or radiotherapy.[217] We followed 51 term pregnancies in patients with macroprolactinomas.[218,219] Of those, 21 were in patients with previous surgery, and none of the patients presented with symptoms or signs of tumor growth. Of the 30 patients treated with pregestational bromocriptine only, 11 (37%) manifested complaints related to tumor growth: all of them presented with headaches, and seven had visual alterations (Fig. 11-18). Pituitary imaging after delivery was performed in 23 other patients, and an asymptomatic growth of the tumor was observed in 4 more cases.

These data show the higher risk of tumor growth in macroprolactinomas during pregnancy, necessitating a stricter follow-up (Fig. 11-19). The first recommendation should be the use of a nonhormonal contraceptive along with a dopamine agonist until tumor shrinkage has been shown within sellar boundaries. The duration of previous treatment with dopamine also might be important. A follow-up study of 37 pregnancies showed signs of tumor growth in 7, all of them treated with bromocriptine for less than 1 year. No tumor enlargement was found in the 14 macroprolactinoma patients treated for a longer time, suggesting

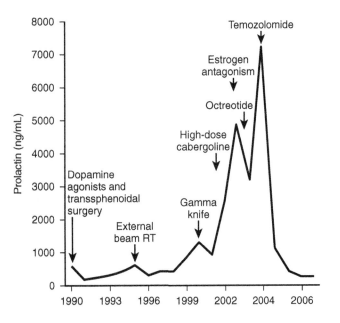

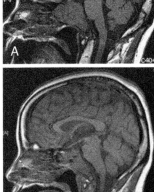

FIGURE 11-17. *Left:* Serum PRL levels over the course of several treatment modalities for an invasive prolactinoma resistant to dopamine agonists, showing a remarkable decrease when temozolomide was introduced. *Right:* Magnetic resonance imaging (sagittal views) before **(A)** and after **(B)** temozolomide therapy of the patient harboring the invasive prolactinoma. A marked reduction in size is depicted. (From Neff LM, Weil M, Cole A et al: Temozolomide in the treatment of an invasive prolactinoma resistant to dopamine agonists. Pituitary 10:81–86, 2007.)

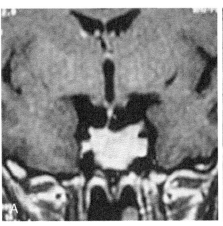
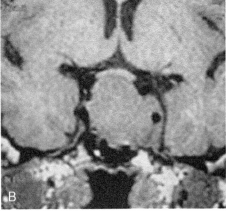

FIGURE 11-18. Magnetic resonance imaging (coronal views) of a patient with macroprolactinoma. **A,** Tumor is limited to sellar boundaries during bromocriptine treatment, before pregnancy. **B,** Tumor growth during the 4th month of pregnancy without bromocriptine use. (From Musolino NRC, Bronstein MD: Prolactinomas and pregnancy. In Bronstein MD [ed]: Pituitary Tumors in Pregnancy. Boston: Kluwer Academic Publishers, 2001, pp 91–108.)

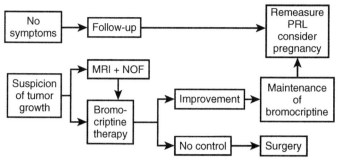

FIGURE 11-19. Suggested algorithm for the follow-up of patients with macroprolactinoma during pregnancy. *NOF*, Neuroophthalmologic examination; *PRL*, prolactin. (From Musolino NRC, Bronstein MD: Prolactinomas and pregnancy. In Bronstein MD [ed]: Pituitary Tumors in Pregnancy. Boston: Kluwer Academic Publishers, 2001, pp 91–108.)

Table 11-8. Effect of Bromocriptine on Pregnancies

	Bromocriptine		Normal Population (%)
	n	%	
Pregnancies	6239	100	100
Spontaneous abortion	620	9.9	10-15
Terminations	75	1.25	
Ectopic	31	0.5	0.5-1
Hydatidiform moles	11	0.2	0.05-0.7
Deliveries (known duration)	4139	100	100
At term (≥38 wk)	3620	87.5	85
Preterm (<38 wk)	519	12.5	15
Deliveries (known outcome)	5120	100	100
Single births	5031	9.3	8.7
Multiple births	89	1.7	1.3
Infants (known details)	5213	100	100
Normal	5030	96.5	95.0
With malformations	93	1.8	3-4
With perinatal disorders	90	1.7	≥2

Data from Krupp P, Monka C, Richter K: Program of the Second World Congress of Gynecology and Obstetrics, Rio de Janeiro, 1988, p 9.

that the duration of bromocriptine use before conception might be a good prognostic factor in pregnancy.[220]

After pregnancy has been confirmed, the dopamine agonist can be withdrawn, and the patient must be monitored closely for symptoms related to tumor growth. If there is a suspected tumor expansion, the confirmation can be made through MRI, after the fourth month of gestation, and by visual field testing (see Fig. 11-19). Monitoring serum PRL levels during pregnancy does not seem to be useful, because they are not always related to tumor behavior during gestation. The reintroduction of bromocriptine in such cases often leads to clinical amelioration and tumor reduction. In 9 of 11 patients who exhibited complications during pregnancy, bromocriptine reintroduction brought complete resolution of the symptoms related to tumor growth.[219] Surgery also can be employed as treatment for symptomatic tumor growth in pregnancy. Several authors have reported good results, although the increased risk of spontaneous abortion in patients who undergo surgery is well known.[219]

The safety of bromocriptine reintroduction or even maintenance during pregnancy is supported by a large experience with this dopamine agonist reported in the literature. A large review[221] consisted of 2587 pregnancies and did not show an increase of maternal or fetal morbidity or mortality. Since then, some authors have favored the maintenance of bromocriptine in pregnancy to prevent complications in patients with macroprolactinomas without previous surgery or radiotherapy.[222] It is our policy to indicate such an approach only when the patient gets pregnant after a short treatment period, mainly without confirmation of tumor shrinkage or when the tumor is outside sellar boundaries. Surgery is indicated before pregnancy in cases without tumor reduction during treatment with dopamine agonists or in patients who developed tumor growth in previous gestations.[219]

Pregnancy and Other Dopamine Agonist Drugs

In recent years, the use of new dopamine agonists such as quinagolide, cabergoline, and pergolide for the treatment of hyperprolactinemia has increased, and pregnancies have been described. Data were obtained on 176 pregnancies in which quinagolide was used, on average, for 37 days. Miscarriages occurred in 14% of the cases, with one ectopic pregnancy. Fetal malformation was described in nine cases, although other drugs had been used in three patients.[223] Quinagolide was used successfully during pregnancy in two bromocriptine-resistant patients who presented symptoms of tumor growth.[178] Cabergoline has been the most used medication among the more recent dopamine agonist drugs, and reports on pregnancies during

cabergoline therapy are emerging. We followed six full-term gestations in patients who withdrew cabergoline as soon as pregnancy was confirmed and did not observe malformations, but two premature births occurred.[219] A review from 1996, with 204 gestations, did not observe an increase of spontaneous abortion (12%) or malformations (four cases).[224] A recent multicenter study encompassing 329 pregnancies in hyperprolactinemic women also suggests that fetal exposure to cabergoline through early pregnancy does not induce any increase in the risk of miscarriage or fetal malformation.[225] Nevertheless, the drug's long action, which persists 3 weeks after its withdrawal, associated with fewer data compared with bromocriptine (around 700 versus >6000 pregnancies) (Table 11-8), still limits (albeit not so strictly) its indication for patients who wish to conceive or its use during pregnancy. Regarding pergolide, animal data point to its safety in pregnancy.[226] No human data are available to date.

Follow-Up After Delivery

Breastfeeding does not increase the risk of tumor growth in patients who progressed well during pregnancy.[219] Breastfeeding is contraindicated only when patients need to maintain the dopamine agonist after delivery, owing to tumor-growth signs.

There have been several reports in the literature regarding reduction or normalization of serum PRL levels after delivery.[219,227] In our hands, 60% and 72% of patients with microprolactinomas and macroprolactinomas showed a decrease in PRL levels after delivery compared with pregestational levels. In 11% of all patients who conceived, PRL levels normalized after pregnancy, some with a new gestation without therapy. On average, PRL levels decreased from 336 ± 105 ng/mL to 133 ± 20 ng/mL in 62 patients who were available for comparison.[218] These results are similar to ones reported by other authors. A study reported PRL normalization after pregnancy in 29% of women.[227] Tumor reduction after pregnancy also has been described. A study with 16 patients harboring prolactinomas found 27% of tumor reduction or disappearance after delivery.[228] We also observed tumor reduction in 8 of 23 patients with macroprolactinomas, assessed by imaging before and after delivery. Two other patients developed asymptomatic apoplexy. The explanation for this "curative" effect of pregnancy is to be clarified. It may be related partly to modifications in the vasculature

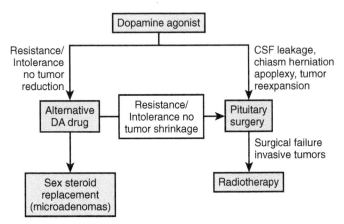

FIGURE 11-20. Suggested algorithm for treatment of prolactinomas. *CSF,* Cerebrospinal fluid; *DA,* dopamine.

of the adenoma due to the estrogen stimulation, resulting in necrosis or microinfarctions of the adenomatous tissue. Hemorrhagic zones in prolactinoma patients receiving estrogen therapy already have been described.[229]

Another issue of concern is the outcome of the children whose mothers took dopamine agonist drugs during pregnancy. One study reported the follow-up spanning 4 months to 9 years in 546 children exposed to intrauterine bromocriptine.[221] The authors did not find any developmental impairment in the children. We followed 70 children born to mothers who conceived on bromocriptine.[219] At a mean follow-up of 67 months (range, 12 to 240 months), only two children presented with disorders of neuropsychomotor development: one case of idiopathic hydrocephaly and another of tuberous sclerosis. We did not find any similar reports in the literature. Fifteen of these children already had started puberty, one of them precociously.

TREATMENT PLANNING AND FOLLOW-UP

Based on the previously described evidence, to date the gold-standard therapy for either microprolactinomas or macroprolactinomas is medical treatment with dopamine agonist drugs (Fig. 11-20). Physicians must motivate patients to embark on such long-term treatment based on the overall better results compared with surgery and, mainly based on more recent data,[147,191] the possibility of drug withdrawal for a substantial number of patients with maintenance of normoprolactinemia. Surgical treatment of prolactinomas is indicated for patients with persistent intolerance or hormonal or tumor resistance to more than one dopamine agonist drug—in particular if pregnancy is desired—or if the tumor has grown during medical treatment. In cases of resistance, rare conditions, such as acidophil stem cell adenoma or PRL-secreting carcinomas, must be considered. Malignant prolactinomas respond only temporarily, if they respond at all, when patients are switched to another dopamine

agonist drug or undergo surgery. Surgical therapy also is indicated frequently in pituitary apoplexy, in dopamine agonist–induced CSF leakage occurring in invasive macroprolactinomas, and in the exceedingly rare occurrence of visual loss secondary to optic chiasm herniation during medical therapy. Additionally, surgery in skilled hands may be considered for patients not willing to be submitted to long-term medical therapy, especially patients harboring microprolactinomas and serum PRL levels less than 100 ng/mL. Radiotherapy, either conventional or stereotactic, is reserved for prolactinomas not responsive to medical or surgical treatment, particularly regarding the invasive ones.

There is evidence that, in general, estrogen replacement is not harmful for women harboring microprolactinomas. This approach may be used when fertility is not an issue for patients with intolerance or resistance to medical therapy and not cured by or not willing to undergo pituitary surgery. In addition, women successfully treated medically may use hormonal contraceptives if they have not adapted to barrier methods. Menopausal women bearing microprolactinomas can interrupt dopamine agonist drug use and are allowed to start hormone replacement therapy if it is indicated.[203] Although there is evidence of a PRL role in carcinogenesis in animal models, mainly carcinoma of the mammary gland, human data are still highly controversial.[230-233] It is now apparent that human mammary epithelial cells can synthesize PRL endogenously, permitting autocrine/paracrine actions within the mammary gland that are independent of pituitary PRL and probably not affected by dopamine agonist drugs. To date, the maintenance of high serum PRL levels in premenopausal and postmenopausal women is not a concern with regard to carcinogenesis. Finally, for macroprolactinomas that are not adequately controlled, the use of estrogens is generally discouraged, given their potential for inducing growth.

There are many therapeutic perspectives for resistant/aggressive prolactinomas: specific somatostatin or somatostatin/dopamine analogues, selective anti-estrogen drugs, cytotoxic drugs such as temozolomide, and PRL-receptor antagonists. Nevertheless, more studies are needed in order to assess their places in the treatment algorithm.

The follow-up planning for patients with prolactinomas depends on the tumor size and clinical, laboratory, and imaging response to therapy. Many patients are clinically controlled even if serum PRL levels are still above the normal range and do not need further drug dose increases. For microprolactinomas and especially for macroprolactinomas, significant tumor shrinkage or "disappearance" on MRI is a good prognostic marker, and in such cases, imaging reassessment can be performed sporadically. Medically or surgically controlled patients must be reassessed periodically, clinically and hormonally, to identify patients who may discontinue the dopamine agonist drug with maintenance of normoprolactinemia or patients with recurrence of hyperprolactinemia.

REFERENCES

1. Miyai K, Ichibara K, Kondo L, et al: Asymptomatic hyperprolactinemia and prolactinoma in the general population mass screening by paired assays of serum prolactin, Clin Endocrinol (Oxf) 25:549–554, 1986.
2. Hardy J: Transsphenoidal microsurgery of the normal and pathological pituitary, Clin Neurosurg 16:185–217, 1969.
3. Kars M, Roelfsema F, Romijn JA, et al: Malignant prolactinoma: case report and review of the literature, Eur J Endocrinol 155:523–534. 2006

4. Glezer A, D'Alva CB, Salgado LR, et al: Pitfalls in pituitary diagnosis: peculiarities of three cases, Clin Endocrinol (Oxf) 57:135–139, 2002.
5. Striker P, Grueter F: Action du lobe antérieur de l'hypophyse sur la montée laiteuse, C R Soc Biol Paris 99:1978–1980, 1929.
6. Riddle O, Bartes RW, Dykshorn DW: The preparation, identification and assay of prolactin—a hormone of the anterior pituitary, Am J Physiol 105:191–216, 1933.

7. Mendel EB: Chiari-Frommel syndrome, Am J Obstet Gynecol 51:889–892, 1946.
8. Argonz J, del Castillo EB: A syndrome characterized by estrogenic insufficiency, galactorrhea and decreased urinary gonadotropin, J Clin Endocrinol Metab 13:79–87, 1953.
9. Forbes AP, Henneman PH, Griswold GC, et al: Syndrome characterized by galactorrhea, amenorrhea and low urinary FSH: comparison with acromegaly and normal lactation, J Clin Endocrinol Metab 14:264–271, 1954.

10. Hwang P, Guyda H, Friesen H: A radioimmunoassay for human prolactin, Proc Natl Acad Sci U S A 68:1902–1906, 1971.

11. Burrow GN, Wortzman G, Rewcastle NB, et al: Micro-adenomas of the pituitary and abnormal sellar tomograms in an unselected autopsy series, N Engl J Med 304:156–158, 1981.

12. Ciccarelli A, Daly AF, Beckers A: The epidemiology of prolactinomas, Pituitary 8:3–6, 2005

13. Berezin M, Karasik A: Familial prolactinoma, Clin Endocrinol (Oxf) 42:483–486, 1995.

14. Herman V, Fagin J, Gonsky R, et al: Clonal origin of pituitary adenomas, J Clin Endocrinol Metab 71:1427–1433, 1990.

15. Zhang X, Horwitz GA, Heaney AP, et al: Pituitary tumor transforming gene (PTTG) expression in pituitary adenomas, J Clin Endocrinol Metab 84:761–767, 1999.

16. Shimon I, Hinton DR, Weiss MH, et al: Prolactinomas express human heparin-binding secretory transforming gene (HST) protein product: marker of tumour invasiveness, Clin Endocrinol (Oxf) 48:23–29, 1998.

17. Heaney AP, Fernando M, Melmed S: Functional role of estrogen in pituitary tumor pathogenesis, J Clin Invest 109:277–283, 2002.

18. Ben-Shlomo A, Miklovsky I, Ren SG, et al: Leukemia inhibitory factor regulates prolactin secretion in prolactinoma and lactotroph cells, J Clin Endocrinol Metab 88:858–863, 2003.

19. Fiorentini C, Guerra N, Facchetti M, et al: Nerve growth factor regulates dopamine D(2) receptor expression in prolactinoma cell lines via p75(NGFR)-mediated activation of nuclear factor-kappaB, Mol Endocrinol 16:353–366, 2002.

20. Paez-Pereda M, Giacomini D, Refojo D, et al: Involvement of bone morphogenetic protein 4 (BMP-4) in pituitary prolactinoma pathogenesis through a Smad/estrogen receptor crosstalk, Proc Natl Acad Sci U S A 100:1034–1039, 2003.

21. Finelli P, Pierantoni GM, Giardino D, et al: The high-mobility group A2 gene is amplified and overexpressed in human prolactinomas, Cancer Res 62:2398–2405, 2002.

22. Turner HE, Harris AL, Melmed S, et al: Angiogenesis in endocrine tumors, Endocr Rev 24:600–632, 2003.

23. Sarkar DK, Gottschall PE, Meites J: Damage to hypothalamic dopaminergic neurons is associated with development of prolactin-secreting pituitary tumors, Science 218:684–686, 1982.

24. Schuff KG, Hentges ST, Kelly MA, et al: Lack of prolactin receptor signaling in mice results in lactotroph proliferation and prolactinomas by dopamine-dependent and -independent mechanisms, J Clin Invest 110:973–981, 2002.

25. Cruz-Soto ME, Scheiber MD, Gregerson KA, et al: Pituitary tumorigenesis in prolactin gene-disrupted mice, Endocrinology 143:4429–4436, 2002.

26. Friedman E, Adams EF, Hoog A, et al: Normal structural dopamine type 2 receptor gene in prolactin-secreting and other pituitary tumors, J Clin Endocrinol Metab 78:568–574, 1994.

27. Prezant TR, Levine J, Melmed S: Molecular characterization of the MEN1 tumor suppressor gene in sporadic pituitary tumors, J Clin Endocrinol Metab 83:1388–1391, 1998.

28. Daly AF, Vanbellinghen JF, Khoo SK, et al: Aryl hydrocarbon receptor-interacting protein gene mutations in familial isolated pituitary adenomas: analysis in 73 families, J Clin Endocrinol Metab 92:1891–1896, 2007.

29. Yu R, Bonert V, Saporta I, Raffel LJ, et al: Aryl hydrocarbon receptor interacting protein variants in sporadic pituitary adenomas, J Clin Endocrinol Metab 91:5126–5129, 2006

30. Hardy J: Transsphenoidal surgery of hypersecreting pituitary tumors. In Kolhler G, Ross GT, editors: Diagnosis and Treatment of Pituitary Tumors, New York, 1973, Elsevier, pp 179–194.

31. Scheithauer BW, Kovacs KT, Laws ER Jr, et al: Pathology of invasive pituitary tumors with special reference to functional classification, J Neurosurg 65:733–744, 1986.

32. Horvath E, Kovacs K: Pathology of prolactin cell adenomas of the human pituitary, Semin Diagn Pathol 3:4–17, 1986.

33. Bevan JS, Burke CW, Esiri MM, et al: Misinterpretation of prolactin levels leading to management errors in patients with sellar enlargement, Am J Med 82:29–32, 1987.

34. Horvath E, Kovacs K, Singer W, et al: Acidophil stem cell adenoma of the human pituitary: clinicopathologic analysis of 15 cases, Cancer 47:761–771, 1981.

35. Ozbey N, Sariyildiz E, Yilmaz L, et al: Primary hypothyroidism with hyperprolactinaemia and pituitary enlargement mimicking a pituitary macroadenoma, Int J Clin Pract 51:409–411, 1997.

36. Bellastella A, Bizzarro A, Coronella C, et al: Lymphocytic hypophysitis: a rare or underestimated disease? Eur J Endocrinol 149:363–376, 2003.

37. Bihan H, Christozova V, Dumas JL, et al: Sarcoidosis: clinical, hormonal, and magnetic resonance imaging (MRI) manifestations of hypothalamic-pituitary disease in 9 patients and review of the literature, Medicine (Baltimore) 86:259–268, 2007.

38. Gonzalez JG, Elizondo G, Saldivar D, et al: Pituitary gland growth during normal pregnancy: an in-vivo study using magnetic resonance imaging, Am J Med 85:217–220, 1988.

39. Scheithauer BW, Sano T, Kovacs KT, et al: The pituitary gland in pregnancy: a clinic pathologic and immunohistochemical study of 69 cases, Mayo Clin Proc 65:461–474, 1990.

40. Morris LF, Braunstein GD: Impact of pregnancy on normal pituitary function. In Bronstein MD, editor: Pituitary Tumors in Pregnancy, Boston, 2001, Kluwer Academic Publishers, pp 1–32.

41. Vieira JG, Oliveira JH, Tachibana T, et al: Evaluation of plasma prolactin levels: is it necessary to rest before the collection? Arq Bras Endocrinol Metabol 50:569–702, 2006.

42. Molitch ME: Drugs and prolactin, Pituitary 11:209–218, 2008.

43. Kelley SR, Kamal TJ, Molitch ME: Mechanism of verapamil calcium channel blockade-induced hyperprolactinemia, Am J Physiol 270:96–100, 1996.

44. Hutchinson J, Murphy M, Harries R, et al: Galactorrhoea and hyperprolactinaemia associated with protease inhibitors, Lancet 356:1003–1004, 2000.

45. Drange MR, Fram NR, Herman-Bonert V, et al: Pituitary tumor registry: a novel clinical resource, J Clin Endocrinol Metab 85:168–174, 2000

46. Karavitaki N, Thanabalasingham G, Shore HC, et al: Do the limits of serum prolactin in disconnection hyperprolactinaemia need re-definition? A study of 226 patients with histologically verified non-functioning pituitary macroadenoma, Clin Endocrinol (Oxf) 65:524–529, 2006.

47. Glezer A, Paraiba DB, Bronstein MD: Rare sellar lesions, Endocrinol Metab Clin North Am 37:195–211, 2008

48. Greenman Y: Dopaminergic treatment of nonfunctioning pituitary adenomas, Nat Clin Pract Endocrinol Metab 3:554–555, 2007

49. Barbetta L, Dall'Asta C, Ambrosi B: Hyperprolactinemia preceding Cushing's disease, J Endocrinol Invest 23:491–492, 2000.

50. Stryker TD, Molitch ME: Reversible hyperthyrotropinemia, hyperthyroxinemia, and hyperprolactinemia due to adrenal insufficiency, Am J Med 79:271–276, 1985.

51. Estopinan Garcia V, Martinez Burgui JA, Ballester Ferrer A, et al: Prolactin and polycystic ovary sindrome. Med Clin (Barc) 116:759, 2001.

52. Saha MT, Saha HH, Niskanen LK, et al: Time course of serum prolactin and sex hormones following successful renal transplantation, Nephron 92:735–737, 2002.

53. Zietz B, Lock G, Plach B, et al: Dysfunction of the hypothalamic-pituitary-glandular axes and relation to Child-Pugh classification in male patients with alcoholic and virus-related cirrhosis, Eur J Gastroenterol Hepatol 15:495–501, 2003

54. Leung AK, Pacaud D: Diagnosis and management of galactorrhea, Am Fam Physician 70:543–550, 2004

55. Molitch ME, Schwartz S, Mukherji B: Is prolactin secreted ectopically? Am J Med 70:803–807, 1981.

56. Martin TL, Kim M, Malarkey WB: The natural history of idiopathic hyperprolactinemia, J Clin Endocrinol Metab 60:855–858, 1985.

57. De Bellis A, Colao A, Pivonello R, et al: Antipituitary antibodies in idiopathic hyperprolactinemic patients, Ann N Y Acad Sc 1107:129–135, 2007.

58. Mah PM, Webster J: Hyperprolactinemia: etiology, diagnosis, and management, Semin Reprod Med 20:365–374, 2002.

59. Abe T, Matsumoto K, Kuwazawa J, et al: Headache associated with pituitary adenomas, Headache 38:782–786, 1998.

60. Matharu MS, Levy MJ, Merry RT, et al: SUNCT syndrome secondary to prolactinoma, J Neurol Neurosurg Psychiatry 74:1590–1592, 2003.

61. Zikel OM, Atkinson JL, Hurley DL: Prolactinoma manifesting with symptomatic hydrocephalus, Mayo Clin Proc 74:475–477, 1999.

62. Minniti G, Jaffrain-Rea ML, Santoro A, et al: Giant prolactinomas presenting as skull-base tumors, Surg Neurol 57:99–103, 2002.

63. Bronstein MD, Musolino NR, Cardim CS, et al: Treatment of macroprolactinomas with a long-acting, parenteral and repeatable new form of bromocriptine. In Landolt AM, Heitz PU, Zapf J, et al, editors: Advances in Pituitary Adenoma Research, Oxford, 1988, Pergamon Press.

64. Franks S, Murray MA, Jequier AM, et al: Incidence and significance of hyperprolactinaemia in women with amenorrhea, Clin Endocrinol (Oxf) 4:597–607, 1975.

65. Hattori N: Macroprolactinemia: a new cause of hyperprolactinemia, J Pharmacol Sci 92:171–177, 2003.

66. Serri O, Chik CL, Ur E, Ezzat S: Diagnosis and management of hyperprolactinemia, Can Med Assoc J 169:575–581, 2003.

67. Kars M, van der Klaauw AA, Onstein CS, et al: Quality of life is decreased in female patients treated for microprolactinoma, Eur J Endocrinol 157:133–139, 2007.

68. Vartej P, Poiana C, Vartej I: Effects of hyperprolactinemia on osteoporotic fracture risk in premenopausal women, Gynecol Endocrinol 15:3–7, 2001.

69. Ciccarelli E, Savino L, Carlevatto V: Vertebral bone density in non-amenorrhoeic hyperprolactinaemic women, Clin Endocrinol (Oxf) 28:1–6, 1988.

70. Bronstein MD, Marino R Jr, Pereira DHM: Therapeutic alternatives for hyperprolactinemia: the role of bromoergocriptine, Rev Bras Ginecol Obstet 5:193, 1983.

71. Kleinberg DL, Noel GL, Frantz AG: Galactorrhea: a study of 235 cases, including 48 with pituitary tumors, N Engl J Med 296:589–600, 1977.

72. Asano S, Ueki K, Suzuki I, et al: Clinical features and medical treatment of male prolactinomas, Acta Neurochir (Wien) 143:465–470, 2001.

73. Bronstein MD: Prolactinoma in men. Arq Bras Endocrinol Metab 43:338, 1999.

74. Drago F, Scapagnini U: Side effects of drugs stimulating prolactin secretion on the behavior of male rats, Arch Int Pharmacodyn Ther 276:271–278, 1985.

75. Molitch ME, Thorner MO, Wilson C: Management of prolactinomas, J Clin Endocrinol Metab 82:996–1000, 1997.

76. Naliato EC, Farias ML, Braucks GR, et al: Prevalence of osteopenia in men with prolactinoma, J Endocrinol Invest 28:12–17, 2005.

77. Cannavo S, Venturino M, Curto L, et al: Clinical presentation and outcome of pituitary adenomas in teenagers, Clin Endocrinol (Oxf) 58:519–527, 2003.

78. Colao A, Loche S, Cappa M, et al: Prolactinomas in children and adolescents: clinical presentation and long-term follow-up, J Clin Endocrinol Metab 83:2777–2780, 1998.

79. Jallad RS, Goic MSZ, Musolino NR, et al: Prolactinomas in children and adolescents: retrospective study on 47 patients, Arq Bras Endocrinol Metabol 44:300, 2000.

80. Di Sarno A, Rota F, Auriemma R, et al: An evaluation of patients with hyperprolactinemia: have dynamic tests had their day? J Endocrinol Invest 26:39–47, 2003.

81. Frieze TW, Mong DP, Koops MK: "Hook effect" in prolactinomas: case report and review of literature, Endocr Pract 8:296–303, 2003.

82. Sinha YN: Structural variants of prolactin: occurrence and physiological significance, Endocr Rev 16:354–369, 1995.

83. Jackson RD, Wortsman J, Malarkey WB: Macroprolactinemia presenting like a pituitary tumor, Am J Med 78:346–350, 1985.

84. Tritos NA, Guay AT, Malarkey WB: Asymptomatic "big" hyperprolactinemia in two men with pituitary adenomas, Eur J Endocrinol 138:82–85, 1998.

85. Glezer A, Vieira JG, Giannella-Neto D, et al: Clinical asymptomatic hyperprolactinemia is not always linked

to macroprolactinemia: peculiarities of two cases. ENDO Society 85th Annual Meeting, Philadelphia, 2003, P3-649, p 630.

86. Vallette-Kasic S, Morange-Ramos I, Selim A, et al: Macroprolactinemia revisited: a study on 106 patients, J Clin Endocrinol Metab 87:581–588, 2002.
87. Vieira JG, Tachibana TT, Obara LH, et al: Extensive experience and validation of polyethylene glycol precipitation as a screening method for macroprolactinemia, Clin Chem 44:1758–1759, 1998.
88. Cavaco B, Leite V, Santos MA, et al: Some forms of big-big prolactin behave as a complex of monomeric prolactin with an immunoglobulin G in patients with macroprolactinemia or prolactinoma, J Clin Endocrinol Metab 80:2342–2346, 1995.
89. Hattori N, Nakayama Y, Kitagawa K, et al: Anti-prolactin (PRL) autoantibodies suppress PRL bioactivity in patients with macroprolactinaemia, Clin Endocrinol (Oxf) 68:72–76, 2008.
90. Glezer A, Soares CR, Vieira JG, et al: Human macroprolactin displays low biological activity via its homologous receptor in a new sensitive bioassay, J Clin Endocrinol Metab 91:1048–1055, 2006.
91. Andersen M, Hagen C, Frystyk J, et al: Development of acromegaly in patients with prolactinomas, Eur J Endocrinol 149:17–22, 2003.
92. George LD, Nicolau N, Scanlon MF, et al: Recovery of growth hormone secretion following cabergoline treatment of macroprolactinomas, Clin Endocrinol (Oxf) 53:595–599, 2000.
93. Sibal L, Ugwu P, Kendall-Taylor P, et al: Medical therapy of macroprolactinomas in males: I. Prevalence of hypopituitarism at diagnosis. II. Proportion of cases exhibiting recovery of pituitary function, Pituitary 5:243–246, 2002.
94. Rennert J, Doerfler A: Imaging of sellar and parasellar lesions, Clin Neurol Neurosurg 109:111–124, 2007.
95. Buchfelder M, Nistor R, Fahlbusch R, et al: The accuracy of CT and MR evaluation of the sella turcica for detection of adrenocorticotropic hormone-secreting adenomas in Cushing disease. Am J Neuroradiol 14:1183–1190, 1993.
96. Patronas N, Bulakbasi N, Stratakis CA, et al: Spoiled gradient recalled acquisition in the steady state technique is superior to conventional postcontrast spin echo technique for magnetic resonance imaging detection of adrenocorticotropin-secreting pituitary tumors, J Clin Endocrinol Metab 88:1565–1569, 2003.
97. Aron DC, Howlett TA: Pituitary incidentalomas, Endocrinol Metab Clin North Am 29:205–221, 2000.
98. Molitch ME: Pituitary incidentalomas, Endocrinol Metab Clin North Am 26:725–740, 1997.
99. Hall WA, Luciano MG, Doppman JL, et al: Pituitary magnetic resonance imaging in normal human volunteers: occult adenomas in the general population, Ann Intern Med 120:817–820, 1994.
100. Chanson P, Daujat F, Young J, et al: Normal pituitary hypertrophy as a frequent cause of pituitary incidentaloma: a follow-up study, J Clin Endocrinol Metab 86:3009–3015, 2001.
101. Dinç H, Esen F, Demirci A, et al: Pituitary dimensions and volume measurements in pregnancy and post partum. MR assessment, Acta Radiol 39:64–69, 1998.
102. Krishnan KRR, Doraiswamy PM, Lurie SN, et al: Pituitary size in depression, J Clin Endocrinol Metab 72:256–259, 1991.
103. Scillitani A, Dicembrino F, Di Fazio P, et al: In-vivo visualization of pituitary dopaminergic receptors by ^{123}iodine methoxybenzamide (IBZM) correlates with sensitivity to dopamine agonists in two patients with macroprolactinomas, J Clin Endocrinol Metab 80:2523–2525, 1995.
104. de Herder WW, Reijs AE, de Swart J, et al: Comparison of iodine-123 epidepride and iodine-123 IBZM for dopamine D2 receptor imaging in clinically non-functioning pituitary macroadenomas and macroprolactinomas, Eur J Nucl Med 26:46–50, 1999.
105. Muhr C: Positron emission tomography in acromegaly and other pituitary adenoma patients, Neuroendocrinology 83:205–210, 2006.
106. Petrossians P, de Herder W, Kwekkeboom D, et al: Malignant prolactinoma discovered by D2 receptor imaging, J Clin Endocrinol Metab 85:398–401, 2000.
107. Fluckiger E, Wagner HR: 2-Br-alpha-ergokryptin: influence on fertility and lactation in the rat, Experientia 24:1130–1131, 1968.
108. Grosvenor AE, Laws ER: The evolution of extracranial approaches to the pituitary and anterior skull base, Pituitary 11(4):337–345, 2008.
109. Cho DY, Liau WR: Comparison of endonasal endoscopic surgery and sublabial microsurgery for prolactinomas, Surg Neurol 58:371–375, 2002.
110. Prevedello DM, Doglietto F, Jane JA Jr, et al: History of endoscopic skull base surgery: its evolution and current reality, J Neurosurg 107:206–213, 2007.
111. Ciric I, Ragin A, Baumgartner C, et al: Complications of transsphenoidal surgery: results of a national survey, review of the literature, and personal experience, Neurosurgery 40:225–236, 1997.
112. Chandler WF, Barkan AL: Treatment of pituitary tumors: a surgical perspective, Endocrinol Metab Clin North Am 37:51–66, 2008.
113. Tyrrell JB, Lamborn KR, Hannegan LT, et al: Transsphenoidal microsurgical therapy of prolactinomas: initial outcomes and long-term results, Neurosurgery 44:254–261, 1999.
114. Losa M, Mortini P, Barzaghi R, et al: Surgical treatment of prolactin-secreting pituitary adenomas: early results and long-term outcome, J Clin Endocrinol Metab 87:3180–3186, 2002.
115. Gillam MP, Molitch ME, Lombardi G, et al: Advances in the treatment of prolactinomas, Endocr Rev 27:485–534, 2006.
116. Bronstein M, Musolino N, Cunha-Neto M, et al: Hyperprolactinemia therapy: lessons learned from long-term follow-up, Eur J Endocrinol 130:116, 1994.
117. Landolt AM, Keller PJ, Froesch ER, et al: Bromocriptine: does it jeopardise the result of later surgery for prolactinomas? Lancet 2:657–658, 1982.
118. Soule SG, Farhi J, Conway GS, et al: The outcome of hypophysectomy for prolactinomas in the era of dopamine agonist therapy, Clin Endocrinol (Oxf) 44:711–716, 1996.
119. Perrin G, Treluyer C, Trouillas J, et al: Surgical outcome and pathological effects of bromocriptine preoperative treatment in prolactinomas, Pathol Res Pract 187:587–592, 1991.
120. Sughrue ME, Chang EF, Tyrell JB, et al: Pre-operative dopamine agonist therapy improves post-operative tumor control following prolactinoma resection, Pituitary 2008 Jul 24 [Epub ahead of print] doi: 10.1007/s11102-008-0135-1.
121. Serri O, Rasio E, Beauregard H, et al: Recurrence of hyperprolactinemia after selective transsphenoidal adenomectomy in women with prolactinoma, N Engl J Med 309:280–283, 1983.
122. Amar AP, Couldwell WT, Chen JC, et al: Predictive value of serum prolactin levels measured immediately after transsphenoidal surgery, J Neurosurg 97:307–314, 2002.
123. Maira G, Anile C, De Marinis L, et al: Prolactin-secreting adenomas: surgical results and long-term follow-up, Neurosurgery 24:736–743, 1989.
124. Massoud F, Serri O, Hardy J, et al: Transsphenoidal adenomectomy for microprolactinomas: 10 to 20 years of follow-up, Surg Neurol 45:341–346, 1996.
125. Thomson JA, Gray CE, Teasdale GM: Relapse of hyperprolactinemia after transsphenoidal surgery for microprolactinoma: lessons from long-term follow-up, Neurosurgery 50:36–39, 2002.
126. Nawar RN, AbdelMannan D, Selman WR, et al: Pituitary tumor apoplexy: a review, Intensive Care Med 23:75–90. 2008
127. Adler I, Barsi P, Czirják S, et al: Rapid re-enlargement of a macroprolactinoma after initial shrinkage in a young woman treated with bromocriptine, Gynecol Endocrinol 20:317–321,2005.
128. Bronstein MD, Musolino NR, Benabou S, et al: Cerebrospinal fluid rhinorrhea occurring in long-term bromocriptine treatment for macroprolactinomas, Surg Neurol 32:346–349, 1989.
129. Suliman SG, Gurlek A, Byrne JV, et al: Nonsurgical cerebrospinal fluid rhinorrhea in invasive macroprolactinoma: incidence, radiological, and clinicopathological features, J Clin Endocrinol Metab 92:3829–3835, 2007.
130. Jones SE, James RA, Hall K, et al: Optic chiasmal herniation—an under-recognized complication of dopamine agonist therapy for macroprolactinoma, Clin Endocrinol (Oxf) 53:529–534, 2000.
131. Kreutzer J, Buslei R, Wallaschofski H, et al: Operative treatment of prolactinomas: indications and results in a current consecutive series of 212 patients, Eur J Endocrinol 158(1):11–18, 2008.
132. Besser GM, Parke L, Edwards CR, et al: Galactorrhoea: successful treatment with reduction of plasma prolactin levels by brom-ergocryptine, Br Med J 3:669–672, 1972.
133. Ben-Jonathan N: Regulation of prolactin secretion. In Imura H, editor: The Pituitary Gland, New York, 1994, Raven Press, p 261.
134. Vance ML, Evans WS, Thorner MO: Bromocriptine, Ann Intern Med 100:78–91, 1984.
135. Pinzone JJ, Katznelson L, Danila DC, et al: Primary medical therapy of micro- and macroprolactinomas in men, J Clin Endocrinol Metab 85:3053–3057, 2000.
136. Corenblum B, Webster BR, Mortimer CB, et al: Possible antitumour effect of bromoergocryptine in 2 patients with large prolactin-secreting pituitary adenomas, Clin Res 23:614A, 1975.
137. Molitch ME, Elton RL, Blackwell RE, et al: Bromocriptine as primary therapy for prolactin-secreting macroadenomas: results of a prospective multicenter study, J Clin Endocrinol Metab 60:698–705, 1985.
138. Essais O, Bouguerra R, Hamzaoui J, et al: Efficacy and safety of bromocriptine in the treatment of macroprolactinomas, Ann Endocrinol (Paris) 63:524–531, 2002.
139. Wu ZB, Yu CJ, Su ZP, et al: Bromocriptine treatment of invasive giant prolactinomas involving the cavernous sinus: results of a long-term follow up, J Neurosurg 104:54–61, 2006.
140. Tindall GT, Kovacs K, Horvath E, et al: Human prolactin-producing adenomas and bromocriptine: a histological, immunocytochemical, ultrastructural, and morphometric study, J Clin Endocrinol Metab 55:178–183, 1982.
141. Gruszka A, Pawlikowski M, Kunert-Radek J: Antitumoral action of octreotide and bromocriptine on the experimental rat prolactinoma: anti-proliferative and pro-apoptotic effects, Neuroendocrinol Lett 22:343–348, 2001.
142. Kovacs K, Stefaneanu L, Horvath E, et al: Effect of dopamine agonist medication on prolactin producing pituitary adenomas: a morphological study including immunocytochemistry, electron microscopy and in-situ hybridization, Virchows Arch 418:439–446, 1991.
143. Orrego JJ, Chandler WF, Barkan AL: Rapid re-expansion of a macroprolactinoma after early discontinuation of bromocriptine, Pituitary 3:189–192, 2000.
144. van't Verlaat JW, Croughs RJ: Withdrawal of bromocriptine after long-term therapy for macroprolactinomas: effect on plasma prolactin and tumour size, Clin Endocrinol (Oxf) 34:175–178, 1991.
145. Bevan JS, Webster J, Burke CW, et al: Dopamine agonists and pituitary tumor shrinkage, Endocr Rev 13:220–240, 1992.
146. Molitch ME: Medical management of prolactin-secreting pituitary adenomas, Pituitary 5:55–65, 2002.
147. Passos VQ, Souza JJ, Musolino NR, et al: Long-term follow-up of prolactinomas: normoprolactinemia after bromocriptine withdrawal, J Clin Endocrinol Metab 87:3578–3582, 2002.
148. Biswas M, Smith J, Jadon D, et al: Long-term remission following withdrawal of dopamine agonist therapy in subjects with microprolactinomas, Clin Endocrinol (Oxf) 63:26–31, 2005.
149. Gen M, Uozumi T, Ohta M, et al: Necrotic changes in prolactinomas after long term administration of bromocriptine, J Clin Endocrinol Metab 59:463–470, 1984.
150. Koppelman MC, Jaffe MJ, Rieth KG, et al: Hyperprolactinemia, amenorrhea, and galactorrhea: a retrospective assessment of 25 cases, Ann Intern Med 100:115–121, 1984.
151. Schlechte J, Dolan K, Sherman B, et al: The natural history of untreated hyperprolactinemia: a prospective analysis, J Clin Endocrinol Metab 68:412–418, 1989.
152. Sisam DA, Sheehan JP, Sheeler LR: The natural history of untreated microprolactinomas, Fertil Steril 48:67–71, 1987.
153. Karunakaran S, Page RC, Wass JA: The effect of the menopause on prolactin levels in patients with hyperprolactinaemia, Clin Endocrinol (Oxf) 54:295–300, 2001.
154. Pinto G, Zerah M, Trivin C, et al: Pituitary apoplexy in an adolescent with prolactin-secreting adenoma, Horm Res 50:38–41, 1998.

155. Turner TH, Cookson JC, Wass JA, et al: Psychotic reactions during treatment of pituitary tumours with dopamine agonists, Br Med J 289:1101–1103, 1984.
156. Ciubotaru V, Poinsignon Y, Brunet-Bourgin F, et al: Severe pleuropericarditis induced by long-term bromocriptine therapy, report of a case and review of the literature, Rev Med Interne 25:310–314, 2004
157. Liuzzi A, Dallabonzana D, Oppizzi G, et al: Low doses of dopamine agonists in the long-term treatment of macroprolactinomas, N Engl J Med 313:656–659, 1985.
158. Merola B, Colao A, Caruso E, et al: Effectiveness and long-term tolerability of the slow release oral form of bromocriptine on tumoral and non-tumoral hyperprolactinemia, J Endocrinol Invest 15:173–176, 1992.
159. Bronstein MD, Cardim CS, Marino R Jr: Short-term management of macroprolactinomas with a new injectable form of bromocriptine, Surg Neurol 28:31–37, 1987.
160. Beckers A, Petrossians P, Abs R, et al: Treatment of macroprolactinomas with the long-acting and repeatable form of bromocriptine: a report on 29 cases, J Clin Endocrinol Metab 75:275–280, 1992.
161. Darwish AM, Farah E, Gadallah WA, et al: Superiority of newly developed vaginal suppositories over vaginal use of commercial bromocriptine tablets: a randomized controlled clinical trial, Reprod Sci 14:280–285, 2007.
162. Brue T, Pellegrini I, Priou A, et al: Prolactinomas and resistance to dopamine agonists, Horm Res 38:84–89, 1992.
163. Pellegrini I, Rasolonjanahary R, Gunz G, et al: Resistance to bromocriptine in prolactinomas, J Clin Endocrinol Metab 69:500–509, 1989.
164. Passos VQ, Fortes MA, Giannella-Neto D, et al: Genes differentially expressed in prolactinomas responsive and resistant to dopaminergic agonists, Neuroendocrinology, 89(2):163–170, 2009.
165. Caccavelli L, Feron F, Morange I, et al: Decreased expression of the two D2 dopamine receptor isoforms in bromocriptine-resistant prolactinomas, Neuroendocrinology 60:314–322, 1994.
166. Delgrange E, Duprez T, Maiter D: Influence of parasellar extension of macroprolactinomas defined by magnetic resonance imaging on their responsiveness to dopamine agonist therapy, Clin Endocrinol (Oxf) 64:456–462, 2006
167. Delgrange E, Crabbe J, Donckier J: Late development of resistance to bromocriptine in a patient with macroprolactinoma, Horm Res 49:250–253, 1998.
168. Lamberts SW, Quik RF: A comparison of the efficacy and safety of pergolide and bromocriptine in the treatment of hyperprolactinemia, J Clin Endocrinol Metab 72:635, 1991.
169. Berezin M, Avidan D, Baron E: Long-term pergolide treatment of hyperprolactinemic patients previously unsuccessfully treated with dopaminergic drugs, Isr J Med Sci 27:375–379, 1991.
170. Freda PU, Andreadis CI, Khandji AG, et al: Long-term treatment of prolactin-secreting macroadenomas with pergolide, J Clin Endocrinol Metab 85:8–13, 2000.
171. Orrego JJ, Chandler WF, Barkan AL: Pergolide as primary therapy for macroprolactinomas, Pituitary 3:251–256, 2000.
172. Vance ML, Lipper M, Klibanski A, et al: Treatment of prolactin-secreting pituitary macroadenomas with the long-acting non-ergot dopamine agonist CV 205-502, Ann Intern Med 112:668–673, 1990.
173. Serri O, Beauregard H, Lesage J, et al: Long term treatment with CV 205-502 in patients with prolactin-secreting pituitary macroadenomas, J Clin Endocrinol Metab 71:682–687, 1990.
174. van der Lely AJ, Brownell J, Lamberts SW: The efficacy and tolerability of CV 205-502 (a nonergot dopaminergic drug) in macroprolactinoma patients and in prolactinoma patients intolerant to bromocriptine, J Clin Endocrinol Metab 72:1136–1141, 1991.
175. Kvistborg A, Halse J, Bakke S, et al: Long-term treatment of macroprolactinomas with CV 205-502, Acta Endocrinol (Copenh) 128:301–307, 1993.
176. Glaser B, Nesher Y, Barziliai S: Long-term treatment of bromocriptine-intolerant prolactinoma patients with CV 205-502, J Reprod Med 39:449–454, 1994.
177. Brue T, Pellegrini I, Gunz G, et al: Effects of the dopamine agonist CV 205-502 in human prolactinomas resistant to bromocriptine, J Clin Endocrinol Metab 74:577–584, 1992.
178. Morange I, Barlier A, Pellegrini I, et al: Prolactinomas resistant to bromocriptine: long-term efficacy of quinagolide and outcome of pregnancy, Eur J Endocrinol 135:413–420, 1996.
179. Del Dotto P, Bonuccelli U: Clinical pharmacokinetics of cabergoline, Clin Pharmacokinet 42:633–645, 2003.
180. Ferrari C, Paracchi A, Mattei AM, et al: Cabergoline in the long-term therapy of hyperprolactinemic disorders, Acta Endocrinol (Copenh) 126:489–494, 1992.
181. Cannavo S, Curto L, Squadrito S, et al: Cabergoline: a first-choice treatment in patients with previously untreated prolactin-secreting pituitary adenoma, J Endocrinol Invest 22:354–359, 1999.
182. Biller BM, Molitch ME, Vance ML, et al: Treatment of prolactin-secreting macroadenomas with the once-weekly dopamine agonist cabergoline, J Clin Endocrinol Metab 81:2338–2343, 1996.
183. Colao A, Vitale G, Cappabianca P, et al: Outcome of cabergoline treatment in men with prolactinoma: effects of a 24-month treatment on prolactin levels, tumor mass, recovery of pituitary function, and semen analysis, J Clin Endocrinol Metab 89:1704–1711, 2004.
184. Vilar L, Freitas MC, Naves LA, et al: Diagnosis and management of hyperprolactinemia: results of a Brazilian multicenter study with 1234 patients—intolerance/resistance, J Endocrinol Invest 31:436–444, 2008.
185. Webster J, Piscitelli G, Polli A, et al, Cabergoline Comparative Study Group: A comparison of cabergoline and bromocriptine in the treatment of hyperprolactinemic amenorrhea, N Engl J Med 331:904–909, 1994.
186. Pascal-Vigneron V, Weryha G, Bosc M, et al: Hyperprolactinemic amenorrhea: treatment with cabergoline versus bromocriptine: results of a national multicenter randomized double-blind study, Presse Med 24:753–757, 1995.
187. Verhelst J, Abs R, Maiter D, et al: Cabergoline in the treatment of hyperprolactinemia: A study in 455 patients, J Clin Endocrinol Metab 84:2518–2522, 1999.
188. Sabuncu T, Arikan E, Tasan E, et al: Comparison of the effects of cabergoline and bromocriptine on prolactin levels in hyperprolactinemic patients, Intern Med 40:857–861, 2001.
189. Colao A, Di Sarno A, Landi ML, et al: Macroprolactinoma shrinkage during cabergoline treatment is greater in naive patients than in patients pretreated with other dopamine agonists: a prospective study in 110 patients, J Clin Endocrinol Metab 85:2247–2252, 2000.
190. Colao A, Di Sarno A, Sarnacchiaro F, et al: Prolactinomas resistant to standard dopamine agonists respond to chronic cabergoline treatment, J Clin Endocrinol Metab 82:876–883, 1997.
191. Colao A, Di Sarno A, Cappabianca P, et al: Withdrawal of long-term cabergoline therapy for tumoral and nontumoral hyperprolactinemia, N Engl J Med 349:2023–2033, 2003.
192. Schade R, Andersohn F, Suissa S, et al: Dopamine agonists and the risk of cardiac valve regurgitation, N Engl J Med 356:29–38, 2007.
193. Zanettini R, Antonini A, Gatto G, et al: Valvular heart disease and the use of dopamine agonists for Parkinson's disease, N Engl J Med 356:39–46, 2007.
194. Bogazzi F, Buralli S, Manetti L, et al: Treatment with low doses of cabergoline is not associated with increased prevalence of cardiac valve regurgitation in patients with hyperprolactinaemia, Int J Clin Pract 62:1865–1869, 2008.
195. Vallette S, Serri K, Rivera J, et al: Long-term cabergoline therapy is not associated with valvular heart disease in patients with prolactinomas, Pituitary Jul 2, 2008. [Epub ahead of print.]
196. Kars M, Delgado V, Holman ER, et al: Aortic valve calcification and mild tricuspid regurgitation, but no clinical heart disease after 8 years of dopamine agonist therapy for prolactinoma, J Clin Endocrinol Metab Jun 17, 2008. [Epub ahead of print].
197. Acquati S, Pizzocaro A, Tomei G, et al: A comparative evaluation of effectiveness of medical and surgical therapy in patients with macroprolactinoma, J Neurosurg Sci 45:65–69, 2001.
198. Tsang RW, Brierley JD, Panzarella T, et al: Role of radiation therapy in clinical hormonally active pituitary adenomas, Radiother Oncol 41:45–53, 1996.
199. Molitch ME: Pathologic hyperprolactinemia, Endocrinol Metab Clin North Am 21:877–901, 1992.
200. Landolt AM, Lomax N: Gamma-knife radiosurgery for prolactinomas, J Neurosurg 93:14–18, 2000.
201. Pouratian N, Sheehan J, Jagannathan J, et al: Gamma-knife radiosurgery for medically and surgically refractory prolactinomas, Neurosurgery 59:255–266, 2006.
202. Pan L, Zhang N, Wang EM, et al: Gamma-knife radiosurgery as a primary treatment for prolactinomas, J Neurosurg 93:10–13, 2000.
203. Testa G, Vegetti W, Motta T, et al: Two-year treatment with oral contraceptives in hyperprolactinemic patients, Contraception 58:69–73, 1998.
204. Gillam MP, Middler S, Freed DJ, et al: The novel use of very high doses of cabergoline and a combination of testosterone and an aromatase inhibitor in the treatment of a giant prolactinoma, J Clin Endocrinol Metab 87:4447–4451, 2002.
205. Bronstein MD, Knoepfelmacher M, Liberman B, et al: Absence of suppressive effect of somatostatin on prolactin levels in patients with hyperprolactinemia, Horm Metab Res 19:271–274, 1987.
206. Shimon I, Yan X, Taylor JE, et al: Somatostatin receptor (SSTR) subtype-selective analogues differentially suppress in vitro growth hormone and prolactin in human pituitary adenomas: Novel potential therapy for functional pituitary tumors, J Clin Invest 100:2386–2392, 1997.
207. Jaquet P, Ouafik L, Saveanu A, et al: Quantitative and functional expression of somatostatin receptor subtypes in human prolactinomas, J Clin Endocrinol Metab 84:3268–3276, 1999.
208. Fusco A, Gunz G, Jaquet P, et al: Somatostatinergic ligands in dopamine-sensitive and resistant prolactinomas, Eur J Endocrinol 158:595–603, 2008
209. Ishikawa H, Heaney AP, Yu R, et al: Human pituitary tumor-transforming gene induces angiogenesis, J Clin Endocrinol Metab 86:867–874, 2001.
210. Goffin V, Bernichtein S, Touraine P, et al: Development and Potential Clinical Uses of Human Prolactin Receptor Antagonists, Endocrine Reviews 26:400–422, 2005.
211. Neff LM, Weil M, Cole A, et al: Temozolomide in the treatment of an invasive prolactinoma resistant to dopamine agonists, Pituitary 10:81–86, 2007.
212. Kovacs K, Horvath E, Syro LV, et al: Temozolomide therapy in a man with an aggressive prolactin-secreting pituitary neoplasm: Morphological findings, Hum Pathol 38:185–189,2007.
213. Fadul CE, Kominsky AL, Meyer LP, et al: Long-term response of pituitary carcinoma to temozolomide. Report of two cases, J Neurosurg 105:621–626, 2006..
214. Facchetti M, Uberti D, Memo M, et al: Nerve growth factor restores p53 function in pituitary tumor cell lines via trkA-mediated activation of phosphatidylinositol 3-kinase, Mol Endocrinol 18:162–172, 2004.
215. Missale C, Losa M, Boroni F, et al: Nerve growth factor and bromocriptine: a sequential therapy for human bromocriptine-resistant prolactinomas, Br J Cancer 72:1397–1399, 1995.
216. Gemzell C, Wang CF: Outcome of pregnancy in women with pituitary adenoma, Fertil Steril 31:363–372, 1979.
217. Molitch ME: Pregnancy and the hyperprolactinemic woman, N Engl J Med 312:1364–1370, 1985.
218. Musolino NRC, Bronstein MD: Prolactinomas and pregnancy. In Bronstein MD, editor: Pituitary Tumors in Pregnancy, Boston, 2001, Kluwer Academic Publishers, pp 91–108.
219. Bronstein MD: Prolactinomas and pregnancy, Pituitary 8:31–38, 2005.
220. Holmgren U, Bergstrand G, Hagenfeldt K, et al: Women with prolactinoma-effect of pregnancy and lactation on serum prolactin and on tumour growth, Acta Endocrinol (Copenh) 111:452–459, 1986.
221. Krupp P, Monka C: Bromocriptine in pregnancy: safety aspects, Klin Wochenschr 65:823–827, 1987.
222. Konopka P, Raymond JP, Merceron RE, et al: Continuous administration of bromocriptine in the prevention of neurological complications in pregnant women with prolactinomas, Am J Obstet Gynecol 146:935–938, 1983.
223. Webster J: A comparative review of the tolerability profiles of dopamine agonists in the treatment of hyperprolactinaemia and inhibition of lactation, Drug Saf 14:228–238,1996
224. Robert E, Musatti L, Piscitelli G, et al: Pregnancy outcome after treatment with the ergot derivative, cabergoline, Reprod Toxicol 10:333–337, 1996.

225. Colao A, Abs R, Bárcena DG, et al: Pregnancy outcomes following cabergoline treatment: extended results from a 12-year observational study, Clin Endocrinol (Oxf) 68:66–71, 2008.

226. Buelke-Sam J, Cohen IR, Tizzano JP, et al: Developmental toxicity of the dopamine agonist pergolide mesylate in CD-1 mice: II. Perinatal and postnatal exposure, Neurotoxicol Teratol 13:297–306, 1991.

227. Crosignani PG, Mattei AM, Severini V, et al: Long-term effects of time, medical treatment and pregnancy in 176 hyperprolactinemic women, Eur J Obstet Gynaecol Reprod Biol 44:175–180, 1992.

228. Badawy SZ, Marziale JC, Rosenbaum AE, et al: The long-term effects of pregnancy and bromocriptine treatment on prolactinomas—the value of radiologic studies, Early Pregnancy 3:306–311, 1997.

229. Peillon F, Racadot J, Moussy D, et al: Prolactin-secreting adenomas: a correlative study of morphological and clinical data. In Fahlbuch R, von Werder K, editors: Treatment of Pituitary Adenomas. Stuttgart, 1978, Thieme, p 114.

230. Wang PS, Walker AM, Tsuang MT, et al: Dopamine antagonists and the development of breast cancer, Arch Gen Psychiatry 59:1147–1154, 2002.

231. Manjer J, Johansson R, Berglund G, et al: Postmenopausal breast cancer risk in relation to sex steroid hormones, prolactin and SHBG (Sweden), Cancer Causes Control 14:599–607, 2003.

232. Rose-Hellekant TA, Arendt LM, Schroeder MD, et al: Prolactin induces ERα-positive and ERα-negative mammary cancer in transgenic mice, Oncogene 22:4664–4674, 2003.

233. Liby K, Neltner B, Mohamet L, et al: Prolactin overexpression by MDA-MB-435 human breast cancer cells accelerates tumor growth, Breast Cancer Res Treat 79:241–252, 2003.

PITUITARY SURGERY

PAOLO CAPPABIANCA, LUIGI M. CAVALLO, ORESTE DE DIVITIIS, and FELICE ESPOSITO

Pituitary surgery is a distinct subspecialty of neurosurgery that demands precise knowledge of basic neurosurgical techniques and associated skills, together with specific knowledge, interest, and appreciation of pituitary pathophysiology, allowing the surgeon to make the right choice at the right moment. It is currently possible to manage many of the different pituitary syndromes with more than one option, including medical, surgical, and radiotherapeutic, alone or in various combinations. Pituitary surgery yields the best outcomes when performed in centers where the entire range of pituitary specialties is offered in an environment of effective teamwork. Such teamwork demands a "teamwork attitude," which is not just the addition of the expertise of the single contributors, but rather a cultural and psychological attitude, with the single units working with a goal of true exchange and sincere collaboration; this allows a cooperative effort for the benefit of the patient and positive feedback for physicians and surgeons. Pituitary surgery, perhaps more than other areas of neurosurgery, requires careful and specific postoperative management and long-term patient follow-up, which can make the difference between a satisfactory result and a poor result. A patient can be operated on successfully, but the outcome may not be as brilliant as the surgical procedure if mutual exchange between specialists such as the pathologist, the ophthalmologist, the neuroradiologist, and the endocrinologist is not established. If teamwork logic is established, each participant contributes to the final outcome of the patient while promoting growth of the other components, which calls for further work and better allocation of competencies and effectiveness: A virtuous circuit develops.

It is in such a context that pituitary surgery should exist today, where the neurosurgeon dealing with techniques, indications, and results is a member of an orchestra who is playing a refined instrument. The neurosurgeon must have keen perception, good instincts, steady hands, and the ability to perform an operation made to measure for the individual patient and not mass produced. To realize these goals, the neurosurgeon must know detailed anatomy, learned in the laboratory before working in an operating room; he or she must be experienced in neuroimaging, must know pathophysiology and the natural history of pituitary disease, and must be familiar with the various therapeutic options. The neurosurgeon plays a crucial role and in the interest of the patient and of the institution where the operation is done must be fully informed about current therapeutic possibilities.

Historical Background

Pituitary surgery was developed and has advanced on the basis of repeated innovations and exchanges between Europe and the New World. The first operation on a pituitary tumor was performed by Horsley in 1889, who published in 1906[1] the results obtained on a series of 10 patients, first by means of a frontal craniotomy and later through a temporal approach.[2] The first surgeon who reported on an operation specifically for a pituitary tumor was a British general surgeon, Paul; in 1893, he performed a temporal decompression in an acromegalic patient without actually reaching the tumor.[3,4]

The next milestone was the first transsphenoidal approach achieved by the Viennese surgeon Schloffer in Innsbruck, Austria, in 1907.[5] The use of a direct route through the nose toward the brain was not absolutely new: Many centuries ago, the Egyptians used to extract cerebral tissue transnasally in the mummification process by means of special hooked instruments, without disfiguring the face. Based on anatomic studies of the Italian physician Giordano, chief surgeon of the Hospital of Venice,[6,7] Schloffer performed a lateral rhinotomy, reflecting the nose to the right; removed the turbinates; and opened the maxillary, ethmoid, and sphenoid sinuses before reaching the sella. In the same year, von Eiselsberg,[8] in Vienna, performed a similar, if even more extended, procedure. The next evolutionary step, approaching the modern transsphenoidal approach, was realized in 1909 by Kocher, professor of surgery in Berne, Switzerland, who was awarded the Nobel Prize for Medicine and Physiology in 1909 for his contributions concerning the thyroid; he performed a transseptal submucosal approach by means of an external midline incision on the nasal bridge,[9,10] but without exenteration of frontal, ethmoidal, and maxillary sinuses. Another remarkable contribution was that of Kanavel,[11,12] who proposed an approach through an infranasal skin incision. The first totally endonasal procedure, without complete dislocation of the nose, was achieved in 1910 in five stages with the patient under local anesthesia by Hirsch, a Viennese rhinologist, who was the first to incorporate a nasal speculum.[13] He used the technique of his teacher Hajek,[14] which was used previously for purulent infections of the sphenoid sinus, first opening the posterior ethmoid sinus, then enlarging the opening into the sphenoid sinus after a submucosal resection of the septum, according to Kocher's and Kilian's techniques,[9,15] beginning with a hemitransfixion incision in the right nasal cavity. Hirsch moved to the United States in 1938 to escape the Nazis, and worked in Boston with the neurosurgeon Hamlin.[16]

In 1910, Halstead[17,18] was a pioneer of the sublabial approach, which initially was performed as a multistage operation in Chicago. Cushing performed his first transsphenoidal procedure in 1909,[19] but his classic sublabial, transseptal, transsphenoidal approach[20] was the evolution of his technique and a combination of different methods reported by other authors, such as Halstead, Hirsch, Kanavel, and Kocher (i.e., sublabial incision + submucosal paraseptal approach to the sphenoid sinus + use of the nasal speculum + use of an electric headlamp). Cushing later abandoned this procedure,[10,21,22] likely because of better recovery of vision in patients operated transcranially owing to difficulty with hemostasis and completeness of tumor removal in large suprasellar tumors and owing to difficulty in preoperative differential diagnosis. His advocacy of the transcranial option prompted most neurosurgeons to follow his recommendations. Another leading American neurosurgeon, Dandy, stated, "The nasal route is impractical and can never be otherwise."[23] In 1918, at the Johns Hopkins Medical Society, Dandy had presented his experience in about 20 cases operated on through an intracranial intradural approach to the chiasm, according to a frontotemporal route to the pituitary along the sylvian fissure, originally conceived by Heuer in 1914.[24,25] The two main transcranial options—subfrontal and frontotemporal—are still used today, together with more recent skull base approaches.

The late 1920s to the 1960s was a relatively dark period for transsphenoidal surgery, because of the absence of antibiotics and replacement therapy for adrenocortical hormones, the lack of adequate illumination, and the opinions of the most authoritative opinion leader, Cushing. The only pupil of Cushing who did not abandon the transsphenoidal method was Dott, neurosurgeon of the Royal Infirmary at Edinburgh.[10,26] He had learned the method from Cushing when he had been awarded a 1 year Rockefeller Fellowship at the Peter Bent Brigham Hospital in 1923. It is not clear why Dott did not publish his results, but he kept the procedure alive, improved the technique by adding two light bulbs to the speculum designed by Cushing, and taught the method to the French neurosurgeon Guiot during his visit to the Royal Infirmary in 1956. Guiot at the Hôpital Foch in Paris and Guiot's trainee Hardy in Montreal deserve credit for the "transsphenoidal renaissance" in the late 1960s and 1970s. Modern transsphenoidal surgery takes advantage of the innovations of intraoperative image intensification and fluoroscopy, introduced by Guiot, and the use of the operating microscope according to Hardy,[27] who introduced the concept of microadenoma and selective microsurgical resection.

No new progress was made until the 1990s, when the latest innovation, the endoscope, was introduced. By analogy with the evolution of Picasso's painting, the "cubist evolution" of transsphenoidal surgery occurred, from devastating transfacial approaches to minimally invasive contemporary procedures,[28] and with the endoscope used as a visualizing instrument for pituitary surgery. Used for the first time by Guiot in 1963[29] as an adjunct to the microscope to expand the field of vision (endoscope-assisted microneurosurgery), then abandoned for

many years because it still was technically insufficient, the endoscope has come into regular use as a stand-alone visualizing and operating tool (pure endoscopic transsphenoidal surgery), thanks primarily to the work of Jho in Pittsburgh[30,31] and of our group in Naples, Italy[32,33]; these workers standardized a unilateral endonasal anterior sphenoidotomy approach to the sella, without the use of the operating microscope or of a transsphenoidal retractor. Further advancement and evolution of the technique are expected through intraoperative magnetic resonance imaging (MRI), robotics, and miniaturization, as well as the rapidly emerging biomolecular frontiers, which are expected to change the world of pituitary surgery.

Surgical Anatomy

The pituitary gland, or the hypophysis cerebri, is situated within the hypophyseal fossa, a fibro-osseous compartment near the center of the cranial base (Fig. 12-1). This fossa is limited laterally and superiorly by reflections of dura mater, and anteriorly, posteriorly, and inferiorly by the sella turcica, a depression in the body of the sphenoid bone. At the superior edge of the anterior wall of the sella turcica is a bony protrusion called the tuberculum sellae, and its posterior wall is the dorsum sellae.

The degree of pneumatization of the sphenoid bone and the thickness of the bone separating the sphenoid sinus from the hypophyseal fossa are highly variable. Three sinus types are distinguished by their shape and size: In the conchal type ($\approx$3%), the area below the sella is a solid block of bone without an air cavity; in the presellar type ($\approx$17%), the air cavity does not penetrate beyond a vertical plane parallel to the anterior sellar wall; and in the sellar type ($\approx$80%), the air cavity extends into the body of the sphenoid below the sella and as far posteriorly as the clivus. The conchal type is most common in children before the age of 12 years, at which time pneumatization progresses within the sphenoid sinus. The greater the degree of pneumatization of the sphenoid sinus, the easier is the access to the sellar region through the transsphenoidal approach.

The space within the sphenoid sinus is subdivided by one or more septa. Single septa are not always located in the midline, and in 20% of cases, the posterior attachment of the sphenoid septum to the sphenoid sinus is on the carotid protuberance, serving as an important landmark for preventing injury to the carotid artery.

The diaphragma sellae, a fold of dura with a central aperture, forms an incomplete roof above the sella turcica. The diaphragma separates the anterior lobe from the overlying optic chiasm. The central opening of the diaphragma is of variable size and transmits the pituitary stalk and its blood supply. The subarachnoid space of the chiasmatic cistern can extend through the aperture of the diaphragma and into the sella turcica for varying distances above the gland. When there is an incompetent diaphragma sellae (i.e., wide central aperture of the diaphragma), the chiasmatic cistern herniates to fill the sella turcica partially, leading to remodeling and enlargement of the hypophyseal fossa and flattening of the pituitary gland, a condition called empty sella,[34] which is found in 5% to 23% of cases at autopsy.[35] When this condition is associated with the presence of an adenoma, usually a microadenoma, the surgeon must be careful to avoid entering the subarachnoid space (i.e., the chiasmatic cistern herniated into the sella), to prevent an intraoperative cerebrospinal fluid (CSF) leak, which could increase the difficulty of resecting the lesion.

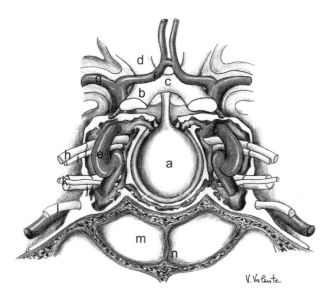

FIGURE 12-1. Frontal view: schematic drawing of the sellar region. *a*, Pituitary gland. *b*, Optic nerve. *c*, Optic chiasm. *d*, Optic tract. *e*, Internal carotid artery. *f*, Anterior cerebral artery. *g*, Middle cerebral artery. *h*, Oculomotor nerve. *i*, Trochlear nerve. *j*, Ophthalmic branch (V1) of the trigeminal nerve. *k*, Abducent nerve. *l*, Maxillary branch (V2) of the trigeminal nerve. *m*, Sphenoid sinus. *n*, Sphenoid septum. (Courtesy V. Valente, MD.)

The folds of the dura mater form the lateral walls of the hypophyseal fossa and the medial wall of the so-called cavernous sinuses, these latter consisting of a series of compartmentalized venous channels separated by fibrous trabeculae and communicating with each other by means of the anterior and posterior intercavernous sinuses.[36-40] The oculomotor nerve, the trochlear nerve, and the first two divisions of the trigeminal nerve are embedded in the lateral wall of the cavernous sinus, lying between the endothelial lining and the dura mater, whereas the abducens nerve is contained within the sinus itself. The cavernous sinus also envelops a portion of the internal carotid artery (ICA) and the sympathetic nerve plexus encircling it. The intracavernous segment of the ICA extends forward, adjacent to the superolateral surface of the body of the sphenoid bone, in a groove called the carotid sulcus. The carotid arteries and the bone layers overlying them in the sphenoid sinus form two protuberances, which represent important landmarks in the transsphenoidal approach, particularly at the level of the sellar floor, where they are considered the lateral margins of a correct opening of the sella.

The pituitary gland derives its blood supply from two groups of arteries. The superior hypophyseal artery primarily supplies the anterior lobe, the pituitary stalk, and the inferior surface of the optic nerve and chiasm, whereas the inferior hypophyseal artery is related primarily to the pars nervosa. The superior hypophyseal artery can arise from the supraclinoid portion of the ICA or from the posterior communicating artery, whereas the inferior hypophyseal artery arises from the meningohypophyseal trunk, a branch of the cavernous segment of the ICA.

The pituitary gland is overlaid by the visual pathways and the hypothalamus. The relationships between the pituitary gland, diaphragma sellae, sulcus chiasmatis, and optic apparatus are important determinants of the visual deficits produced by an expanding pituitary tumor.[41] In some cases, the anterior border of the optic chiasm is closely applied to the sulcus chiasmatis of the sphenoid bone; this leads to a lower position of the optic chiasm, which is much nearer to the diaphragma sellae. This condition, called prefixed chiasm and present in 5% to 10% of cases,[42,43] must be considered during transcranial approaches and in the transsphenoidal opening of the upper portion of the sellar floor, as in the extended approaches to the planum sphenoidale, because of the possibility of producing iatrogenic damage to the optic chiasm. In other cases, the optic chiasm is located above the anterior part of the diaphragma sellae, making it extremely vulnerable to the suprasellar extension of a pituitary tumor. This pattern is found in about 12% of cases.[42,43] In most cases (75%), the optic chiasm is placed more posteriorly, lying over the posterior aspect of the diaphragma sellae, near the dorsum sellae,[42,43] which is a more favorable relationship for the removal of a sellar lesion because in such a circumstance, the suprasellar region is free from the optic chiasm. The remaining pattern is that of an optic chiasm located on and behind the dorsum sellae, called postfixed chiasm (4% to 11% of cases).[42,43] In such cases, the intracranial course of the optic nerves is longer, and the medial aspects of the optic nerves are more vulnerable to the suprasellar extension of the pituitary tumor.

Anatomy should represent an uninterrupted line in the surgeon's mind. The surgeon must have a thorough knowledge of anatomy and must refer to it before, during, and after performing the surgical procedure. Only in this way can the surgeon determine the correct surgical approach, that is, the exact plan for each operation; perform the necessary intraoperative controls; and check the ultimate results of the intervention.

Progress in diagnostic imaging techniques (computed tomography [CT] and MRI) has given the neurosurgeon preoperative detailed knowledge of the anatomy of each patient and of the surgical route to follow, rendering the surgical procedure safer and more comfortable for the patient and the surgeon. CT of the nasal and paranasal structures provides precise information on the surgical route to follow, which is particularly useful for the endoscopic transsphenoidal procedure and reveals the possible presence of turbinate hypertrophy; nasal septal deviation; concha bullosa; unusual sphenoid sinus type (sellar, presellar, or conchal type); single or multiple sphenoid septa; presence of an Onodi cell, which represents a potential risk for the optic nerve; and any bone structure alteration caused by the sellar lesion, such as thinning or erosion or both of the sellar floor. MRI of the sellar area, before and after intravenous administration of a paramagnetic contrast medium (gadolinium-diethylene-triaminepentaacetic acid), is fundamental. Imaging permits precise localization of the lesion with its peculiar characteristics, localization of the anatomic endosellar and parasellar structures (cisterns, optic nerves, medial wall of the cavernous sinus with the ICA), and knowledge of their mutual relationships. In clinical practice, MRI is performed in the sagittal and coronal planes: The sagittal sections give good definition of the morphology and size of the lesion; of the pituitary gland and of the pituitary stalk, when recognizable; of the suprasellar cisterns; and of the optic chiasm. The coronal slices add an evaluation of symmetry at the sellar and parasellar level. In the axial plane, the images are obtained as completion, to define better the anterosellar and retrosellar extensions of the lesion.

The need to define intraoperatively the exact location of a lesion and its relationships with surrounding vascular and nervous structures has led to the development of neuronavigation and intraoperative MRI, which provide continuous anatomic information. The neuronavigator is a computer-based system that offers the surgeon real-time information related to the operating site. The basic function of the navigator is to determine the location of a probe tip within the surgical field and to translate it into CT/MRI coordinates. The patient's head is related initially to the CT/MRI coordinates; this relationship is established preoperatively by a set of fiducial markers on the patient's head. During transsphenoidal surgery, this relationship can obviate the need for intraoperative fluoroscopy, avoiding exposure of the operating room staff and the patient to radiation. Its employment is particularly useful in the presence of a conchal or presellar type of sphenoid sinus, in identifying the boundaries of the sella, and in some cases of recurrence in which prior surgery has altered the landmarks needed to reach the sella safely.[44-49]

Intraoperative MRI, with the use of a magnetic resonance magnet positioned in a specially designed operating room with a movable operating table that allows translation of the patient from the surgical equipment to the MRI imager, offers the opportunity of a second look during the same surgical procedure. In transsphenoidal surgery, intraoperative MRI allows documentation of the extent of surgical resection of the sellar lesion, and removal of the suprasellar portion of the tumor can be evaluated reliably.[50-55]

Surgery

Therapy for pituitary adenomas is targeted to achieve multiple goals, as follows:
- Normalization of excess hormone secretion
- Preservation or restoration of normal pituitary function
- Elimination of mass effect
- Preservation or restoration of normal neurologic function, usually with visual acuity or visual field (or both) affected more frequently
- Prevention of tumor recurrence
- Achievement of a complete histologic diagnosis
- Gathering of tissue for scientific studies

Despite advances in medical treatment for pituitary adenoma, most of these tumors are managed surgically. Indications for surgery for pituitary adenomas are as follows:
- Pituitary apoplexy, a relatively rare condition presenting with sudden headache, abrupt visual loss, ophthalmoplegia, altered level of consciousness, and collapse from acute adrenal insufficiency. It is caused by a hemorrhage into the tumor or its acute necrosis, with subsequent swelling and frequent spreading into the subarachnoid space, leading to other signs of meningeal irritation; the related acute and severe clinical syndrome demands glucocorticoid replacement and surgical decompression, usually transsphenoidal, if visual loss is severe and progressive.[56-59] If the patient has a mild form of apoplexy and is clinically stable, it is prudent to measure the serum prolactin because some patients with prolactinoma present in this fashion and can be treated successfully with medical therapy.
- Progressive mass effect, producing compression of surrounding neurovascular structures and usually causing visual deficit (due to compression of the optic chiasm) or less frequently cranial nerve palsy (due to compression of cranial nerves inside the cavernous sinus). In cases of prolactin-secreting macroadenomas, dopamine agonist administration can be considered as the first treatment option because of predictable dramatic shrinkage of the lesion, with rapid recovery of neurologic deficits. In such circumstances, frequent visual field and imaging controls are necessary to monitor the clinical evolution.

Because pituitary tumors are biologically, endocrinologically, and pathologically a heterogeneous group of lesions, the role of surgery differs for the different pituitary tumor subtypes. The primary role of surgery is established in the following conditions:
- Nonfunctioning pituitary tumors
- Cushing's disease, because of the present inadequacy of pharmacologic agents
- Acromegaly, in combination with medical treatment (preoperative and postoperative, if necessary)
- Thyroid-stimulating hormone–secreting adenomas

The role of surgery in prolactinoma is secondary, but it still is necessary in selected conditions. Indications for surgery include the following:
- Failure of or resistance to medical treatment or intolerable side effects of medical therapy
- Recurrence, in combination or in association with the other therapeutic options, medical or radiotherapeutic or both

Indications for surgery have changed over time and with the refinement of surgical techniques and according to the evaluation of results and experiences, the development of knowledge about the biology of pituitary tumors, and the use of effective new pharmacologic agents[60-62] and radiation techniques. Large invasive pituitary tumors are difficult to cure regardless of the approach because removal of every fragment of the tumor is often impossible. Extended transsphenoidal approaches sometimes can represent a valid alternative to transcranial options; excellent visual outcomes derive from the transsphenoidal method.[58,63] Visual impairment does not indicate the need for a transcranial operation, as Cushing believed at one time.[64]

The surgical approach, with respect to basic principles for resecting pituitary adenomas, can be performed by two main approaches, each of them with several subcategories:
1. Transsphenoidal
   a. Microsurgical
      (1) Transnasal
      (2) Sublabial
      (3) Endonasal
   b. Endoscopic
2. Transcranial
   a. Subfrontal unilateral
   b. Frontolateral or pterional
   c. Subfrontal bilateral interhemispheric

After an initial flourishing of transsphenoidal surgery in the early 1900s, transcranial approaches attained success and were popular in the first half of the twentieth century. This fundamental debate lasted for decades, until the introduction of intraoperative fluoroscopy and microscopy effectively put it to rest. With these new imaging techniques, adequate exposure and thorough exploration of the sella turcica became possible without the need for a craniotomy and associated brain retraction. As a result, the transseptal transsphenoidal approach came to be accepted as the procedure of choice for the surgical management of most pituitary lesions.[65,66]

The success of the transsphenoidal approach is based on solid foundations: It is the least traumatic route to the sella, it lacks visible scars, it provides excellent visualization of the pituitary gland and adjacent pathology, it offers lower morbidity and mortality rates compared with transcranial procedures, and it requires only a brief hospital stay. Indications for transsphenoidal surgery today include more than 95% of the surgical indications in the sellar area and approximately 96% of all pituitary adenomas.[67] The well-established indications for this route are as follows:

- Almost all adenomatous lesions[68]
- Non-neoplastic intrasellar cysts[34,69-71]
- Craniopharyngiomas, preferably cystic, extra-arachnoidal,[72] and infradiaphragmatic,[73] with an enlarged sella[74-76]

Absolute indications were established in the 1970s and still are valid today; they include the following[77]:

- Elevated surgical risk of the transcranial route
  - In the elderly
  - In long-standing compression of the chiasm, not able to tolerate additional trauma
  - In cases of acute endosellar hypertension
  - In most cases of pituitary apoplexy
  - In pan-invasive, not radically removable adenomas
- Adenomas with downward development
- Microadenomas

To these classic guidelines for the transsphenoidal option, in more recent decades the following can be added:

- The extended transsphenoidal approaches to the spheno-ethmoid planum, for suprasellar craniopharyngiomas, Rathke's cleft cysts, some tuberculum sellae meningiomas, and anterior cranial base CSF leaks[78-88]; to the clival area, for chordomas[79,89-93]; and to the parasellar compartment,[37,79,91,94-99] for invasive adenomas and chordomas. The development of extended transsphenoidal approaches has provided transsphenoidal access to several lesions that previously would have been considered accessible by transcranial approaches only. The spectrum of lesions accessible to transsphenoidal surgery is widening. Extended approaches today represent standard procedures in selected centers and in experienced hands and are expected to progress further in the near future with additional technical and instrumental development.
- A sequential transsphenoidal approach, in intrasuprasellar adenomas, as an intentionally two-staged transsphenoidal operation. This operation is designed to encourage the descent of a suprasellar remnant of the adenoma incompletely removed in the first step, to limit the risks for brisk decompression of huge lesions, and to manage lesions with a second surgery.[100]

The striking figure indicating that 19% of primary brain tumors treated in academic centers in the United States are operated transsphenoidally provides testimony to what we have reported about evolving modern and contemporary indications for the transsphenoidal approach. Conditions may limit and sometimes contraindicate the choice of the transsphenoidal approach in favor of the transcranial, because of either the anatomy of the surgical pathway or the morphology and consistency of the lesion. The size of the sella, its degree of mineralization, the size and pneumatization of the sphenoid sinus, and the position and tortuosity of the carotid arteries can increase remarkably the difficulty of the transsphenoidal procedure and the final surgical result and may determine the opportunity or even the necessity for the transcranial alternative.

Indications for transcranial surgery include the following[68,73]:

- Tumors with extensive intracranial invasion, into the anterior cranial fossa or lateral or posterior extension, into the middle and posterior cranial fossae[101]
- Tumors with asymmetric suprasellar development, particularly if major vessel involvement is present

- Tumors with intracranial extension separated from the intrasellar portion by a narrow neck (dumbbell adenoma) and showing an hourglass configuration[102]
- Suprasellar tumors not completely resectable through the transsphenoidal route[103]
- Recurrent or residual pituitary tumors in patients who already have had unsuccessful transsphenoidal surgery
- When preoperative MRI assessment, on the basis of long repetition time (TR) signal, suggests a firm consistency of the adenoma, preventing easy debulking with subsequent collapse and descent into the sella, when resected from below.[104-106] This may occur after radiotherapy[107]; increased fibrosis also has been reported after treatment with dopamine agonists[108] or somatostatin analogues,[109,110] but these reports do not reflect our experience.
- When the sphenoid sinus is not pneumatized and the sella is small or does not make it easy to reach the suprasellar extension of the tumor[111]
- When coexisting vascular[96,112] and tumoral surgical pathology is evident and one-time surgical treatment for both conditions is chosen

TRANSSPHENOIDAL APPROACHES

One or another variation of the transsphenoidal approach represents the most physiologic and minimally traumatic corridor of surgical access to the sella, providing direct and superior visualization of the pituitary gland and adjacent pathology.[92,113] The transsphenoidal approach represents a midline approach that has been performed since the 1960s with use of the operating microscope as a visualizing tool, through transnasal transseptal, sublabial transseptal, or endonasal procedures (microsurgical transsphenoidal procedures). The transsphenoidal approach also can be performed by using the endoscope as the sole visualizing tool during the entire surgical procedure, realizing a "pure" endoscopic endonasal transsphenoidal approach. The combined use of the microscope and the endoscope during the same approach defines the condition of endoscope-assisted microsurgery.

Microsurgical Transsphenoidal Approaches

Although many different transsphenoidal procedures and variations have been described, three basic microsurgical transsphenoidal approaches to pituitary tumors are used: the transnasal transseptal transsphenoidal approach, the sublabial transseptal transsphenoidal approach, and the endonasal transsphenoidal approach. The patient can be positioned on the operating table supine, as originally proposed by Cushing, with the surgeon behind the patient's head, or in the semisitting position, as favored by Guiot, with the surgeon standing in front of the patient. The procedure is performed with an operating microscope for visualization, illumination, and magnification of the surgical field. Intermittent fluoroscopy is used for trajectory guidance, or, more recently, neuronavigational systems permit the surgeon to gather information about the current position of anatomic structures or instruments during the procedure itself.[44-49] Intraoperative MRI is capable of enhancing safety and providing additional knowledge about the completeness of lesion removal.[50,51,53-55] The three main transsphenoidal methods differ slightly one from each other primarily in the initial phase up to the exposure of the sphenoid sinus; they then follow the same surgical sphenoidal and sellar steps.

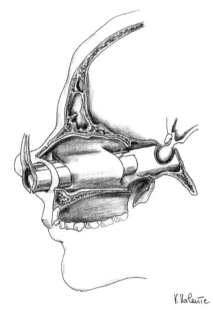

FIGURE 12-2. Sagittal view: schematic drawing of the microsurgical transnasal transseptal transsphenoidal approach. (Courtesy V. Valente, MD.)

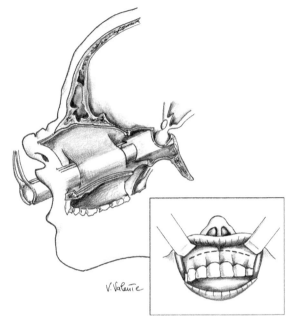

FIGURE 12-3. Sagittal view: schematic drawing of the microsurgical sublabial transseptal transsphenoidal approach. See detail of the sublabial incision on the right. (Courtesy V. Valente, MD.)

Microsurgical Transnasal Transseptal Transsphenoidal Approach

In a diffused version of the transnasal approach (Fig. 12-2), the operation starts in the right nostril, with retraction of the columella to the patient's left to expose through the incision in the nostril the anterior edge of the septal cartilage, 2 to 3 cm behind the mucosal-cutaneous junction. The nasal mucosa usually adheres tightly to the most anterior region of the septum: Its dense, fibrous strands are divided through a combination of sharp and blunt dissection. The submucosal dissection is extended posteriorly, elevating the nasal mucosa away from the septal cartilage up to its junction with the bony septum. The cartilaginous septum is dissected from the mucoperichondrium along its right side, then is laterally pushed on the left side, at the junction point, to free the cartilaginous septum from the bony septum. Posterior submucosal tunnels are created along both sides of the bony septum, which is partially removed to facilitate the introduction of a self-retaining transsphenoidal retractor, following the use of a nasal speculum in the dissection of the nasal septum. Care must be taken to avoid mucosal perforation during these maneuvers.

Microsurgical Sublabial Transseptal Transsphenoidal Approach

The upper lip is retracted, and an incision is made along the buccogingival junction, between the two canine fossae (Fig. 12-3). The upper lip and the periosteum are elevated to expose the anterior nasal spine and the inferior border of the pyriform aperture of the nasal cavities. The mucosa of the floor of the nose is elevated first on both sides with a small periosteal elevator, which is introduced along the nasal septum to detach the mucosa from the cartilage. The elevated mucosa is held in place by a nasal speculum, which allows further mucosal elevation from the bony nasal septum. The inferior and posterior portion of the cartilaginous septum is dissected from the bony nasal septum and is deflected laterally. The self-retaining nasal speculum is introduced and opened widely to hold the retracted mucosa out of the field. The sublabial approach permits a more anterior trajectory with respect to the transnasal option; this can be useful in lesions that extend into the suprasellar area or toward the planum sphenoidale.

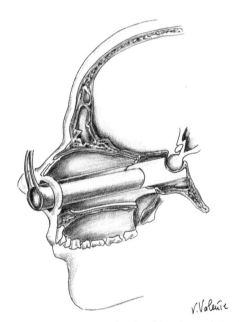

FIGURE 12-4. Sagittal view: schematic drawing of the microsurgical endonasal transsphenoidal approach. (Courtesy V. Valente, MD.)

Microsurgical Endonasal Transsphenoidal Approach

A handheld speculum is inserted into the nostril along the middle turbinate, which reliably leads to the sphenoid sinus (Fig. 12-4). In the posterior nasal cavity, an elevator is used to make a vertical mucosal incision at the junction of the keel of the sphenoid bone and the posterior nasal septum. The septum, with its intact mucosa, is pushed off the midline by the medial blade of the handheld speculum. Bilateral mucosal flaps over the keel of the sphenoid bone are elevated and reflected laterally, with identification of the sphenoid ostia. The handheld speculum is replaced by a thin nasal speculum, which is placed up to the face of the sphenoid bone. After lesion removal, the speculum is withdrawn, the nasal septum is returned to the midline, and the ipsilateral outfractured middle turbinate may be moved toward the midline to prevent a maxillary sinus mucocele. Nasal packing is placed for 24 hours in selected cases but is not used routinely.[114,115]

When the anterior wall of the sphenoid sinus has been reached by one of the aforementioned three routes, bone punches are used to make a large opening in the anterior wall of the sphenoid sinus, which extends beyond the sphenoid ostia to provide adequate sellar floor exposure. After the anterior wall of the sphenoid sinus has been opened, one or more septa can be identified. The surgeon should review the anatomy of the sphenoid sinus on preoperative nasal and paranasal cavity CT scans and should compare them with the intraoperative scans, particularly when the septa are implanted on one of the carotid prominences and the sphenoid sinus is of a presellar type. Insertion of the septum along the posterior wall of the sphenoid sinus may produce a useful anatomic landmark for identifying the sellar floor and for defining the medial extent of the cavernous sinus. Even if in selected cases it is not necessary to remove all the sphenoid septa, their removal must allow exposure of all crucial anatomic findings that are visible inside the sphenoid cavity.

Usually, the sphenoid mucosa is displaced laterally as much as necessary to open the sellar floor, unless adenomatous infiltration is evident or suspected, and the mucosa is resected in such cases. Its preservation is thought to ensure adequate mucociliary transport, along with its associated function in maintaining the physiology of nasosinusal ventilation.

After the sphenoid septa have been removed completely, the sella is recognizable on the posterior wall of the sphenoid sinus; its anatomic boundaries, when not clearly visible, are confirmed by C-arm fluoroscopy or neuronavigation. Adequate bony exposure of the sellar floor is crucial to the success of the approach, particularly when one is dealing with large tumors.

With a presellar or a conchal type of sphenoid sinus, the sphenoidotomy calls for some precautions.[116] With these two variants of incomplete sphenoid sinus pneumatization, a microdrill is used to open the sellar floor. In these cases, fluoroscopy or neuronavigation is extremely useful, if not essential, for identification of the superior and inferior edges of the sella, even in experienced hands. The method used to open the sellar floor depends on its consistency: If it is intact, opening is achieved by means of a microdrill or bone punches or both; if it is eroded or thinned, opening is achieved by means of a dissector, sometimes realizing an osteoplastic opening useful for sellar repair.[117]

The dura is incised in a midline position, in a linear or cross fashion, and a fragment of dura can be taken for histologic examination if it appears infiltrated.[118] When the dura is incised, the surgeon must keep in mind that the perisellar sinuses,[119] and particularly the superior and inferior intercavernous sinuses, are compressed and usually are obliterated by macroadenomas, making the dural incision bloodless. The situation is different with microadenomas, particularly in cases of Cushing's disease, in which it is not unusual to find the entire sellar dura covered by one or two venous channels that can bleed during tumor resection. Caution is necessary when incising the dura in microadenomas to avoid damaging a possibly ectatic carotid artery, which may be located within the sella, especially in acromegalic patients.

Before removing an adenoma, the surgeon must keep in mind that the pituitary gland is an extra-arachnoid structure, situated below the diaphragma sellae. During the removal of a pituitary adenoma, surgical maneuvers must respect these structures, to avoid postoperative CSF leaks and other major complications. Concerning the removal of a microadenoma, if it is visible on the surface of the gland, a cleavage plane between the microadenoma and the residual anterior pituitary should be found, with the aim of delimiting the lesion. When the microadenoma is not superficial, and no change in the appearance of the overlying anterior pituitary is evident, such as discoloration or attenuated texture, a small incision can be made in the normal pituitary gland on the same side of the microadenoma, and the lesion can be removed with the help of small ring curettes. After curettage of the adenoma, a small cottonoid is inserted inside the tumor cavity and with a forceps is turned in alternate directions to mobilize fragments of the lesion or of the neoplastic capsule. Concerning the removal of macroadenomas, the surgeon first must try to remove the tumor tissue from the interior of the sella and from any lateral extension, to avoid cumbersome obstruction of the surgical field by a down-hanging, inverted diaphragma sella. If a gradual descent of the suprasellar portion of the lesion is not observed, it is useful to ask the anesthetist to perform the Valsalva maneuver, which may cause protrusion into the sellar cavity of a part of the dura and arachnoid covering the suprasellar tumor extension (suprasellar cistern), or to inject air through a lumbar drain preoperatively positioned for the same purpose.[120]

After intracapsular emptying of the adenoma, its capsule can be dissected from the suprasellar cistern, when possible. As the macroadenoma grows, it sometimes distends the residual normal anterior pituitary, which appears as a thin layer of tissue surrounding the adenoma capsule, sometimes seen on MRI, the removal of which could cause postoperative hypopituitarism. It is also important to recognize the neurohypophysis, sometimes present in front of the dorsum sellae, where curettage or aspiration must be avoided, to prevent the development of postoperative diabetes insipidus.

After lesion removal, closure of the sellar floor is performed, especially when an intraoperative CSF leak has occurred, using a variety of techniques (intradural or extradural closure of the sella, packing of the sella with or without packing of the sphenoid sinus) and different autologous and synthetic materials.[121,122] Overpacking of the sella must be avoided to prevent compression of the optic system.

As with removal of lesions that often originate or develop inside the intra-arachnoid compartment, such as craniopharyngiomas or Rathke's cleft cysts, additional considerations are appropriate. These lesions develop primarily in the suprasellar region, with an intact or only slightly enlarged sellar cavity. In such cases, an extended approach is often necessary to manage the lesion. The anterior sellar wall, the tuberculum sellae, and the posterior portion of the planum sphenoidale are drilled away, according to the circumstances, with the use of a microdrill with a diamond bur. The superior intercavernous sinus is identified, coagulated, and divided in a midline position. When the lesion is exposed, it is removed, with as much respect as possible given to the arachnoid membrane, to avoid intraoperative and postoperative complications, which seem to be more frequent than with conventional transsphenoidal surgery.[83]

Endoscopic Endonasal Transsphenoidal Approach

Endoscopic endonasal transsphenoidal surgery (Fig. 12-5) is a novel, minimally invasive transsphenoidal approach performed with the endoscope as a stand-alone visualizing and operating instrument, without the need for the transsphenoidal retractor. It has the same indications as the conventional microsurgical technique,[33,123] and since the 1990s, it has enjoyed progressive

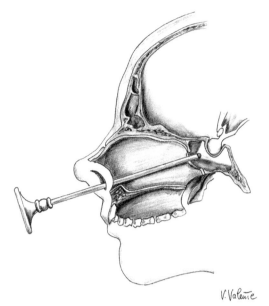

FIGURE 12-5. Sagittal view: schematic drawing of the endoscopic endonasal transsphenoidal approach. (Courtesy V. Valente, MD.)

acceptance among surgeons and patients for its minimal invasiveness and for the excellent surgical view it provides.[30-33,124-127] This procedure requires specific endoscopic skills and is based on a different concept because the endoscopic view that the surgeon receives on the video monitor is not a transposition of the real image, as it would be if looking through the eyepiece of a microscope, but is the result of a microprocessor's elaboration.

The procedure consists of three main aspects: exposure of the lesion, management of the relevant pathology, and reconstruction of the sella; these proceed through three different steps: the nasal, sphenoid, and sellar phases. In the first two steps, the corridor to the lesion and the room in which to work comfortably are identified and adapted to the need of each single case; in the sellar phase, the lesion is removed, and tailored reconstruction of the sellar area is realized.

The patient is positioned supine with the trunk elevated 10 degrees and the head turned 10 degrees toward the surgeon, not fixed in a Mayfield headrest with pins, but just in a horseshoe-type headrest. The endoscopic equipment (monitor, light source, video camera, video recorder) is positioned ergonomically behind the head of the patient and in front of the operator, who is on the patient's right. The anesthetist with his or her equipment is positioned on the left of the patient at the level of the head, the assistant is positioned on the patient's left, and the nurse is positioned at the level of the patient's legs. The table-mounted endoscope holder, which holds the endoscope in the sphenoid and sellar phases of the operation, allowing the surgeon to work with two hands, is fixed next to the patient's shoulder and is tilted so as not to interfere with the maneuvers of the surgical instruments. Before beginning the surgical procedure, the anesthesiologist helps to ensure bloodless nasal cavities, sometimes by means of slightly controlled hypotension and always with excellent analgesia, to minimize mucosal bleeding, especially until the anterior sphenoidotomy has been performed.

The endoscope (4 mm in diameter, 0 degree angled lens, 18 cm in length) is introduced through the chosen nostril, tangential to the floor of the nasal cavity. The first structures to be identified are the inferior turbinate laterally and the nasal septum medially. Above the inferior turbinate, one can see the head of middle turbinate, usually close to the nasal septum. As the endoscope advances along the floor of the nasal cavity, it reaches the choana. Cottonoids soaked with diluted epinephrine (1:100,000) or with xylometazoline hydrochloride are positioned between the middle turbinate and the nasal septum to enlarge the space between them and to obtain decongestion of the nasal mucosa (which has a rich innervation and vascularization). The head of the middle turbinate is delicately dislocated laterally to widen further the virtual space between the middle turbinate and the nasal septum and to create an adequate surgical pathway. After suitable space has been created between the middle turbinate and the nasal septum, the endoscope is angled upward along the roof of the choana and the sphenoethmoid recess, until it reaches the sphenoid ostium, which usually is located about 1.5 cm above the roof of the choana. When the sphenoid cavity is reached, coagulation of the sphenoethmoid recess and of the area around the sphenoid ostium is performed, starting about 0.5 cm from the top of the choana up to the superior border of the nasal cavity, to avoid arterial bleeding originating from septal branches of the sphenopalatine artery.

At this point, a microdrill with a cutting burr separates the nasal septum from the sphenoid rostrum. The whole anterior wall of the sphenoid sinus is now visible and is enlarged circumferentially, with the use of bone punches or a microdrill; care must be taken in the inferolateral direction, where the sphenopalatine artery or its major branches lie. To avoid these vessels, it is sufficient to cut away the nasal mucosa slightly in an inferolateral direction and to coagulate it with the bipolar forceps to expose the sphenoid rostrum completely. The sphenoid rostrum is removed in fragments and not en bloc, because this last maneuver could cause lacerations and bleeding in the nasal mucosa while passing through the nasal cavity. It is mandatory to remove widely the anterior wall of the sphenoid sinus, especially downward, before reaching the sella; otherwise, the instruments would not be able to reach all the areas visible via the endoscope. When the anterior sphenoidotomy has been completed, small amounts of bleeding originating from the edges of the sphenoidotomy must be controlled to avoid occluding the lens of the endoscope during the next phases.

The sphenoid and sellar phases of the endoscopic procedure are performed according to the same rules and principles as the microsurgical transsphenoidal approach. Nevertheless, because of the characteristics of the endoscopic approach and owing to intrinsic properties of the endoscope itself, some procedural considerations should be noted, as follows:

- After the sphenoid septa have been removed, thanks to the wider view offered by the endoscope, the posterior and lateral walls of the sphenoid sinus are visible, with the sellar floor at the center, the sphenoethmoid planum above it, and the clival indentation below; lateral to the sellar floor, the bony prominences of the ICA and of the optic nerves can be seen and between them the optocarotid recess, molded by pneumatization of the optic strut of the anterior clinoid process. These prominences and depressions, especially in a well-pneumatized sphenoid sinus not invaded by a sellar lesion, define a sort of "fetal face," where the forehead corresponds to the sphenoid planum, the eyes to the two optocarotid recesses, the eyebrows to the two optic nerve protuberances, the nose to the sella, and the mouth to the clivus, laterally limited by the two paraclival carotid artery protuberances that represent the cheeks. Nevertheless, in most sellar-type sphenoid sinuses, all these landmarks may not be clearly recognizable because of the different degree of sphenoid sinus pneumatization or extension of the lesion, but identification of the sphenoethmoid planum, of the clival indentation, and of the bony protuberances of the ICA can be considered sufficient to determine safely the edges of the sellar floor. Because of the paucity of anatomic landmarks, only in the presence of a presellar or a conchal sphenoid sinus or in some recurrences, a neuronavigation system or C-arm fluoroscopy is needed to avoid lateral misdirection, close to the parasellar and paraclival courses of the ICAs.

- Before the sellar floor is opened, a longer endoscope (4 mm in diameter, 0 degree angled lens, 30 cm in length), fixed to the holder, is positioned inside the upper portion of the nasal cavity to free both of the surgeon's hands and to allow comfortable introduction of two instruments under the endoscope, without coming into conflict with it.
- Opening of the sellar floor, a dural incision, and lesion removal are performed in accordance with the already well-defined rules of the microsurgical transsphenoidal approach. If enough space is present in the sellar cavity, during or after lesion removal, angled endoscopes (30 degree and 45 degree) can be advanced to verify the presence of possible tumor remnants, which often are imprisoned in the recesses created by the descent of the suprasellar cistern. When the lesion extends toward the medial wall of the cavernous sinus, its removal can be accomplished under direct endoscopic vision, with the use of curved instruments and suction cannulas.
- After removal of the tumor, if evidence or risk for a CSF leak is noted, closure of the sella is performed according to common guidelines. Sellar reconstruction is performed also with the purpose of creating a barrier outward, of reducing the dead space, and of preventing the descent of the chiasm into the sellar cavity[122]; in certain other cases, no plugging is used.[121] Because of the minimal invasiveness of the endoscopic procedure, no autologous bone or cartilage from the nasal septum is usually available, and different synthetic or resorbable materials,[128] when necessary,[121] must be employed to effect a safe and effective repair of the sella. Lumbar drainage is adopted in cases of intraoperative CSF leakage, only when the closure is not judged absolutely watertight, in extended approaches, or when minimal unexpected postoperative CSF leakage occurs.
- At the end of the procedure, hemostasis is obtained; final irrigation is performed; the endoscope is gradually removed; and the middle turbinate is gently restored in a medial direction, while avoiding contact with the nasal septum to prevent the formation of synechiae. Packing of the nasal cavity is not commonly considered necessary except in cases of diffuse intraoperative bleeding from the nasal mucosa, as can occur in some acromegalic patients or in poorly controlled hypertensive patients, in whom it is applied for a few hours.

Because transsphenoidal endoscopy is a more recent contribution to pituitary surgery, some advantages, pitfalls, and peculiar aspects related to this technique must be highlighted:

- The main advantages of the endoscopic procedure compared with microsurgical procedures are related to the properties of the endoscope itself and to the absence of the nasal speculum.[33,125] While avoiding use of the nasal speculum, which creates a "fixed tunnel" and an almost coaxial restriction of the microinstruments, the endoscope discloses its superior properties, permitting a wider vision of the surgical field, with a close-up "look" inside the anatomy. Angled lens endoscopes enable the surgeon to work on tumors located in suprasellar and parasellar regions under direct visual control.
- The whole procedure seems to be less traumatic, and the percentage of many complications is reduced compared with the traditional microsurgical approach.[129] Because the real operation starts from the natural ostium of the sphenoid sinus and the submucosal nasal phase is avoided, septal perforations, nasal scars, damage to the nasal spine, and orodental complications due to the incision in the buccogingival junction are prevented.
- In almost all cases, no nasal packing is employed, and postoperative breathing difficulties are reduced.
- The use of an endoscopic approach is particularly advantageous in the case of recurrent or residual tumor already treated by a transsphenoidal operation,[130] in which the surgeon usually finds distorted anatomy and may encounter nasal synechiae, septal perforations, mucoceles, and intrasellar scarring. With the endoscopic procedure, thanks to avoidance of the submucosal nasal phase of the microsurgical operation, the real beginning of the operation occurs at the sphenoid sinus, which already is enlarged by the former approach, rendering the procedure faster and more straightforward compared with the microsurgical transsphenoidal method. The wide anatomic view of the surgical field that the endoscope offers in the sphenoid and sellar areas minimizes the chance of a misdirected orientation when the midline anatomic landmarks are not recognizable or are absent, thus reducing the possibility of injury to the intrasellar and parasellar structures.
- The endoscopic endonasal approach can be employed in cases of intentionally two-staged transsphenoidal operations[100] because of its excellent ability in reaching the sellar region during the second operation.

Disadvantages of the endoscopic approach include the requirement of a steep learning curve to enhance confidence with the unfamiliar anatomy of the nasal cavities and with specific endoscopic dexterity. Nevertheless, after adequate experience has been attained, the operating time becomes the same as or shorter than that required for transsphenoidal microsurgery, especially in cases of recurrence. The endoscope offers only bidimensional vision on the video monitor. A sense of depth can be gained by the surgeon's experience, and the endoscope can be made to execute in and out movements, while looking for many useful different anatomic landmarks and referring to many protuberances and depressions in the sphenoid sinus, which represent reflections and shadows that correspond to different structures. Dedicated microsurgical endoscopic instruments with secure grip, straight and not bayonet shaped, which are provided with different and variably angled tips, are necessary to reach the surgical targets, particularly targets that the angled endoscopes are able to show.[131,132]

Extended Endoscopic Endonasal Approach to the Suprasellar Area

Lesions located in the suprasellar area historically have been approached through different extensive transcranial and/or nasofacial approaches, such as anterior, anterolateral, and/or pterional techniques.[133-137] Such surgical routes often cause tissue disruption related to brain retraction and neurovascular manipulation, with sometimes aesthetically disfiguring results, and lead to higher rates of surgical morbidity and mortality.

Over past decades, the evolution of endoscopic surgical techniques and technological developments have boosted the progressive reduction in invasiveness of transcranial approaches,[134,138-141] as well as of transsphenoidal surgery, in which endoscopic variance represents the last evolution of the technique. Nevertheless, the transsphenoidal route has been used historically only for sellar lesions, especially for pituitary adenomas. It was Guiot, in the early 1960s, who first renewed and fixed the indications for the transsphenoidal route[142]; he proposed that such a technique could be used as treatment for craniopharyngiomas and advised practitioners to consider the transsphenoidal approach, preferably for those lesions with a cystic component, with a minimal supradiaphragmatic extension and with an enlarged sella. These suggestions have lasted for over three decades,[143,144] so that such a route most often was indicated for sellar or intra-suprasellar intradiaphragmatic lesions.[142,144,145] An enormous contribution to the widespread use of the transsphenoidal technique is attributed to Jules Hardy, who introduced technical innovations such as the operating microscope and the concept of microadenoma. He improved the effectiveness of such approaches and, at the same time, conceived their application for the management of different sellar and skull base lesions, such as "a chordoma or a meningioma."[146]

In 1987, Weiss[147] termed and originally defined the *extended transsphenoidal approach,* while describing a transsphenoidal approach with removal of additional bone along the tuberculum sellae and the posterior planum sphenoidale between the optic canals. As a matter of fact, the dural opening was completely above the diaphragma sellae.

This approach, which initially was performed via microsurgical technique[147,148] through a transnasal or sublabial route, provides midline access and direct visualization of the suprasellar space, thus offering the possibility of treatment for small, midline suprasellar lesions, which traditionally have been approached transcranially, without brain manipulation.

Besides, the possibility of reaching the suprasellar compartment via a different route—through the sellar cavity (i.e., via the transsellar/transdiaphragmatic approach)—has been reported.[149,150] Nevertheless, the supradiaphragmatic structures become visible only after the intrasellar portion of the lesion has been removed. Again, it should be kept in mind that the exposure provided by such an approach most often depends on the sellar dimensions; therefore, this approach seems to be more easily amenable for those lesions that already have enlarged the sella and the diaphragma.

To achieve a more comfortable route to the supradiaphragmatic space, other authors[138,148,151-160] have described a modified transsphenoidal microsurgical approach, the so-called transsphenoidal transtuberculum approach. As a matter of fact, this technique definitively overcame Guiot's paradigm, providing enough exposure for the removal of suprasellar/supradiaphragmatic tumors. Indeed, thanks to additional bone removal from the anterior cranial base (tuberculum and posterior planum sphenoidale), such a modified extended transsphenoidal approach makes available excellent direct access to the suprasellar/supradiaphragmatic area, regardless of sellar size (even with a sella that is not enlarged), and avoids the risk for pituitary tissue injury.

More recently, widespread use of the endoscope in transsphenoidal surgery has led to new interest in this surgical technique,

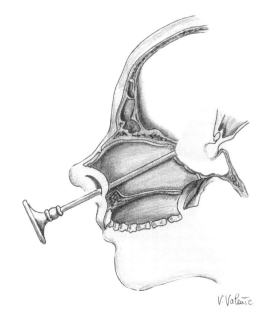

FIGURE 12-6. Sagittal view: schematic drawing of the extended endoscopic endonasal approach to the suprasellar area. (Courtesy V. Valente, MD.)

affording extension of the transsphenoidal approach.[138,161-167] The wider and panoramic view offered by the endoscope has improved the safety of the transsphenoidal approach with the possibility of passing through a less noble structure (nasal cavity) to reach a more noble one (the brain with its neurovascular structures). Because of the enormous contributions of many groups all around the world, the applicability of such a route has been expanded to the removal of different "pure" supradiaphragmatic lesions.[128,155,157,165,168-180] Indeed, the extended endoscopic approach has been adopted in many centers as treatment for pathologies such as craniopharyngiomas (intraventricular or extraventricular), tuberculum sellae, planum sphenoidale or olfactory groove meningiomas, Rathke's cleft cysts, or even pituitary macroadenomas with suprasellar symmetric and/or asymmetric extension—all of which were once considered amenable to open transcranial surgery only (Fig. 12-6). Credit should be given to Kassam and his group in Pittsburgh for having provided the main guidelines for extended endonasal transsphenoidal management of the skull base (i.e., a binostril approach), removal of the middle turbinate on one side (usually the right one), lateralization of the middle turbinate in the other nostril (sometimes even this turbinate can be removed), removal of the posterior portion of the nasal septum, and wider sphenoidotomy, and furthermore for having systematized this strategy according to strict anatomic principles along the coronal and sagittal planes.[180,181] In this way, it is possible to use two or three instruments plus the endoscope when working through both nostrils.

An extended endoscopic approach to the suprasellar area requires the use of additional tools that could be useful in rendering the procedure safer and more effective:

- Detailed, complete preoperative planning, integrated with three-dimensional (3D) reconstructions, so as to tailor the skull base opening with the 3D volume of the lesion
- An image-guided system (neuronavigator), which is used to intraoperatively identify the limits of the lesion, the midline, and the trajectory, and which offers better precision in defining the boundaries of bone removal and neurovascular relationships

- Dedicated instruments (i.e., high-speed low-profile micro-drills, micro-Doppler probes, bipolar forceps with angled tips, low-profile ultrasonic aspirators, or radiofrequency cavitron-like coagulation) to manage properly lesions involving such a delicate environment

As a matter of fact, the extended approaches require a wider surgical corridor, as compared with standard endoscopic approaches, increased work space, and greater maneuverability of instruments.

During the nasal phase, in contrast to the standard approach, the middle turbinate on one side (usually on the right) is removed, whereas the middle turbinate in the other nostril (sometimes even this turbinate can be removed) is pushed laterally. Finally, the posterior portion of the nasal septum is removed to create adequate conditions for the use of two or three instruments plus the endoscope through both nostrils.

An anterior sphenoidotomy, wider than that required for the standard approach, is performed; furthermore, it is useful to remove the superior turbinate and the posterior ethmoid air cells (bilaterally) to create enough space. As usual, all septa inside the sphenoid sinus are removed, and every irregularity of the bone and/or the mucosa, especially those covering the limit between the sphenoidal and the ethmoidal planum, is flattened to allow better maneuverability of the endoscope and of surgical instruments while working above the sella and later permitting better reconstruction.

Although complete exposure of the posterior wall of the sphenoid sinus is achieved, a series of protuberances and depressions (according to the grade of pneumatization) become visible[182]; again, it is extremely important to keep in mind perfect knowledge of such anatomic landmarks so as to preserve correct orientation and better refine the bone opening.

From this point forward, the surgeon could proceed in performing a bimanual dissection while a "tuned" coworker holds the endoscope, moving it dynamically, and as requested inserts another surgical instrument.[138] This so-called 3 to 4 hands technique[183] requires good collaboration between two surgeons that should be tuned as if they were running a rally car race, with one—the "navigator"—holding the endoscope, and another—the "pilot"—handling two surgical instruments inside the surgical field. The pilot and the navigator therefore can pass continuously between the close-up view, as during dissecting maneuvers, and a panoramic view of neurovascular structures. However, it is possible to fix the endoscope to an autostatic holder, which can be settled by a single surgeon.

Once such preliminary staging has been performed, which is common to all extended approaches to the skull base, additional bone removal from the cranial base (i.e., the tuberculum sellae and the planum sphenoidale) is required (transtuberculum-transplanum approach) to reach the suprasellar area. First, the sellar floor and the tuberculum sellae are drilled (with a 2 mm diameter burr), with consideration of the two medial optocarotid recesses as lateral limits; hence, the bone opening is enlarged along the planum sphenoidale with a Kerrison rongeur. It is essential to keep in mind that it is possible to extend more laterally the bone opening above the medial optocarotid recesses, so that it may resemble a chef's hat. Indeed, in its inferior part, the osteodural opening is narrower, because it is limited by the parasellar portion of the intracavernous carotid arteries and the optic nerves at their entrance into the optic canals; however, it can be wider in its superior half, since the optic nerves diverge toward the orbits. Again, during each step of the procedure, the role of the neuronavigator is to assist in better defining the limits

of bone removal. It has to be remembered that when bone removal is performed, it is not rare that bleeding occurs in the superior intercavernous sinus; as a matter of fact, the bleeding sometimes can be difficult to manage, requiring the use of different hemostatic agents with temporary gentle compression with cottonoids and/or bipolar coagulation.

At this point in the procedure, management of the lesion can begin: Its fundamental steps of dissection and removal are tailored to each lesion, according to the principles of transcranial microsurgery. Furthermore, it has to be said that through the transsphenoidal route, because of the closer-up and wider view offered by the endoscope, it is possible to easily perform a subdural extra-arachnoidal dissection of the lesion, thus enormously favoring its removal through such an extracranial corridor.

Because of the conspicuous intraoperative CSF leakage caused by the larger osteodural opening required to approach the suprasellar area, accurate reconstruction of the skull base defect is needed after lesion removal. Reconstruction has to be watertight to prevent postoperative CSF leakage, which could occur even more frequently in cases of a large opening of the arachnoid cistern, or of the third ventricle. First of all, a thin layer of fibrin glue is placed within the intradural space to seal the arachnoid space and create a first barrier against the CSF, thus filling the dead space. Thereafter, the osteodural defect is closed with a heterologous dural substitute combined with an autologous septal or turbinate bone, or even an easy-to-shape, synthetic bone substitute. The reconstruction is performed according to different techniques (i.e., intradural, extradural, and intra-extradural), even though the most effective seems to be the extradural approach.[184] In this latter procedure, termed a gasket seal,[185] or "grandma's cap,"[184] a single large layer of dural substitute is positioned within the extradural space, covering the dural opening, and a conformed sheath of resorbable solid material then is overlapped with the dural substitute and embedded in the extradural space, dragging the dural substitute in overlay position.

Once closure of the defect has been completed, achieving a watertight barrier, multiple layers of dural substitute are placed over to support the reconstruction; this is reinforced by the mucoperichondrium of the middle turbinate and/or a pedicled flap of septal mucosa (i.e., the Hadad-Carrau flap).[186,187] This latter approach, recently introduced into clinical practice, has proved helpful in improving healing of the skull base defect.[179] Finally, the sphenoid sinus is filled with cellulose gelatin (Surgicel), surgical glue (Tisseel), and/or Duraseal, to reduce dead spaces and to hold reconstruction material in place.[188,189] No lumbar drainage is required at the end of the procedure; nevertheless, we advise our patients to have bed rest for 3 to 5 days, according to the grade of pneumoencephalus (especially in cases of third ventricle craniopharyngioma), while medical therapy with acetazolamide, laxatives, and wide-spectrum antibiotics is administered.

As compared with the transcranial route, the extended transsphenoidal approach provides a direct view of the neurovascular structures of the suprasellar region from below; as a matter of fact, through this "low route," no brain manipulation is required, and furthermore, because of the wider view provided by the endoscope, median and bilateral exposure is gained. Thus, it is undisguised how the risk for postoperative visual loss, which is strictly related to the integrity of the vascularization of the optic chiasm, is minimal. In fact, at this level, most of the blood supply to the optic system comes from its superior surface, from the branches of the anterior cerebral and anterior communicating arteries, thus rendering the inferior approaches less dangerous than the transcranial routes in such regard.

The extended endoscopic endonasal approach to the supradiaphragmatic area does not differ consistently from the microscopic one; nevertheless, some advantages related to the inner properties of the endoscope should be considered. With the endoscope, a wider, close-up view of the surgical field is attained; thus identification of many surgical landmarks in the sphenoid sinus and even intradurally, in the suprasellar area, is improved. Again, this allows the surgeon to perform a safer dissection of the tumor from the neurovascular structures, thus avoiding brain retraction and optic apparatus manipulation. In some cases, such as tuberculum sellae meningioma, this surgical route from below offers the possibility of performing early devascularization, permitting an easier and almost bloodless tumor debulking.

On the other hand, it should be recalled that the extended endoscopic endonasal approach to the suprasellar area is more technically demanding and requires additional skills related to use of the endoscope itself and to the opposite anatomic point of view.[190,191] Besides, it is crucial to focus on some parameters related to the lesion and its anatomy, which could affect lesion management via such a route.[138] Indeed, a well-pneumatized sphenoid sinus allows better visualization of all important landmarks on its posterior wall, which, again, is needed to maintain surgical orientation while bone is removed.[157] On the contrary, a conchal-type sphenoid sinus could hinder the extended endonasal approach, while a small sella, with two close intracavernous carotids, could require a narrower approach.

In terms of lesion-related conditions, it has to be said that the effectiveness of the extended transsphenoidal approach could be reduced in cases of lesions with an eccentric shape and/or a wider lateral extension, with encasement of one or both ICAs and/or of the AcomA complex. Moreover, lesions that displace the optic chiasm posteriorly or that cause this latter structure to be postfixed are easily removed through this route; indeed, internal debulking of the mass from below provides enough space for dissection from the chiasm and from the optic nerves. More limited access to the suprasellar and supradiaphragmatic areas is achieved if the chiasm is prefixed or anteriorly displaced.[138,168]

It should be recalled that greater risk for postoperative CSF leak,[173] as compared with transcranial approaches, remains a challenging matter.[179,192,193] Nevertheless, improvements in reconstruction techniques and the use of new, dedicated instruments seem to significantly reduce such risks.[184,186,188]

The transsphenoidal-transtuberculum approach seems to be a minimally invasive, direct route to the suprasellar area that could be used in cases of small and medium-size suprasellar midline lesions, with or without limited parasellar extension and without involvement of vascular structures such as craniopharyngiomas, tuberculum sellae meningiomas, suprasellar Rathke's cleft cysts, or large fibrotic pituitary adenomas in which extracapsular dissection is required. It could be considered also as treatment for recurrent lesions, already operated on transcranially, and/or for suprasellar lesions with an unclear preoperative diagnosis, for bioptic or partial removal purposes.

TRANSCRANIAL APPROACHES

With the selected indications described previously, many different standard transcranial or alternative skull base approaches are used routinely, depending on the direction of the extrasellar growth of the lesion. Most surgeons become familiar with one or two approaches and tend to use them in most cases. We describe just the major variations of transcranial techniques that

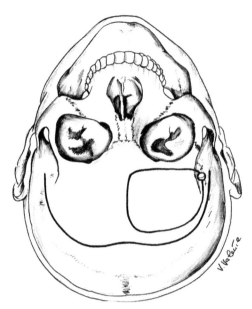

FIGURE 12-7. Schematic drawing of the unilateral subfrontal approach (seen from a surgical point of view). The bottom, curved line shows the skin incision, and the circular line shows the border of the craniotomy. (Courtesy V. Valente, MD.)

remain in popular use for the resection of pituitary tumors with extensive suprasellar and parasellar extension: the unilateral subfrontal approach, the pterional approach, and the bilateral subfrontal interhemispheric approach. Depending on the particular compartment where the tumor is located, the size of the opening must be commensurate with the best and safest removal of the tumor—"as small as possible, as large as necessary, but cosmetically optimal."[194] With all variations, the operating microscope and dedicated microinstruments are employed, according to the general principles of central nervous system microneurosurgery, and in more recent times, the condition of endoscope-assisted microsurgery sometimes is realized.

The unilateral subfrontal approach (Fig. 12-7), described for the first time with an extradural version by McArthur in 1912,[195] then by Frazier in 1913,[196] and by Krause in Berlin in 1914, with a right frontal osteoplastic flap,[197] was adopted by Cushing[21,64] and is still in current use. This approach is indicated mainly for large suprasellar adenomas with an asymmetric supraparasellar extension and for tumors that have expanded into the upper prepontine cistern. It gives excellent bilateral access to the optic nerves and the chiasm.[198]

The patient is placed on the surgical table in a supine position with the head slightly elevated, rotated to the contralateral side, and extended 20 to 40 degrees to facilitate spontaneous movement of the frontal lobes away from the orbital roof. Different skin incisions fit the purpose, but usually a bicoronal skin incision is adopted that begins less than 1 cm anterior to the tragus and proceeds in a curvilinear fashion to the superior temporal line near the opposite tragus behind the hairline. The craniotomy usually is performed through a single keyhole, made on the right side, positioned in the anterosuperior margin of the right temporalis muscle, immediately below the superior orbital ridge, for cosmetic purposes. If a correct dissection of the dura cannot be accomplished from a single burr hole, a second burr hole is made, and dural separation from the bone is completed by means of a blunt dissector, minimizing injury to the subjacent brain. The craniotome is introduced, and a quadrangular craniotomy is performed, keeping the basal cut as low as possible. Preopera-

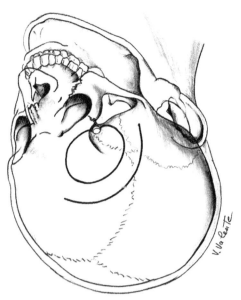

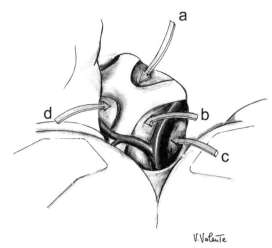

FIGURE 12-8. Schematic drawing of the pterional approach (seen from a surgical point of view). The curved line shows the skin incision, and the circle shows the border of the craniotomy. (Courtesy V. Valente, MD.)

FIGURE 12-9. Schematic drawing of the different surgical corridors available by means of the pterional approach. *a*, Interoptic corridor. *b*, Optocarotid corridor. *c*, Corridor lateral to the internal carotid artery. *d*, Translamina terminalis corridor. (Courtesy V. Valente, MD.)

tively, the surgeon should have a clear idea of the size of the frontal sinuses to avoid entering them with the craniotome. If the frontal sinus is opened before the dural opening is made, it should be stripped of mucosa—a procedure called cranialization—and packed, then covered in a layer of galea capitis, temporalis fascia, tensor fascia lata, or dural substitute, which then is fixed in a position to prevent the leakage of CSF.

After the dural opening has been made, the olfactory nerve is microscopically freed from its arachnoid attachments; care must be taken to avoid damage to the small vascular feeders. The frontal lobe is retracted gently so that the parachiasmatic cisterns can be opened carefully until the optic nerves, the chiasm, the A1 segments, and the anterior communicating artery are well exposed. The lesion is identified. After bipolar coagulation and incision of the capsule between the optic nerves, the adenoma is debulked and can be removed gently, preserving the pituitary stalk. During retrochiasmatic removal, care must be taken to minimize manipulations, thus avoiding damage to the optic pathways.

The frontolateral craniotomy, initially reported by Dandy in 1918,[23,199] and subsequently modified and popularized by Yasargil[194] as the pterional approach (Fig. 12-8), is a versatile craniotomy that gives good exposure of the inferolateral portion of the frontal lobe and the anterior temporal lobe. The pterional approach provides a short distance to the suprasellar region and is the craniotomy of choice for adenomas with unilateral extrasellar parasellar extension, when it is necessary to expose the compartment between the optic nerve and the ICA, or between the ICA and the third cranial nerve. It may be useful when cavernous sinus area invasion[39] or a significant retrochiasmatic component is present. The opening of the basal cisterns early in the approach is used to minimize brain retraction; mannitol is used when further cerebral relaxation is necessary.

For a pterional scalp and bone flap, the patient is positioned supine on a standard operating table. The head is secured with a three-point pin fixation system, directed 20 degrees vertex down and rotated 30 degrees toward the side where the craniotomy will be done. The incision starts posterior to the frontal

branch of the facial nerve, just anterior to the tragus; swings forward with a large radius arc; and terminates at the midline, posterior to the hairline, high on the forehead. Burr holes in a pterional craniotomy usually are placed at the intersection of the zygomatic bone, the superior temporal line, and the supraorbital ridge (keyhole), and just superior to the zygoma 1 cm anterior to the tragus. The two craniotome cut segments when joined together create a relatively circular pterional craniotomy bone flap.

The laterobasal frontal and anteromedial temporal lobes lie within the perimeter of the craniotomy bone flap. The dura is opened in a curvilinear fashion, centered over the sphenoid wing, draped inferiorly, and fixed with dural stitches. The sylvian fissure should be opened on the frontal side of the sylvian vein to dissect free the M1 segment, by splitting the arachnoid spanning from the surface of the basal frontal to the temporal lobes; the frontal lobe must be mobilized, giving the surgeon access to the sellar and parasellar regions, in a basic extracerebral approach (Yasargil's pterional-transsylvian approach).

At this time, the sequence of cisternal openings depends on the extension of the lesion: The carotid cistern is completely opened, revealing the carotid artery and its branches. The tumor can be found in the optochiasmatic cistern, the interpeduncular cistern (Liliequist's membrane), and the cistern of the lamina terminalis. In the case of intraventricular extension, the adenoma can be reached through the translamina terminalis corridor (Fig. 12-9).[200-203]

The optimal technique is to decompress the tumor between the optic nerves and mobilize it from the opticocarotid space to the interoptic space. Intracapsular debulking starts between the two optic nerves with suction, ring curettes, or ultrasonic aspirator, according to the consistency. With the surgeon working within and without the tumor capsule, the adenoma is removed from the surrounding neurovascular structures.

When a large pituitary tumor invades the parasellar-cavernous sinus area and the adjacent central skull base regions, this approach can be modified in keeping with Dolenc's technique.[39] A transbasal approach is performed: It is extradural and consists of an osteoplastic frontotemporoparietal craniotomy; unroofing of the orbit; resection of the sphenoid wing and the

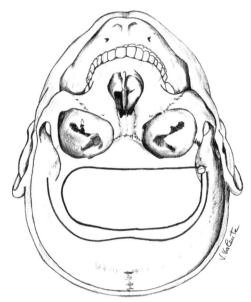

FIGURE 12-10. Schematic drawing of the bilateral subfrontal approach (seen from a surgical point of view). The bottom, curved line shows the skin incision, and the circular line shows the border of the craniotomy. (Courtesy V. Valente, MD.)

anterior clinoid process; opening of the optic canal; and exposure of cranial nerves III, IV, and VI.

The bilateral interhemispheric subfrontal approach (Fig. 12-10), initially described by Killiani[204] in 1904 for the removal of chiasmatic lesions, and variously used by many neurosurgeons for selected anterior cranial fossa lesions, such as large olfactory groove meningiomas, is not used today as frequently as the other two options described here. It has been revised recently[205-207] as treatment for large craniopharyngiomas with retrochiasmatic extension. It offers wide exposure of the anterior cranial base with a good overview of the sellar, suprasellar, and parasellar areas. It affords an excellent midline orientation and may be used as treatment for huge pituitary adenomas with large bilateral suprasellar extension because occasionally, a unilateral approach is insufficient for adequate bilateral management of the lesion. This technique requires patience and time, which can be rewarded fully by the technical advantages provided by excellent exposure of the surgical field.

The extracranial steps of the bilateral interhemispheric subfrontal approach are identical to the steps described earlier, except that the craniotomy is extended on both sides. Two burr holes are made on each side with a high-speed drill. With the use of a craniotome, an osteoplastic osteotomy or a free bone flap is performed, extending close to the orbital roof anteriorly and along the cranial convexity posteriorly. If the frontal sinus is entered, it must be treated before the dura is opened, as was already described. The dura is opened frontobasally, the sagittal sinus is ligated in its most anterior extremity and is divided with proper technique, and the falx is transected up to its insertion on the crista galli and is retracted with the frontal lobes. The interhemispheric and bilateral olfactory cisternae are opened to drain CSF and to avoid excessive retraction. Both olfactory nerves should be dissected symmetrically, as is done in the unilateral subfrontal approach. After that, the surgical overview allows better visualization of both olfactory nerves and both optic nerves. The tumor capsule can be seen, and dissection between the carotid artery and the capsule is performed on both sides. After this step, the tumor can be debulked and the resection

performed. The tumor is removed with sharp and blunt dissection from beneath and around the optic nerves and chiasm and from surrounding brain and blood vessels.

These craniotomy approaches, which at first sight might seem traumatic, often provide excellent results for the patient, especially when more modern technological advances (i.e., microscopic magnification, ultrasonic aspiration, bipolar coagulation, and neuronavigation) are employed by suitably trained neurosurgeons.

RADIOSURGERY

In addition to traditional forms of pituitary surgery, either transsphenoidal or transcranial, a third kind of "surgery" should be considered—radiosurgery. It is a way of treating brain disorders through precise delivery of a single high dose of radiation, usually given in a 1 day session. Treatment, which involves the use of focused radiation beams delivered stereotactically to a specific area of the brain, has such a dramatic effect on the target zone that the changes are considered "surgical." Through the use of three-dimensional, computer-aided planning and the high degree of immobilization provided by stereotactic head fixation, the amount of radiation to healthy brain tissue can be minimized. The patient's head is secured to a stereotactic frame and is positioned so that the tumor is centered in the spot where all the beams intersect. In this way, the tumor receives a great deal of radiation, while the surrounding brain tissue receives very little radiation. Each low-energy radiation beam passes harmlessly through scalp, skull, and overlying brain, but all beams focus on the tumor.

Radiosurgery usually is proposed as second-line therapy after surgery, if the tumor volume is small and the distance from the adenoma surface to the optic pathways is broad enough to allow a safe procedure (5 mm). It is indicated in some patients with recurrent adenomas that are known to be locally invasive in the cavernous sinus, bone, or dura, or when the recurrence is clearly manifested by a return of symptoms, and the tumor is considered unlikely to respond to additional resection.

Three basic forms of radiosurgery are delivered by three different technological instruments: the gamma knife, the linear accelerator (LINAC), and the cyclotron. Each instrument operates differently, with a different source of radiation—gamma rays or x-rays for the gamma knife, the LINAC, and charged particles (protons or helium ions) for the cyclotron.

With the gamma knife, radiation is produced from decay of Cobalt-60 radiation sources; 201 beams from fixed radiation sources intersect at the center of the unit. The Cobalt-60–based machines provide extremely accurate targeting and precise treatment for brain lesions. They are dedicated mainly to treating brain tumors and arteriovenous malformations via 1 day treatment.

In the LINAC, the radiation beam is produced electronically by a linear accelerator, resulting in a similar type of energy. The beam is moving constantly around its isocenter in a spherical arc, but only one beam intersects itself from many different directions. LINAC-based machines can perform radiosurgery on larger tumors and can fractionate treatments over several days. Treatments that are given over time are referred to as fractionated stereotactic radiotherapy.

Because the main limitation of gamma knife or LINAC radiosurgery is the distance between the tumor margin and the optic chiasm, appropriate candidates for these treatments[208] are patients with a small residual tumor or a tumor confined to the cavernous sinus, in whom the risk for damage to vision is minimized. The delay in reducing excessive hormone secretion to normal is shorter than with conventional radiotherapy.[209-211]

The particle beam or cyclotron is in limited use in the United States; in addition to brain tumors, it treats other cancers in a fractionated manner. Dedicated neurosurgeons with specific expertise and close cooperation with physicists and radiation oncologists are involved in this special field, which is not yet fully developed.

Complications

Complications of pituitary surgery depend on the surgical route employed to reach the sella. We refer to transsphenoidal (microsurgical and endoscopic) and transcranial complications. Microsurgical transsphenoidal surgery, with its lack of visible scars and lower mortality and morbidity compared with conventional transcranial approaches, is appealing to patients and physicians. Serious complications of transsphenoidal surgery are uncommon and seem to be related to the size of the tumor and the experience of the surgeon. Nevertheless, even if the mortality rate is low (usually <1%),[212-215] complications still occur.[216] Major morbidity (CSF leak, meningitis, stroke, intracranial hemorrage, and visual loss) occurs in 3.4% of cases, whereas minor complications (sinus disease, nasal septal perforations) are present in approximately 4.6% of procedures.[67] Microsurgical transsphenoidal approach complications can be divided into different groups, according to the anatomic structures and the systems that may be involved. The following categories have been identified:

1. Nasofacial complications (approach complications)
2. Sphenoid sinus complications
3. Sella turcica complications
4. Suprasellar and parasellar complications
5. Endocrine complications

Nasofacial complications, including nasal septal perforations, bleeding from the mucosal branches of the sphenopalatine artery, injury or fracture of the cribriform plate with subsequent CSF leak, anesthesia of the upper lip and of the anterior maxillary teeth, saddle nose, anosmia caused by undue superior nasal septum dissection, diastasis of the maxilla, and fracture of the hard palate due to overspreading of the speculum, have been reported. Sphenoid sinus complications that occur more frequently are sinusitis and mucocele, a rare and usually late-onset disorder caused by obstruction of airflow at the osteomeatal complex. Fracture of the sphenoid body with injury to the optic nerves and the carotid arteries, sometimes due to thin or absent bone, is exceptional but must be kept in mind. Sella turcica complications that may occur include CSF leak due to violation of the arachnoid membrane, subarachnoid hemorrhage, vasospasm, and tension pneumocephalus. A wide range of suprasellar and parasellar complications have been reported: hypothalamic injury, resulting from direct surgical injury or from hemorrage or ischemia provoked by the procedure; visual damage, caused by direct surgical trauma, hemorrhage, or ischemia; vascular injury to one of the vessels of the circle of Willis, which represents one of the main sources of operative mortality[66,217]; meningitis, related to a CSF leak or to contamination; cavernous sinus injury (ICA; sixth, thirth, and fourth cranial nerve injury), resulting from surgical maneuvers performed to remove the lesion extending into the parasellar area; and brain stem injury, caused by a misdirected approach to the clivus. These complications occur infrequently. The endocrine sequelae are the most

frequent complications after a transsphenoidal procedure. Loss of one or more anterior pituitary functional axes occurs in approximately 3% of microadenomas, whereas in macroadenomas, this occurs in about 5% of cases.[67] Permanent diabetes insipidus occurs in 3% of cases.[67]

For the endoscopic transsphenoidal approach, differences in the type of complications are noted compared with complications described with the microsurgical transsphenoidal approach. These differences arise from the different type of approach used and from the absence of a nasal speculum in the endoscopic procedure. The endoscopic approach is endonasal, whereas the microsurgical approach has a phase in which the oral mucosa or nasal septum or both are dissected; this, even if rarely, can be the reason for anesthesia of the upper lip and of the anterior maxillary teeth, nasal septal perforations, saddle nose, and anosmia. The lack of a nasal speculum avoids the development of other rare complications, such as diastasis of the maxilla and fracture of the hard palate, which are due to overspreading of the speculum; fracture of the orbit; and injury or fracture of the cribriform plate and subsequent CSF leak. Bleeding from the mucosal branches of the sphenopalatine artery[218] also is possible with the endoscopic approach. Series of endoscopic operations[125,127,129] showed an overall decreased incidence of complications compared with historical microsurgical transsphenoidal series.[213] In addition to a decrease in functional and esthetic nasofacial complications, a correlated decrease is seen in all the other complications described in the literature. The explanation for the reduced complication rate might be found in the wider "overview inside the anatomy," facilitated by the endoscope, and in decreased surgical trauma with the endoscopic approach itself.

Transcranial approaches are associated with significantly higher morbidity and mortality compared with the transsphenoidal route; morbidity and mortality have decreased in the microsurgical era. Direct comparison of the complications between the two groups is not possible because the respective inclusion criteria have changed over the years. One aspect that should not be underestimated is that nowadays transcranial surgery usually is employed for giant and invasive pituitary adenomas,[73,219,220] or for adenomas invading the parasellar compartment or the central skull base,[221] and representing a cohort of subjects with the most difficult surgical management and intricate surgical problems. Despite these considerations, a surprisingly high total tumor resection rate (63% to 96%) has been reported more recently.[221] In a similar subset of patients, the recurrence rate has been 15.2%.[73]

Specific complications, common to any supratentorial craniotomy, are related to traction on the frontal and temporal lobes, dissection of major or perforating vessels, and manipulation of the optic or oculomotor nerves.[222] The most feared complication is postoperative hematoma in the sellar and suprasellar region, leading to coma and autonomic deterioration. The most common postoperative complication is diabetes insipidus, immediate, delayed (4 to 5 days), or triphasic; transient (31.8%) or permanent (21.1%); followed by hemiparesis, transient (33.3%), or permanent (9.1%).[73] Loss of vision can occur, most commonly as the result of disruption of the blood supply to the chiasm or the optic nerves. Other complications, such as worsening of anterior pituitary function, epilepsy, infection, and CSF leak, also can occur. The strict operative mortality (5%) or mortality from disease-related complications (11.3%) is not negligible.[73]

Surgery, either transsphenoidal or transcranial, should accomplish the goal of total removal of the lesion during the first operation, if possible, for the patient's best chance of "cure." Only a reasonable risk can be borne by the patient in terms of complications and postoperative deficits, however, because long-term benefits optimizing the results of surgery can be obtained by means of additional medical or radiotherapeutic treatment. The surgeon always must attempt to attain a complete and radical result, but at the same time always must remember that a wide variety of options—medical, surgical, and radiotherapeutic—are now available. What is crucial, regardless of the surgical option selected for a single case, whether transsphenoidal or transcranial, is for the surgeon to relate the goal of surgery to the patient's needs. Never is there a reason to take unnecessary risks. What is most important is the concept that one must be able to select the best option for the actual condition of the patient among all the options available, surgical or otherwise.

Another aspect that has major importance in the general perspective is the necessity for long-term postoperative follow-up, together with the attitude of teamwork of the entire neuroendocrine unit. This has equal value to the surgical/technical aspects and indications discussed in this chapter.

Acknowledgments

We wish to thank our teacher, Professor Enrico de Divitiis, for his constant guidance; Professor Edward R. Laws, Jr., for his encouragement and support; all the colleagues of our team, especially the endocrinologists and AnnaMaria Colao, MD, PhD, for their extraordinary partnership; and Vinicio Valente, MD, for the artwork.

REFERENCES

1. Fahlbusch R, Buchfelder M, Nomikos P: Pituitary Surgery. In Melmed S, editor: The Pituitary. Malden, MA, 2002, Blackwell, pp 405–417.
2. Horsley V: Address in surgery on the technic of operation on the central nervous system, Br Med J 2:411–423, 1906.
3. Caton R, Paul FT: Notes on a case of acromegaly treated by operation, Br Med J 2:1421–1423, 1893.
4. Jane JA Jr, Thapar K, Laws ER Jr: A history of pituitary surgery, Oper Tech Neurosurg 5:200–209, 2002.
5. Schloffer H: Erfolgreiche Operationen eines Hypophysentumors auf Nasalem Wege, Wien Clin Wochenschr 20:621–624, 1907.
6. Artico M, Pastore FS, Fraioli B, et al: The contribution of Davide Giordano (1864–1954) to pituitary surgery: the transglabellar-nasal approach, Neurosurgery 42:909–912, 1998.
7. Giordano D: Compendio di Chirurgia Operativa Italiana, Torino, 1911, UTET, pp 100–103.
8. von Eiselsberg A, von Frankl-Hochwart L: Uber die operative Behandlung der Tumoren der Hypophysisgegend, Neurol Centralblatt 26:994–1001, 1907.
9. Kocher T: Ein Fall von Hypophysis-Tumor mit Operativer Heilung, Dtsch Zeitschrift Chir 100:13–37, 1909.
10. Lanzino G, Laws ER Jr: Pioneers in the development of transsphenoidal surgery: Theodor Kocher, Oskar Hirsch, and Norman Dott, J Neurosurg 95:1097–1103, 2001.
11. Kanavel AB: The removal of tumors of the pituitary body by an infranasal route: a proposed operation with a description of the technique, JAMA 53:1704–1707, 1909.
12. Kanavel AB, Grinker J: Removal of tumors of the pituitary body with a suggestion as to a two-step route, and a report of a case with a malignant tumor operated upon with primary recovery, Surg Gynecol Obstet 10:414–418, 1910.
13. Hirsch O: Uber Methoden der Behandlung von Hypophysistumoren auf endonasalem Wege, Arch Laryngol Rhinol 24:129–177, 1911.
14. Hajek M: Zur Diagnose und intranasalen chirurgischen Behandlung der Eiterungen der Keilbeinhöhle und des hinteren Siebbeinlabyrinthes, Arch Laryngol Rhinol 16:105–143, 1904.
15. Kilian G: Die submuköse Fensterresektion der Nasenscheidewand, Arch Laryngol Rhinol 16:362–387, 1904.
16. Hamlin H: Oskar Hirsch, Surg Neurol 16:391–393, 1981.
17. Halstead AE: The operative treatment of tumors of the hypophysis, Surg Gynecol Obstet 10:494, 1910.
18. Halstead AE: Remarks on the operative treatment of tumors of the hypophysis: with the report of two cases operated on by an oronasal method, Tran Am Surg Assoc 28:73–93, 1910.
19. Cushing H: Partial hypophysectomy for acromegaly: with remarks on the functions on the hypophysis, Ann Surg 30:1002–1017, 1909.
20. Cushing H: Surgical experiences with pituitary disorders, JAMA 63:1515–1525, 1914.
21. Cushing H: Intracranial Tumors: Notes upon a Series of Two Thousand Verified Cases with Surgical-Mortality Percentages Pertaining Thereto, Springfield, IL, 1932, Charles C Thomas, pp 69–79.
22. Rosegay H: Cushing's legacy to transsphenoidal surgery, J Neurosurg 54:448–454, 1981.
23. Dandy WE: The brain. In Lewis D, editor: Practice of Surgery, Hagerstown, MD, 1934, WF Prior, pp 556–605.
24. Heuer GJ: Surgical experiences with an intracranial approach to chiasmal lesions, Arch Surg 1:368–381, 1920.
25. Heuer GJ: The surgical approach and the treatment of tumors and other lesions about the optic chiasm, Surg Gynecol Obstet 53:489–518, 1931.
26. Liu JK, Das K, Weiss MH, et al: The history and evolution of transsphenoidal surgery, J Neurosurg 95:1083–1096, 2001.
27. Hardy J: Transsphenoidal microsurgery of the normal and pathological pituitary, Clin Neurosurg 16:185–217, 1969.
28. Cappabianca P, de Divitiis O, Maiuri F: Evolution of transsphenoidal surgery. In de Divitiis E, Cappabianca P, editors: Endoscopic Endonasal Transsphenoidal Surgery, New York, Springer, 2003, pp 1–7.
29. Guiot G, Rougerie J, Fourestier M, et al: Explorations endoscopiques intracraniennes, Presse Med 71:1225–1228, 1963.
30. Carrau R, Jho HD, Ko Y: Transnasal-transsphenoidal endoscopic surgery of the pituitary gland, Laryngoscope 106:914–918, 1996.
31. Jho HD, Carrau RL, Ko Y: Endoscopic pituitary surgery. In Wilkins H, Rengachary S, editors: Neurosurgical Operative Atlas, Park Ridge, IL, 1996, American Association of Neurological Surgeons, pp 1–12.
32. Cappabianca P, Alfieri A, de Divitiis E: Endoscopic endonasal transsphenoidal approach to the sella: towards functional endoscopic pituitary surgery (FEPS), Minim Invasive Neurosurg 41:66–73, 1998.
33. de Divitiis E, Cappabianca P, Cavallo LM: Endoscopic endonasal transsphenoidal approach to the sellar region. In de Divitiis E, Cappabianca P, editors: Endoscopic Endonasal T Transsphenoidal Surgery, New York, 2003, Springer, pp 91–130.
34. de Divitiis E, Spaziante R, Stella L: Empty sella and benign intrasellar cysts. In Krayenbühl H, editor: Advances and Technical Standards in Neurosurgery. New York, 1981, Springer-Verlag, pp 3–74.
35. Aron DC, Findling JW, Tyrell JB: Hypothalamus and pituitary. In Greenspan FS, Strewler GJ, editors: Basic and Clinical Endocrinology. Stanford, 1997, Appleton & Lange, pp 95–156.
36. Alfieri A, Jho HD: Endoscopic endonasal cavernous sinus surgery: an anatomical study, Neurosurgery 48:827–837, 2001.
37. Alfieri A, Jho HD: Endoscopic endonasal approaches to the cavernous sinus: surgical approaches, Neurosurgery 49:354–362, 2001.
38. Cavallo LM, Cappabianca P, Galzio R, et al: Endoscopic transnasal approach to the cavernous sinus versus transcranial route: anatomic study, Neurosurgery 56(2 suppl):379–389, 2005.
39. Dolenc VV: Transcranial epidural approach to pituitary tumors extending beyond the sella, Neurosurgery 41:542–550, 1997.
40. Partington M, Davis DH, Laws ER, et al: Pituitary adenomas in childhood and adolescence, J Neurosurg 80:209–216, 1994.
41. Amar AP, Weiss MH: Pituitary anatomy and physiology, Neurosurg Clin North Am 13:11–23, 2003.
42. Kirgis HD, Locke W: Anatomy and embriology. In Locke W, Schally AV, editors: The Hypothalamus and Pituitary in Health and Disease, Springfield, IL, 1972, Charles C Thomas, pp 3–65.
43. Schaeffer JP: Some points in the regional anatomy of the optic pathway, with special reference to tumors of the hypophysis cerebri and resulting ocular changes, Anat Rec 28:243–279, 1924.
44. Elias WJ, Chadduck JB, Alden TD, et al: Frameless stereotaxy for transsphenoidal surgery, Neurosurgery 45:271–277, 1999.
45. Jane JA Jr, Thapar K, Alden TD, et al: Fluoroscopic frameless stereotaxy for transsphenoidal surgery, Neurosurgery 48:1302–1308, 2001.
46. Kajiwara K, Nishikazi T, Ohmoto Y, et al: Image-guided transsphenoidal surgery for pituitary lesions using Mehrkoordinaten Manipulator (MKM) navigation system, Minim Invasive Neurosurg 46:78–81, 2003.
47. Lasio G, Ferroli P, Felisati G, et al: Image-guided endoscopic transnasal removal of recurrent pituitary adenomas, Neurosurgery 51:132–137, 2002.
48. Ohhashi G, Kamio M, Abe T, et al: Endoscopic transnasal approach to the pituitary lesions using a navigation system (Insta Trak system): technical note, Minim Invasive Neurosurg 45:120–123, 2002.
49. Sandeman D, Moufid A: Interactive image-guided pituitary surgery: an experience of 101 procedures, Neurochirurgie 44:331–338, 1998.
50. Bohinski RJ, Warnick RE, Gaskill-Shipley MF, et al: Intraoperative magnetic resonance imaging to determine the extent of resection of pituitary macroadenomas during transsphenoidal microsurgery, Neurosurgery 49:1133–1144, 2001.
51. Fahlbusch R, Ganslandt O, Buchfelder M, et al: Intraoperative magnetic resonance imaging during transsphenoidal surgery, J Neurosurg 95:381–390, 2001.
52. Lewin JS, Metzger A, Selman WR: Intraoperative magnetic resonance image guidance in neurosurgery, J Magn Reson Imaging 12:512–524, 2000.
53. Martin CH, Schwartz R, Jolesz F, et al: Transsphenoidal resection of pituitary adenomas in an intraoperative MRI unit, Pituitary 2:155–162, 1999.
54. Nimsky C, Ganslandt O, Hofmann B, et al: Limited benefit of intraoperative low-field magnetic resonance imaging in craniopharyngioma surgery, Neurosurgery 53:72–81, 2003.
55. Steinmeier R, Fahlbusch R, Ganslandt O, et al: Intraoperative magnetic resonance imaging with the magnetom open scanner: Concepts, neurosurgical indications,

and procedures: a preliminary report, Neurosurgery 43:739–748, 1998.

56. Bills D, Meyer F, Laws ER Jr, et al: A retrospective analysis of pituitary apoplexy, Neurosurgery 33:602–609, 1993.

57. Ebersold MJ, Laws ER Jr, Scheithauer BW, et al: Pituitary apoplexy treated by transsphenoidal surgery: a clinicopathological and immunocytochemical study, J Neurosurg 58:315–320, 1983.

58. Laws ER Jr, Trautmann JC, Hollenhorst RW Jr: Transsphenoidal decompression of the optic nerve and chiasm: visual results in 62 patients, J Neurosurg 46:717–722, 1977.

59. Laws ER Jr: Surgical management of pituitary apoplexy. In Welch K, Caplan L, Reis D, editors: Primer on Cerebrovascular Diseases, New York, 1997, Academic Press, pp 508–510.

60. Colao A, Ferone D, Marzullo P, et al: Long-term effect of depot long-acting somatostatin analog octreotide on hormone levels and tumor mass in acromegaly, J Clin Endocrinol Metab 86:2779–2786, 2001.

61. Colao A, Di Sarno A, Cappabianca P, et al: Withdrawal of long-term cabergoline therapy for tumoral and nontumoral hyperprolactinemia, N Engl J Med 349:2023–2033, 2003.

62. Di Sarno A, Landi ML, Cappabianca P, et al: Resistance to cabergoline as compared with bromocriptine in hyperprolactinemia: prevalence, clinical definition, and therapeutic strategy, J Clin Endocrinol Metab 86:5256–5261, 2001.

63. Cohen AR, Cooper PR, Kupersmith MJ, et al: Visual recovery after transsphenoidal removal of pituiatry adenomas, Neurosurgery 17:446–452, 1985.

64. Henderson WR: The pituitary adenomata: a follow-up study of the surgical results in 338 cases (Dr Harvey Cushing's series), Br J Surg 26:811–921, 1939.

65. Laws ER Jr: Pituitary surgery, Endocrinol Metab Clin North Am 16:647–665, 1987.

66. Laws ER Jr, Thapar K: Pituitary surgery, Endocrinol Metab Clin North Am 28:119–131, 1999.

67. Thapar K, Laws ER Jr: Pituitary tumors. In Kaye AW, Laws ER Jr, editors: Brain Tumors, London, 2001, Churchill Livingstone, pp 804–854.

68. Wilson CB: Role of surgery in the management of pituitary tumors, Neurosurg Clin North Am 1:139–159, 1990.

69. Baskin DS, Wilson CB: Transsphenoidal treatment of non-neoplastic intrasellar cysts: a report of 38 cases, J Neurosurg 60:8–13, 1984.

70. El-Mahdy W, Powell M: Transsphenoidal management of 28 symptomatic Rathke's cleft cysts, with special reference to visual and hormonal recovery, Neurosurgery 42:7–17, 1998.

71. Ross DA, Norman D, Wilson CB: Radiologic characteristics and results of surgical management of Rathke's cysts in 43 patients, Neurosurgery 30:173–179, 1992.

72. Ciric IS, Cozzens JW: Craniopharyngiomas: transsphenoidal method of approach—for the virtuoso only? Clin Neurosurg 27:169–187, 1980.

73. Yasargil MG: Transcranial surgery for large pituitary adenomas. In Yasargil MG, editor: Microneurosurgery: Microneurosurgery of CNS Tumors. Stuttgart, 1996, Georg Thieme Verlag, pp 200–204, 1997.

74. Abe T, Lüdecke DK: Transnasal surgery for infradiaphragmatic craniopharyngiomas in pediatric patients, Neurosurgery 44:957–966, 1999.

75. Laws ER Jr: Transsphenoidal microsurgery in the management of craniopharyngioma, J Neurosurg 52:661–666, 1980.

76. Spaziante R, de Divitiis E: Drainage techniques for cystic craniopharyngiomas, Neurosurg Quart 7:183–208, 1997.

77. Guiot G: Transsphenoidal approach in surgical treatment of pituitary adenomas: general principles and indications in non-functioning adenomas. In Kohler PO, Ross GT, editors: Diagnosis and Treatment of Pituitary Adenomas, Amsterdam, 1973, Excerpta Medica, pp 159–178.

78. Castelnuovo P, Locatelli D, Mauri S, et al: Extended endoscopic approaches to the skull base. Anterior cranial base CSF leaks. In de Divitiis E, Cappabianca P, editors: Endoscopic Endonasal Transsphenoidal Surgery, New York, 2003, Springer, pp 137–158.

79. de Divitiis E, Cappabianca P, Cavallo LM: Endoscopic transsphenoidal approach: adaptability of the procedure to different sella lesions, Neurosurgery 51:699–707, 2002.

80. Jane JA Jr, Thapar K, Kaptain GJ, et al: Pituitary surgery: transsphenoidal approach, Neurosurgery 51:435–444, 2002.

81. Jho HD: The expanding role of endoscopy in skull-base surgery: indications and instruments, Clin Neurosurg 48:287–305, 2001.

82. Jho HD: Endoscopic endonasal approach to the optic nerve: a technical note, Minim Invasive Neurosurg 44:190–193, 2001.

83. Kaptain GJ, Vincent DA, Sheehan JP, et al: Transsphenoidal approaches for extracapsular resection of midline suprasellar and anterior cranial base lesions, Neurosurgery 49:94–101, 2001.

84. Kato T, Sawamura J, Abe H, et al: Transsphenoidal-transtuberculum sellae approach for supradiaphragmatic tumours: technical note, Acta Neurochir 140:715–719, 1998.

85. Kim J, Choe I, Bak K, et al: Transsphenoidal supradiaphragmatic intradural approach: technical note, Minim Invasive Neurosurg 43:33–37, 2000.

86. Kouri JG, Chen MY, Watson JC, et al: Resection of suprasellar tumors by using a modified transsphenoidal approach, J Neurosurg 92:1028–1035, 2000.

87. Mason RB, Nieman LK, Doppman JL, et al: Selective excision of adenomas originating in or extending into the pituitary stalk with preservation of pituitary function, J Neurosurg 87:343–351, 1997.

88. Weiss WH: The transnasal transsphenoidal approach. In Apuzzo MLJ, editor: Surgery of the Third Ventricle. Baltimore, 1987, Williams & Wilkins, pp 476–494.

89. Jho HD, Carrau RL, McLaughlin ML, et al: Endoscopic transsphenoidal resection of a large chordoma in the posterior fossa, Acta Neurochir 139:343–348, 1997.

90. Kelley TF, Stankiewicz JA, Chow JM, et al: Endoscopic closure of postsurgical anterior cranial fossa cerebrospinal fluid leaks, Neurosurgery 39:743–746, 1996.

91. Lalwani AK, Kaplan MJ, Gutin PH: The transsphenoethmoid approach to the sphenoid sinus and clivus, Neurosurgery 31:1008–1014, 1992.

92. Laws ER Jr: Transsphenoidal surgery. In Apuzzo MLJ, editor: Brain Surgery: Complications Avoidance and Management. New York, 1993, Churchill Livingstone, pp 357–362.

93. Maira G, Pallini R, Anile C, et al: Surgical treatment of clival chordomas: the transsphenoidal approach revisited, Neurosurgery 85:784–792, 1996.

94. Fraioli B, Esposito V, Santoro A, et al: Transmaxillosphenoidal approach to tumors invading the medial compartment of the cavernous sinus, J Neurosurg 82:63–69, 1995.

95. Frank G, Pasquini E: Extended endoscopic approaches to the skull base: approach to the cavernous sinus. In de Divitiis E, Cappabianca P, editors: Endoscopic Endonasal Transsphenoidal Surgery, New York, 2003, Springer, pp 159–175.

96. Hermier M, Turjman F, Tournut P, et al: Intracranial aneurysm associated with pituitary adenoma shown by MR angiography: case report, Neuroradiology 36:115–116, 1994.

97. Inoue T, Rhoton AL Jr, Theele D, et al: Surgical approaches to the cavernous sinus: a microsurgical study, Neurosurgery 26:903–932, 1990.

98. Kitano M, Taneda M: Extended transsphenoidal approach with submucosal posterior ethmoidectomy for parasellar tumors: technical note, J Neurosurg 94:999–1004, 2001.

99. Sabit I, Schaefer SD, Couldwell T: Extradural extranasal combined transmaxillary transsphenoidal approach to the cavernous sinus: A minimally invasive microsurgical model, Laryngoscope 110:286–291, 2000.

100. Saito K, Kuwayama A, Yamamoto N, et al: The transsphenoidal removal of non functioning pituitary adenomas with suprasellar extension: the open sella method and intentionally staged operation, Neurosurgery 36:668–676, 1995.

101. Mortini P, Giovanelli M: Transcranial approaches to pituitary tumors, Oper Tech Neurosurg 5:1–13, 2002.

102. Van Alpen HA: Microsurgical fronto-temporal approach to pituitary adenomas with extrasellar extension, Clin Neurol Neurosurg 78:246–256, 1975.

103. Alleyne CH Jr, Barrow DL, Oyesiku NM: Combined transsphenoidal and pterional craniotomy approach to giant pituitary tumors, Surg Neurol 57:380–390, 2002.

104. Ishii K, Ikeda H, Takahashi S, et al: MR imaging of pituitary adenomas with sphenoid sinus invasion: characteristic MR findings indicating fibrosis, Radiat Med 14:173–178, 1996.

105. Iuchi T, Saeki N, Tanaka M, et al: MRI prediction of fibrous pituitary adenomas, Acta Neurochir 140:779–786, 1998.

106. Snow RB, Johnson CE, Morgello S, et al: Is magnetic resonance imaging useful in guiding the operative approach to large pituitary tumors? Neurosurgery 26:801–803, 1990.

107. Patterson RH: The role of transcranial surgery in the management of pituitary adenoma, Acta Neurochir 65(Suppl):16–17, 1996.

108. Esiri M, Bevan JS, Burke CW, et al: Effect of bromocriptine treatment on the fibrous tissue content of prolactin-secreting and nonfunctioning macroadenomas of the pituitary gland, J Clin Endocrinol Metab 63:383–388, 1986.

109. Barkan AL, Lloyd RV, Chandler WF, et al: Preoperative treatment of acromegaly with long-acting somatostatin analog SMS 201-995: Shrinkage of invasive pituitary macroadenomas and improved surgical remission rate, J Clin Endocrinol Metab 67:1040–1048, 1988.

110. Ezzat S, Horvath E, Harris AG, et al: Morphological effects of octreotide on growth hormone-producing pituitary adenomas, J Clin Endocrinol Metab 79:113–118, 1994.

111. Rhoton AL Jr: Operative techniques and instrumentation for neurosurgery, Neurosurgery 53:907–934, 2003.

112. Revuelta R, Arriada-Mendicoa N, Ramirez-Alba J, et al: Simultaneous treatment of a pituitary adenoma and an internal carotid artery aneurysm through a supraorbital keyhole approach, Minim Invasive Neurosurg 45:109–111, 2002.

113. Elias WJ, Laws ER Jr: Transsphenoidal approach to lesions of the sella. In Schmidek HH, editor: Schmidek and Sweet Operative Neurosurgical Techniques, Philadelphia, 2000, WB Saunders, pp 373–384.

114. Rhoton AL Jr: The supratentorial cranial space: microsurgical anatomy and surgical approaches, Neurosurgery 51(Suppl 1):335–374, 2002.

115. Zada G, Kelly DF, Cohan P, et al: The endonasal transsphenoidal approach for pituitary adenomas and other sellar lesions: an assessment of efficacy, safety and patient impressions, J Neurosurg 98:350–358, 2003.

116. Landolt AM, Schiller Z: Surgical technique: transsphenoidal approach. In Landolt AM, Vanve ML, Reilly PR, editors: Pituitary Adenomas, New York, 1996, Churchill Livingstone, pp 315–331.

117. de Divitiis E, Spaziante R: Osteoplastic opening of the sellar floor in transsphenoidal surgery: technical note, Neurosurgery 20:445–446, 1987.

118. Meij B, Lopes MB, Ellegala DB, et al: The long term significance of microscopic dural invasion in 354 patients with pituitary adenomas treated with transsphenoidal surgery, J Neurosurg 96:195–208, 2002.

119. de Divitiis E, Spaziante R, Iaccarino V, et al: Phlebography of the cavernous and intercavernous sinuses, Surg Neurol 15:306–312, 1981.

120. Spaziante R, de Divitiis E: Forced subarachnoid air in transsphenoidal excision of pituitary tumours (pumping technique), J Neurosurg 71:864–867, 1989.

121. Cappabianca P, Cavallo LM, Esposito F, et al: Sellar repair in endoscopic endonasal transsphenoidal surgery: results of 170 cases, Neurosurgery 51:1365–1372, 2002.

122. Spaziante R, de Divitiis E, Cappabianca P: Repair of the sella after transsphenoidal surgery. In Schmideck HH, editor: Schmidek and Sweet Operative Neurosurgical Techniques, Philadelphia, 2000, WB Saunders, pp 398–416.

123. Jho HD: Endoscopic surgery of pituitary adenomas. In Krisht AF, Tindall GT, editors: Comprehensive Management of Pituitary Disorders. Hagerstown, MD, 1999, Lippincott Williams & Wilkins, pp 389–403.

124. Cappabianca P, Cavallo LM, Colao A, et al: Endoscopic endonasal transsphenoidal approach: Outcome analysis of 100 consecutive procedures, Minim Invasive Neurosurg 45:1–8, 2002.

125. de Divitiis E, Cappabianca P: Endoscopic endonasal transsphenoidal surgery. In Pickard JD, editor: Advances and Technical Standards in Neurosurgery, New York, 2002, Springer Verlag, pp 137–177.

126. Jho HD, Carrau RL: Endoscopic endonasal transsphenoidal surgery: experience with 50 patients, J Neurosurg 87:44–51, 1997.

127. Jho HD: Endoscopic transsphenoidal surgery. In Schmidek HH, editor: Schmidek and Sweet Operative Neurosurgical Techniques, Philadelphia, 2000, WB Saunders, pp 385–397.

128. Cappabianca P, Cavallo LM, Mariniello G, et al: Easy sellar reconstruction in endoscopic transsphenoidal surgery with polyester-silicone dural substitute and fibrin glue: technical note, Neurosurgery 49:473–476, 2001.

129. Cappabianca P, Cavallo LM, Colao A, et al: Surgical complications of the endoscopic endonasal transsphenoidal approach for pituitary adenomas, J Neurosurg 97:293–298, 2002.

130. Cappabianca P, Alfieri A, Colao A, et al: Endoscopic endonasal transsphenoidal surgery in recurrent and residual pituitary adenomas: technical note, Minim Invasive Neurosurg 43:38–43, 2000.

131. Cappabianca P, Alfieri A, Thermes S, et al: Instruments for endoscopic endonasal transsphenoidal surgery, Neurosurgery 45:392–396, 1999.

132. Leonhard M, Cappabianca P, de Divitiis E: The endoscope, endoscopic equipment and instrumentation. In de Divitiis E, Cappabianca P, editors: Endoscopic Endonasal Transsphenoidal Surgery, New York, 2003, Springer, pp 9–19.

133. Fahlbusch R, Schott W: Pterional surgery of meningiomas of the tuberculum sellae and planum sphenoidale: surgical results with special consideration of ophthalmological and endocrinological outcomes, J Neurosurg 96:235–243, 2002.

134. Goel A, Muzumdar D, Desai KI: Tuberculum sellae meningioma: a report on management on the basis of a surgical experience with 70 patients, Neurosurgery 51:1358–1363; discussion 1363–1354, 2002.

135. Hakuba A, Liu S, Nishimura S: The orbitozygomatic infratemporal approach: a new surgical technique, Surg Neurol 26:271–276, 1986.

136. Hakuba A, Tanaka K, Suzuki T, et al: A combined orbitozygomatic infratemporal epidural and subdural approach for lesions involving the entire cavernous sinus, J Neurosurg 71:699–704, 1989.

137. Kawase T, Shiobara R, Toya S: Anterior transpetrosal-transtentorial approach for sphenopetroclival meningiomas: surgical method and results in 10 patients, Neurosurgery 28:869–875; discussion 875–866, 1991.

138. de Divitiis E, Cavallo LM, Cappabianca P, et al: Extended endoscopic endonasal transsphenoidal approach for the removal of suprasellar tumors: Part 2, Neurosurgery 60:46–58; discussion 58–59, 2007.

139. Delashaw JB Jr, Tedeschi H, Rhoton AL: Modified supraorbital craniotomy: technical note, Neurosurgery 30:954–956, 1992.

140. Jallo GI, Benjamin V: Tuberculum sellae meningiomas: microsurgical anatomy and surgical technique, Neurosurgery 51:1432–1439; discussion 1439–1440, 2002.

141. Reisch R, Perneczky A: Ten-year experience with the supraorbital subfrontal approach through an eyebrow skin incision, Neurosurgery 57:242–255, 2005.

142. Guiot G: Transsphenoidal approach in surgical treatment of pituitary adenomas: general principles and indications in non-functioning adenomas. In Kohler PO, Ross GT, editors: Diagnosis and treatment of pituitary adenomas. Amsterdam, 1973, Excerpta Medica, pp 159–178.

143. Liu JK, Das K, Weiss MH, et al: The history and evolution of transsphenoidal surgery, J Neurosurg 95:1083–1096, 2001.

144. McDonald TJ, Laws ER Jr: Historical aspects of the management of pituitary disorders with emphasis on transsphenoidal surgery. In Laws ER Jr, Randall RV, Kern EB, Abboud CF, editors: The Management of Pituitary Adenomas and Related Lesions with Emphasis on Transsphenoidal Microsurgery, New York, 1982, Appleton-Century-Crofts, pp 1–13.

145. Laws ERJ: Transsphenoidal surgery. In Apuzzo MLJ, editor: Brain surgery: Complications Avoidance and Management, Vol 1, New York, 1993, Churchill Livingstone, pp 357–362.

146. Hardy J: Transsphenoidal hypophysectomy, J Neurosurg 34:582–594, 1971.

147. Weiss MH: The transnasal transsphenoidal approach. In Apuzzo MLJ, editor: Surgery of the third ventricle, Baltimore, 1987, Williams & Wilkins, pp 476–494.

148. Kato T, Sawamura Y, Abe H, et al: Transsphenoidal-transtuberculum sellae approach for supradiaphragmatic tumours: technical note, Acta Neurochir (Wien) 140:715–719, 1998.

149. Mason RB, Nieman LK, Doppman JL, et al: Selective excision of adenomas originating in or extending into the pituitary stalk with preservation of pituitary function, J Neurosurg 87:343–351, 1997.

150. Laws ER, Kanter AS, Jane JA Jr, et al: Extended transsphenoidal approach, J Neurosurg 102:825–827; discussion 827–828, 2005.

151. Cook SW, Smith Z, Kelly DF: Endonasal transsphenoidal removal of tuberculum sellae meningiomas: technical note, Neurosurgery 55:239–244, 2004.

152. Couldwell WT, Weiss MH, Rabb C, et al: Variations on the standard transsphenoidal approach to the sellar region, with emphasis on the extended approaches and parasellar approaches: surgical experience in 105 cases, Neurosurgery 55:539–550, 2004.

153. Kim J, Choe I, Bak K, et al: Transsphenoidal supradiaphragmatic intradural approach: technical note, Minim Invasive Neurosurg 43:33–37, 2000.

154. Kouri JG, Chen MY, Watson JC, et al: Resection of suprasellar tumors by using a modified transsphenoidal approach. Report of four cases, J Neurosurg 92:1028–1035, 2000.

155. Dusick JR, Esposito F, Kelly DF, et al: The extended direct endonasal transsphenoidal approach for nonadenomatous suprasellar tumors, J Neurosurg 102:832–841, 2005.

156. Kaptain GJ, Vincent DA, Sheehan JP, et al: Transsphenoidal approaches for the extracapsular resection of midline suprasellar and anterior cranial base lesions, Neurosurgery 49:94–101, 2001.

157. Cappabianca P, Frank G, Pasquini E, et al: Extended endoscopic endonasal transsphenoidal approaches to the suprasellar region, planum sphenoidale and clivus. In de Divitiis E, Cappabianca P, editors: Endoscopic endonasal transsphenoidal surgery, Wien - New York, 2003, Springer, pp 176–187.

158. Laufer I, Anand VK, Schwartz TH: Endoscopic, endonasal extended transsphenoidal, transplanum transtuberculum approach for resection of suprasellar lesions, J Neurosurg 106:400–406, 2007.

159. Kitano M, Taneda M: Extended transsphenoidal surgery for suprasellar craniopharyngiomas: infrachiasmatic radical resection combined with or without a suprachiasmatic trans-lamina terminalis approach, Surg Neurol, 71:290–298, 2009.

160. Kitano M, Taneda M, Nakao Y: Postoperative improvement in visual function in patients with tuberculum sellae meningiomas: results of the extended transsphenoidal and transcranial approaches, J Neurosurg 107:337–346, 2007.

161. Cappabianca P, Alfieri A, de Divitiis E: Endoscopic endonasal transsphenoidal approach to the sella: towards functional endoscopic pituitary surgery (FEPS), Minim Invasive Neurosurg 41:66–73, 1998.

162. Cappabianca P, de Divitiis E: Endoscopic pituitary surgery. Anatomy and surgery of the transsphenoidal approach to the sellar region, Tuttlingen, 2001, Endo-Press.

163. Cappabianca P, de Divitiis E: Endoscopy and transsphenoidal surgery, Neurosurgery 54:1043–1048; discussions 1048–1050, 2004.

164. Cappabianca P, de Divitiis E: Back to the Egyptians: neurosurgery via the nose. A five-thousand year history and the recent contribution of the endoscope, Neurosurg Rev 30:1–7; discussion 7, 2007.

165. Cavallo LM, Messina A, Cappabianca P, et al: Endoscopic endonasal surgery of the midline skull base: anatomical study and clinical considerations, Neurosurg Focus 19:E2, 2005.

166. Maroon JC: Skull base surgery: past, present, and future trends, Neurosurg Focus 19:E1, 2005.

167. Prevedello DM, Doglietto F, Jane JA Jr, et al: History of endoscopic skull base surgery: its evolution and current reality, J Neurosurg 107:206–213, 2007.

168. Cavallo LM, de Divitiis O, Aydin S, et al: Extended endoscopic endonasal transsphenoidal approach to the suprasellar area: anatomic considerations—part 1, Neurosurgery 61:ONS-24–ONS-34, 2007.

169. Frank G, Pasquini E, Mazzatenta D: Extended transsphenoidal approach, J Neurosurg 95:917–918, 2001.

170. Kassam A, Snyderman CH, Mintz A, et al: Expanded endonasal approach: the rostrocaudal axis. Part II. Posterior clinoids to the foramen magnum, Neurosurg Focus 19:E4, 2005.

171. Kassam A, Snyderman CH, Mintz A, et al: Expanded endonasal approach: the rostrocaudal axis. Part I. Crista galli to the sella turcica, Neurosurg Focus 19:E3, 2005.

172. de Divitiis E, Cappabianca P, Cavallo LM: Endoscopic transsphenoidal approach: adaptability of the procedure to different sellar lesions, Neurosurgery 51:699–705; discussion 705–707, 2002.

173. Cappabianca P, Cavallo LM, Esposito F, et al: Extended endoscopic endonasal approach to the midline skull base: the evolving role of transsphenoidal surgery. In Pickard JD, Akalan N, Di Rocco C, Dolenc VV, Lobo Antunes J, Mooij JJA, Schramm J, Sindou M, editors: Advances and Technical Standards in Neurosurgery, Wien New York, 2008, Springer, pp 152–199.

174. Frank G, Pasquini E, Doglietto F, et al: The endoscopic extended transsphenoidal approach for craniopharyngiomas, Neurosurgery 59 (suppl 1):ONS75–ONS83, 2006.

175. de Divitiis E, Cappabianca P, Cavallo LM, et al: Extended endoscopic transsphenoidal approach for extrasellar craniopharyngiomas, Neurosurgery 61:219–227; discussion 228, 2007.

176. Kassam AB, Gardner PA, Snyderman CH, et al: Expanded endonasal approach, a fully endoscopic transnasal approach for the resection of midline suprasellar craniopharyngiomas: a new classification based on the infundibulum, J Neurosurg 108:715–728, 2008.

177. de Divitiis E, Cappabianca P, Esposito F, et al: Tuberculum sellae meningiomas: High route or low route? A series of 51 consecutive cases, Neurosurgery 62:556–563; discussion 556–563, 2008.

178. Gardner PA, Prevedello DM, Kassam AB, et al: The evolution of the endonasal approach for craniopharyngiomas, J Neurosurg 108:1043–1047, 2008.

179. Gardner PA, Kassam AB, Snyderman CH, et al: Outcomes following endoscopic, expanded endonasal resection of suprasellar craniopharyngiomas: a case series, J Neurosurg 109:6–16, 2008.

180. Kassam A, Thomas AJ, Snyderman C, et al: Fully endoscopic expanded endonasal approach treating skull base lesions in pediatric patients, J Neurosurg 106:75–86, 2007.

181. Kassam A, Snyderman C, Carrau R: An evolving paradigm to the ventral skull base, Skull Base 14(suppl 1), February, 2004.

182. Cappabianca P, Cavallo LM, de Divitiis E: Endoscopic endonasal transsphenoidal surgery, Neurosurgery 55:933–940; discussion 940–941, 2004.

183. Castelnuovo P, Pistochini A, Locatelli D: Different surgical approaches to the sellar region: focusing on the "two nostrils four hands technique", Rhinology 44:2–7, 2006.

184. Cavallo LM, Messina A, Esposito F, et al: Skull base reconstruction in the extended endoscopic transsphenoidal approach for suprasellar lesions, J Neurosurg 107:713–720, 2007.

185. Leng LZ, Brown S, Anand VK, et al: "Gasket-seal" watertight closure in minimal-access endoscopic cranial base surgery, Neurosurgery 62:5(suppl 2):ONSE342–343; discussion ONSE343, 2008.

186. Hadad G, Bassagasteguy L, Carrau RL, et al: A novel reconstructive technique after endoscopic expanded endonasal approaches: vascular pedicle nasoseptal flap, Laryngoscope 116:1882–1886, 2006.

187. Pinheiro-Neto CD, Prevedello DM, Carrau RL, et al: Improving the design of the pedicled nasoseptal flap for skull base reconstruction: a radioanatomic study, Laryngoscope 117:1560–1569, 2007.

188. Kassam A, Carrau RL, Snyderman CH, et al: Evolution of reconstructive techniques following endoscopic expanded endonasal approaches, Neurosurg Focus 19:E8, 2005.

189. Cappabianca P, Cavallo LM, de Divitiis E: Endoscopic pituitary and skull base surgery. Anatomy and surgery of the endoscopic endonasal approach. Tuttlingen, 2008, Endo-Press.

190. Snyderman C, Kassam A, Carrau R, et al: Acquisition of surgical skills for endonasal skull base surgery: a training program, Laryngoscope 117:699–705, 2007.

191. Prevedello DM, Kassam AB, Snyderman C, et al: Endoscopic cranial base surgery: ready for prime time? Clin Neurosurg 54:48–57, 2007.
192. Cappabianca P, Cavallo LM, Esposito F, et al: Craniopharyngiomas, J Neurosurg 109:1–3, 2008.
193. Rutka JT: Endonasal resection of craniopharyngiomas, J Neurosurg 109:1; reply 3–5, 2008.
194. Yasargil MG: General operative techniques. In Yasargil MG, editor: Microneurosurgery: Microsurgical Anatomy of the Basal Cisterns and Vessels of the Brain, Diagnostic Studies, General Operative Techniques and Pathological Considerations of the Intracranial Aneurysms, vol I, New York, 1984, Georg Thieme Verlag, pp 215–233.
195. McArthur LL: An aseptic surgical access to the pituitary body and its neighbourhood, JAMA 58:2009–2011, 1912.
196. Frazier CH: Lesions of the hypophysis from the viewpoint of the surgeon, Surg Gynecol Obstet 17:724–736, 1913.
197. Krause F: Freilegung der Hypophyse. In Krause F, editor: Chirurgie der Gehirnkrankheiten, Stuttgart, 1914, Ferdinand Enke, pp 465–470.
198. Powell MP, Pollock JR: Transcranial surgery. In Powell MP, Lightman SL, Laws ER Jr, editors: Management of Pituitary Tumors, Totowa, NJ, 2003, Humana Press, pp 147–159.
199. Dandy WE: A new hypophysis operation, Bull Johns Hopkins Hosp 29:154–155, 1918.
200. Bhagwati SN, Deopujari CE, Parulekar GD: Lamina terminalis approach for retrochiasmal craniopharyngiomas, Childs Nerv Syst 6:425–429, 1990.
201. de Divitiis O, Angileri F, d'Avella D, et al: Microsurgical anatomic features of the lamina terminalis, Neurosurgery 50:563–570, 2002.
202. King TT: Removal of intraventricular craniopharyngiomas through the lamina terminalis, Acta Neurochir 45:277–286, 1979.
203. Maira G, Anile C, Colosimo C, et al: Craniopharyngiomas of the third ventricle: trans-lamina terminalis approach, Neurosurgery 47:563–570, 2000.
204. Killiani OGT: Some remarks on tumors of the chiasm, with a proposal how to reach the same by operation, Ann Surg 40:35–43, 1904.
205. Fahlbusch R, Honegger J, Paulus W, et al: Surgical treatment of craniopharyngiomas: experience with 168 patients, J Neurosurg 90:237–250, 1999.
206. Samii M, Tatagiba M: Craniopharyngioma. In Kaye AW, Laws ER Jr, editors: Brain Tumors, London, 1995, Churchill Livingstone, pp 873–894.
207. Suzuki J: The bifrontal anterior interhemispheric approach. In Apuzzo MLJ, editor: Surgery of the Third Ventricle, Baltimore, 1998, Williams & Wilkins, pp 489–515.
208. Ganz JC: Gamma knife treatment of pituitary adenomas. In Landolt A, Vance M, Reilly P, editors: Pituitary Adenomas, Edinburgh, 1996, Churchill Livingstone, pp 461–474.
209. Degerblad M, Rahn T, Bergstrand G, et al: Long-term results of stereotactic radiosurgery to the pituitary gland in Cushing's disease, Acta Endocrinol 112:310–314, 1986.
210. Landolt A, Haller D, Lomax N, et al: Stereotactic radiosurgery for recurrent surgically treated acromegaly: comparison with fractionated radiotherapy, J Neurosurg 88:1002–1008, 1998.
211. Vance ML, Laws ER Jr: Gamma Knife radiosurgery for secretory pituitary adenomas. In Powell SL, Lightman SL, Laws ER Jr, editors: Management of Pituitary Tumors, Totowa, NJ, 2003, Humana Press, pp 221–229.
212. Black PMcL, Zervas NT, Candia GL: Incidence and management of complications of transsphenoidal operation for pituitary adenomas, Neurosurgery 20:920–924, 1987.
213. Ciric I, Ragin A, Baumgartner C, et al: Complications of transsphenoidal surgery: results of a national survey, review of the literature, and personal experience, Neurosurgery 40:225–237, 1997.
214. Laws ER Jr, Kern EB: Complications of trans-sphenoidal surgery, Clin Neurosurg 23:401–416, 1976.
215. Zervas NT: Surgical results in pituitary adenomas: Results of an international survey. In Black PMcL, Zervas NT, Ridgway EC Jr, Martin JB, editors: Secretory Tumors of the Pituitary Gland, New York, 1984, Raven Press, pp 377–385.
216. Laws ER Jr, Kern EB: Complications of trans-sphenoidal surgery. In Laws ER Jr, Randall RV, Kern EB, editors: Management of Adenomas and Related Lesions, New York, 1982, Appleton-Century-Crofts, pp 329–346.
217. Laws ER Jr: Vascular complications of transsphenoidal surgery, Pituitary 2:163–170, 1999.
218. Cockroft KM, Carew JF, Trost D, et al: Delayed epistaxis resulting from external carotid artery injury requiring embolization: a rare complication of transsphenoidal surgery: Case report, Neurosurgery 47:236–239, 2000.
219. Guiot G, Derome P: Surgical problems of pituitary adenomas. In Krayenbühl H, editor: Advances and Technical Standards in Neurosurgery, New York, 1976, Springer Verlag, pp 3–33.
220. Mohr G, Hardy J, Comtois R, et al: Surgical management of giant adenomas, Can J Neurol Sci 17:62–66, 1990.
221. Dolenc VV: Pituitary tumors extending beyond the sella. In Microsurgical Anatomy and Surgery of the Central Skull Base, New York, 2003, Springer, pp 236–252.
222. Fahlbusch R, Buchfelder M: Surgical complications. In Landolt AM, Vance ML, Reilly PR, editors: Pituitary Adenomas, New York, 1996, Churchill Livingstone, pp 395–408.

Chapter 13

EVALUATION AND MANAGEMENT OF CHILDHOOD HYPOTHALAMIC AND PITUITARY TUMORS

CRISTINA TRAGGIAI and RICHARD STANHOPE

Intracranial and spinal cord tumors are the most frequent type of childhood cancer after leukemia. Tumors in the pediatric age group differ from adults in the types and location of tumors, the value of extensive surgical resection of malignant tumors, the importance of chemotherapy, improved prognosis, and the delay in using radiotherapy. The relationship between tumor location and tumor type is close. Advances in the therapy of malignant brain tumors in children have led to a significant improvement in survival rates over the last few years. Radiation therapy still plays a major role in the management of intracranial malignancies. Together with surgical resection and, more recently, chemotherapy, this has led to improvement in the outcomes of several tumor types. Endocrine symptoms are well recognized as sequelae of the treatment of intracranial tumors. Much less commonly, hypothalamic tumors can result in children presenting with growth failure and/or endocrine dysfunction. Endocrinopathies are significant consequences of childhood intracranial tumors and their treatment. The risk of developing these adverse events is related to the underlying tumor, as well as surgery, chemotherapy, and irradiation therapy.

Epidemiology

Intracranial and spinal cord tumors are the second most frequent type of childhood malignancy after leukemia, accounting for approximately 20% of cases.[1] While much is known about the epidemiology of malignant intracranial tumors in childhood, there is a paucity of information about benign tumors. The incidence of brain tumors in childhood is 3 per 100,000. The highest age-adjusted incidence, 31.4 per million, was observed in the Nordic countries, and rates between 24 and 27 per million were found in most other predominantly white populations. In the United States, the age-adjusted incidence rate was 36% higher in males and 68% higher in females than the rate based on malignant tumors alone. Black children had a significantly lower incidence than white children. Lower rates were seen in South America, Africa, and Asia; the lowest rates were for Chinese populations and for blacks in Africa, both below 15 per million. Among white populations, astrocytoma was the most common histologic type, often with an incidence of at least 10 per million, followed by medulloblastoma, 5 to 6 per million, and ependymoma, 2 to 4 per million. In other regions with lower incidence rates, these three types accounted for similar proportions of the total. Black children in the United States had a higher incidence of craniopharyngioma than white children, and there was an unusually high incidence of pineal tumors in Japan, 0.9 per million compared with 0.3 to 0.4 in many other countries. An incidence rate of 2.76 per 100,000 people younger than 18 years of age was found. Tumors in the suprasellar/hypothalamic region are unusual, the most common being craniopharyngiomas, which are approximately 9% of childhood intracranial tumors; other tumors are much rarer. The incidence of intracranial germinoma is only 0.26 cases per million children per year.[1,2] Considerable progress has been made toward improving survival for children with brain tumors, and yet there is still relatively little known regarding the molecular genetic events that contribute to tumor initiation or progression. Nonrandom patterns of chromosomal deletions in several types of childhood brain tumors suggest that the loss or inactivation of tumor suppressor genes is a critical event in tumorigenesis. Deletions of chromosomal regions 10q, 11, and 17p, for example, are frequent events in medulloblastoma, whereas loss of a region within 22q11.2, which contains the *INI1* gene, is

Table 13-1. Histologic Classification of Intracranial Tumors

Supratentorial midline tumors	Low-grade glioma
	Craniopharyngioma
	Germ cell tumor
	Pineal cell tumors (pineocytoma/
	pineoblastoma)
Supratentorial hemispheric tumors	
Infratentorial tumors	

involved in the development of atypical teratoid and rhabdoid tumors.

Classification

Intracranial tumors are most commonly situated in the posterior fossa in 70% of cases, in the supratentorial region in 30%, and can occur at any age, although the most frequent age is between 2 and 5 years. The classification can be made either on the basis of histology or on the location of tumor site (Table 13-1). Many sellar and suprasellar tumors in childhood, such as craniopharyngiomas and Rathke's cysts, do not originate from the central nervous system and are not "brain tumors." Hypothalamic tumors are usually hypothalamic hamartoma, low-grade astrocytoma, Langerhans' cell histiocytosis (LCH), and dermoid and epidermoid tumors. Tumors such as craniopharyngiomas and germinomas tend to affect the hypothalamus indirectly, originating in the peripituitary or pituitary region and extending upward. The pituitary stalk is typically affected from lesions such as germinomas, LCH, and craniopharyngiomas. LCH commonly affects the middle of the pituitary stalk, in a similar appearance to tuberculosis and sarcoidosis, which may be related to LCH cells involving the cerebrospinal fluid. The anterior pituitary is frequently affected by benign pituitary adenoma, whereas the posterior pituitary is the common location of pilocytic astrocytoma and LCH. Malignant glioma, meningioma, Schwann cell, and pituitary tumors, as well as metastases (which are the most common intracranial tumors in adults), are comparatively uncommon in children.[3] In contrast, benign glioma, primitive neuroectodermal tumors, and craniopharyngiomas account for a substantially higher percentage of intracranial tumors in children than in adults.[4,5] Classification of primitive neuroepithelial cells is based on appearance of the tumor as determined by light microscopy, immunocytochemical techniques, and ultrastructural features without consideration for site of origin.[6]

Symptoms and Signs

The mode of presentation depends on the age of the child and the location of the tumor. Symptoms and signs can be usefully divided into those from raised intracranial pressure, focal neurologic signs, and endocrinopathy. Nonspecific symptoms of increased intracranial pressure are repeated and frequent headaches, especially if they are worsening and associated with nausea or vomiting, often occurring in the early morning; irritability; listlessness; vomiting; failure to thrive; macrocephaly; and loss of developmental milestones.[7] Epilepsy may be the initial presenting feature of an intracranial tumor. This may be due to the structural abnormality caused by the space-occupying lesion but may be secondary to the associated endocrinopathies of hypoglycemia (secondary to growth hormone and/or cortisol insuf-

ficiency) or hyponatremia (from the syndrome of inappropriate antidiuretic hormone secretion). Although young children are more likely than infants to manifest localizing neurologic abnormalities, these are by no means uniformly present. In older children, a larger percentage of tumors manifest with localizing symptoms and signs that often suggest the location as well as the histologic identity of the tumor. Midline tumors often present in an insidious onset with various symptoms and signs: visual defects such as nystagmus, complete loss of vision, and diplopia because of paralysis of the lateral rectus muscles due to a sixth nerve palsy or due to raised intracranial pressure because of obstruction of the cerebrospinal fluid pathways; neuroendocrine dysfunction, behavioral and appetite disturbances, and regression of motor skills; or they may reflect the compression or infiltration of adjacent structures. Pineal region tumors typically manifest with eye movement abnormalities, such as Parinaud's syndrome or hydrocephalus and alteration of consciousness.[8]

ENDOCRINE DYSFUNCTION

For both benign and malignant tumors, presenting symptoms usually reflect the age of the child and the position of the tumor. Growth failure in children with occult intracranial tumors is characteristic. In idiopathic (congenital) growth hormone deficiency (GHD), birth length is relatively short, but growth rate is normal until approximately 18 months of age, when a gradual deceleration occurs. Idiopathic GHD is usually easily distinguished from the growth failure associated with an occult intracranial tumor, in which growth is initially normal and height is appropriate for the parental percentiles, followed by a marked growth deceleration. This is usually due to GHD but may exceptionally be due to the presence of the intracranial tumor with normal endocrine function. Absence of puberty of more than 2 standard deviations (SD) will require neuroradiologic imaging, but delayed puberty with growth deceleration is usually due to constitutional delay of growth and puberty. Even a child with suspected constitutional delay who does not respond to sex-steroid therapy should be investigated endocrinologically and neuroradiologically. Craniopharyngiomas commonly present with failure to enter puberty or arrested puberty associated with an abnormal growth spurt; they usually demonstrate an absence of the normal consonance of puberty.[9]

The idiopathic form of central precocious puberty (CPP) occurs in 74% of affected girls, and in 60% of affected boys, who are more likely to have an occult intracranial tumor than girls.[10,11] Although it is commonly recognized that gonadotropin-dependent precocious puberty (or CPP) in boys is usually caused by an intracranial lesion, it used to be believed that girls had an idiopathic etiology and did not require neuroradiologic imaging. Recent large series of girls with gonadotropin-dependent precocious puberty have shown that both girls and boys should have neuroradiologic imaging. Although in girls with CPP, hypothalamic hamartoma is the most common lesion, other tumors such as astrocytomas may present in this fashion; it is important not to miss the opportunity for an early diagnosis. Intracranial tumors causing CPP in girls are histologically specific, despite being in the same anatomic site involving the hypothalamus between the mamillary bodies and the median eminence, and may be related to the secretion of specific local growth factors. CPP may be caused by hypothalamic hamartomas, astrocytomas, optic gliomas, pineal tumors, and arachnoid cysts. Interestingly, some other suprasellar tumors such as craniopharyngiomas, germinomas, and LCH are only rarely associated with the development of gonadotropin-dependent precocious puberty, despite the lesion being in the same anatomic site. High-risk factors for the presence of an intracranial tumor in children with CPP are: a young age of onset (under age 3), high serum luteinizing hormone concentrations not associated with the development of a luteinizing hormone surge, and high serum leptin concentrations. However, it is impossible to exclude an intracranial lesion in a child with CPP without performing a magnetic resonance imaging (MRI) scan.[12,13] Diencephalic syndrome is a rare cause of failure to thrive in infancy and early childhood. The syndrome is characterized by profound emaciation despite normal or increased caloric intake, absence of cutaneous adipose tissue, locomotor hyperactivity, euphoria, and alertness. It commonly occurs in association with chiasmatic and hypothalamic gliomas. It has also been described in association with other lesions, such as midline cerebellar astrocytomas, suprasellar ependymomas, suprasellar spongioblastomas, and thalamic tumors.[14] Such children may even present to an eating disorder clinic, their growth failure attributed to an anorexic illness.[15]

The onset of diabetes insipidus (DI) with or without an evolving anterior pituitary endocrinopathy is suspicious of a space-occupying lesion. DI followed by an evolving anterior pituitary deficiency, including growth failure from GHD, is usually due to a sella/suprasellar tumor. Although DI is also common in midline cerebral malformations (such as septo-optic dysplasia), this usually follows or is contemporaneous with anterior pituitary failure.[16]

The term *Cushing's disease* describes the symptoms and signs of hypercortisolism due to a pituitary overproduction of adrenocorticotropic hormone. It must be distinguished from *Cushing's syndrome*, which results from any etiology causing glucocorticoid excess. Symptoms and signs of childhood Cushing's disease are similar to those of adults and have often been present for many years prior to the diagnosis: obesity, hirsutism, acne, moon facies, hypertension, buffalo hump on the back of the neck, muscular weakness, psychiatric disturbance, depression, and osteoporosis. However, the initial and most characteristic symptom in childhood is growth arrest; this combined with rapid weight gain should point to the diagnosis. In young children, Cushing's syndrome is usually of adrenal etiology, including McCune-Albright syndrome. However, in older children and adolescents, it is more likely to be Cushing's disease with excessive adrenocorticotropic hormone production from a tumor of the anterior pituitary.

Pituitary gigantism is a rare disorder due to growth hormone (GH) hypersecretion, usually secondary to an adenoma of the anterior pituitary. Overproduction of GH secretion is responsible for gigantism in a patient with open epiphyses and for acromegaly in a patient with closed epiphyses. The physical signs of GH excess are common to both disorders, but the signs in pituitary gigantism are usually less obvious because of the shorter duration of the endocrinopathy. From what data are available, surprisingly, such children appear to continue to grow for many years even after epiphyseal closure. GH-secreting tumors may occur in multiple endocrine neoplasia type 1 and McCune-Albright syndrome. Pituitary gigantism is a rare component of McCune-Albright syndrome, whereas the more usual manifestations are characteristic cutaneous pigmentation, polyostotic fibrous dysplasia, and gonadotropin-independent precocious puberty. Rarely, endocrine manifestations are adrenal dependent, Cushing's syndrome, thyrotoxicosis, and hyperparathyroidism.

The most common endocrine presentation of macroprolactinoma (more common in children and adolescents than micro-prolactinoma) is delayed/absent puberty due to prolactin (PRL) suppression of gonadotropin pulsatility, combined with gynecomastia in boys and galactorrhea in girls. The presentation may be part of multiple endocrine neoplasia type 1. Macroprolactinomas usually extend upward and encroach on the visual pathway and are often accompanied by visual field defects. It is important to measure the serum PRL in every child with pituitary enlargement, particularly before any surgery is contemplated.[17]

Isolated adrenocorticotropic hormone insufficiency may occur in lymphocytic hypophysitis, although this condition is not a malignant tumor but presents as the differential diagnosis of a central pituitary mass. This tumor usually occurs in the puerperium and is extremely rare in childhood.[18]

Patients with arachnoid cyst tended to be older at initial diagnosis than those with craniopharyngioma or Rathke's cleft cyst. Patients with craniopharyngioma generally present with a long duration of symptoms, especially visual symptoms. Mass effects, such as visual problems and headaches, are common symptoms of all three cystic lesions, but psychiatric symptoms, eating disorders, and calcification of solid tumor components on neuroimaging are characteristic of craniopharyngioma. Children are more likely to present with neurologic symptoms than adults.

Diagnosis

MRI scans have become the preferred diagnostic study for pediatric intracranial tumors. MRI is preferred under most circumstances, providing superior resolution and multiplanar imaging capabilities and avoiding the "spray" artifact from the petrous ridge that may obscure computed tomographic images of the base of the brain, without a radiation burden to the child. The administration of gadolinium diethylenetriamine-pentaacetic acid appears to be a safe and effective contrast agent for MRI and provides a more accurate method of imaging in the follow-up of brain tumors in pediatric patients. Where clinical suspicion remains (normal neuroradiologic imaging in patients with DI), scans reported as normal should be sent for expert review and consideration of repeat imaging with time. The intervals for scanning should also be guided clinically, since any set interval is empirical. MRI scan should be performed at a minimum of yearly intervals.[19] For lesions with a high frequency of cerebrospinal fluid dissemination, such as primitive neuroectodermal tumors and germ cell tumors, a neuraxis staging evaluation by spinal MRI, if not obtained preoperatively, should be performed approximately 2 weeks after surgery. In children with pineal region tumors, measurement of α-fetoprotein and β–human chorionic gonadotropin in the blood is useful for the diagnosis of malignant germ cell tumors (pineoblastomas); however, cerebrospinal fluid markers are of limited assistance. Placental alkaline phosphatase is a clinically useful tumor marker for primary intracranial germinoma.[20]

Thyroid function tests (as well as serum PRL concentration) are always required prior to surgery of a suspected pituitary tumor.[17] An elevated serum PRL concentration requires the distinction between stalk compression with moderate rise in PRL from the very high PRL concentrations associated with a PRL-secreting tumor. Macroprolactinomas usually have very high PRL secretion, and there is little ambiguity about the diagnosis. It is important to distinguish thyroid-stimulating hormone–secreting adenomas, which are extremely rare, from the pituitary hyperplasia associated with longstanding primary hypothyroidism. After prolonged, severe primary hypothyroidism with increased secretion of thyroid-stimulating hormone, the pituitary gland is usually increased in size and may attain a suprasellar extension and compression of the optic chiasm/nerves. This may be accompanied by a gonadal form of premature sexual maturation which is not true puberty (isolated breast development in girls and large testicular volumes with minimal virilization in boys).[21] These signs of premature maturation and pituitary enlargement decrease or resolve following the decrease in secretion of thyroid-stimulating hormone within 6 months of commencing appropriate thyroxin replacement.

Therapy

GENERAL PRINCIPLES OF TREATMENT

In general, the aim of therapy is to eradicate the tumor, with minimal morbidity and mortality, since prognosis is correlated with the extent of resection. If no biopsy has been obtained, histology will be undertaken postoperatively. Because the details of treatment for many types have evolved over time and likely will continue to evolve, treatment decisions for individual patients are best made in the context of a multidisciplinary "team" approach (Table 13-2). The neurosurgeons estimate the extent of resection, but it must be confirmed by computed tomography or MRI examination, preferably within the first 48 hours postoperatively. Postoperatively, computed tomography or MRI provides an objective assessment of the volume of residual tumor. These studies should be performed within 48 hours of surgery if possible to minimize the confounding effect of postsurgical enhancement around the operative bed. After diagnosis and initiation of treatment, follow-up imaging studies in children with malignant tumors are generally obtained every 3 months for 1 year, every 6 months for up to 5 years, and periodically thereafter. Imaging in benign tumors is typically obtained 3 to 6 months postoperatively and every 12 to 24 months thereafter for at least 5 years, the frequency largely depending on whether or not a complete resection has been confirmed on the initial postoperative scan. However, the optimal frequency of follow-up studies remains uncertain.

PERIOPERATIVE MANAGEMENT

Use of glucocorticoids to reduce peritumoral edema, cerebrospinal fluid diversion to treat hydrocephalus, anticonvulsants to prevent seizures, and hormonal replacement for patients with tumors in the hypothalamic-pituitary region are essential components of the perioperative management. Since edema commonly exacerbates the neurologic impairment produced by the tumor, glucocorticoids (e.g., dexamethasone 0.1 mg/kg/6 hours) are generally started preoperatively, continued intraoperatively, and then discontinued within 5 to 7 days postoperatively. In patients with pineal region tumors, a third ventriculostomy is a useful alternative to external ventricular drainage or shunt insertion. In patients with hypothalamic tumors, high doses of corticosteroids (e.g., hydrocortisone) are administered in the perioperative period unless dexamethasone is being used.

SURGICAL THERAPY

For the majority of pediatric brain tumors, direct open biopsy coupled with tumor resection is preferred. Although complete tumor removal is often feasible only for well-circumscribed benign tumors, a "near-complete" resection can be achieved with many parenchymal tumors, affording substantial cytoreduction and relieving symptoms of mass effect. Transsphenoidal approach for hypothalamic-pituitary tumors is possible over the age of approximately 8 years. In younger children, this approach is not usually possible due to the small size of the nasal passages and the nonaeration of the sphenoid sinus.

CHEMOTHERAPY

A radiosensitizing effect of certain drugs is often postulated. Among patients with malignant brain tumors, infants and very young children have the worst prognosis and the most severe treatment-related neurotoxic effects. Chemotherapy appears to be an effective primary postoperative treatment for many malignant brain tumors in young children. Disease control for 1 or 2 years in a large minority of patients permits a delay in the delivery of radiation and, on the basis of preliminary results, a reduction in neurotoxicity. For patients who had undergone total surgical resection or who had a complete response to chemotherapy, the results are sufficiently encouraging to suggest that radiation therapy may not be needed in this subgroup of children after at least 1 year of chemotherapy.[22] Also, a significant proportion of children with malignant brain tumors can avoid radiotherapy and prolonged maintenance chemotherapy yet still achieve durable remission by administering myeloablative consolidation chemotherapy with autologous bone marrow reconstitution after maximal surgical resection and conventional induction chemotherapy.[23] No long-term side effects on height, bone mineral density, body composition, and bone maturation were found in patients with leukemia treated with chemotherapy alone. It causes growth retardation, but catch-up growth occurs after cessation of treatment.[24] Gonadal damage after cyclophosphamide (dose related; may be reversible) and busulfan (the

Table 13-2. Management Scheme for Pediatric Intracranial Tumors

Tumor Type	Surgery	Radiotherapy	Chemotherapy
Chiasmatic-hypothalamic glioma	Exophytic lesions	Progressive lesions (older children)	Progressive lesions (young children)
Craniopharyngioma	Gross total resection Subtotal resection Stereotaxic approaches	Improves disease control after subtotal resection	No proven benefit (except for local cyst control)
Germinoma	Biopsy to establish diagnosis to determine if results equal those of radiotherapy with less morbidity	Effective therapy	Studies ongoing
Malignant germ cell tumors	Biopsy Gross total resection	Craniospinal	Platinum-based, appear beneficial
Pineal parenchymal tumors (pineoblastoma, pineocytoma)	Biopsy Gross total resection	Craniospinal for pineoblastoma	Probably beneficial for local or stereotaxic therapy for nondisseminated pineocytoma

association may cause permanent ovarian failure) is well documented in adults; it seems that prepubertal and pubertal ovaries are more resistant than ovaries of adults. Ovaries are more resistant than testes, and seminiferous tubules are more sensitive.[25]

RADIOTHERAPY

The indications for radiotherapy of pediatric intracranial tumors and the parameters for radiation delivery have evolved in several ways during the last decade. Tumors have conventionally been treated with 5000 to 6000 cGy in 180 to 200 cGy/day fractions using multiple portals. Newer approaches, such as hyperfractionated irradiation and interstitial irradiation (stereotactic radiosurgery and interstitial brachytherapy) attempt to improve therapeutic efficacy while minimizing irradiation of surrounding brain and correspondingly reduce toxicity. Nevertheless, because more children are surviving brain tumors following surgery and radiation therapy, the price of the successful therapy is being increasingly realized in terms of adverse effects, particularly in the very young child. Chemotherapy is increasingly used to delay or avoid using irradiation in children younger than 3 years of age with high-grade and incompletely resected low-grade tumors. Improvements in imaging and dose-delivery techniques have allowed radiotherapy administration to be tailored to the geometry of the tumor. Hyperfractionated irradiation technique is based on the premise that normal cells are better able than tumor cells to repair sublethal damage between doses and that multiple fractions are more likely to irradiate proliferating cells in a sensitive part of the cell cycle.[26] Finally, novel approaches for focal irradiation, such as stereotactic radiosurgery and interstitial brachytherapy, are increasingly being employed in selected unresectable lesions to provide high doses of radiation to the tumor while minimizing irradiation of surrounding brain.[27,28] Radiosurgery is ideally suited to the treatment of small foci of unresectable disease and has led to long-term disease control in well-circumscribed benign lesions. In addition, ongoing studies in older children with selected lesions, such as "standard-risk" medulloblastoma and germinoma, use reduced doses of radiotherapy in conjunction with chemotherapy to minimize radiation-induced neurotoxicity. For many low-grade gliomas that have been extensively resected, adjuvant therapy often is deferred because these tumors may remain quiescent for extended periods.

Sequelae of Treatment

The small increase in incidence noted over the past 2 decades most likely represents advancements in diagnostic technology rather than true changes in disease frequency, though this is controversial. Survivors of childhood intracranial tumors are 13 times more likely to die than healthy age- and sex-matched peers.[29] Disease recurrence remains the single most common cause of late deaths. The sequelae of surgical treatment are evident soon after the operation, but the sequelae of irradiation and chemotherapy become apparent over many decades. Neurologic, neurocognitive, and endocrine disturbances are the most prevalent disabilities observed among the long-term survivors of pediatric intracranial tumors. Maximum quality of life for the individual patient can only be achieved by long-term care and close cooperation of specialists in the different medical disciplines involved. It has been demonstrated that cranial irradiation has been implicated as the major cause for cognitive dysfunction. In that study, intellectual functioning was significantly lower in children whose treatment included cranial irradiation than in

those treated without cranial irradiation, and this effect was more pronounced in nonverbal than in verbal intellectual abilities.[30] Some authors also showed that children younger than 7 years at diagnosis had a mean IQ loss of 27 points, whereas children older than 7 years at diagnosis showed no significant decrease in IQ. They also demonstrated that decline in IQ occurred between baseline and year 2 of follow-up; none could be documented between years 2 and 4. All children younger than 7 years at diagnosis were receiving special education at follow-up; 50% of the children older than 7 years at diagnosis were receiving supplemental educational services.[30] In Packer's study, children demonstrated a wide range of dysfunction, including deficits in fine-motor, visual-motor, and visual-spatial skills and memory difficulties; although not retarded, they had a multitude of neurocognitive deficits that detrimentally affected school performance after 2 years from treatment. The younger the child is at the time of treatment, the greater is the likelihood and severity of damage.[31] Reimers and colleagues tried to identify subgroups of children who are at increased risk for cognitive deficits; they showed that younger age at diagnosis, tumor site in the cerebral hemisphere, hydrocephalus treated with a shunt, and treatment with radiation therapy were found to be significant predictors of lower cognitive function. Radiation therapy was the most important risk factor for impaired intellectual outcome. The mean observed full-scale IQ was 97 for the nonirradiated patients and 79 for the irradiated patients. Verbal IQ, but not performance and full-scale IQ, had a significant negative correlation to biological effective dose of irradiation to the tumor site.[32] Tumor involving the hypothalamic-pituitary area often produces a loss of endocrine function during a characteristic sequence in time, an evolving endocrinopathy. The risk of developing these adverse events is related to the underlying disease and its treatment with cytotoxic drugs and radiation therapy. The incidence and time course of disorders and the number of anterior pituitary hormones that are deficient depend on the sensitivity of the hormone itself to such therapy, on the dose, fractionation, and time elapsed since irradiation. Early detection and appropriate replacement therapy before clinical manifestations occur may carry important benefits in terms of normal pubertal and social development, growth, fertility, and bone mineralization.[33] The GH axis is the most sensitive and the adrenal axis the most resistant to the effects of direct irradiation to the hypothalamic-pituitary region. Patients who have received high doses (>30 Gy) of cranial, craniospinal, or total body irradiation are likely to develop GHD within 2 to 5 years from cessation of treatment.[34] Growth may be further impaired by spinal irradiation which directly interferes with spinal growth and is not due to an endocrinopathy.

In the rare syndrome of "growth without GH," normal or accelerated growth continues despite the patient having GHD, and this occurs at the expense of hyperphagia and rapid weight gain. It is considered that the etiology of this condition is related to insulin and insulin-like peptides, which allow growth in the presence of GH insufficiency. This phenomenon usually occurs after craniopharyngioma surgery. Indeed, the first sign of a recurrence of a treated intracranial tumor while on GH therapy may be growth deceleration.[35] GHD newborns can have a length within the normal range, which suggests that other growth factors dominate longitudinal gain during gestation. Obese children grow at a normal rate despite their low serum GH levels and reduced response to pharmacologic stimulation tests. Children with hypopituitarism secondary to craniopharyngioma resection may continue to grow and may even show growth rate acceleration if their weight increases significantly. Several possible mechanisms might underlie the growth stimulation in obese children, such as elevated levels of insulin and reduced levels of insulin-like growth factor binding protein 11. Recently, elevated sex hormone levels and elevated leptin levels in obese children were found to affect epiphyseal growth, and it may be that leptin also participates in the growth without GH observed in obesity, especially after craniopharyngioma removal. In the absence of GH, the sex hormones stimulate growth through a direct GH-independent effect on the epiphyses. Leptin, insulin, and sex hormones locally activate the insulin-like growth factor system in the epiphyseal growth plate.[36]

There is a correlation between the age at diagnosis (the immature hypothalamus may be more sensitive to irradiation), the dose of radiation given, different regimens, fractionation of irradiation, and pubertal development. Gonadal dysfunction can be induced by a direct injury to the gonads (hypergonadotropic hypogonadism) and less frequently by neuroendocrine injury to the hypothalamic-pituitary axis (hypogonadotropic hypogonadism).[37] Low doses of cranial irradiation (18 to 24 Gy) can cause precocious puberty, especially in girls, with a compromised growth spurt leading to a loss in final height, whereas delayed puberty has been reported after high doses (>40 Gy) used to treat solid tumors adjacent to the hypothalamus. Either low-dose cranial irradiation given as prophylaxis in the treatment of acute lymphoblastic leukemia, or high-dose irradiation for tumors distant from the hypothalamic-pituitary axis can cause hypogonadism.[38] The irradiation to the gonads from the spinal irradiation could potentially cause oligo/azoospermia with total doses of 6 Gy; the Leydig cell damage is common after total doses greater than 20 Gy.[39,40] Early menopause has been reported as well.[41] The possibility of using gonadotropin-releasing hormone agonists to prevent ovarian damage has been proposed. A number of treatment options for preserving fertility are available for cancer survivors. Sperm banking should be offered even to young adolescent boys. Sperm are present in urine from the early teens onward and can be obtained and banked. Ovary banking will be a technique in the future as some centers develop the procedures. Concern that residual cancer cells are not also banked with the ovarian cells is an issue still to be addressed. Cryopreservation of embryos is part of current practice and is useful in cases when couples desire it.[42] Further information on the ability of both ovary and uterus to sustain a pregnancy is crucial in deciding which treatment option to pursue. Pregnancy presents a cardiorespiratory stress; peripartum heart failure in women treated as children with anthracycline chemotherapy is a known complication.[43] Survivors who have been exposed to anthracycline therapy with or without radiation to the heart and those who received therapy known to induce pulmonary fibrosis or cardiopulmonary radiation therapy may benefit from a cardiac evaluation or pulmonary function test before pregnancy.[44] Delayed puberty development was reported in boys and girls after a total body irradiation (TBI) containing conditioning regimen, whereas patients given bone marrow transplantation for severe aplastic anemia (without total body irradiation) presented a normal puberty.[45] Other authors demonstrated that children who have been treated with a dose of 25 Gy for acute lymphoblastic leukemia at an early age (<7 years) had normal pubertal development. Girls who had a late presentation of acute lymphoblastic leukemia and a late treatment had delayed puberty.[37] Deficiency of thyroid-stimulating hormone, adrenocorticotropic hormone, and hyperprolactinemia can be seen following high-dose radiotherapy (>40 Gy) of the hypothalamic-pituitary axis, especially among young women.[46,47]

Patients in whom the pituitary stalk is injured during surgery often manifest a triphasic response of impaired fluid regulation characterized by an initial period of vasopressin insufficiency lasting 1 to 2 days, a subsequent period of inappropriate antidiuretic hormone release lasting several days, and a final phase of persistent DI. In view of the rapid changes in vasopressin secretion in the perioperative period, careful attention to fluid replacement and cautious administration of synthetic vasopressin, if needed, are essential to avoid electrolyte and fluid imbalance. The presence of DI may be masked by cortisol insufficiency and not revealed until glucocorticoids have been administered. One of the most difficult hypothalamic diseases to treat during childhood is hypoadipsia combined with DI. This usually results in difficult management of DI and repeated episodes of hypernatremia or hyponatremia associated with intercurrent infections, especially with gastroenteritis. The condition is usually managed by training the child to take a fixed fluid intake by mouth every hour, and then titrate the dose of vasopressin that is required. Although it is relatively easy to achieve homoeostasis when the child is well, the predominant problems revolve around intercurrent illnesses, especially if the child has concurrent anterior pituitary failure and has seizures treated with carbamazepine and/or lamotrigine; both interfere with fluid secretion from the renal tubules. It is unusual for children with adipsia and DI to survive childhood.

The incidence of second malignancies ranges from 1% to more than 3%. The majority of second tumors are thyroid cancer, malignant gliomas, meningiomas, and sarcomas that occur within radiotherapy treatment fields 10 to 20 years after irradiation. An increased incidence of hematologic malignancies has been noted after chemotherapy.[48] Thyroid ultrasound scan should be performed once a year. Cranial radiation has also been associated with carotid occlusive disease, which often manifests as Moyamoya syndrome with progressive ischemic cerebrovascular symptoms. This syndrome is particularly common in patients irradiated for parasellar lesions such as chiasmatic-hypothalamic gliomas.[49]

Treatment of Specific Tumors

The treatment of hypothalamic hamartoma is generally pharmacologic; surgical intervention is difficult and does not usually lead to resolution of the early puberty. The hamartoma usually remains the same size. Surgery would be very unlikely to be successful for the resolution of CPP. However, surgical resection, especially if the hamartoma is pedunculated, would be an option for frequent and inadequately controlled gelastic seizures.[50]

Lateralization using petrosal sinus sampling, as well as transsphenoidal surgical approach, is difficult in young children with adrenocorticotropic hormone–secreting adenoma. Plasma cortisol measurements the day after surgery will confirm surgical cure.

The treatment of a macroprolactinoma is medical and does not usually require surgery. However, in the occasional child who presents with chiasmal compression from a large mass lesion, resection may be performed urgently. Treatment with dopamine agonists, such as bromocriptine and cabergoline, usually results in rapid tumor shrinkage; additional treatment of surgery and/or radiotherapy may not be necessary. In a child who is awake and alert, with a large mass lesion that is producing substantial mass effect, resection is performed on the next operating day.

OPTIC CHIASMATIC–HYPOTHALAMIC GLIOMAS

Optic chiasmatic–hypothalamic gliomas have been considered benign tumors and self-limiting in growth potential because of their histologic appearance. Chiasmatic and chiasmatic-hypothalamic tumors are different entities. Most clinical series have reported significant morbidity and mortality, especially with the more extensive, posteriorly positioned tumors. The biological behavior of optic chiasmatic–hypothalamic gliomas is age dependent, with patients younger than 5 years and older than 20 years typically having tumors that exhibit aggressive growth. There are no specific pathologic features to help differentiate the clinical behavior of such tumors. The emergence of modern imaging techniques, including MRI, has facilitated the monitoring of the natural history of the disease and the determination of the effects of therapy. Most patients with optic chiasmatic–hypothalamic gliomas survive for many years. Management is controversial, partly related to failure to separate out those tumors involving the optic chiasm only (chiasmatic tumors) from those also involving the hypothalamus (chiasmatic-hypothalamic tumors). Some authors suggested a conservative treatment for patients with optic chiasmatic–hypothalamic gliomas in the context of neurofibromatosis type 1 (NF-1) without visual failure, with cerebrospinal fluid shunting for hydrocephalus, if present, and medical therapy for endocrine dysfunction.[51,52] For the chiasmatic-hypothalamic tumors, there was more morbidity and no prolongation of time to progression when radical resections were compared to more limited resections. However, over 90% of children with optic glioma without NF-1 will require some form of therapy.[53] Therefore, if surgery is performed, it may be appropriate to do a surgical procedure that strives only to provide a tissue diagnosis and to decompress the optic apparatus and/or ventricular system.[54] After tumor resection, patients whose vision is significantly compromised or who show progression of their disease on serial neuroimaging scans receive chemotherapy. A variety of regimens have been employed (e.g., carboplatinum, vincristine; and 6-thioguanine, procarbazine, dibromodulcitol), with response or stabilization rates of 75% to 100%.[55] Radiation therapy is effective in stabilization or improvement of vision and prevention of tumor progression in both optic pathway and chiasmatic-hypothalamic gliomas to children older than 5 years.[56] Optic chiasmatic–hypothalamic gliomas have an excellent long-term prognosis, with a 10-year survival of over 85%.[57]

Chemotherapy is an increasing component of the management of diencephalic gliomas. It can result in tumor shrinkage and significant disease control in some patients. However, decisions concerning the initiation of treatment should be based on the goals of treatment. Factors include age of the patient, whether the child has NF-1, tumor size and location, potential sequelae of radiotherapy, and the acute and long-term toxicity of the chemotherapeutic approach used. The erratic natural history of diencephalic tumors confounds evaluation of efficacy of the regimen chosen.

CYSTIC SELLA TUMORS

The distinction among craniopharyngioma, Rathke's cleft cyst, and intrasellar arachnoid cyst remains a difficult preoperative problem, although the presence of calcification makes the diagnosis of the former more likely. Accurate diagnosis of these rare pituitary lesions is important to determine the type of treatment and predict prognostic outcome. Only 10% of craniopharyngiomas are completely solid. The treatment of craniopharyngioma remains controversial. Although craniopharyngioma is a benign

tumor, its location makes even advanced microsurgical techniques difficult to perform because of its adherence to the optic chiasm, hypothalamus, and vessels of the circle of Willis. Despite advances in microsurgical techniques, the complete removal of the tumor is possible in only 66% to 90% of patients.[58] Radiosurgery avoids the shortcoming of surgical resection near the hypothalamic-pituitary axis, without the morbidity of open surgery.[59-61] In tumors with a large cystic component, stereotactic drainage or instillation of radioactive and/or chemotherapeutic agents have been used. Only several authors have reported the use of bleomycin for the treatment of recurrent cystic craniopharyngioma, although there is not an established protocol for using it. However, the risk of local complications after the administration of intratumoral bleomycin in these patients is around 10%, and some fatal toxic reactions have been recently reported.[62] Intracystic administration of bleomycin is a valid option as adjuvant therapy for craniopharyngioma in patients with recurrences that are not surgical candidates because of the high risk of complications. Other authors suggest that cystic lesions may be treated with intracavitary instillation of phosphorus-32 to deliver a cyst wall radiation dose of approximately 20,000 cGy.[63] If a treatment algorithm has been devised and followed that combines both surgery (radical and conservative) and radiotherapy (both external fractionated and intracyst instillations), long-term tumor control and minor disability are achieved. Endocrinologic deficits had the worst prognosis after surgery, especially DI combined with absent thirst. Tumor recurrence occurred both radiographically and clinically, typically in the first 3 to 4 years after surgery; this suggests a need for close surveillance initially with neuroimaging, particularly in younger children, and also clinical examination. Lack of calcification at diagnosis is associated with a tendency to remain free of relapse. Predictors of high morbidity included severe hydrocephalus, intraoperative adverse events, and age younger than 5 years at presentation. Large tumor size, young age, and severe hydrocephalus were predictors of tumor recurrence, whereas complete tumor resection (as determined by postoperative neuroimaging) and radiotherapy given electively after subtotal excision were less likely to be associated with recurrent disease. However, patients treated with surgery alone have a significantly worse freedom from progression when compared to patients treated with surgery and radiation therapy or radiation therapy alone.[58] In the extensive experience of Yasargil and colleagues from the University of Zurich, using an aggressive surgical approach, total resection was achieved in 90% of 144 patients, with an operative mortality rate of 16% and a good functional outcome in 67%.[59] In general, if total resection can be obtained, long-term control rate is between 50% and 80%; however, after subtotal resection, 50% to 100% of children experience local recurrence.[64,65] Since craniopharyngioma is potentially radioresponsive, external beam radiation therapy has long been used in the treatment of craniopharyngioma following incomplete surgical resection. Regine and Kramer reported a 60% 20-year survival rate in these patients.[66] In the series from the Royal Marsden Hospital, in 25 patients treated with salvage radiotherapy, the 15-year progression-free survival rate was 72%.[67] Recommended doses have ranged from 50 to 60 Gy in 180 to 200 cGy daily fractions.[68] Although the addition of fractionated postoperative radiation therapy has shown to reduce the recurrence rate, the incidence of hypothalamic and pituitary disorders is increased as seen with radical surgery.[58,69] Merchant and colleagues concluded that DI was the only endocrine deficiency that differed substantially in frequency between the groups treated with surgery and with radiotherapy, respectively.[70] Other complications of conventional radiation therapy include radiation necrosis, optic neuritis, and dementia. Obesity and the metabolic syndrome secondary to hypothalamic dysfunction seem to be important complications of craniopharyngioma treatment.[71]

PINEAL TUMORS

It is now recognized that the wide variety of tumor types found in the pineal region necessitates different modes of treatment; improved microsurgical and stereotactic surgical techniques have made mortality and morbidity rates acceptably low. The secondary deposits from pineal tumors, especially germinomas, are common in the suprasellar region. Benign teratomas, if resected totally, may require no further therapy; lesions that have been resected subtotally are treated with local radiotherapy.

Nondisseminated germinomas are highly radiosensitive. Nongerminomatous germ cell tumors are treated with craniospinal radiation and chemotherapy, but even with aggressive therapy, 5-year survival is less than 50%.[72-74] Pineoblastomas are considered to be primitive neuroectodermal tumors, and their treatment and outcome are comparable to those of high-risk medulloblastomas. Chemotherapy without radiotherapy appears to be ineffective therapy for young children and for children older than 18 months of age at diagnosis treated with craniospinal radiation therapy and chemotherapy.[75,76] Some authors concluded that most pineal cysts are clinically benign, and they should be followed up for many years.[77] Pineocytomas, although benign histologically, show a propensity for local recurrence and cerebrospinal fluid dissemination; these lesions have been treated with local or craniospinal radiotherapy and, in some cases, chemotherapy.

REFERENCES

1. Stiller CA, Nectoux J: International incidence of childhood brain and spinal tumours, Int J Epidemiol 23:458–464, 1994.
2. Keene DL, Hsu E, Ventureyra E: Brain tumors in childhood and adolescence, Pediatr Neurol 20:198–203, 1999.
3. Reed UC, Rosemberg S, Gherpelli JL, et al: Brain tumors in the first two years of life: a review of forty cases, Pediatr Neurosurg 19:180–185, 1993.
4. Rickert CH, Probst-Cousin S, Gullotta F: Primary intracranial neoplasms of infancy and early childhood, Childs Nerv Syst 13:507–513, 1997.
5. Pollack IF: Brain tumors in children [Review], N Engl J Med 331:1501–1507, 1994.
6. Rorke LB: The cerebellar medulloblastoma and its relationship to primitive neuroectodermal tumors, J Neuropathol Exp Neurol 42:1–15, 1983.
7. Albright AL: Pediatric brain tumors, CA Cancer J Clin 43:272–288, 1993.
8. Pollack IF: Pediatric brain tumors [Review], Semin Surg Oncol 16:73–90, 1999.
9. Stanhope R, Adams J, Brook CG: Disturbances of puberty, Clin Obstet Gynaecol 12:557–577, 1985.
10. De Sanctis V, Corrias A, Rizzo V, et al: Etiology of central precocious puberty in males: The results of the Italian Study Group for Physiopathology of Puberty, J Pediatr Endocrinol Metab 13:687–693, 2000.
11. Cisternino M, Arrigo T, Pasquino AM, et al: Etiology and age incidence of precocious puberty in girls: a multicentric study, J Pediatr Endocrinol Metab 13:695–701, 2000.
12. Chemaitilly W, Trivin C, Adan L, et al: Central precocious puberty: clinical and laboratory features, Clin Endocrinol (Oxf) 54:289–294, 2001.
13. Stanhope R: Central precocious puberty and occult intracranial tumours, Clin Endocrinol (Oxf) 54:287–288, 2001.
14. Russell A: A diencephalic syndrome of emaciation in infancy and childhood, Arch Dis Child 26:274, 1951.
15. De Vile CJ, Sufraz R, Lask BD, et al: Occult intracranial tumours masquerading as early onset anorexia nervosa, Br Med J 311:1359–1360, 1995.
16. Mootha SL, Barkovich AJ, Grumbach MM, et al: Idiopathic hypothalamic diabetes insipidus, pituitary stalk thickening, and the occult intracranial germinoma in children and adolescents, J Clin Endocrinol Metab 82:1362–1367, 1997.
17. Torpiano J, Vanderpump M, Stanhope R: The management of sellar masses: not all pituitary tumours require surgery for diagnosis and/or therapy, J Pediatr Endocrinol Metab 17:663–664, 2004.
18. Cemeroglu AP, Blaivas M, Muraszko KM, et al: Lymphocytic hypophysitis presenting with diabetes insipidus in a 14-year-old girl: case report and review of the literature, Eur J Pediatr 156:684–688, 1997.
19. Sherwood MC, Stanhope R, Preece MA, et al: Diabetes insipidus and occult intracranial tumours, Arch Dis Child 61:1222–1224, 1986.
20. Shinoda J, Yamada H, Sakai N, et al: Placental alkaline phosphatase as a tumor marker for primary intracranial germinoma, J Neurosurg 68:710–720, 1988.
21. Pringle PJ, Stanhope R, Hindmarsh P, et al: Abnormal pubertal development in primary hypothyroidism, Clin Endocrinol (Oxf) 28:479–486, 1988.
22. Duffner PK, Horowitz ME, Krischer JP, et al: Postoperative chemotherapy and delayed radiation in children less than three years of age with malignant brain tumors, N Engl J Med 328:1725–1731, 1993.
23. Mason WP, Grovas A, Halpern S, et al: Intensive chemotherapy and bone marrow rescue for young children with newly diagnosed malignant brain tumors, J Clin Oncol 16:210–221, 1998.
24. Van der Sluis I, van der Heuvel-Eibrink MM, Hahlen K, et al: Bone mineral density, body composition, and height in long term survivors of acute lymphoblastic leukemia in childhood, Med Pediatr Oncol 35:415–420, 2000.
25. Kumar R, Biggart JD, McEvoy J, et al: Cyclophosphamide and reproductive function, Lancet 1:1212–1214, 1972.
26. Packer RJ, Boyett JM, Zimmerman RA, et al: Hyperfractionated radiotherapy (72 Gy) for children with brain stem gliomas. A Children's Cancer Group Phase I/II Trial, Cancer 72:1414–1421, 1993.
27. Grabb PA, Lunsford LD, Albright AL, et al: Stereotactic radiosurgery for glial neoplasms of childhood, Neurosurgery 38:696–702, 1996.
28. McDermott MW, Gutin PH, Larson DA, et al: Interstitial brachytherapy [Review], Neurosurg Clin North Am 1:801–824, 1990.
29. Sklar CA: Childhood brain tumors, J Pediatr Endocrinol Metab 15(Suppl):669, 2002.
30. Radcliffe J, Packer RJ, Atkins TE, et al: Three- and four-year cognitive outcome in children with noncortical brain tumors treated with whole-brain radiotherapy, Ann Neurol 32:551–554, 1992.
31. Packer RJ, Sutton LN, Atkins TE, et al: A prospective study of cognitive function in children receiving whole-brain radiotherapy and chemotherapy: 2-year results, J Neurosurg 70:707–713, 1989.
32. Reimers TS, Ehrenfels S, Mortensen EL, et al: Cognitive deficits in long-term survivors of childhood brain tumors: identification of predictive factors, Med Pediatr Oncol 40:26–34, 2003.
33. Cohen LE: Endocrine late effects of cancer treatment, Curr Opin Pediatr 15:3–9, 2003.
34. Livesey EA, Hindmarsh PC, Brook CG, et al: Endocrine disorders following treatment of childhood brain tumours, Br J Cancer 61:622–625, 1990.
35. Locatelli F, Giorgiani G, Pession A, et al: Late effects in children after bone marrow transplantation: a review, Haematologica 78:319–328, 1993.
36. Phillip M, Moran O, Lazar L: Growth without growth hormone, J Pediatr Endocrinol Metab 15(Suppl):1267–1272, 2002.
37. Hughes IA, Napier A, Thompson EN: Pituitary-gonadal function in children treated for acute lymphoblastic leukaemia, Acta Paediatr Scand 69:691–692, 1980.
38. Rappaport R, Brauner R, Czernichow P, et al: Effect of hypothalamic and pituitary irradiation on pubertal development in children with cranial tumors, J Clin Endocrinol Metab 54:1164–1168, 1982.
39. Castillo LA, Craft AW, Kernahan J, et al: Gonadal function after 12-Gy testicular irradiation in childhood acute lymphoblastic leukaemia, Med Pediatr Oncol 18:185–189, 1990.
40. Leiper AD, Grant DB, Chessells JM: Gonadal function after testicular radiation for acute lymphoblastic leukaemia, Arch Dis Child 61:53–56, 1986.
41. Byrne J: Infertility and premature menopause in childhood cancer survivors, Med Pediatr Oncol 33:24–28, 1999.
42. Edwards RG, Morcos S, Macnamee M, et al: High fecundity of amenorrhoeic women in embryo-transfer programmes, Lancet 338:292–294, 1991.
43. Katz A, Goldenberg I, Maoz C, et al: Peripartum cardiomyopathy occurring in a patient previously treated with doxorubicin, Am J Med Sci 314:399–400, 1997.
44. Collis CH: Chemotherapy-related morbidity to the lungs. In Plowman PN, McElwain TJ, Meadows AT, editors: Complications of Cancer Management, Guildford, England, 1991, Butterworth Scientific Ltd, pp 250–271.
45. Sanders JE: The impact of marrow transplant preparative regimens on subsequent growth and development. The Seattle Marrow Transplant team, Semin Hematol 28:244–249, 1991.
46. Ogilvy-Stuart AL, Clark DJ, Wallace WH, et al: Endocrine deficit after fractionated total body irradiation, Arch Dis Child 67:1107–1110, 1992.
47. Wittert G, Donald RA, Espiner EA, et al: The hormonal effects of pituitary surgery and irradiation: a review of 59 cases, N Z Med J 98:93–97, 1985.
48. Hawkins MM, Draper GJ, Kingston JE: Incidence of second primary tumours among childhood cancer survivors, Br J Cancer 56:339–347, 1987.
49. Bitzer M, Topka H: Progressive cerebral occlusive disease after radiation therapy, Stroke 26:131–136, 1995.
50. de Brito VN, Latronico AC, Arnhold IJ, et al: Treatment of gonadotropin dependent precocious puberty due to hypothalamic hamartoma with gonadotropin releasing hormone agonist depot, Arch Dis Child 80:231–234, 1999.
51. Alshail E, Rutka JT, Becker LE, et al: Optic chiasmatic-hypothalamic glioma, Brain Pathol 7:799–806, 1997.
52. Wisoff JH, Abbott R, Epstein F: Surgical management of exophytic chiasmatic-hypothalamic tumors of childhood, J Neurosurg 73:661–667, 1990.
53. Jenkin D, Angyalfi S, Becker L, et al: Optic glioma in children: surveillance, resection or irradiation? Int J Radiat Oncol Biol Phys 25:215–225, 1993.
54. Steinbok P, Hentschel S, Almqvist P, et al: Management of optic chiasmatic/hypothalamic astrocytomas in children, Can J Neurol Sci 29:132–138, 2002.

55. Gajjar A, Heideman RL, Kovnar EH, et al: Response of pediatric low grade gliomas to chemotherapy [Review], Pediatr Neurosurg 19:113–120, 1993.
56. Erkal HS, Serin M, Cakmak A: Management of optic pathway and chiasmatic-hypothalamic gliomas in children with radiation therapy, Radiother Oncol 45:11–15, 1997.
57. Pollack IF, Claassen D, al-Shboul Q, et al: Low-grade gliomas of the cerebral hemispheres in children: an analysis of 71 cases, J Neurosurg 82:536–547, 1995.
58. De Vile CJ, Grant DB, Kendall BE, et al: Management of childhood craniopharyngioma: Can the morbidity of radical surgery be predicted? Neurosurg 85:73–81, 1996.
59. Yasargil MG, Curcic M, Kis M, et al: Total removal of craniopharyngiomas. Approaches and long-term results in 144 patients, J Neurosurg 73:3–11, 1990.
60. Carmel PW: Craniopharyngiomas. In Wilkins RH, Rengachary SS, editors: Neurosurgery, New York, 1985, McGraw-Hill, pp 905–916.
61. Pang D: Surgical management of craniopharyngioma. In Sekhar LN, Janecka IP, editors: Surgery of Cranial Base Tumors, New York, 1993, Raven Press, pp 787–807.
62. Hader WJ, Steinbok P, Hukin J, et al: Intratumoral therapy with bleomycin for cystic craniopharyngiomas in children, Pediatr Neurosurg 33:211–218, 2000.

63. Pollock BE, Lunsford LD, Kondziolka D, et al: Phosphorus-32 intracavitary irradiation of cystic craniopharyngiomas: current technique and long-term results, Int J Radiat Oncol Biol Phys 33:437–446, 1995.
64. Kalapurakal JA, Goldman S, Hsieh YC, et al: Clinical outcome in children with craniopharyngioma treated with primary surgery and radiotherapy deferred until relapse, Med Pediatr Oncol 40:214–218, 2003.
65. Kalapurakal JA, Goldman S, Hsieh YC, et al: Clinical outcome in children with recurrent craniopharyngioma after primary surgery, Cancer J 6:388–393, 2000.
66. Regine WF, Kramer S: Pediatric craniopharyngiomas: long term results of combined treatment with surgery and radiation, Int J Radiat Oncol Biol Phys 24:611–617, 1992.
67. Bloom HJG: Combined modality therapy for intracranial tumors, Cancer 35:111–120, 1975.
68. Tarbell N, Barnes P, Scott RM, et al: Advances in radiation therapy for craniopharyngiomas, Pediatr Neurosurg 21(Suppl):101–107, 1994.
69. Honegger J, Buchfelder M, Fahlbusch R: Surgical treatment of craniopharyngiomas: endocrinological results, J Neurosurg 90:251–257, 1999.
70. Merchant TE, Kiehna EN, Sanford RA, et al: Craniopharyngioma: the St. Jude Children's Research Hospital experience 1984–2001, Int J Radiat Oncol Biol Phys 53:533–542, 2002.

71. Harz KJ, Muller HL, Waldeck E, et al: Obesity in patients with craniopharyngioma: assessment of food intake and movement counts indicating physical activity, J Clin Endocrinol Metab 88:5227–5231, 2003.
72. Regis J, Bouillot P, Rouby-Volot F, et al: Pineal region tumors and the role of stereotactic biopsy: review of the mortality, morbidity, and diagnostic rate in 370 cases, Neurosurgery 39:907–914, 1996.
73. Edwards MS, Hudgins RJ, Wilson CB, et al: Pineal region tumors in children, J Neurosurg 68:689–697, 1988.
74. Balmaceda C, Heller G, Rosenblum M, et al: Chemotherapy without irradiation—a novel approach for newly diagnosed CNS germ cell tumors: results of an international cooperative trial, J Clin Oncol 14:2908–2915, 1996.
75. Jakacki RI, Zeltzer PM, Boyett JM, et al: Survival and prognostic factors following radiation and/or chemotherapy for primitive neuroectodermal tumors of the pineal region in infants and children: a report of the Children's Cancer Group, J Clin Oncol 13:1377–1383, 1995.
76. Dirks PB, Harris L, Hoffman HJ, et al: Supratentorial primitive neuroectodermal tumors in children, J Neurooncol 29:75–84, 1996.
77. Mandera M, Marcol W, Bierzynska-Macyszyn G, et al: Pineal cysts in childhood, Childs Nerv Syst 19:750–775, 2003.

Chapter 14

VASOPRESSIN, DIABETES INSIPIDUS, AND THE SYNDROME OF INAPPROPRIATE ANTIDIURETIC HORMONE SECRETION

DAVID CARMODY, MARK JOHN HANNON, and CHRIS THOMPSON

In humans, normal cellular function is dependent on normal tonicity of the extracellular fluid. To maintain normal extracellular tonicity, sophisticated regulation of water homeostasis—the process of osmoregulation—is needed. Osmoregulation is dependent on the integration of the production and action of vasopressin, the antidiuretic actions of vasopressin on the renal collecting ducts, and normal regulation of thirst and fluid intake.

In this chapter, we discuss the physiologic production and action of vasopressin and its interaction with the regulation of thirst. We then apply these physiologic principles to the pathophysiologic mechanisms that serve as the basis for diabetes insipidus and the syndrome of inappropriate antidiuretic hormone.

Vasopressin

SYNTHESIS AND SECRETION

Arginine vasopressin (AVP) is a polypeptide that contains nine amino acids, with a disulfide bridge between cysteine residues, and considerable structural homology with oxytocin, which also is secreted from the posterior pituitary (Fig. 14-1).[1] Vasopressin is synthesized predominantly in the magnocellular neurons in the paraventricular (PVN) and supraoptic (SON) nuclei of the anterior hypothalamus (Fig. 14-2). The cell bodies of the vasopressinergic neurons in the PVN and SON have axonal projections that connect to the posterior pituitary gland.

In addition to magnocellular neurons, which project from the SON and the PVN to the posterior pituitary, parvocellular vasopressinergic neurons are present in the PVN and the suprachiasmatic nucleus.[2] These smaller neurons project via the median eminence to the portal vascular system of the anterior pituitary while secreting vasopressin and corticotropin-releasing factor (CRF); they stimulate secretion of adrenocorticotropic hormone (ACTH) from the anterior pituitary gland. Some parvocellular vasopressinergic neurons also project from the PVN to the forebrain, brain stem, and spinal cord. Vasopressin is released into the central nervous system, where it acts as a neurotransmitter and/or a neuromodulator.[3]

The gene that encodes the AVP precursor is expressed mainly in the hypothalamus but also in other tissues, including adrenal glands, gonads, cerebellum, and pituicytes in the posterior pituitary. It is structurally closely related to the gene that codes for the oxytocin (OT) precursor, which is expressed in different populations of hypothalamic magnocellular neurons. The vasopressin and oxytocin genes are closely linked in a tail-to-tail orientation on chromosome 20 with an intergenic region of 12 kb.[4] Significant posttranslational processing is needed to form

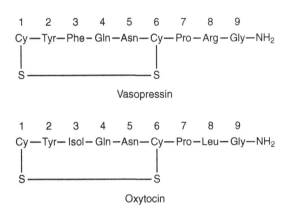

FIGURE 14-1. Amino acid structure of vasopressin and oxytocin. Note that only positions 3 and 8 have different amino acids.

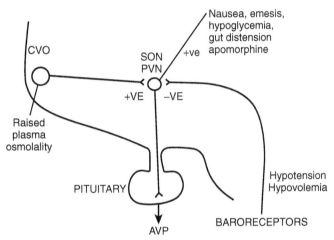

FIGURE 14-2. Factors governing arginine vasopressin (AVP) secretion. *CVO,* Circumventricular organ (site of osmoreceptors); *PVN,* paraventricular nuclei; *SON,* supraoptic nuclei.

the mature hormone. The posttranslational product prepro-AVP-NPII is the precursor from which AVP is derived.[4] The precursor consists of a signal peptide, AVP, neurophysin II (NPII; 95 amino acids), and a glycopeptide, copeptin (39 amino acids).

Neurophysin II is cleaved from prepro-AVP-NPII but remains complexed together with AVP before it is secreted into the bloodstream by exocytosis. Vasopressinergic neurons open voltage-gated calcium channels in nerve terminal membranes. This transient calcium ion influx results in fusion of neurosecretory granules with the nerve terminal membrane, as well as release of AVP and NPII in equimolar amounts into the circulation.[5] Copeptin, although of unknown biological significance, may be a stable indirect marker of AVP release.

Magnocellular neurons in the supraoptic and paraventricular nuclei synthesize vasopressin within their cell bodies. The hormone is carried within neurosecretory granules down the predominantly unmyelinated axons of the magnocellular neurons, in the supraoptic-hypophyseal tract, at a speed of 2 mm per hour. The precursor undergoes successive cleavage by basic endopeptidases.[6] These axons terminate in the posterior pituitary, which is rich in fenestrated capillaries.

CELLULAR ACTION OF VASOPRESSIN

Vasopressin binds to seven transmembrane, G-protein–coupled receptors on the plasma membrane of target cells. Three sub-

types of vasopressin receptor exist (V1-V3) with distinct distribution, actions, and signal transduction.[7,8]

The V1 Receptor

The V1 receptor is found in vascular smooth muscle, liver, platelets, and multiple sites in the central nervous system. It is a 418 amino acid protein linked to the phosphinositol signaling pathway. Binding of AVP to the receptor causes activation of Gq/11-mediated phospholipase C, resulting in an increase in intracellular calcium.

Binding of AVP to V1 receptors at physiologic plasma concentrations has been shown to exert a weak pressor effect.[8a] The vasocontriction seen with vasopressin is most notable in the splanchnic, renal, and hepatic artery beds[9-11] and has given rise to the successful use of the hormone in the treatment of bleeding esophageal varicies. At higher plasma concentrations, for instance, in response to significant hypotension or hypovolemia, vasopressin has been shown to have a significant pressor effect.[12] A highly selective V1 vasopressin analogue has been shown to have similar effects in patients with sepsis.[13] Rebound hypotension on withdrawal of treatment coupled with concerns regarding reduced cardiac output, pulmonary hypertension, hyponatremia, and bowel ischemia, has limited the widespread use of vasopressin in the setting of septic shock.

The V2 Receptor

The V2 receptor is predominantly expressed on the basolateral membrane of the distal convoluting tubule and collecting ducts. Binding of AVP to renal V2 receptors stimulates the recruitment of selective water channels (aquaporins), which allow reabsorption of renal tubular water and concentration of urine. Extrarenal effects of V2 activation include factor VII release from hepatocytes and release of von Willebrand factor from vascular endothelium. AVP also causes activation of liver glycogen phosphorylase with release of glucose into the circulation.

When AVP binds to the V2 receptors on the basolateral membrane of the cells of the collecting ducts, it triggers an increase in cytoplasmic cyclic adenosine monophosphate (cAMP), which activates protein kinase (Fig. 14-3). Subsequently, movement of stored aquaporin-2 to the luminal membrane of the cell occurs. Aquaporin-2 forms tetramers in the cell membrane, with each monomer acting as a water channel[14]; this allows passage of tubular water into the cell. Free water reabsorption from the distal nephron and thus urine concentration are directly influenced by serum vasopressin levels. This relationship was established prior to the discovery of aquaporins. The AVP/V2 receptor interaction also simultaneously causes an increase in expression of the aquaporin-2 gene, with increased generation of mRNA for aquaporin-2.

The V3 Receptor

The V3 receptor is found on corticotropic cells in the anterior pituitary. In isolation, AVP is a weak ACTH secretagogue, but when it acts synergistically with CRF, it causes significant secretion of ACTH, which is physiologically important. Parvocellular neurons, which coexpress AVP and CRF, project via the median eminence and terminate in the hypophyseal portal bed, which provides circulation to the anterior pituitary. AVP and CRF expression by these parvocellular neurons is subject to negative feedback control by glucocorticoids.[15-17] AVP has no secretagogue properties with respect to the other anterior pituitary hormones.

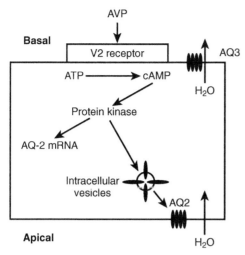

FIGURE 14-3. Arginine vasopressin (AVP) binds to the V2 receptor and stimulates movement of aquaporin-2 (AQ2) to the apical membrane, where it forms a water channel for reabsorption of water (H_2O). Water moves through the apical membrane to the blood via aquaporin-3 (AQ3).

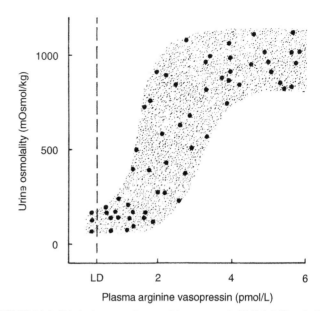

FIGURE 14-4. Relation between plasma arginine vasopressin (AVP) (pAVP) and urine osmolality. Data were obtained during water loading and fluid restriction in a group of healthy adults. Maximal urine concentration is achieved by pAVP values of 3 to 4 pmol/L. LD, Limit of detection of the AVP assay, 0.3 pmol/L.

Regulation of Vasopressin Release

OSMOREGULATION OF VASOPRESSIN RELEASE

Plasma osmolality in healthy man varies by only 1% to 2% in physiologic conditions where there is free access to water. This precise regulation of plasma osmolality is maintained by the homeostatic process of osmoregulation.[18]

Changes in plasma osmolality are detected by specialized osmoreceptor cells in the anterior hypothalamus (see Fig. 14-2). Fenestrations in the blood-brain barrier cause the magnocellular cells of the circumventricular organs—the subfornical organ and the organum vasculosum lamina terminalis—to be bathed in plasma. Changes in plasma osmolality cause these hypothalamic nuclei to depolarize, sending neural signals, via the nucleus medianus, to the supraoptic and paraventricular nuclei. Elevation in plasma osmolality causes depolarization of these nuclei, leading to increased synthesis of AVP and secretion of AVP from the posterior pituitary. The osmoreceptor cells are solute specific, in that they respond vigorously to changes in plasma sodium concentration but less so to variations in blood urea.[19] They respond to mannitol but are completely insensitive to changes in blood glucose concentration in experimental situations.

A linear relationship has been noted between plasma osmolality and plasma AVP concentrations throughout the physiologic range of plasma tonicity.[20-22] If plasma concentrations are lowered by excessive ingestion of hypotonic fluid to below 280 to 285 mOsm/kg, secretion of AVP is suppressed, and plasma concentrations of the hormone are undetectable on radioimmunoassay measurement. In the absence of AVP-mediated water reabsorption from the kidney, hypotonic polyuria develops.[22] The increase in free water clearance allows plasma osmolality to rise into the normal range. If plasma osmolality rises, owing to dehydration, plasma concentrations of AVP increase in proportion to the rise in plasma osmolality. The action of AVP in concentrating the urine and allowing reabsorption of water restores plasma osmolality to normal. This homeostatic process occurs continuously to maintain plasma osmolality within a narrow reference range. The relationship between plasma AVP concentration and urine osmolality is shown in Fig. 14-4.

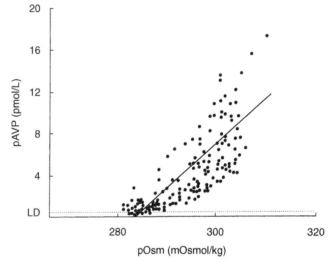

FIGURE 14-5. Relation between plasma osmolality (pOsm) and plasma arginine vasopressin (AVP) (pAVP). Increases in pAVP in response to hypertonicity induced by infusion of 855 mmol/L saline in a group of healthy adults. The mean regression line (dashed line) is defined by the following equation: pAVP = 0.43 (pOsm 284); r = 0.96; P < .001. LD, Limit of detection of the AVP assay, 0.3 pmol/L.

The development of sensitive radioimmunoassays has allowed the nature of this relationship to be studied experimentally. When intravenous infusion of hypertonic sodium chloride solution is used to increase plasma osmolality in healthy volunteers, plasma AVP can be shown to increase in a linear fashion. Application of linear regression analysis to the data shows that a direct correlation defines the relationship between plasma osmolality and plasma AVP concentration (Fig. 14-5). The qualitative relationship is expressed by the following equation:

$$pAVP = 0.43(pOsm - 284)$$

where pAVP indicates plasma AVP concentration, and pOsm indicates plasma osmolality.[23]

This mathematical formula describes two important physiologic characteristics of the relationship between plasma osmolality and plasma AVP that are clinically relevant. The first of these is the osmotic threshold for AVP release, which is defined by the abscissal intercept of the regression line. At a mean plasma osmolality of 284 mOsm/kg, plasma AVP is secreted, with increments in secretion as plasma osmolality rises. This represents the "set point," or the osmotic threshold for AVP release, which is identical in man to the osmotic threshold for the onset of thirst.[23] This is an important physiologic concept, as hypotonic polyuria develops when plasma osmolality is suppressed by water ingestion to concentrations below this "set point." Therefore, AVP detectable in the plasma by radioimmunoassay at plasma osmolalities below this is, by definition, "inappropriately" elevated. Measurements of plasma AVP with ultrasensitive cytochemical methods at plasma osmolalities below the physiologic threshold have led to suggestions that secretion cannot be completely suppressed by hypotonicity,[24] although the very low concentrations demonstrated experimentally could equally represent incomplete clearance of pre-secreted AVP.

The slope of the regression line, which represents the change in plasma AVP concentration per unit change in plasma osmolality, is the second important characteristic of the formula. This defines the sensitivity of the osmoreceptor-AVP releasing unit. Steeper slopes indicate a larger rise in plasma AVP concentrations after osmotic stimulation. Shallow slopes indicate lower rates of AVP secretion in response to hyperosmolality; a pathologic example of this can be seen in partial hypothalamic diabetes insipidus.[25]

In a few rare cases, complete disconnection of AVP-secreting neurons from their osmoreceptors has been described. The pathologic abnormality is persistent low-grade AVP release, despite plasma osmolalities that may fall below the osmotic threshold.[26] AVP secretion can be increased to above this "basal" rate by stimulation of osmoreceptors, but secretion is never switched off entirely. It is hypothesized that some cells exert an inhibitory effect on AVP release, and if these cells malfunction, AVP secretion is abnormally continuous.

The osmotic threshold and sensitivity of AVP release vary significantly between individuals, but repeat testing has shown good reproducibility of these parameters within individuals.[27] Studies in twins have suggested that the characteristics of the osmoregulatory line may be genetically determined, given that they are similar in monozygous but not dizygous twins.[28]

Although physiologic control of AVP secretion and thirst is almost entirely osmotic, the switch-off of the two is nonosmotic and is triggered by the act of drinking. In studies in healthy men who have been rendered hyperosmolar by hypertonic saline infusion[29] or by dehydration,[30] drinking is associated with an immediate fall in plasma AVP and thirst, before any changes in plasma osmolality can be measured. The fall in plasma AVP is so rapid that it mimics the half-life of AVP,[29] suggesting that a neuroendocrine reflex, stimulated by oropharyngeal distention, switches off AVP secretion.

The conventional relationship between plasma osmolality and plasma AVP concentration is altered in a number of physiologic and pathophysiologic situations. Pregnancy causes a lowering of the threshold for AVP secretion in both rats[31] and humans,[32] which is responsible for the fall in basal plasma sodium concentration during pregnancy. The sensitivity of the osmoregulatory line remains unchanged. The mechanism is unclear but may be related to increased plasma concentrations of human chorionic gonadotropin (hCG). In the luteal phase of the ovulatory cycle, a small but significant decrease in plasma osmolality also occurs as a result of downward resetting of the osmotic thresholds for thirst and AVP release.[33]

Normal physiologic aging is associated with complex changes in osmoregulation.[34] Basal circulating AVP concentrations increase with age, and the AVP response to osmotic stimulation has been shown to be enhanced in comparison with that in younger subjects.[35,36] Thirst, as measured by visual analogue scales, is attenuated, however, and measured water intake after osmotic stimulation intake is reduced.[37] This makes elderly humans more vulnerable to hypernatremia; many elderly patients in long-term care institutions exhibit permanent hypernatremia, although cognitive impairment may contribute to reduced thirst in these individuals.[38]

Osmoregulation in diabetes mellitus seems normal,[39] even in the presence of hypernatremia,[40] with preserved solute specificity of both AVP release and thirst; hyperglycemia stimulates neither thirst nor AVP secretion. Chronic hyperglycemia renders the renal tubules resistant to the antidiuretic effects of AVP, however, as the result of failure of recruitment of aquaporin-2.[41] Improved glycemic control reverses the state of partial nephrogenic diabetes insipidus.[41] Survivors of HONK, however, show typical osmoregulatory changes of aging, with exaggerated AVP secretion and attenuated thirst in response to dehydration.[42]

BAROREGULATION OF VASOPRESSIN RELEASE

Although small variations in plasma osmolality can have profound effects on AVP secretion, physiologic fluctuations in blood pressure have almost no effect on plasma AVP secretion. However, pathophysiologic falls in both blood volume and pressure can stimulate AVP secretion. Although small falls in arterial blood pressure (on the order of 10%) have been shown to slightly increase plasma AVP concentrations (see Fig. 14-5), larger falls of 20% to 30% are required to stimulate sufficient AVP to exert a compensatory pressor effect.[43,44] This makes teleologic sense as falls in blood pressure of up to 10% are common during a daily cycle, and if AVP were stimulated by these small falls, humans would be in a permanent state of antidiuresis. The relationship between blood pressure and plasma AVP is shown in Fig. 14-6.

The baroreceptors are situated in the cardiac atria, the carotid sinus, and the aortic arch. They exert a tonic inhibitory effect on AVP secretion in normal circumstances, but when they are unloaded during hypotension or hypovolemia, they can stimulate very high plasma concentrations of AVP via pathways that are separate from the osmoreceptors. The relation between blood pressure and AVP is exponential rather than linear and can be modified by neurohumoral influences such as atrial natriuretic peptides, which inhibit AVP responses, and norepinephrine, which augments baroregulatory AVP responses.[45] Baroregulatory inputs also modify osmotic AVP secretion, in that hypovolemia augments the AVP response to hypernatremia.[46,47]

OTHER MECHANISMS REGULATING VASOPRESSIN RELEASE

In addition to osmotic and baroregulatory stimuli, AVP secretion occurs in response to nausea,[48,49] manipulation of abdominal contents at surgery,[50] and hypoglycemia.[51] All of these secretagogues stimulate AVP secretion independently of the osmotic pathways.

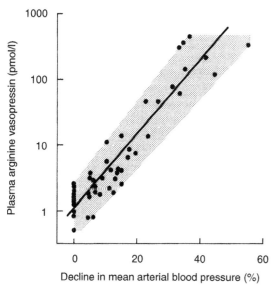

FIGURE 14-6. Relation of plasma arginine vasopressin (AVP) (pAVP) to the percentage decline in mean arterial blood pressure (MABP). Arterial blood pressure was reduced by infusing increasing doses of trimetaphan in healthy men. The regression line is defined by the following equation: log (pAVP) = 0.06 (MABP 0.67); r = 0.98; P < .001; N = 48.

Table 14-1. Causes of Diabetes Insipidus

Hypothalamic DI

Congenital	Hereditary (X-linked or AD)
	DIDMOAD
Acquired	Pituitary surgery
	Tumors (craniopharyngioma, germinoma, pinealoma, metastases)
	Traumatic brain injury
	Granuloma (TB, sarcoid, histiocytosis X)
	Infection (encephalitis, meningitis)
	Vascular disorder (Sheehan's syndrome, aneurysms, subarachnoid hemorrhage, GI bleed)
	Hypophysitis (A/immune, lymphocytic)
	Idiopathic
	Pregnancy

Nephrogenic DI

Congenital	Hereditary (X-linked recessive or AD)
Acquired	Chronic renal disease
	(polycystic kidneys, obstructive uropathy)
	Metabolic disease (hypercalcemia, hypokalemia)
	Drugs (lithium, demeclocycline)
	Osmotic diuresis (glucose, mannitol)
	Amyloidosis
	Myelomatosis

Dipsogenic DI

Compulsive water drinking
Affective disorders (e.g., schizophrenia)
Craniopharyngioma/Rathke's cleft cyst
Sarcoidosis

AD, Autosomal dominant; DI, diabetes insipidus; DIDMOAD, diabetes insipidus, diabetes mellitus, optic atrophy, and deafness; GI, gastrointestinal; TB, tuberculosis.

Diabetes Insipidus

Diabetes insipidus is a clinical syndrome characterized by hypotonic polyuria due to failure to concentrate urine. Urine flow rates in excess of 40 mL/kg per 24 hours in adults, or more than 100 mL/kg per 24 hours in infants, are suggestive of diabetes insipidus. Three major categories of diabetes insipidus have been identified.[52]

Polyuria is caused by insufficient AVP secretion, so that there is no effective antidiuretic hormone. There needs to be a loss of at least 80% of the magnocellular neurons that synthesize and secrete AVP before polyuria develops.

In nephrogenic diabetes insipidus, AVP secretion is normal, but renal insensitivity to the antidiuretic effects of the hormone is present.

In dipsogenic diabetes insipidus, excessive fluid intake reflects abnormal perception of thirst.

A full list of causes of diabetes insipidus is shown in Table 14-1.

HYPOTHALAMIC DIABETES INSIPIDUS

HDI (also known as neurogenic, central, or cranial DI) occurs when AVP secretion is insufficient to prevent the development of a hypotonic diuresis, such that the patient presents with polyuria and nocturia. The lesion in the vast majority of cases spares the thirst mechanism[53]; therefore, because thirst appreciation is intact, patients respond to the polyuria with appropriate polydipsia. The increase in fluid intake is nearly always sufficient to maintain normonatremia; hypernatremia in which fluid is freely available should always raise the suspicion of associated thirst abnormalities. The AVP deficiency may be complete, with no detectable plasma AVP, or partial, where AVP is detectable in the plasma at low concentrations inappropriate to the ambient plasma osmolality.

HDI is rare in the general population with an estimated prevalence of 1:25,000 but is common in certain subgroups, such as patients undergoing pituitary surgery, or transiently in other forms of neurosurgical intervention.

Most cases of HDI are acquired during adult life, and the most common cause of DI in most endocrine practices is surgery for pituitary tumors. Pituitary adenomas rarely cause DI, and when a pituitary mass is associated with polyuria, then craniopharyngioma, granuloma, and hypophysitis are far more likely diagnoses.

DI occurs in the immediate postoperative period in 18% to 30% of cases,[54-57] with most cases presenting in the first 2 days following surgery. The most common natural history is spontaneous resolution over the next 2 to 5 days. The pathophysiology of acute transient DI is thought to be surgical contusion injury to the magnocellular neurons projecting from the supraoptic and paraventricular nuclei to the posterior pituitary. In some patients however, DI persists and AVP deficiency becomes permanent. Most neurosurgical series report a low incidence of 1% to 8% for permanent DI, following transsphenoidal surgery.[54,56-58] Many published studies are retrospective, however, and use polyuria alone as the criteria for diagnosis of DI. We found that formal water deprivation testing identified permanent DI in 30% of patients who had transcranial surgery for pituitary adenoma and much higher figures of over 90% following craniopharyngioma surgery.[55]

In a small minority of patients, post-hypophysectomy DI follows the triple phase response. Initially, classical postoperative DI presents in the first 2 days following surgery. However, after 4 to 8 days of hypotonic polyuria, urine output drops and plasma sodium begins to fall, even after discontinuation of desmopressin therapy. This second, antidiuretic phase is characterized by a rise in plasma AVP concentrations, presumably from uncontrolled release of pre-stored peptide from damaged magnocellular neurons. If hypotonic intravenous fluids continue to be administered, the fall in plasma sodium concentration can be abrupt.

The antidiuretic phase of the triple phase response usually lasts 5 to 7 days, but considerable variation is noted, from 2 to 14 days, before progression to the final phase, the development of permanent DI. It is thought that permanent DI occurs when gliosis of damaged neurons prevents further AVP release.

The major factor influencing the risk of developing diabetes insipidus following pituitary surgery is tumor type. Craniopharyngioma is associated with preoperative DI, but in addition, surgical intervention is far more commonly associated with the development of DI than is surgery for any other intracranial tumor.[55] Surgery for ACTH-secreting pituitary adenomas has been associated with a higher risk of developing DI in a number of series.[54,56,58] Data from the literature are conflicting regarding the influence of tumor size on the risk of postoperative diabetes insipidus. Although pituitary adenomas rarely cause HDI, metastatic deposits in the hypothalamus, or more often the pituitary stalk, can result in HDI. Metastatic deposits usually have no endocrine effects, even when they are found in the stalk or the pituitary itself, but some, particularly from carcinoma of the breast or bronchus, produce HDI. Other tumors such as germinoma, pinealoma, and parasellar meningioma can cause HDI. It is interesting to note that although radiotherapy for nonpituitary cranial tumors commonly causes anterior pituitary dysfunction, it does not seem to cause DI.[59]

Lymphocytic infiltration of the neurohypophysis (infundibulo-neurohypophysitis), recognized by a thickened pituitary stalk and inflammatory infiltrates of T lymphocytes and plasma cells with eosinophils, is a well-described cause of HDI.[60] HDI is present in up to 30% of adult patients with Langerhans' cell histiocytosis (LCH).[61]

Idiopathic DI is diagnosed less often, as better imaging techniques have been introduced and awareness of autoimmune causes has increased.[62,63] It has been estimated that one third of patients previously diagnosed to have idiopathic HDI may an autoimmune origin of the condition. The characteristics of autoimmune DI include the presence of circulating antibodies against AVP-secreting cells, young age of onset, and thickened pituitary stalk T1-weighted magnetic resonance imaging (MRI).[64] Patients with autoimmune DI have an increased incidence of other organ-specific autoimmune endocrine disease, particularly thyroid disease.

Traumatic brain injury causes acute diabetes insipidus in 20% of cases,[65] some of which result in a triple phase response similar to that seen after pituitary surgery. DI following brain injury is nearly always transient,[66] however, and only 7% of long-term survivors of head injury have permanent DI when formally tested with water deprivation.[67]

Sheehan's syndrome is now rare and is not usually associated with HDI, even when anterior hypopituitarism is widespread, but maximal urine-concentrating ability is impaired in some patients.[68] HDI can occasionally occur in normal pregnancy as the result of increased activity of circulating vasopressinase, the placental aminopeptidase.[69] Symptoms resolve post partum. The actions of vasopressinase can unmask partial HDI in patients with pituitary disease or can worsen symptoms in undiagnosed partial HDI. HDI in pregnancy must be differentiated from the transient NDI that is seen very occasionally.[70]

Familial HDI is extremely rare. Autosomal dominant HDI (adHDI) is associated with loss-of-function mutations in the *AVP* gene, resulting in the production of a folding-incompetent peptide precursor that accumulates in the secretory pathway apparatus of magnocellular neurons.[71,72] This mutant precursor is responsible for an autophagocytic process that causes progressive damage and loss of VP neurons. A single mutant allele is sufficient for this process to occur. Most mutations affect exons 1 and 2 of the *AVP* gene.[73-75] Familial HDI almost always presents in childhood.[76]

The Wolfram, or DIDMOAD, syndrome (diabetes insipidus, diabetes mellitus, optic atrophy, and deafness) is a rare autosomal recessive, progressive neurodegenerative disorder characterized by the association of HDI with diabetes mellitus, optic atrophy, and bilateral sensorineural deafness, although other manifestations may include gonadal failure, renal outflow tract dilatation (secondary to reduced nerve fibers in the bladder wall), and progressive ataxia with brain stem atrophy.[77] The syndrome is associated with premature death, usually due to ascending renal tract infection secondary to atonic bladder and hydronephrosis. Although DI is often reported to occur in only one third of cases, in one series where careful testing with AVP responses to hypertonic saline was performed, subnormal responses were seen in all patients.[78] WS is associated with loss-of-function mutations in the *WFS1* gene on Ch.4p16.1, which encodes an 890 amino acid glycoprotein (wolframin) found in the endoplasmic reticulum. An additional locus for WS has been identified recently at Ch.4q22-24, suggesting that the syndrome may be genetically heterogeneous.[79]

NEPHROGENIC DIABETES INSIPIDUS

Nephrogenic diabetes insipidus (NDI) occurs when renal resistance to the antidiuretic effects of VP allows hypotonic diuresis to develop. An outline of potential causes is given in Table 14-1. Lithium therapy is the most common cause of NDI in clinical practice, occurring in up to 30% of patients. Although polyuria usually disappears with cessation of treatment, a minority of patients develop interstitial nephritis, and permanent NDI occurs. Hypokalemia and hypercalcemia can produce acquired NDI, which is reversible with correction of the metabolic abnormality. Poorly controlled diabetes mellitus causes renal resistance to AVP, which seems to be due to failure to recruit aquaporin-2. The reversibility of the metabolic causes of NDI shows how the generation of aquaporins can be vulnerable to metabolic and pharmacologic insults.

Familial NDI is rare. X-linked recessive familial NDI (X-FNDI) is caused by inherited loss-of-function mutations in the V2-R. More than 70 different mutations have been described, affecting all aspects of receptor physiology, including expression, ligand binding, and G protein coupling. A vast majority cause complete loss of function and present in infancy, although some mutations are associated with partial loss of function.[80] A minority of FNDI families have autosomal recessive (AR-FNDI), loss-of-function mutations of the gene encoding AQP2. Most mutations occur in the region of the gene that encodes the transmembrane domain of the water channel protein. Other kindreds have been described with an autosomal dominant NDI (AD-NDI) caused by loss-of-function mutations in *AQP2* affecting the carboxyl-terminal intracellular domain of the protein. NDI is expressed in these kindreds because the protein product of the mutant allele forms mixed oligomers with the product of the wild-type allele, resulting in sequestration within the Golgi or mistargeting to the basolateral rather than the apical membrane in a dominant negative manner.[81,82]

DIPSOGENIC DIABETES INSIPIDUS

Dipsogenic diabetes insipidus (DDI) occurs when excessive fluid intake lowers plasma osmolality to levels below the osmotic threshold for vasopressin secretion.[83] In the absence of circulating AVP, hypotonic polyuria develops. Many patients seem to have no underlying illness, but careful osmoregulatory studies have identified a number of abnormalities of thirst regulation. Patients typically have a low osmotic threshold for thirst, which compels them to drink, even when plasma osmolality is lowered below the usual physiologic thirst threshold. In addition, they have an exaggerated thirst response to osmotic challenge and an inability to suppress thirst in response to drinking, so the volume of fluid drunk is in excess of that required for normal hydration.[84] Some forms of DDI are associated with psychiatric disorders, and up to 20% of patients with chronic schizophrenia have DDI. If these patients are simultaneously prescribed drugs that can cause syndrome of inappropriate antidiuretic hormone secretion (SIADH), hyponatremia is inevitable and occasionally severe. Rarely, the problem may be associated with irritative structural abnormalities in the hypothalamus or posterior pituitary, such as hypothalamic sarcoidosis or craniopharyngioma, but usually brain imaging is normal.

INVESTIGATION OF DIABETES INSIPIDUS

A careful history is always valuable in the investigation of a polyuric patient. Although the history is less often diagnostic than in other conditions, useful clinical clues can be obtained. Daytime polyuria without nocturia is a pointer toward dipsogenic DI. Frequent passage of small volumes of urine may suggest prostatism, urinary tract infection, or bladder instability. A history of lithium or diuretic therapy is relevant. Knowledge that a sellar mass is present raises the diagnosis of craniopharyngioma or germinoma. A strong family history of autoimmune thyroid disease might suggest an autoimmune origin.

Initial investigations should aim to confirm that the patient is polyuric; 15% of patients who are referred to our service for investigation of polyuria have normal urine volumes, with frequency of micturition due to urinary tract disease. A 24-hour urine volume less than 3 liters makes osmotic studies unnecessary. Simple ambulatory investigations include electrolytes, calcium, midstream specimen of urine (MSU), and urinalysis; if the patient does not have glycosuria, polyuria is not due to diabetes mellitus. Clinic plasma and urine osmolality are rarely diagnostic unless the urine osmolality exceeds 700 mOsm/kg, at which point further investigation is not necessary. Urine osmolality is low in all three forms of DI. However, an elevated plasma osmolality is more likely with HDI or NDI, whereas a plasma osmolality at the low end of the reference range is suggestive of DDI.

In most patients, it is necessary to proceed to a water deprivation test.[52] This is a two-step test of osmoregulatory function. The first step consists of an 8-hour period of dehydration. The normal physiologic response is to respond to the rise in plasma osmolality with secretion of AVP and concentration of urine to more than 750 mOsm/kg. Theoretically, patients with DDI have a normal osmoregulatory mechanism and should respond to dehydration with appropriate urine concentration. In the simplest use of this test, therefore, the key measurement is final urine osmolality, and the result answers the key question, "Does the patient have true DI, or not?" In patients who are being investigated for post-hypophysectomy HDI, only this step is needed to make the diagnosis.

The second step is the response to desmopressin. Urine osmolality is measured at intervals after intramuscular desmopressin; in patients with HDI, a normal concentrating response should occur, with a rise in urine osmolality to >750 mOsm/kg. In contrast, patients with NDI will fail to respond to desmopressin. Step 2 therefore involves distinguishing between HDI and NDI.

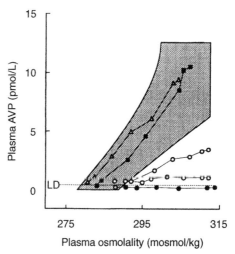

FIGURE 14-7. Dynamic tests of the arginine vasopressin (AVP) axis in patients with polyuria. Plasma AVP (pAVP) and osmolality (pOsm) responses to hypertonic (855 mmol/L) saline infusion. pAVP and urine osmolality (uOsm) responses to a period of fluid restriction in the same group of patients. *Shaded areas*, Range of the normal response. *I and I*, Patients with hypothalamic diabetes insipidus (HDI); *n*, patients with nephrogenic diabetes insipidus (NDI); *s*, patients with dipsogenic diabetes insipidus (DDI).

In practice, the water deprivation test does not always produce straightforward results. Surreptitious water intake can give spurious results, so the test should be undertaken with strict supervision; results are best expressed in units and are optimal when attained by the clinician who has experience in performing the test. Partial forms of HDI and NDI cannot be differentiated from DDI.[85] Furthermore, prolonged polyuria from any cause leads to partial resistance to the antidiuretic action of vasopressin (VP), caused by dilution of the renal medullary interstitium.[86] This can mean that patients with severe polyuria due to dipsogenic DI may appear to have partial NDI. The accuracy of the test can be enhanced by the incorporation of AVP measurement with a reliable radioimmunoassay, if available. We incorporate measurement of thirst by visual analogue scale, which gives valuable information in the diagnosis of specific thirst problems.

The most accurate diagnosis of HDI is attained by direct measurement of plasma AVP concentration during intravenous infusion of hypertonic saline[86,87] (Fig. 14-7). Patients with HDI are identified by undetectable or subnormal plasma AVP concentrations with respect to plasma osmolalities, whereas patients with DDI and NDI have plasma AVP responses in the normal range. DDI and NDI can be distinguished by relating plasma AVP concentration to urine osmolality at the end of the test. NDI is characterized by inappropriately high plasma AVP values for concomitant urine osmolality, whereas DDI patients show an appropriate relation. A visual analogue scale[53] is equally useful in this form of osmotic stimulation.

Because the concentrations of AVP in urine are higher than those in plasma, and thus are detectable by a wider range of available assays, measurement of urinary AVP concentration during osmotic stress has been proposed as an additional alternative to the measurement of plasma AVP in the diagnosis of HDI, but this method needs further evaluation.[88]

Once the diagnosis of HDI has been confirmed, imaging of the hypothalamic-pituitary region with MRI scanning is mandatory to exclude structural lesions. Sellar tumors in patients with HDI most often are craniopharyngiomas. A stalk mass has a wider differential diagnosis, including craniopharyngioma, germinoma, metastasis, lymphocytic hypophysitis, and stalk thickening in autoimmune HDI. Typical appearances may be found in sarcoid, hemochromatosis, and other inflammatory conditions. The posterior pituitary has as a characteristic bright signal on T1-weighted MRI, which is absent in most patients with HDI.[89] The posterior lobe signal is also diminished in the elderly and in patients with anorexia nervosa, septic shock, and poorly controlled diabetes mellitus, and those on hemodialysis. It is thought that this may represent persistent hypersecretion and thus decreased VP-NPII complex content.

If the diagnosis is thought to be idiopathic DI, awareness of the possibility of an autoimmune origin is important. Routine measurement of thyroid function, vitamin B_{12}, and autoantibodies is worthwhile, whereas tests for primary adrenal failure should be considered when clinically indicated. Serum angiotensin-converting enzyme concentration and chest films should be considered if sarcoid is suspected. It is important to repeat MRI imaging when initial films are normal, as some parasellar tumors such as germinomas can present with DI prior to the development of radiologic abnormalities. If stalk lesions are present, serum hCG and α-fetoprotein measurements may give a clue to the presence of germinoma, and early repeat MRI is important for assessing tumor growth. Biopsy should be considered early, as germinomas are best treated with chemotherapy and radiotherapy rather than surgical intervention. Dynamic tests of anterior pituitary function should be considered in cases in which structural pituitary lesions exist. Data in children suggest that growth hormone deficiency commonly accompanies autoimmune HDI,[90] although anecdotal evidence suggests that this is not the case in adults.

Patients with NDI should undergo renal investigations as appropriate, including urine microscopy and renal tract ultrasound to exclude obstruction, and tests of other aspects of tubular function. Genetic studies in suspected familial disease remain research tools.

ADIPSIC DIABETES INSIPIDUS

Although diabetes insipidus is almost always associated with normal thirst and drinking appropriate to clinical needs, adipsic diabetes insipidus (ADI) is a rare but highly complex condition. It is seen most commonly after clipping of anterior communicating artery aneurysms, following subarachnoid hemorrhage[91,92];

the vascular supply to the osmoreceptors is derived from small arteries arising from the anterior communicating artery, and it is assumed that these vessels are damaged during aneurysm clipping, and that infarction of the circumventricular organs occurs where the osmoreceptors are sited. The osmoregulatory defect is almost always permanent, although anecdotal, unpublished reports have described recovery. Extensive hypothalamic surgery for craniopharyngioma,[92] or, rarely, pituitary macroadenoma,[93] have been reported to cause ADI.

In ADI secondary to clipping of the anterior communicating artery, a pure osmoreceptor defect is present. Osmotic stimulation with hypertonic saline causes no rise in plasma AVP or in thirst ratings, despite marked hyperosmolality. In contrast, non-osmotic baroregulated AVP secretion is completely normal, with secretion of AVP to produce plasma concentrations a hundred-fold higher than those needed for maximal urine concentration.[94] The AVP synthesis/secretion unit of the SON/PVN/posterior pituitary is thus intact, but is not innervated by the osmoreceptors. In patients who undergo destructive surgery to the pituitary, all secretory function is lost.[94]

The diagnosis of ADI presents a management dilemma.[95] Patients are unable to perceive changes in plasma tonicity via the usual thirst mechanisms and are vulnerable to marked swings in plasma sodium concentration. Severe hypernatremia is a particular hazard. Management requires regular desmopressin, fixed fluid intakes that may vary with climatic conditions, and regular review for measurement of plasma sodium. Recent data have also highlighted associated hypothalamic abnormalities that are often seen with ADI (Table 14-2), including hypothalamic obesity, seizure disorders, sleep apnea, and thermoregulatory disorders.[92] Episodes of dehydration are often complicated by thrombotic complications, including pulmonary thromboembolism.[92,96] Many patients die prematurely owing to postsurgical complications, electrolyte abnormalities, or sleep apnea.

TREATMENT FOR DIABETES INSIPIDUS

Although the intact thirst mechanism prevents dehydration in DI, the need to continually seek fluids and facilities for polyuria is a great inconvenience. The treatment of choice is DDAVP (desmopressin), a synthetic, long-acting VP analogue that possesses minimal pressor activity and has twice the antidiuretic potency of AVP. It can be administered as an intranasal spray, but more often is given orally in two to three daily doses. The

Table 14-2. Comorbidities Associated With Adipsic Diabetes Insipidus

Pt	Diagnosis	Baroreg AVP Release	Sleep Apnea	DVT	BMI, kg/m²	Other Morbidity	Death
A	ACAA	Yes	No	No	24.8	Nil	
B	ACAA	Yes	No	No	24.2	Hemiparesis	
C	ACAA	Yes	No	No	27.6	Seizures, hypothermia	
D	ACAA	Yes	Yes	Yes	37.2	Nil	
E	ACAA	Yes	No	Yes	32.9	Nil	
F	TBI	Yes	No	No	25.5	Nil	
G	Toluene	Yes	Yes	No	35.7	Hypothermia, hypothalamic seizures, abnormal thermoregulation	
H	Cranio	No	No	No	56.9	Hypercholesterolemia	
I	Cranio	No	Yes	Yes	33.5	Seizures, hydrocephalus	24 yr
J	Cranio	No	No	No	34.7	Seizures	
K	Cranio	No	Yes	No	28.2	Hypernatremic seizure	
L	Cranio	No	Yes	Yes PTE	41.3	Abnormal thermoregulation	48 yr
M	PRLoma	No	Yes	Yes	53.0	Nil	
N	Sarcoid	Yes	Yes	No	57.1	Diabetes mellitus, seizures	36 yr
O	Congenital	Yes	Yes	Yes PTE	32.4	Behavioral disorder, acute pancreatitis, seizures	18 yr

ACAA, Post clipping of anterior communicating artery aneurysm; *Baroreg*, baroregulated; *AVP,* arginine vasopressin; *Cranio*, craniopharyngioma (all post surgery);
   DVT, deep venous thrombosis; *PRLoma*, prolactinoma; *PTE*, pulmonary thromboembolism; *TBI*, traumatic brain injury.
Based on previously unpublished data from authors' lab.

Table 14-3. Origin of SIADH

Malignancy	Drugs	Pulmonary	Intracranial Pathology	Miscellaneous
SCC lung	DDAVP	Pneumonia (esp *Mycoplasma*)	Tumor	Multiple sclerosis
Mesothelioma	PGs	TB	Meningitis	Guillain-Barré syndrome
GI tract	SSRIs	Abscess	Encephalitis	Acute intermittent porphyria
Pancreas	TCAs	Vasculitis	Abscess	HIV
GU tract	Phenothiazines	Positive-pressure ventilation	Vasculitis	Idiopathic causes
Nasopharyngeal	Haloperidol		Subarachnoid hemorrhage	
Lymphoma	MDMA		Subdural hemorrhage	
Sarcoma	Quinolones		Traumatic brain injury	
	Levetiracetam			
	Carbamazepine			
	Cyclophosphamide			
	Vincristine			

DDAVP, Desmopressin; *GI,* gastrointestinal; *GU,* genitourinary; *HIV,* human immunodeficiency virus; *MDMA,* 3,4-methylenedioxymethamphetamine; *PG,* prostaglandin; *SCC,* squamous cell carcinoma; *SSRI,* selective serotonin reuptake inhibitor; *TB,* tuberculosis; *TCA,* tricyclic antidepressant.

main complication is dilutional hyponatremia, which can produce headaches, bloating, and occasionally seizures. Dilutional hyponatremia is minimized by omission of DDAVP once weekly, to allow a hypotonic diuresis that prevents water intoxication. Partial HDI (urine volume <4 L per 24 hours) can be managed with adequate fluids to quench thirst with a nocturnal dose of DDAVP to prevent loss of sleep due to nocturia. Plasma electrolytes should be measured at regular intervals after the introduction of treatment to look for hyponatremia; a decrease in plasma sodium concentration should prompt a therapy review.

NDI due to an acquired metabolic problem is best managed by addressing the underlying cause and maintaining adequate hydration while function recovers. For those patients with congenital NDI or in whom the acquired defect is irreversible, a number of additional measures including thiazide diuretics (hydrochlorothiazide, 25 mg/24 hours) may be used; prostaglandin inhibitors such as nonsteroidal antiinflammatory drugs (ibuprofen, 200 mg/24 hours) and dietary salt restriction also can be used. All work probably via a combination of reducing glomerular filtration rate and interfering with the diluting capacity of the distal nephron. Occasionally, DDAVP can produce some benefit.

As with other causes of DI, the approach to DDI should try to address the underlying cause. This may be difficult. Switching treatment to alternative agents may help those patients with chronic schizophrenia and a history of hyponatremia. Individuals with persistent DDI are at risk for hyponatremia if treated with DDAVP. Reduction in fluid intake is the only rational treatment.

The Syndrome of Inappropriate Antidiuretic Hormone

INTRODUCTION

In 1956, in a presentation to the American Society for Clinical Investigation, Frederic Bartter and William Schwartz first described the syndrome of inappropriate antidiuretic hormone secretion (SIADH) as it occurred in two patients with lung carcinoma who had severe hyponatremia at presentation.[97] By alternating fluid restriction with fluid loading, the investigators demonstrated a state of antidiuresis and hypothesized that their patients manifested a clinical syndrome of inappropriate antidiuresis secondary to excess circulating antidiuretic hormone. Once radioimmunoassays for the measurement of plasma AVP became available, their index clinic description and pathophysi-

ologic hypothesis were substantiated by papers that reported elevated plasma vasopressin concentrations in the syndrome,[98] which is now recognized to occur in a wide spectrum of disease states. However, differentiation of SIADH from other causes of hyponatremia remains important to the prescription of appropriate treatment regimens.

CAUSES OF SIADH

SIADH is associated with a great number of illnesses and most often presents as a coincidental biochemical manifestation of the causative disease. The most common causes of SIADH are summarized in Table 14-3. The origin of SIADH is clinically divided into four categories: malignant, pulmonary, pharmacologic, and neurologic causes.

Bartter and Schwartz first described SIADH in association with bronchogenic lung carcinoma. In small cell carcinoma of the lung, SIADH is relatively common, occasionally occurring as the presenting abnormality that prompts a search for the tumor.[99] Most neoplasms have been reported to cause SIADH, and the association between malignant disease and SIADH is so strong that a patient presenting with SIADH, general malaise, and unexplained weight loss should be considered to have an underlying malignancy until proven otherwise.

SIADH is commonly associated with intracranial diseases, particularly traumatic brain injury,[65-67] in which almost all cases resolve spontaneously with recovery from brain injury. More than 50% of patients with subarachnoid hemorrhage develop hyponatremia in the first week following the bleed, and 70% of these events are due to SIADH.[100] SIADH also commonly occurs after hypophysectomy and after surgery for primary brain tumor.

Many drugs are important clinical causes of hyponatremia. The selective serotonin reuptake inhibitors (SSRIs) are thought to cause SIADH by direct stimulation of AVP secretion by serotonin.[101] SIADH usually occurs in the first few weeks after SSRIs are introduced, particularly in elderly patients.[102] It has been estimated that 12% of hospitalized patients on SSRI therapy develop SIADH.[103] Psychotropic medications such as phenothiazines, haloperidol, and tricyclic antidepressants all cause SIADH. Many patients who have conditions treated with psychotropic drugs also have abnormal thirst; if these patients develop drug-induced SIADH, they can develop very significant hyponatremia. For instance, up to 20% of patients with chronic schizophrenia have psychogenic polydipsia, and excess fluid intake can precipitate severe hyponatremia. MDMA ("Ecstasy") is thought to stimulate both AVP release and thirst as a result of hyperthermia, and this has been implicated in the development of cases of life-threatening hyponatremia.[104]

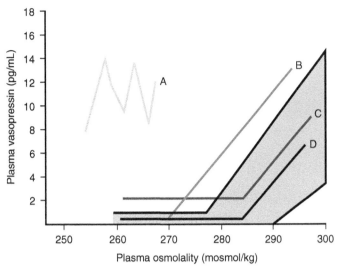

FIGURE 14-8. Summary of the four different patterns of arginine vasopressin (AVP) secretion in syndrome of inappropriate antidiuretic hormone secretion (SIADH).

SIADH must be distinguished from exercise-associated hyponatremia (EAH),[105] in which the electrolyte profile mimics SIADH. The pathophysiology is different, however. EAH occurs in athletes who ingest excessive hypotonic fluid during exercise, with resultant dilutional hyponatremia. Women, marathon runners racing for longer than 4 hours, and athletes of low body mass index are at greatest risk.[106] Although some athletes with EAH fail to suppress AVP, EAH probably should be considered to be distinct from SIADH.

PATHOPHYSIOLOGY OF SIADH

SIADH occurs by definition when AVP secretion is not suppressed when plasma sodium concentration falls below the osmotic threshold for SIADH. However, Zerbe and colleagues were able to differentiate four different types of SIADH, depending on the pattern of AVP secretion [98] (Fig. 14-8).

Type A is the most common form of SIADH (40%). Characteristically, Type A patients exhibit excessive, random secretion of AVP, with loss of the close linear relationship between plasma osmolality and plasma AVP. Plasma AVP concentrations fluctuate widely in this variant, with no relationship to ambient plasma osmolality, but with consistent antidiuresis and inappropriate urine concentration despite hyponatremia. Type A is common in lung cancer; in vitro studies have demonstrated that some lung tumors synthesize AVP,[107] and tumor tissue stains positive for AVP messenger RNA.[108] However, Type A SIADH also occurs in non-neoplastic disease, for which ectopic AVP secretion could not be implicated. Plasma AVP concentrations in Type A SIADH are not suppressed by drinking,[109] which makes patients vulnerable to the development of severe hyponatremia.

Type B is also common (40%). The osmotic threshold for AVP release is lowered—a "reset osmostat"—in such a way that secretion of AVP occurs at lower plasma osmolalities than normal. At plasma osmolalities above this reset threshold, the linear relationship between plasma AVP and plasma osmolality is preserved. Equally, because AVP is suppressed at plasma osmolalities below the lower, reset threshold, overhydration leads to suppression of AVP release. A hypotonic diuresis then develops, which protects against the progression to severe hyponatremia. Similar lowering of the osmotic threshold occurs in hypovolemia and

hypotension, leading to speculation that the function of afferent baroregulatory pathways is disturbed in these patients.

Type C is a rare condition characterized by failure to suppress AVP secretion at plasma osmolalities below the osmotic threshold. Plasma AVP concentrations are thus inappropriately high at low plasma osmolalities, but a normal relationship is noted between plasma osmolality and plasma AVP at physiologic plasma osmolalities. This variant may be due to dysfunction of inhibitory neurons in the hypothalamus, leading to persistent low-grade basal AVP secretion.

Type D provides a rare clinical picture of SIADH without detectable circulating AVP.[110] It is postulated that a nephrogenic syndrome of inappropriate antidiuresis (NSIAD) may be responsible for the Type D picture of SIADH.[111] Recent reports described two male infants in whom gain-of-function mutations in the V2 receptor led to a clinical picture of SIADH, with undetectable AVP levels. Both children were diagnosed in infancy. Identified mutations had different nucleotide substitution with different levels of V2 receptor activation.[111]

Studies in rat models of SIADH have demonstrated that the increase in water reabsorption is secondary to AVP-mediated expression of renal aquaporin-2,[112] with a consequent increase in AQP protein excretion in the urine.[113] Aquaporin-2 recruitment has been shown to be reversible through administration of a V2 receptor antagonist[112,114] that provides the scientific rationale for the use of AVP antagonists in the treatment of this condition. Prolonged SIADH is associated with "escape" from antidiuresis, with downregulation of AQP2 mRNA and protein expression.

Although patients with SIADH have ambient plasma osmolalities that are below the physiologic osmotic threshold for thirst, they continue to drink apparently normal fluid volumes. In experiments in which patients with SIADH of mixed causes were infused intravenously with hypertonic sodium chloride solution, the osmotic threshold for thirst was lowered to a setting that was identical to that for AVP.[109] Parallel lowering of the thresholds for thirst and AVP release ensured the maintenance of fluid intake, predisposing to persistent hyponatremia.

As fluid intake is maintained in the face of reduced free water clearance, patients with SIADH can develop severe hyponatremia. However, hyponatremia is often limited by "escape from antidiuresis." This protective homeostatic mechanism occurs when the kidney begins to increase free water clearance despite inappropriate plasma AVP concentrations.[115] Initial natriuresis is followed by an increase in urine flow[116] with consequent water loss; this allows plasma sodium to stabilize and, occasionally, to rise. Although plasma sodium concentration does not usually rise into the normal physiologic range during escape from antidiuresis, the development of severe hyponatremia is prevented.

Experimental models of SIADH, in which hyponatremia was induced in Sprague-Dawley rats by the injection of subcutaneous desmopressin, showed that desmopressin administration alone did not lead to hyponatremia.[117] Plasma volume expansion due to water loading, leading to increased renal perfusion pressure, was vital for initiation of escape from antidiuresis.[118] A decrease in AQP2 protein expression and V2 receptor binding capacity[119,120] has been postulated to cause the renal resistance to AVP observed during escape from antidiuresis.

In normal physiology, AVP has long-term effects on AQP2 via mRNA and protein expression, but it has short-term effects via the V2 receptor, leading to increased cyclic adenosine monophosphate (cAMP). It is likely that this short-term AVP action is also altered in escape, because reduced levels of cAMP in the

Table 14-4. Essential Criteria for the Diagnosis of SIADH

Decreased plasma osmolality of the ECF (pOsm <280 mOsm/kg H_2O)
Inappropriate urinary concentration during hypo-osmolality
  (uOsm >100 mOsm/kg H_2O, normal renal function)
Clinical euvolemia
Elevated urinary sodium excretion (>30 mmol/L) on normal salt and water
  intake
Absence of other potential causes of euvolemic hypo-osmolality, particularly
  hypothyroidism, hypocortisolism, and diuretic use

ECF, Extracellular fluid; *SIADH,* syndrome of inappropriate antidiuretic hormone
secretion.

collecting ducts of "escaped" rats have been demonstrated.[121] This finding of reduced cAMP activity suggests both the short-term regulation of AQP activity by reduced vesicle "shuttling" and the long-term downregulation of AQP mRNA expression in the genesis of "escape from antidiuresis."

DIAGNOSIS OF SIADH

Essential criteria for the diagnosis of SIADH are presented in Table 14-4. Two additional supplemental criteria—raised plasma vasopressin concentration and abnormal water load test—are rarely used in clinical practice. Water loading of a patient with SIADH runs the risk of symptomatic hyponatremia; therefore, this procedure should be restricted to centers with considerable experience in managing disorders of water balance. Plasma AVP concentrations are elevated in almost all causes of hyponatremia and therefore are rarely of diagnostic benefit in hyponatremic patients; lack of access to local radioimmunoassays dictates that the results of tests may take weeks to come back, which further diminishes their clinical value.

The minimum data set for the diagnosis of SIADH is hyponatremia in a euvolemic patient with inappropriate concentrated urine (osmolality >100 mOsm/kg), elevated urine sodium (>30 mmol/L), and exclusion of cortisol and thyroid hormone insufficiency. Older textbooks dictate that urine osmolality should exceed plasma osmolality for the diagnosis to be secure, but osmoregulatory physiology indicates that this criterion is redundant. If plasma osmolality is below the osmotic threshold for AVP secretion, plasma AVP levels should be suppressed, allowing hypotonic diuresis with urine osmolality <100 mOsm/kg. Urine osmolalities in excess of 100 mOsm/kg indicate inappropriate urine concentration and are compatible with the diagnosis of SIADH. Many hyponatremic patients do not undergo the requisite tests and may be misdiagnosed with SIADH without satisfying the diagnostic criteria.

DIFFERENTIAL DIAGNOSIS OF SIADH

Glucocorticoid Deficiency

ACTH deficiency causes hyponatremia with a biochemical profile identical to classical SIADH. Hyponatremia responds to glucocorticoid replacement.[122] Fluid restriction, which constitutes first-line therapy for SIADH, is deleterious and worsens hypovolemia.[123] Measurement of plasma cortisol therefore is essential, as clinical signs are not always sufficiently reliable to differentiate between glucocorticoid deficiency and SIADH.[124] Glucocorticoid-deficient patients have impairment of free water clearance, causing a relative excess of body water to sodium.[125,126] Glucocorticoids are thought to suppress AVP release, and elevation of plasma AVP concentrations has been reported in ACTH-deficient patients who develop hyponatremia.[127]

The differentiation of SIADH from glucocorticoid deficiency is particularly important in patients with neurosurgical condi-

tions, who commonly present with hyponatremia, which is traditionally ascribed to SIADH.[128] Recent evidence indicates that acute pituitary dysfunction occurs commonly following traumatic brain injury and subarachnoid hemorrhage, with ACTH deficiency reported in 16% of patients with acute[65] and 12.7% of patients with chronic head injury[129] and in 2.5% of patients after subarachnoid hemorrhage.[130] Glucocorticoid deficiency may present with hyponatremia; coexistent hypoglycemia or hypotension suggests the diagnosis of hypopituitarism.[131] We have seen acute ACTH deficiency severe enough to cause a biochemical picture, which mimics SIADH in traumatic brain injury, subarachnoid hemorrhage, and intracranial hemorrhage. Therefore, in patients presenting with SIADH against a background of sudden intracerebral catastrophe, we consider that the possibility of acute hypopituitarism should be considered in the differential diagnosis.

Hypothyroidism

Hyponatremia in hypothyroidism is rare, but life-threatening hyponatremia is occasionally reported.[132,133] Hypothyroid patients have elevated AVP responses to subtle volume contraction, with increased recruitment of AQP2.[134] However, the hyponatremia is probably multifactorial. Thyroxine has direct effects on sodium reabsorption from the tubule and on renal ability to excrete free water[135,136]; decreased glomerular filtration rate also occurs in hypothyroidism, which corrects with thyroid hormone replacement.[137]

TREATMENT FOR SIADH

Factors Affecting Therapy

Symptomatic cerebral irritation is the most important factor in determining that hyponatremia should be treated. However, the degree of hyponatremia is also important in that symptoms, morbidity, and mortality are all related to the degree of hyponatremia. Modest falls in plasma sodium to 130 mmol/L are unlikely to be symptomatic or to require any intervention. However, the likelihood of symptoms increases as the plasma sodium concentration falls.[138] At plasma sodium concentrations below 120 mmol/L, morbidity and mortality are more common. Two other factors increase the likelihood of symptoms. The first of these is the coexistence of other structural or biochemical abnormalities; the likelihood of seizures, for instance, is increased at any plasma sodium concentration in the presence of intracerebral lesions such as tumor or hemorrhage. In addition, cerebral irritation due to hyponatremia is increased if the patient is hypoxic, hypotensive, or dehydrated.

The second important factor is the rate of development of hyponatremia, which is even more important than comorbidity in determining the likelihood and severity of cerebral symptoms. Patients with chronic hyponatremia (>48 hours' duration) are much less likely to develop symptoms than those in whom the fall in plasma sodium concentration occurs rapidly (acute hyponatremia, <48 hours' duration) and may have no symptoms at all despite marked hyponatremia. For instance, many patients can withstand chronic hyponatremia due to diuretics for long periods with no symptoms other than postural dizziness due to hypotension. These patients undergo cerebral adaptation by extruding solutes such as potassium and organic osmolytes into the plasma. This prevents osmotic movement of water into the brain, where it can cause cerebral edema. In contrast, in acute hyponatremia, for instance, in neurosurgical conditions, this time-dependent process does not occur with the subsequent development of brain edema and cerebral irritation.[139] Rapid treatment therefore is more likely to be necessary when hyponatremia has developed quickly, as serious symptoms are more likely, and failure to treat can be fatal.[138]

Treatment for Chronic Hyponatremia

Modest hyponatremia of >130 mmol/L will rarely need treatment, but the frequency of symptoms and adverse effects, such as seizures, increases with plasma sodium concentrations below this. After careful exclusion of treatable underlying conditions such as glucocorticoid deficiency, water restriction is the treatment of choice. Fluid restriction of 1 L per day is occasionally sufficient to correct hyponatremia,[140] with a slow, steady rise in plasma sodium. If the patient has been polydipsic, however, fluid restriction can cause a more rapid rise in plasma sodium concentration. Fluid restriction is difficult to maintain in patients with cognitive difficulties, in those with a history of polydipsia, and in patients receiving intravenous medications. In addition, in more severe hyponatremia, the degree of fluid restriction necessary to correct hypo-osmolality may be too difficult to maintain.

Pharmacologic therapy tends to be reserved for more severe hyponatremia and for cases that are unresponsive to fluid restriction. Demeclocycline, a tetracycline antibiotic that induces nephrogenic diabetes insipidus by a postreceptor effect, can be effective in this situation. Side effects, including photosensitivity and nephrotoxicity, particularly in patients with liver disease, complicate long-term therapy. Occasionally, hypernatremic dehydration can develop if polyuria is marked. Urea has been used, but it is unpleasant and is contraindicated in renal failure.

The development of specific V2 receptor antagonists offers a specific antidote to AVP-mediated hyponatremia.[141] These agents act as "aquaretics," which increase free water excretion without a natriuresis and offer a therapeutic effect regardless of the cause of raised AVP.

Selective V2 antagonists (e.g., tolvaptan, lixivaptan) and combined V1a/V2 antagonists (e.g., conivaptan) may be used.[142] Pure V2 antagonism may be suitable for patients with SIADH but may lead to a rise in AVP levels. Few clinical data are available for this group of patients. V2 antagonists appear to be more effective in SIADH than in cirrhosis.[143]

REFERENCES

1. Schally AV: Hormones of the neurohypophysis. In Lock W, Schally AV, editors: The Hypothalamus and Pituitary in Health and Disease, Springfield, IL, 1972, Charles C Thomas, pp 154–171.
2. Zimmerman EA, Nilaver G, Hou-ya A, et al: Vasopressinergic and oxytocinergic pathways in the central nervous system, Fed Proc 43:91–96, 1984.
3. Sofroniew MV: Projections from vasopressin, oxytocin and neurophysin neurones to neural targets in the rat and human, J Histochem Cytochem 28:475–478, 1980.
4. Mohr E, Schmitz E, Richter D: A single rat genomic cDNA fragment encodes both the oxytocin and vasopressin genes separated by 11 kilobases and orientated in opposite transcriptional directions, Biochemie 70:649–654, 1988.
5. Dutton A, Dyball REJ: Phasic firing enhances vasopressin release from the rat neurohypophysis, J Physiol 290:433–440, 1979.
6. Russell JT, Brownstein MJ, Gainer H: Biosynthesis of vasopressin, oxytocin and neurophysins: isolation and characterization of two common precursors (propressophysin and prooxyphysin), Endocrinology 107:1880–1891, 1980.
7. Zing HH: Vasopressin and oxytocin receptors, Ballieres Clin Endocrinol Metab 10:75–96, 1996.
8. Thibonnier M, Conarty DM, Preston JA, et al: Molecular pharmacology of human vasopressin receptors, Adv Exp Med Biol 449:251–276, 1988.
8a. Montani JP, Liard JF, Schoun J, et al: Hemodynamic effects of exogenous and endogenous vasopressin at low plasma concentrations in conscious dogs, Circ Res 47:346–355, 1980.
9. Altura BM, Altura BT: Actions of vasopressin, oxytocin, and synthethic analogs on vascular smooth muscle, Fed Proc 43:80–86, 1984.
10. Liard J-F: Acute hemodynamic effects of antidiuretic agents. In Comley AW, Liard J-F, Ausiello DA, editors: Vasopressin: Cellular and Integrative Functions, New York, 1988, Raven Press, pp 461–466.
11. Aisenbrey GA, Handelman WA, Arnold P, et al: Vascular effects of arginine vasopressin during fluid deprivation in the rat, J Clin Invest 67:961–968, 1981.
12. Dunser MW, Mayr AJ, Ulmer H, et al: Arginine vasopressin in advanced vasodilatory shock: a prospective, randomized, controlled study, Circulation 107(18):2313–2319, 2003 May 13.
13. Morelli A, Rocco M, Conti G, et al: Effects of terlipressin on systemic and regional haemodynamics in cate-

cholamine-treated patients, Intensive Care Med 30(4):597–604, 2004 Apr.
14. Gonen T, Walz T: The structure of aquaporins, Q Rev Biophys 39(4):361–396, 2006.
15. Du Pasquier D, Dreifuss JJ, Dubois-Dauphin M, et al: Binding sites for vasopressin in the human pituitary are associated with corticotrophs and may differ from other known vasopressin receptors, J Neuroendocrinol 3:237–247, 1991.
16. Sawchenko PE, Swanson LW, Vale WW: Co-expression of corticotrophin releasing factor and vasopressin immunoreactivity in parvocellular neurosecretory neurons of the adrenalectomized rat, Proc Natl Acad Sci U S A 81:1877–1883, 1984.
17. Baldino F, Davis LG: Glucocorticoid regulation of vasopressin messenger RNA. In Uhl GR, editor: In Situ Hybridization in the Brain, New York, 1986, Plenum Press, p 97.
18. Robertson GL, Aycitema P, Zerbe RL: Neurogenic disorders of osmoregulation. Am J Med 72(2):339–353, 1982 Feb.
19. Zerbe RL, Robertson GL: Osmoregulation of thirst and vasopressin secretion in human subjects: effect of various solutes, Am J Physiol 244:E607–E614, 1983.
20. Robertson GL, Shelton RL, Athar S: The osmoregulation of vasopressin, Kidney Int 10:25–37, 1976.
21. Hammer M, Ladefoged J, Olgaard K: Relationship between plasma osmolality and plasma vasopressin in human subjects, Am J Physiol 238:E313–E317, 1980.
22. Baylis PH, Thompson CJ: Osmoregulation of vasopressin secretion and thirst in health and disease, Clin Endocrinol 29:549–576, 1988.
23. Thompson CJ, Bland J, Burd J, et al: The osmotic thresholds for thirst and vasopressin release are similar in a healthy man, Clin Sci 71:651–656, 1986.
24. Baylis PH, Pippard C, Gill GV, et al: Development of a cytochemical assay for plasma vasopressin: application to studies on water loading normal man, Clin Endocrinol 24:383–392, 1986.
25. Baylis PH, Gill GV: Investigation of polyuria, Clin Endocrinol Metab 13:295–310, 1984.
26. Robertson GL: Physiology of ADH secretion, Kidney Int 32(Suppl 21):S20–S26, 1987.
27. Thompson CJ, Selby P, Baylis PH: Reproducibility of osmotic and non-osmotic tests of vasopressin secretion in man, Am J Physiol 60:R533–R539, 1991.
28. Zerbe RL: Genetic factors in normal and abnormal regulation of vasopressin secretion. In Schrier RW, editor: Vasopressin, New York, 1985, Raven Press, pp 213–220.

29. Thompson CJ, Burd JM, Baylis PH: Acute suppression of plasma vasopressin and thirst after drinking in hypernatraemic man, Am J Physiol 252:R1138–R1142, 1986.
30. Seckl JR, Williams TD, Lightman SL: Oral hypertonic saline causes transient fall in vasopressin in humans, Am J Physiol 251:R214–R217, 1986.
31. Durr JA, Stamoutsos BA, Lindheimer MD: Osmoregulation during pregnancy in the rat: evidence for resetting of the threshold for vasopressin secretion during gestation, J Clin Invest 68:337–346, 1981.
32. Davison JM, Gilmore EA, Durr J, et al: Altered threshold for vasopressin secretion and thirst in human pregnancy, Am J Physiol 246:F105–F109, 1984.
33. Spruce BA, Baylis PH, Burd J, et al: Variation in osmoregulation of arginine vasopressin during the human menstrual cycle, Clin Endocrinol 22:37–42, 1985.
34. Miller M: Fluid and electrolyte homeostasis in the elderly: physiological changes of ageing and clinical consequences, Baillieres Clin Endocrinol Metab 11:367–387, 1997.
35. Johnson AG, Crawford GA, Kelly D: Arginine vasopressin and osmolality in the elderly, J Am Geriatr Soc 42:399–404, 1994.
36. Helderman JH, Vestal RE, Rowe JW, et al: The response of arginine vasopressin to intravenous alcohol and hypertonic saline in man: The impact of ageing, J Gerontol 33:39–47, 1978.
37. Phillips PA, Rolls BJ, Ledingham JGG: Reduced thirst after water deprivation in healthy elderly men, N Engl J Med 311:753–759, 1984.
38. Crowe MJ, Forsling ML, Rolls BJ: Altered water excretion in healthy elderly men, Age Ageing 16:285–293, 1987.
39. Thompson CJ, David SN, Butler PC, et al: Osmoregulation of thirst and vasopressin secretion in insulin dependent diabetes mellitus, Clin Sci 74:599–606, 1988.
40. Thompson CJ, Davis SN, Baylis PH: Effects of blood glucose concentration on osmoregulation in insulin dependent diabetes mellitus, Am J Physiol 256:R597–R604, 1989.
41. McKenna K, Morris AD, Newton RW, et al: Renal resistance to vasopressin in poorly controlled insulin dependent diabetes, Am J Physiol 279:E155–E160, 2000.
42. McKenna K, Morris AD, Azam H, et al: Exaggerated vasopressin secretion and attenuated osmoregulated thirst in human survivors of hyperosmolar coma, Diabetologia 42(5):534–538, 1999 May.

43. Johnson JA, Zehr JE, Moore WW: Effects of separate and concurrent osmotic and volume stimuli on plasma ADH in sheep, Am J Physiol 218:1273–1280, 1970.

44. Baylis PH: Posterior pituitary function in health and disease, Clin Endocrinol Metab 12:747–770, 1983.

45. Goetz KL, Zhu JL, Leadley RJ, et al: Hemodynamic and hormonal influences on the secretion of vasopressin. In Jard S, Jamison R, editors: Vasopressin, Montrouge, France, 1991, John Libbey, pp 279–286.

46. Dunn FL, Brennan TJ, Nelson AE, et al: The role of blood osmolality and volume in regulating vasopressin secretion in the rat, J Clin Invest 52:3212–3219, 1973.

47. Goldsmith SR, Dodge D, Cowley AW: Nonosmotic influences on osmotic stimulation of vasopressin in humans, Am J Physiol 252:H85–H88, 1987.

48. Rowe JW, Shelton RL, Helderman JH, et al: Influence of the emetic reflex on vasopressin release in man, Kidney Int 16:729–735, 1979.

49. Verbalis JG, Richardson DW, Stricker EM: Vasopressin release in response to nausea-producing agents and cholecystokinin in monkeys, Am J Physiol 252:R749–R753, 1987.

50. Ukei M, Moran WH, Zimmerman B: The role of visceral afferent pathways on vasopressin secretion and urinary excretory patterns during surgical stress, Ann Surg 168:16–28, 1968.

51. Baylis PH, Robertson GL: Arginine vasopressin response to insulin induced hypoglycemia in man, J Clin Endocrinol Metab 53:935–940, 1981.

52. Thompson CJ: Polyuric states in man. In Baylis PH, editor: Water and salt homeostasis in health and disease, London, 1989, Bailliere Tindall, pp 473–497.

53. Thompson CJ, Baylis PH: Thirst in diabetes insipidus: clinical relevance of quantitative assessment, Q J Med 56:853–862, 1987.

54. Hensen J, Henig A, Fahlbusch R, et al: Prevalence, predictors and patterns of postoperative polyuria and hyponatraemia in the immediate course after transsphenoidal surgery for pituitary adenomas, Clin Endocrinol 50:431–439, 1999.

55. Smith D, Finucane F, Phillips J, et al: Abnormal regulation of thirst and vasopressin secretion following surgery for craniopharyngioma, Clin Endocrinol 61:273–279, 2004.

56. Nemergut EC, Zuo Z, Jane JA Jr, et al: Predictors of diabetes insipidus after transsphenoidal surgery: a review of 881 patients, J Neurosurg 103:403–454, 2005.

57. Adams JR, Blevins LS Jr, Allen GS, et al: Disorders of water metabolism following transsphenoidal pituitary surgery: a single institution's experience, Pituitary 9:93–99, 2006.

58. Sudhakar N, Ray A, Vafidis JA: Complications after trans-sphenoidal surgery: our experience and a review of the Literature, Br J Neurosurg 18 (5):507–512, 2004 October.

59. Agha A, Sherlock M, Brennan S, et al: Hypothalamic-pituitary dysfunction following irradiation of non-pituitary brain tumours in adults, J Clin Endocrinol Metab 90(12):6355–6360, 2005 Dec.

60. Imura H, Nakao K, Shimatsu A: Lymphocytic infundibuloneurohypophysitis as a cause of central diabetes insipidus, N Engl J Med 329:683–689, 1993.

61. Arico M, Girschikofsky M, Genereau T: Langerhans cell histiocytosis in adults: report from the International Registry of the Histiocyte Society, Eur J Cancer 39:2341–2348, 2003.

62. Blotner H: Primary or idiopathic diabetes insipidus: a system disease, Metabolism 7:191–206, 1958.

63. Baylis PH: Understanding the cause of idiopathic cranial diabetes insipidus: a step forward, Clin Endocrinol 40:171–172, 1994.

64. Pivoello R, De Bellis A, Faggiano A, et al: Central diabetes insipidus and autoimmunity: relationship between the occurrence of antibodies to arginine vasopressin-secreting cells and clinical, immunological, and radiological features in a large cohort of patients with central diabetes insipidus of known and unknown etiology, J Clin Endocrinol Metab 88:1629–1636, 2003.

65. Agha A, Rogers B, Mylotte D, et al: Neuroendocrine dysfunction in the acute phase of traumatic brain injury, Clin Endocrinol 60:584–591, 2004.

66. Agha A, Sherlock M, Phillips J, et al: The natural history of post-traumatic neurohypophysial dysfunction, Eur J Endocrinol 152:371–377, 2005.

67. Agha A, Thornton E, O'Kelly P, et al: Posterior pituitary dysfunction following traumatic brain injury, J Clin Endocrinol Metab 89:5987–5992, 2004.

68. Jialal I, Desai K, Rajput MC: An assessment of posterior pituitary function in patients with Sheehan's syndrome, Clin Endocrinol 27:91–95, 1987.

69. Baylis PH, Thompson CJ, Burd JM, et al: Recurrent pregnancy-induced polyuria and thirst due to hypothalamic diabetes insipidus: An investigation into possible mechanisms responsible for polyuria, Clin Endocrinol 24:459–466, 1986.

70. Barron WM, Cohen LH, Ulland LA: Transient vasopressin-resistant diabetes insipidus of pregnancy, N Engl J Med 310:442–444, 1984.

71. Ito M, Jameson JL, Ito M: Molecular basis of autosomal dominant neurohypophyseal diabetes insipidus: cellular toxicity caused by the accumulation of mutant vasopressin precursors within the endoplasmic reticulum, J Clin Invest 99:2897–2905, 1997.

72. Eubank S, Nguyen TL, Deeb R: Effects of diabetes insipidus mutations on neurophysin folding and function, J Biol Chem 276:29671–29680, 2001.

73. Davies J, Murphy D: Autophagy in hypothalamic neurones of rats expressing a familial neurohypophyseal diabetes insipidus transgene, J Neuroendocrinol 14:629–637, 2002.

74. Rittig S, Sigaard C, Ozata M: Autosomal dominant neurohypophyseal diabetes insipidus due to substitution of histidine for tyrosine-2 in the vasopressin moiety of the hormone precursor, J Clin Endocrinol Metab 87:3351–3355, 2002.

75. Christenson JH, Sigaard C, Corydon TJ: Impaired trafficking of mutated AVP prohormone in cells expressing rare disease genes causing autosomal dominant familial neurohypophyseal diabetes insipidus, Clin Endocrinol 60:125–136, 2004.

76. Elias PCL, Ellias LLK, Torres N: Progressive decline of vasopressin secretion in familial autosomal dominant neurohypophyseal diabetes insipidus presenting a novel mutation in the vasopressin-neurophysin II gene, Clin Endocrinol 59:511–518, 2003.

77. Barrett TG, Bundey SE: Wolfram (DIDMOAD) syndrome, J Med Genet 34:838–841, 1997.

78. Thompson CJ, Charlton J, Walford S, et al: Vasopressin secretion in the DIDMOAD (Wolfram) syndrome, Q J Med 71:333–345, 1989.

79. Cryns K, Sivakumaran TA, Van den Ouweland JMW: Mutational spectrum of the WFS1 gene in Wolfram syndrome, non-syndromic hearing impairment, diabetes mellitus and psychiatric disease, Hum Mutat 22:275–287, 2003.

80. Barbieris C, Mouillac B, Durroux T: Structural basis of vasopressin/oxytocin receptor function, J Endocrinol 156:223–229, 1998.

81. Mulders SM, Bichet DG, Rijss JPL: An aquaporin-2 water channel mutant which causes autosomal dominant nephrogenic diabetes insipidus is retained in the Golgi complex, J Clin Invest 102:57–66, 1998.

82. Asai T, Kuwahara M, Kurihara H: Pathogenesis of nephrogenic diabetes insipidus by aquaporin-2 C-terminus mutations, Kidney Int 64:2–10, 2003.

83. McKenna K, Thompson C: Osmoregulation in clinical disorders of thirst and thirst appreciation, Clin Endocrinol 49:139–152, 1998.

84. Thompson CJ, Edwards CRW, Baylis PH: Osmotic and non-osmotic regulation of thirst and vasopressin secretion in patients with compulsive water drinking, Clin Endocrinol 35:221–228, 1991.

85. Zerbe RL, Robertson GL: A comparison of plasma vasopressin measurements with a standard indirect test in the differential diagnosis of polyuria, N Engl J Med 305:1539–1546, 1981.

86. Robertson GL: Diagnosis of diabetes insipidus. In Czernichow P, Robinson AG, ediotrs: Diabetes Insipidus in Man: Frontiers of Hormone Research, vol 13, Basel, 1985, S. Karger, pp 176–189.

87. Baylis PH, Robertson GL: Vasopressin response to hypertonic saline infusion to assess posterior pituitary function, J R Soc Med 73:255–260, 1980.

88. Diedrich S, Eckmanns T, Exner P: Differential diagnosis of polyuric/polydipsic syndromes with the aid of urinary vasopressin measurement in adults, Clin Endocrinol 54:665–671, 2001.

89. Fujisawa I: Magnetic resonance imaging of hypothalamic-neurohypophyseal system, J Neuroendocrinol 16:297–302, 2004.

90. Ghirardello S, Garrè ML, Rossi A, et al: The diagnosis of children with central diabetes insipidus, J Pediatr Endocrinol Metab 20(3):359–375, 2007 Mar.

91. McIver B, Connacher A, Whittle I, et al: Adipsic hypothalamic diabetes insipidus after clipping of anterior communicating artery aneurysm, BMJ 303(6815):1465–1467, 1991.

92. Crowley RK, Sherlock M, Agha A, et al: Clinical insights into adipsic diabetes insipidus: a large case series, Clin Endocrinol 66:475–482, 2007.

93. Sherlock M, Agha A, Crowley R, et al: Adipsic diabetes after surgery for macroprolactinoma, Pituitary 9:59–64, 2006.

94. Smith D, McKenna K, Moore K, et al: Baroregulation of vasopressin release in adipsic diabetes insipidus, J Clin Endocrinol Metab 87(10):4564–4568, 2002.

95. Ball SG, Vaidja B, Baylis PH: Hypothalamic adipsic syndrome: diagnosis and management, Clin Endocrinol 47(4):405–409, 1997.

96. Bergada I, Aversa L, Heinrich JJ: Peripheral venous thrombosis in children and adolescents with adipsic hypernatraemia secondary to hypothalamic tumours, Horm Res 61(3):108–110, 2004.

97. Schwartz WB, Bennett W, Curelop S, et al: A syndrome of renal sodium loss and hyponatremia probably resulting from inappropriate secretion of antidiuretic hormone, Am J Med 23(4):529–542, 1957.

98. Zerbe R, Stropes L, Robertson G: Vasopressin function in the syndrome of inappropriate antidiuresis, Annu Rev Med 31:315–327, 1980.

99. Seute T, Leffers P, ten Velde GP, et al: Neurologic disorders in 432 consecutive patients with small cell lung carcinoma, Cancer 100(4):801–806, 2004.

100. Sherlock M, O'Sullivan E, Agha A, et al: The incidence and pathophysiology of hyponatraemia after subarachnoid haemorrhage, Clin Endocrinol (Oxf) 64(3):250–254, 2006 Mar.

101. Matsumoto H: Hyponatremia associated with selective serotonin reuptake inhibitors, Intern Med 44(3):173–174, 2005.

102. Miehle K, Paschke R, Koch CA: Citalopram therapy as a risk factor for symptomatic hyponatremia caused by the syndrome of inappropriate secretion of antidiuretic hormone (SIADH): a case report, Pharmacopsychiatry 38(4):181–182, 2005.

103. Bouman WP, Pinner G, Johnson H: Incidence of selective serotonin reuptake inhibitor induced hyponatraemia due to the syndrome of inappropriate antidiuretic hormone secretion in the elderly, Int J Geriatr Psychiatry 13:123–125, 1998.

104. Budisavljevic MN, Stewart L, Sahn SA: Hyponatremia associated with 3,4-methylenedioxymethylamphetamine ("Ecstasy") abuse, Am J Med Sci 326(2):89–93, 2003.

105. Hew-Butler T, Almond C, Ayus JC, et al: Consensus Statement of the 1st International Exercise-Associated Hyponatraemia Consensus Development Conference, Cape Town, South Africa 2005, Clin J Sport Med 15(4):208–213, 2005.

106. Almond CSD, Shin AY, Fortescue EB: Hyponatraemia among runners in the Boston Marathon, N Engl J Med 352(15):1550–1556, 2005.

107. George JM, Capen CC, Philips AS: Biosynthesis of vasopressin in vitro and ultrastructure of a bronchogenic cancer, J Clin Invest 51:141–148, 1972.

108. Gross AJ, Steinberg SM, Reilly JG: Atrial natriuretic factor and arginine vasopressin production in tumor cell lines from patients with lung cancer and their relationship to serum sodium, Cancer Res 53(1):67–74, 1993 Jan 1.

109. Smith D, Moore K, Tormey W, et al: Downward resetting of the osmotic threshold for thirst in patients with SIADH, Am J Physiol Endocrinol Metab 287(5):E1019–E1023, 2004.

110. Baylis PH: The syndrome of inappropriate antidiuretic hormone secretion, Int J Biochem Cell Biol 35(11):1495–1499, 2003.

111. Feldman BJ, Rosenthal SM, Vargas GA: Nephrogenic syndrome of inappropriate antidiuresis, N Engl J Med 352(18):1884–1890, 2005.

112. Ishikawa S, Saito T, Kasono K: Pathological role of aquaporin-2 in impaired water excretion and hyponatremia, J Neuroendocrinol 16(4):293–296, 2004.

113. Saito T, Higashiyama M, Nagasaka S, et al: Role of aquaporin-2 gene expression in hyponatremic rats with

chronic vasopressin-induced antidiuresis, Kidney Int 60(4):1266–1276, 2001.

114. Ishikawa SE, Schrier RW: Pathophysiological roles of arginine vasopressin and aquaporin-2 in impaired water excretion, Clin Endocrinol 58(1):1–17, 2003.

115. Verbalis JG, Murase T, Ecelbarger CA, et al: Studies of renal aquaporin-2 expression during renal escape from vasopressin-induced antidiuresis, Adv Exp Med Biol 449:395–406, 1998.

116. Levinsky NG, Davidson DG, Berliner RW: Changes in urine concentration during prolonged administration of vasopressin and water, Am J Physiol 196(2):451–456, 1959.

117. Verbalis JG: Escape from vasopressin-induced antidiuresis: insights at the molecular level, News Physiol Sci 14:221, 1999.

118. Verbalis JG: Escape from antidiuresis: a good story, Kidney Int 60(4):1608–1610, 2001.

119. Ecelbarger CA, Nielsen S, Olson BR: Role of renal aquaporins in escape from vasopressin-induced antidiuresis in rat, J Clin Invest 99(8):1852–1863, 1997.

120. Tian Y, Sandberg K, Murase T, et al: Vasopressin V2 receptor binding is down-regulated during renal escape from vasopressin-induced antidiuresis, Endocrinology 141(1):307–314, 2000.

121. Ecelbarger CA, Chou CL, Lee AJ, et al: Escape from vasopressin-induced antidiuresis: role of vasopressin resistance of the collecting duct, Am J Physiol 274(6 Pt 2):F1161–F1166, 1998.

122. Diederich S, Franzen NF, Bahr V, et al: Severe hyponatremia due to hypopituitarism with adrenal insufficiency: report on 28 cases, Eur J Endocrinol 148(6):609–617, 2003.

123. Chen YC, Cadnapaphornchai MA, Summer SN: Molecular mechanisms of impaired urinary concentrating ability in glucocorticoid-deficient rats, J Am Soc Nephrol 16(10):2864–2871, 2005.

124. Olchovsky D, Ezra D, Vered I, et al: Symptomatic hyponatremia as a presenting sign of hypothalamic-pituitary disease: a syndrome of inappropriate secretion of antidiuretic hormone (SIADH)-like glucocorticosteroid responsive condition, J Endocrinol Invest 28(2):151–156, 2005.

125. Saito T, Ishikawa SE, Ando F, et al: Vasopressin-dependent upregulation of aquaporin-2 gene expression in glucocorticoid-deficient rats, Am J Physiol Renal Physiol 279(3):F502–F508, 2000.

126. Okada K, Nomura M, Furusuyo N, et al: Amelioration of extrapontine myelinolysis and reversible parkinsonism in a patient with asymptomatic hypopituitarism, Intern Med 44(7):739–742, 2005.

127. Oelkers W: Hyponatraemia and inappropriate secretion of vasopressin (antidiuretic hormone) in patients with hypopituitarism, N Engl J Med 321:492–496, 1989.

128. Fox J, Falik JL, Shalboub RJ: Neurosurgical hyponatraemia: the role of inappropriate antidiuresis, J Neurosurg 34:506–514, 1971.

129. Agha A, Rogers B, Sherlock M, et al: Anterior pituitary dysfunction in survivors of traumatic brain injury, J Clin Endocrinol Metab 89(10):4929–4936, 2004.

130. Aimaretti G, Ambrosio MR, Di Somma C, et al: Traumatic brain injury and subarachnoid haemorrhage are conditions at high risk for hypopituitarism: screening study at 3 months after the brain injury, Clin Endocrinol (Oxf) 61(3):320–326, 2004.

131. Agha A, Sherlock M, Thompson CJ: Post-traumatic hyponatraemia due to acute hypopituitarism, QJM 98(6):463–464, 2005.

132. Sari R, Sevinc A: Life-threatening hyponatremia due to cessation of L-thyroxine, J Natl Med Assoc 95(10):991–994, 2003.

133. Taskapan C, Sahin I, Taskapan H, et al: Possible malignant neuroleptic syndrome that is associated with hypothyroidism, Prog Neuropsychopharmacol Biol Psychiatry 29(5):745–748, 2005.

134. Chen YC, Cadnapaphornchai MA, Yang J, et al: Nonosmotic release of vasopressin and renal aquaporins in impaired urinary dilution in hypothyroidism, Am J Physiol Renal Physiol 289(4):F672–F678, 2005.

135. Hanna FW, Scanlon MF: Hyponatraemia, hypothyroidism and role of arginine-vasopressin, Lancet 350:755–756, 1997.

136. Schmitz PH, de Meijer PH, Meinders AE: Hyponatremia due to hypothyroidism: a pure renal mechanism, Neth J Med 58(3):143–149, 2001.

137. Montenegro J, Gonzalez O, Saracho R, et al: Changes in renal function in primary hypothyroidism, Am J Kidney Dis 27(2):195–198, 1996.

138. Adrogue HJ: Consequences of inadequate management of hyponatremia, Am J Nephrol 25(3):240–249, 2005.

139. Verbalis JG: Disorders of body water homeostasis, Best Pract Res Clin Endocrinol Metab 17(4):471–503, 2003.

140. Yeates KE, Singer M, Morton AR: Salt and water: a simple approach to hyponatremia, CMAJ 170(3):365–369, 2004.

141. Verbalis JG: Vasopressin V2 receptor antagonists, J Mol Endocrinol 29(1):1–9, 2002.

142. Serradeil-Le Gal C, Wagnon J, Valette G, et al: Nonpeptide vasopressin receptor antagonists: development of selective and orally active V1a, V2 and V1b receptor ligands, Prog Brain Res 139:197–210, 2002.

143. Palm C, Reimann D, Gross P: The role of V2 vasopressin antagonists in hyponatremia, Cardiovasc Res 51(3):403–408, 2001.

Chapter 15

THE PINEAL GLAND AND MELATONIN

GARY WAND

The human pineal gland is the most poorly understood endocrine organ. Although it has been described as a dispensable gland in humans, the pineal gland converts light information into a hormonal signal in the form of melatonin. Melatonin is a chronobiotic hormone with multiple pleomorphic actions. The hormone transmits information regarding day length which helps organize circadian and seasonal rhythms. The mammalian pineal gland plays numerous modulatory roles in the regulation of sleep, body temperature, reproductive, and immune function. However, there is still little evidence that the pineal gland has a vital regulatory role in human biology. For example, there is no clearly documented severe morbid phenotype produced following pinealectomy. Despite the lack of evidence that the pineal gland is essential in human biology, there is growing evidence that exogenously administered melatonin may have therapeutic value in treating several disorders. Moreover, there are a variety of tumors of the pineal gland region that can impose substantial morbidity and mortality for the patient if not quickly diagnosed and appropriately treated.

Pineal Gland

The human pineal gland weighs approximately 100 to 200 mg and is roughly 5 to 9 mm in length, 1 to 5 mm in width, and 3 to 5 mm in thickness. The name *pineal* is derived from the pinecone-like structure of the gland. The pineal gland is formed by a central core of lobules surrounded by a cortex with a diffuse distribution of neurons. The gland is an embryologic outgrowth of the roof of the third ventricle and at birth is attached to the posterior roof of the third ventricle between the posterior commissure and the dorsal habenula, located on top of and between the superior colliculi.

Histologically, the pineal gland is composed of pinealocytes, which have endocrine cell properties that include cytoplasmic processes terminating on fenestrated capillaries. Neuroglia are found unevenly distributed surrounding the pinealocytes. The pineal gland belongs to circumventricular organs of the CNS that surround the third ventricle and thus are not protected by the blood-brain barrier.

Calcareous deposits are a common radiographic characteristic of the gland. This material is composed of calcium and magnesium salts, hydroxyapatite, and trace elements. These deposits can be present at birth but increase in density with age. The impact of these deposits on pineal gland function is uncertain.

NEURAL INNERVATION OF THE PINEAL GLAND

Phylogenetically, the pineal gland is derived from photoreceptor cells; however, these properties have been lost in humans. The mammalian pineal gland does not have photoreceptor activity but rather receives photosensory information from the neuroretina. This information is relayed through the retinohypothalamic tract to the suprachiasmatic nucleus (SCN) of the hypothalamus, which functions as a circadian oscillator or clock (Fig. 15-1). Fibers from the SCN then descend to the spinal cord, projecting to the superior cervical ganglia, from which postganglionic adrenergic neurons return to innervate the pineal gland. These fibers contain norepinephrine and neuropeptide Y. Through this pathway, melatonin synthesis is controlled and its

THE PINEAL GLAND

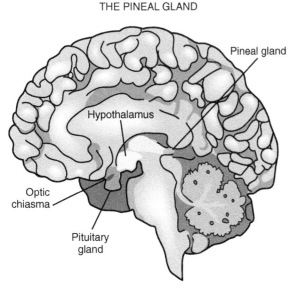

FIGURE 15-1. Anatomic relationship among the pineal gland, hypothalamus, and pituitary gland.

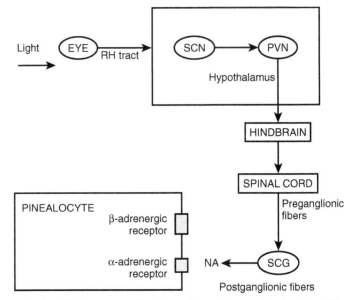

FIGURE 15-2. Pathways providing light and neural input to the pineal gland. The melatonin rhythm is synchronized to a 24-hour light/dark cycle primarily by the retina and retinohypothalamic projections to the SCN. *RH*, retinohypothalamic; *SCN*, suprachiasmatic nucleus; *PVN*, paraventricular nucleus; *SCG*, superior cervical ganglion; *NA*, norepinephrine.

rhythm entrained (synchronized) to the 24-hour light/dark cycle (see below). It is generated in the SCN by a closed loop of negative feedback of clock gene expression.[1]

The pineal gland also receives parasympathetic and peptidergic innervation originating in the hypothalamus, mesolimbic system, and visual structures. These fibers contain a number of neurotransmitters such as somatostatin, serotonin, and histamine. The pineal gland also contains gonadotropin-releasing hormone (GnRH), thyrotropin-releasing hormone (TRH), vasotocin, and other peptides whose roles are yet to be defined.

Melatonin

The word *melatonin* is a derivative of the Greek words *melas* and *tonein*, coined because of the property of melatonin to lighten amphibian skin.[2] Melatonin is *N*-acetyl-5-methoxytryptamine, an indolamine derivative of tryptophan. The molecule is extremely well conserved across the phyla and has been identified in all major taxa, including bacteria, unicellular eukaryotes, many plants species, and all animals.[3] In the vertebrate, melatonin is primarily secreted by the pineal gland, although a variety of other tissues, including the retina, bone marrow, skin, lymphocytes, and gastrointestinal tract, also synthesize the hormone. Melatonin derived from the gastrointestinal tract can be released into the circulation after ingestion of high dietary tryptophan.[4]

SYNTHESIS AND SECRETION OF MELATONIN

Through the neuroretinal pathways described above, the pineal gland becomes a neuroendocrine transducer, transmitting the SCN message into a hormonal code which signals that light or darkness has arrived. Indeed, the main function of the pineal gland is to translate SCN activity into the rhythmic release of melatonin, which in turn helps synchronize several daily and seasonal cycles. The synthesis of melatonin is presented in Fig. 15-2. The hormone is synthesized from the amino acid tryptophan, which is converted into serotonin prior to being processed into melatonin. Melatonin synthesis and secretion are greater during the dark phase compared to the light phase of the cycle. During the light phase of the photoperiod, SCN activity is high,

resulting in low norepinephrine levels. Under reduced adrenergic activity, tryptophan is converted into serotonin in a two-step process via the intermediary, 5-hydroxytryptophan. At this point, serotonin does not come into contact with the enzyme responsible for converting it into melatonin. Therefore, plasma levels of melatonin are low during the light phase. However, with the arrival of the dark period, SCN activity becomes quiescent, and noradrenergic activity increases, resulting in activation of β-adrenergic receptors (and to a lesser extent α-adrenergic receptors) on the pinealocyte. The β-adrenergic receptors are coupled to cyclic adenosine monophosphate (cAMP)/protein kinase A signaling pathways that stimulate melatonin synthesis (Fig. 15-3). Stimulation of α-adrenergic receptors potentiates β-adrenergic function, resulting in a cascade that mobilizes calcium ions, phosphatidylinositol, diacylglycerol, and protein kinase C.[5] This process requires serotonin to be first converted into *N*-acetyl serotonin by the enzyme serotonin-*N*-acetyltransferase, which in turn is converted into melatonin after coming into contact with the enzyme hydroxyindole-*O*-methyltransferase (HIOMT).[6] The longer the dark phase, the longer the duration of melatonin secretion.

Melatonin is not stored after synthesis but merely diffuses out of the pineal gland into the blood stream and cerebrospinal fluid. In the transition from light to dark, plasma melatonin concentrations increase from 2 to 10 pg/mL to 100 to 200 pg/mL.[7] Melatonin levels start to rise during the evening, reach maximum levels in the middle of the night, and start decreasing in the early morning before sunrise. Although the melatonin rhythm is highly responsive to the light cycle, it does persist when people are placed for a few days in a dark room and does not immediately phase shift when the light schedule is altered.[7] This indicates that the rhythm is not simply generated by the light/dark cycle but is free running and modulated by endogenous signals probably arising in the SCN. Indeed, the rhythm is abolished by lesioning of the SCN and persists, albeit in modified form, in the blind.[8] The day-to-day pattern of melatonin secretion is extremely stable within an individual.[9] However, the melatonin rhythm varies widely among individuals, in part owing to genetic determinants.[9a] In fact, a small number of healthy persons have no detectable melatonin in plasma at any time of day.[10]

Melatonin has a bi-exponential half-life, with a first distribution $T_{1/2}$ of 2 minutes and a second of 20 minutes. The hormone is lipophilic and enters tissues rapidly. Up to 70% of melatonin is bound to albumin in plasma.[11] In addition to blood, saliva, and urine, melatonin is also found in cerebrospinal fluid (CSF), the anterior chamber of the eye, and in many reproductive fluids, including semen, amniotic fluid, and breast milk.[12] Melatonin levels in plasma, CSF, saliva, and urine become undetectable following removal of the pineal gland, demonstrating that the pineal gland is the main source of melatonin in these compartments.[13]

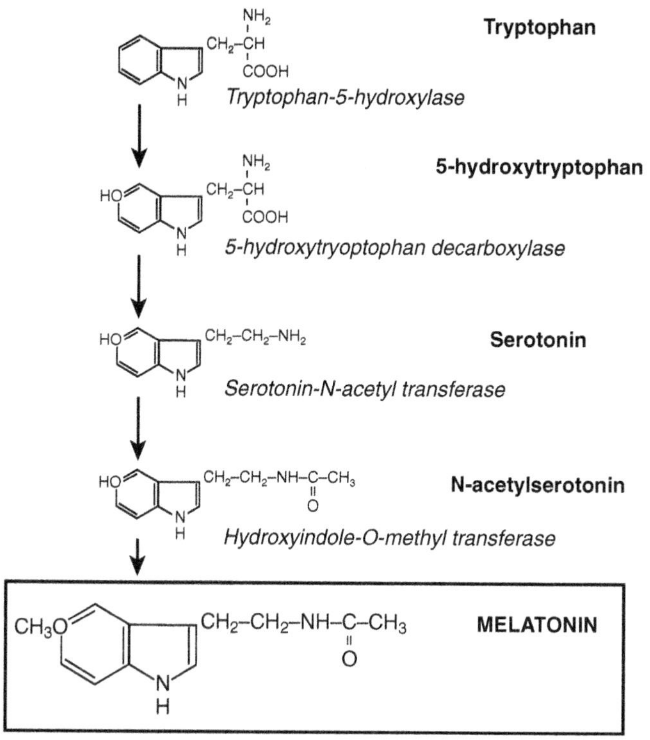

Melatonin secretion varies across the life cycle. Secretion of the hormone begins in the fourth month of postnatal life and then increases rapidly, peaking between the ages of 1 and 3. Nocturnal melatonin secretion then starts a marked decline over each decade of life[14] (Fig. 15-4). Nocturnal melatonin concentrations can also be affected by drugs that interfere with the transmission of neurotransmitter signals to the pineal gland. These drugs include β-blockers, caffeine, and ethanol.[15-17] Nocturnal melatonin secretion is also suppressed by exposure to environmental lighting. Indeed, there is a dose-dependent and spectral-sensitive acute suppressive effect of light on melatonin.[18,19] Even low light levels found indoors can suppress nocturnal melatonin production. In addition to light, exercise and postural changes decrease plasma melatonin levels.[20,21]

Melatonin Receptors

In the mammal, there are at least two melatonin receptors, designated MT1 and MT2, which belong to the superfamily of G protein–coupled receptors containing the usual seven transmembrane domains. A third melatonin binding site, MT3, was found to be the enzyme quinone reductase 2.[22] These receptors have distinct structures, chromosomal localization, and pharmacologic properties.[23] The MT1 and MT2 receptors are differentially expressed across the nervous system. The highest density is found in the SCN, followed by the anterior pituitary and the retina.[24] Studies have shown that the MT1 receptor in the SCN allows melatonin to inhibit firing of SCN neurons during the nighttime.[24] The SCN MT2 receptor possibly mediates the effect of melatonin on SCN circadian rhythms.[24] Both receptors are co-localized within the SCN and are coupled to multiple signaling pathways, with suppression of cyclic AMP production through a Gi-dependent process being the most common.[23] The receptors can also stimulate phospholipase C, affecting various ion channels, as well as stimulating the mitogen-activated protein kinase cascade and the estrogen-dependent signaling cascade.[25] Melatonin is a small, lipophilic compound which easily crosses membranes. In this regard, melatonin has been shown to bind to specific nuclear receptors of the retinoic acid receptor family[26,27] and to calmodulin. Melatonin receptors have also been identified in the heart, kidney, liver, and many other peripheral tissues.[28,29]

The MT1 and MT2 receptors have different profiles for receptor desensitization. Exposure of the MT1 receptor to supraphysi-

FIGURE 15-3. Melatonin biosynthetic pathway.

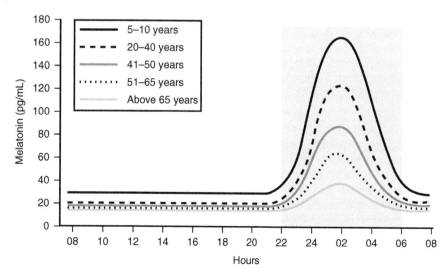

FIGURE 15-4. Circadian profile of serum melatonin across the life cycle; gray area indicates darkness.

ologic concentrations of melatonin causes an increase in MT1 receptor density, with a concurrent decrease in affinity and functional sensitivity.[24] In contrast, exposure of the MT2 receptor to physiologic concentrations of melatonin can induce a concentration and time-dependent receptor desensitization and internalization.[30] The interplay between desensitization of the MT1 and MT2 receptors to daytime and nighttime physiologic concentrations of melatonin may promote changes in melatonin receptor function throughout the human circadian cycle. With the SCN ultimately controlling the production of melatonin, a feedback loop is created that may use melatonin as the regulatory control of SCN firing and phase-shifting functions.[31] Desensitization of MT1 and MT2 receptors needs to be taken into account when administering melatonin to patients.

Melatonin Metabolism

Melatonin in the circulation is mainly inactivated by the liver's cytochrome P450-specific mono-oxygenase, which first hydroxylates position C6 and then conjugates the product to a sulfate excreted into urine and feces as 6-sulfatooxymelatonin.[32] The metabolism in nonhepatic tissue is different and is mainly through deacetylation. Melatonin can also be nonenzymatically metabolized in all cells and also extracellularly by free radicals.

Approximately 2% of circulating melatonin is excreted unchanged into urine and saliva. These body fluids can be assayed for melatonin.

Actions of Endogenous and Exogenous Melatonin

Seasonal and circadian rhythms serve an essential function in all living organisms. In conjunction with the SCN, melatonin signals the time of day and time of year to cells throughout the body and in so doing, modulates seasonal and circadian rhythms.

Seasonal variations in day length have reciprocal effects on melatonin secretion and can thus differentially affect plasma melatonin levels, depending on the location of the human population. For example, individuals living at high northern latitudes have a lengthening of melatonin secretion during winter nights.[33] This may help explain how changes in the seasons affect reproductive vitality. In the laboratory setting, artificial shorting or lengthening of "night" will also adjust the duration of melatonin secretion.[34]

Circadian rhythms are biological processes that have a 24-hour periodicity even in the absence of external cues. Melatonin is involved in regulating several circadian cycles, including core body temperature and the sleep/wake cycle. The temporal organization of human circadian rhythms has been assigned the following terms: "biological day," "biological night," "biological dawn," and "biological dusk."[35] During this 24-hour cycle, rising melatonin levels are associated with decreasing core body temperature, cortisol levels, and alertness. As melatonin levels wane, core body temperature, REM sleep propensity, and cortisol levels increase. It remains unclear whether there is a causal relationship between melatonin and these changes in the sleep/wake cycle. However, exogenously administered melatonin can phase shift body temperature, sleep timing, and the endogenous melatonin cycle.[32] The ability of melatonin to phase shift circadian cycles has been exploited in the treatment of jet lag and shift-work disorders (see below).

SLEEP

The evening rise in melatonin precedes bedtime by about 2 hours and suggests a causal relationship. Indeed, the peak in plasma melatonin occurs when alertness is at its nadir. However, the sleep/wake cycle is regulated by both homeostatic and circadian processes and is only partially influenced by melatonin. The Smith-Magenis syndrome illustrates the association between melatonin and the sleep/wake cycle. The manifestations of this disorder include excessive daytime sleepiness and insomnia at night. Treatment of these patients with a β-adrenergic blocker decreases daytime melatonin levels and diminishes daytime sleepiness.[36] Administration of physiologic and pharmacologic doses of melatonin to normal sleepers induces soporific symptoms. However, evidence of a direct relationship between endogenous melatonin and insomnia has been mixed.[37,38] The number of reports that have measured plasma melatonin concentrations in sleep disorders is surprisingly low, considering its use as sleep-promoting agent for insomnia. Sleep disturbances have been described in some but not all pinealectomized patients, and administration of melatonin has sometimes been found to be efficacious in this setting.[39]

Although the exact role of endogenous melatonin in regulating human sleep remains to be fully elucidated, exogenous melatonin administration (0.1 to 0.3 mg) resulting in physiologic levels of melatonin will promote the onset and maintenance of sleep.[32] Both a 1997 and a 2005 meta-analysis showed that melatonin administration decreases sleep latency, increases sleep efficiency, and increases total sleep duration in patients with primary insomnia.[40,41] However, a meta-analysis published in 2006 which included patients with secondary causes of insomnia produced less clear-cut results.[42]

The sleep-promoting effect of melatonin has been linked to the inhibition of neuronal activity through activation of SCN MT1 receptors.[43] A synthetic melatonin agonist, Ramelteon, which selectively activates MT1 and MT2 melatonin receptors, has been approved for the treatment of insomnia. Ramelteon shows 10-fold higher binding affinity for the MT1 compared to the MT2 receptor and 17 times higher affinity than melatonin for either receptor. The drug shows no affinity for a large number of other G protein–coupled receptors, enzymes, and neurotransmitter channels. In addition to Ramelteon, there are several other melatonin agonists under development.[24]

JET LAG

Jet lag is a syndrome associated with transmeridian travel resulting in disturbances to circadian rhythms. Manifestations of jet lag include problems sleeping, malaise, fatigue, and reduced performance. A similar syndrome may result from shift work and rarely from the transition to daylight savings time. Eastbound travel is generally associated with worse symptoms than westbound travel. The severity of jet lag is also proportional to the number of time zones crossed. Left untreated, the relationship between endogenous rhythms and environmental cues will come back into synchrony over several days to a week. The ability of melatonin to speed up the process of resynchronization accounts for its efficacy in the treatment of jet lag. Phase shifting of the neuronal firing rhythms has been linked to activation of the MT2 receptor at dusk, although MT1 may also be involved.[44]

For air travelers crossing five or more time zones going in the eastward direction, melatonin has been found to be effective in treating jet lag when administered close to the target bedtime at the travel destination.[45] Doses from 0.5 to 5 mg are found to be effective. Treatment should begin the first evening upon arrival to the destination. Side effects of melatonin in this setting include daytime sleepiness, especially with the higher doses, dizziness, headaches, and loss of appetite.[45] In addition to melatonin administration, proper nutrition, going to sleep according to the new time zone, exercising, and maximizing light exposure when awake can help alleviate jet lag symptoms.

Similar to individuals with jet lag, shift workers often have symptoms of fatigue, sleep disturbances, and gastrointestinal problems.[46] Studies have observed marked variability in circadian melatonin profile in these workers.[47] When administered at the desired bedtime during a night shift, melatonin seems to improve sleep and increase daytime alertness.[46]

Disorders in the sleep/wake cycle, core body temperature, and cortisol secretion are very common in blind people with no significant light perception.[48] Many blind individuals have abnormal melatonin or 6-sulfatoxymelatonin circadian profiles.[49,50] In these settings, melatonin has proven effective in phase-shifting the circadian clock and in so doing, stabilizing sleep onset and sometimes improving quality and duration of sleep.[49,51]

REPRODUCTION

In seasonal-breeding mammals, melatonin is involved in regulating the breeding cycle.[52] The effects of melatonin on the reproductive system are generally antigonadotropic. Melatonin inhibits secretion of the gonadotropin hormones LH and FSH. This inhibitory affect is most likely due to inhibition of GnRH from the hypothalamus.[53] For seasonal-breeding animals, seasonal changes in day length and thus melatonin secretion will up-regulate or down-regulate the gonadal axis. For example, during the shorter period of daylight that accompanies the nonbreeding season, melatonin levels are increased and down-regulate the gonadal axis. As the breeding season approaches and length of daylight increases, melatonin levels fall, allowing rejuvenation of the gonads.

Humans are not seasonal breeders, but melatonin may mediate the moderate seasonal fluctuations observed in human reproductive function.[3] The increased conception rate seen in northern latitudes during the summer season has been reported to be caused by changes in gonadotropin induced by changes in melatonin secretion. Melatonin levels have been reported elevated in male infertility[54] and in men with hypogonadotropic hypogonadism.[55,56] Moreover, elevated melatonin levels have been reported in women with stress- and exercise-induced amenorrhea and in men with infertility.[57] Exogenous melatonin administration has been shown to suppress LH levels in men and women and to reduce sperm motility in men.[58]

Melatonin has also been implicated in sexual maturation, where it may have inhibitory action on the onset of puberty. It has been proposed that a decline of melatonin below a threshold value may be a signal that activates GnRH pulsation in early puberty.[3] Circumstantial evidence that melatonin is involved in sexual maturation includes the observation that children with precocious puberty have lower plasma melatonin levels, whereas children with delayed puberty exhibit higher nocturnal melatonin concentrations. However, a causal relationship between the pineal gland and human reproductive function is far from clear.

TEMPERATURE

Body temperature and plasma melatonin levels have a reciprocal profile; the 24-hour temperature nadir correlates with peak plasma melatonin levels.[59] It has been estimated that approximately half of the nighttime decline in core temperature is induced by melatonin.[60] Supporting a causal relationship between melatonin and body temperature are studies showing that exogenously administered melatonin will decrease body temperature in humans.[61]

BLOOD PRESSURE

There is circumstantial evidence that melatonin may be involved in the regulation of blood pressure. During the night, humans have lower blood pressure, heart rate, and cardiac output which are all associated with increases in plasma melatonin levels. There is an increased risk of myocardial infarction and stroke in the early morning when melatonin levels are low. Moreover, patients with coronary heart disease have lower melatonin levels and higher norepinephrine levels compared to persons without cardiac disease. It is known that the nocturnal surge in melatonin is blunted in patients with hypertension, especially nocturnal hypertension.[62] To this end, studies have shown that melatonin (~2 mg) can lower nighttime blood pressure.[63]

IMMUNE SYSTEM AND CANCER

In animal models, melatonin has immunoenhancing properties and can reverse the immunosuppressive effects of acute stress, cancer drug therapy, and viral infections.[64] Surgical and functional pinealectomy has been shown to reduce thymic and splenic weights in mice, rats, and hamsters corresponding to a reduction in B and T cells.[65] Pinealectomy alters the activity of thymic enzymes and in the newborn rodent is associated with disorganization of thymic structures. In the rodent, neonatal pinealectomy also impairs immune function. Conversely, the administration of melatonin to rodents increases thymic and splenic weight, provides protection against the catabolic effects of dexamethasone on body weight and atrophy of the thymus and adrenal glands, and enhances immune responses to certain infectious agents.[66] Melatonin administration increases the number of natural killer (NK) cells and monocytes in bone marrow and increases helper T-cell activity and interleukin-2 (IL-2) production in human lymphocytes.[66] In general, these observations show that melatonin's stimulatory effects on the immune system are best observed in states of immunosuppression. The role of pineal-derived and immune cell–derived melatonin on human immunity is not clear.

Melatonin is also reported to have oncostatic actions.[3] Pinealectomized rats and hamsters have accelerated growth in a variety of transplanted cancers. Although chronic melatonin administration has oncostatic effects in breast and ovarian cancer in rodent models, high-dose melatonin did not alter survival in human melanoma patients.[67] However, co-administration of melatonin and interferon gamma improved tumor regression in patients with metastatic renal cell carcinoma.[68] Melatonin has also been shown to protect the host from negative effects of IL-2 while synergizing with the anticancer action of the cytokine.[69] Much more information is needed to prove that melatonin will serve as a useful oncostatic medication in humans.

ANTIOXIDANT AND ANTI-AGING

At supraphysiologic concentrations, melatonin has antioxidant properties. Melatonin's free-radical scavenging properties are due in part to its ability to modulate catalase, superoxide dismutase, and glutathione peroxidase. Compared to two well-known scavengers, glutathione and mannitol, melatonin is 4 times and 14 times more effective, respectively.[70] The small molecule is both lipophilic and hydrophilic and easily enters the cytosol and nucleus, thus making it a potentially efficient antioxidant.[71] However, the question still remains whether in physiologic concentrations, melatonin is an efficient free-radical scavenger. In a meta-analysis of three trials of melatonin treatment for the cognitive impairment associated with dementia, no evidence of benefit was seen.[72]

PSYCHIATRIC DISORDERS

Altered melatonin rhythms and levels have been observed in depression, mania, schizophrenia, anorexia nervosa, and other psychiatric disorders.[73] However, there is no compelling evidence that melatonin contributes to the symptomatology associated with these psychiatric disorders.

Lesions of the Pineal Gland and Pineal Region

The pineal region can give rise to cysts and many types of neoplastic masses, including pineal cell tumors, germ cell tumors, gliomas, meningiomas, and metastases. Early detection and appropriate treatment of the neoplastic syndromes maximizes chances for better outcomes.

PINEAL GLAND CYSTS

A pineal cyst is a benign lesion lined by normal pineal parenchymal and glial cells. It is not uncommon for the endocrinologist to order a magnetic resonance imaging (MRI) scan of the brain during the evaluation of a pituitary disorder and also find an incidental pineal cyst. Indeed, the asymptomatic pineal cyst is a common neuroimaging finding seen on approximately 4% of MRI scans and observed in up to 40% of routine autopsies.[74] The main importance in identifying a pineal cyst is to distinguish it from cystic tumors that also occur in this region and require treatment.

On computerized tomography (CT) images, pineal cysts are hypodense; occasionally there is evidence of hemorrhage. Cyst walls may or may not show contrast enhancement, and calcifications within the wall are found in about half of cases. On MRI images, the pineal cyst is round and smooth without intracystic trabeculations. It has low signal intensity on both T1WI and T2WI.[75] Occasionally the imaging appearance of a benign pineal cyst is indistinguishable from small cystic neoplasms. For example, similar to pineal cysts, pineocytomas may be isointense with respect to CSF, but the latter usually have intratumoral trabeculations.

Pathologic analysis occasionally misdiagnoses benign pineal gland cysts as pineocytoma or pilocytic astrocytoma. This is an important error to avoid, since misdiagnosis could lead to inappropriate therapies. Errors are more likely to be made when small specimens were obtained at biopsy, making it difficult to determine whether the pineal tissue is normal or neoplastic.

Most pineal cysts are small, and patients are asymptomatic. Some cysts spontaneously resolve. One study observed that in 32 patients with pineal cysts, 75% remained stable over time, 16% decreased in size or resolved, whereas only 8% increased in size.[76] Small, asymptomatic cysts require no intervention.

Rarely, a pineal cyst becomes symptomatic.[77] Symptomatic cysts tend to be larger than their asymptomatic counterparts. Although symptomatic pineal cysts have been reported in patients from 7 to 69 years of age, most occur be between 21

and 30 years of age. There is a 3:1 female predominance. Patients generally present with headaches as a result of acute hydrocephalus. A high degree of clinical suspicion is needed, because headache may be the only symptom. Headache may have either a prolonged intermittent or acute course.

The symptomatic patient is generally treated with either an open procedure or endoscopic stereotactic resection. Either procedure can cure the patient and eliminate the need for CSF shunting. Both procedures allow for both histologic sampling and relief of symptoms. Some surgeons prefer the stereotactic technique because morbidity is lower compared to an open procedure.

TUMORS IN THE PINEAL GLAND REGION

Meningiomas

Meningiomas constitute about 8% of lesions in the pineal gland region, and pineal meningiomas account for less than 1% of all meningiomas.[78] They tend to occur in middle age and have a female predominance. Patients with meningiomas in the pineal region usually present with headaches and the other signs related to acute hydrocephalus.

Pineal meningiomas usually present with dural attachment, which can compromise venous flow. Less commonly, the tumor is not attached to dura. Peripheral calcification is commonly observed on CT imaging. On MRI, meningiomas have well-defined margins, and attachments to the falx can be appreciated on sagittal images.[75] Cerebral angiography should be performed to outline the relationship between tumor and the surrounding vasculature. The main therapy is surgical resection.

Pineal Parenchymal Tumors

Approximately 10% to 28% of pineal-region tumors are of pineal parenchymal origin.[79] Pineal parenchymal tumors occur throughout the life cycle but are 10 times more common in children than in adults.[80] These tumors originate from parenchymal cells showing varying degrees of differentiation, from primitive parenchymal cells through tumors consisting of well-differentiated pinealocytes. Some experts classify this histologic continuum into three types of pineal cell neoplasms: (1) pineocytoma (most differentiated), (2) pineal parenchymal tumors of intermediate differentiation, and (3) pineoblastoma (least differentiated).[81] The less differentiated tumors are more aggressive, more apt to metastasize, and are associated with a worse prognosis. Adults are more likely to present with pineocytoma, whereas children are more likely to develop pineoblastoma.[82]

Pineocytoma

Pineocytomas are slow-growing lesions containing mature cells that are histologically almost indistinguishable from normal pineal parenchyma. Pineocytomas correspond histologically to World Health Organization (WHO) grade II. These tumors can occur in any age but tend to affect young adults, with a peak incidence at age 30 to 35.[83] Pineocytomas often have calcifications that are peripherally displaced. These well-circumscribed lesions account for 45% of pineal parenchymal tumors.[84] They usually do not seed the CSF.

Microscopically, pineocytomas are composed of sheets of non-pleomorphic, mature-appearing cells containing pseudorosettes arranged in lobules with occasional or absent mitotic figures.[85] Necrosis is absent. The pseudorosettes are separated by fibrovascular septa. The absence of rosettes (i.e., lack of neuronal differentiation) is associated with a poorer prognosis. The cells almost always stain positive for neuron-specific enolase, retinal S-antigen and rhodopsin and sometimes for neurofilament protein, chromogranin A, β-tubulin III and αB crystalline.[85] Staining for neuron-specific enolase can be used to distinguish pineocytomas and pineoblastomas from astrocytic tumors.

Pineoblastoma

The pineoblastoma is a neoplasm composed of poorly differentiated, primitive cells with significant potential for leptomeningeal and extracranial spread. This tumor is a variant of primitive neuroectodermal tumors and is similar to medulloblastoma and retinoblastinoma.[85] The tumors correspond histologically to WHO grade IV.[81] Pineoblastomas usually occur in the first 2 decades of life. They constitute approximately 45% of pineal parenchymal tumors.[86] The 5-year prognosis is approximately 58% or less.

Microscopically, pineoblastomas are highly cellular tumors composed of irregular sheets of pleomorphic, small, undifferentiated cells without lobular architecture. Necrosis is common. Pineoblastomas lack the pseudorosettes found in pineocytomas but can have Homer-Wright or Flexner-Wintersteiner rosettes, which are markers of retinoblastic differentiation.[85] This tumor is indistinguishable from medulloblastoma. Pineoblastomas express neuronal and photosensory markers similar to pineocytomas, but staining is more variable.[87]

Intermediate Pineal Parenchymal Tumors

Approximately 10% of pineal parenchymal tumors are of intermediate differentiation. These types of tumor can be divided into two kinds: (1) tumors composed of both poorly differentiated pineoblastoma-like cells and well-differentiated pineocyte-like cells or (2) tumors consisting of cells with intermediate histologic features between pineocytoma and pineoblastoma cells. The clinical behavior of the intermediate tumor is variable, usually more aggressive than a pineocytoma and less aggressive than a pineoblastoma.

Germ Cell Tumors

Germ cell tumors account for approximately 30% to 85% of tumors in the pineal region.[82] Males are twice as likely as females to develop germ cell lesions in the pineal region, with evidence of an even higher male-to-female ratio for nongerminomatous germ cell tumors. Germ cell tumors account for approximately 1% to 2% of intracranial tumors in adults and 10% in children. For unclear reasons, pineal germ cell tumors have a relatively higher incidence in Japan and East Asia than in the West. Most patients with germ cell tumors are between 10 and 30 years of age, with a peak age of presentation in the second decade.

Similar to germ cell tumors in the periphery, central nervous system germ cell tumors occur in midline locations and most commonly occur in the pineal region and in the hypothalamic-neurohypophyseal region. In several series, approximately 15% of germ cell tumors were located in both the pineal and neurohypophyseal regions.[88] These bifocal lesions are often brought to attention with the onset of diabetes insipidus. Imaging typically shows a small pineal-region mass and thickening of the infundibulum.

Germ cell tumors are derived from embryonal cells and are generally classified into six types: germinoma, teratoma, mixed germ cell tumors, embryonal carcinoma, choriocarcinoma, and yolk sack tumor. The exact incidence of the specific types of germ cell tumors is difficult to determine, but approximately a third are germinomas, a third are teratomas, and a fifth are mixed germ cell lesions, with the remainder subtypes accounting for the rest. Mixed germ cell tumors have multiple subtypes; the prognosis is determined by the most malignant cell type.[89] Teratomas have the capacity to differentiate from ectoderm, mesoderm, or endoderm, and mature tumors do not metastasize. Yolk sack tumors, choriocarcinoma, and embryonal cell tumors are the least common of the germ cell tumors and are generally aggressive. Germ cell tumors frequently metastasize and disseminate into the CSF. Most nongerminomatous germ cell tumors and some germinomas are associated with tumor markers in CSF. Beta human chorionic gonadotropin (β-hCG) is elevated in choriocarcinomas, whereas α-fetoprotein (AFP) is elevated in yolk sac and embryonic tumors.[90] High elevation of these markers is diagnostic of nongerminomatous germ cell tumors, and the degree of elevation correlates with aggressiveness of the tumor.[91] Although markers can be elevated in blood, the CSF compartment is a much more sensitive indicator of disease. Germinomas are much less likely than nongerminomatous tumors to be associated with high elevations in CSF, AFP, or β-hCG.

Clinical Presentation for All Tumors in the Pineal Region

Pineal regional tumors share a clinical presentation because all tumors in this region cause symptoms by compression or invasion of local surrounding structures. This often results in blockage of CSF flow at the level of the third ventricle or aqueduct, resulting in hydrocephalus. The most common symptoms are headaches, visual abnormalities, nausea, vomiting, and difficulty walking (Table 15-1).

The most common presenting signs seen in patients with pineal body lesions are papilledema, ataxia, loss of upward gaze, tremor, altered papillary reflexes, and hyperactive deep tendon reflexes (see Table 15-1). Owing to pressure placed on the pretectal area of the brain, many patients present with abnormalities in vertical gaze, especially upward gaze, nystagmus, and impaired convergence and divergence. This is known as *Parinaud's Syndrome* (Table 15-2). Patients may also have leptomeningeal symptoms, which are common in pineoblastomas and germ cell tumors.

Because 10% to 15% of germinomas are simultaneously located in both the pineal and suprasellar region, patients with bifocal tumors usually present with evidence of hypothalamic and/or pituitary dysfunction, including diabetes insipidus. An interesting phenomenon has been observed where diabetes

Table 15-1. Symptoms and Signs Associated With Lesions in the Pineal Region

Symptoms
Headaches
Vision abnormalities
Nausea and vomiting
Impaired ambulation

Signs
Papilledema
Ataxia
Loss of upward gaze
Tremor
Altered pupillary reflexes

Table 15-2. Parinaud's Syndrome

Symptoms

Difficulty looking up
Double vision
Blurred vision
Oscillopsia

Signs

Vertical gaze abnormalities, especially upgaze
Convergence retraction nystagmus
Lid retraction (Collier's "tucked lid" sign)
Impaired convergence and divergence
Excessive convergence tone
Bilateral ptosis
Pupillary abnormalities (large with light-near dissociation)

insipidus has been found in patients for whom the tumor is restricted to the pineal region. It has been posited that the presence of diabetes insipidus in patients with pineal germinomas indicates that germinomatous tissue is also present on the floor of the third ventricle despite negative neuroradiographic findings.[92] Patients with bifocal disease may also present with precocious puberty with or without elevations in LH and/or β-hCG.[92]

IMAGING

Although imaging alone cannot determine tumor histology, it can help the clinician narrow down the rather extensive differential diagnosis of masses in this region, as well as clarify the degree of obstructive hydrocephalous that may be present. Moreover, imaging is crucial in the staging process (see below).

Magnetic Resonance Imaging

On MRI, pineal neoplasms are often lobulated, solid tumors.[93] Generally, pineoblastomas are isointense to gray matter on T2WI (weighted image) and may also show brain edema or invasion in the surrounding brain parenchyma.[94] Pineocytomas, with a higher degree of cytoplasm, have relatively higher signal intensity on T2WI.[95]

Small germ cell lesions may be difficult to identify on MRI, and therefore gadolinium should always be used. Almost all germ cell tumors show heterogeneous enhancement. Cystic lesions are observed in about 50% of germinomas and 90% of other germ cell tumors and can contain either multiple microcysts or several large cystic components. Teratomas often show a honeycomb-like appearance.

The solid components of germ cell tumors range from iso- to hypointense, relative to the gray matter on T1-weighted image (T1WI), and mixed iso- and hyperintense onT2-weighted image (T2WI).[75] Germinomas are usually mildly hypointense on T1WI and mildly hyperintense on T2WI and may be isointense on both pulse sequence.[96]

Teratomas of the pineal are extremely heterogeneous, contain multiple cystic regions, and often have dense calcification.[97] These tumors show high intensity on both T1WI and T2WI.

Computer Axial Tomography

On computer axial tomography (CAT; or computed tomography [CT]) scan, pineocytomas are typically isodense and enhance homogeneously with contrast.[75] Cysts and calcifications are present in approximately 50% of pineocytomas, with peripheral calcifications more suggestive of pineocytoma than germi-

noma.[98,99] Pineoblastomas are hyperintense on CT and are not generally calcified.[98] Calcifications can be identified in two thirds of pineal gliomas.

Germ cell tumors, especially germinomas, appear as a hyperintense mass on precontrast CT imaging. Most germ cell tumors will surround pineal gland calcifications, whereas there is an exploded appearance to the calcification in pineocytomas.

STAGING WORKUP AND HISTOLOGIC DIAGNOSIS

A staging workup for patients with suspected pineal tumors is mandatory in order to customize therapy for the various types of neoplasms that grow in this brain region. Staging includes a contrast-enhanced MRI of the brain and the entire spine, an examination of CSF for cytology and tumor markers, as well as a biopsy.

After imaging and CSF analysis, histologic diagnosis is required for optimal management of pineal-region tumors. Biopsy is usually necessary because histology predicts tumor behavior and will also determine the therapeutic approaches. Either stereotactic or open biopsy can be completed.[100,101] Although the stereotactic approach has minimal morbidity, an open procedure allows for greater diagnostic accuracy, since more tissue is procured. The exception to the biopsy requirement are nongerminomatous germ cells tumors where their presence is assumed when imaging studies are consistent with the diagnosis and when CSF levels of AFP and/or β-hCG are elevated.

Although approximately a third of pineal and germ cell tumors may be cured by surgery alone, it is generally recommended that biopsy for histologic determination be completed before gross total resection is attempted.[101] This recommendation is based on the fact that many tumors arising in this area are sensitive to both radiation therapy (RT) and chemotherapy, and under certain circumstances these treatments may be preferred over surgery. For example, over 90% of germinomas are cured with RT alone, and the procedure is associated with lower morbidity and mortality compared to surgery.[102]

Historically, empirical RT was employed as the initial approach to pineal lesions without performing a biopsy. This was especially true in Asia, where there is a high incidence of radiosensitive pineal lesions. This empirical approach to treatment is considered obsolete and is not recommended.

General Treatment Remarks

Tumors of the pineal region are not common. As a result, there is a paucity of well-designed, prospective trials of sufficient sample size to inform the clinician of the best treatment modalities. Indeed, there is no unanimity concerning treatment for this group of tumors. However, it is clear that the variables that most significantly influence survival are extent of disease at presentation, tumor histology, degree of cellular differentiation, and residual disease following therapy.[103]

Most germinomas can be treated with only radiotherapy, but most other germ cell tumors, pineoblastomas, and intermediate tumors will require a combination of radiotherapy and/or chemotherapy with or without surgery. The exception is nongerminomatous germ cell tumors where chemotherapy is first-line therapy, providing there is no CSF obstruction. The most differentiated of the tumors (pineocytoma and mature teratoma) are generally cured by surgery alone and have the best prognosis.

In addition to the ability of surgery to help determine tumor histology and to debulk or remove the lesion, another role for surgery is to treat the frequent occurrence of hydrocephalus. This can be accomplished with placement of a ventriculoperitoneal (VP) shunt or a third ventriculostomy.[101] An endoscopic third ventriculostomy can be completed when the diagnostic biopsy is performed. This procedure is preferred over VP shunts, which can be complicated by infection, injury, and malfunction.

Craniospinal radiation is often employed to treat local and disseminated disease, but it can also be used prophylactically when histology predicts aggressive behavior. For example, prophylactic postoperative craniospinal radiation is frequently recommended for pineoblastomas and germ cell tumors where leptomeningeal spread is more likely to occur compared to pineocytomas.[104] The best overall cure rates have been reported in series where craniospinal radiation has been utilized. However, the use of prophylactic radiation (and all forms of radiation) must be balanced with its potential for inducing cognitive deficits in the young, as well as neuroendocrine dysfunction in all patients. Arguments remain regarding optimal dosing and volume of treatment (lesion versus brain versus craniospinal) when radiation is employed.

There is a growing role for multimodality strategies combining radiation, chemotherapy, and surgery to treat aggressive tumors.[82]

Specific Treatments

Pineocytoma

Pineocytomas do not metastasize, and therefore surgery is first-line treatment.[104a] For most pineocytomas, complete surgical resection is often possible and provides excellent long-term, recurrence-free survival; no further treatment is required. The 5-year survival rate is greater than 86%. Based on this data, adjuvant radiotherapy is not typically recommended after gross total resection of a pineocytoma. Many advocate adjuvant RT for only those pineocytomas which lack neuronal differentiation and which behave more like pineoblastomas.

The role of stereotactic radiosurgery to replace surgery as first-line treatment of pineocytomas is being studied; however, experience remains limited.[105-107] The focused beam minimizes radiation exposure to the surrounding CNS. This form of therapy avoids the risks of general anesthesia and craniotomy. In the largest series of 30 pineal tumors treated with stereotactic radiation, all patients with pineocytomas remained disease-free.[106] More studies are needed to decide whether stereotactic radiotherapy, like surgery, can be considered first-line therapy for pineocytomas.

Pineoblastoma

The aggressive nature of pineoblastoma and many intermediate pineal parenchymal tumors requires a combination of several treatment modalities. Generally, surgery is performed first to debulk or for total gross resection. The benefits of aggressive surgical resection among pineoblastoma and the other more malignant tumors are not clear. Some but not all studies show that the degree of tumor removal correlates with improved outcome.[82] Regardless of the aggressiveness of the surgical procedure, patients with pineoblastomas will require additional therapy following resection.

Radiation is always employed following surgery to treat pineoblastoma. In a study of pineoblastoma patients drawn from the Brain Tumor Registry of Japan, cranial irradiation (>40 Gy) and total gross resection were associated with improved survival compared to surgery with lower doses of radiation or treatment with only surgery.[103] In the uncommon situation when a pineoblastoma is discovered before evidence of metastasis, prophylactic craniospinal radiation can be employed; however, as stated above, this must be weighed against the side effects of radiation.

The most aggressive pineal tumors are not generally effectively treated with surgery and radiation. Therefore, various chemotherapy regiments have been attempted.[108-110] Unfortunately, most studies have shown that chemotherapy alone is not effective compared to radiation alone or radiation with chemotherapy. This is especially disappointing, since infants can be treated with chemotherapy without incurring significant cognitive impairment, whereas radiation is contraindicated. Recent studies have employed high-dose chemotherapy supported by autologous hematopoietic stem cell transplantation, showing improved treatment outcomes.[111]

Germinomas

Germinomas are extremely sensitive to radiation and 5-year survival is greater than 90%.[112] However, there is still uncertainty concerning the optimal dose and volume of radiation. Given the potential for radiation to induce significant cognitive impairment in children, there are multiple small studies being conducted examining the efficacy of either reducing the dose of radiation or eliminating it altogether by substituting chemotherapy in its place,[82] but a study that employed only chemotherapy had a relapse rate that was considerably higher than studies utilizing only radiation therapy.[113] This has prompted studies to employ combination therapy (chemo and radiation), where patients who respond to chemotherapy receive reduced-dose radiation therapy. This approach appears to be more promising.[82]

There is no solid evidence to support the use of prophylactic craniospinal radiation to treat germinomas, since the likelihood of CSF seeding is remote.

Teratomas

Surgery is first-line treatment for the mature teratomas, and a relatively favorable outcome is observed. In contrast, immature teratomas have a less favorable prognosis, with survival rates ranging between 50% and 70%.[114] Both radiation and chemotherapy, alone or combination, have been used in this setting.[115]

Nongerminomatous Germ Cell Tumors

Similar to the pineoblastoma, nongerminomatous germ cells tumors are extremely aggressive, requiring multiple treatment modalities. These tumors are markedly less sensitive to radiation compared to germinomas. Generally, nongerminomatous germ cells tumors are diagnosed by evidence of high CSF tumor markers and then treated with radiation and/or chemotherapy. Surgery is performed when there is residual mass. This has been dubbed the "second look" strategy.[82] In this setting of residual tumor, surgery is both diagnostic and therapeutic.

Craniospinal radiation is almost uniformly recommended for patients with evidence of disseminated disease at the time of diagnosis; however, it is rarely curative as a single treatment modality. Recent results suggest that chemotherapy can improve the overall duration and rate of survival when used in conjunction with craniospinal radiotherapy as part of initial treatment, with survival rates of up to 60%.[116] Similar to pineoblastoma, the rationale for chemotherapy is to improve survival in those patients with disseminated disease or reduce consequences from radiation in patients with localized disease. Several platinum-based regiments have been employed with varying degrees of success.[117,118]

Although all nongerminomatous germ cell tumors are partially sensitive to radiation and chemotherapy, the relative roles of surgery, radiotherapy, and chemotherapy in the management of such lesions remain controversial. There is no general consensus concerning the dose or volume of irradiation or of a particular chemotherapy regimen needed for any form of germ cell tumor. Nongerminomatous germ cell tumors, including mixed germ cell tumors and embryonal cell carcinomas or tumors that have been termed *yolk sac tumors*, have a poorer prognosis, with reported survival rates ranging between 40% and 70%.[92] The efficacy of prophylactic craniospinal radiation in patients without disseminated disease at the time of diagnosis remains unclear, but it is generally administered.

Trilateral Retinoblastoma

Uncommonly, patients with hereditary retinoblastoma develop a midline neuroblastic tumor referred to as a *trilateral retinoblastoma*.[119] Approximately three fourths of reported cases arise in the pineal gland. The mean age at diagnosis is 31 months. Despite aggressive therapy, this is ultimately a fatal disease. The average survival from diagnosis is 6 to 11 months.

REFERENCES

1. Reppert SM, Weaver DR: Molecular analysis of mammalian circadian rhythms, Annu Rev Physiol 63:647–676, 2001.
2. Lerner AB, Case JD, Takahashi Y: Isolation of melatonin, a pineal factor that lightens melanocytes, J Am Chem Soc 80:2057–2058, 1958a.
3. Pandi-Perumal SR, Srinivassan V, Maestroni GJM, et al: Melatonin: Nature's most versatile biological signal? FEBS J 273:2813–2836, 2006.
4. Bubenik GA: Gastrointestinal melatonin: Localization, function, and clinical relevance, Dig Dis Sci 47:2336–2348, 2002.
5. Sugden D: Melatonin biosynthesis in the mammalian pineal gland, Experientia 45:922–931, 1989.
6. Hardeland R, Pandi-Perumal SR, Cardinali DP: Melatonin, Int J Biochem Cell Biol 38:313–316, 2006.
7. Lynch JH, Jimerson DC, Ozaki Y, et al: Entrainment of rhythmic melatonin secretion in man to a 12-hour phase shift in the light/dark cycle, Life Sci 23:1557, 1978.
8. Klein DC, Moore RY: Pineal N-acetyltransferase and hydroxyindole-O-methyltransferase: control by the retino-hypothalamic tract and the suprachiasmatic nucleus, Brain Res 174:245–262, 1979.
9. Arendt J: Melatonin, Clin Endocrinol 29:205–229, 1988.
9a. Bergiannaki J-D, Paparrigopoulos TJ, Syrengela M, et al: Low and high melatonin excretors among healthy individuals, J Pineal Res 18:159–164, 1995.
10. Arendt J: Mammalian pineal rhythms, Pineal Res Rev 3:161–213, 1985.
11. Cardinali DP, Lynch HJ, Wurtman RJ: Binding of melatonin to human and rat plasma proteins, Endocrinology 91:1213–1218, 1972.
12. Martin XD, Malina HZ, Brennan MC, et al: The ciliary body: The third organ found to synthesize indole amines in humans, Eur J Ophthalmol 2:76–72, 1992.
13. Nelson RJ, Drazen DL: Melatonin mediates seasonal adjustments in immune function, Reprod Nutr Devel 39:383–398, 1999.
14. Karasek M, Winczyk K: Melatonin in humans, J Physiol and Pharmacol 57(5):19–39, 2006.
15. Mayeda A, Mannon S, Hofstetter J, et al: Effects of indirect light and propranolol on melatonin levels in normal human subjects, Psychiatry Res 81:9, 1998.
16. Wright KP Jr, Badia P, Myers BL, et al: Caffeine and light effects on nighttime melatonin and temperature levels in sleep-deprived humans, Brain Res 747:78, 1997.
17. Ekman AC, Leppaluoto J, Huttunen P, et al: Ethanol inhibits melatonin secretion in healthy volunteers in a dose-dependent randomized double blind cross-over study, J Clin Endocrinol Metab 77:780, 1993.
18. Brainard GC, Hanifin JP, Greeson JM, et al: Action spectrum for melatonin regulation in humans: Evidence for a novel circadian photoreceptor, J Neurosci 21:6405–6412, 2001.
19. McIntyre IM, Normal TR, Burrows GD: Human melatonin suppression by light is intensity dependent, J Pineal Res 6:151–156, 1989.
20. Buxton OM, L'Hermite-Baleriaux, M, Hirshfeld U, et al: Acute and delayed effects of exercise on human melatonin secretion, J Biol Rhythms 12:568–574, 1997.
21. Kräuchi K, Cajochen C, Wirz-Justice A: A relationship between heat loss and sleepiness: Effects of postural change and melatonin administration, J Appl Physiol 83:134–139, 1997.

22. Nosjean O, Ferro M, Coge F, et al: Identification of the melatonin binding site MT3 as the quinine reductase 2, J Biol Chem 275:31311–31317, 2000.
23. Dubocovich ML, Markowska M, et al: Molecular pharmacology, regulation and function of mammalian melatonin receptors, Front Biosci 8:d1093–d1108, 2003.
24. Dubocovich ML: Melatonin receptors: Role on sleep and circadian rhythm regulation, Sleep Medicine 8:S34–S42, 2007.
25. Sanchez-Barcelo EJ, Cos S, Mediavilla D, et al: Melatonin-estrogen interactions in breast cancer, J Pineal Res 38:217–222, 2005.
26. Benitez-King G: Melatonin as a cytoskeletal modulator: Implications for cell physiology and disease, J Pineal Res 40:1–9, 2006.
27. Carlberg C: Gene regulation by melatonin, Ann YY Acad Sci 917:387–396, 2000.
28. Ekmekcioglu C: Melatonin receptors in humans: biological role and clinical relevance, Biomed Pharmacother 60:97–108, 2006.
29. Poon AMS, Mak ASY, Luk HT: Melatonin and 2[125] iodomelatonin binding sites in the human colon, Endocrinol Res 22:77–94, 1996.
30. Gerdin MJ, Masana MI, Dubocovich ML: Melotonin-mediated regulation of human MT(1) melatonin receptors expressed in mammalian cells, Biochem Pharmacol 67:2023–2030, 2004.
31. Hastings MH, Reddy AB, Maywood ES: A clockwork web: circadian timing in brain and periphery, in health and disease, Nat Rev Neurosci 4:649–661, 2003.
32. Macchi MM, Bruce JN: Human pineal physiology and functional significance of melatonin, Frontiers in Neuroendocrinol 25:177–195, 2004.
33. Lacoste L, Wetterberg L: Individual variations of rhythms in morning and evening types with special emphasis on seasonal differences In: Wetterberg L, editor: Light and Biological Rhythms in Man, New York, 1993, Pergamon Press, pp 287–304.
34. Vondrasová-Jel.'ková D, Hájek H, Illnerová H: Adjustment of the human melatonin and cortisol rhythms to shortening of the natural summer photoperiod, Brain Res 816:249–253, 1999.
35. Wehr TA, Aeschback D, Duncan WC Jr: Evidence for a biological dawn and dusk in the human circadian timing system, J Physiol 535:937–951, 2001.
36. De Leersnyder H, de Blois MC, Bresson JL, et al: Inversion of the circadian melatonin rhythm in Smith-Magenis syndrome, Rev Neurol (Paris) 159(6):S21–S26, 2003.
37. Riemann D, Klein T, Rodenbeck A, et al: Nocturnal cortisol and melatonin secretion in primary insomnia, Psychiatry Res 113:17–27, 2002.
38. Lavie P: Melatonin: Role in gating nocturnal rise in sleep propensity, J Biol Rhythms 12:657–665, 1997.
39. Ates O, Cayli S, Gurses I, et al: Effect of pinealectomy and melatonin replacement on morphological and biochemical recovery after traumatic brain injury, Int J Dev Neurosci 24(6):357–363, 2006.
40. Zhdanova IV, Wurtman RJ: Efficacy of melatonin as a sleep-promoting agent, J Biol Rhythms 12:644, 1997.
41. Brzezinski A, Vangel MG, Wurtman RJ, et al: Effects of exogenous melatonin on sleep: A meta-analysis, Sleep Med Rev 9:41, 2005.
42. Buscemi N, Vandermeer B, Hooton N, et al: Efficacy and safety of exogenous melatonin for secondary sleep disorders and sleep disorders accompanying sleep restriction: Meta-analysis, BMJ 332:385, 2006.

43. Liu C, Weaver DR, Jin X, et al: Molecular dissection of two distinct actions of melatonin on the suprachiasmatic circadian clock, Neuron 19:91–102, 1997.
44. Dubocovich M, Hudson RL, Sumaya IC, et al: Effect of MT melatonin receptor deletion on melatonin-mediated phase shift of circadian rhythms in the C57BL/6 mouse, J Pineal Res 39:113–120, 2005.
45. Herxheimer A, Petrie KH: Melatonin for the prevention and treatment of jet lag. Cochrane Database Syst Rev:CD001520, 2002.
46. Arendt J, Deacon S: Treatment of circadian rhythm disorders—Melatonin, Chronobiol Int 14:185–204, 1997.
47. Wiebel L, Spiegel K, Gfonfier C, et al: Twenty-four-hour melatonin and core body temperature rhythms: Their adaption in night workers, Am J Physiol 272:R948–R954, 1997.
48. Skene DJ, Lockley SW, Arendt J: Melatonin in circadian sleep disorders in the blind, Biol Signals Recept 8:90–95, 1999.
49. Lewy AJ, Newsom DA: Different types of melatonin circadian secretory rhythms in some blind people, J Clin Endocrinol Metab 56:1103–1107, 1983.
50. Lockley SW, Skene DJ, Arendt T, et al: Relationship between melatonin rhythms and visual loss in the blind, J Clin Endocrinol Metab 82:3763–3770, 1997.
51. Lockley SW, Skene DJ, James K, et al: Melatonin administration can entrain the free-running circadian system in blind subjects, J Endocrinol 164:R1–R6, 2000.
52. Goldman BD, Elliott JA: Photoperiodism and seasonality in hamsters: Role of the pineal gland. In Stetson MH, editor: Processing of Environmental Information in Vertebrates, New York, 1988, Springer Verlag, pp 203–218.
53. Roy D, Belsham DD: Melatonin receptor activation regulates GnRH gene expression and secretion in GT1–7 GnRH neurons: Signal transduction mechanisms, J Biol Chem 277:251–258, 2001.
54. Karasek M, Pawlikowski M, Nowakowska-Jankiewicz B, et al: Circadian variations in plasma melatonin, FSH, LH, prolactin and testosterone levels in infertile men, J Pineal Res 9:149–157, 1990.
55. Puig-Domingo M, Webb SM, Serrano J, et al: Melatonin-related hypogonadotropic hypogonadism, N Engl J Med 327:1356–1359, 1992.
56. Luboshitzky R, Lavi S, Thuma I, et al: Increased nocturnal melatonin secretion in male patients with hypogonadotropic hypogonadism and delayed puberty, J Clin Endocrinol Metab 80:2144–2148, 1995.
57. Berga SL, Yen SSC: Amplification of nocturnal melatonin secretion in women with functional hypothalamic amenorrhea, J Clin Endocrinol Metab 66:242–244, 1988.
58. Voordouw BCG, Euser R, Verdonk RER, et al: Melatonin and melatonin-progestin combinations alter pituitary-ovarian function in women and can inhibit ovulation, J Clin Endocrinol Metab 74:10817, 1992.
59. Akerstedt T, Froberg JE, Friberg W, et al: Melatonin excretion, body temperature and subjective arousal during 64 hours of sleep deprivation, Psychoneuroendocrinology 4:219,1979.
60. Cagnacci A, Elliot JA, Yen SS: Melatonin: A major regulator of the circadian rhythm of core body temperature in humans, J Clin Endocrinol Metab 75:447–452, 1992.

61. Deacon S, English J, Arendt J: Acute phase-shifting effects of melatonin associated with suppression of core body temperature in humans, Neurosci Lett 178:32–34, 1994.

62. Jones M, Garfinkel D, Zisapel N, et al: Impaired nocturnal melatonin secretion in non-dipper hypertensive patients, Blood Press 12:19, 2003.

63. Grossman E, Laudon M, Yalcin R, et al: Melatonin reduces night blood pressure in patients with nocturnal hypertension, Am J Med 119:898, 2006.

64. Conti A: Oncology in neuroimmunology. What progress has been made? In Conti A, Maestroni GJM, Cann SMM, et al, editors: Neuroimmunomodulation: Perspectives at the New Millennium, New York, 2000, The New York Academy of Sciences, pp 68–83.

65. Carrillo-Vico A, Guerrero JM, Lardone PJ, et al: A review of the multiple actions of melatonin on the immune system, Endocrine 27(2):189–200, 2005.

66. Maestroni GJM: The immunoendocrine role of melatonin, J Pineal Res 14:1–10, 1993.

67. Robinson WA: Melatonin in the treatment of the human malignant metastatic melanoma. In: Proceedings of the NATO workshop. The Pineal Gland and its hormones: Fundamentals and Clinical Perspectives, Italy, 1994, Erice.

68. Neri B, Fiorelli C, Moroni F, et al: Modulation of human lymphoblastoid interferon activity by melatonin in metastatic renal cell carcinoma. A phase II study, Cancer 73:3015–3019, 1994.

69. Lissoni P: Efficacy of melatonin in immunotherapy. In Bartsch C, Bartsch H, Blask DE, et al, editors: The Pineal Gland and Cancer: Neuroendocrine Mechanisms in Malignancy, Berlin, 2001, Springer-Verlag, pp 465–475.

70. Tan DX, Chen LD, Peoggeler B, et al: A potent, endogenous hydroxyradical scavenger, Endocrine J 1:57–60, 1993.

71. Reiter RJ: Oxidative damage in the central nervous system: protection by melatonin, Progr Neurobiol 56:359–384, 1998.

72. Jansen SL, Forbes DA, Duncan V, et al: Melatonin for cognitive impairment. Cochrane Database Syst Rev :CD003802, 2006.

73. Brown GM: Melatonin in psychiatric and sleep disorders: Therapeutic implications, CNS Drugs 3:209–226, 1995.

74. Michielsen G, Benoit Y, Baert E, et al: Symptomatic pineal cysts: Clinical manifestations and management, Acta Neurochir (Wien) 144:233–242, 2002.

75. Korogi Y, Takahashi M, Ushio Y: MRI of pineal region tumors, J Neuro-Oncology 54:251–261, 2001.

76. Barboriak DP, Lee L, Provenzale JM: Serial MR imaging of pineal cysts: Implications for natural history and follow-up, AJR Am J Roentgenol 176:737, 2001.

77. Patel AJ, Fuller GN, Wildrick DM, et al: Clinicopatho-Pineal cyst apoplexy: Case report and review of the literature, Neurosurgery 57:1066, 2005.

78. Konovalov AN, Spallone A, Pitzkhelauri DI: Meningioma of the pineal region: A surgical series of 10 cases, J Neurosurg 85:586, 1996.

79. Lantos PL, VandenBerg SR, Dleihues P: Tumors of the nervous system. In: Graham DI, Lantos PL, editors: Greenfield's neuropathology, 6th ed., Vol 2. London, 1997, Arnold, pp 677–682.

80. Mena H, Nakazato Y, Jouvet A, et al: Pineocytoma. In: Kleihues P, Cavenee WK, editors: Pathology and Genetics: Tumors of the Nervous System, Lyon, 2000,

81. Mena H, Nakazato Y, Jouvet A, et al: Pineoblastoma. In: Kleihues P, Cavenee WK, editors: Pathology and Genetics: Tumors of the Nervous System, Lyon, 2000, International Agency for Research on Cancer, p. 116.

82. Blakeley JO, Grossman SA: Management of pineal region tumors, Curr Treat Options Oncol 7:505–516, 2006.

83. Nomura K: Epidemiology of germ cell tumors in Asia of pineal region tumor, J Neuro-Oncology 54:211–217, 2001.

84. Konovalov AN, Pitskhelauri DI: Principles of treatment of the pineal region tumors, Surg Neurol 59:250–268, 2003.

85. Hirato J, Nakazato Y: Pathology of pineal region tumors, J Neuro-Oncol 54:239–249, 2001.

86. Brain Tumor Registry of Japan, Vol 9, 1969–1990. The Committee of Brain Tumor Registry of Japan, Tokyo, 1996.

87. Mena H, Rushing EJ, Ribas JL, et al: Tumors of pineal parenchymal cells: A correlation of histological features, including nucleolar organizer regions, with survival in 35 cases, Hum Pathol 26:20–30, 1995.

88. Jennings MT, Gelman R, Hochberg F: Intracranial germ-cell tumors: Natural history and pathogenesis, J Neurosurg 63:155–167, 1985.

89. Brandes AA, Pasetto LM, Monfardini S: The treatment of cranial germ cell tumours, Cancer Treat Rev 26:23–242, 2000.

90. Matsutani M: Clinical management of primary central nervous system germ cell tumors, Semin Oncol 31:676–683, 2004.

91. Choi JU, Kim DS, Chung SS, et al: Treatment of germ cell tumors in the pineal region, Childs Nerv Syst 14:41–48, 1998.

92. Packer RJ, Cohen BH, Coney K: Intracranial Germ Cell Tumors, The Oncologist 5:312–320, 2000.

93. Lambrinides K, Reichert M: MR imaging of pineoblastomas, Radiol Technol 66:106, 1994.

94. Nakamura M, Saeki N, Iwadate Y, et al: Neuroadiological characteristics of pineocytoma and pineoblastoma, Neuroradiology 42:509, 2000.

95. Ganti SR, Hilal SK, Stein BM, et al: CT of the pineal region tumors, AJR Am J Roentgenol 146:451, 1986.

96. Sumida M, Uozumi T, Kiya K, et al: MRI of intracranial germ cell tumors, Neuroradiology 37:32–37, 1995.

97. Satoh H, Uozumi T, Kiya K, Juris K, et al: MRI of pineal region tumors: Relationship between tumors and adjacent structures, Neuroradiology 37:624–630, 1995.

98. Chiechi MV, Smirniotopoulos JG, Mena H: Pineal parenchymal tumors: CT and MR features, J Comput Assist Tomogr 19:509, 1995.

99. Vaquero J, Ramiro J, Martinez R, et al: Clinicopathological experience with pineocytomas: Report of five surgically treated cases, Neurosurgery 27:612, 1990.

100. Little KM, Friedman AH, Fukushima T: Surgical approaches to pineal region tumors, J Neuro-Oncology 54:287–299, 2001.

101. Bruce JN, Ogden AT: Surgical strategies for treating patients with pineal region tumors, J Neuro-Oncology 69:221–236, 2004.

102. Endo H, Kumabe T, Jokura H, et al: Stereotactic radiosurgery followed by whole ventricular irradiation for primary intracranial germinoma of the pineal region, Minim Invasive Neurosurg 48:186–190, 2005.

103. Lee JYK, Wakabayashi T, Yoshida J: Management and survival of pineoblastoma: An analysis of 34 adults from the Brain Tumor Registry of Japan, Neurol Med Chir (Tokyo) 45:132–142, 2005.

104. Hasegawa T, Kondziolka D, hadjipanayis CG, et al: The role of radiosurgery for the treatment of pineal parenchymal tumors, Neurosurgery 51:880–889, 2002.

104a. Bruce JN, Ogden AT: Surgical strategies for treating patients with pineal region tumors, J Neurooncol 69:221–236, 2004.

105. Dempsey PK, Lunsford LD: Streotactic radiosurgery for pineal region tumors, Neurosurg Clin N Am 3:245, 1992.

106. Kobayashi T, Kida Y, Mori Y: Stereotactic gamma radiosurgery for pineal and related tumors, J Neuro-Oncology 54:301, 2001.

107. Kondziolka D, Hadjipanayis CG, Flickinger JC, et al: The role of radiosurgery for the treatment of pineal parenchymal tumors, Neurosurgery 51:880, 2002.

108. Jackson ASN, Plowman PN: Pineal parenchymal tumors. I. Pineocytoma: A tumor responsive to platinum-based chemotherapy, Clin Oncol 16:238–243, 2004.

109. Lutterbach J, Fauchon F, Schild SE, et al: Malignant pineal parenchymal tumors in adult patients: patterns of care and prognostic factors, Neurosurgery 51:44–56, 2002.

110. Fauchon F, Jouvet A, Paquis P, et al: Parenchymal pineal tumors: A clinicopathological study of 76 cases, Int J Radiat Oncol Biol Phys 46:959–968, 2000.

111. Gururangan S, McLaughlin C, Quinn J, et al: High-dose chemotherapy with autologous stem-cell rescue in children and adults with newly diagnosed pineoblastomas, J Clin Oncol 21:2187, 2003.

112. Hussain SA, Ma YT, Cullen MH: Management of metastatic germ cell tumors, Expert Rev Anticancer Ther 8(5):771–784, 2008.

113. Balmaceda C, Heller G, Rosenblum M, et al: Chemotherapy without irradiation: A novel approach for newly-diagnosed central nervous system (CNS) germ-cell tumors (GCT), Results of an international cooperative trial, J Clin Oncol 14:2908–2915, 1994.

114. Gobel U, Schneider DT, Calaminus G, et al: Germ cell tumors in childhood and adolescence, Ann Oncol 11:263–271, 2000.

115. Garre ML, El-Hossainy MO, Fonelli P, et al: Is chemotherapy effective therapy for intracranial immature teratoma? A case report, Cancer 77:97–982, 1996.

116. Baranzelli MC, Patte C, Bouffet E, et al: An attempt to treat pediatric intracranial alphaFP and beta HCG secreting germ cell tumors with chemotherapy alone. SFOP experience with 18 cases. Societe Francaise d'Oncologic Pediatrique, J Neuro-Oncology 37:229–239, 1998.

117. Buckner JC, Peethambaram PP, Smithson WA, et al: Phase II trial of primary chemotherapy followed by reduced-dose radiation for CNS germ cell tumors, J Clin Oncol 17:933–940, 1999.

118. Kretschmar C, Kleinberg L, Greenberg M, et al: Pre-radiation chemotherapy with response-based radiation therapy in children with central nervous system germ cell tumors: A report from the Children's Oncology Group, Pediatr Blood Cancer, 2006.

119. Marcus DM, Brooks SE, Leff G, et al: Trilateral retinoblastoma: Insights into histogenesis and management, Surv Ophthalmol 43:59, 1998.

Chapter 16

REGULATION OF GROWTH HORMONE AND ACTION (SECRETAGOGUES)

JOHN J. KOPCHICK, GABRIEL Á. MARTOS-MORENO, MÁRTA KORBONITS, BRUCE D. GAYLINN, RALF NASS, and MICHAEL O. THORNER

Since the initial discovery of a growth-promoting principle from the pituitary gland in 1921,[1] human growth hormone (hGH) has been identified and isolated and has entered clinical use in growth hormone (GH)-deficient patients. In 1979, hGH complementary DNA (cDNA) was cloned and expressed[2]; subsequently (in 1985), recombinant (r)hGH was generated and approved for clinical use, which has increased its availability and utilization, even in non–GH-deficient states.

Major scientific goals during the past few decades have been to establish the mechanism by which GH interacts with its recep-

tor (GHR) and to identify downstream intracellular signaling pathways. Another important goal has been to understand the regulation of pulsatile GH secretion from the pituitary. In the 1960s, Reichlin[3,4] proposed the existence of a hypothalamic GH-releasing hormone (GHRH) that regulates the release of GH. GHRH was characterized, isolated, and sequenced using a single human pancreatic tumor. The receptor for GHRH was cloned from a cDNA library derived from the tumor of an acromegalic patient, through proposed homology to the secretin/vasoactive intestinal polypeptide (VIP) receptor family.

Distinct from GHRH, GH-releasing peptides (GHRPs) that act as GH secretagogues to stimulate GH release through a separate mechanism were developed from the neuropeptide enkephalin by a process of reverse pharmacology. Then stable small molecule GHRP mimetics were developed and utilized to expression clone the GH secretagogue receptor. Cell lines overexpressing this receptor allowed Kojima and colleagues to identify ghrelin as an endogenous ligand that could stimulate GH release. This has assisted our understanding of the intricate control of GH secretion, which involves somatostatin (SS) and GHRH coming from the hypothalamus, and ghrelin from the stomach, together with feedback of insulin-like growth factor-1 (IGF-1) at both pituitary and hypothalamus.

This chapter summarizes the most recent and significant findings in the GH field and provides pertinent background information and references to more detailed reviews of earlier work.

Growth Hormone

Growth hormone (GH), chorionic somatomammotropin (CS), placental lactogen (PL), and prolactin (PRL) belong to a family of hormones thought to have evolved from a common precursor.[5] The hGH family members are encoded by genes located in the long arm of chromosome 17 that span ≈2.0 kilobases (kb) and contain five exons and four intervening sequences. The translation start and stop codons are located in exons 1 and 5, respectively.[5]

Each member of the GH family of proteins contains ≈200 amino acids, with two (GH) or three (PRL) disulfide bonds and a molecular mass of ≈22,000, with similar sedimentation and diffusion coefficients. The amino acid composition and sequence of the molecules are comparable, ranging from ≈60% to 90% in amino acid sequence identity.[6] GHs are synthesized as precursor proteins, that is, they contain aminoterminal secretory signal peptides.[5]

The hGH gene family consists of hGH, a GH variant termed hGH-V, hCS, and hPRL. Unlike hGH, which is expressed primarily (although not exclusively) in the pituitary, hGH-V encodes a glycosylated protein that is expressed in the placenta and is found in the serum during pregnancy. It differs from pituitary hGH in 13 of 191 amino acid residues[5] and, like hGH, it promotes growth. Another variant of hGH, termed 20 kDa (20K), has been found in the pituitary and blood. It is produced by alternative splicing of the hGH precursor messenger RNA (mRNA) and lacks amino acids 32 to 46 (Fig. 16-1).[7]

A family of genes that encodes several transcription factors, including *POU1F1* (POU domain, class 1, transcription factor 1, formerly called *PIT1*) and *PROP1* (prophet of *PIT1*), have been identified and cloned, and have been found to have a major influence on the development of GH-producing cells. Expression of these genes is important in differentiation of pituitary cell lines to somatotrophs that ultimately synthesize and release GH.[8] Expression and secretion of GH by somatotrophs are controlled by nutrition, sleep, exercise, and several hormones, as well as by hypothalamic peptides such as GHRH and SS, and GH secretagogues, including ghrelin. This topic is thoroughly covered in this chapter.

GH ACTIVITIES

As the name implies, the major function of GH is growth promotion, regardless of the heterogeneity of *GH* genes and isoforms and variants of the respective hormones. However, several non–growth-promoting GH actions have been demonstrated, most of which relate to the role of GH in metabolism. We will briefly mention some of these activities.

Hyposecretion of GH during childhood and adolescence leads to a GH-deficient state associated with dwarfism, whereas hypersecretion of GH before the end of puberty leads to gigantism. These disorders are due to the lack or excess of the growth-promoting action of GH on the bone growth plate. In contrast, during adulthood, when linear growth has already been completed, GH deficiency does not affect growth; however, it does affect body composition, carbohydrate and lipid metabolism, cardiovascular risk profile, and quality of life.[9,10] Hypersecretion of GH in adults, mainly derived from pituitary adenomas, results in a clinical condition known as acromegaly that is characterized by soft tissue enlargement, most of which occurs in the acral regions, and involves abnormal growth of several organs, including the heart, liver, and kidneys. Together, these pathologic changes lead to life-threatening conditions, including diabetes mellitus, cardiovascular disease, and sleep apnea.[11]

In healthy adults, GH displays several metabolic effects, including those noted on protein and fat, although its major effects are exerted on carbohydrate metabolism. Insulin is the main hormone that controls substrate metabolism during the fed state; however, during fasting, when insulin secretion is suppressed, this function shifts to GH.[12] Nevertheless, the specific impact of GH on carbohydrate metabolism is not fully understood, with two contradictory actions described: acute or early insulin-like activities, and chronic or late anti-insulin effects. The chronic effect is also described as the diabetogenic activity of GH; acute insulin-like activities include hypoglycemia and increased glucose and amino acid transport and metabolism, with increased protein synthesis,[13] increased glycogenesis, and increased lipogenesis.[10] These insulin-like activities are seen primarily in vitro or under special in vivo circumstances, and have been suggested to be secondary to an immediate increase in pancreatic insulin release caused by GH.[14]

The anti-insulin activities of GH in animals were discovered many decades ago,[15] when GH was found to inhibit the action of insulin, with associated rises in serum glucose levels. This activity was also shown in humans in the 1960s,[16] and 19% to 56% of individuals with acromegaly develop type 2 diabetes that results from chronically elevated circulating insulin levels and subsequent insulin resistance. This increase in insulin results in an increased rate of triglyceride production, along with an altered lipoprotein profile.[11]

The anti-insulin effect of GH has been found to occur after relatively long periods of GH treatment, that is, after chronic exposure, both in cultured cells and in vivo, or in acromegalic patients who overproduce GH. This diabetogenic effect, which is thought to represent a major physiologic effect of GH, includes hyperglycemia secondary to an increase in hepatic glucose output following enhanced gluconeogenesis and glycolysis, hyperinsulinemia, and decreased glucose transport, as well as increased lipolysis. This last effect results in an increase in serum levels of nonesterified fatty acids, which further enhances the insulin-resistant state.[10,17,18]

The diabetogenic effect of GH is exerted directly by GH-induced intracellular signaling through the Janus kinase (JAK)/signal transducer and activator of transcription (STAT) pathway in humans, as well as in rodents and cultured cell lines. Indeed, GH was recently shown to upregulate the p85α regulatory

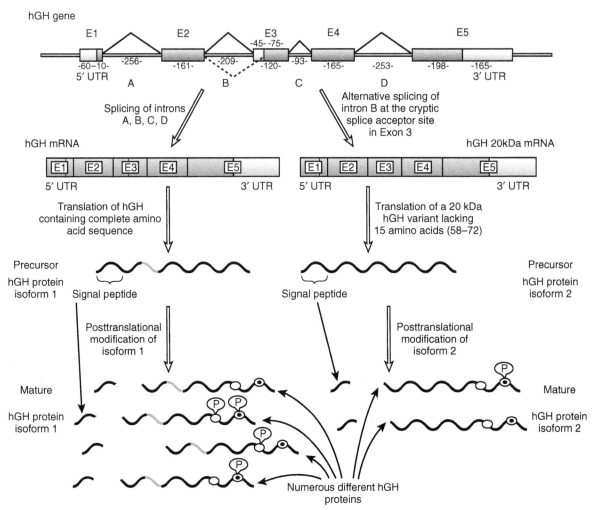

FIGURE 16-1. Schematic representation of the human *GH1* gene showing the alternative splicing of exon 3. This gene contains five exons and four introns; exons are numbered *E1* through *E5* and introns are shown as *A* through *D*. Lengths of these introns and exons are shown in kilobases. As is shown on the left-hand side, normal gene transcription and precursor RNA splicing produces a messenger RNA that is translated to produce a growth hormone (GH) precursor of 217 amino acids (isoform 1). The mature protein, as a result of post-translational cleavage of the signal peptide (which allows it to exit the cell), contains 191 amino acids and has a molecular weight of 22 kDa. As is shown on the right-hand side, alternative precursor RNA splicing gives rise to a variant GH of 20 kDa (isoform 2) that lacks 15 amino acids from the beginning of exon 3 (amino acid residues 58 through 72). This alternative splicing reaction (indicated by the *dashed line*) takes place because of the presence of a 3′ cryptic alternative splice acceptor site in exon 3. Each GH isoform can undergo further post-translational modification. Several such variants of human (h)GH have been described, including variable phosphorylation of residues Ser132 (*white circles*) and Ser176 (*white circles with black dots*). mRNA, Messenger RNA; *UTR*, untranslated region; *P*, phosphate group. (From Kopchick JJ, Sackmann-Sala L, Ding J: Primer: molecular tools used for the understanding of endocrinology, Nat Clin Pract Endocrinol Metab 3[4]:355–368, 2007.)

subunit of phosphoinositide (PI)-3 kinase expression and, thus, the activity of PI-3 kinase in white adipose tissue (WAT),[19] skeletal muscle, and liver.[20] This upregulation of p85α results in relative inhibition of the insulin signaling pathway, and ultimately insulin resistance accompanied by low levels of adiponectin, an insulin-sensitizing adipokine.[19,20] However, other studies have questioned the role of PI-3 kinase in GH-induced insulin resistance in human muscle tissue.[21]

Mouse models of GH action have added significantly to the understanding of the physiologic effects of GH. These models include giant GH transgenic mice, dwarf GH antagonist (GHA) transgenic mice, and GHR gene deleted or knockout mice (GHR–/–) (Fig. 16-2). GH transgenic mice are giant, lean, and insulin resistant, and die prematurely as the result of kidney, liver, and heart problems. GHA transgenic mice are dwarf, have low levels of IGF-1, are somewhat insulin sensitive, and possess normal life spans. GHR–/– mice are dwarf and obese, express extremely low levels of IGF-1, are extremely insulin sensitive, and

have extended longevity.[22-24] The fact that GHR–/– mice are obese and yet insulin sensitive challenges the dogmatic notion that obesity is directly related to insulin resistance. However, contrary to what has been found in these mouse models, lipolysis induction by GH and its effect on body composition can indirectly exert a beneficial effect on insulin sensitivity, as is seen in GH-deficient patients treated with rGH.[25] The effect of obesity on insulin resistance therefore may reside in the fat depot affected by GH.

One of the major physiologic effects of GH is its influence on body composition and adipose tissue distribution. As stated above, GH transgenic mice are giant and possess a lean phenotype. In contrast, GHR–/– mice are dwarf and obese.[26,27] It is surprising that a nonuniform distribution of adipose tissue in these mouse models was discovered. In GHR–/– mice, the subcutaneous and retroperitoneal depots are increased relative to control mice.[26,28] Also, GHR–/– mice exhibit major decreases in the numbers of intraperitoneal adipocytes, whereas subcutaneous adipocyte number is increased relative to controls.[26,28] This

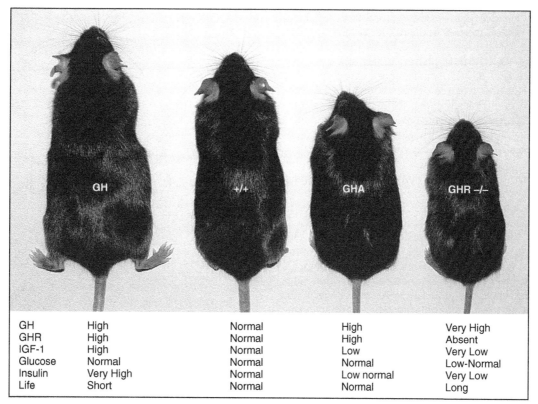

	GH	+/+	GHA	GHR -/-
GH	High	Normal	High	Very High
GHR	High	Normal	High	Absent
IGF-1	High	Normal	Low	Very Low
Glucose	Normal	Normal	Normal	Low-Normal
Insulin	Very High	Normal	Low normal	Very Low
Life	Short	Normal	Normal	Long

FIGURE 16-2. GH transgenic, wild-type (+/+), GH antagonist (GHA) transgenic, and GHR/BP gene-disrupted (GHR–/–) mice. A wild-type mouse is shown second from the left (+/+). The GHR/BP (–/–) mouse is approximately half the size of the normal, wild-type (+/+) mouse and is slightly smaller than the GHA transgenic mice. General endocrine values, including life span (life), are noted.

differential effect of GH on adipose depots is an exciting new finding in the GH field that may help to resolve the mechanisms of GH-induced insulin resistance.

Many of the functional effects of GH may result from the autocrine, paracrine, and endocrine actions of IGF-1, production of which is directly stimulated by GH, as well as other modulators. Nevertheless, determining which of the GH-associated physiologic effects are the direct outcomes of GH action and which are caused indirectly by IGF-1 has been and continues to be an active area of research.

The non–growth-related roles of GH have widened the clinical utilization of recombinant (r)hGH. Initially, rhGH was indicated for GH-deficient children. In addition, rhGH is now indicated for growth promotion during childhood and adolescence in several conditions associated with growth impairment in the absence of GH deficiency. These indications include Turner's and Prader-Willi syndromes, chronic renal insufficiency, *SHOX* gene defects, and children born small for gestational age (SGA) without catch-up growth. Two further indications—idiopathic short stature and Noonan's syndrome—have been approved in the United States, but not in Europe, for specific brands of rhGH. In addition, rhGH treatment has been approved for GH-deficient adults, after its beneficial effects on body composition, metabolic parameters, and quality of life in these individuals were documented.[29]

Involvement of GH in cancer was, and still is, a controversial issue. Data from the Pfizer International Metabolic Database (KIMS) database provide no evidence that administration of rhGH to humans causes or promotes cancer.[30] In addition, in a long-term study in mice and rats, administration of rGH had no effect on the incidence of cancer.[31] However, Swanson and col-

leagues have shown that GH signaling is important in mouse prostate[32] and mammary[33] carcinogenesis. These investigators crossed the GHR–/– mouse with the C3(1)/TAg mouse, in which males develop prostatic intraepithelial neoplasia (PIN) and females develop mammary carcinomas driven by the large T antigen (TAg). (In both sexes, carcinogenesis is known to progress to invasive prostate carcinoma in a manner similar to the process observed in humans.) Progeny of this cross were genotyped, and TAg/GHR+/+ and TAg/GHR–/– mice were compared. In both prostate and mammary cancer models, carcinogenesis was significantly slowed in animals harboring TAg but lacking GHR (TAg/GHR–/–) compared with TAg mice expressing wild-type GHR (TAg/GHR+/+).

Swanson's group has also shown that the spontaneous dwarf rat (SDR), which lacks GH as the result of a point mutation in the *GH* gene, is resistant to chemically induced mammary carcinogenesis or TAg-driven prostate cancer.[34] This model is significant in that the SDR differs from the Sprague-Dawley rat only by this single point mutation. Exposure of the Sprague-Dawley rat to *N*-methyl-*N*-nitrosourea (MNU) is one of the most commonly used and thoroughly characterized models for human breast cancer, particularly for the ability of hormones to regulate tumor growth, and is considered to be an excellent model of human breast cancer. Finally, this group has reported that the SDR can be made vulnerable to MNU-induced mammary carcinogenesis by treatment with GH, and that once mammary tumors were established, cessation of GH treatment induced rapid and dramatic regression of mammary tumors.[35]

Through analysis of converging results from epidemiologic research and in vivo carcinogenesis models, Pollak and coworkers have established an association between the GH/IGF-1 axis and cancer, showing that high levels of circulating IGF-1 are associated with a modest increase in the risk for several common cancers, such as colorectal, prostate, and breast cancer.[36] Based on these findings, experimental pharmacologic strategies that reduce IGF-1 receptor (IGF-1R) signaling are currently under development. In addition, when mice that express a GH antagonist were exposed to chemically induced breast cancer, significant suppression of the development of breast cancer was noted.[37] Finally, a GH antagonist inhibited the growth of human meningiomas and colorectal and breast carcinomas in xenograft experiments in mice, suggesting this class of drugs as potential therapeutic agents through blockade of GHR-mediated signal transduction pathways.[38]

Recently, Lobie and colleagues have shown that hGH is synthesized at a number of extrapituitary sites, with autocrine hGH expression found in certain human carcinoma cell lines. This autocrine GH was found to stimulate survival, proliferation, migration, and invasion of human microvascular endothelial cells. Furthermore, recent studies have demonstrated that autocrine hGH is a wild-type orthotopically expressed oncogene for immortalized human mammary epithelial cells. Thus, autocrine and paracrine hGH may play a key role in angiogenic and lymphangiogenic processes in tumor neovascularization.[39] It is important to note that the GH antagonist (described above) inhibits some of these processes.[40] Thus, the association of GH with the initiation and progression of a variety of cancers is controversial, requiring further study before any conclusions can be drawn. Nonetheless, the GH antagonist (Pegvisomant) and any interventions that downregulate the GH-IGF axis may be possible treatment options for several types of cancer.

To explain these various GH actions, several hypotheses have been presented, including (1) the existence of multiple GHRs; (2) the presence of multiple "active centers" in the GH molecule; and (3) the presence of small, active GH fragments (≈90 fragments have been studied) with a variety of activities.[41] Data related to these hypotheses are presented in the following section.

STRUCTURE OF GH

The crystal structure of the GH molecule, in particular, porcine (p)GH, was solved in 1987 (Fig. 16-3).[42] GH was found to be an elongated molecule with approximate dimensions of $55 \times 35 \times 35$ Å. The molecule contains four α helices, which are tightly packed as antiparallel bundles aligned in an up-up-down-down orientation, and contain 54% of the 191 amino acids of GH. The molecule also contains a "large loop" between residues 33 and 75, a "smaller loop" between residues 129 and 154, and a "small loop" located at the carboxyterminus.[42] In 1992, the crystal structure of hGH, along with the GH binding protein (GHBP), was solved.[43] Again, four GH α helices were detected: α helix I (residues 9 through 34), α helix II (residues 72 through 92), α helix III (residues 106 through 128), and α helix IV (residues 155 through 184). Two small mini-helices, residues 38 through 47 and 64 through 79, were also found in the large loop between α helices I and II.[43]

The third α helix possesses amphiphilic characteristics, that is, the hydrophobic residues are geographically separated from the hydrophilic ones. Nevertheless, the third α helix of bovine (b)GH is imperfect in that Glu 117 (a hydophilic residue) is found in the hydrophobic one half of the α helix, while Ala 122 and Gly 119 (hydophobic residues) are positioned in the hydrophilic portion of the α helix. Amphiphilic secondary structures have been proposed to be important functional

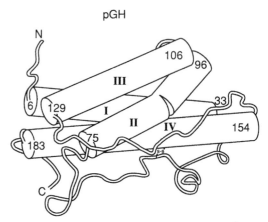

pGH

FIGURE 16-3. Crystal representation of porcine (pGH) at the 2.8 Å resolution level. Four α helices are depicted (cylindrical rods). The nonhelical region is shown as a thin tube. Also, one of the two disulfide bonds is shown; the other is hidden behind helix IV. The amino (A) and carboxyl (C) termini are located in the upper left and lower left corners, respectively. (Modified from Abdel-Meguid SS, et al: Three-dimensional structure of a genetically engineered variant of porcine growth hormone, Proc Natl Acad Sci U S A 84[18]:6434–6437, 1987.)

domains for many peptide hormones, as well as for transcriptional activators.

Bovine GH has four Cys residues located at positions 53, 164, 181, and 189, which are conserved among all GH, PRL, and placental lactogen molecules.[6] The four Cys residues form two disulfide bridges in bGH (three in PRL) that are located between Cys 53 and Cys 164, which results in a large loop, and between Cys 181 and Cys 189, which forms a small C-terminal loop. Conservation of the Cys residues among members of the GH family may indicate that these residues are important for the structural integrity and biological activity of the molecules. Thus, disulfide bonds, as well as the third α helix, constitute potentially important elements for the activity of this molecule.

STRUCTURE/FUNCTION STUDIES OF GH

Multiple studies have been developed to assess the importance of the disulfide bonds in the activity of GH, including bond splitting and site-directed mutagenesis techniques targeting the Cys residues involved in disulfide bond formation. Results derived from these experiments were contrasting but suggested that the biological significance of the disulfide bond integrity may be species specific, and that the integrity of the large loop, but not that of the small loop, is essential for the growth-enhancing activity of GH.[44] However, the effect of GH on lipid metabolism was unchanged.[45]

Information about functional domains of GH obtained through fragment experiments was limited because the overall conformation of the protein is not maintained. In the early 1990s, a novel approach toward understanding the structure of GH was employed using recombinant DNA techniques termed "homologue scanning." Cloned DNA sequences encoding hPRL, which possess minimal GHR binding affinity, were substituted for corresponding regions of hGH, and the PRL/GH chimeric molecules were assayed for their ability to bind PRLR or GHR. This approach was very effective in defining the receptor binding domains of hGH.[46] It was found that the GHR binding domains in hGH are located mainly in the NH_2-terminal portion of α helix I, a loop region between amino acid residues 54 and 74, and the COOH-terminal portion of α helix IV.[46] However, these experiments could not identify the specific residues involved in the ligand/receptor interaction.

Following the GH homologue scanning studies, a more refined approach was applied to the structure/binding relationships of GH and GHR. In this approach, Ala codons were systematically substituted for many codons in the *GH* gene, including those encoding residues found in α helix I, the large loop, and α helix IV. This "alanine scanning" approach was used to define specific amino acids residues important for GHR binding.[47] It was reported that amino acid residues 10, 54, 56, 58, 64, and 68, which were in the loop region, and 171, 172, 175, 178, 182, and 185, in the C terminus, are involved in GHR binding.[46,47] The scanning mutagenesis studies largely ignored the third α helix of GH because of the fact that amino acid substitutions in this region resulted in little change in receptor binding affinity.

THE THIRD α HELIX OF GH

The search for a growth-related domain in GH was pioneered by Sonenberg's group in the late 60s and early 70s. Their main finding was that a short sequence, generated by tryptic digestion of bGH and containing residues 96 through 133, retained low but significant bone growth–stimulating activity, whereas segments 1 through 95 and 134 through 191 had much less activity. It is interesting to note that the tryptic peptide, 96-133, contains the third α helix of GH. Subsequently, it was reported that an hGH fragment (1-134) was fully active in an assay using the IM-9 strain of human lymphocyte assay.[48]

Recombinant hormones possessing different portions of GH, PRL, or PL also have been generated and analyzed. hGH 1-134 was linked to hPL 141-191 and hPL 1-134 was linked to hGH 141-191 through a Cys53-Cys165 disulfide bond.[49] These recombinant hormones then were tested for both their immunoreactivities and their receptor binding properties; recombinant hGH (1-134)-hPL (141-191) retained hGH immunoreactivity and full GHR binding ability but had little hPL activity; on the other hand, recombinant hPL (1-134)-hGH (141-191) possessed a large quantity of hPL immunoreactivity and PRLR binding characteristics, with negligible hGH activity. These observations showed that the immunoreactivity and biological activity of hormones were determined primarily by the NH_2-terminal fragment (residues 1 through 134), while the carboxyl-terminus appears to have little effect in determining the specificity of biological activity. Together these results suggested that GH activity could be ascribed to different regions of the GH molecule, and that the 96-133 segment might be an "active core" required for growth promotion.[49]

These two lines of evidence laid the foundation for the structure/function studies of the third α helix of GH. By combining site-specific mutagenesis of the *GH* gene with the ability of resulting bGH analogues to enhance the growth of transgenic mice, we have reported a growth-promoting region of GH localized in the third α helix (50-55), which is not a perfectly amphiphilic helix because of the presence of Glu 117, Gly 119, and Ala 122, as stated previously. To convert the imperfect third amphiphilic α helix of GH to a "perfectly amphiphilic" α helix, we substituted Glu 117, Gly 119, and Ala 122 with Leu, Arg, and Asp, respectively.[50] The resulting GH analogue was bound to GHRs with the same affinity as native GH. However, when the Glu117Leu, Gly119Arg, Ala122Asp GH analogue (termed M8) was assayed for its ability to enhance growth in transgenic mice, this GH analogue did not enhance growth but suppressed it, resulting in mice with a dwarf phenotype. This was the first

report of a GH analogue that antagonized the action of endogenous GH and, thus, the first report of a GHR antagonist.[50]

In a subsequent study, we extended this observation by performing individual amino acid substitutions. Substitution of Leu 117 for Glu resulted in a GH analogue that behaved identically to native GH,[51] so we concluded that residue 117 of bGH is not likely to be involved in growth-promoting activity. In contrast, the bGH analogue Gly119Arg was found to bind to GHRs with the same affinity as native GH, but transgenic mice that expressed this analogue were about one-half the size of their non-transgenic littermates.[51] This was the second report of a GHR antagonist. We further confirmed this observation by generating hGH-Gly120Arg dwarf transgenic mice.[54] Also, several other amino acids were substituted for bGH Gly119 and were found to act as GHR antagonists.[55] Finally, substitution of Asp for Ala at residue 122 results in a bGH analogue that binds to GHRs but does not enhance (or suppress) growth in transgenic mice and may be acting as a partial agonist. Together, these studies were the first to document the discovery of GHR antagonists.[51-53]

It is important to note that GH analogues with amino acid substitutions that resulted in changes in growth-promoting activity are located within a region of nine amino acids, that is, between Asp 115 and Leu 123,[55] which form two turns of third helix. In viewing the side chains of these potentially important amino acids, it appears that Gly 119 and Ala 122, two amino acids with relatively small side chains, form a "hinge-like" or "cleft" structure that, as stated previously, has been shown to exist in the crystal structure of hGH,[43] near the center of this α helix, primarily as the result of Gly 119 (Fig. 16-4). We postulated that this cleft is important for the growth-promoting activity of the GH molecule, and that Gly may be the only residue that is tolerable at this position.[51] Extension of this model would yield the prediction that any other amino acid substitution at this position would decrease the flexibility of the molecule and/or "fill" the cleft, which ultimately would result in decreased biological activity. Finally, Asp 115 and Leu 123, amino acids with negatively charged (Asp) and long (Leu) side chains, respectively, flank the cleft and may be involved in the interaction with GHR.

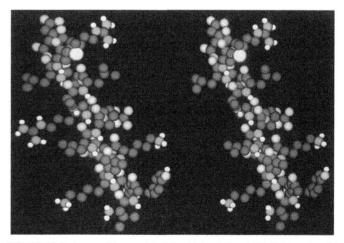

FIGURE 16-4. A space-filling model of the third α helix of GH *(right)* and a GH antagonist *(left)*. The amino terminal of the helices is located on the top of the figure, and the COOH end at the bottom. Note the cleft that is located in the middle of the wild-type helix *(right)* and the occupancy of this cleft with the side chain of Arg *(left)*. (From Chen WY, et al: Glycine 119 of bovine growth hormone is critical for growth-promoting activity, Mol Endocrinol 5[12]:1845–1852, 1991.)

To further substantiate the importance of the cleft in the third α helix, we designed a bGH analogue with a deletion at Gly 119 (Δ119). Transgenic mice that expressed this analogue demonstrated a phenotype similar to that of their littermates.[55] These data provide supportive evidence for the importance of the cleft structure in the third α helix. It is interesting to point out that all bGH analogues tested in this study were able to bind to the GHR with an affinity similar to bGH, including Δ119 (deletion mutation, inactive analog), SAP (scrambled helix, weak antagonist), and Gly119Arg (potent antagonist).

To accommodate all of the data related to amino acid substitutions in GH, including those derived from the alanine scanning studies[47] and those directed at the third α helix of GH,[50] we proposed the *second target hypothesis* for GH action.[50] In this model, residues in α helices I and IV and the large loop region interact with the GHR, as reported by Cunningham.[47] Additionally, we postulated that the cleft region in the third α helix interacts with an unidentified target, and the tripartite complex is the functional unit responsible for the induction of GH action.[49]

GH ANTAGONISTS

Gly 119 is conserved among all members of the GH family, including PRL and PL.[6] Gly is unique among amino acids in that it possesses a single hydrogen atom as a side chain. The absolute conservation of this amino acid within a strong α-helical forming region of helix III of GH implies a crucial role for this residue.

As stated above, when bGH Gly 119 or hGH Gly 120 was replaced with a variety of amino acids and the mutated genes were expressed in transgenic mice, dwarf animals resulted.[50,51,54] We also tested for the ability of the GH-substituted molecules to inhibit GH-dependent conversion of mouse preadipocytes to adipocytes. The bGH Gly119Arg or hGH Gly120Arg analogues were found to inhibit this reaction by 50% at equal molar concentrations of GH and analogues, thereby defining them as GHR antagonists.[56,57] A confirmatory study on the generation of a GH antagonist by substitution of arginine for glycine at position 120 in hGH was subsequently reported.[58]

Later, Chihara and coworkers reported that another *hGH* gene mutation resulted in a "natural" GH antagonist.[59] They also reported another *hGH* gene mutation that encoded an inactive GH[60] in patients with reduced growth and short stature. In the first case, the codon for Arg 77 was found to be mutated so as to encode Cys, and the resulting molecule inhibited GH-stimulated JAK2 phosphorylation in vitro.[59] Unexpectedly, the expression of this GH analogue, hGH Arg77Cys, in transgenic mice resulted in giant animals (Stevens and Kopchick, unpublished results). In the second case, the mutation resulted in the substitution of Gly for Asp acid at codon 112, found to be within Site 2 of the GH molecule[60] (see later). No additional data have been reported on these *GH* gene mutations, which may encode a GHR antagonist and/or inactive GH.

In vitro and in vivo studies of hGH antagonists (GHAs) have demonstrated that they possess great potential to counteract the pathologic conditions of excess hGH in clinical settings, which include acromegaly, diabetic nephropathy, diabetic retinopathy, and, as stated before, certain cancers. Additionally, when GH (giant) and GHA (dwarf) mice are crossed, the resulting offspring are intermediate in size, suggesting that GHAs may overcome the growth-enhancing properties of GH.[61]

The GHA (hGH-Gly120Lys), like wild-type GH, has a short half-life,[62] which limits its utility in the clinical setting. To increase the serum half-life of the molecule, the hGH antagonist has been modified by the addition of polyethylene-glycol (PEG);

hGH-Gly120Lys with four to six PEGs has a half-life of approximately 18 hours after single intravenous (iv), intraperitoneal (ip), or subcutaneous (sc) injection.[62] When mice received a daily sc single injection of various doses (0.25 to 4 mg/kg) of Gly120Lys-PEG or vehicle for 5 days, a significant, dose-dependent suppression of IGF-1 became obvious, starting at day 3. The maximum suppression (up to 70%) of IGF-1 production was achieved by 1 mg/kg dosing at day 6 after the first injection. Hepatic GHRs were significantly increased on day 8, also in a dose-dependent manner (Chen et al., unpublished data). These results suggest that exogenous administration of Gly120Lys-PEG can dramatically decrease serum IGF-1 levels.

These mouse data led to the development of the first hGH antagonist for the treatment of individuals with acromegaly. This hGH antagonist included eight amino acid substitutions at Site 1 of GH and the original G120K substitution at Site 2, along with four to five PEG additions. This molecule was termed B2036-PEG and was also called Pegvisomant. Pegylation of the molecule reduces clearance and therefore increases the serum half life and reduces immunogenicity, as well as its interaction with the GHBP.[63] Thus, relatively high doses of Pegvisomant are required to lower serum IGF-1. Also, Pegvisomant binds to a pre-formed receptor dimer[64] with an affinity similar to wild-type G120K and induces internalization but not subsequent GH-dependent intracellular signaling[63,65] (Fig. 16-5). Thus, the importance of the eight amino acid substitutions in Pegvisomant is not one of increased GHR binding characteristics. However, because two of the amino acid substitutions at GH Site 1 involved Lys residues, and because Lys are potential pegylation sites, the importance of the changes may be that GH Site 1 cannot be pegylated. Thus, the molecule would be able to interact with the GHR.[63]

Debate has occurred over the mechanism of action of the GH antagonist. Fuh et al.[58] suggested that the antagonist prevented the formation of the receptor dimer. However, because the GHR is pre-dimerized,[63-65] the GHAs do not prevent GHR dimerization but prevent proper or functional GHR dimerization and subsequent signal transduction that ultimately results in decreased IGF-1 levels.[66]

Somavert (Pegvisomant for injection) has been approved for use in acromegalic individuals in the United States, Europe, and

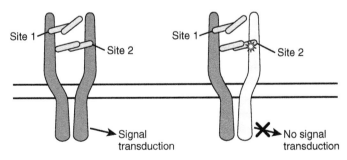

FIGURE 16-5. A, The one-GH/two-GHR model of GH action. The GH molecule and its four α helices are represented by the horizontal cylinders. The pre-formed GHR is shown as crossing the cellular membrane (*dark horizontal lines*). The interaction of GH with the pre-formed GHR at Site 1 and Site 2 is indicated. Not shown are the several N-linked glycosylation sites on the GHR. **B,** The interaction of a GH antagonist (A) with the pre-formed GHR dimer. The GHA and its four α helices are represented by horizontal cylinders. The Gly-to-Lys change in the third α helix is depicted by a star. The interaction of GHA with the pre-formed GHR at Site 1 and Site 2 is indicated. An improper or nonfunctional GHA/GHR dimer is indicated by the *light shade of gray* in the second GHR molecule found in the pre-formed dimer. Not shown are the several N-linked glycosylation sites on the GHR.

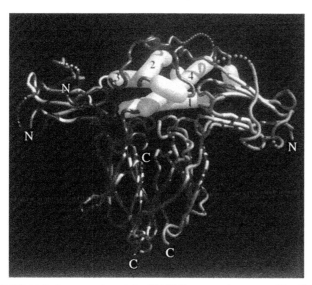

FIGURE 16-6. Representation of the GH/GHR co-crystal structure. The GH α helices are indicated as cylinders and are labeled 1, 2, 3, and 4. α helices 1 and 4 (Site 1) are shown interacting with one GHBP; α helix 3 (Site 2) is shown interacting with a second GHBP. (From de Vos AM, Ultsch M, Kossiakoff AA: Human growth hormone and extracellular domain of its receptor: crystal structure of the complex, Science 255[5042]:306–312, 1992.)

Japan. Data describing the results of Pegvisomant in acromegalic individuals, as well as their quality of life after treatment, have been put forth.[67,68]

CO-CRYSTALLIZATION OF GH WITH THE GHR

As was stated previously, when the crystal structure of hGH complexed with GHBP was solved,[43] two identical GHBP molecules were found to interact with one GH molecule. This observation of two GHRs interacting with one GH molecule (Fig. 16-6) is one of the most fundamental findings in the GH molecular endocrinology field. Thus, the co-crystallization of one GH molecule with two GHBPs supported the GH *second target hypothesis* of GH action,[50] that is, the "second target" was another GHR. It should be pointed out that reagents used in these co-crystallization studies include non-glycosylated, bacterially synthesized GHBP, and not a membrane-associated and glycosylated full-length GHR. Also, GH has not been found in a GHBP dimer in vivo.

Growth Hormone Receptor

GHR AND GHBP

Growth hormone receptors (GHRs) have been found on the cell surfaces of many tissues throughout the body, including liver, muscle, adipose, and kidney, and in early embryonic and fetal tissue. Although most GHRs reside on the cell surface and in the endoplasmic reticulum, pronounced nuclear localization is noted in many cells.[69] Evidence for the importance of the GHR in growth has come from studies on individuals expressing different mutations located throughout the *GHR* gene that result in the dwarf phenotype and a GH-insensitive state, also termed Laron syndrome. Later, another proof of the importance of the GHR in growth was shown with disruption of the *GHR* and *GHBP* genes in mice.[70] These mice are approximately half the

size of wild-type mice and are obese; they express very low levels of IGF-1 and insulin and high levels of GH, and they have an extended life span.[24,71] Whether data on extended life span from GHR-/- mice extends to humans is not known. More research on this controversial subject will ensue.

The GHR is a member of the class 1 hematopoietic cytokine family. The human *GHR* gene encompasses 10 exons and approximately 90 kb, and encodes an extracellular domain, a small transmembrane domain, and an intracellular domain. The protein-coding region of the *GHR* gene is encoded by exons 2 through 10. Exon 2 of the *GHR* gene encodes the secretory signal peptide and the first six amino acids of the mature form of the protein; exons 3 through 7 encode the extracellular domain, exon 8 the transmembrane domain, and exons 9 and 10 the intracellular domain.

The extracellular portion of the GHR consists of two fibronectin type III domains, each containing seven β-strands, arranged to form a sandwich of two antiparallel β-sheets.[43] Stabilizing the GHR structure is a salt bridge between Arg 39 and Asp 132, and hydrogen bonds between Arg 43 and Glu 169.[43] Also, the GHR contains seven cysteine residues in its extracellular domain[43]; the six in the GH binding domain form three disulfide bonds in the active signaling conformation, and help the receptor to maintain its correct three-dimensional structure.[72] Van den Eijnden and coworkers have suggested, after studying the effects of replacing the Cys with Ser and Ala residues, that the middle disulfide bond, Cys83-Cys94, is important for ligand binding, whereas removal of disulfide bond Cys108-Cys122 has little effect on GH-induced intracellular signaling.[72] The GHR has a half-life of approximately 1 hour and is degraded continuously even in the absence of GH through two known mechanisms: endocytosis and ectodomain cleavage. The reader is referred to excellent reviews on the GHR.[69,73,74]

In addition to the membrane-bound GHR, a soluble form exists that is composed of a portion of the extracellular domain, GHBP. In mice and rats, it is encoded by an additional exon, Exon 8A, and is produced by alternative splicing of the GHR precursor mRNA. In other vertebrates, it is believed that it is generated by proteolytic cleavage of the extracellular domain of the GHR. A metalloprotease tumor necrosis factor (TNF)-α converting enzyme (TACE/ADAM-17) acts on surface GHR to generate the GHBP.[75] The function of the GHBP is not fully understood, but it may modulate GH activity by enhancing its half-life or reducing its availability to bind the GHR. The reader is referred to a review paper on GHBPs for further information.[76]

GH/GHR INTERACTION

Examination of the 2.8 Å crystal structure of the complex between GH and the extracellular domain of the GHR produced by *Escherichia coli* (hGHBP) demonstrated that the complex consisted of one molecule of GH and two molecules of the GHR (Fig. 16-6).[43] Furthermore, the crystal structure reveals how a nonsymmetrical molecule, that is, GH, binds to two copies of the GHR, with one of the GHRs binding with high affinity to the GH molecule at Site 1, and with a weaker binding between Site 2 of GH and a second GHR.

Amino acid residues in the hGHR (actually hGHBP) involved in contact with hGH have been determined from co-crystallization analyses of the GH/GHR complex.[43] The major binding determinants in the GH molecule (Site 1), located in the two mini-helices between α helices 1 and 2 (amino acids 60 through 63) and between the center and carboxyterminus of helix IV (amino acids 168 through 174), match to GHR amino acids 40 through 45 and 101 through 106, respectively, and with GHR Trp 169 interacting with hGH residues 171 through 179 in α helix IV. Site 2 GH residues are important for contact and dimerization and only Phe 1, Ile 4, and Asp 116, whereas the significant binding determinants in the GHR are similar as for GHR Site 1, especially Trp 104 and Trp 109.[77] Of particular interest is the close encounter with hGH Gly 120 and GHR Trp 104 in this Site 2 interaction.

The model for GHR activation postulates that GH induces GHR dimerization and, consequently, activation and signaling in which most amino acid residues in the two binding interfaces act in an additive fashion.[78] In addition, the GHR contains a GH-induced dimerization domain in which Cys 241 undergoes GH-induced intermolecular disulfide bonding, thus bridging together two GHRs. Eight hGHR amino acid residues are involved in the salt bridge and the hydrogen bond interactions across the extracellular dimerization domain.[43] Of these eight residues, five are important for GH/GHR-mediated signal transduction, namely, Ser 145, His 150, Asp 152, Try 200, and Ser 201, but not Leu 146 or Thr 147. This study, as well as others using monoclonal antibodies to induce a GH response,[79] suggests that a GH-induced conformational change in the GHR is required for a full biological response. Additionally, subtle but significant differences between the 1hGH/2GHR[43] and 1hGH/1GHR[80] co-crystal structures suggest that a conformational change does occur in the one ligand/two receptor complex.

Although most if not all of these GH/GHBP interactive studies use a non-glycosylated, bacterially expressed GHBP, and not the membrane bound GHR, the interaction of one GH with two GHBPs has been extrapolated to the in vivo interaction of GH with the GHR. This finding has led to the theory of a sequential binding mechanism in which hGH binds to two GHRs.[77] In this model, hGH must first bind to one GHR using a high-affinity receptor binding site, which subsequently allows binding of the second receptor. The binding Site 1 of hGH is located at residues identified by Ala scanning mutagenesis studies,[47] that is, α helix I, the loop between amino acids 54 through 74 and α helix four. Binding Site 2 is located at the N-terminus (Ile 4), and the third α helix, namely, Gly 120. The model predicts that a Typ 104 residue of the GHR "fits" into the "cleft" of the third α helix of GH. Chen et al.[56,57] have proposed that the reason that hGH-Gly120Arg acts as a GH antagonist is because substitution of Arg for Gly at position 120 blocked or inhibited the "second" GHR from properly interacting with binding Site 2 on the GH molecule. This would inhibit proper or functional GH-induced GHR dimerization. These data nicely supported the "cleft" theory pertaining to the interaction of hGH Gly 120 with a second target.[56,57] The importance of GH-induced GHR dimerization in humans has been supported by the finding of an adenine-to-guanine mutation in the *hGH* gene that results in the conversion of Asp112 to Gly. In the heterozygous state, this mutation is believed to be the cause of dwarfism in a female child, with the encoded hGH analogue binding to hGHR in vitro, but not inducing GHR dimerization and JAK2 and STAT5 activation.[60]

Later studies have dramatically changed the GH-induced dimerization theory. The work of Gent et al.,[64] who used coimmunoprecipitation and epitope-tagged truncated GHRs, conclusively showed that ligand-independent GHR dimerization occurs in the endoplasmic reticulum and on cell membranes independent of GH binding.[64] In addition, studies with GHAs (bGH Gly119Arg, hGH Gly120Lys; B2036 and Pegvisomant) have demonstrated that these antagonists exist in a complex with two

GHRs and are internalized properly.[63,65] Thus, results showed that GHAs prevent neither GHR dimerization nor internalization, but they interfere with proper GHR dimerization. This has led to the proposed model of GH binding to a constitutively homodimerized GHR, causing a structural change that results in activation of JAK2 and signal transduction.[69]

The mechanism by which GH binding converts the inactive pre-dimerized GHR to its active conformation remains uncertain. However, it has been shown that the composition and/or length of the transmembrane domain does not affect GH-induced GHR dimerization.[81] Also, through the mutation of Site 2 in GHR, this site has been shown to be not essential for GHR to achieve its active conformation (identified by GHR disulfide linkages) and to trigger signal transduction. Additionally, the extracellular domain of GHR shows substantial flexibility to achieve active conformation in response to GH and will even accommodate GH-GH dimers.[82] The interaction of GH with the GHR has been proposed to cause repositioning of the intracellular domain of GHR, in which rotation of individual GHR molecules ultimately triggers GH-induced intracellular signal transduction.[83] This model, developed by Waters and colleagues over the past few years, has greatly influenced and stimulated research on the interaction of GH with GHRs and represents a seminal finding in the GH field.[83]

Finally, the mechanisms responsible for GHR turnover (proteolysis) have been shown to influence GH sensitivity. As was stated before, cleavage of the extracellular domain of the GHR is catalyzed by a transmembrane ectoenzyme termed TACE (tumor necrosis-α cleaving enzyme, also known as ADAM-17).[75] GHR proteolysis renders cells less sensitive to subsequent GH-induced signaling by downregulating GHR abundance. Recent in vivo studies indicate that this mechanism of receptor downregulation may also mediate desensitization to GH in vivo[84] and in pathophysiologic states in which it may be advantageous to limit the anabolic effects of GH (e.g., sepsis). It is interesting to note that the GHR remnant that results from metalloproteolysis is further cleaved within the transmembrane domain by an enzyme termed γ-secretase, leading to release of the intracellular domain into the cytosol and its accumulation in the nucleus. The consequences of this inducible nuclear localization of the GHR intracellular domain are as yet unknown, but may suggest novel GHR-dependent signaling pathways.

We have only touched on a few of the structural characteristics of the GHR. For a more exhaustive review of this subject, the reader is referred to an excellent review by Brooks, Waters, and coworkers.[69]

CLINICAL MANISFESTATIONS OF MUTATIONS IN THE GHR

GH-insensitive individuals with a dwarf phenotype were first described by Laron. The molecular defect in these Laron syndrome (LS) individuals has been found in the GHR. Since the initial series of *GHR* mutations was documented in LS individuals, many other sites of GHR mutation have been documented.[85] Because these individuals are GH insensitive, treatment with IGF-1 is the only option.[85,86]

In 2004, Dos Santos et al.[87] reported that a rather frequent polymorphism of the *GHR* gene was associated with increased responsiveness to GH. This *GHR* gene mutation resulted in removal of exon 3 and has been termed the d3 GHR allele.[87] Children born SGA, children with idiopathic short stature, girls with Turner's syndrome, and children with severe GH deficiency all in the presence of a d3 GHR polymorphism have a greater response to exogenous rhGH administration than do similar individuals who express the full-length GHR. These findings suggest that a subpopulation of individuals with the d3 GHR allele may have increased sensitivity to GH. Also, in a study of acromegalic individuals,[88] the wild-type, full-length GHR was found to be homozygous in 50% of patients, while 50% had at least one d3 GHR allele. The GHR genotype (specifically, the deletion of exon 3) was hypothesized to modulate the relationship between GH and IGF-1 serum concentrations in these acromegalic individuals.[88]

GH-Induced Signal Transduction

The molecular mechanisms by which GH transmits its signals via its receptor have been largely elucidated by experiments in cultured cells or hypophysectomized rats. However, GH-induced in vivo tissue-specific signal transduction systems are still largely unknown, although data are beginning to emerge in this area, as is knowledge about modulators of GHR.[21,89,90] Several GH-mediated intracellular signal transduction pathways are summarized below, some of which may overlap with signal transduction intermediates induced by insulin and other hormones, thus providing opportunities for "biological cross-talk" between these molecules. Several reviews on the subject have been presented.[89,90] It is interesting to note that one of the hormones involved in this cross-talk is GH-induced IGF-1. Recently, examination of GH signaling in murine 3T3-F442A preadipocytes revealed that GH induces formation of a complex that includes the GHR, JAK2, and the IGF-1 receptor (IGF-1R).[91] Even though both the GHR and JAK2 in the complex are tyrosine phosphorylated, formation of this complex does not depend on tyrosine phosphorylation of any of the partners. It is interesting to note that co-treatment of cells with the combination of GH and IGF-1 resulted in enhancement of downstream signals compared with GH alone. This suggests functional consequences of the complex formation. Further evidence for the idea that the GHR and the IGF-1R may function in parallel has come from studies in primary mouse osteoblasts in which the *IGF-1R* gene is flanked by loxP sites that enable excision of the gene when Cre recombinase is expressed. When IGF-1R was deleted from these cells, GH-induced STAT5 activation was substantially diminished, suggesting that the IGF-1R, even when not engaged by IGF-1, contributes to optimal GH-induced GHR signaling.[92]

JANUS KINASE ACTIVATION

In the early 1990s, GH treatment of responsive cells was found to induce association of a tyrosine kinase with the GHR. This kinase was later identified as a 121 kDA protein and was found to be a member of the Janus kinase (JAK) family of proteins, in particular JAK2. Activation of JAKs appears to be an initial step in one of the GH-induced signal transduction systems. Although three JAK molecules are involved in GH/GHR signal transduction, JAK2 exhibits the greatest degree of activation. GH-dependent JAK2 activation requires interaction between JAK2 and the membrane-proximal, proline-rich motif (termed Box 1) located in the intracellular region of GHR. Because the GHR itself has no intrinsic kinase activity, it is thought that co-localization of two JAK2 molecules by the dimerized GHR results in transphosphorylation of one JAK2 by the other, leading to JAK2 activation. Activated JAK2, in turn, is thought to phosphorylate GHR on multiple tyrosine residues, providing docking sites for cytosolic components of at least three distinct signaling pathways: the STAT, MAPK, and PI3K pathways.[90,93,94] An overview of these pathways is presented in Fig. 16-7.

SIGNAL TRANSDUCERS AND ACTIVATORS OF THE TRANSCRIPTION SIGNALING PATHWAY

Many of the physiologic effects of GH result from transcriptional regulation of a variety of genes. Several different signaling pathways contribute to this regulation, but the pathway that was discovered in the mid-1990s, and perhaps the most universal pathway implicated in GH action, involves signal transducers and activators of transcription (STAT) proteins. Upon phosphorylation, cytoplasmic STAT proteins form homodimers or heterodimers, translocate into the nucleus, bind DNA, and activate transcription.[95]

GH-dependent tyrosyl phosphorylation requiring JAK2 activation has been demonstrated for STAT1, STAT3, and STAT5 (a and b). In addition, STAT5 activation requires regions of GHR not involved in JAK2 activation, suggesting that STAT5 also interacts directly with GHR. As was previously stated, the docking of STAT5 with the GHR requires phosphorylated tyrosine residues presumably mediated by JAK2. The tyrosine residues found to be phosphorylated and important in STAT5 docking and subsequent activation have been reported. Although STAT5 has been found to directly associate with the GHR, STAT1 and STAT3 probably do not interact with the GHR but with JAK2 instead. STAT1, STAT3, STAT5, and possibly STAT4 have also been identified in GH-induced DNA binding complexes of several genes, and their presence is required for maximum transcriptional gene activation.[90,94]

In liver and other GH-responsive tissues, STAT5 activation following the stimulation of cell surface GHRs by plasma GH occurs intermittently, reflecting the pulsatile nature of pituitary GH secretion. GH secretion and consequently the temporal patterns of plasma GH levels differ between males and females, with more frequent episodes of pituitary GH release and shorter plasma GH interpulse intervals in females as compared with males, both in rodents and in humans.[96] This sex difference or dimorphism in plasma GH profiles leads to sex differences in hepatic STAT5 signaling and liver gene expression. Thus, in male rat liver, intracellular STAT5 signaling is intermittent and is followed by downregulation of hepatic STAT5 signaling and resetting of the intracellular signaling apparatus in time for STAT5 to respond to the next plasma GH pulse. In females, more frequent plasma GH pulsation leads to partial desensitization of hepatic STAT5 activation, with the peak level of active STAT5 in the nucleus being substantially lower than in males.[97]

Additional studies of these gender differences have shown that male mice with a targeted disruption of the STAT5b gene display two striking phenotypes that are not seen (or are much less dramatic) in female mice: (1) Body growth rates are reduced in STAT5b-deficient males beginning just prior to puberty; and (2) sex-specific liver gene expression is abolished, with more than 1000 STAT5b-dependent, sex-specific genes identified in the liver.[98] These genes are important for physiologic processes such as lipid metabolism and steroid hormone metabolism, and include genes that code for phenomone-binding proteins, cytochromes P-450, and other enzymes that metabolize steroids, drugs, and environmental chemicals. The loss of liver sexual dimorphism that is seen in global STAT5b-knockout male mice and in liver-specific STAT5a/STAT5b–double knockout male mice involves downregulation of ≈90% of male-specific genes and upregulation (de-repression) of ≈60% of female-specific genes.[98,99] The mechanisms that underlie these effects of STAT5b

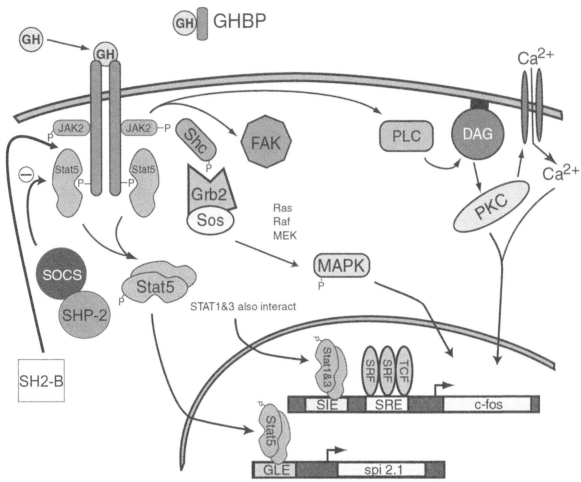

FIGURE 16-7. A model depicting intracellular signaling intermediates induced by binding of GH with the GHR. (Modified from Kopchick JJ, Andry JM: Growth hormone [GH], GH receptor, and signal transduction, Mol Genet Metab 71[1-2]:293–314, 2000.)

on liver sexual dimorphism are complex and most likely involve both direct and indirect effects of STAT5b on sex-specific genes.[100] Sex-dependent effects of GH on liver gene expression may be important in humans as well, as CYP3A4, the major catalyst of human hepatic drug metabolism, shows sex-specific expression (female > male)[101] and a pattern of GH regulation similar to that of several mouse *Cyp3a* genes. These findings have important implications for the sex-dependent metabolism and pharmacokinetics observed with a wide range of drugs in humans.

MITOGEN-ACTIVATED PROTEIN KINASE SIGNALING PATHWAY

Another GH-inducible pathway that ultimately culminates in transcriptional regulation of a number of genes involves activation of two mitogen-activated protein kinases (MAPKs), termed extracellular signal regulated kinase (ERK) 1 and ERK2.[102] This pathway was first described for insulin-mediated signal transduction. The pathway most likely begins with GH-stimulated binding of adapter protein (SHC) family members to phosphorylated residues in both GHR and JAK2, followed by phosphorylation of the SHCs by JAK2. Subsequently, the tyrosyl phosphorylated SHC proteins interact with growth factor receptor bound 2 (GRB2) that, in turn, interacts with *son of sevenless* (SOS).[103] Finally, GH activates RAS GTPase, RAF kinase, and MAP-ERK kinase (MEK).[103] These studies, as well as those by Winston and

Hunter,[104] implicate GH as the inducer of the SHC-GRB2-SOS-RAS-RAF-MEK pathway for activation of MAPK. GH also activates insulin receptor substrates (IRS)-1 and IRS-2,[105] which can lead to activation of the RAS-MEK signaling pathway.

GH activates the S6 kinase, p90[RSK], most likely via MAPK. p90[RSK], in turn, can phosphorylate a transcription factor, termed serum response factor (SRF), that binds to the GH-responsive serum response element (SRE) of the c-*fos* promoter/enhancer.[106] GH may activate another protein, the ternary complex factor p62[TCF]/ELK1, which interacts with SRF to bind SRE but is directly activated by ERKs 1 and 2.[107] Further evidence that MAPKs are involved in the GH-dependent transcriptional regulation of c-*fos* comes from the observation that the same regions of GHR required for activation of MAPK are also required for c-*fos* gene induction.[108] As mentioned earlier, STAT proteins are also involved in c-*fos* gene regulation, demonstrating a convergence of at least two divergent GH signaling pathways in the regulation of a single gene. MAPK activation, also inducible by a number of growth factors, may represent a common signal transduction system, whereas activation of STAT proteins (in particular STAT5) may be more specific to GH.[102]

Based on recent mutational studies, disruption of the conformational change induced by GH on the F'G' loop of the GHR (residues 216 through 221) causes specific impairment of ERK signaling without affecting STAT activation in FDC-P1 cells.[109] This finding suggests that movements of this F'G' loop could determine the signaling choice after GH binding to GHR. It is interesting to note that this conformational change in the GHR is not induced after binding of the human GH antagonist (hGHA) to the GHR.

INSULIN RECEPTOR SUBSTRATE/PI3K-AKT SIGNALING PATHWAY

In addition to sharing some MAPK pathway intermediates with insulin, GH activates members of an additional insulin signaling pathway: insulin receptor substrate (IRS)-1 and IRS-2. Although the nature of the interaction between the IRS molecules and the GHR/JAK2 complex is not clear, it does appear that JAK2 activation results in tyrosyl phosphorylation of IRS-1 and IRS-2, which is involved in the insulin-like effects of GH. Phosphoinositol-3-kinase (PI3K) is also involved in the insulin-like effects of GH, in that a GH-induced interaction between the regulatory subunit of PI3K and tyrosyl phosphorylated IRS-1 and IRS-2 has been demonstrated in adipocytes.[19] The ability of the PI3K-AKT pathway to promote cell proliferation and differentiation and to prevent apoptosis has been well documented.

A role for GH induction of the PI3K-AKT pathway in GH regulation of IGF-1 expression cannot be ruled out, because inhibition of this pathway results in reduction of GH-induced IGF-1 expression in mouse cells. Nevertheless, targeted gene disruption studies of the p85α regulatory subunit of PI3K, as well as the downstream effector of PI3K-AKT, indicate that, although the PI3K-AKT pathway is essential for survival and normal growth, its effects are not necessarily direct functions of GH action.[110] In contrast, and as stated previously, upregulation of the p85α regulatory subunit of PI3K by GH has been suggested as the possible mechanism of its diabetogenic effect in adipose tissue, skeletal muscle, and liver,[19,20] although this mechanism is not unanimously accepted in human tissue.[21]

PROTEIN KINASE C SIGNALING PATHWAY

Experiments designed to inhibit or deplete protein kinase C (PKC) activity have suggested the involvement of this family of enzymes in a number of physiologic responses to GH. These responses include the insulin-like stimulation of lipogenesis, induction of c-*fos* gene expression, and stimulation of Ca^{2+} uptake.

One pathway for PKC activation involves GH-induced 1,2-diacylglycerol (DAG) production by phospholipase C (PLC) that is possibly coupled to GHR via a G protein.[111] Another proposed pathway for PKC activation involves the IRS/PI3K.[111] This proposal is supported by our finding that GH promotes activation and translocation of a PK isoform, PKC-ε, from the cytosol to plasma membrane, suggesting that GH-dependent activation of PKC may involve the IRS/PI3′-kinase pathway.[112]

SUPPRESSORS OF CYTOKINE SIGNALING, PROTEIN TYROSINE PHOSPHATASES, AND SRC KINASES

Several molecules have been implicated as inhibiting GH-induced intracellular signaling. Suppressors of cytokine signaling (SOCS) proteins are important in the regulation of GHR/JAK2 signaling. The SOCS family has eight members, and GH induces SOCS 1, 2, and 3; conversely, SOCS 1, 2, 3, and 7 proteins downregulate GH signaling by inhibiting JAK2 and STAT molecules, and have been postulated as the intracellular mediators of cytokine inhibition of GH action.[113] In addition to SOCS proteins, several protein tyrosine phosphatases are involved in termination of GH-activated STAT signaling. PTP-H1 modulates GHR signaling

and systemic growth through IGF-1 secretion.[114] Finally, the possible involvement of another family of kinases (Src kinases) in GH signaling and STAT/ERK activation has been ruled out recently through the absence of signs of impairment in GH-induced STAT/ERK activation after blockage of Src kinase.[115] Work continues in the area of GH-induced signaling, and, as stated earlier, data generated from human tissue are desperately needed.

GHRH, Ghrelin, and GH Secretagogues

GH is secreted from the anterior pituitary somatotrophs in a pulsatile pattern consisting of 20 to 25 secretion pulses per 24 hours in man. The minute-to-minute regulation of secretion is mediated through both hypothalamic and peripheral inputs. Hypothalamic GHRH and somatostatin are responsible for the timing and regulation of synthesis and secretion of GH. GHRH and somatostatin regulate GH directly at the pituitary level, while somatostatin also modulates GH secretion by inhibiting hypothalamic GHRH neurons. Insulin-like growth factor (IGF-1) provides negative feedback on GH release at the level of the hypothalamus and pituitary.

Ghrelin, a 28 amino acid peptide, was discovered as an endogenous ligand for the GH secretagogue receptor. It is secreted predominantly into the circulation from the stomach and has strong GH-releasing effects. It amplifies the spontaneous secretion of GH. Ghrelin exerts its central GH-releasing effects via stimulation of GHRH secreting neurons and by functional somatostatin antagonism at both the hypothalamic and pituitary levels. Ghrelin has also been shown to play a significant role in energy homeostasis. It is present in hypothalamic neurons in the arcuate nucleus, and it activates NPY- and AGRP-containing neurons, as well as the midbrain dopamine reward circuitry, to stimulate orexigenesis. Clinical studies suggest that under fed conditions, the acylated form of circulating ghrelin increases the amplitude of GH secretion pulses. Based on its orexigenic and GH-releasing effects, ghrelin has emerged as a crucial factor, connecting physiologic systems that regulate energy balance, nutritional partitioning, and growth (Fig. 16-8).

Growth Hormone–Releasing Hormone

HISTORY

In 1982, growth hormone–releasing hormone (GHRH) became the last of the originally proposed hypophysiotropic factors to be identified structurally. Its existence had been proposed by Reichlin because selective hypothalamic lesions yielded a GH deficiency state and growth failure,[3,4] although it was finally isolated from GHRH-producing abdominal tumors rather than from the hypothalamus. In a patient with acromegaly and Turner's syndrome, the acromegaly was due to somatotroph hyperplasia, as it persisted despite transsphenoidal surgery.[116] Two different teams isolated a 40 amino acid peptide from a 5 cm tumor in the tail of the patient's pancreas, GHRH(1-40)-OH, then designated GH-releasing factor (GH-RF or GRF).[117-119] Simultaneously, the Guillemin laboratory sequenced three GHRH peptides from a different tumor: GHRH(1-44)-NH₂, GHRH(1-40)-OH, and GHRH(1-37)-OH.[120,121] Complete amino acid sequence identity occurred apart from varying C-terminal extensions, indicating possible peptide processing prior to release. The full biological activity resided in residues 1 to 29,[122] and by sequence

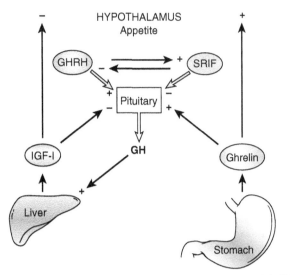

FIGURE 16-8. Schematic depicting the feedback network through which GHRH, SRIF, ghrelin, and IGF-1 regulate GH.

homology, the peptides were members of the glucagon-secretin family. These peptides eventually were demonstrated to fulfill all the requirements of a hypophysiotropic growth hormone–releasing hormone.

MOLECULAR AND CELLULAR BIOLOGY

GHRH is produced predominantly by neurons in the arcuate nucleus of the hypothalamus, which send processes to the median eminence, where GHRH is released into the pituitary portal circulation. GHRH then stimulates the pulsatile release of GH from somatotrophs of the anterior pituitary.[123] Both GHRH(1-44)-NH$_2$ and GHRH(1-40)-OH can be found in the human hypothalamus[124] and in pituitary tumors of acromegalic patients.[125] GHRH is also produced in other tissues, where it may serve autocrine or paracrine roles.

GHRH Peptide

GHRH is a member of a family of homologous peptides that in humans includes secretin, glucagon, glucagon-like peptides (GLP-1, GLP-2), vasoactive intestinal peptide (VIP), pituitary adenylate cyclase–activating peptide (PACAP), PACAP-related peptide (PRP), peptide histidine-methionine (PHM, known as PHI in other species where the C-terminal residue is isoleucine), and glucose-dependent insulinotrophic polypeptide (GIP, also called gastric inhibitory peptide).[126,127] These peptides are thought to have arisen from a common ancestor through a series of gene duplications[127]; as the result of sequence and structural similarities, they can interact at each other's receptors to a varying extent.[126] The N-terminal (1-29) residues of GHRH are required for receptor binding in the human[122] and are 62% identical in the mouse (the most divergent known mammal) and are less conserved in more distant species, including birds, fish, and even protochordate invertebrates.[128-130] This is in contrast to related peptides such as PACAP, VIP, and glucagon, which are 100% identical in many mammals and better than 90% identical in more distant vertebrates.[127,130] Indeed, because of sequence similarities between PRP and GHRH in non-mammalian vertebrates, some of the peptides from non-mammalian species originally named as GHRH or GHRH-like are now seen to be orthologues of PRP, and not GHRH.[131,132] The relative activities of these PRPs at GHRH receptors appear to differ between species[131,133];

specific receptors that respond preferentially to PRPs have been identified in fish,[134] but a corresponding *PRP receptor* gene appears to be absent in mammals,[134] and human PRP has no activity at the human GHRH receptor.

It has been proposed that the active tertiary structure of the GHRH peptide is an amphiphilic α helix that runs from residue 4 onward.[135,136] This helical structure, with polar and hydrophobic faces, is presumably stabilized when the peptide is bound to its receptor but is not stable in aqueous solution.[137] Circulating GHRH is inactivated rapidly in vivo by dipeptidylaminopeptidase IV (DPP-IV) acting at Ala2,[138] and more slowly by oxidation at Met27.[122] Medicinal chemists have used the GHRH scaffold to develop peptidic GHRH analogues with increased stability and potency. These efforts have utilized combinations of strategies that include increasing the stability of the α helix with helix-forming residues or ring structures; prolonging the half-life of the peptide in the circulation by introducing unnatural amino acids or polyethylene glycol (PEG) residues to decrease DPP, tryptic, and chymotryptic protease susceptibility; and replacing the oxidizable methionine.[122,139-143] An analogue of GHRH has also been developed that couples to endogenous circulating albumin when injected, thus conferring an extended half-life,[144,145] and modified GHRH sequences have been expressed in muscle tissue by electrophoration of injected plasmids.[146] Substituting the alanine at position 2 with D-arginine was found to produce a GHRH antagonist,[147] and subsequently, more stable, higher-affinity versions of this type of antagonist have been developed[148] that may prove useful in blocking the mitogenic effects of GHRH.[149] Although GHRH acts as a low-affinity agonist at the VIP receptor, GHRH analogues such as N-Ac-Tyr[1] and D-Phe[2]GHRH(1-29)-NH$_2$ have been developed as VIP antagonists.[150]

Gene and mRNA

Complementary DNA (cDNA) probes have allowed identification of the single-copy *GHRH* gene on human chromosome 20. Human, rat, and mouse genes span approximately 10 kb of DNA and include five exons. The third exon encodes residues 1 through 31, which are sufficient for the known biological activities of GHRH. However, the human mRNA encodes a 108 amino acid precursor protein, the middle region of which is processed to form the mature GHRH peptide. Brain-, placenta-, and gonad-specific forms of GHRH mRNA have been isolated,[151-153] the messages for which are initiated at different gene promotors and result in mRNAs of different sizes, although the encoded precursor protein remains identical. Immunologic evidence shows that the C-terminal fragment of the precursor protein is processed into an additional peptide known as GHRH-related peptide (GHRH-RP), which is expressed in the human hypothalamus,[154] where its role is not known, and in rat testis, where it is reported to regulate Sertoli cell function.[155] An additional, alternatively spliced mRNA found in rat placenta but not hypothalamus encodes the normal GHRH but includes an altered GHRH-RP.[156]

Tissue Distribution

In humans and a number of other species, GHRH immunoreactivity is present in the basal hypothalamus, appropriate anatomically for release into the pituitary portal vessels.[157] GHRH cell bodies directing processes to the median eminence originate from both the perifornical nucleus[158] and the arcuate (rat) or infundibular (human) nucleus.[157] GHRH perikarya are also found in the ventromedial nucleus,[159] electrical stimulation of which can induce increased release of GH.[160] A reciprocal innervation occurs between GHRH and somatostatin neurons in the rat hypothalamus,[161] providing the potential for direct communication between the major stimulatory and inhibitory neurons governing GH release. This relationship may participate in the ultradian oscillation of hypothalamic GHRH and somatostatin mRNA.[162] GHRH neurons also directly express somatostatin receptors.[163] A number of other brain regions outside of the hypothalamus contain immunoreactive GHRH.[158,164,165] The ontogeny of GHRH neurons suggests that they appear in the human fetus at between 18 and 29 weeks' gestation,[166] and in the rat on embryonic day 18, reaching adult levels by postnatal day 30.[167]

Much evidence for GHRH is evident outside the central nervous system in a number of cell types and tissues in humans and in rodents, but its function outside the GH axis remains to be established. mRNA for GHRH, immunoactive GHRH, or bioactive GHRH content is reported in the anterior pituitary, ovaries, testes, placenta, leukocytes, adrenal medulla, pancreas, and gastrointestinal tract,[168] and in tumors associated with the GH axis,[125,169-171] as well as many other tumor types, including human breast, endometrium, and ovarian.[172] Indeed, trace amounts of GHRH mRNA have been found in most rat tissues examined by reverse transcriptase polymerase chain reaction (RT-PCR).[173] Studies in the somatotrope found immunoreactive GHRH in secretory granules and in the cell nuclei.[174] Additional data demonstrate somatotrope uptake of labeled GHRH into secretory granules, lysosomes, and the nuclear membrane.[175]

GHRH RECEPTOR

GHRH acts through a high-affinity G protein–coupled receptor (GHRH-R) found on the anterior pituitary somatotroph and coupled to cyclic adenosine monophosphate (cAMP).[176] The receptor was cloned from human pituitary tumor and from rat and mouse pituitary,[177-179] and it was found to be a member of the G protein–coupled receptor family B, also called the secretin family; the rat and human protein sequences are 82% identical.[177] The GHRH-R protein has 47%, 42%, 35%, and 28% sequence identity with receptors for VIP, secretin, calcitonin, and parathyroid hormone, respectively.[177,178] The isolated cDNAs encoded a 423 amino acid protein that has seven putative transmembrane domains and a 108 residue extracellular N-terminal domain (after signal peptide cleavage) containing one glycosylation site. The GHRH-R sequence predicts ten extracellular cysteine residues that also are found in the secretin, VIP, and PACAP receptor subgroup; eight of these ten are also conserved in most members of the wider receptor family B. These cysteine residues are proposed to form sulfhydral cross-links that stabilize an extracellular domain involved in hormone binding.[180]

Cloned pituitary GHRH-R expressed in cell lines demonstrated saturable, high-affinity, GHRH-specific binding and stimulated the accumulation of intracellular cAMP in response to physiologic concentrations of GHRH.[177-179] Unlike some related receptors that could signal through both cAMP : PKA and phospholipase C : IP3 : PKC pathways, only cAMP activation could be detected, although stimulation of phospholipid turnover was noted in somatotrope cells. A specific GHRH antagonist blocked both binding and second messenger responses.

Data from the cloned receptor were consistent with photoaffinity cross-linking studies of GHRH-R in sheep pituitary membranes that revealed high-affinity binding sites with an apparent molecular weight of 55 kDa and one glycosylation site. After deglycosylation and taking into account the mass of the coupled GHRH analogue, the molecular weight (MW) of the native ovine

receptor protein was estimated at 42 kDa,[181] in agreement with the prediction from the human cDNA sequence of 45 kDa, assuming cleavage of a signal peptide.[178] Further, the binding characteristics of the natural sheep receptor and the cloned human receptor are largely in agreement with a single high-affinity site with a K_d of $\approx$0.2 nM.

Various radiolabeled forms of GHRH bind to membranes of the pituitary, thymus, and spleen. The dissociation constants estimated in these studies vary wildly from 41 pM[182] to 590 nM.[183] No binding was measurable in three nonfunctional pituitary adenomas, although consistent GHRH binding to five acromegalic adenomas was seen, with dissociation constants averaging 0.3 nM.[184]

Studies that attempted to delineate the receptor's GHRH binding domains using chimeric receptor constructs[180] or GHRH cross-linking[185] suggest that although the large N-terminal extracellular domain plays a major role in GHRH binding, other domains are also essential for ligand selectivity and binding. In vitro studies of a naturally occurring receptor truncation mutant[186] and a receptor truncation resulting from alternative splicing[187] show a dominant negative effect on GHRH signaling, suggesting that the receptor may function as a dimer .

GHRH Receptor mRNA and Gene

Two GHRH-R mRNA transcripts of approximately 2.5 and 4 kb were identified in rat pituitary, as were 2.0 and 2.1 kb in mouse and 3.5 kb in ovine pituitary.[177-179] Further, in mouse, the receptor is expressed in a spatial and temporal pattern that corresponds to expression of GH.[179] In the mouse, the first evidence of POU1F1 (a pituitary specific transcription factor, also called Pit-1 or GHF1) expression occurred at embryonic day 14.5, while transcripts encoding the cloned receptor first appeared on embryonic day 16.5.[179] Mutations that cause a loss of POU1F1 expression, such as in dw/dw mice, lead to a lack of GHRH-R gene expression and somatotrope hypoplasia.[179]

The human GHRH-R gene is divided into 13 exons separated by variably sized introns that spread its length to over 15 kb, the complete sequence of which is known.[188] Fluorescent in situ hybridization localized the gene to human chromosome 7p14-15.[189,190] Studies of the promoter region of the receptor gene found no traditional initiator motifs such as a TATA box.[191,192] Putative binding sites for several transcription factors, including POU1F1, Oct-1, Brn-2, NF-1, cAMP response element (CRE), and estrogen receptor response elements (EREs), were identified. An in vitro reporter system demonstrated that expression was enhanced by POU1F1 and glucocorticoids, and was inhibited by estrogen.[191] POU1F1 stimulation is consistent with previous studies in Snell and Jackson dwarf mice showing POU1F1 dependence of receptor expression[179]; five different POU1F1 sites have been shown to contribute to this POU1F1 dependence.[193] The glucocorticoid effect on the promotor may be the mechanism for glucocorticoid upregulation of GHRH binding sites[194] and receptor mRNA[195,196] in rats. The estrogen inhibition of promotor transcription is consistent with observed sexual dimorphism in receptor mRNA expression.[197] Studies have suggested that GHRH-R expression is upregulated by GHRH itself[198-200]; although a putative CRE that could explain this effect was found in the receptor gene promoter, in vitro regulation of the promoter by forskolin could not be demonstrated.[191]

The structure of the rat GHRH-R gene[201] closely matches that of the human but includes an additional exon that would predict an alternatively spliced receptor message that encodes 41 additional amino acids in the third intracellular loop. Indeed, both rat and mouse GHRH-R cDNA clones for this long form have been isolated,[177,179] although analysis of rat pituitary mRNA by PCR found evidence of the shorter form only.[177] Alternative splicing at the homologous site in the PACAP receptor results in functional receptors that differ in their relative signaling through cAMP and phospholipase C second messenger pathways.[202] When the long form of the rat GHRH-R is stably expressed in cell lines, it binds GHRH, but no intracellular signaling could be detected.[201]

In mice, evidence is seen of an alternative splice variant that encodes a receptor devoid of the first transmembrane domain.[179] Alternatively spliced GHRH mRNA encoding a receptor lacking the last two transmembrane domains has been reported in human pituitary tumors and in normal pituitary.[203] In the rat, an alternative splice replacing the last five amino acid residues at the C terminus with a new 17-residue sequence has been found by PCR[204]; this receptor variant appears to signal cAMP normally. No functional role for any of these alternatively spliced GHRH-R messages has been established, although it has been proposed that a truncated receptor variant expressed in tumors can act as a dominant negative in inhibiting GHRH signaling.[187,205]

Synthetic GHRH antagonists can inhibit the growth and proliferation of a variety of human tumors and tumor cell lines,[206-208] which is consistent both with the hypothesis that GHRH can act as a local autocrine/paracrine factor in the stimulation of cell growth[209] and with the mitogenic actions of GHRH at the somatotroph.[210] The mechanism underlying this action has been unclear because a full-length GHRH receptor could not be detected in the cell lines that responded to GHRH antagonist.[208] However, many tumor cells and also normal human prostate express low levels of alternatively spliced forms of GHRH receptor messages not found in the pituitary.[208,211] Indeed, a receptor splice variant with an alternative N-terminal domain (SV1) may be the site of action for the antiproliferative effects of GHRH antagonists,[212-214] as well as for ligand-independent stimulation of tumor growth.[215]

GHRH-R mutations resulting in dwarfism have been identified in mouse and humans. The first such mutation was found in the *little* mouse, a dwarf strain that has an inherited autosomal defect resulting in low levels of GH and pituitary hypoplasia, but is still responsive to exogenous GH. Pituitary cells from these mice would not respond to GHRH but could release GH in response to other activators of cAMP, suggesting a receptor defect.[216] After cloning of the GHRH-R cDNA, the mouse gene was localized to the midregion of chromosome 6.[217,218] Subsequent sequencing of the receptor demonstrated an Asp-to-Gly point mutation at residue 60 of the receptor's extracellular domain, which is highly conserved in related receptors, mutation of which resulted in complete loss of cAMP signaling. Additional studies demonstrated that this mutant receptor was properly expressed and localized in the cell membrane, but was unable to bind GHRH.[219]

In humans, a variety of loss-of-function GHRH-R mutations have been identified in patients with GH deficiency and proportionate short stature.[220] Two such mutations have been found in large kindreds—one in three distantly related families from India, Pakistan, and Sri Lanka, and another in a Brazilian kindred with more than 100 affected individuals.[221] Additional receptor mutations continue to be identified, and it is now suggested that 10% of all human familial isolated GH deficiency type 1 is caused by GHRH-R defects.[222] Affected individuals are homozygous for point mutations or deletions in the receptor protein coding region, at an intron splice junction, or in the gene's promoter. In addition, some affected individuals are compound heterozygotes with two different loss-of-function mutations. Individuals

heterozygous for an inactivating missense point mutation of the *GHRH-R* gene did not show a significant reduction in adult stature or in serum IGF-1, but changes in body composition and possibly an increase in insulin sensitivity were reported.[223] In contrast to this, two different receptor truncations have been shown to have dominant negative properties in vitro[186,187]; thus truncation mutations could potentially affect heterozygotes. It is proposed that activating receptor mutations could be associated with acromegaly or adenoma, but screening of pituitary tumors for activating mutations so far has yielded only ambiguous[224] or negative results.[225,226]

GHRH INTRACELLULAR SIGNALING

At the somatotrope, GHRH activates many of the classical signaling systems, including cAMP, calmodulin, calcium mobilization, and phospholipid pathways, indicating a significant commitment of the somatotrope to respond to GHRH. As with many secretory cells, GHRH-accelerated GH release requires both calcium[227] and calmodulin.[228,229] Intracellular calcium is elevated within seconds of a GHRH stimulus, both in pituitary cells[230] and in thymocytes.[231] This calcium response is dependent on influx of extracellular calcium rather than on the release of intracellular stores.[232] cAMP also signals to the cell nucleus, regulating gene expression via multiple transcription factors.[233]

cAMP Metabolism

At the somatotrope, GHRH stimulates cAMP accumulation and GH release, and these responses are blocked by somatostatin.[234,235] Glucococorticoid pretreatment enhances both the potency and the efficacy of GHRH in driving cAMP accumulation and GH release[236]; this steroid is necessary for GHRH-induced cAMP accumulation after several days in culture. Adenylate cyclase activity in membranes of normal rat pituitary or human acromegalic tumor[237] is enhanced by GHRH in a guanine nucleotide– and calmodulin-sensitive manner.[229] Pertussis toxin enhances GHRH-initiated cAMP accumulation and GH release.[234] The spontaneous reduction in GHRH-stimulated cAMP levels that occurs over time can be blocked by cycloheximide,[234] and the stimulatory ability of GHRH is potentiated by protein kinase C activation.[238,239] This indicates that another receptor system that stimulates C kinase may directly enhance the productivity of the GHRH-R–coupling protein-adenylate cyclase complex,[240] a candidate for which is the ghrelin (growth hormone secretagogue) receptor.[239]

Phospholipids

GHRH increases phosphatidylinositol labeling[241] and free arachidonate levels[242] in the pituitary. Although in most systems, no effect of GHRH on polyphosphoinositide hydrolysis is detectable,[243] a report shows that in a specific subclass of porcine somatotropes (low-density somatotropes), GHRH stimulates both cAMP- and inositol phosphate–dependent second messenger pathways.[244] Other metabolic pathways involving phospholipid metabolism may be activated by or may modulate GHRH activity.[238,245] cAMP metabolism can be dissociated from GH release after GHRH with some phospholipid metabolic enzyme inhibitors, indicating that they may act distal to the cAMP system to evoke exocytosis.[238]

Mitogenic Signaling

In vivo, insufficient GHRH signaling during development through a GHRH-R defect[218] or as the result of GHRH antisera administration[246] results in somatotrope hypoplasia. Excess

GHRH signaling through tumor expression,[116] Gs mutation,[247] or transgenic overexpression[248] stimulates somatotrope hyperplasia. In vitro, GHRH is a mitogenic signal for somatotrope proliferation.[210] The MAPK pathway is a potential mechanism for this action. GHRH dose dependently stimulates tyrosine phosphorylation of MAPK.[249-251]

GH mRNA and Release Dynamics in Culture

GHRH stimulates the level of GH mRNA,[252] the release of newly synthesized GH[253] and total GH (stored plus released),[254] and the proliferation of somatotropes in vitro.[210] The GHRH effect on the somatotrope varies according to the anatomic location of the somatotrope within the pituitary,[255] and the GH-releasing effect is further enhanced by acute administration of glucocorticoids,[256] possibly through increased GHRH binding.[194] Like glucocorticoids, triiodothyronine,[257] ghrelin,[258] and ghrelin mimetics[239] can amplify GHRH-stimulated GH secretion. In contrast, IGF-1[256] and somatostatin[259] are noncompetitive inhibitors of GHRH-accelerated GH release in vitro.

Accelerated GH release occurs immediately after exposure to GHRH[234] and remains elevated for the duration of the GHRH pulse,[234] albeit at declining rates of release after about 10 minutes.[260] This spontaneous decline could occur without GH content depletion[260] and could be blocked by cycloheximide, suggesting the participation of a rapidly turning over inhibitory protein.[229] The reciprocal interaction of GHRH and somatostatin, as suggested neuroanatomically and by pituitary portal blood measurements,[168] results in a greater mass of GH release per GHRH pulse. This has been demonstrated in perifusion culture.[261]

Picomolar to nanomolar concentrations of GHRH that likely are present in pituitary portal blood[262,263] regulate a graded GH response from the somatotrope.[118] GHRH also stimulates modest prolactin release at low GHRH concentrations in vitro,[264,265] as well as the secretion of a protein known as peptide 23 (identical to pancreatitis-associated protein and a member of the C-type lectin supergene family).[266,267] Because GHRH can interact with VIP receptors in intestinal epithelium[268] and GH$_3$ cells,[269] it is possible that pharmacologic or pathologic levels of GHRH can activate this and other receptor types.

ANIMAL STUDIES

GHRH Release

The pulsatile release of GH is influenced by numerous factors, including nutrition, body composition, metabolism, age, sex steroids, adrenal corticoids, thyroid hormones, and renal and hepatic functions.[168] A major common pathway for these factors is seen in their effects on GHRH release from the hypothalamus through direct actions on GHRH neurons, and also through interplay with somatostatin neurons. These effects may be mediated through other factors such as ghrelin, catecholamines, interleukin-1, somatostatin, opioids, leptin, inhibin, and neuropeptide Y (NPY).[270,271]

GHRH Effects on the GH Axis

GHRH was first demonstrated to stimulate GH release in vivo in anesthetized rats.[272,273] These GH responses to GHRH could be enhanced by passive immunization against somatostatin or blocked by passive immunization against rat GHRH.[168] It was soon found that GHRH could enhance GH secretion in every vertebrate species tested, including mammals, birds, and fish.

GHRH is necessary for endogenous pulsatile GH secretion, as anti-GHRH antisera treatment eliminated these pulses in rats and

sheep.[168] However, rhythmic GH secretion persists in an amplitude-miniaturized version in the absence of a GHRH-R signal, at least in men.[274] This observation is supported by a gender-specific difference after administration of a GHRH antagonist, with no change in basal secretion in men but a significant decrease in women.[275] Antisera to GHRH also decreased statural growth[276] and GHRH-R mRNA expression[199] in the rat. Conversely, GHRH administered over several days to weeks enhanced body or organ growth and function in experimental animals.[277] The effect is particularly striking in mice transgenic for GHRH.[278,279] Pulses of GHRH are measured in pituitary portal plasma of unanesthetized sheep with peak values of 25 to 40 pg/mL for a period of 71 minutes.[263] Temporal analysis of GH pulses in sheep suggested a complex regulation that can be explained only partially by GHRH and somatostatin pulses and ghrelin.[239,280]

During development, basal GH responses to exogenous GHRH decrease from postnatal day 1 to day 28 in the rhesus monkey.[281] Passive immunization against GHRH shows that endogenous GHRH is an active secretagogue up to day 9.[282] In the rat, GHRH injections do not increase GH levels at postnatal day 2,[283] whereas stimulatory responses of similar magnitude are measured at postnatal days 10, 30, and 75, as well as at 14 months.[284] Likewise, GHRH injections given over 5 days elevate GH biosynthesis in rat pituitaries at postnatal day 10.[285] Rat pituitary GHRH-R mRNA expression was highest in early gestation, declined to a nadir at 12 days of age, increased at the onset of sexual maturation, and then declined with aging.[286]

Significant changes in GHRH status are noted during aging. In the hypothalamus, a reduction in *GHRH* gene expression and content is seen,[287] as is a decrease in GHRH binding to pituitary in 18-month-old rats.[288] GHRH-R mRNA is correspondingly decreased in 18-month-old rats but can be brought back toward levels observed in younger animals through treatment with GHRH.[289] Decreased GHRH-R expression may contribute to the diminished pituitary response to GHRH in aged male rats[290] and humans.[291]

The GHRH system is also strongly influenced by gender (or gonadal steroids). Hypothalamic GHRH mRNA levels are greater in male than female rats[292,293] and are reduced by orchidectomy and increased by testosterone treatment in intact[294] or castrated[295] male rats. Estradiol has no effect on hypothalamic GHRH mRNA.[296] The ability of GHRH to elicit a GH response in vivo varies during the rat estrous cycle[297]; it is of greater magnitude in the male than in the female[284,298] and is strongly sex steroid dependent.[298] Somatotropes from male rats likewise have greater cAMP and GH responses to GHRH than do those from female rats when studied in static[299] or perifusion[298] cultures. Furthermore, the intact and castrate male rat treated with testosterone yields the greatest quantity of GHRH-responsive somatotropes,[298] as does direct testosterone treatment of cultured somatotropes.[300] Gender differences can be measured at the level of the single somatotrope using the hemolytic plaque assay[301]; testosterone (administered in vivo) increases secretory capacity and recruits a subpopulation of somatotropes, while estradiol has the opposite effects.[302] GHRH receptor message levels are dramatically lower in female than in male rats,[168] and estrogen acts at the receptor gene to inhibit GHRH-R mRNA expression.[191]

In addition to sex steroid effects, free fatty acids[303] and GH itself[304] reduce the in vivo release of GH in response to GHRH. GH treatment decreases hypothalamic GHRH content in intact rats[293] and after hypophysectomy GHRH levels in the hypothalamus rise,[305] suggesting feedback regulation of GHRH by GH. Thyroxine replacement can restore hypothalamic immunoreactive GHRH levels reduced by thyroidectomy in rats,[168] and triiodothyronine and cortisol can protect against reduced GHRH-stimulated GH release in hypothyroid[306] or adrenalectomized rats,[307] respectively. Indeed, long-term glucocorticoids in vivo decrease GHRH expression in GHRH neurons of the arcuate nucleus.[308]

Months of excess GHRH exposure in transgenic mice is associated with increased pituitary mass and mammosomatotrope hyperplasia[278] that eventually results in adenoma formation after 12 months.[309] This is reminiscent of the clinical findings in patients with ectopic GHRH secretion. What was surprising was the rapidity of this effect; GHRH infusions were capable of inducing enlargement of the anterior pituitary within days in intact, normal rats.[310] The dose range of this acute effect has yet to be defined, and this observation does not address the potential risks of replacement of GHRH in deficiency states. In pituitary allograph studies, in orchidectomized hamsters, exogenous GHRH maintains somatotrope size without affecting the percent of GH cells.[311]

GHRH Effects on Functions Outside of the GH Axis

GHRH stimulates gastrin release and epithelial cell proliferation in the digestive tract.[312] It also stimulates insulin, glucagon, and somatostatin secretion from the pancreas.[313-315] GHRH enhances non–rapid eye movement sleep in rats.[316] GHRH antisera[317] or GHRH antagonists[318] inhibit sleep, and sleep deprivation enhances hypothalamic GHRH mRNA levels.[319] GHRH-Ab treatment of female rats results in osteopenic effects,[320] and plasmid-mediated GHRH expression in an animal model of cancer cachexia was able to prevent weight loss.[321] Most of these activities, including control of GH status, suggest that GHRH predominantly acts as a nutrient-partitioning hormone, to regulate body composition.

Circulating GHRH in Humans

Following the initial synthesis of GHRH, radioimmunoassays (RIAs) were used to demonstrate that, contrary to hopes that GHRH in the peripheral circulation would be principally of hypothalamic origin and its measurement would thus serve as an index of hypothalamic secretion, most circulating GHRH is not of hypothalamic origin, but instead comes from the gut.[322] Further, an RIA ideally would measure intact biologically active hormone. However, as the result of cleavage by DPP-IV, GHRH(1-44)-NH$_2$ has a very short half-life in the circulation of 6.8 minutes, and the metabolite GHRH(3-44)NH$_2$ appears within 1 minute of an IV injection of GHRH(1-44)NH$_2$.[323] The biological activity of GHRH(3-44)NH$_2$ is less than 10^{-3} that of GHRH(1-44) NH$_2$.[138] Unfortunately, most RIAs measure GHRH(1-44)-NH$_2$ and GHRH(3-44)-NH$_2$ with equal efficiency, and measurements therefore do not reflect biological activity in the circulation. Most assays are directed to the midportion of the GHRH molecule and therefore do not distinguish between different circulating forms. Besides the RIA, more sensitive enzyme immunoassays for GHRH measurement have been developed.[324] One of the few indications for measuring serum GHRH is a GHRH-producing tumor.

GHRH Levels in Acromegaly

Interest in the frequency of ectopic GHRH as a cause of acromegaly has been intense. Two extensive studies have addressed this issue. In a study of 80 patients with acromegaly, 76 had GHRH levels in the normal range[325]; of the four with elevated levels, one was known to harbor a GHRH-secreting tumor. Extensive evaluation of the other three failed to determine a source for the GHRH. In a second study, 3 of 177 patients with

acromegaly exhibited elevated serum levels of GHRH.[326] In all cases, GHRH levels were markedly elevated (i.e., in the nanogram per milliliter range), and patients were known to have had previous GHRH-secreting tumors. Thus, although apparently rare, ectopic secretion of GHRH must be considered as a possible cause of acromegaly, and measurement of peripheral GHRH seems prudent as a part of the evaluation. Because it is known that the release of ectopic hormones may be intermittent, and because only 300 pg/mL of GHRH is necessary to stimulate GH release in normal subjects, a single normal or modestly elevated GHRH determination may not exclude ectopic GHRH-associated acromegaly.

The subject of GHRH-producing tumors has been reviewed previously.[327,328] GHRH-producing tumors associated with acromegaly are rare. Unique features of patients with acromegaly harboring tumors secreting GHRH included young age, female preponderance, foregut derivation of the tumors, benign biological behavior, small secretory granules in the tumor, and frequent association with multiple endocrine neoplasia type 1 (MEN-1) syndrome. The pancreas and the lung are common primary sites. GHRH-containing tumors that are not associated with acromegaly include those of the gut and thymus, small cell carcinoma of the lung, and medullary carcinoma of the thyroid. Several tumors are plurihormonal. In contrast to somatotroph adenoma as seen in patients with classic acromegaly, the hypophyseal lesion represents somatotroph hyperplasia in acromegalic patients with GHRH-producing tumor. This finding indicates that GHRH not only increases somatotroph secretory activity, but causes somatotroph proliferation. Studies of GHRH-producing tumors are of fundamental importance for obtaining insight into endocrine activity of pituitary somatotrophs and the pathogenesis of GH-secreting pituitary adenomas associated with acromegaly; the importance of GHRH in the origin of acromegaly is still unresolved. Preliminary evidence suggests that the amount of GHRH mRNA expression seen in somatotroph adenomas is associated with the progression and aggressiveness of these tumors.[171] The GHRH receptor mRNA is specifically expressed in GH-producing adenomas and somatotrophs.[170] To address whether GHRH can produce tumors, transgenic mice expressing the human *GHRH* gene have been developed. These animals, which had been exposed to excessive quantities of GHRH throughout development and life, developed mammosomatotrope or somatotrope adenomas.[329] The significance of these observations in terms of human disease is unclear, and additional studies are needed. Early studies have investigated the beneficial effects of GHRH antagonists in animals and humans. It is interesting to note that in one single reported clinical case, ectopic GHRH secretion was associated with empty sella syndrome.[330]

Treatment of transgenic mice overexpressing the human *GHRH* gene with GHRH antagonists resulted in suppression of GH and secretion of IGF-1.[331] The relationship between GHRH-secreting tumors and MEN-1 syndrome is controversial; additional studies are required to elucidate whether they represent two distinct entities, or whether GHRH-producing tumors accompanied by acromegaly are only forme fruste manifestations of MEN-1 syndrome. Several cases of acromegaly due to ectopic GHRH secretion associated with MEN-1 syndrome have been described.[332-336]

Eutopic GHRH Secretion

Occasionally, hypothalamic gangliocytomas may be associated with acromegaly; immunocytochemical staining of such tumors for GHRH has been described. It has been suggested that these tumors should be considered as an unusual cause of acromegaly.[337] On occasion, these tumors are intrasellar; in such cases, the observation that somatotrophs are in close anatomic association with neurons suggests that GHRH not only stimulates GH secretion but may also cause adenoma formation. An intrasellar gangliocytoma with somatotroph adenoma has been described, which was strongly positive for gastrin and weakly positive for GHRH. Because gastrin administered intracerebroventricularly increases GH secretion, it has been suggested that gastrin release may act in a paracrine fashion on gangliocytoma to enhance GHRH secretion and thus cause somatotrope adenoma.[338]

GHRH Levels in GH-Deficient Children

Many reports describing serum and cerebrospinal fluid (CSF) concentrations of GHRH in children with various forms of growth deficiency have appeared. In 22 children with the diagnosis of constitutional short stature (defined as 2 to 3 SD below the predicted mean height for age, peak levels of GH in excess of 10 µg/L during at least one provocation test, and bone age approximating chronological age), basal GHRH levels (8 to 148 pg/mL) were no different from those noted in normal children.[339] In addition, in five of nine children, GHRH levels rose twofold 15 minutes after administration of levodopa (500 mg po). In another study of 16 children with idiopathic delayed puberty, the peak serum GHRH concentration following levodopa was 41 ± 10 pg/mL, and this compared with 96 ± 25 pg/mL in children with constitutional short stature.[340] Similarly, in patients with hypothalamic hypopituitarism, no increase in circulating GHRH levels was seen after levodopa, a finding that contrasts with responses in normal subjects.[341,342] These patients with hypothalamic hypopituitarism do respond to exogenous GHRH administration. Insulin-induced hypoglycemia increased circulating GHRH levels in normal subjects, but not in six patients with isolated GH deficiency.[343] In ten children with short stature, GHRH levels increased at 15 minutes after hypoglycemia from 10 ± 0.5 to 17.1 ± 3.1 pg/mL.[344] No increase in GHRH was evident after arginine, even though hypoglycemia alone or arginine alone increased GH concentrations.

However, in contrast to children with constitutional short stature, five children with GH deficiency associated with hypothalamic germinomas were reported to have undetectable concentrations of GHRH in the CSF.[345] In addition, children with idiopathic GH deficiency have GHRH present in the CSF but at concentrations lower than those in normal children (15.1 ± 1.0 vs. 29.3 ± 2.0 pg/mL; mean ± SEM).

GHRH AS A DIAGNOSTIC AGENT

Until 1985, the use of cadaveric GH was strictly controlled and was limited to use in children with short stature due to severe GH deficiency. Dynamic tests of GH reserve were therefore of clinical significance in pediatric endocrinology and were performed primarily for academic interest in adults with hypothalamic-pituitary disease. With the advent of recombinant human GH, now available in unrestricted quantities, and its approval for use in adults with GH deficiency resulting from hypothalamic-pituitary disease in the United States, Europe, and Australia, the need to diagnose GH deficiency safely and effectively has become an important issue in adult endocrinology.[346]

Many of the tests used to determine GH status are hazardous under certain circumstances (the insulin tolerance test [ITT] is contraindicated in the elderly and in patients with ischemic heart disease or a history of seizures) or are associated with unpleasant side effects (glucagon causes nausea and delayed hypoglycemia, clonidine is associated with drowsiness and hypotension, and arginine causes dizziness and phlebitis). Tests that are effective in children, such as those using arginine or clonidine as the stimulus, are less effective at releasing GH in adults.[347] The ITT is frequently quoted as the gold standard investigation for diagnosing GH deficiency in children and adults, but many endocrinologists shy away from this procedure because of concerns about the effects of hypoglycemia in their patients, and because the test has to be supervised by a physician for its duration.

Growth hormone–releasing hormone (GHRH) and the GH-releasing substances (e.g., growth hormone–releasing peptide 6 (GHRP-6), growth hormone–releasing peptide 1 (GHRP-1), growth hormone–releasing peptide 2 (GHRP-2), hexarelin, MK-0677) are powerful GHSs that are safe and well tolerated in both adults and children. These agents have attracted increasing attention as stimuli used to determine GH status in both adults and children. Typically, tests of GH reserve in both children and adults have utilized procedures that depend on effects mediated by the hypothalamus. For example, agents such as arginine, glucagon, clonidine, or levodopa and insulin-induced hypoglycemia are assumed to elicit a hypothalamic signal that acts upon the somatotrophs to stimulate the release of GH. A lesion of the hypothalamus or the pituitary may produce an abnormal GH response to these stimuli. The use of GHRH to stimulate GH release directly from the somatotrophs allows a theoretical distinction to be made between patients with a pituitary abnormality, who will have an abnormal response to GHRH, and those with hypothalamic lesions, who may respond normally to GHRH. This may be important when the therapeutic strategy for an individual patient is determined.

Administration of GHRH to Normal Individuals

The effects of GHRH and its analogues given as a bolus have been studied in healthy men, women, and children.[348-358] Following an IV injection of GHRH, GH levels begin to rise within 5 minutes and reach a peak at between 30 and 60 minutes. The ability of GHRH to release GH is dose dependent,[357] the maximal response being observed following a dose of 1 µg/kg or higher.[352] In adults, the GH response to GHRH is similar in men and women, although women are more sensitive to GHRH than men; the dose of GHRH required for half-maximal GH secretion is 0.4 µg/kg in men and 0.2 µg/kg in women. The GH response to GHRH in women is not altered by the changes in sex steroid hormones that occur during the menstrual cycle.[356]

The effect of pubertal development on the GH response to GHRH is slight.[359,360] When 68 prepubertal children were compared with 66 children at various stages of puberty, no overall difference in GH response to GHRH was observed.[359] In a more detailed study that examined children at each stage of puberty, a slight decrease in GH response to GHRH was seen in boys during midpuberty. Although a similar decrease was not observed in girls, the GH response to GHRH did not differ significantly between the sexes during puberty.[360] In prepubertal children who are being evaluated for poor growth, priming the hypothalamic-pituitary-GH axis with sex steroids can normalize a suboptimal GH response to some stimuli. The GH response to GHRH is not affected by priming with estrogen,[361] suggesting that sex steroids assert their effects at the hypothalamus, either reducing somatostatin tone or increasing GHRH release—not at the pituitary.

The ability of GHRH to release GH is similar in prepubertal and pubertal children, and in young adults. However, over the course of the adult life span, the magnitude of the GH peak following GHRH declines with increasing age.[348,362] The likely mechanism for the age-related decline in response to GHRH is an increase in somatostatin tone.[363] Support for this is found in studies that utilize GHRH in combination with pyridostigmine or arginine.[364,365] These agents have been used alone as diagnostic tests for GH deficiency, producing a GH pulse by reducing somatostatin tone.[366,367] Arginine and pyridostigmine act synergistically with GHRH, producing large GH pulses similar to those seen in younger adults.

The GHRH Test

With any test used in clinical practice, it is important to determine what constitutes a normal response. Accordingly, several studies have addressed this question for the GHRH test. Ranke et al.[368] defined the normal range of GH responses to GHRH in 86 children with a normal GH axis as 11.8 to 172.4 μg/L, by determining the mean response ±2 SD. This study also concluded that a GH response of less than 10 μg/L should be used as the diagnostic threshold for GH deficiency in children.

The diagnostic threshold of 10 μg/L has been used in other studies utilizing the GHRH test[369-371] and now is generally accepted in pediatric practice. This peak is similar to that used to define GH deficiency when most stimuli are used in children, although it is recognized that different stimuli are not equal in their ability to release GH.[359] Such thresholds are defined arbitrarily, despite attempts to rationalize them.[372] This may reflect the fact that the diagnosis of GH deficiency in a child depends primarily on the clinical finding of poor growth, and that the stimulation test is used to confirm the presence of GH deficiency.

In adults, the diagnostic threshold used to identify patients with GH deficiency is lower than that used in pediatric practice. For example, a GH peak of less than 3 μg/L during an ITT is considered to be indicative of severe GH deficiency that warrants therapy with exogenous GH. If arginine were to be used as the stimulus, the diagnostic cutoff would be even lower than this.[373] In adults, the GHRH test is generally a more potent stimulus of GH secretion, resulting in higher pulses than those seen following ITT, arginine, or glucagon.[374] This would suggest that the diagnostic cutoff for severe GH deficiency might be higher than 3 μg/L when the GHRH test is used in adults, but this has not been determined.

The GHRH Test in Children With Short Stature

Normal Hypothalamic-Pituitary-GH Axis. The GH response elicited by GHRH in children with short stature due to a variety of causes has been well characterized.[368,369,375-383] Children who have constitutional short stature with no underlying pathology have a normal GH peak following GHRH administration,[377,383] but the timing of that peak may be delayed.[378] Children who are short as a result of intrauterine growth retardation also have a normal GH response to GHRH.

GH Deficiency. Children with GH deficiency defined by the use of conventional tests frequently have a greater response to GHRH than to other tests of GH status.[375] In a study of prepubertal children undergoing investigation of abnormal growth, subjects were divided into groups according to their responses to conventional tests. GH status was considered normal if the peak GH response to a conventional test was greater than 10 μg/L; partial and severe GH deficiency were defined as a peak GH response of between 5 and 10 μg/L and less than 5 μg/L, respectively. When a diagnostic cutoff of 10 μg/L is assumed for the GHRH test, 76% of children with partial and 39% with severe GH deficiency had a GH peak greater than 10 μg/L during the GHRH test. Conversely, 10% of children considered to have a

normal GH axis had a peak GH response less than 10 μg/L—a figure consistent with the findings of other studies. This study demonstrated a considerable discordance between conventional tests of GH status and the GHRH test. It also indicated that, in a significant proportion of children with GH deficiency diagnosed clinically and confirmed by conventional tests, somatotroph function may be preserved, with the cause of impaired GH status being hypothalamic rather than pituitary dysfunction.

Patients who develop GH deficiency following cranial irradiation also exhibit discordance between the GHRH test and conventional tests of GH status. The GH response to GHRH in such patients was greater than the response to the ITT and the arginine test in 80% of patients in one study.[384] This suggests that radiation primarily affects the hypothalamic mechanisms that regulate GH secretion from the anterior pituitary. The magnitude of the GH peak during the GHRH test decreases as time from radiation increases. This may be a direct effect of radiation on the somatotrophs or the indirect effect of long-standing GHRH deficiency, which depletes the available GH pool within the somatotroph. The latter is supported by the observation that priming with GHRH for several days prior to the GHRH test can significantly increase the GH response to GHRH.[385]

GHRH and the Diagnosis of GH Deficiency in Adults

The few published studies that examined GHRH as a diagnostic test in GH-deficient adults were performed on small numbers of patients, most of whom had childhood-onset GH deficiency. More recently, studies that have investigated GHRH as a diagnostic agent in adults have utilized it in combination with other agents, with the aim of normalizing the GH response across the adult life span (see later).

Limitations of the GHRH Test

The use of GHRH alone as a diagnostic test for GH deficiency is limited by several factors. The discordance observed between the results of the GHRH test and the results of other stimulation tests such as the ITT can lead to difficulties in interpreting the results of the GHRH test. Considerable interindividual and intraindividual variation has been noted in results of the GHRH test. The coefficient of variation for the GHRH test has been reported as 60% for children[386] and 45% for adults,[374] although the variability diminishes with increasing age in adults.[387] The sensitivity of the GHRH test is relatively poor in children with short stature and varies with the severity of the GH deficiency as determined by other tests of GH status. In one study, the sensitivity of the GHRH test was 24% in patients with GH insufficiency (GH peak 5.0 to 10.0 μg/L to conventional tests) and 61% in patients with severe GH deficiency (GH peak <5.0 μg/L).[375] The specificity of the GHRH test has been reported to be 85% to 90%.[359,375] The ability to interpret the GHRH test is confounded further by the inhibition of the GH response in obese subjects.[388,389] This may be particularly important when patients with GH deficiency are assessed, because they have abnormal body composition with a propensity to abdominal obesity. The GH response to GHRH in obese patients with pituitary tumors is reduced, making it difficult to define their GH status accurately, particularly when the GH deficiency is isolated.[390]

The GHRH test is safe, is associated with few side effects, and requires minimal medical supervision, making it an attractive test for use in the outpatient setting. However, the problems outlined above make it difficult to interpret the results of the GHRH test in clinical practice; therefore, it must be used with caution. A GH peak greater than 10 μg/L does not exclude GH deficiency in a child with poor growth, and further evaluation of the hypothalamic-pituitary axis should be undertaken. A positive result (i.e., a GH peak <10 µg/L) will be indicative of GH deficiency, but because 10% to 15% of normal children fall into this group, further evaluation to confirm the diagnosis of GH deficiency will be necessary. The relatively good specificity of the GHRH test suggests that a positive result is significant, such that the child should be evaluated further with additional investigations and monitoring. At the present time, the primary role of the GHRH test is to determine which children are candidates for GHRH therapy.

Tests Utilizing GHRH in Combination With Other Agents

The observation that GHRH acts synergistically with agents that reduce somatostatin tone has led to the development of tests combining GHRH with arginine, pyridostigmine, or clonidine. GHRH acts synergistically with these agents, producing large GH pulses, the magnitude of which frequently exceeds 50 µg/L in healthy subjects.[359,374,391] The addition of these agents to GHRH increases the reproducibility of the test and improves diagnostic accuracy.

GHRH in combination with pyridostigmine or arginine causes profound release of GH. In one study of normal children and adolescents, the normal range for GHRH plus pyridostigmine was 22.6 to 90.0 µg/L (n = 94), and that of GHRH plus arginine, 22.4 to 108 µg/L (n = 81).[359] The results of these tests were not influenced by pubertal stage in either girls or boys.[359,392] However, a study by Maghnie et al.[393] concludes that in patients with acquired childhood-onset GH deficiency, the number of pituitary hormone deficits and patient age affect the GH response to the combined GHRH and arginine test. Additional study suggests that body mass index (BMI) and age do have an impact on the GHRH arginine test in children with idiopathic GH deficiency.[394] Both studies were conducted with a small number of patients.

In children with GH deficiency, the GHRH-pyridostigmine test, used with the diagnostic threshold of 20 µg/L, confirmed the diagnosis in 100% of patients with organic GH deficiency (caused by craniopharyngioma) and in 80% of patients with idiopathic GH deficiency.[395] GHRH in combination with arginine has been extensively evaluated in adults with pituitary disease in the hope that it will provide a safer alternative to the ITT, which currently is considered to be the gold standard investigation of GH status in adults. In assessing GH secretion, no difference in sensitivity and specificity has been noted in young adults among the Arg + GHRH test, the PD + GHRH test, and the ITT.[396] The combination of GHRH with arginine was chosen over pyridostigmine because the side effects with pyridostigmine were unpleasant and the GH response to GHRH plus arginine is not affected by age.[397] In adults, the GH response to GHRH and arginine is not affected by gender or age, as similar results are achieved in male and female subjects and in young and old adults.[391,397,398] Across the adult life span, the third percentile limit of GH response to GHRH plus arginine is 16.5 µg/L, and the first percentile limit is 9 µg/L.

Adults with GH deficiency all had a peak GH response to GHRH plus arginine that fell below 16.5 µg/L, and 92% of patients had a peak below 9 µg/L. GH peaks achieved during the GHRH-arginine test correlate well with those obtained during the ITT, although the absolute GH response to GHRH plus arginine is considerably greater than that to the ITT. Of seven patients who had achieved a peak GH greater than 9 µg/L during the GHRH-arginine test, six had achieved a GH peak greater than

the diagnostic threshold for the ITT (3 µg/L). Thus, the authors proposed that the diagnostic cutoff for the GHRH-arginine test should be 9 µg/L for severe GH deficiency in adults and 16.5 µg/L for GH insufficiency. Comparison of the sensitivity and specificity of six different tests—ITT, arginine (ARG), levodopa (L-DOPA), ARG + L-DOPA, ARG + GHRH, and IGF-I measurement—in the diagnosis of GH deficiency found the greatest diagnostic accuracy with the ARG + GHRH test and the ITT. The former was preferred over the latter because it produced fewer side effects.[399] The GRS consensus of 2007[400] suggested that GHRH + Arg, GHRH + Ghrelin, and glucagon tests are as sensitive as the ITT in GHD, provided that appropriate cutoff limits are considered. Clinical practice guidelines of the Endocrine Society[401] suggest that ITT and the GHRH-arginine tests have sufficient sensitivity and specificity to establish the diagnosis of GHD. In the clinical situation of radiation-induced GH deficiency, ITT should be used instead of the GHRH-arginine test.[402] GHRH directly stimulates the pituitary; therefore it can give a falsely normal GH response in patients with GHD of hypothalamic origin (e.g., those having received irradiation of the hypothalamic-pituitary region). In patients with new-onset GHD (within 10 years) (e.g., that due to irradiation), testing with GHRH-arginine may be misleading. The guidelines also suggest that in the presence of deficiencies of three or more pituitary axes, the occurrence of GHD is very likely, and provocative testing is optional. The validated cutoff level for GHD in adults for the ITT and the glucagon test is a peak GH response <3 µg/L; this has not been validated in obesity. For the GHRH + Arg test, the following cutoff levels have been validated, depending on the BMI: <25 kg/m^2, peak GH <11 µg/L; 25 to 30 kg/m^2, peak GH <8 µg/L; >30 kg/m^2, peak GH <4 µg/L.[403] The cutoff level validated for the GHRH + GHRP-6 is 10 µg/L in lean patients and 5.0 µg/L in obese patients.[404,405]

GHRH THERAPY IN GH-DEFICIENT CHILDREN

The potential of GHRH as a therapeutic agent for GH-deficient children has been examined in several studies. Most GH-deficient children with short stature and growth failure have a disorder of hypothalamic regulation of the pituitary rather than a defect of the somatotroph. In these children, injections of GHRH, as well as other GHSs, might be a useful treatment option. One of the first studies published in 1985 reported the use of GHRH (1-40)-OH administered sc with a peristaltic pump every 3 hours to two children with organic hypopituitarism (post-traumatic, hydrocephalus).[406] Children received 3-hourly doses of 1 or 3 µg/kg GHRH for 6 months. Both children increased their growth rate by 1.5- to 6.0-fold compared with the growth rate before administration of GHRH(1-40)-OH. The rationale for using this dose regimen was based on the observation that, in growing children, five to nine pulses of GH are detected every 24 hours.

Since that time, several studies have been performed to evaluate the benefits of GHRH therapy in GH-deficient children with different GHRH injection regimens and different doses.[385,407-423] However, the groups of children who were treated were not homogeneous, and their diagnoses varied from GH deficiency and short stature to normal variant short stature without GH deficiency. The GHRH preparations used included GHRH(1-40)-OH, GHRH(1-44)-NH$_2$, and GHRH(1-29)-NH$_2$.

GHRH Given by Pump

Response to the administration of GH with a pump varied from 71% to 100%. The growth rate on GHRH therapy varied from

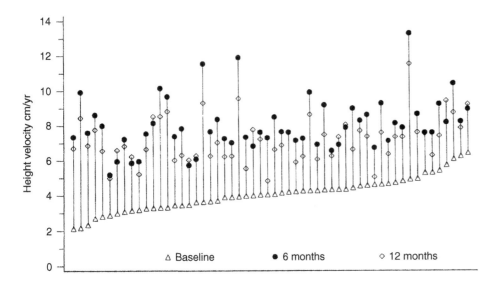

FIGURE 16-9. The effect of 6 and 12 months' growth hormone–releasing hormone (1-29) treatment in growth hormone–deficient children. The height velocities at baseline *(triangle)* and after 6 months *(circle)* and 12 months *(diamond)* of treatment are plotted by increasing baseline values. (From Thorner M, et al: Once daily subcutaneous growth hormone–releasing hormone therapy accelerates growth in growth hormone-deficient children during the first year of therapy. Geref International Study Group, J Clin Endocrinol Metab 81[3]:1189–1196, 1996.)

6.2 to 10 cm/yr over the first 6 months and was maintained for up to 5 years. Growth velocity appears to be related to the total daily dosage, which ranged from 10 to 2150 μg/day. So far, no studies have evaluated whether it is the frequency of administration or the total daily dose that has the greatest impact on therapeutic outcome. The first study that looked at administration by pump or single injections of GHRH was published in 1988.[407] It described the effects of different routes of GHRH administration in 24 GH-deficient children. GHRH (1-40) was given either by pump every 3 hours sc or every 3 hours sc overnight only. Alternatively, GHRH was given twice daily at a dose of 1 to 4 μg/kg per dose for 6 months. In all three circumstances, the growth velocity increased between 1.8- and 2.9-fold, with greatest effects seen during pump therapy with injections given every 3 hours.

Unfortunately, no long-term comparative studies have examined the growth-promoting effects of GHRH with GH. Two short-term studies (6 months' treatment) provided conflicting results: One suggested a comparable growth response with GHRH similar to that with GH treatment,[408] whereas the other suggested that GHRH was less effective.[409]

GHRH Given sc Twice a Day[407,410-417]

The most impressive results with GHRH injections given twice daily were achieved in a multicenter study using GHRH(1-44)-NH$_2$ in 20 GH-deficient children.[414] All children responded with accelerated growth velocity, which increased from 3.6 cm/yr before treatment to 8.6 cm after 6 months and decreased to 8.1 cm after 12 months. Ogilvy-Stuart et al.[417] reported a significant beneficial effect of GHRH(1-29) given at a dose of 30 μg/kg/day over 1 year, which resulted in a 1.8-fold increase in growth velocity per year in nine children with radiation-induced GH deficiency.

The effects of GHRH(1-29) therapy in growth retardation caused by chronic renal failure were examined in nine children by Pasqualini and coworkers.[416] Children were treated conservatively or with dialysis, or underwent renal transplantation, and GHRH(1-29) 52 μg/kg/day was administered for 3 to 6 months. Growth velocity increased from 3.8 to 8 cm/yr.

GHRH Given sc Once a Day

Several groups have investigated the effects of GHRH given sc by once-daily injection.[385,418-423] A study investigating 110 GH-deficient children treated with a dose of 30 μg/kg/day of GHRH(1-29)[423] showed a significant increase in linear growth velocity, with 4.1 cm/yr measured before treatment and 7.2 cm/yr after 1 year of treatment (Fig. 16-9). The largest number of children was investigated in the GHRH European Multicenter Study,[420] which reported on the treatment of 111 GH-deficient children. Height velocity increased from 3.8 cm/yr before to 6 cm/yr during 6 months of treatment. The group of Bozzola[419] reported an increase in growth velocity from 3.5 cm/yr to 7.3 cm/yr after 6 months of treatment in 10 GH-deficient children with GHRH(1-44). Optimal growth velocity was observed during the first 9 months of therapy in most studies.[418] Lanes and Carrillo[422] reported that therapy with GHRH(1-29) in 16 prepubertal GH-deficient children given once daily sc over 12 to 24 months resulted in a significant increase in growth velocity.

Which Children Should be Considered for GHRH Therapy?

The use of GHRH(1-29)-NH$_2$ in the treatment of idiopathic GH deficiency in children with growth failure was approved by the U.S. Food and Drug Administration (FDA), but due to lack of relative efficacy compared to pharmacologic doses of growth hormone it was withdrawn and is not currently being used. The development of long acting preparations may reverse this.

Adverse Effects

Development of antibodies during GHRH treatment has been described.[407,420,423] Treatment-related adverse events, including local injection reactions characterized by pain, swelling, or redness, and headache, flushing, dysphagia, dizziness, hyperactivity, and urticaria, have been reported. Few data on thyroid function have been reported in children with GH deficiency. One study reported an increase in thyroid replacement requirements in one of seven patients[424]; another study reported a 5% incidence of hypothyroidism.[407] The mechanism underlying the change in thyroid function is unclear, but it has been hypothesized that an increase in GH levels results in an increase in somatostatin tone with subsequent inhibition of TSH secretion.[425]

GHRH TREATMENT IN ADULTS

Optimal GHRH therapy requires the functional integrity of somatotroph cells.[426] Although in GH-deficient adults this is no longer the case, older adults in whom somatotroph hyposecretion is thought to be caused by decreased activity of GHRH-secreting neurons[427] still have an intact hypothalamic-pituitary axis. In addition, the pituitary GH-releasable pool in the elderly is comparable with that in young adults.

In fact, the few available studies dealing with the administration of GHRH in adults have been performed in the elderly to investigate whether GHRH treatment could counteract the age-dependent decline in GH. Twice-daily injections of GHRH(1-29) for 2 weeks,[428] as well as continuous GHRH(1-44) infusions for 2 weeks, in healthy older men[429] partially reversed the age-related decrease in GH, as well as IGF-1 levels. Another study, performed over 6 weeks,[430] suggested that administration of GHRH to the elderly might attenuate some effects of aging on muscle strength.

The half-life of GHRH after iv injection is about 10 to 12 minutes, which is one of the limitations of the use of GHRH as a therapeutic. The long-acting analogue of GHRH, CJC-1295, contains full biological activity of GHRH(1-44)NH$_2$. It binds to endogenous serum albumin after sc administration, which prolongs its duration of action, and it is modified by substitution of four amino acids, which makes the compound resistant to proteolytic cleavage. Subcutaneous injection of CJC-1293, another GHRH analogue, in healthy adults resulted in increased GH and IGF-1 levels 1 week after injection, which was explained mainly by the increase in trough levels.[431] Another study[432] showed that in healthy volunteers aged 21 to 61 years, elevated GH and IGF-1 serum concentrations were present for 6 and 14 days, and that tachyphylaxis did not occur with this compound. The sc administration of another compound, PEG-GHRH, increased GH levels in healthy adults, an effect that was present for 12 hours.[433] Overall, additional studies are necessary to assess the safety profile of these compounds and its short-term and long-term effects on body composition.

Ghrelin and Growth Hormone Secretagogues (GHS)

Opiates have long been recognized to stimulate GH secretion. The GHS story evolved from the seminal observation by Bowers and colleagues that met-enkephalin analogues, such as GH-releasing peptide-6, which lacked analgesic activity, preserved their GH-releasing activity.[434] Numerous peptide and non-peptide analogues active in GH release were developed (for reviews on analogues see references 435 and 436), and a group at Merck, using one of its synthetic compounds (MK-0677), succeeded in cloning the GHS receptor, at that point an orphan receptor.[437] A natural ligand for this receptor, ghrelin, was identified in 1999 as the result of a "reverse pharmacology" process.[438] Although the highest concentration of the receptor is found in the hypothalamus and the pituitary, ghrelin was identified from the stomach. At the same time, the ghrelin mRNA sequence was identified from the stomach by another group and was named motilin-related peptide m46.[439] Ghrelin, well conserved over 400 million years, has been detected in a number of tissues, including small amounts in the pituitary and hypothalamus, and is a new member of the brain-gut peptides.[440] Following earlier reports on positive effects on the appetite of some GHSs, the profound GH-independent orexigenic effects of ghrelin were recognized.[441]

Another peptide has been identified arising from the proghrelin molecule (Fig. 16-10) named obestatin.[442] Considerable controversy surrounds the physiologic effects and the target receptor of this circulating peptide,[443] with suggestions of having anorectic effects and inhibitory effects on gastric motility, and GPR39 being the obestatin receptor. Later studies could not reproduce the originally published obestatin activities, and the controversy remains unresolved.

GHRELIN STRUCTURE

Ghrelin is a 28 amino acid peptide with a unique fatty acid chain modification on the N-terminal third amino acid (see Fig. 16-10). The acylation of the hydroxyl group of Ser3 is necessary for the activities mediated by the GHS-R1a receptor such as calcium mobilization, GH release, and appetite effects. In contrast, the proliferative, anti-apoptotic, lipogenic, and cardiovascular effects of ghrelin do not appear to require acylation.[440] As is shown in Fig. 16-10, several forms of ghrelin are found in the circulation. Amino acid Gln14 may be omitted owing to variations in intron splicing, and Arg28 may be removed as the result of variations in cleavage from the prohormone. Also, the acylation at Ser3 can be 8 or 10 carbons long and occasionally includes one double bond. Yet, all of these acylated variants appear to have comparable biological activity.

Studies of ghrelin processing have shown that prohormone convertase 1/3 (PC1/3) is the endoprotease responsible for the production of ghrelin from proghrelin.[444] It is interesting to note that in the absence of PC1/3, ghrelin was still acylated normally, consistent with a model in which acylation takes place on the nascent peptide before cleavage. The enzyme that acylates ghrelin has been identified recently[445,446] and is a member of the family of membrane-bound O-acyl transferases (MBOATs) that was named GOAT (ghrelin O-acyl transferase). The mRNA for GOAT was found in stomach, intestine, and pancreas, consistent with the place where ghrelin is found. GOAT was the only MBOAT capable of acylating ghrelin in vitro, and a GOAT knockout animal had no detectable circulating acyl-ghrelin,[446] suggesting that GOAT is the physiologic mechanism of ghrelin acylation. Because no substrate for GOAT other than ghrelin is known, GOAT is being investigated as a specific pharmacologic target for the modulation of ghrelin activity.[447]

ASSAYS FOR GHRELIN

Most published studies have used single-antibody ghrelin assays that recognize an epitope unique to acyl-ghrelin (active ghrelin), or common to both acyl- and des-acyl ghrelin (total ghrelin). Akamizu et al.[448] report that 40% to 60% of the signal detected at a single-site, total ghrelin assay is due to inactive ghrelin fragments. Two-site sandwich assays can have greater specificity and can avoid cross-reactivity with peptide fragments.[449] These two-site assays report lower levels of ghrelin but see greater percent suppression upon eating,[450] suggesting greater physiologic relevance.

Acyl-ghrelin is deacylated quickly by esterase activity in the blood, and it is likely that it is also degraded by other mechanisms. For assay of acyl-ghrelin, blood samples should be collected to chilled tubes with esterase inhibitor, and cold plasma should be separated and acidified promptly.[450] Acidification to pH ≈3 inhibits esterase, but if insufficient acid is used, the esterase activitys returns upon neutralization for assay, and if too

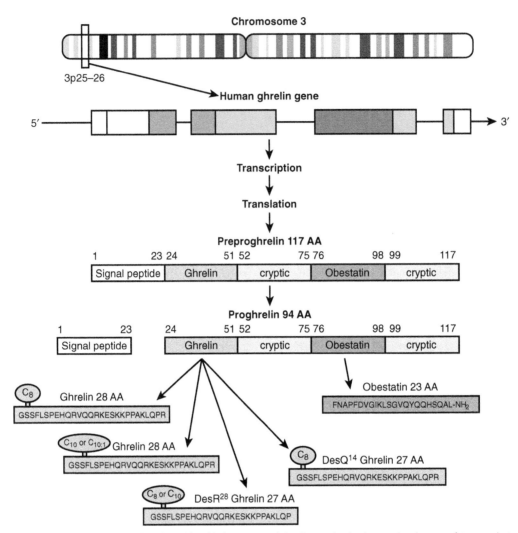

FIGURE 16-10. Schematic diagram of the preproghrelin polypeptide with the post-translational steps that lead up to the cleavage of two products, ghrelin and obestatin. Variants of the ghrelin peptide and its lipid modification are also shown (see text). Numbers represent amino acids (AA); subscript number next to C represents the length of the lipid moiety.

much acid is used (pH ≤2), the acylation can be chemically cleaved.[451]

Ghrelin measurement is further complicated by the strong basic charge and hydrophobic acylation of ghrelin, which can cause it to stick to surfaces. In the circulation, ghrelin, but not des-acyl ghrelin, may be predominantly bound to carrier proteins, with ghrelin having specific lipoprotein interactions not seen with des-acyl ghrelin; ghrelin antisera differ in their ability to detect these bound forms. Together, these factors can affect the assay of ghrelin, as when two popular commercial RIA kits were compared on the same sample set, a 10-fold difference in measured total ghrelin levels was observed.[452]

Serious concerns have also been expressed about the specificity of available acyl-ghrelin assays. In one study examining patients with anorexia nervosa,[453] the acyl-ghrelin levels measured in the same sample set were increased, decreased, or unchanged in subjects with anorexia relative to normal controls, depending on which of three different active ghrelin assays was used.

Sites of Ghrelin Synthesis

In the stomach, ghrelin is synthethized in the X/A-like cells, which represent about 20% of the chromogranin A–immunore-

active endocrine cells. Circulating ghrelin levels are reduced after gastrectomy in rats and humans, but levels increase over time postoperatively.[440] Outside the intestinal tract, ghrelin expression has been identified in a number of tissues, at the mRNA or protein level, or both. In the hypothalamus, ghrelin peptide has been detected by immunostaining and was localized in the internuclear space between the hypothalamic nuclei and the ependymal layer of the third ventricle.[440] Ghrelin was also seen in the axon terminals, and these axons innervated the arcuate, ventromedial, paraventricular, and dorsomedial nucleus and the lateral hypothalamus, as well as outside the hypothalamus in the bed nucleus of the stria terminalis, amygdala, thalamus, and habenula.[454] Circulating ghrelin might reach the hypothalamic nuclei directly from the bloodstream (arcuate nucleus) or by crossing the blood-brain barrier,[455] but peripheral (vagal) connections to the brain stem may also play an important role in the effects of ghrelin (Fig. 16-11). Within the pituitary, ghrelin immunostaining was co-localized to prolactin, growth hormone, and thyroid-stimulating hormone (TSH)-secreting cells, but not to adrenocorticotropic hormone (ACTH) or gonadotroph cells. Ghrelin mRNA and/or protein expression has been described in all normal human tissues studied, as well as in different tumors, including pituitary adenomas, neuroendocrine tumors, thyroid

Table 16-1. Regulation of Ghrelin Secretion

Regulation of Ghrelin Secretion	
Increases in Response to	**Decreases in Response to**
Fasting (short term)	Food intake
Low BMI	High BMI
Leptin?	Glucose
GHRH	Insulin
Thyroid hormones	Somatostatin
Testosterone	GH (short term)
Parasympathetic activity	GHS, ghrelin
	PYY3-36

and medullary thyroid carcinomas, and endocrine tumors of the pancreas and lung. Ghrelin peptide has been shown to be expressed in pituitary, immune cells, lung, placenta, testis, and kidney, and by cyclic expression in the ovary. In the pancreas, controversial reports show expression in β and α cells, or in a new islet cell type, the ϵ cell.

REGULATION OF GHRELIN

Factors shown to be important in ghrelin regulation are listed in Table 16-1. In the human, ghrelin levels are high during short-term caloric restriction and fall immediately after food intake. Higher levels are observed during the night.[456,457] However, after prolonged fasting, acyl-ghrelin levels are lower when compared with fed conditions.[450] Similar findings are reported when only total ghrelin is measured.[458] Chronic regulation is influenced by body weight, with high levels in subjects with low BMI and low levels in obese subjects.[459] Insulin appears to be an important regulator of ghrelin levels, as both insulin resistance and hyper-insulinemia predict low ghrelin levels in a population consisting of insulin-resistant and insulin-sensitive subjects who have equal BMI.[460] Several studies suggest that ghrelin levels are similar in males and females, but some data have showed higher ghrelin levels in females. Estrogen elevates the peak overnight production rate of acylated ghrelin. Other studies suggest that combined estrogen-progestin supplementation enhances GH responsiveness to ghrelin in postmenopausal women. In addition, estradiol-dependent augmentation of the orexigenic potency of ghrelin has been reported.

PHYSIOLOGY AND MOLECULAR BIOLOGY

Following the identification of GHRP-6, GHRP-2, and the first non-peptide analogues of Merck, a large number of pharmaceutical companies and research groups started to actively develop GHSs, resulting in the identification of many new peptide and non-peptide compounds.[435,436] Ghrelin effects are similar to a number of recognized effects of GHSs; however, different GHSs seem to differ in their relative potencies for these effects, suggesting differing cross-reactivities at possible known or unknown receptor subtypes, and raising hopes for new compounds tailored specifically for these sites. An example of specific effect is the activity of hexarelin on the lipid scavanger receptor CD36; this is not shared by ghrelin or some other GHSs.[461] Although ghrelin and some GHS compounds are reported to elevate prolactin, ACTH, and cortisol, others may have greater specificity for appetite, sleep, and cardiac function.[462] The effects of GH release and appetite can be separated, as a pharmacologic antagonist of GHS-R1a–induced GH release can still induce appetite and weight increase,[463,464] while des-acyl ghrelin can also stimulate appetite possibly via the orexin pathway.[465]

SITES OF ACTION

Considerable evidence suggests that for their GH-releasing effects, ghrelin and GHSs act at the level primarily of the hypothalamus but also of the pituitary. The dominant role of this hypothalamic action is demonstrated by the fact that GHSs are unable to release GH in children and adults with pituitary stalk transsection, although animal study suggests that this could be due to the lack of GHRH input on GH synthesis, as exogenous GHRH overcomes the effects of stalk transsection and allows GHS responses. The major site of ghrelin action for the appetite effect is more complex. The arcuate nucleus, the ventromedial nucleus, the paraventricular nucleus, and the nucleus tractus solitarius have been shown to express GHS-R1a, and to be involved in the orexogenic effects of ghrelin.

GHS RECEPTOR

With the use of S^{35}-MK-0677, two types of GHS-R cDNA (types 1a and 1b) were identified.[437] The human type 1a cDNA encodes a 366 amino acid seven-transmembrane receptor of the rhodopsin family and has a relatively limited tissue distribution, including the hypothalamus, the hippocampus (dentate gyrus, CA2 and CA3 regions), the pars compacta of the substantia nigra, the ventral tegmental area, the dorsal and medial raphe nuclei, Edinger-Westphal nucleus, and pons and medulla oblongata, as well as peripheral tissues, such as the thyroid gland, intestine, pancreas, kidney, heart, and aorta, and various endocrine tumors of the pituitary, pancreas, lung, and stomach.[462] Growth hormone secretagogue receptor (GHS-R) established a new branch in the rhodopsin family of G protein–coupled receptors, with other related receptors later identified, including the motilin receptor. The type 1b GHS-R cDNA represented an alternatively spliced message from the same gene but encoded only 289 amino acids, representing the first five transmembrane domains, and appeared to be nonfunctional.[437] Although the mRNA of the type 1b form is widely detectable in tissues, it is unclear whether the type 1b receptor is expressed as a protein, although it is conceivable that this truncated form could interact with the full-length receptor and modulate its activity.

Ghrelin is bound primarily on presynaptic axon terminals, suggesting that the receptor is regulating neurotransmission via presynaptic localization. Ghrelin and the GHSs act on somatotrophs through a phospholipase C–inositol triphosphate–PKC signaling pathway distinct from the cAMP-protein kinase A (PKA) pathway activated by GHRH.[438] Data suggest, however, that cAMP levels are elevated when ghrelin and GH secretagogues are co-administered with GHRH, but the exact mechanism of this synergism is not known. The GHS-R, similar to other G protein–coupled receptors, shows desensitization in its calcium and GH effects, although long-term human studies with ghrelin mimetics showed sustained elevation of IGF-1 levels for 1 to 2 years.[466,467]

The GHS-R was found to be highly constitutively active in a ligand-independent manner in transfected COS-7 and HEK293 cells. Although ghrelin and GHSs further increased inositol phosphate turnover, a low-potency antagonist (substance P antagonist) was found to be a high-affinity inverse agonist.[468] These data open the possibility for development of inverse agonist compounds to oppose the effects of activation of the receptor.

Regulation of the GHS Receptor

Studies using the dw/dw rat model or normal rats to investigate the effects of GH on hypothalamic and pituitary GHS-R expression suggested that GHS-Rs are involved in feedback regulation of GH. Whether these effects occur directly at the pituitary level or are mediated indirectly through the hypothalamus has yet to be determined. In addition, expression of the pituitary GHS-R mRNA seems to be sex dependent, whereas the hypothalamic expression of this receptor showed no significant sex difference. GHRH appears to positively regulate the pituitary GHS-R in rats. GHS-R has been found to be upregulated by GHRH, GH deficiency, estrogen, glucocorticoids, and thyroid hormones.[462]

Evidence for Alternative Ligands and Receptor Subtypes

Evidence for alternative ligands for the GHS receptor is controversial. Adenosine has been proposed to act as a partial agonist at the GHS-R,[469,470] although others refute this.[471,472] Cortistatin, a 14 amino acid peptide neuropeptide with similarity to somatostatin, has been reported to bind to GHR-Rs in the pituitary.[473] Recently, it was proposed that GHRH binds directly to the GHS-R expressed in vitro, activating calcium mobilization and enhancing ghrelin binding. The authors suggest positive cooperativity between two distinct binding sites on the GHS-R—one for ghrelin and one for GHRH.[474]

Animals with the known GHS-R knocked out showed neither an appetite change nor GH release in response to acyl-ghrelin.[475] However, these GHS-R knockout animals continue to respond to des-acyl ghrelin, and it is possible that other actions of acyl-ghrelin may be transduced at additional sites. Alternative binding sites for ghrelin, des-acyl ghrelin, and some GHSs have been identified in the pituitary, thyroid, heart, and other tissues, and ghrelin has been found to be associated with a high-density lipoprotein in plasma.[462] Hexarelin-like GHSs but not ghrelin can act at a macrophage scavenger receptor CD36.[476]

EFFECTS OF GHRELIN AND GHSs

In recent years, the metabolic effects of ghrelin came to the forefront of research as opposed to the originally described classical pituitary hormone effects on GH, ACTH, and prolactin release. Ghrelin has been described to have effects on feeding, glucose and lipid metabolism, gastric acid secretion, gastric motility, and cell proliferation, as well as on sleep, anxiety, and memory (Table 16-2). Data from ghrelin and GHS-R knockout mice suggest that alternative pathways can compensate for a number of the known effects of ghrelin (see later), but subtle abnormalities are detected under various experimental conditions (Table 16-3).

GH-Related Effects

The GH-releasing effect of ghrelin acts via a dual mechanism involving the hypothalamus and the pituitary. In in vitro studies with rat pituitary cultures, ghrelin has been shown to specifically activate the GHS-R and to stimulate GH release[438] via the phospsholipase C–diacylglycerol–IP3–Ca^{2+}–protein kinase 3 pathway. At the level of individual pituitary cells examined with

Table 16-2. A Summary of the Effects of Ghrelin

Hormonal effects	↑ Release of growth hormone in humans and animals[462]
	↑ Release of adrenocorticotrophin (ACTH) and cortisol in humans and animals[462]
	↑ Prolactin release in rats and adult humans but ↓ in prepubertal children[477]
	↓ Secretion of testosterone and luteinising hormone (LH)[477,478]
	↑ Release of antidiuretic hormone[479]
	↑ Secretion of aldosterone in humans[258]
Metabolic effects	↑ Appetite in animals and humans[441,462]
	↑ Insulin resistance independent of GH[480]
	Regulation of metabolic substrates[462]
	↑ Gastric emptying and gastrointestinal (GI) tract motility[462]
	↓ Colonic transit time[481]
	Stimulates glucose output by hepatocytes[482]
	Antilipolytic effects on adipose tissue[483]
Cardiovascular effects	↑ Left ventricular ejection fraction and ↑ cardiac output in humans[462]
	↑ Stroke volume[462]
	↑ Systemic vasodilatation and ↓ systemic vascular resistance[462]
	↓ Blood pressure[462]
	↑ Coronary perfusion pressure via vasoconstriction of coronary arterioles[484]
	Reversal of right ventricular hypertrophy and vascular remodeling in pulmonary hypertension[485]
	Reversal of endothelial dysfunction (the first step in the process of atherosclerosis)[486]
	Improved survival after myocardial infarction[487]
Autonomic nervous system effects	↓ Sympathetic activity[462]
	↓ Thermogenesis[462]
	Possible antiemetic effects[486,488]
	↓ Release of serotonin[489]
Immunologic effects	↓ Expression of various proinflammatory cytokines, including interleukin (IL)1-β, IL-6, and tumor necrosis factor-α (TNF-α)[490]
	↓ Proliferation of anti-CD3 activated T cells and inhibition of both Th1 and Th2 cytokines in rats and mice[490]
	Attenuates the known proinflammatory effects of leptin in human neutrophils and T cells[490]
	↑ Phagocytosis and ↑ superoxide production in trout[491]
	May have a renal-protective effect on kidneys damaged by acute renal failure[492]
	Exerts protective effects on the gastric mucosa when exposed to stress,[493] mediated at least in part by anti-inflammatory effects[494]
	Anti-inflammatory effect in arthritis[495]
	Improves tissue perfusion in severe sepsis[496]
Musculoskeletal system effects	Promotes bone formation[497] and ↑ bone mineral density[498]
	↓ Metabolic activity in chondrocytes[499]
	↑ Spontaneous locomotor activity in goldfish[500] and may affect locomotor activity in rats[501,502]
Other effects	Promotes sleep[462]
	↑ Anxiety[462]
	Protects against depressive symptoms of chronic stress[503]
	Improves memory and learning[504]
	May play a role in embryonic implantation and fetal growth[462]
	May have effects on cell proliferation[462]

Table 16-3. Transgenic and Knockout Models for Ghrelin and GHS-R

Embryonic/Adult	Finding	Reference
Ghrelin		
Embryonic ghrelin KO	No detected difference as compared with wild type (WT)	Sun et al. 2003[510]
Embryonic ghrelin KO	KO animals on a high-fat diet showed preferential use of fat as a metabolic substrate	Wortley et al. 2004[566]
Embryonic ghrelin KO	Males on high-fat diet show less weight gain and higher locomotor activity	Wortley et al. 2005[567]
Embryonic ghrelin KO	Young animals show lower respiratory quotient and higher heat production	De Smet et al. 2006[568]
Adult (given spiegelmer to neutralize effects of ghrelin)	Weight loss occurred in diet-induced obese mice	Shearman et al. 2006[560]
Adult (given ghrelin antibody)	Weight loss and reduced food intake in pigs	Vizcarra et al. 2006[561]
Overexpression of des-acyl-ghrelin in mice	Lower body weight, body length, and GH and insulin-like growth factor (IGF)-1 levels	Ariyasu et al. 2005[569]
Transgenic overexpression of ghrelin	Normal-size animal. No desensitization of the food intake effect of exogenous ghrelin shown, but lower epididymal fat pad growth response and GH response	Wei et al. 2006[570]
Embryonic ghrelin/leptin double KO	Obesity and hyperphagia shown, but with improved insulin sensitivity	Sun et al. 2006[527]
Embryonic ghrelin KO, fully backcrossed for 10 generations	Not resistant to high-fat diet, reduced blood sugar during starvation	Sun et al. 2008[565]
GHS-R		
Embryonic GHS-R KO	Lower IGF-1 and body weight	Sun et al. 2004[475]
Embryonic GHS-R KO	Reduced food intake and weight gain on high-fat diet, increased fat burning	Zigman et al. 2005[563]
Adult (given GHS-R antagonist [D-Lys-3]-GHRP-6)	Reduced food intake in lean, diet-induced obesity and ob/ob mice, and reduced weight gain in ob/ob mice	Asakawa et al. 2003[564]
Embryonic (given antisense GHS-R mRNA, which selectively attenuates GHS-R protein expression in the arcuate nucleus)	Lower body weight and less adipose tissue, reduced food intake, and abolition of the stimulatory effect of GHS on feeding	Shuto et al. 2002[562]
Embryonic GHS-R KO, fully backcrossed for 10 generations	Not resistant to high-fat diet, reduced blood sugar during starvation	Sun et al. 2008[565]

the reverse hemolytic plaque assay, GHSs increase the number of GH-secreting cells without altering the amount of GH released per cell. In contrast, GHRH increases both the amount of GH secreted per cell and the number of GH-secreting cells, while somatostatin predominantly acts to decrease the number of secreting cells; this is the opposite of the effect of GHSs and supports the view that GHSs act as functional antagonists of somatostatin.[462] The effect of GHSs in vivo is much stronger than the in vitro effect; IV administration of ghrelin to freely moving rats caused a dose-dependent increase in GH release, but the effect depends on the presence of GHRH. Although hypothalamic activation can be seen in the *lit/lit* mouse, which has an inactivating mutation of GHRH-R, no GH release is observed. It is interesting to note that in humans with GHRH-R mutations, a very small but significant GH response can be observed with sensitive GH assays, while the ACTH and prolactin-releasing effects of GHSs are intact.[505] The efficacy of GHSs or ghrelin is greatly attenuated following administration of anti-GHRH serum in rats or a GHRH antagonist in humans. Pituitary stalk lesions cause attenuation of GHS or ghrelin effects, but less so if the lesion occurred recently and the pituitary somatotrophs are not atrophic because of long-term GHRH deficiency. Coadministration of GHS with GHRH causes a synergistic GH release, and this effect can be used for diagnostic purposes to diagnose adult GH deficiency. Continuous ghrelin administration leads to attenuation of the effect; intermittent administration causes long-lasting effects. GHSs do not stimulate GH synthesis in adult somatotroph cells, although a positive effect on GH synthesis was shown in infant rat pituitary. Both peripherally and centrally administered GHSs and ghrelin stimulate the hypothalamic arcuate nucleus GHS-R and directly act at the pituitary GHS-R to release GH. However, blockade of the afferent fibers of the vagus nerve abolished peripheral ghrelin-induced GH release. Therefore, the exact mechanism of GH release elucidated by peripheral ghrelin remains to be clarified.

In humans, the GH rise after an equivalent dose (1 μg/kg) of IV bolus GHRH, hexarelin, and ghrelin shows significantly different responses, with ghrelin being the most effective (peak mean GH ± SEM: 26.7 ± 8.7 μg/L, 68.4 ± 14.7 μg/L, and 92.1 ± 16.7 μg/L, respectively). Studies in rodents found no change in the magnitude of the ghrelin-induced GH release with age.[506] No age or gender dependence in the ACTH, cortisol, and prolactin effects and in the glucose (increase) and insulin (decrease) effects of ghrelin have been described.[507] Reduced GH release is observed more often in obese subjects than in normal subjects in response to ghrelin or to GHSs. Food intake decreases the effects of ghrelin on GH release in both animal and human studies.

Ghrelin, a natural ligand for GHS-R, potently stimulates GH release when administered exogenously. An increasing set of data, albeit not all data, suggests that ghrelin not only potently stimulates GH release when administered exogenously, it also plays a role in physiologic GH regulation. Both SC and intracerebroventricular infusions of the rat GHS-R antagonist BIM-28163[508] did not alter the pulsatile pattern of GH secretion but lowered the GH pulse amplitude. In humans, a GHS-R missense mutation, which impairs the constitutive activity of the GHS-R, is associated with short stature.[509] Consistent with these results, GHS-R–null mice have lower IGF-1 levels when compared with wild-type animals,[475] and ghrelin-null mice also show a tendency to lower IGF-1 concentrations when compared with control animals[510]; however, this did not reach statistical significance. This body of data implies that endogenous ghrelin plays a role in GH regulation. In a patient with ghrelin-secreting pancreatic tumor and 50 times higher ghrelin levels, GH and IGF levels were in the normal range, although desensitization and downregulation of the GHS-R are possible in this situation, and it was not tested whether the ghrelin secreted by the tumor was in the active acylated form. Several clinical studies have found a relationship between ghrelin and GH levels[511-513]; others have not.[514-516] All of these studies measured total ghrelin and did not distinguish between acyl-ghrelin, des-acyl ghrelin, and inactive fragments. Studies measuring acyl-ghrelin levels every 20 minutes with a single-site assay found no relationship with GH under fed or fasting conditions.[517] In a study using a two-site ghrelin assay and more frequent sampling (every 10 minutes for 24 hours), a close association between full-length acyl-ghrelin levels and amplitudes of individual GH secretory events was demonstrated, suggesting that acyl-ghrelin modulates GH release.[518]

Other Hormone-Related Effects

Ghrelin stimulates the HPA axis, resulting in increased ACTH and cortisol levels, via hypothalamic corticotropin-releasing hormone (CRH) and vasopressin stimulation, while having no direct pituitary or adrenal effects. Stimulation of the HPA axis is attenuated during prolonged treatment with long-acting GHSs. Ghrelin and GHSs release prolactin by activating the somato-mammotroph cells in the pituitary.

Feeding Effect

Ghrelin stimulates feeding in both animal and human studies.[440] Similar effects were shown earlier for GHSs.[519] Ghrelin acts via stimulating NPY/AGRP cells and orexin cells and indirectly inhibiting pro-opiomelanocortin (POMC) cells in the hypothalamus.[462] The vagus also seems to play an important role in the feeding effects, as vagotomy inhibits the feeding effects of peripheral ghrelin. Therefore, the feeding effect of ghrelin could occur via three possible mechanisms (Fig. 16-11): (1) via peripheral ghrelin reaching the arcuate nucleus and stimulating orexigenic cells; (2) via GHS-R in the peripheral vagal afferents and the nucleus tractus solitarius; or (3) via locally produced ghrelin-stimulating arcuate and lateral hypothalamus orexigenic cells, and or inhibiting anorectic cells, although it has to be emphasized that some studies were not able to detect ghrelin and/or ghrelin cells in the hypothalamus.[520-522] The mechanism of ghrelin effects on appetite involves the metabolic enzyme adenosine monophosphate-induced protein kinase (AMPK).[523] A recently suggested pathway for the orexigenic effect of ghrelin includes the activation of Ca^{2+} signaling in NPY neurones in the arcuate nucleus (ARC). The Ca^{2+} rise leads to CAMKK2 acti-

vation, which can stimulate hypothalamic AMPK. AMPK activation leads to increased mitochondrial oxidation and activation of the uncoupling protein 2 (UCP2), which can regulate NPY/AgRP neuronal activity, and ultimately to stimulation of appetite (see Fig. 16-12 and review[524]).

Other Effects of Ghrelin

Most animal and human studies have observed that ghrelin inhibits insulin levels, leading to increased glucose levels.[525] Ghrelin has been shown to inhibit AMPK activity in liver, which could lead to disinhibition of phosphoenolpyruvate carboxykinase (PEPCK) and activation of gluconeogenesis.[526] The most

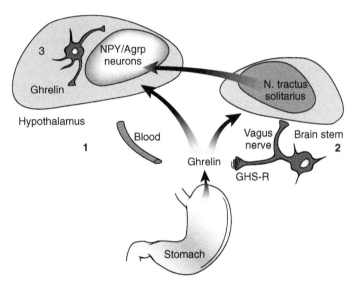

FIGURE 16-11. Ghrelin exerts its effects in the hypothalamus via three different pathways[462]: (1) Ghrelin synthesized in the stomach reaches the arcuate nucleus via the bloodstream and possibly other brain areas via active transport through the blood-brain barrier[438,455]; (2) ghrelin synthesized in the periphery is stimulating vagal afferents, which has been shown to express GHS-R, and vagal connections reach the nucleus tractus solitarius in the brain stem, which then communicates with the hypothalamus[645]; (3) controversy has arisen over whether ghrelin cells are present in the hypothalamus,[521,522,566] but some data suggest that ghrelin is synthesized locally in the hypothalamus and has direct connections with NPY/AGRP and other hypothalamic cells.[454]

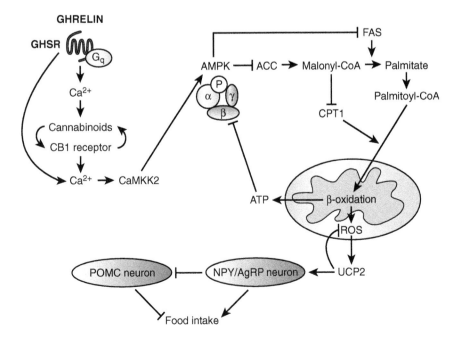

FIGURE 16-12. Schematic diagram showing the proposed molecules involved in the appetite-inducing effect of ghrelin. (*GHS-R,* Growth hormone secretagogue receptor; *CaMKK,* calmodulin kinase kinase; *CB1,* cannabinoid receptor type 1; *AMPK,* AMP-activated protein kinase; *ACC,* acetyl-coenzyme A carboxylase; *malonyl-CoA,* malonyl coenzyme A; *FAS,* fatty acid synthase; *CPT1,* carnitil palmitoyl transferase 1; *ROS,* reactive oxygen species; *UCP2,* uncoupled protein 2; *NPY,* neuropeptide Y; *AgRP,* agouti-related peptide; *POMC,* pro-opiomelanocortin.) (Redrawn based on results from several studies reviewed in Kola and Korbonits 2009.[524])

powerful proof of the important effect of ghrelin on carbohydrate mechanism comes from the double mutant ghrelin/leptin knockout mice, as these mice are obese similar to leptin knockouts, but ablation of ghrelin improves the diabetic phenotype.[527]

That ghrelin analogues increase body fat in rodents, despite their GH-releasing effect, has been elegantly demonstrated by Lall et al.[528] Ghrelin specifically stimulates fat accumulation and has been shown to have a direct stimulatory effect on adipocyte proliferation and on peroxisome-proliferator–activated receptor-γ (PPAR-γ) synthesis. Ghrelin inhibits AMPK activity in fat tissue, which could explain its adipogenic effect.[526]

GHSs and ghrelin have GH-independent effects on the cardiovascular system. Ghrelin is effective in improving cardiac performance in chronic heart failure.[529,530] Ghrelin prevents increased sympathetic tone and reduces mortality after myocardial infarction.[487] Ghrelin stimulates AMPK in cardiac tissue, which could be important in terms of its positive inotropic and anti-ischemic effects.[526] Ghrelin has vasodilator effects, and the density of ghrelin binding is increased in atherosclerosis.[531] Ghrelin inhibits apoptosis via an MAPK- and Akt-dependent pathway in cardiomyocytes. Desoctanoyl ghrelin has also been shown to produce similar effects, and it has been shown to bind to H9c2 cells that do not express GHS-R1a mRNA.[532] It seems that at least some of the cardiovascular effects of ghrelin and hexarelin on cardiac function are different; this is apparently due to the specific actions of hexarelin at the CD36 receptor.[476]

Given the fact that the reproductive axis is highly dependent on nutritional status, ghrelin, acting at central and peripheral levels, could be one of the signaling mechanisms linking nutritional status to the hypothalamo-pituitary-gonadal axis.[533] Both animal and human studies have shown that ghrelin can inhibit luteinizing hormone (LH) pulsatility, possibly via the central nervous system (CNS).[478]

In some cell types (thyroid, breast), ghrelin has been reported to inhibit cell proliferation; in others (prostate, hepatoma, adrenal, pancreatic, cardiac, adipose cells, and pituitary), it has stimulatory effects on cell proliferation.

Ghrelin has an inhibitory effect on cardiovascular sympathetic activity, a stimulatory effect on gastrointestinal parasympathetic activity (gastric acid secretion and gastric motility), and an inhibitory effect on vagal afferent discharge. Ghrelin stimulates gastric motility, similar to motilin, and gastric acid secretion.

Both GHSs and ghrelin have been shown to promote sleep in humans, although GHRP-2 showed an increase in stage 2 sleep, and MK-0677 and ghrelin increase slow wave sleep. It is interesting to note that in *lit/lit* mice with a nonfunctional GHRH receptor, ghrelin increased food intake but had no effect on sleep, suggesting that GHRH is involved in the sleep effect of ghrelin.[534]

GHS-R has been identified in the hippocampus, and ghrelin administration increases anxiety.[535,536] On the other hand, ghrelin defends against depressive symptoms of chronic stress.[503] These findings suggest that ghrelin may have a role in mediating neuroendocrine and behavioral responses to stressors, and that the stomach might play an important role in the regulation of anxiety.

GHRELIN LEVELS IN PATHOLOGIC CONDITIONS
Abnormal Body Weight

Ghrelin is negatively correlated with weight, and higher ghrelin levels were found in patients on a low-calorie diet[457,537] and in patients suffering from anorexia due to cancer,[538,539] cardiac disease,[540] or anorexia nervosa.[541] Patients with anorexia nervosa

have high ghrelin levels, and weight gain decreases ghrelin concentrations.[542,543] Neonates with intrauterine growth retardation have higher ghrelin levels than normal neonates, and the increased orexigenic drive could contribute to postnatal catch-up growth.[544]

Obese subjects have lower ghrelin levels than lean subjects.[545] Weight loss through dieting increases circulating ghrelin levels.[457,537] Data suggest that ghrelin depends on body weight, probably via regulation by insulin, and does not depend on fat mass or fat distribution.

The most effective treatment for morbid obesity is gastric surgery with Roux-en-Y gastric bypass or adjustable gastric banding. It has long been observed that Roux-en-Y gastric bypass has effects beyond restriction of the capacity of the stomach, and long-term reduction in appetite is achieved. It has been suggested that decreased ghrelin levels, probably due to the loss of stomach tissue involved in food processing, could be the cause of loss of appetite after gastric bypass surgery. However, other studies were not able to reproduce uniformly these data. A review of 18 prospective and cross-sectional studies summarized the results so far as being ambiguous and inconsistent, with insufficient evidence to support a firm conclusion of any sort about the relationship between ghrelin levels and bariatric surgery[546]; more recent studies have still resulted in mixed outcomes regarding ghrelin levels.

Diabetes Mellitus and Insulin Resistance

Patients with insulin resistance (type 2 diabetes, polycystic ovary syndrome) have lower ghrelin levels than BMI-matched controls.[440] The relationship between higher insulin concentration (and/or the pathologic process of insulin resistance) and lower ghrelin levels cannot be determined by these data. Low ghrelin levels appeared to be associated with high blood pressure independent of BMI in a population-based study as well as in pregnant women.

Prader-Willi Syndrome

Although all forms of human obesity, including simple obesity, congenital leptin deficiency, leptin receptor or melanocortin-4 receptor mutations, or hypothalamic obesity from craniopharyngioma, show low ghrelin levels, patients with Prader-Willi syndrome (PWS) have inappropriately high ghrelin levels, in the range of patients with anorexia nervosa.[547-550] PWS is the most common syndromal cause of genetic obesity, caused by loss of expression of imprinted genes on the paternally inherited chromosome 15q11-q13, and characterized by life-threatening childhood-onset hyperphagia and obesity, as well as GH deficiency and hypogonadism, thought to be due to hypothalamic abnormalities.[551] Hyperghrelinemia, which is three to four times higher than in BMI-matched controls, is reduced after food intake in parallel to normal subjects.[552] Somatostatin treatment of PWS patients inhibited ghrelin levels, but no change in the hyperphagia was noted.[553] It remains to be determined whether ghrelin is directly involved in the pathogenesis of the different symptoms in PWS.

Acromegaly and Growth Hormone Deficiency

Ghrelin levels increase after surgery in acromegalic subjects in inverse correlation with GH, IGF-1, and insulin levels, suggesting that one or a combination of these hormones results in suppressed ghrelin levels in active acromegaly.[554,555] GH-deficient patients have low or normal ghrelin levels compared with BMI-matched subjects, and again the increased percent body fat can play a role in determining ghrelin levels. GH replacement causes a reduction in ghrelin levels.[556]

Hyperthyroidism

Ghrelin levels are reduced in hyperthyroidism, suggesting that ghrelin is not involved in the hyperphagia of hyperthyroidism.[557] Because known factors suppressing ghrelin levels—high BMI, high insulin, or somatostatin—cannot play a role here, and because the decreased body weight of hyperthyroidism should rather stimulate ghrelin levels, it is assumed that thyroid hormones have a direct inhibitory effect on ghrelin.

Renal Disease

Ghrelin levels are elevated in chronic renal failure and show a reduction after a single course of hemodialysis.[558] Unpublished data (T. Kuppusamy, R. Gupta, J. Patrie, M.O. Thorner, J. Liu, B. Gaylinn, and W.K. Bolton) suggest that the reduction on dialysis is predominantly des-acyl and not acyl-ghrelin, consistent with evidence that acyl- but not des-acyl ghrelin circulates in a bound form.[559]

MODELS OF GHRELIN OR GHRELIN RECEPTOR DEFICIENCY

Research into the functional importance of ghrelin has included animal models that had a genetic or an acquired deficiency of ghrelin or ghrelin receptor (see Table 16-3). The data about ghrelin deficiency are somewhat controversial, depending on the timing of onset of ghrelin deficiency and on appropriate backcrossing of the genetically modified animals. Embryonic knockout animals show very little if any difference in energy metabolism, possibly only in insulin sensitivity, and no difference in pituitary function (see Table 16-3). It is interesting to note that the leptin-ghrelin double knockout model shows obesity and hyperphagia but improved insulin release (via reduction of levels of UCP2) and insulin sensitivity, suggesting an important role for ghrelin in β cell physiology.[527] An acquired ghrelin deficiency resulted in diet-induced obese mice eating less and storing less fat, and ultimately having a lower body weight and body fat mass as compared with control or vehicle groups,[560] while pigs showed reduced food intake and weight loss after ghrelin immunoneutralization.[561] The prominent phenotype in acquired ghrelin deficiency as opposed to the mild phenotype of the embryonic knockouts suggests that prenatal ablation of the ghrelin gene produced more subtle phenotypic effects as a consequence of the plasticity within the system, as other metabolic pathways had been able to develop in a way that enabled them to compensate for loss of ghrelin. However, this compensation was not possible when the effects of ghrelin were neutralized in adult life.[560] This suggests that ghrelin is an important player in the field of energy homeostasis and appetite regulation, as part of a bigger network of regulatory molecules, which can only compensate for its loss if this occurs early in development.

A selective hypothalamic knockout model using antisense GHS-R mRNA expression under the tyrosine hydroxylase control showed lower GH and IGF-1 levels in female animals.[562]

GHS-R knockout mice have lower body weight[475,563] and lower IGF-1 values.[475] In keeping with this, a study into the effects of antagonizing the GHS-R receptor (in adult mice) found that this decreased feeding in both lean and obese mice lowered body weight gain and reduced the rate of gastric emptying.[564] It is interesting to note that a recent study backcrossing knockout animals to 10 generations found that knockout animals are not resistant to high-fat diet–induced obesity,

and the only abnormality described is reduced blood sugar during starvation.[565]

CLINICAL IMPLICATIONS OF GHRELIN AND GHS

Growth Hormone Secretagogues

Since early studies reported the GH-releasing capabilities of GHSs in humans, interest in their potential as diagnostic agents has increased. Peptide and non-peptide GHSs are powerful stimulators of GH release, effective when administered IV, sc, intranasally,[571] or PO.[572] These agents typically cause GH release in excess of that observed following GHRH or during ITT.

GHS ACTIONS IN HEALTHY SUBJECTS

GHSs cause the release of GH in a dose-dependent fashion.[573] They are more potent than GHRH: 1 μg/kg of GHRP-6 peptide results in significantly greater GH release than the same dose of GHRH. The effect of GHSs on GH release is more reproducible than the effect of GHRH. The peptide GHSs (e.g., GHRP-6, GHRP-1, GHRP-2, hexarelin) and the non-peptide GHSs (e.g., MK-0677) differ in terms of their pharmacokinetics. MK-0677 has been developed specifically as an orally active agent. The peptidyl GHSs are active po, but only at doses several hundred times higher than that required when IV is administered.

An intact hypothalamic-pituitary axis is vital in facilitating the maximal effect of GHSs on GH release. GHRH and somatostatin both influence the action of GHSs, augmenting and diminishing the magnitude of the GH pulse, respectively. When GHRH is administered in combination with GHSs, the effect is synergistic, the magnitude of the GH pulse being greater than that obtained from the sum of the two agents administered separately.[574-577] The presence of GHRH is required for GHSs to exert their effects on GH secretion. In a family from the remote Valley of Sind in Pakistan, a missense mutation in the GHRH receptor that changes the glycine at residue 72 in the extracellular domain to a stop codon results in a phenotype analogous to the little mouse.[505] When members of the family that were homozygous for the mutation were challenged with hexarelin, no GH response was detectable. In addition, studies performed in children who are GH deficient as the result of pituitary stalk transsection show that they are unresponsive to GHSs.[578] Thus, somatotroph exposure to GHRH is necessary for GHSs to exert their full action.

Manipulation of somatostatin tone also affects the GH response to GHSs. When hexarelin was given to subjects in combination with somatostatin, the amount of GH released was significantly reduced.[579] When arginine was administered to the elderly, a group proposed to have increased somatostatin tone, GH levels following the administration of GHRP-6 increased significantly, to levels seen in younger subjects.[580]

GHSs demonstrate GH-releasing activity during the neonatal period at a level that persists during prepubertal life.[581] During puberty, increased GH response to GHSs persists into adult life.[582-584] Subsequently, over the course of the adult life span, the GH response to GHSs declines, in line with the reduction in spontaneous GH secretion.[575,580,585]

The response to GHSs does not vary with sex, apart from during puberty, when girls exhibit a greater response to GHSs than do boys.[583] The response in adult women is similar to that observed in men. Women who received GHSs at various times during the menstrual cycle achieved similar peaks, whether studied during the early follicular, late follicular, or luteal phase.[586] Several studies suggest that estrogen and estrogen-progestin supplementation has an impact on the GH response to ghrelin.[587,588]

GHSs AND THE DIAGNOSIS OF GH DEFICIENCY

The combination of GHRH and GHS is the most potent stimulus of GH release known and provides a promising alternative to ITT in the diagnosis of GH deficiency. In normal subjects, the lower limit of the normal range (third percentile) of responses to GHRH and hexarelin was 55.5 µg/L, which was considerably higher than the lower limit of normal following GHRH and arginine (third percentile = 17.5 µg/L). The response to GHS plus GHRH is reproducible within an individual; GH levels attained are similar among individuals and do not appear to decline with age.[577] Similar to GHRH+Arg, the combined GHRH+GHRP-6 is partially refractory to the inhibitory effects of glucose and free fatty acid load, as well as of rGH.[589] Perhaps the most important feature of the GHS-GHRH test is its ability to discriminate GH-deficient patients from normal subjects. In two studies, the combination of GHS and GHRH had a specificity and a sensitivity of 100%.[590,591] The combination of GHS and GHRH is safe and well tolerated; side effects are similar to those seen when the two agents are administered separately. Chihara et al.[592] compared the effects of a single iv GHRP-2 injection versus a classical ITT in patients with severe GHD. Severe GHD could be diagnosed with high reliability in all subjects using a threshold of 15 µg/L. Since the discovery of the natural ligand of the GHS receptor ghrelin in 1999, several studies have been performed to evaluate the acute effects of ghrelin on GH release, while the use of ghrelin or a ghrelin mimetic alone has not been suggested for diagnostic use in GH deficiency, these used in combination with GHRH form a very effective test. Aimaretti et al[593] showed that ghrelin given IV in a dose of 1 µg/kg to adults with isolated GH deficiency increased GH levels significantly higher when compared with the ITT and the combined test of GHRH and arginine. These data suggest that ghrelin itself should be a good agent to be used in a provocative test in the future; however, normative data are still missing.

THE GHRH AND GHS TEST IN DIFFICULT DIAGNOSTIC SITUATIONS

The power of the combined stimulus of GHRH and GHS has resulted in its application to difficult diagnostic situations in which GH release, both spontaneous and stimulated, is reduced by a coexisting process. The problem of aging has already been discussed, but other situations, particularly obesity and syndromes of glucocorticoid excess, may confound the diagnosis of GH deficiency.

Obesity

Spontaneous and stimulated GH secretion is reduced in obese subjects.[389] The exact cause of the hyposomatotropism is uncertain, but a variety of mechanisms have been suggested. Among the hypotheses put forward are increased somatostatin tone, a reduction in the secretion of GHRH or of the natural ligand for the GHS receptor, and any combination of these.[594] What is known for certain is that the GH response to a number of stimuli, including GHRH,[388] GHRH and arginine,[595] GHRP-6,[596] and hexarelin,[597] is inversely correlated with body fat mass, specifically, abdominal fat mass. The diminished GH response can make it difficult to accurately define the GH status of obese patients with hypothalamic-pituitary disease, particularly those in whom GH deficiency may be the only hormone abnormality.

The combination of GHRH with either arginine[598] or GHS[596] administered to an obese subject causes a GH response far greater than any other stimulus, although the GH level does not quite reach that seen in normal controls. These tests are useful tools in the differentiation of true GH deficiency from hyposomatotropism caused by obesity. The validated cutoff level for growth hormone deficiency (GHD) in adults for the ITT and the glucagon test is a peak GH response <3 µg/L, which has not been validated in obesity. For the GHRH+Arg test, the following cutoff levels have been validated, depending on the BMI: <25 kg/m², a peak GH <11 µg/L; 25 to 30 kg/m², a peak GH <8 µg/L; >30 kg/m², a peak GH <4 µg/L.[403] The cutoff level validated for the GHRH+GHRP-6 is 10 µg/L in lean patients and 5.0 µg/L in obese patients.[404,405]

Syndromes of Glucocorticoid Excess

In rats, glucocorticoids potentiate GHRH action and enhance spontaneous GH secretion. In normal humans, a biphasic effect results from pharmacologic doses of glucocorticoids. When normal men were treated with a single IV bolus of dexamethasone 4 mg, and 3 hours later were challenged with a bolus injection of GHRH, the peak GH response to GHRH increased from 9.9 ± 2.0 µg/L to 29.2 ± 5.7 µg/L. When the dexamethasone dose was increased to 8 mg IV 12 hours before a GHRH bolus, the peak GH response to GHRH was attenuated to 3 ± 1.1 µg/L. These results suggest an acute stimulatory response followed by a later inhibitory effect.[599] Pretreatment with pyridostigmine before administration of GHRH partially reversed the effects of 48 hours of dexamethasone therapy, suggesting that somatostatin tone may be increased by glucocorticoids.[600]

Patients with glucocorticoid excess caused by Cushing's syndrome or by exogenous steroids have markedly impaired GH secretion.[601] This may result from the combined effects of chronic exposure to glucocorticoids and the changes in body composition associated with Cushing's syndrome, particularly the central adiposity. The suppression of GH in these patients may persist for up to 1 year after resolution of the glucocorticoid excess,[602] which may give rise to misinterpretation of a patient's GH status. GHRH and GHRP-6 have been administered to patients with Cushing's syndrome separately and in combination. The effect of GHRH in these patients was almost abolished and the response to GHRP-6 was considerably reduced compared with controls. The combination of GHRH and GHRP-6 was considerably more potent than either GHRH or GHRP-6 used alone, but the GH peaks were only 20% of those seen in normal subjects.[603] Similarly, the GH-releasing effects of ghrelin are significantly reduced in patients with Cushing's disease.[604,605] An earlier study had shown that the response to GHRH and pyridostigmine increased threefold following 7 days' priming with GHRH.[606] These data suggest that the effects of chronic glucocorticoid excess are caused primarily by reduced GHRH secretion. Whether the combination of GHRH and GHS will be able to predict which patients with Cushing's disease will recover normal GH secretion is a matter for further study.

Nascif et al.[607] demonstrate that the effects of GHSs, GHRP-6, GHRH, and ghrelin in hyperthyroid patients were significantly greater with ghrelin than with GHRP-6. A significant decrease in GH responsiveness to ghrelin, GHRP-6, and GHRH was also noted in the hyperthyroid group compared with controls.

THERAPEUTIC POTENTIAL OF GHSs

Since the discovery of GHRPs in 1976, 5 years before the discovery of GHRH,[608] several different types of GHSs have been developed, including a series of nonpeptidyl GHSs.[609-613] The concept that these agents amplify the pulsatile GH secretory pathway, instead of overriding normal physiology, has made this group of drugs the target of intensive research. The initial enthusiasm that accompanied the concept of orally available peptidergic and non-peptidergic GHSs, however, has been mitigated by the controversial results of several studies suggesting that no benefits are evident in terms of changes in body composition, as well as a report of tolerance.[614] Others could not find development of tolerance and described beneficial effects on body composition.[615]

Therefore, the area of GHSs as therapeutic agents remains controversial. Some areas are discussed later for which GHSs might be a useful agent, especially under the assumption that new compounds with higher efficacy and better oral availability will be developed. It is essential for the reader to recognize that each GHS is unique in terms of its bioavailability profile, its metabolism, and its specificity of action. Thus no two GHSs may be compared, except on a superficial level. It is not sound to extrapolate from one GHS to another.

Therapeutic Potential of GHSs in Children

The use of GHSs in children with growth retardation has been thought to have therapeutic potential. Several studies have proved the GH-releasing effects of these compounds, peptidergic as well as non-peptidergic, in short-term infusion studies in children. As a GH stimulus, they are as potent as, or even more potent than, GHRH. Loche and coworkers[616] demonstrated that IV bolus infusions of hexarelin, 2 µg/kg body weight, can enhance GH release in short-statured children (familial short stature and constitutional delay of growth).

In a trial performed by Mericq et al.,[617] GHRP-2 was administered subcutaneously to six prepubertal children of short stature with GH deficiency, defined as a GH response of less than 7 µg/L to at least two standard provocative tests and a growth velocity of 4 cm/year or less. Agents were administered for 6 months at increasing doses (0.3, to 1.0, to 3.0 µg/kg/day). At months 7 and 8, the children received GHRP-2, 3 µg/kg/day, together with GHRH, 3 µg/kg/day. The maximal overnight GH and GH peak amplitude showed a progressive increase at the higher doses. Growth velocities were increased when compared with baseline (5.3 ± 0.8 vs. 3.0 ± 0.5 cm/year; $P < .05$). During the long treatment period, GHRP-2 injections were well tolerated. However, the study was not placebo controlled.

To date, only two studies have reported the effects of non-peptidergic GHSs in children.[618,619] In a short-term pilot study of 8 days, MK-0677 increased GH, IGF-1, and IGFBP-3 in some children with GH deficiency. In the following long-term double-blind placebo-controlled study by Yu et al.,[618] with the GHS MK-0677 and 94 previously untreated, prepubertal GH-deficient children (height <5th percentile, growth velocity <25th percentile, peak GH <10 ng/mL on two tests), the GHS was well tolerated. The children were treated for 6 months with 0.4 mg/kg/day or 0.8 mg/kg/day. Mean growth velocity increased by more than 3 cm/year at 6 months.[618]

Similar results have been reported[620] in a group of prepubertal non–GH-deficient children. In this study, eight prepubertal children with constitutional short stature were treated with hexarelin administered three times daily intranasally. After treatment for up to 8 months, the growth velocity increased significantly (mean ± SD) from 5.3 ± 0.8 to 8.3 ± 1.7 cm/year in this group. Whether these changes would translate to increased adult height in these children after a longer therapy period is unclear to date.

Altogether, in preliminary studies, the growth response to GHS in GH-deficient children has been lower than that seen with GH treatment. Whether this is explained by the type of GH-deficient children selected for the trials or by a suboptimal dosing

regimen has yet to be determined. The development of new compounds with improved pharmacodynamic properties might bring improved results.

The use of GHSs in children with non–GH-deficient short stature has to be evaluated very carefully in the future.

Therapeutic Potential of GHSs in Adults

GH therapy has been approved in adults in the United States with organic GH deficiency[346] caused by hypothalamic-pituitary disease and by the AIDS-related wasting syndrome.[621] Because adults with GH deficiency very often do not have an intact hypothalamic-pituitary axis, only some of these patients probably would benefit from the use of GHSs.[622,623] A synthetic GHRH(1-44) analogue that has an increased half-life compared with the native GHRH has been shown to have sustained positive effects on visceral adipose tissue and lipid profiles in patients with HIV.[624,625] Currently, no data have been derived by investigating the potential positive effects of ghrelin or ghrelin mimetics treatment in the AIDS-related wasting syndrome, even though this agent might be a suitable candidate for this type of disease based on the GH-releasing and anorexic effects of ghrelin and ghrelin mimetics.

Another potential field of research is the catabolic state of severe illness. It seems that in the prolonged catabolic state of critical severe illness, a relative hyposomatotropism occurs, which seems to be of hypothalamic origin in part.[626] Infusion studies with GHRP-2 showed that given alone or together with GHRH, the somatotrophs can respond in this condition. In addition, a significant responsiveness to GH seems to occur under GHRP infusion to these patients.[626-628] A 5 day infusion of GHRP-2 and thyrotropin-releasing hormone (TRH) in protracted critical illness not only reactivated the blunted GH and TSH secretion but also showed metabolic effectiveness in this condition.[629] A double-blind placebo-controlled study[630] in a small number of healthy volunteers showed that diet-induced nitrogen wasting can be reduced after 7 days of treatment with an oral GH secretagogue (MK-0677). Studies by Neary et al.[631] suggest that ghrelin is able to increase energy intake in cancer patients. Similar data in animal cancer models support the anticachectic effect of ghrelin.[632] A 3 week preliminary study conducted in patients with pulmonary cachexia showed promising effects on lean body mass and respiratory muscle strength with daily ghrelin IV infusions.[633] However, the study was not blinded and was not placebo controlled. This study also showed that ghrelin administration decreased circulating plasma norepinephrine levels (i.e., sympathetic nerve activity[633]). The same group of researchers found beneficial cardiac and muscle effects in patients with congestive heart failure (CHF) after daily IV ghrelin administration for 3 weeks.[634] These findings support the concept of GHS use in the catabolic state. Further evaluation of the merits of the use of GHSs in adult patients on maintenance hemodialysis is warranted.[635]

The use of GHSs for treatment of critically ill patients has to be evaluated carefully. A previous study[636] showed that treatment with high doses of GH (0.07 to 0.13 mg/kg/day) leads to an increase in morbidity and mortality in these patients.

Another potential field of application for GHSs is seen in the normal older population, as there is an age-dependent decrease in GH secretion.[363] Some of the changes in body composition seen in the elderly resemble those seen in GH-deficient adults.[363] Studies investigating the effects of GH treatment in the elderly have shown that GH treatment in the elderly might have beneficial effects on lean body mass, adipose tissue, and bone mineral density.[637] In addition, the releasable GH pool of the pituitary is preserved in the elderly.

The few existing studies investigating the effects of GHSs in the elderly have shown conflicting results. One study, using the peptidergic GHS hexarelin, could not show a beneficial effect on body composition after 16 weeks of SC treatment. The same investigators reported a partial and reversible attenuation of the GH response to hexarelin, measured 4 weeks after cessation of hexarelin therapy. IGF-1 did not change significantly.[614]

Studies performed with an oral non-peptidergic GHS (MK-0677) resulted in a significant increase in IGF-1 concentration compared with that of young adults after 4 weeks of treatment with 25 mg given once a day. This increase was accompanied by an increase in the mean 24 hour GH concentration, GH pulse height, and interpulse nadir concentrations of these volunteers. No significant changes in pulse number were observed. No desensitization of the hypothalamic-pituitary GH axis occurred. Despite the fact that GHSs have been shown to have ACTH- and PRL-releasing activity, no change in cortisol secretion was found in this study. PRL levels rose slightly but remained within the normal range. Fasting insulin levels, as well as glucose levels, have been reported to increase under MK-0677 treatment. Results of a double-blind placebo-controlled trial show that MK-0677 is able to significantly increase IGF-1 levels in healthy older men and women for 2 years.[467] In the same study, fat-free mass increased by 1.1 kg in the treatment group after 1 year of treatment; however, strength and function did not change significantly.[467] Total appendicular skeletal mass increased significantly after 1 year of treatment, and a small but significant decrease in LDL levels was noted after 1 year of treatment with MK-677.[467] Similar changes in body composition were found with the orally active ghrelin mimetic capromorelin[466] after 6 months of treatment. The group described an improvement in functional parameters after 6 and 12 months. In a randomized, placebo-controlled study with 292 postmenopausal women, the effects of a GHS (MK-0677) on bone mineral density (BMD) alone and in combination with an antiresorptive agent (alendronate) resulted in increased BMD at the femoral neck when given together.[638] In a 6 month study in healthy older adults recovering from hip fracture treatment with MK-0677, greater improvement relative to placebo was noted in some lower extremity measures. Overall performance measures did not show a significant change.[639] The interpretation of such functional data is difficult, and a consensus is needed to define meaningful end points. These divergent results underline once again that each GHS is unique in terms of its bioavailability and specificity profiles.

Whether the use of GHSs in obesity will be of any benefit is questionable and requires further careful evaluation. GH-releasing effects in obesity are decreased when compared with a normal population.[388,640] Eight weeks of treatment with the GHS MK-0677 at a dose of 25 mg/day in 24 obese men showed no change in total or visceral fat.[615] Of interest is the fact that the fat-free mass increased significantly and IGF-1 levels increased by approximately 40% in this study.

Other ghrelin agonists such as TZP-101 and RC-1291, which can be given orally, are currently under evaluation for possible use in gastrointestinal motility.[641] The latter has been evaluated for possible use in cancer cachexia.[642] The compound showed promising effects in animal studies on cisplatin-induced hyperalgesia and cisplatin-induced cachexia. Previous animal studies in an animal melanoma model showed promising anti-cachectic effects of ghrelin.[632] In animal studies, MK-0677

resulted in increased production of cytotoxic T lymphocytes and enhanced resistance to initiation of tumor growth and metastases.[643] EPO1572, another ghrelin agonist, has been shown to effectively release GH.[644] The results of long-term studies with MK-677[467] suggest that this intervention is safe and well tolerated. However, before a final conclusion about the beneficial effects of these compounds can be reached, studies with carefully selected target populations and outcome parameters are recommended.

Summary

The GH axis is crucial not just for its role in initial growth and development, but also because of its complex functions in maintaining the adult body via the regulation of metabolism, nutrient partitioning, appetite, response to starvation, longevity, sleep, and mental, immune, and cardiac function, with additional roles still being uncovered. The identification of pituitary GH has led to the availability of rGH hormone for treatment of patients with GH deficiencies. Studies of the structure of GH and its receptor and their interaction have led to the development of GH antagonists useful for the treatment of GH excess. Improving our knowledge of the GH signaling pathway may allow us to understand its complex interactions with other pathways, and may allow us to intervene intelligently so as to control more selectively specific actions.

Examination of the endogenous pulsatile pattern of GH release has demonstrated that this pulsatile delivery is required for physiologic GH action, and that even low levels of continuous GH can cause symptoms of acromegaly. Hypothalamic GHRH is the major stimulus for pituitary somatotroph proliferation, and for GH synthesis and release. GHRH also may have an autocrine/paracrine role in the proliferation of other cell types. Identification of GHRH and its receptor has led to the use of GHRH to stimulate endogenous pulsatile GH release, to the development of GHRH analogues with prolonged half-life, and to the development of GHRH antagonists that have promising antitumor activity.

Synthetic GHSs, originally developed from enkephalin, stimulate GH release through a mechanism distinct from that of GHRH and act synergistically with GHRH. Identification of the secretagogue receptor led to the identification of its endogenous ligand, ghrelin. Ghrelin acts at the somatotrope to enhance the amplitude of endogenous GH pulses. Because it is secreted primarily from the stomach, ghrelin is in position to tie the GH actions on metabolism and nutrient utilization directly to nutrient availability. Studies of ghrelin have shown that it also has major effects on appetite, adipogenesis, lipid metabolism, gastric motility and secretion, cell proliferation, insulin secretion, blood pressure, mental function, sleep, and more. Ghrelin has a unique hydrophobic modification of Ser3, an acylation that is cleaved by serum esterases, making ghrelin unstable and requiring careful preanalytical processing of samples to assay for the active form. Although the GHS receptor mediates the orexigenic and GH-releasing actions of acyl-ghrelin, many other actions of ghrelin and all the actions of des-acyl ghrelin work through unknown mechanisms, suggesting that additional receptors and possibly additional ligands remain to be discovered. Some GHSs (ghrelin mimetics) appear to differentially affect appetite, gastric motility, or GH release, suggesting the possibility of orally active agents that might specifically target obesity, GI hypomobility, or the sarcopenia of aging.

REFERENCES

1. Evans H, Long J: The effect of the anterior lobe administered intraperitoneally upon growth, maturity, and oestrus cycle of the rat, Anat Rec 21:62–63, 1921.

2. Martial JA, et al: Human growth hormone: complementary DNA cloning and expression in bacteria, Science 205(4406):602–607, 1979.

3. Reichlin S: Growth and the hypothalamus, Endocrinology 67:760–773, 1960.

4. Reichlin S: Growth hormone content of pituitaries from rats with hypothalamic lesions, Endocrinology 69:225–230, 1961.

5. Miller WL, Eberhardt NL: Structure and evolution of the growth hormone gene family, Endocr Rev 4(2):97–130, 1983.

6. Kopchick JJ, Chen WY: Structure function relationships of growth hormone (GH) and other members of the GH gene family, in Handbook of Physiology, Oxford, 2000, Oxford University Press, pp 325–360.

7. Kopchick JJ, Sackmann-Sala L, Ding J: Primer: molecular tools used for the understanding of endocrinology, Nat Clin Pract Endocrinol Metab 3(4):355–368, 2007.

8. Kelberman D, Dattani MT: Hypothalamic and pituitary development: novel insights into the aetiology, Eur J Endocrinol 157(suppl 1):S3–S14, 2007.

9. Svensson J, Johannsson G, Bengtsson BA: Body composition and quality of life as markers of the efficacy of growth hormone replacement therapy in adults, Horm Res 55(suppl 2):55–60, 2001.

10. Jorgensen JO, et al: Effects of growth hormone on glucose and fat metabolism in human subjects, Endocrinol Metab Clin North Am 36(1):75–87, 2007.

11. Ben-Shlomo A, Melmed S: Acromegaly, Endocrinol Metab Clin North Am 37(1):101–122, viii, 2008.

12. Sakharova AA, et al: Role of growth hormone in regulating lipolysis, proteolysis, and hepatic glucose production during fasting, J Clin Endocrinol Metab 93(7):2755–2759, 2008.

13. Cameron CM, et al: The acute effects of growth hormone on amino acid transport and protein synthesis are due to its insulin-like action, Endocrinology 122(2):471–474, 1988.

14. Sirek A, et al: Effect of growth hormone on acute glucagon and insulin release, Am J Physiol 237(2):E107–E112, 1979.

15. Houssay B: The hypophysis and metabolism, N Engl J Med 214:961–985, 1936.

16. Rabinowitz D, Zierler KL: A metabolic regulating device based on the actions of human growth hormone and of insulin, singly and together, on the human forearm, Nature 199:913–915, 1963.

17. Holt RI, Simpson HL, Sonksen PH: The role of the growth hormone-insulin-like growth factor axis in glucose homeostasis, Diabet Med 20(1):3–15, 2003.

18. LeRoith D, Yakar S: Mechanisms of disease: metabolic effects of growth hormone and insulin-like growth factor 1, Nat Clin Pract Endocrinol Metab 3(3):302–310, 2007.

19. del Rincon JP, et al: Growth hormone regulation of p85alpha expression and phosphoinositide 3-kinase activity in adipose tissue: mechanism for growth hormone-mediated insulin resistance, Diabetes 56(6):1638–1646, 2007.

20. Dominici FP, et al: Influence of the crosstalk between growth hormone and insulin signalling on the modulation of insulin sensitivity, Growth Horm IGF Res 15(5):324–336, 2005.

21. Jessen N, et al: Evidence against a role for insulin-signaling proteins PI 3-kinase and Akt in insulin resistance in human skeletal muscle induced by short-term GH infusion, Am J Physiol Endocrinol Metab 288(1):E194–E199, 2005.

22. Kopchick JJ, Bartke A, Berryman DE: Extended life span in mice with reduction in the GH/IGF-1 axis. In Guarente LP, Wallace DC, editors: Molecular Biology of aging, New York, 2008, Cold Spring Harbor Laboratory Press, pp 347–369.

23. Berryman DE, et al: Role of the GH/IGF-1 axis in lifespan and healthspan: lessons from animal models, Growth Horm IGF Res 18(6):455–471, 2008.

24. Coschigano KT, et al: Deletion, but not antagonism, of the mouse growth hormone receptor results in severely decreased body weights, insulin, and insulin-like growth factor I levels and increased life span, Endocrinology 144(9):3799–3810, 2003.

25. Yuen KC, Dunger DB: Therapeutic aspects of growth hormone and insulin-like growth factor-I treatment on visceral fat and insulin sensitivity in adults, Diabetes Obes Metab 9(1):11–22, 2007.

26. Berryman DE, et al: Comparing adiposity profiles in three mouse models with altered GH signaling, Growth Horm IGF Res 14(4):309–318, 2004.

27. Berryman DE, et al: Effect of growth hormone on susceptibility to diet-induced obesity, Endocrinology 147(6):2801–2808, 2006.

28. Flint DJ, et al: Developmental aspects of adipose tissue in GH receptor and prolactin receptor gene disrupted mice: site-specific effects upon proliferation, differentiation and hormone sensitivity, J Endocrinol 191(1):101–111, 2006.

29. Quigley CA: Growth hormone treatment of non-growth hormone-deficient growth disorders, Endocrinol Metab Clin North Am 36(1):131–186, 2007.

30. Banerjee I, Clayton PE: Growth hormone treatment and cancer risk, Endocrinol Metab Clin North Am 36(1):247–263, 2007.

31. Farris GM, et al: Recombinant rat and mouse growth hormones: risk assessment of carcinogenic potential in 2-year bioassays in rats and mice, Toxicol Sci 97(2):548–561, 2007.

32. Wang Z, et al: Disruption of growth hormone signaling retards early stages of prostate carcinogenesis in the C3(1)/T antigen mouse, Endocrinology 146(12):5188–5196, 2005.

33. Zhang X, et al: Inhibition of estrogen-independent mammary carcinogenesis by disruption of growth hormone signaling, Carcinogenesis 28(1):143–150, 2007.

34. Wang Z, et al: Disruption of growth hormone signaling retards prostate carcinogenesis in the Probasin/TAg rat, Endocrinology 149(3):1366–1376, 2008.

35. Shen Q, et al: Advanced rat mammary cancers are growth hormone dependent, Endocrinology 148(10):4536–4544, 2007.

36. Pollak MN, Schernhammer ES, Hankinson SE: Insulin-like growth factors and neoplasia, Nat Rev Cancer 4(7):505–518, 2004.

37. Pollak M, et al: Reduced mammary gland carcinogenesis in transgenic mice expressing a growth hormone antagonist, Br J Cancer 85(3):428–430, 2001.

38. Yin D, et al: Clinical pharmacodynamic effects of the growth hormone receptor antagonist pegvisomant: implications for cancer therapy, Clin Cancer Res 13(3):1000–1009, 2007.

39. Perry JK, et al: The contribution of growth hormone to mammary neoplasia, J Mammary Gland Biol Neoplasia 13(1):131–145, 2008.

40. Kaulsay KK, et al: The effects of autocrine human growth hormone (hGH) on human mammary carcinoma cell behavior are mediated via the hGH receptor, Endocrinology 142(2):767–777, 2001.

41. De Palo EF, et al: Growth hormone isoforms, segments/fragments: does a link exist with multifunctionality? Clin Chim Acta 364(1-2):77–81, 2006.

42. Abdel-Meguid SS, et al: Three-dimensional structure of a genetically engineered variant of porcine growth hormone, Proc Natl Acad Sci U S A 84(18):6434–6437, 1987.

43. de Vos AM, Ultsch M, Kossiakoff AA: Human growth hormone and extracellular domain of its receptor: crystal structure of the complex, Science 255(5042):306–312, 1992.

44. Chen XZ, et al: Conversion of bovine growth hormone cysteine residues to serine affects secretion by cultured cells and growth rates in transgenic mice, Mol Endocrinol 6(4):598–606, 1992.

45. Campbell RM, Kostyo JL, Scanes CG: Lipolytic and antilipolytic effects of human growth hormone, its 20-kilodalton variant, a reduced and carboxymethylated derivative, and human placental lactogen on chicken adipose tissue in vitro, Proc Soc Exp Biol Med 193(4):269–273, 1990.

46. Cunningham BC, et al: Receptor and antibody epitopes in human growth hormone identified by homolog-scanning mutagenesis, Science 243(4896):1330–1336, 1989.

47. Cunningham BC, Wells JA: High-resolution epitope mapping of hGH-receptor interactions by alanine-scanning mutagenesis, Science 244(4908):1081–1085, 1989.

48. Aston R, Ivanyi J: Antigenic, receptor-binding and mitogenic activity of proteolytic fragments of human growth hormone, EMBO J 2(4):493–497, 1983.

49. Russell J, et al: Recombinant hormones from fragments of human growth hormone and human placental lactogen, J Biol Chem 256(1):296–300, 1981.

50. Chen WY, et al: Expression of a mutated bovine growth hormone gene suppresses growth of transgenic mice, Proc Natl Acad Sci U S A 87(13):5061–5065, 1990.

51. Chen WY, et al: Glycine 119 of bovine growth hormone is critical for growth-promoting activity, Mol Endocrinol 5(12):1845–1852, 1991.

52. Chen WY, et al: Functional antagonism between endogenous mouse growth hormone (GH) and a GH analog results in dwarf transgenic mice, Endocrinology 129(3):1402–1408, 1991.

53. Chen WY, et al: Mutations in the third alpha-helix of bovine growth hormone dramatically affect its intracellular distribution in vitro and growth enhancement in transgenic mice, J Biol Chem 266(4):2252–2258, 1991.

54. Chen WY, et al: In vitro and in vivo studies of the antagonistic effects of human growth hormone analogs, J Biol Chem 269(32):15892–15897, 1994.

55. Chen WY, et al: Amino acid residues in the third alpha-helix of growth hormone involved in growth promoting activity, Mol Endocrinol 9(3):292–302, 1995.

56. Okada S, et al: A growth hormone (GH) analog can antagonize the ability of native GH to promote differentiation of 3T3-F442A preadipocytes and stimulate insulin-like and lipolytic activities in primary rat adipocytes, Endocrinology 130(4):2284–2290, 1992.

57. Okada S, Kopchick JJ: Effects of growth hormone antagonist (hGH-G120R) on 3T3-F442A adipocytes, Diabetes 44(suppl 1):135A, 1995.

58. Fuh G, et al: Rational design of potent antagonists to the human growth hormone receptor, Science 256(5064):1677–1680, 1992.

59. Chihara K, et al: Short stature caused by a natural growth hormone antagonist, Horm Res 49(suppl 1):41–45, 1998.

60. Takahashi Y, et al: Biologically inactive growth hormone caused by an amino acid substitution, J Clin Invest 100(5):1159–1165, 1997.

61. Chen NY, et al: Co-expression of bovine growth hormone (GH) and human GH antagonist genes in transgenic mice, Endocrinology 138(2):851–854, 1997.

62. Chen WY, et al: Pharmacokinetic and pharmacodynamic studies of human growth hormone antagonist G120K-PEG in mice, 21, 10th International Congress of Endocrinology, San Francisco, CA, 1996, International Congress of Endocrinology, p 275.

63. Ross RJ, et al: Binding and functional studies with the growth hormone receptor antagonist, B2036-PEG (pegvisomant), reveal effects of pegylation and evidence that it binds to a receptor dimer, J Clin Endocrinol Metab 86(4):1716–1723, 2001.

64. Gent J, et al: Ligand-independent growth hormone receptor dimerization occurs in the endoplasmic reticulum and is required for ubiquitin system-dependent endocytosis, Proc Natl Acad Sci U S A 99(15):9858–9863, 2002.

65. Harding PA, et al: Growth hormone (GH) and a GH antagonist promote GH receptor dimerization and internalization, J Biol Chem 271(12):6708–6712, 1996.

66. Thorner MO, et al: Growth hormone (GH) receptor blockade with a PEG-modified GH (B2036- PEG) lowers serum insulin-like growth factor-I but does not acutely stimulate serum GH, J Clin Endocrinol Metab 84(6):2098–2103, 1999.

67. Kopchick JJ, et al: Growth hormone receptor antagonists: discovery, development, and use in patients with acromegaly, Endocr Rev 23(5):623–646, 2002.

68. Neggers SJ, et al: Quality of life in acromegalic patients during long-term somatostatin analog treatment with and without pegvisomant, J Clin Endocrinol Metab 93(10):3853–3859, 2008.

69. Brooks AJ, et al: Growth hormone receptor; mechanism of action, Int J Biochem Cell Biol 40(10):1984–1989, 2008.

70. Zhou Y, et al: A mammalian model for Laron syndrome produced by targeted disruption of the mouse growth hormone receptor/binding protein gene (the Laron mouse), Proc Natl Acad Sci U S A 94(24):13215–13220, 1997.

71. Coschigano KT, et al: Assessment of growth parameters and life span of GHR/BP gene-disrupted mice, Endocrinology 141(7):2608–2613, 2000.

72. van den Eijnden MJ, Lahaye LL, Strous GJ: Disulfide bonds determine growth hormone receptor folding, dimerisation and ligand binding, J Cell Sci 119(Pt 15):3078–3086, 2006.

73. Bougneres P, Goffin V: The growth hormone receptor in growth, Endocrinol Metab Clin North Am 36(1):1–16, 2007.

74. Kelly PA, et al: The prolactin/growth hormone receptor family, Endocr Rev 12(3):235–251, 1991.

75. Zhang Y, et al: Tumor necrosis factor-alpha converting enzyme (TACE) is a growth hormone binding protein (GHBP) sheddase: the metalloprotease TACE/ADAM-17 is critical for (PMA-induced) GH receptor proteolysis and GHBP generation, Endocrinology 141(12):4342–4348, 2000.

76. Fisker S: Physiology and pathophysiology of growth hormone-binding protein: methodological and clinical aspects, Growth Horm IGF Res 16(1):1–28, 2006.

77. Cunningham BC, et al: Dimerization of the extracellular domain of the human growth hormone receptor by a single hormone molecule, Science 254(5033):821–825, 1991.

78. Waters MJ, et al: New insights into growth hormone action, J Mol Endocrinol 36(1):1–7, 2006.

79. Rowlinson SW, et al: Activation of chimeric and full-length growth hormone receptors by growth hormone receptor monoclonal antibodies: a specific conformational change may be required for full-length receptor signaling, J Biol Chem 273(9):5307–5314, 1998.

80. Ultsch MH, et al: The crystal structure of affinity-matured human growth hormone at 2 A resolution, J Mol Biol 236(1):286–299, 1994.

81. Yang N, et al: Role of the growth hormone (GH) receptor transmembrane domain in receptor predimerization and GH-induced activation, Mol Endocrinol 21(7):1642–1655, 2007.

82. Yang N, et al: Activation of growth hormone receptors by growth hormone and growth hormone antagonist dimers: insights into receptor triggering, Mol Endocrinol 22(4):978–988, 2008.

83. Brown RJ, et al: Model for growth hormone receptor activation based on subunit rotation within a receptor dimer, Nat Struct Mol Biol 12(9):814–821, 2005.

84. Wang X, et al: Endotoxin-induced proteolytic reduction in hepatic growth hormone (GH) receptor: a novel mechanism for GH insensitivity, Mol Endocrinol 22(6):1427–1437, 2008.

85. Savage MO, et al: Endocrine assessment, molecular characterization and treatment of growth hormone insensitivity disorders, Nat Clin Pract Endocrinol Metab 2(7):395–407, 2006.

86. Chernausek SD, et al: Long-term treatment with recombinant insulin-like growth factor (IGF)-I in children with severe IGF-I deficiency due to growth hormone insensitivity, J Clin Endocrinol Metab 92(3):902–910, 2007.

87. Dos Santos C, et al: A common polymorphism of the growth hormone receptor is associated with increased responsiveness to growth hormone, Nat Genet 36(7):720–724, 2004.

88. Schmid C, et al: Growth hormone (GH) receptor isoform in acromegaly: lower concentrations of GH but not insulin-like growth factor-1 in patients with a genomic deletion of exon 3 in the GH receptor gene, Clin Chem 53(8):1484–1488, 2007.

89. Birzniece V, Sata A, Ho KK: Growth hormone receptor modulators, Rev Endocr Metab Disord 10(2):145–156, 2008.

90. Lanning NJ, Carter-Su C: Recent advances in growth hormone signaling, Rev Endocr Metab Disord 7(4):225–235, 2006.

91. Huang Y, et al: Physical and functional interaction of growth hormone and insulin-like growth factor-I signaling elements, Mol Endocrinol 18(6):1471–1485, 2004.

92. DiGirolamo DJ, et al: Mode of growth hormone action in osteoblasts, J Biol Chem 282(43):31666–31674, 2007.

93. Kopchick JJ, Andry JM: Growth hormone (GH), GH receptor, and signal transduction, Mol Genet Metab 71(1–2):293–314, 2000.

94. Chilton BS, Hewetson A, Gerald PS: Prolactin and growth hormone signaling, in current topics in developmental biology, New York, 2005, Academic Press, pp 1–23.

95. Schindler C, Darnell JE Jr: Transcriptional responses to polypeptide ligands: the JAK-STAT pathway, Annu Rev Biochem 64:621–651, 1995.

96. Veldhuis JD, Bowers CY: Human GH pulsatility: an ensemble property regulated by age and gender, J Endocrinol Invest 26(9):799–813, 2003.

97. Gebert CA, Park SH, Waxman DJ: Down-regulation of liver JAK2-STAT5b signaling by the female plasma pattern of continuous growth hormone stimulation, Mol Endocrinol 13(2):213–227, 1999.

98. Clodfelter KH, et al: Sex-dependent liver gene expression is extensive and largely dependent upon signal transducer and activator of transcription 5b (STAT5b): STAT5b-dependent activation of male genes and repression of female genes revealed by microarray analysis, Mol Endocrinol 20(6):1333–1351, 2006.

99. Holloway MG, et al: Loss of sexually dimorphic liver gene expression upon hepatocyte-specific deletion of Stat5a-Stat5b locus, Endocrinology 148(5):1977–1986, 2007.

100. Waxman DJ, O'Connor C: Growth hormone regulation of sex-dependent liver gene expression, Mol Endocrinol 20(11):2613–2629, 2006.

101. Wolbold R, et al: Sex is a major determinant of CYP3A4 expression in human liver, Hepatology 38(4):978–988, 2003.

102. Harding PA, Wang XZ, Kopchick JJ: Growth hormone (GH)-induced tyrosine-phosphorylated proteins in cells that express GH receptors, Receptor 5(2):81–92, 1995.

103. VanderKuur JA, et al: Signaling molecules involved in coupling growth hormone receptor to mitogen-activated protein kinase activation, Endocrinology 138(10):4301–4307, 1997.

104. Winston LA, Hunter T: JAK2, Ras, and Raf are required for activation of extracellular signal-regulated kinase/mitogen-activated protein kinase by growth hormone, J Biol Chem 270(52):30837–30840, 1995.

105. Argetsinger LS, et al: Growth hormone, interferon-gamma, and leukemia inhibitory factor utilize insulin receptor substrate-2 in intracellular signaling, J Biol Chem 271(46):29415–29421, 1996.

106. Rivera VM, et al: A growth factor-induced kinase phosphorylates the serum response factor at a site that regulates its DNA-binding activity, Mol Cell Biol 13(10):6260–6273, 1993.

107. Hill CS, Treisman R: Transcriptional regulation by extracellular signals: mechanisms and specificity, Cell 80(2):199–211, 1995.

108. Gong TW, et al: Regulation of glucose transport and c-fos and egr-1 expression in cells with mutated or endogenous growth hormone receptors, Endocrinology 139(4):1863–1871, 1998.

109. Rowlinson SW, et al: An agonist-induced conformational change in the growth hormone receptor determines the choice of signalling pathway, Nat Cell Biol 10(6):740–747, 2008.

110. Rosenfeld RG, et al: Defects in growth hormone receptor signaling, Trends Endocrinol Metab 18(4):134–141, 2007.

111. Catalioto RM, Ailhaud G, Negrel R: Diacylglycerol production induced by growth hormone in Ob1771 pre-adipocytes arises from phosphatidylcholine breakdown, Biochem Biophys Res Commun 173(3):840–848, 1990.

112. Okada S, Kopchick JJ: Growth hormone inhibits translocation of protein kinase C-α and -γ stimulated by insulin in 3T3-F422A cells. in 10th International Congress of Endocrinology. San Francisco, USA, 1996.

113. Greenhalgh CJ, Alexander WS: Suppressors of cytokine signalling and regulation of growth hormone action, Growth Horm IGF Res 14(3):200–206, 2004.

114. Pilecka I, et al: Protein-tyrosine phosphatase H1 controls growth hormone receptor signaling and systemic growth, J Biol Chem 282(48):35405–35415, 2007.

115. Jin H, Lanning NJ, Carter-Su C: JAK2, but not Src family kinases, is required for STAT, ERK, and Akt signaling in response to growth hormone in preadipo-cytes and hepatoma cells, Mol Endocrinol 22(8):1825–1841, 2008.

116. Thorner MO, et al: Somatotroph hyperplasia: successful treatment of acromegaly by removal of a pancreatic islet tumor secreting a growth hormone-releasing factor, Trans Assoc Am Physicians 95:177–187, 1992.

117. Spiess J, et al: Sequence analysis of a growth hormone releasing factor from a human pancreatic islet tumor, Biochemistry 21(24):6037–6040, 1982.

118. Rivier J, et al: Characterization of a growth-releasing factor from a human pancreatic islet cell tumour, Nature 300:276–278, 1982.

119. Esch FS, et al: Characterization of a 40 residue peptide from a human pancreatic tumor with growth hormone releasing activity, Biochem Biophys Res Commun 109:152–158, 1982.

120. Sassolas G, et al: Acromegaly, clinical expression of the production of growth hormone releasing factor in pancreatic tumors, Ann Endocrinol 44(6):347–354, 1983.

121. Guillemin R, et al: Growth hormone-releasing factor from a human pancreatic tumor that caused acromegaly, Science 218(4572):585–587, 1982.

122. Campbell RM, et al: GRF analogs and fragments: correlation between receptor binding, activity and structure, Peptides 12(3):569–574, 1991.

123. Frohman LA, Jansson JO: Growth hormone-releasing hormone, Endocr Rev 7(3):223–253, 1986.

124. Bohlen P, et al: Human hypothalamic growth hormone releasing factor (GRF): evidence for two forms identical to tumor derived GRF-44-NH2 and GRF-40, Biochem Biophys Res Commun 114(3):930–936, 1983.

125. Asa SL, et al: Immunohistological localization of growth hormone-releasing hormone in human tumors, J Clin Endocrinol Metab 60(3):423–427, 1985.

126. Christophe J, et al: The VIP/PHI/secretin/helodermin/helospectin/GRF family: structure-function relationships of the natural peptides, their precursors and synthetic analogues as tested in vitro on receptors and adenylate cyclase in a panel of tissue membranes. In Martinez J, editor: Peptide hormones as prohormones: processing, biological activity, Pharmacology, Chichester [England] New York, 1989, E. Horwood; Halsted Press, pp 211–243.

127. Campbell RM, Scanes CG: Evolution of the growth hormone-releasing factor (GRF) family of peptides, Growth Regul 2(4):175–191, 1992.

128. McRory JE, Parker RL, Sherwood NM: Expression and alternative processing of a chicken gene encoding both growth hormone-releasing hormone and pituitary adenylate cyclase-activating polypeptide, DNA Cell Biol 16(1):95–102, 1997.

129. Vaughan JM, et al: Isolation and characterization of hypothalamic growth-hormone releasing factor from common carp, Cyprinus carpio, Neuroendocrinology 56(4):539–549, 1992.

130. McRory J, Sherwood NM: Two protochordate genes encode pituitary adenylate cyclase-activating polypeptide and related family members, Endocrinology 138(6):2380–2390, 1997.

131. Toogood AA, et al: Cloning of the chicken pituitary receptor for growth hormone-releasing hormone, Endocrinology 147(4):1838–1846, 2006.

132. Lee LTO, et al: Discovery of growth hormone-releasing hormones and receptors in nonmammalian vertebrates, Proc Natl Acad Sci 104(7):2133–2138, 2007.

133. Wang Y, et al: Identification of the endogenous ligands for chicken growth hormone-releasing hormone (GHRH) receptor: evidence for a separate gene encoding GHRH in submammalian vertebrates, Endocrinology 148(5):2405–2416, 2007.

134. Wu S, et al: Newly-identified receptors for PHI and GHRH-like peptide in zebrafish help to elucidate the mammalian secretin superfamily, J Mol Endocrinol 41(5):343–366, 2008.

135. Kaiser ET, Kezdy FJ: Amphiphilic secondary structure: design of peptide hormones, Science 223(4633):249–255, 1984.

136. Campbell RM, Bongers J, Felix AM: Rational design, synthesis, and biological evaluation of novel growth hormone releasing factor analogues, Biopolymers 37(2):67–88, 1995.

137. Clore GM, Martin SR, Gronenborn AM: Solution structure of human growth hormone releasing factor: combined use of circular dichroism and nuclear magnetic resonance spectroscopy, J Mol Biol 191(3):553–561, 1986.

138. Frohman LA, et al: Dipeptidylpeptidase IV and trypsin-like enzymatic degradation of human growth hormone-releasing hormone in plasma, J Clin Invest 83(5):1533–1540, 1989.

139. Kovacs M, et al: An evaluation of intravenous, subcutaneous, and in vitro activity of new agmatine analogs of growth hormone-releasing hormone hGH-RH (1-29) NH2, Life Sci 42(1):27–35, 1988.

140. Coy DH, Hocart SJ, Murphy WA: Human growth hormone-releasing hormone analogues with much improved in vitro growth hormone-releasing potencies in rat pituitary cells, Eur J Pharmacol 204(2):179–185, 1991.

141. Zarandi M, et al: Potent agonists of growth hormone-releasing hormone. Part I, Int J Pept Protein Res 39(3):211–217, 1992.

142. Campbell RM, et al: Pegylated peptides. V. Carboxy-terminal PEGylated analogs of growth hormone-releasing factor (GRF) display enhanced duration of biological activity in vivo, J Pept Res 49(6):527–537, 1997.

143. Cervini LA, et al: Human growth hormone-releasing hormone hGHRH(1–29)-NH2: systematic structure-activity relationship studies, J Med Chem 41(5):717–727, 1998.

144. Jette L, et al: Human growth hormone-releasing factor (hGRF)1–29-albumin bioconjugates activate the GRF receptor on the anterior pituitary in rats: identification of CJC-1295 as a long-lasting GRF analog, Endocrinology 146(7):3052–3058, 2005.

145. Alba M, et al: Once-daily administration of CJC-1295, a long-acting growth hormone-releasing hormone (GHRH) analog, normalizes growth in the GHRH knockout mouse, Am J Physiol Endocrinol Metab 291(6):E1290–E1294, 2006.

146. Draghia-Akli R, Li X, Schwartz RJ: Enhanced growth by ectopic expression of growth hormone releasing hormone using an injectable myogenic vector, Nature Biotechnol 15(12):1285–1289, 1997.

147. Coy DH, et al: Structure-activity studies on the N-terminal region of growth hormone releasing factor, J Med Chem 28(2):181–185, 1985.

148. Toth K, et al: New analogs of human growth hormone-releasing hormone (1–29) with high and prolonged antagonistic activity, J Pept Res 51(2):134–141, 1998.

149. Jungwirth A, et al: Growth hormone-releasing hormone antagonist MZ-4-71 inhibits in vivo proliferation of Caki-I renal adenocarcinoma, Proc Natl Acad Sci U S A 94(11):5810–5813, 1997.

150. Waelbroeck M, et al: Interaction of growth hormone-releasing factor (GRF) and 14 GRF analogs with vasoactive intestinal peptide (VIP) receptors of rat pancreas: discovery of (N-Ac-Tyr1, D-Phe2)-GRF(1–29)-NH2 as a VIP antagonist, Endocrinology 116(6):2643–2649, 1985.

151. Mayo KE, et al: Characterization of cDNA and genomic clones encoding the precursor to rat hypothalamic growth hormone-releasing factor, Nature 314(6010):464–467, 1985.

152. Gonzalez-Crespo S, Boronat A: Expression of the rat growth hormone-releasing hormone gene in placenta is directed by an alternative promoter, Proc Natl Acad Sci U S A 88(19):8749–8753, 1991.

153. Berry SA: Growth hormone-releasing hormone-like messenger ribonucleic acid and immunoreactive peptide are present in human testis and placenta, J Clin Endocrinol Metab 75(1):281–284, 1992.

154. Bloch B, et al: Immunohistochemical evidence that growth hormone-releasing factor (GRF) neurons contain an amidated peptide derived from cleavage of the carboxyl-terminal end of the GRF precursor, Endocrinology 118(1):156–162, 1986.

155. Breyer PR, et al: A novel peptide from the growth hormone releasing hormone gene stimulates Sertoli cell activity, Endocrinology 137(5):2159–2162, 1996.

156. Perez-Riba M, Gonzalez-Crespo S, Boronat A: Differential splicing of the growth hormone-releasing hormone gene in rat placenta generates a novel pre-proGHRH mRNA that encodes a different C-terminal flanking peptide, FEBS Lett 402(2-3):273–276, 1997.

157. Lin HD, et al: Immunoreactive growth hormone-releasing factor in human stalk median eminence, J Clin Endocrinol Metab 58(6):1197–1199, 1984.

158. Merchenthaler I, et al: Immunocytochemical localization of growth hormone-releasing factor in the rat hypothalamus, Endocrinology 114(4):1082–1085, 1984.

159. Bloch B, et al: Topographical study of the neurons containing hpGRF immunoreactivity in monkey hypothalamus, Neurosci Lett 37(1):23–28, 1983.

160. Leveston SA, et al: Acromegaly and Cushing's syndrome associated with a foregut carcinoid tumor, J Clin Endocrinol Metab 53(4):682–689, 1981.

161. Horvath S, et al: Electron microscopic immunocytochemical evidence for the existence of bidirectional synaptic connections between growth hormone-releasing hormone- and somatostatin-containing neurons in the hypothalamus of the rat, Brain Research 481(1):8–15, 1989.

162. Zeitler P, et al: Ultradian oscillations in somatostatin and growth hormone-releasing hormone mRNAs in the brains of adult male rats, [Erratum appears in Proc Natl Acad Sci U S A 89(5):1997.] Proc Natl Acad Sci U S A 88(20):8920–8924, 1991.

163. Tannenbaum GS, et al: Growth hormone-releasing hormone neurons in the arcuate nucleus express both Sst1 and Sst2 somatostatin receptor genes, Endocrinology 139(3):1450–1453, 1998.

164. Bugnon C, et al: Immunocytochemical demonstration of a novel peptidergic neurone system in the cat brain with an anti-growth hormone-releasing factor serum, Neurosci Lett 38(2):131–137, 1983.

165. Jacobowitz DM, et al: Localization of GRF-like immunoreactive neurons in the rat brain, Peptides 4(4):521–524, 1983.

166. Bloch B, et al: Topographical and ontogenetic study of the neurons producing growth hormone-releasing factor in human hypothalamus, Regul Peptides 8(1):21–31, 1984.

167. Ishikawa K, et al: Ontogenesis of growth hormone-releasing hormone neurons in the rat hypothalamus, Neuroendocrinology 43(5):537–542, 1986.

168. Muller EE, Locatelli V, Cocchi D: Neuroendocrine control of growth hormone secretion, Physiol Rev 79(2):511–607, 1999.

169. Joubert D, et al: Normal and growth hormone (GH)-secreting adenomatous human pituitaries release somatostatin and GH-releasing hormone, J Clin Endocrinol Metab 68:572–577, 1989.

170. Lopes MB, et al: Growth hormone-releasing hormone receptor mRNA in acromegalic pituitary tumors, Am J Pathol 150(6):1885–1891, 1997.

171. Thapar K, et al: Overexpression of the growth-hormone-releasing hormone gene in acromegaly-associated pituitary tumors: an event associated with neoplastic progression and aggressive behavior, Am J Pathol 151(3):769–784, 1997.

172. Kahan Z, et al: Expression of growth hormone-releasing hormone (GHRH) messenger ribonucleic acid and the presence of biologically active GHRH in human breast, endometrial, and ovarian cancers, J Clin Endocrinol Metab 84(2):582–589, 1999.

173. Matsubara S, et al: Differential gene expression of growth hormone (GH)-releasing hormone (GRH) and GRH receptor in various rat tissues, Endocrinology 136(9):4147–4150, 1995.

174. Morel G, et al: Ultrastructural evidence for endogenous growth hormone-releasing factor-like immunoreactivity in the monkey pituitary gland, Neuroendocrinology 38:123–133, 1984.

175. Mentlein R, Buchholz C, Krisch B: Binding and internalization of gold-conjugated somatostatin and growth hormone-releasing hormone in cultured rat somatotropes, Cell Tissue Res 258:309–317, 1989.

176. Mayo KE, et al: The growth-hormone-releasing hormone receptor: signal transduction, gene expression, and physiological function in growth regulation, Ann N Y Acad Sci 805:184–203, 1996.

177. Mayo KE: Molecular cloning and expression of a pituitary-specific receptor for growth hormone-releasing hormone, Mol Endocrinol 6(10):1734–1744, 1992.

178. Gaylinn BD, et al: Molecular cloning and expression of a human anterior pituitary receptor for growth hormone-releasing hormone, Mol Endocrinol 7(1):77–84, 1993.

179. Lin C, et al: Pit-1-dependent expression of the receptor for growth hormone releasing factor mediates pituitary cell growth [see comments], Nature 360(6406):765–768, 1992.

180. DeAlmeida VI, Mayo KE: Identification of binding domains of the growth hormone-releasing hormone receptor by analysis of mutant and chimeric receptor proteins, Mol Endocrinol 12(5):750–765, 1998.

181. Gaylinn BD, et al: Photoaffinity cross-linking to the pituitary receptor for growth hormone-releasing factor, Endocrinology 135(3):950–955, 1994.

182. Seifert H, et al: Binding sites for growth hormone releasing factor on rat anterior pituitary cells, Nature 313:487–489, 1985.

183. Abribat T, Boulanger L, Gaudreau P: Characterization of [125I-Tyr10] human growth hormone-releasing factor (1–44) amide binding to rat pituitary: evidence for high and low affinity classes of sites, Brain Res 528(2):291–299, 1990.

184. Ikuyama S, et al: Characterization of growth hormone-releasing hormone receptors in pituitary adenomas from patients with acromegaly, J Clin Endocrinol Metab 66(6):1265–1271, 1988.

185. Gaylinn BD, Lyons CE, Thorner MO: Mapping of the GHRH receptor binding site by photoaffinity crosslinking from different residues of GHRH, in 79th Annual Meeting of the Endocrine Society, 1997, Minneapolis, MN.

186. Horikawa R, et al: A growth hormone-releasing hormone (GHRH) receptor mutation that acts as a dominant negative, in Endocrine Society, 83rd Annual Meeting, 2001, Denver, CO, USA.

187. McElvaine AT, Mayo KE: A dominant-negative human growth hormone-releasing hormone (GHRH) receptor splice variant inhibits GHRH binding, Endocrinology 2006:147(4):1884–1894.

188. Andrews S, Dubbelde C, Ryan E: The sequence of Homo sapiens PAC clone DJ0877J02, 1998, U.S. National Center for Biotechnology Information, National Library of Medicine: GenBank accession AC005155. Available at: http://www.ncbi.nlm.gov/.

189. Gaylinn BD, et al: Assignment of the human growth hormone-releasing hormone receptor gene (GHRHR) to 7p14 by in situ hybridization, Genomics 19(1):193–195, 1994.

190. Wajnrajch MP, et al: Human growth hormone-releasing hormone receptor (GHRHR) maps to a YAC at chromosome 7p15, Mamm Genome 5(9):595, 1994.

191. Petersenn S, et al: Structure and regulation of the human growth hormone-releasing hormone receptor gene, Mol Endocrinol 12(2):233–247, 1998.

192. Iguchi G, et al: Cloning and characterization of the 5′-flanking region of the human growth hormone-releasing hormone receptor gene, J Biol Chem 274(17):12108–12114, 1999.

193. McElvaine AT, et al: Pituitary-specific expression and Pit-1 regulation of the rat growth hormone-releasing hormone receptor gene, Mol Endocrinol 21(8):1969–1983, 2007.

194. Seifert H, et al: Growth hormone-releasing factor binding sites in rat anterior pituitary membrane homogenates: modulation by glucocorticoids, Endocrinology 117(1):424–426, 1985.

195. Tamaki M, et al: Dexamethasone increases growth hormone (GH)-releasing hormone (GRH) receptor mRNA levels in cultured rat anterior pituitary cells, J Neuroendocrinol 8(6):475–480, 1996.

196. Miller TL, Mayo KE: Glucocorticoids regulate pituitary growth hormone-releasing hormone receptor messenger ribonucleic acid expression, Endocrinology 138(6):2458–2465, 1997.

197. Ono M, et al: Sexually dimorphic expression of pituitary growth hormone-releasing factor receptor in the rat, Biochem Biophys Res Commun 216(3):1060–1066, 1995.

198. Bilezikjian LM, Seifert H, Vale W: Desensitization to growth hormone-releasing factor (GRF) is associated with down-regulation of GRF-binding sites, Endocrinology 118(5):2045–2052, 1986.

199. Horikawa R, et al: Growth hormone-releasing factor (GRF) regulates expression of its own receptor, Endocrinology 137(6):2642–2645, 1996.

200. Aleppo G, et al: Homologous down-regulation of growth hormone-releasing hormone receptor messenger ribonucleic acid levels, Endocrinology 138:1058–1065, 1997.

201. Miller TL, et al: The rat growth hormone-releasing hormone receptor gene: structure, regulation, and generation of receptor isoforms with different signaling properties, Endocrinology 140(9):4152–4165, 1999.

202. Journot L, et al: Differential signal transduction by six splice variants of the pituitary adenylate cyclase-

activating peptide (PACAP) receptor, Biochem Soc Trans 23(1):133–137, 1995.

203. Tang J, et al: Identification of human growth hormone-releasing hormone receptor splicing variants, J Clin Endocrinol Metab 80(8):2381–2387, 1995.

204. Zeitler P, Stevens P, Siriwardana G: Functional GHRH receptor carboxyl terminal isoforms in normal and dwarf (dw) rats, J Mol Endocrinol 21(3):363–371, 1998.

205. Motomura T, et al: Inhibition of signal transduction by a splice variant of the growth hormone-releasing hormone receptor expressed in human pituitary adenomas, Metabolism 47(7):804–808, 1998.

206. Halmos G, et al: Human renal cell carcinoma expresses distinct binding sites for growth hormone-releasing hormone, Proc Natl Acad Sci U S A 97(19):10555–10560, 2000.

207. Kiaris H, et al: Growth hormone-releasing hormone: an autocrine growth factor for small cell lung carcinoma [see comments], Proc Natl Acad Sci U S A 96(26):14894–14898, 1999.

208. Rekasi Z, et al: Isolation and sequencing of cDNAs for splice variants of growth hormone-releasing hormone receptors from human cancers, Proc Natl Acad Sci U S A 97(19):10561–10566, 2000.

209. Kineman RD: Antitumorigenic actions of growth hormone-releasing hormone antagonists, Proc Natl Acad Sci U S A 97(2):532–534, 2000.

210. Billestrup N, Swanson LW, Vale W: Growth hormone-releasing factor stimulates proliferation of somatotrophs in vitro, Proc Natl Acad Sci U S A 83:6854–6857, 1986.

211. Chopin LK: A potential autocrine pathway for growth hormone releasing hormone (GHRH) and its receptor in human prostate cancer cell lines, Prostate 49(2):116–121, 2001.

212. Kiaris H, et al: Expression of a splice variant of the receptor for GHRH in 3T3 fibroblasts activates cell proliferation responses to GHRH analogs, Proc Natl Acad Sci U S A 99(1):196–200, 2002.

213. Halmos G, et al: Expression of growth hormone-releasing hormone and its receptor splice variants in human prostate cancer, J Clin Endocrinol Metab 87(10):4707–4714, 2002.

214. Garcia-Fernandez MO, et al: The expression of growth hormone-releasing hormone (GHRH) and its receptor splice variants in human breast cancer lines: the evaluation of signaling mechanisms in the stimulation of cell proliferation, Breast Cancer Res Treat 77(1):15–26, 2003.

215. Kiaris H, et al: Ligand-dependent and -independent effects of splice variant 1 of growth hormone-releasing hormone receptor, Proc Natl Acad Sci U S A 100(16):9512–9517, 2003.

216. Jansson JO, et al: Receptor-associated resistance to growth hormone-releasing factor in dwarf "little" mice, Science 232(4749):511–512, 1986.

217. Godfrey P, et al: GHRH receptor of little mice contains a missense mutation in the extracellular domain that disrupts receptor function, Nat Genet 4(3):227–232, 1993.

218. Lin SC, et al: Molecular basis of the little mouse phenotype and implications for cell type-specific growth, Nature 364(6434):208–213, 1993.

219. Gaylinn BD, et al: The mutant growth hormone-releasing hormone (GHRH) receptor of the little mouse does not bind GHRH, Endocrinology 140(11):5066–5074, 1999.

220. Baumann G: Mutations in the growth hormone releasing hormone receptor: a new form of dwarfism in humans, Growth Horm IGF Res 9(suppl B):24–29, 1999; discussion 29–30.

221. Salvatori R, et al: Familial dwarfism due to a novel mutation of the growth hormone-releasing hormone receptor gene, J Clin Endocrinol Metab 84(3):917–923, 1999.

222. Salvatori R: Isolated growth hormone (GH) deficiency due to compound heterozygosity for two new mutations in the GH-releasing hormone receptor gene, Clin Endocrinol 54(5):681–687, 2001.

223. Pereira RM, et al: Heterozygosity for a mutation in the growth hormone-releasing hormone receptor gene does not influence adult stature, but affects body composition, J Clin Endocrinol Metab 92(6):2353–2357, 2007.

224. Adams EF, et al: A polymorphism in the growth hormone (GH)-releasing hormone (GHRH) receptor gene is associated with elevated response to GHRH by human pituitary somatotrophinomas in vitro, Biochem Biophys Res Commun 275(1):33–36, 2000.

225. Lee EJ, et al: Absence of constitutively activating mutations in the GHRH receptor in GH-producing pituitary tumors, J Clin Endocrinol Metab 86(8):3989–3995, 2001.

226. Salvatori R, et al: Absence of mutations in the growth hormone (GH)-releasing hormone receptor gene in GH-secreting pituitary adenomas, Clin Endocrinol 54(3):301–307, 2001.

227. Bilezikjian LM, Vale WW: Stimulation of adenosine 3′,5′-monophosphate production by growth hormone-releasing factor and its inhibition by somatostatin in anterior pituitary cells in vitro, Endocrinology 113(5):1726–1731, 1983.

228. Mougin C, et al: Roles of cyclic AMP and calcium in the mechanism of the release of growth hormone by somatocrinin, Comp Rendus Acad Sci 299:83–88, 1984.

229. Schettini G, et al: Human pancreatic tumor growth hormone-releasing factor stimulates anterior pituitary adenylate cyclase activity, adenosine 3′,5′-monophosphate accumulation, and growth hormone release in a calmodulin-dependent manner, Endocrinology 115(4):1308–1314, 1984.

230. Holl RW, Thorner MO, Leong DA: Intracellular calcium concentration and growth hormone secretion in individual somatotropes: effects of growth hormone-releasing factor and somatostatin, Endocrinology 122(6):2927–2932, 1988.

231. Guarcello V, Weigent DA, Blalock JE: Growth hormone releasing hormone receptors on thymocytes and splenocytes from rats, Cell Immunol 136:291–302, 1991.

232. Thorner MO, Holl RW, Leong DA: The somatotrope: an endocrine cell with functional calcium transients, J Exp Biol 139:169–179, 1988.

233. Bertherat J: Nuclear effects of the cAMP pathway activation in somatotrophs, Horm Res 47(4-6):245–250, 1997.

234. Cronin MJ, et al: Human pancreatic tumor growth hormone (GH)-releasing factor and cyclic adenosine 3′,5′- monophosphate evoke GH release from anterior pituitary cells: the effects of pertussis toxin, cholera toxin, forskolin, and cycloheximide, Endocrinology 114(3):904–913, 1984.

235. Ray KP, Wallis M: Regulation of growth hormone secretion and cyclic AMP metabolism in ovine pituitary cells: interactions involved in activation induced by growth hormone-releasing hormone and phorbol esters, Mol Cell Endocrinol 58:243–252, 1988.

236. Michel D, Lefevre G, Labrie F: Dexamethasone is a potent stimulator of growth hormone-releasing factor-induced cyclic AMP accumulation in the adenohypophysis, Life Sci 35:597–602, 1984.

237. Spada A, Vallar L, Giannattasio G: Presence of an adenylate cyclase dually regulated by somatostatin and human pancreatic growth hormone (GH)-releasing factor in GH-secreting cells, Endocrinology 115:1203–1209, 1984.

238. Cronin MJ, MacLeod RM, Canonico PL: Modification of basal and GRF-stimulated cyclic AMP levels and growth hormone release by phospholipid metabolic enzyme inhibitors, Neuroendocrinology 40:332–338, 1985.

239. Cheng K, et al: The synergistic effects of His-D-Trp-Ala-Trp-D-Phe-Lys-NH2 on growth hormone (GH)-releasing factor-stimulated GH release and intracellular adenosine 3′,5′-monophosphate accumulation in rat primary pituitary cell culture, Endocrinology 124(6):2791–2798, 1998.

240. Summers ST, Cronin MJ: Phorbol esters induce two distinct changes in GH3 pituitary cell adenylate cyclase activity, Arch Biochem Biophys 262:12–18, 1988.

241. Canonico PL, et al: Human pancreatic GRF stimulates phosphatidylinositol labeling in cultured anterior pituitary cells, Am J Physiol 245:E587–E590, 1983.

242. Canonico PL, et al: Growth hormone releasing factor (GRF) increases free arachidonate levels in the pituitary: a role for lipoxygenase products, Life Sci 38:267–272, 1986.

243. Dobson PRM, et al: The effect of growth hormone releasing factor on cyclic AMP accumulation and phos-

phatidylinositol breakdown, in 5th Internatl Conf Cyclic Nucleotides Protein Phosphorylation, Milan, Italy, 1983.

244. Ramirez JL, et al: Growth hormone-releasing factor mobilizes cytosolic free calcium through different mechanisms in two somatotrope subpopulations from porcine pituitary, Cell Calcium 23(4):207–217, 1998.

245. Snyder GD, Yadagiri P, Falck JR: Effect of epoxyeicosatrienoic acids on growth hormone release from somatotrophs, Am J Physiol 256:E221–E226, 1989.

246. Cella SG, et al: Long-term changes of somatotrophic function induced by deprivation of growth hormone-releasing hormone during the fetal life of the rat, J Endocrinol 140(1):111–117, 1994.

247. Landis CA, et al: GTPase inhibiting mutations activate the alpha chain of Gs and stimulate adenylyl cyclase in human pituitary tumours, Nature 340(6236):692–696, 1989.

248. Lloyd RV, et al: Morphologic effects of hGRH gene expression on the pituitary, liver, and pancreas of MT-hGRH transgenic mice: an in situ hybridization analysis, Am J Pathol 141(4):895–906, 1992.

249. Pombo CM, et al: Growth hormone-releasing hormone stimulates mitogen-activated protein kinase, Endocrinology 141(6):2113–2119, 2000.

250. Mayo KE, et al: Regulation of the pituitary somatotroph cell by GHRH and its receptor, Recent Prog Horm Res 55:237–266, 2000; discussion 266–267.

251. Zeitler P, Siriwardana G: Stimulation of mitogen-activated protein kinase pathway in rat somatotrophs by growth hormone-releasing hormone, Endocrine 12(3):257–264, 2000.

252. Barinaga M, et al: Transcriptional regulation of growth hormone gene expression by growth hormone-releasing factor, Nature 306(5938):84–85, 1983.

253. Stachura ME, Tyler JM, Farmer PK: Fractional reduction of somatostatin concentration interacted with rat growth hormone releasing hormone to titrate the magnitude of pulsatile growth hormone and prolactin release in perifusion, Neuroendocrinology 48:500–506, 1988.

254. Dieguez C, et al: The effects of long term growth hormone releasing factor (GRF 1- 40) administration on growth hormone secretion and synthesis in vitro, Biochem Biophys Res Commun 121:111–117, 1984.

255. Perez FM, Hymer WC: A new tissue-slicing method for the study of function and position of somatotrophs contained within the male rat pituitary gland, Endocrinology 127:1877–1886, 1990.

256. Brazeau P, et al: Growth hormone releasing factor, somatocrinin, releases pituitary growth hormone in vitro, Proc Natl Acad Sci U S A 79:7909–7913, 1982.

257. Vale W, et al: Effects of synthetic human pancreatic (tumor) GH releasing factor and somatostatin, triiodothyronine and dexamethasone on GH secretion in vitro, Endocrinology 112:1553–1555, 1983.

258. Arvat E, et al: Endocrine activities of ghrelin, a natural growth hormone secretagogue (GHS), in humans: comparison and interactions with hexarelin, a nonnatural peptidyl GHS, and GH-releasing hormone, J Clin Endocrinol Metab 86(3):1169–1174, 2001.

259. Arimura A, et al: In vitro pituitary hormone releasing activity of 40 residue human pancreatic tumor growth hormone releasing factor, Peptides 4(1):107–110, 1983.

260. Zafar MS, et al: Acromegaly associated with a bronchial carcinoid tumor: evidence for ectopic production of growth hormone-releasing activity, J Clin Endocrinol Metab 48:66–71, 1979.

261. Weiss J, Cronin MJ, Thorner MO: Periodic interactions of GH-releasing factor and somatostatin can augment GH release in vitro, Am J Physiol 253(5 Pt 1):E508–E514, 1987.

262. Plotsky PM, Vale W: Patterns of growth hormone-releasing factor and somatostatin secretion into the hypophysial-portal circulation of the rat, Science 230(4724):461–463, 1985.

263. Frohman LA, et al: Measurement of growth hormone-releasing hormone and somatostatin in hypothalamic-portal plasma of unanesthetized sheep: spontaneous secretion and response to insulin-induced hypoglycemia, J Clin Invest 86(1):17–24, 1990.

264. Law GJ, Ray KP, Wallis M: Effects of growth hormone-releasing factor, somatostatin and dopamine on growth hormone and prolactin secretion from cultured ovine pituitary cells, FEBS Lett 166:189–193, 1984.

265. Stachura ME, Tyler JM, Farmer PK: Human pancreatic growth hormone-releasing factor-44 differentially stimulates release of stored and newly synthesized rat growth hormone in vitro, Endocrinology 116:698–706, 1985.

266. Tachibana K, et al: Growth hormone-releasing hormone stimulates and somatostatin inhibits the release of a novel protein by cultured rat pituitary cells, Mol Endocrinol 2:973–978, 1988.

267. Katsumata N, et al: Molecular cloning and expression of peptide 23, a growth hormone-releasing hormone-inducible pituitary protein, Endocrinology 136(4):1332–1339, 1995.

268. Bergstrom RW, et al: Hypogonadotropic hypogonadism and anosmia (Kallmann's syndrome) associated with a marker chromosome, J Androl 8(1):55–60, 1987.

269. Zeytin FN, et al: Growth hormone (GH)-releasing factor does not regulate GH release or GH mRNA levels in GH3 cells, Endocrinology 114(6):2054–2059, 1984.

270. Giustina A, Veldhuis JD: Pathophysiology of the neuroregulation of growth hormone secretion in experimental animals and the human, Endocr Rev 19(6):717–797, 1998.

271. Smith RG, et al: Peptidomimetic regulation of growth hormone secretion, Endocr Rev 18(5):621–645, 1997.

272. Wehrenberg WB, et al: Physiological roles of somatocrinin and somatostatin in the regulation of growth hormone secretion, Biochem Biophys Res Commun 109:562–567, 1982.

273. Wehrenberg WB, et al: Somatocrinin, growth hormone releasing factor, stimulates secretion of growth hormone in anesthetized rats, Biochem Biophys Res Commun 109:382–387, 1982.

274. Maheshwari HG, et al: Pulsatile growth hormone secretion persists in genetic growth hormone-releasing hormone resistance, Am J Physiol Endocrinol Metab 282(4):E943–E951, 2002.

275. Jessup SK, et al: Sexual dimorphism of growth hormone (GH) regulation in humans: endogenous GH-releasing hormone maintains basal GH in women but not in men [see comment], J Clin Endocrinol Metab 88(10):4776–4780, 2003.

276. Cella SG, et al: Deprivation of growth hormone-releasing hormone early in the rat's neonatal life permanently affects somatotropic function, Endocrinology 127:1625–1634, 1990.

277. Thorner MO, Cronin MJ: Growth hormone-releasing factor: clinical and basic studies, In Mueller EE, MacLeod RM, Frohman LA, editors: Neuroendocrine perspectives, Amsterdam, 1985, Elsevier, pp 95–144.

278. Mayo KE, et al: Dramatic pituitary hyperplasia in transgenic mice expressing a human growth hormone-releasing factor gene, Mol Endocrinol 2:606–612, 1988.

279. Stefaneanu L, et al: Adenohypophysial changes in mice transgenic for human growth hormone-releasing factor: a histological, immunocytochemical, and electron microscopic investigation, Endocrinology 125(5):2710–2718, 1989.

280. Sugino T, et al: A transient ghrelin surge occurs just before feeding in a scheduled meal-fed sheep, Biochem Biophys Res Commun 295(2):255–260, 2002.

281. Wheeler MD, Wehrenberg WW, Styne DM: Growth hormone regulation by growth hormone-releasing hormone in infant rhesus monkeys, Biol Neonate 60:19–28, 1991.

282. Wheeler MD, Styne DM: Longitudinal changes in growth hormone response to growth hormone-releasing hormone in neonatal rhesus monkeys, Pediatr Res 28:15–18, 1990.

283. Acs Z, Lonart G, Makara GB: Role of hypothalamic factors (growth-hormone-releasing hormone and gamma-aminobutyric acid) in the regulation of growth hormone secretion in the neonatal and adult rat, Neuroendocrinology 52(2):156–160, 1990.

284. Ge F, et al: Relationship between growth hormone-releasing hormone and somatostatin in the rat: effects of age and sex on content and in-vitro release from hypothalamic explants, J Endocrinol 123(1):53–58, 1989.

285. Cozzi MG, et al: Growth hormone-releasing hormone and clonidine stimulate biosynthesis of growth hormone in neonatal pituitaries, Biochem Biophys Res Commun 138:1223–1230, 1986.

286. Korytko AI, Zeitler P, Cuttler L: Developmental regulation of pituitary growth hormone-releasing hormone receptor gene expression in the rat, Endocrinology 137(4):1326–1331, 1996.

287. Colonna VD, et al: Reduced growth hormone releasing factor (GHRF)-like immunoreactivity and GHRF gene expression in the hypothalamus of aged rats, Peptides 10:705–708, 1989.

288. Abribat T, et al: Alterations of pituitary growth hormone-releasing factor binding sites in aging rats, Endocrinology 128(1):633–635, 1991.

289. Girard N, et al: Differential in vivo regulation of the pituitary growth hormone-releasing hormone (GHRH) receptor by GHRH in young and aged rats, Endocrinology 140(6):2836–2842, 1999.

290. Sonntag WE, Gough MA: Growth hormone releasing hormone induced release of growth hormone in aging male rats: dependence on pharmacological manipulation and endogenous somatostatin release, Neuroendocrinology 47:482–488, 1988.

291. Pavlov EP, et al: Responses of growth hormone (GH) and somatomedin-C to GH-releasing hormone in healthy aging men, J Clin Endocrinol Metab 62(3):595–600, 1986.

292. Argente J, et al: Sexual dimorphism of growth hormone-releasing hormone and somatostatin gene expression in the hypothalamus of the rat during development, Endocrinology 128(5):2369–2375, 1991.

293. Maiter DM, et al: Sexual differentiation of growth hormone feedback effects on hypothalamic growth hormone-releasing hormone and somatostatin, Neuroendocrinology 51:174–180, 1990.

294. Zeitler P, et al: Growth hormone-releasing hormone messenger ribonucleic acid in the hypothalamus of the adult male rat is increased by testosterone, Endocrinology 127(3):1362–1368, 1990.

295. Zeitler P, et al: Regulation of somatostatin and growth hormone-releasing hormone gene expression in the rat brain, Metab Clin Exp 39(9 suppl 2):46–49, 1990.

296. Maiter D, Koenig JI, Kaplan LM: Sexually dimorphic expression of the growth hormone-releasing hormone gene is not mediated by circulating gonadal hormones in the adult rat, Endocrinology 128:1709–1716, 1991.

297. Aguilar E, Pinilla L: Ovarian role in the modulation of pituitary responsiveness to growth hormone-releasing hormone in rats, Neuroendocrinology 54(3):286–290, 1991.

298. Evans WS, et al: Effects of in vivo gonadal hormone environment on in vitro hGRF-40-stimulated GH release, Am J Physiol 249(3 Pt 1):E276–E280, 1985.

299. Cronin MJ, et al: Biological activity of a growth hormone-releasing factor secreted by a human tumor, Am J Physiol 244(4):E346–E353, 1983.

300. Hertz P, et al: Effects of sex steroids on the response of cultured rat pituitary cells to growth hormone-releasing hormone and somatostatin, Endocrinology 125:581–585, 1989.

301. Leong DA, et al: Enumeration of lactotropes and somatotropes among male and female pituitary cells in culture: evidence in favor of a mammosomatotrope subpopulation in the rat, Endocrinology 116(4):1371–1378, 1985.

302. Ho KY, et al: Effects of gonadal steroids on somatotroph function in the rat: analysis by the reverse hemolytic plaque assay, Endocrinology 123(3):1405–1411, 1988.

303. Alvarez CV, et al: Evidence for a direct pituitary inhibition by free fatty acids of in vivo growth hormone responses to growth hormone-releasing hormone in the rat, Neuroendocrinology 53(2):185–189, 1991.

304. Grings EE, et al: Response to a growth hormone-releasing hormone analog in heifers treated with recombinant growth hormone, Domestic Anim Endocrinol 5:47–53, 1988.

305. Levy A, et al: The effects of pituitary stalk transection, hypophysectomy and thyroid hormone status on insulin-like growth factor 2-, growth hormone releasing hormone-, and somatostatin mRNA prevalence in rat brain, Brain Res 579(1):1–7, 1992.

306. Edwards CA, Dieguez C, Scanlon MF: Effects of hypothyroidism, tri-iodothyronine and glucocorticoids on growth hormone responses to growth hormone-releasing hormone and His-D-Trp-Ala-Trp-D-Phe-Lys-NH2, J Endocrinol 121:31–36, 1989.

307. Wehrenberg WB, et al: Interactions between growth hormone-releasing hormone and glucocorticoids in male rats, Regul Pept 25:147–155, 1989.

308. Senaris RM, et al: Regulation of hypothalamic somatostatin, growth hormone-releasing hormone, and growth hormone receptor messenger ribonucleic acid by glucocorticoids, Endocrinology 137(12):5236–5241, 1996.

309. Asa SL: The role of hypothalamic hormones in the pathogenesis of pituitary adenomas, Pathol Res Pract 187:581–583, 1991.

310. Cronin MJ, Burnier J, Clarke RG: Growth hormone releasing hormone infusion in normal rats enlarges the pituitary within days, J Endocrinol Invest 14(1):34, 1991.

311. Horacek MJ, Campbell GT, Blake CA: Effects of growth hormone-releasing hormone on somatotrophs in anterior pituitary gland allografts in hypophysectomized, orchidectomized hamsters, Cell Tissue Res 253:287–290, 1988.

312. Lehy T, et al: Growth hormone-releasing factor (somatocrinin) stimulates epithelial cell proliferation in the rat digestive tract, Gastroenterology 90(3):646–653, 1986.

313. Hermansen K, Kappelgaard AM: Characterization of growth hormone-releasing hormone stimulation of the endocrine pancreas: studies with alpha- and beta-adrenergic and cholinergic antagonists, Acta Endocrinol 114(4):589–594, 1987.

314. Bailey CJ, et al: Effects of growth hormone-releasing hormone on the secretion of islet hormones and on glucose homeostasis in lean and genetically obese-diabetic (ob/ob) mice and normal rats, J Endocrinol 123(1):19–24, 1989.

315. Green IC, Southern C, Ray K: Mechanism of action of growth-hormone-releasing hormone in stimulating insulin secretion in vitro from isolated rat islets and dispersed islet cells, Horm Res 33(5):199–204, 1990.

316. Wehrenberg WB, Ehlers CL: Effects of growth hormone-releasing factor in the brain, Science 232(4755):1271–1273, 1986.

317. Obal F Jr, et al: Growth hormone-releasing hormone antibodies suppress sleep and prevent enhancement of sleep after sleep deprivation, Am J Physiol 263(5 Pt 2):R1078–R1085, 1992.

318. Zhang J, et al: Intrapreoptic microinjection of GHRH or its antagonist alters sleep in rats, J Neurosci 19(6):2187–2194, 1999.

319. Toppila J, et al: Sleep deprivation increases somatostatin and growth hormone-releasing hormone messenger RNA in the rat hypothalamus, J Sleep Res 6(3):171–178, 1997.

320. Sibilia V, et al: Long-term effects on bone of postnatal immunization against GHRH in female and male rats, J Endocrinol 177(1):93–100, 2003.

321. Draghia-Akli R, et al: Effects of plasmid-mediated growth hormone-releasing hormone in severely debilitated dogs with cancer, Mol Ther 6(6):830–836, 2002.

322. Inoue S, et al: Peripheral plasma levels of human growth hormone releasing hormone (GHRH) during the sleep test in short children, Endocr J 45(suppl):S71–S75, 1998.

323. Frohman LA, et al: Rapid enzymatic degradation of growth hormone-releasing hormone by plasma in vitro and in vivo to a biologically inactive product cleaved at the NH2 terminus, J Clin Invest 78:906–913, 1986.

324. Katakami H, et al: Development and clinical application of a highly sensitive enzyme immunoassay (EIA) for human growth hormone-releasing hormone (hGHRH) in plasma, Endocr J 45(suppl):S67–S70, 1998.

325. Penny ES, et al: Circulating growth hormone releasing factor concentrations in normal subjects and patients with acromegaly, Br Med J 289(6443):453–455, 1984.

326. Thorner MO, et al: Extrahypothalamic growth-hormone-releasing factor (GRF) secretion is a rare cause of acromegaly: plasma GRF levels in 177 acromegalic patients, J Clin Endocrinol Metab 59(5):846–849, 1984.

327. Sano T, Asa SL, Kovacs K: Growth hormone-releasing hormone-producing tumors: clinical, biochemical, and morphological manifestations, Endocr Rev 9(3):357–373, 1988.

328. Faglia G, Arosio M, Bazzoni N: Ectopic acromegaly, Endocrinol Metab Clin North Am 21(3):575–595, 1992.

329. Miell J, et al: Effects of glucocorticoid treatment and acute passive immunization with growth hormone-releasing hormone and somatostatin antibodies on endogenous and stimulated growth hormone secretion in the male rat, J Endocrinol 131:75–86, 1991.

330. Osella G, et al: Acromegaly due to ectopic secretion of GHRH by bronchial carcinoid in a patient with empty sella [see comment], J Endocrinol Invest 26(2):163–169, 2003.

331. Kovacs M, et al: Effects of antagonists of growth hormone-releasing hormone (GHRH) on GH and insulin-like growth factor I levels in transgenic mice overexpressing the human GHRH gene, an animal model of acromegaly, Endocrinology 138(11):4536–4542, 1997.

332. Sano T, et al: Growth hormone-releasing hormone (GHRH)-secreting pancreatic tumor in a patient with multiple endocrine neoplasia type I, Am J Surg Pathol 11(10):810–819, 1987.

333. Asa SL, et al: Pancreatic endocrine tumour producing growth hormone-releasing hormone associated with multiple endocrine neoplasia type I syndrome, Acta Endocrinol 115(3):331–337, 1987.

334. Ramsay JA, et al: Reversible sellar enlargement due to growth hormone-releasing hormone production by pancreatic endocrine tumors in an acromegalic patient with multiple endocrine neoplasia type I syndrome, Cancer 62(2):445–450, 1988.

335. Yamasaki R, et al: Ectopic growth hormone-releasing hormone (GHRH) syndrome in a case with multiple endocrine neoplasia type I, Endocrinol Japon 35(1):97–109, 1988.

336. Liu SW, et al: Acromegaly caused by growth hormone-relating hormone in a patient with multiple endocrine neoplasia type I, Jpn J Clin Oncol 26(1):49–52, 1996.

337. Asa SL, et al: A case for hypothalamic acromegaly: a clinicopathological study of six patients with hypothalamic gangliocytomas producing growth hormone-releasing factor, J Clin Endocrinol Metab 58(5):796–803, 1984.

338. Kojima K, et al: Multiple gastric carcinoids and pituitary adenoma in type A gastritis, Intern Med 36(11):787–789, 1997.

339. Donnadieu M, et al: Variations of plasma growth hormone (GH)-releasing factor levels during GH stimulation tests in children, J Clin Endocrinol Metab 60:1132–1134, 1985.

340. Argente J, et al: Impaired response of growth hormone-releasing hormone (GHRH) measured in plasma after L-dopa stimulation in patients with idiopathic delayed puberty, Acta Paediatr Scand 76(2):266–270, 1987.

341. Mitsuhashi S, et al: Effect of oral administration of L-dopa on the plasma levels of growth hormone-releasing hormone (GHRH) in normal subjects and patients with various endocrine and metabolic diseases, Nippon Naib Gakkai Zasshi Fol Endocrinol Japon 63:934–946, 1987.

342. Chihara K, et al: L-dopa stimulates release of hypothalamic growth hormone-releasing hormone in humans, J Clin Endocrinol Metab 62:466–473, 1986.

343. Kashio Y, et al: Effect of oral glucose administration on plasma growth hormone-releasing hormone (GHRH)-like immunoreactivity levels in normal subjects and patients with idiopathic GH deficiency: evidence that GHRH is released not only from the hypothalamus but also from extrahypothalamic tissue, J Clin Endocrinol Metab 64(1):92–97, 1987.

344. Rosskamp R, et al: Effect of insulin-induced hypoglycemia on circulating levels of plasma growth hormone-releasing hormone and somatostatin in children, Horm Res 27:121–125, 1987.

345. Kashio Y, et al: Presence of growth hormone-releasing factor-like immunoreactivity in human cerebrospinal fluid, J Clin Endocrinol Metab 60:396–398, 1985.

346. Growth Hormone Research Society: Consensus guidelines for the diagnosis and treatment of adults with growth hormone deficiency: summary statement of the Growth Hormone Research society workshop on adult growth hormone deficiency, J Clin Endocrinol Metab 83:379–381, 1998.

347. Rahim A, Toogood AA, Shalet SM: The assessment of growth hormone status in normal young adult males using a variety of provocative tests, Clin Endocrinol 45:557–562, 1996.

348. Shibasaki T, et al: Age-related changes in plasma growth hormone response to growth hormone-releasing factor in man, J Clin Endocrinol Metab 58(1):212–214, 1984.

349. Thorner MO, et al: Human pancreatic growth-hormone-releasing factor selectively stimulates growth-hormone secretion in man, Lancet 1(8314-8315):24–28, 1983.

350. Wood SM, et al: Abnormalities of growth hormone release in response to human pancreatic growth hormone releasing factor (GRF [1-44]) in acromegaly and hypopituitarism, Br Med J 286:1687–1691, 1983.

351. Rosenthal SM, et al: Synthetic human pancreas growth hormone-releasing factor (hpGRF1-44-NH2) stimulates growth hormone secretion in normal men, J Clin Endocrinol Metab 57:677–679, 1983.

352. Gelato MC, et al: Dose-response relationships for the effects of growth hormone- releasing factor-(1-44)-NH2 in young adult men and women, J Clin Endocrinol Metab 59:197–201, 1994.

353. Sassolas G, et al: Effects of human pancreatic tumor growth hormone-releasing hormone (hpGRH1-44-NH2) on immunoreactive and bioactive plasma growth hormone in normal young men, J Clin Endocrinol Metab 59:705–709, 1984.

354. Lang I, et al: Effects of sex and age on growth hormone response to growth hormone-releasing hormone in healthy individuals, J Clin Endocrinol Metab 65:535–540, 1987.

355. Chihara K, et al: Idiopathic growth hormone (GH) deficiency, and GH deficiency secondary to hypothalamic germinoma: effect of single and repeated administration of human GH-releasing factor (hGRF) on plasma GH level and endogenous hGRF-like immunoreactivity level in cerebrospinal fluid, J Clin Endocrinol Metab 60:269–278, 1985.

356. Evans WS, et al: Effects of human pancreatic growth hormone-releasing factor-40 on serum growth hormone, prolactin, luteinizing hormone, follicle-stimulating hormone, and somatomedin-C concentrations in normal women throughout the menstrual cycle, J Clin Endocrinol Metab 59(5):1006–1010, 1984.

357. Vance ML, et al: Human pancreatic tumor growth hormone-releasing factor: dose-response relationships in normal man, J Clin Endocrinol Metab 58(5):838–844, 1984.

358. Gelato M, Malozowski S, Nicoletti M: Responses to growth hormone releasing hormone during development and puberty in normal boys and girls. In symposium on recent developments in the study of growth factors: GRF and somatomedin, Paris, 1985.

359. Ghigo E, et al: Reliability of provocative tests to assess growth hormone secretory status: study in 472 normally growing children, J Clin Endocrinol Metab 81(9):3323–3327, 1996.

360. Gelato MC, et al: Growth hormone (GH) responses to GH-releasing hormone during pubertal development in normal boys and girls: comparison to idiopathic short stature and GH deficiency, J Clin Endocrinol Metab 63:174–179, 1986.

361. Ross RJ, et al: Stilbestrol pretreatment of children with short stature does not affect the growth hormone response to growth hormone-releasing hormone, Clin Endocrinol 27:155–161, 1987.

362. Lang I, et al: The influence of age on human pancreatic growth hormone releasing hormone stimulated growth hormone secretion, Horm Metab Res 20(9):574–578, 1988.

363. Corpas E, Harman SM, Blackman MR: Human growth hormone and human aging, Endocr Rev 14:20–39, 1993.

364. Ghigo E, et al: Growth hormone (GH) responsiveness to combined administration of arginine and GH-releasing hormone does not vary with age in man, J Clin Endocrinol Metab 71(6):1481–1485, 1990.

365. Ghigo E, et al: Pyridostigmine partially restores the GH responsiveness to GHRH in normal aging, Acta Endocrinol 123(2):169–173, 1990.

366. Alba-Roth J, et al: Arginine stimulates growth hormone secretion by suppressing endogenous somatostatin secretion, J Clin Endocrinol Metab 67(6):1186–1189, 1988.

367. Ross RJ, et al: GH feedback occurs through modulation of hypothalamic somatostatin under cholinergic control: studies with pyridostigmine and GHRH, Clin Endocrinol 27(6):727–733, 1987.

368. Ranke MB, et al: Testing with growth hormone-releasing factor (GRF(1-29)NH2) and somatomedin C measurements for the evaluation of growth hormone deficiency, Eur J Pediatr 145(6):485–492, 1986.

369. Bozzola M, et al: Synthetic growth hormone-releasing hormone (GHRH 1-44) in the differential diagnosis between hypothalamic and pituitary GH deficiency, J Endocrinol Invest 9:503–506, 1986.

370. Takano K, et al: Plasma growth hormone (GH) response to GH-releasing factor in normal children with short stature and patients with pituitary dwarfism, J Clin Endocrinol Metab 58:236–241, 1984.

371. Schonberg D: Diagnosis of growth hormone deficiency, Baillieres Clin Endocrinol Metab 6(3):527–546, 1992.

372. Shalet S, et al: The diagnosis of growth hormone deficiency in children and adults, Endocr Rev 19:203–223, 1998.

373. Toogood A, et al: The diagnosis of severe growth hormone deficiency in elderly patients with hypothalamic-pituitary disease, Clin Endocrinol 48:569–576, 1998.

374. Hoeck HC, et al: Differences in reproducibility and peak growth hormone responses to repeated testing with various stimulators in healthy adults, Growth Horm IGF Res 9(1):18–24, 1999.

375. Chatelain P, et al: Growth hormone (GH) response to a single intravenous injection of synthetic GH-releasing hormone in prepubertal children with growth failure, J Clin Endocrinol Metab 65(3):387–394, 1987.

376. Schriock EA, et al: Effect of growth hormone (GH)-releasing hormone (GRH) on plasma GH in relation to magnitude and duration of GH deficiency in 26 children and adults with isolated GH deficiency or multiple pituitary hormone deficiencies: evidence for hypothalamic GRH deficiency, J Clin Endocrinol Metab 58:1043–1049, 1984.

377. Laron Z, et al: Differential diagnosis between hypothalamic and pituitary hGH deficiency with the aid of synthetic GH-RH 1-44, Clin Endocrinol 21:9–12, 1984.

378. Pintor C, et al: Growth-hormone releasing factor and clonidine in children with constitutional growth delay: evidence for defective pituitary growth hormone reserve, J Endocrinol Invest 7:253–256, 1984.

379. Reiter JC, Craen M, van Vliet G: Decreased growth hormone response to growth hormone-releasing hormone in Turner's syndrome: relation to body weight and adiposity, Acta Endocrinol 125:38–42, 1991.

380. Lannering B, Albertsson-Wikland K: Growth hormone release in children after cranial irradiation, Horm Res 27(1):13–22, 1987.

381. Takano K, et al: Plasma growth hormone (GH) response to GH-releasing factor (SM-8144) in children of short stature and patients with GH deficiency, Endocrinol Japon 34(1):117–128, 1987.

382. Cappa M, et al: Growth hormone response to growth hormone releasing hormone 1–40 in Turner's syndrome, Horm Res 27(1):1–6, 1987.

383. Rogol AD, et al: Growth hormone release in response to human pancreatic tumor growth hormone-releasing hormone 1–40 in children with short stature, J Clin Endocrinol Metab 59(4):580–586, 1984.

384. Ahmed SR, Shalet SM: Hypothalamic growth hormone releasing factor deficiency following cranial irradiation, Clin Endocrinol 21:483–488, 1984.

385. Romer TE, et al: Growth hormone-releasing hormone reverses secondary somatotroph unresponsiveness, J Clin Endocrinol Metab 72:503–506, 1991.

386. Hindmarsh PC, Swift PG: An assessment of growth hormone provocation tests, Arch Dis Child 72(4):362–367, 1995; discussion 367–368.

387. Dysken MW, et al: Intrasubject reproducibility of growth hormone-releasing hormone-stimulated growth hormone in older women, older men, and younger men, Biol Psychiatry 33(8-9):610–617, 1993.

388. Williams T, et al: Impaired growth hormone responses to growth hormone-releasing factor in obesity: a pituitary defect reversed with weight reduction, N Engl J M 311(22):1403–1407, 1984.

389. Scacchi M, Pincelli AI, Cavagnini F: Growth hormone in obesity, Int J Obes Rel Metab Dis 23(3):260–271, 1999.

390. Bing-You RG, Bigos ST, Oppenheim DS: Serum growth hormone response to growth hormone-releasing hormone in non-obese and obese adults with hypopituitarism, Metab Clin Exp 42(6):790–794, 1993.

391. Valetto MR, et al: Reproducibility of the growth hormone response to stimulation with growth hormone-releasing hormone plus arginine during lifespan, Eur J Endocrinol 135(5):568–572, 1996.

392. Cappa M, et al: The growth hormone response to pyridostigmine plus growth hormone releasing hormone is not influenced by pubertal maturation, J Endocrinol Invest 14(1):41–45, 1991.

393. Maghnie M, et al: GHRH plus arginine in the diagnosis of acquired GH deficiency of childhood-onset, J Clin Endocrinol Metab 87(6):2740–2744, 2007.

394. Groisne C, et al: Factors influencing the growth hormone response to growth hormone-releasing hormone in children with idiopathic growth hormone deficiency, Horm Res 58(2):94–98, 2002.

395. Ghigo E, et al: A new test for the diagnosis of growth hormone deficiency due to primary pituitary impairment: combined administration of pyridostigmine and growth hormone-releasing hormone, J Endocrinol Invest 13(4):307–316, 1990.

396. Donaubauer J, et al: Re-assessment of growth hormone secretion in young adult patients with childhood-onset growth hormone deficiency, Clin Endocrinol 58(4):456–463, 2003.

397. Ghigo E, et al: New approach to the diagnosis of growth hormone deficiency in adults, Eur J Endocrinol 134(3):352–356, 1996.

398. Aimaretti G, et al: Comparison between insulin-induced hypoglycaemia and growth hormone (GH)-releasing hormone + arginine as provocative tests for the diagnosis of GH deficiency in adults, J Clin Endocrinol Metab 83:1615–1618, 1998.

399. Biller BM, et al: Sensitivity and specificity of six tests for the diagnosis of adult GH deficiency, J Clin Endocrinol Metab 87(5):2067–2079, 2002.

400. Ho KK: Consensus guidelines for the diagnosis and treatment of adults with GH deficiency II: a statement of the GH Research Society in association with the European Society for Pediatric Endocrinology, Lawson Wilkins Society, European Society of Endocrinology, Japan Endocrine Society, and Endocrine Society of Australia, Eur J Endocrinol 157(6):695–700, 2007.

401. Molitch ME, et al: Evaluation and treatment of adult growth hormone deficiency: an Endocrine Society Clinical Practice Guideline, J Clin Endocrinol Metab 91(5):1621–1634, 2006.

402. Darzy KH, et al: The usefulness of the combined growth hormone (GH)-releasing hormone and arginine stimulation test in the diagnosis of radiation-induced GH deficiency is dependent on the post-irradiation time interval, J Clin Endocrinol Metab 88(1):95–102, 2003.

403. Corneli G, et al: The cut-off limits of the GH response to GH-releasing hormone-arginine test related to body mass index, Eur J Endocrinol 153(2):257–264, 2005.

404. Popovic V, et al: GH-releasing hormone and GH-releasing peptide-6 for diagnostic testing in GH-deficient adults [see comments], Lancet 356(9236):1137–1142, 2000.

405. Kelestimur F, et al: Effect of obesity and morbid obesity on the growth hormone (GH) secretion elicited by the combined GHRH + GHRP-6 test, Clin Endocrinol (Oxf) 64(6):667–671, 2006.

406. Thorner MO, et al: Acceleration of growth in two children treated with human growth hormone-releasing factor, N Engl J Med 312(1):4–9, 1985.

407. Thorner MO, et al: Acceleration of growth rate in growth hormone-deficient children treated with human growth hormone-releasing hormone, Pediatr Res 24(2):145–151, 1988.

408. Neyzi O, et al: Growth response to growth hormone-releasing hormone(1-29)-NH2 compared with growth hormone, Acta Paediatr 388(suppl):16–21, 1993; discussion 22.

409. Chen RG, et al: A comparative study of growth hormone (GH) and GH-releasing hormone(1-29)-NH2 for stimulation of growth in children with GH deficiency, Acta Paediatr Suppl 388:32–35, 1993; discussion 36.

410. Ross RJ, et al: Treatment of growth-hormone deficiency with growth-hormone-releasing hormone, Lancet 1(8523):5–8, 1987.

411. Takano K, et al: Human growth hormone-releasing hormone (hGH-RH; hGRF) treatment of four patients with GH deficiency, Endocrinol Japon 35:775–781, 1988.

412. Smith PJ, Brook CG: Growth hormone releasing hormone or growth hormone treatment in growth hormone insufficiency? Arch Dis Child 63(6):629–634, 1988.

413. Butenandt O, Staudt B: Comparison of growth hormone releasing hormone therapy and growth hormone therapy in growth hormone deficiency, Eur J Pediatr 148(5):393–395, 1989.

414. Duck SC, et al: Subcutaneous growth hormone-releasing hormone therapy in growth hormone-deficient children: first year of therapy, J Clin Endocrinol Metab 75(4):1115–1120, 1992.

415. Kirk JM, et al: Treatment with GHRH(1-29)NH2 in children with idiopathic short stature induces a sustained increase in growth velocity, Clin Endocrinol 41(4):487–493, 1994.

416. Pasqualini T, et al: Growth acceleration in children with chronic renal failure treated with growth-hormone-releasing hormone (GHRH), Medicina 56(3):241–246, 1996.

417. Ogilvy-Stuart AL, et al: Treatment of radiation-induced growth hormone deficiency with growth hormone-releasing hormone, Clin Endocrinol 46(5):571–578, 1997.

418. Rochiccioli PE, et al: Results of 1-year growth hormone (GH)-releasing hormone-(1-44) treatment on growth, somatomedin-C, and 24-hour GH secretion in six children with partial GH deficiency, J Clin Endocrinol Metab 65:268–274, 1987.

419. Bozzola M, et al: Long term growth hormone (GH)-releasing hormone and biosynthetic GH therapy in GH-deficient children: comparison of therapeutic effectiveness, J Endocrinol Invest 13(3):235–239, 1990.

420. Lievre M, et al: Treatment with growth hormone-releasing hormone (GHRH) 1-44 in children with idiopathic growth hormone deficiency: a randomized double-blind dose-effect study. The GHRH European Multicenter Study (GEMS) Group, Fundam Clin Pharmacol 6(8-9):359–366, 1992.

421. Wit JM, et al: Short-term effect on growth of two doses of GRF 1-44 in children with growth hormone deficiency: comparison with growth induced by methionyl-GH administration, Horm Res 27:181–189, 1987.

422. Lanes R, Carrillo E: Long-term therapy with a single daily subcutaneous dose of growth hormone releasing hormone (1-29) in prepubertal growth hormone deficient children. Venezuelan Collaborative Study Group, J Pediatr Endocrinol 7(4):303–308, 1994.

423. Thorner M, et al: Once daily subcutaneous growth hormone-releasing hormone therapy accelerates growth in growth hormone-deficient children during the first year of therapy. Geref International Study Group, J Clin Endocrinol Metab 81(3):1189–1196, 1996.

424. Low LC, et al: Long term pulsatile growth hormone (GH)-releasing hormone therapy in children with GH deficiency, J Clin Endocrinol Metab 66(3):611–617, 1988.

425. Lippe BM, et al: Reversible hypothyroidism in growth hormone-deficient children treated with human growth hormone, J Clin Endocrinol Metab 40(4):612–618, 1975.

426. Ghigo E, et al: Diagnostic and therapeutic uses of growth hormone-releasing substances in adult and elderly subjects, Baillieres Clin Endocrinol Metab 12(2):341–358, 1998.

427. Nakamura S, et al: Aging-related changes in in vivo release of growth hormone-releasing hormone and somatostatin from the stalk-median eminence in female rhesus monkeys (Macaca mulatta), J Clin Endocrinol Metab 88(2):827–833, 2003.

428. Corpas E, et al: Growth hormone (GH)-releasing hormone-(1-29) twice daily reverses the decreased GH and insulin-like growth factor-I levels in old men, J Clin Endocrinol Metab 75(2):530–535, 1992.

429. Corpas E, et al: Continuous subcutaneous infusions of growth hormone (GH) releasing hormone 1-44 for 14 days increase GH and insulin-like growth factor-I levels in old men, J Clin Endocrinol Metab 76(1):134–138, 1993.

430. Vittone J, et al: Effects of single nightly injections of growth hormone-releasing hormone (GHRH 1-29) in healthy elderly men, Metab Clin Exp 46(1):89–96, 1997.

431. Ionescu M, Frohman LA: Pulsatile secretion of growth hormone (GH) persists during continuous stimulation by CJC-1295, a long-acting GH-releasing hormone analog, J Clin Endocrinol Metab 91(12):4792–4797, 2006.

432. Teichman SL, et al: Prolonged stimulation of growth hormone (GH) and insulin-like growth factor I secretion by CJC-1295, a long-acting analog of GH-releasing hormone, in healthy adults, J Clin Endocrinol Metab 91(3):799–805, 2006.

433. Munafo A, et al: Polyethylene glycol-conjugated growth hormone-releasing hormone is long acting and stimulates GH in healthy young and elderly subjects, Eur J Endocrinol 153(2):249–256, 2005.

434. Bowers CY, et al: Structure-activity relationships of a synthetic pentapeptide that specifically releases growth hormone in vitro, Endocrinology 106(3):663–667, 1980.

435. Kamiji MM, Inui A: The role of ghrelin and ghrelin analogues in wasting disease, Curr Opin Clin Nutr Metab Care 11(4):443–451, 2008.

436. Smith RG: Development of growth hormone secretagogues, Endocr Rev 26(3):346–360, 2005.

437. Howard AD, et al: A receptor in pituitary and hypothalamus that functions in growth hormone release, Science 273(5277):974–977, 1996.

438. Kojima M, et al: Ghrelin is a growth-hormone-releasing acylated peptide from stomach, Nature 402(6762):656–660, 1999.

439. Tomasetto C, et al: Identification and characterization of a novel gastric peptide hormone: the motilin-related peptide, Gastroenterology 119:395–405, 2000.

440. Higgins SC, Gueorguiev M, Korbonits M: Ghrelin, the peripheral hunger hormone, Ann Med 39(2):116–136, 2007.

441. Tschöp M, Smiley DL, Heiman ML: Ghrelin induces adiposity in rodents, Nature 407:908–913, 2000.

442. Zhang JV, et al: Obestatin, a peptide encoded by the ghrelin gene, opposes ghrelin's effects on food intake, Science 310(5750):996–999, 2005.

443. Gibson C, Korbonits M: The yin and yang of the ghrelin gene products, Immunol Endocr Metabol Agents Med Chem 8(4):292–302, 2008.

444. Zhu X, et al: On the processing of proghrelin to ghrelin, J Biol Chem 281(50):38867–38870, 2006.

445. Yang J, et al: Identification of the acyltransferase that octanoylates ghrelin, an appetite-stimulating peptide hormone, Cell 132(3):387–396, 2008.

446. Gutierrez JA, et al: Ghrelin octanoylation mediated by an orphan lipid transferase, Proc Natl Acad Sci U S A 105(17):6320–6325, 2008.

447. Yang J, et al: Inhibition of ghrelin O-acyltransferase (GOAT) by octanoylated pentapeptides, Proc Natl Acad Sci U S A 105(31):10750–10755, 2008.

448. Akamizu T, et al: Separate measurement of plasma levels of acylated and desacyl ghrelin in healthy subjects using a new direct ELISA assay, J Clin Endocrinol Metab 90(1):6–9, 2005.

449. Nussbaum SR, et al: Highly sensitive two-site immunoradiometric assay of parathyrin, and its clinical utility in evaluating patients with hypercalcemia, Clin Chem 33(8):1364–1367, 1987.

450. Liu J, et al: Novel ghrelin assays provide evidence for independent regulation of ghrelin acylation and secretion in healthy young men, J Clin Endocrinol Metab 93(5):1980–1987, 2008.

451. Hosoda H, et al: Optimum collection and storage conditions for ghrelin measurements: octanoyl modification of ghrelin is rapidly hydrolyzed to desacyl ghrelin in blood samples, Clin Chem 50(6):1077–1080, 2004.

452. Groschl M, Uhr M, Kraus T: Evaluation of the comparability of commercial ghrelin assays [comment], Clin Chem 50(2):457–458, 2004.

453. Hotta M, et al: Plasma levels of intact and degraded ghrelin and their responses to glucose infusion in anorexia nervosa, J Clin Endocrinol Metab 89(11):5707–5712, 2004.

454. Cowley MA, et al: The distribution and mechanism of action of ghrelin in the CNS demonstrates a novel hypothalamic circuit regulating energy homeostasis, Neuron 37:649–661, 2003.

455. Banks WA, et al: Extent and direction of ghrelin transport across the blood-brain barrier is determined by its unique primary structure, J Pharmacol Exp Ther 302:822–827, 2002.

456. Cummings DE, et al: A preprandial rise in plasma ghrelin levels suggests a role in meal initiation in humans, Diabetes 50:1714–1719, 2001.

457. Cummings DE, et al: Plasma ghrelin levels after diet-induced weight loss or gastric bypass surgery, N Engl J Med 346:1623–1630, 2002.

458. Chan JL, et al: Ghrelin levels are not regulated by recombinant leptin administration and/or three days of fasting in healthy subjects, J Clin Endocrinol Metab 89(1):335–343, 2004.

459. Ariyasu H, et al: Stomach is a major source of circulating ghrelin, and feeding state determines plasma ghrelin-like immunoreactivity levels in humans, J Clin Endocrinol Metab 86:4753–4758, 2001.

460. McLaughlin T, et al: Plasma ghrelin concentrations are decreased in insulin-resistant obese adults relative to equally obese insulin-sensitive controls, J Clin Endocrinol Metab 89(4):1630–1635, 2004.

461. Marleau S, et al: EP 80317, a ligand of the CD36 scavenger receptor, protects apolipoprotein E-deficient mice from developing atherosclerotic lesions, FASEB J 19(13):1869–1871, 2005.

462. Korbonits M, et al: Ghrelin—a hormone with multiple functions, Frontiers Neuroendocrinol 25(1):27–68, 2004.

463. Halem HA, et al: Novel analogs of ghrelin: physiological and clinical implications, Eur J Endocrinol 151(suppl 2):S071–S075, 2004.

464. Halem HA, et al: A novel growth hormone secretagogue-1a receptor antagonist that blocks ghrelin-induced growth hormone secretion but induces increased body weight gain, Neuroendocrinology 81(5):339–349, 2005.

465. Toshinai K, et al: Des-acyl ghrelin induces food intake by a mechanism independent of the growth hormone secretagogue receptor, Endocrinology 147(5):2306–2314, 2006.

466. White HK, et al: Effects of an oral growth hormone secretagogue in older adults, J Clin Endocrinol Metab 94(4):1198–1206, 2009.

467. Nass R, et al: Effects of an oral ghrelin mimetic on body composition and clinical outcomes in healthy older adults: a randomized trial, Ann Intern Med 149(9):601–611, 2008.

468. Holst B, et al: High constitutive signaling of the ghrelin receptor—identification of a potent inverse agonist, Mol Endocrinol 17:2201–2210, 2003.

469. Smith RG, et al: Adenosine: a partial agonist of the growth hormone secretagogue receptor, Biochem Biophys Res Commun 276:1306–1313, 2003.

470. Tullin S, et al: Adenosine is an agonist of the growth hormone secretagogue receptor, Endocrinology 141:3397–3402, 2000.

471. Carreira MC, et al: Adenosine does not bind to the growth hormone secretagogue receptor type-1a (GHS-R1a), J Endocrinol 191(1):147–157, 2006.

472. Hermansson N-O, et al: Adenosine is not a direct GHSR agonist—artificial cross-talk between GHSR and adenosine receptor pathways, Acta Physiol 190(1):77–86, 2007.

473. Deghenghi R, et al: Cortistatin, but not somatostatin, binds to growth hormone secretagogue (GHS) receptors of human pituitary gland, J Endocrinol Invest 24:RC1–RC3, 2001.

474. Casanueva FF, et al: Growth hormone-releasing hormone as an agonist of the ghrelin receptor GHS-R1a, Proc Natl Acad Sci U S A 105(51):20452–20457, 2008.

475. Sun Y, et al: Ghrelin stimulation of growth hormone release and appetite is mediated through the growth hormone secretagogue receptor, Proc Natl Acad Sci U S A 101(13):4679–4684, 2004.

476. Bodart V, et al: CD36 mediates the cardiovascular action of growth hormone-releasing peptides in the heart, Circ Res 90(8):844–849, 2002.

477. Tena-Sempere M: Exploring the role of ghrelin as novel regulator of gonadal function, Growth Horm IGF Res 15(2):83–88, 2005.

478. Lanfranco F, et al: Acylated ghrelin inhibits spontaneous luteinizing hormone pulsatility and responsiveness to naloxone but not that to gonadotropin-releasing hormone in young men: evidence for a central inhibitory action of ghrelin on the gonadal axis, J Clin Endocrinol Metab 93(9):3633–3639, 2008.

479. Hosoda H, Kojima M, Kangawa K: Biological, physiological, and pharmacological aspects of ghrelin, J Pharmacol Sci 100(5):398–410, 2006.

480. Vestergaard ET, et al: Ghrelin infusion in humans induces acute insulin resistance and lipolysis independent of growth hormone signaling, Diabetes 57(12):3205–3210, 2008.

481. Tebbe JJ, et al: Ghrelin-induced stimulation of colonic propulsion is dependent on hypothalamic neuropeptide Y1- and corticotrophin-releasing factor 1 receptor activation, J Neuroendocrinol 17(9):570–576, 2005.

482. Gauna C, et al: Ghrelin stimulates, whereas des-octanoyl ghrelin inhibits, glucose output by primary hepatocytes, J Clin Endocrinol Metab 90(2):1055–1060, 2005.

483. Muccioli G, et al: Ghrelin and des-acyl ghrelin both inhibit isoproterenol-induced lipolysis in rat adipocytes via a non-type 1a growth hormone secretagogue receptor, Eur J Pharmacol 498(1–3):27–35, 2004.

484. Cao JM, Ong H, Chen C: Effects of ghrelin and synthetic GH secretagogues on the cardiovascular system, Trends Endocrinol Metab 17(1):13–18, 2006.

485. Henriques-Coelho T, et al: Ghrelin reverses molecular, structural and hemodynamic alterations of the right ventricle in pulmonary hypertension, Rev Port Cardiol 25(1):55–63, 2006.

486. Tesauro M, et al: Ghrelin improves endothelial function in patients with metabolic syndrome, Circulation 112(19):2986–2992, 2005.

487. Schwenke DO, et al: Early ghrelin treatment after myocardial infarction prevents an increase in cardiac sympathetic tone and reduces mortality, Endocrinology 149(10):5172–5176, 2008.

488. Rudd JA, et al: Anti-emetic activity of ghrelin in ferrets exposed to the cytotoxic anti-cancer agent cisplatin, Neurosci Lett 392(1-2):79–83, 2006.

489. Brunetti L, et al: Effects of ghrelin and amylin on dopamine, norepinephrine and serotonin release in the hypothalamus, Eur J Pharmacol 454(2-3):189–192, 2002.

490. Dixit VD, Taub DD: Ghrelin and immunity: a young player in an old field, Exp Gerontol 40(11):900–910, 2005.

491. Yada T, et al: Ghrelin stimulates phagocytosis and superoxide production in fish leukocytes, J Endocrinol 189(1):57–65, 2006.

492. Takeda R, et al: Ghrelin improves renal function in mice with ischemic acute renal failure, J Am Soc Nephrol 17(1):113–121, 2006.

493. Sibilia V, et al: Ghrelin protects against ethanol-induced gastric ulcers in rats: studies on the mechanisms of action, Endocrinology 144(1):353–359, 2003.

494. Konturek PC, et al: Ghrelin—a new gastroprotective factor in gastric mucosa, J Physiol Pharmacol 55(2):325–336, 2004.

495. Granado M, et al: Anti-inflammatory effect of the ghrelin agonist growth hormone-releasing peptide-2 (GHRP-2) in arthritic rats, Am J Physiol Endocrinol Metab 288(3):E486–E492, 2005.

496. Wu R, et al: Ghrelin improves tissue perfusion in severe sepsis via downregulation of endothelin-1, Cardiovasc Res 68(2):318–326, 2005.

497. Svensson J, et al: Treatment with the oral growth hormone secretagogue MK-677 increases markers of bone formation and bone resorption in obese young males, J Bone Miner Res 13:1158–1166, 1998.

498. Fukushima N, et al: Ghrelin directly regulates bone formation, J Bone Miner Res 20(5):790–798, 2005.

499. Caminos JE, et al: The endogenous growth hormone secretagogue (ghrelin) is synthesized and secreted by chondrocytes, Endocrinology 146(3):1285–1292, 2005.

500. Matsuda K, et al: Stimulatory effect of n-octanoylated ghrelin on locomotor activity in the goldfish, Carassius auratus, Peptides 27(6):1335–1340, 2006.

501. Jaszberenyi M, et al: Mediation of the behavioral, endocrine and thermoregulatory actions of ghrelin, Horm Behav 50(2):266–273, 2006.

502. Tang-Christensen M, et al: Central administration of ghrelin and agouti-related protein (83-132) increases food intake and decreases spontaneous locomotor activity in rats, Endocrinology 145(10):4645–4652, 2004.

503. Lutter M, et al: The orexigenic hormone ghrelin defends against depressive symptoms of chronic stress, Nat Neurosci 11(7):752–753, 2008.

504. Diano S, et al: Ghrelin controls hippocampal spine synapse density and memory performance, Nature Neurosci 9(3):381–388, 2006.

505. Maheshwari HG, et al: Selective lack of growth hormone (GH) response to the GH-releasing peptide hexarelin in patients with GH-releasing hormone receptor deficiency, J Clin Endocrinol Metab 84(3):956–959, 1999.

506. Sun Y, Garcia JM, Smith RG: Ghrelin and growth hormone secretagogue receptor expression in mice during aging, Endocrinology 148(3):1323–1329, 2007.

507. Broglio F, et al: The endocrine response to ghrelin as a function of gender in humans in young and elderly subjects, J Clin Endocrinol Metab 88:1537–1542, 2003.

508. Zizzari P, et al: Endogenous ghrelin regulates episodic growth hormone (GH) secretion by amplifying GH pulse amplitude: evidence from antagonism of the GH secretagogue-R1a receptor, Endocrinology 146(9):3836–3842, 2005.

509. Pantel J, et al: Loss of constitutive activity of the growth hormone secretagogue receptor in familial short stature [see comment], J Clin Invest 116(3):760–768, 2006.

510. Sun Y, Ahmed S, Smith RG: Deletion of ghrelin impairs neither growth nor appetite, Mol Cell Biol 23:7973–7981, 2003.

511. Muller AF, et al: Ghrelin drives GH secretion during fasting in man, Eur J Endocrinol 146:203–207, 2002.

512. Koutkia P, et al: Reciprocal changes in endogenous ghrelin and growth hormone during fasting in healthy women, Am J Physiol Endocrinol Metab 289(5):E814–E822, 2005.

513. Misra M, et al: Secretory dynamics of leptin in adolescent girls with anorexia nervosa and healthy adolescents, Am J Physiol Endocrinol Metab 289(3):E373–E381, 2005.

514. Espelund U, et al: Fasting unmasks a strong inverse association between ghrelin and cortisol in serum: studies in obese and normal-weight subjects, J Clin Endocrinol Metab 90(2):741–746, 2005.

515. Norrelund H: The metabolic role of growth hormone in humans with particular reference to fasting, Growth Horm IGF Res 15(2):95–122, 2005.

516. Natalucci G, et al: Spontaneous 24-h ghrelin secretion pattern in fasting subjects: maintenance of a meal-related pattern, Eur J Endocrinol 152(6):845–850, 2005.

517. Avram AM, et al: Endogenous circulating ghrelin does not mediate growth hormone rhythmicity or response to fasting, J Clin Endocrinol Metab 90(5):2982–2987, 2005.

518. Nass R, et al: Evidence for acyl-ghrelin modulation of growth hormone release in the fed state, J Clin Endocrinol Metab 93(5):1988–1994, 2008.

519. Torsello A, et al: Novel hexarelin analogs stimulate feeding in the rat through a mechanism not involving growth hormone release, Eur J Pharmacol 360(2-3):123–129, 1998.

520. Wortley KE, et al: Genetic deletion of ghrelin does not decrease food intake but influences metabolic fuel preference, Proc Natl Acad Sci U S A 101(21):8227–8232, 2004.

521. Nass R, et al: Chronic changes in peripheral growth hormone levels do not affect ghrelin stomach mRNA expression and serum ghrelin levels in three transgenic mouse models, J Neuroendocrinol 16(8):669–675, 2004.

522. Katakami H, et al: Cloning and characterization of ghrelin and GHRH in the rhesus monkey, Macaca mulatto. 86th Annual Meeting of the Endocrine Society, New Orleans, 2004. Abstract OR47-2.

523. Kola B, et al: Expanding role of AMPK in endocrinology, Trends Endocrinol Metab 17(5):205–215, 2006.

524. Kola B, Korbonits M: Shedding light on the intricate puzzle of ghrelin's effects on appetite regulation, J Endocrinol 202(5):191–198, 2009.

525. Broglio F, et al: Ghrelin, a natural GH secretagogue produced by the stomach, induces hyperglycemia and reduces insulin secretion in humans, J Clin Endocrinol Metab 86:5083–5086, 2003.

526. Kola B, et al: Cannabinoids and ghrelin have both central and peripheral metabolic and cardiac effects via AMP-activated protein kinase, J Biol Chem 280(26):25196–25201, 2005.

527. Sun Y, et al: Ablation of ghrelin improves the diabetic but not obese phenotype of ob/ob mice, Cell Metab 3(5):379–386, 2006.
528. Lall S, et al: Growth hormone (GH)-independent stimulation of adiposity by GH secretagogues, Biochem Biophys Res Commun 280:132–138, 2001.
529. Nagaya N, Kangawa K: Ghrelin improves left ventricular dysfunction and cardiac cachexia in heart failure, Curr Opin Pharmacol 3:146–151, 2003.
530. Nagaya N, Kangawa K: Ghrelin, a novel growth hormone-releasing peptide, in the treatment of chronic heart failure, Regul.Pept 114:71–77, 2003.
531. Katugampola SD, Pallikaros Z, Davenport AP: [125I-His(9)]-ghrelin, a novel radioligand for localizing GHS orphan receptors in human and rat tissue: up-regulation of receptors with athersclerosis, Br J Pharmacol 134:143–149, 2001.
532. Baldanzi G, et al: Ghrelin and des-acyl ghrelin inhibit cell death in cardiomyocytes and endothelial cells through ERK1/2 and PI 3-kinase/AKT, J Cell Biol 159:1029–1037, 2002.
533. Caminos JE, et al: Expression of ghrelin in the cyclic and pregnant rat ovary, Endocrinology 144:1594–1602, 2003.
534. Obal F Jr, et al: Sleep in mice with nonfunctional growth hormone-releasing hormone receptors, Am J Physiol Regul Integr Comp Physiol 284(1):R131–R139, 2003.
535. Carlini VP, et al: Ghrelin increases anxiety-like behavior and memory retention in rats, Biochem Biophys Res Commun 299:739–743, 2002.
536. Asakawa A, et al: A role of ghrelin in neuroendocrine and behavioral responses to stress in mice, Neuroendocrinology 74:143–147, 2001.
537. Hansen TK, et al: Weight loss increases circulating levels of ghrelin in human obesity, Clin Endocrinol (Oxf) 56:203–206, 2002.
538. Wisse BE, et al: Reversal of cancer anorexia by blockade of central melanocortin receptors in rats, Endocrinology 142:3292–3301, 2001.
539. Shimizu Y, et al: Increased plasma ghrelin level in lung cancer cachexia, Clin Cancer Res 9:774–778, 2003.
540. Nagaya N, et al: Elevated circulating level of ghrelin in cachexia associated with chronic heart failure: relationships between ghrelin and anabolic/catabolic factors, Circulation 104:2034–2038, 2001.
541. Nakai Y, et al: Plasma levels of active form of ghrelin during oral glucose tolerance test in patients with anorexia nervosa, Eur J Endocrinol 149:R001–R003, 2003.
542. Tanaka M, et al: Fasting plasma ghrelin levels in subtypes of anorexia nervosa, Psychoneuroendocrinology 28:829–835, 2003.
543. Krsek M, et al: Plasma ghrelin levels and malnutrition: a comparison of two etiologies, Eat Weight Disord 8:207–211, 2003.
544. Iniguez G, et al: Fasting and post-glucose ghrelin levels in SGA infants: relationships with size and weight gain at one year of age, J Clin Endocrinol Metab 87:5830–5833, 2002.
545. Tschöp M, et al: Circulating ghrelin levels are decreased in human obesity, Diabetes 50:707–709, 2001.
546. Aylwin SJ: Gastrointestinal surgery and gut hormones, Curr Opin Endocrinol Diabetes 12(1):89–98, 2005.
547. Haqq AM, et al: Serum ghrelin levels are inversely correlated with body mass index, age, and insulin concentrations in normal children and are markedly increased in Prader-Willi syndrome, J Clin Endocrinol Metab 88:174–178, 2003.
548. Cummings DE, et al: Elevated plasma ghrelin levels in Prader-Willi syndrome, Nat Med 8:643–644, 2002.
549. DelParigi A, et al: High circulating ghrelin: a potential cause for hyperphagia and obesity in Prader-Willi syndrome, J Clin Endocrinol Metab 87(12):5461–5464, 2002.
550. Goldstone AP, et al: Elevated fasting plasma ghrelin in Prader-Willi syndrome adults is not solely explained by their reduced visceral adiposity and insulin resistance, J Clin Endocrinol Metab 89:1718–1726, 2004.
551. Goldstone AP: Prader-Willi syndrome: advances in genetics, pathophysiology and treatment, Trends Endocrinol Metab 15:12–20, 2004.
552. Goldstone AP, et al: Fasting and postprandial hyperghrelinemia in Prader-Willi syndrome is partially explained by hypoinsulinemia, and is not due to peptide YY3-36 deficiency or seen in hypothalamic obesity due to craniopharyngioma, J Clin Endocrinol Metab 90(5):2681–2690, 2005.
553. Tan TM, et al: Somatostatin infusion lowers plasma ghrelin without reducing appetite in adults with Prader-Willi syndrome, J Clin Endocrinol Metab 89(8):4162–4165, 2004.
554. Freda PU, et al: Serum ghrelin levels in acromegaly: effects of surgical and long-acting octreotide therapy, J Clin Endocrinol Metab 88:2037–2044, 2003.
555. Cappiello V, et al: Circulating ghrelin levels in basal conditions and during glucose tolerance test in acromegalic patients, Eur J Endocrinol 147:189–194, 2002.
556. Giavoli C, et al: Different effects of short- and long-term recombinant hGH administration on ghrelin and adiponectin levels in GH-deficient adults, Clin Endocrinol 61(1):81–87, 2004.
557. Riis AL, et al: Hyperthyroidism is associated with suppressed circulating ghrelin levels, J Clin Endocrinol Metab 88:853–857, 2003.
558. Jarkovska Z, et al: Plasma levels of active and total ghrelin in renal failure: a relationship with GH/IGF-I axis, Growth Horm IGF Res 15(6):369–376, 2005.
559. Patterson M, et al: Characterization of ghrelin-like immunoreactivity in human plasma, J Clin Endocrinol Metab 90(4):2205–2211, 2005.
560. Shearman LP, et al: Ghrelin neutralization by a ribonucleic acid-SPM ameliorates obesity in diet-induced obese mice, Endocrinology 147(3):1517–1526, 2006.
561. Vizcarra JA, et al: Active immunization against ghrelin decreases weight gain and alters plasma concentrations of growth hormone in growing pigs, Domest Anim Endocrinol 2006.
562. Shuto Y, et al: Hypothalamic growth hormone secretagogue receptor regulates growth hormone secretion, feeding, and adiposity, J Clin Invest 109:1429–1436, 2002.
563. Zigman JM, et al: Mice lacking ghrelin receptors resist the development of diet-induced obesity, J Clin Invest 115(12):3564–3572, 2005.
564. Asakawa A, et al: Antagonism of ghrelin receptor reduces food intake and body weight gain in mice, Gut 52:947–952, 2003.
565. Sun Y, et al: Characterization of adult ghrelin and ghrelin receptor knockout mice under positive and negative energy balance, Endocrinology 149(2):843–850, 2008.
566. Wortley KE, et al: Deletion of ghrelin reveals no effect on food intake, but a primary role in energy balance, Obes Res 12(1):170, 2004.
567. Wortley KE, et al: Absence of ghrelin protects against early-onset obesity [see comment], J Clin Invest 115(12):3573–3578, 2005.
568. De Smet B, et al: Energy homeostasis and gastric emptying in ghrelin knockout mice, J Pharmacol Exp Ther 316(1):431–439, 2006.
569. Ariyasu H, et al: Transgenic mice overexpressing des-acyl ghrelin show small phenotype, Endocrinology 146(1):355–364, 2005.
570. Wei W, et al: Effect of chronic hyperghrelinemia on ingestive action of ghrelin, Am J Physiol Regul Integr Comp Physiol 290(3):R803–R808, 2006.
571. Laron Z, et al: Growth hormone releasing activity by intranasal administration of a synthetic hexapeptide (hexarelin), Clin Endocrinol 41(4):539–541, 1994.
572. Aloi JA, et al: Neuroendocrine responses to a novel growth-hormone secretagogue, L-692,429, in healthy older subjects, J Clin Endocrinol Metab 79:943–949, 1994.
573. Imbimbo BP, et al: Growth hormone-releasing activity of hexarelin in humans: a dose-response study, Eur J Clin Pharmacol 46(5):421–425, 1994.
574. Casanueva FF, et al: Role of the new growth hormone-releasing secretagogues in the diagnosis of some hypothalamopituitary pathologies, Metab Clin Exp 45(8 suppl 1):123–126, 1996.
575. Arvat E, et al: Arginine and growth hormone-releasing hormone restore the blunted growth hormone-releasing activity of hexarelin in elderly subjects, J Clin Endocrinol Metab 79(5):1440–1443, 1994.
576. Bowers CY, et al: Growth hormone (GH)-releasing peptide stimulates GH release in normal men and acts synergistically with GH-releasing hormone, J Clin Endocrinol Metab 70(4):975–982, 1990.
577. Micic D, et al: Preserved growth hormone (GH) secretion in aged and very old subjects after testing with the combined stimulus GH-releasing hormone plus GH-releasing hexapeptide-6, J Clin Endocrinol Metab 83(7):2569–2572, 1998.
578. Maghnie M, et al: The growth hormone response to hexarelin in patients with different hypothalamic-pituitary abnormalities, J Clin Endocrinol Metab 83(11):3886–3889, 1998.
579. Arvat E, et al: Modulation of growth hormone-releasing activity of hexarelin in man, Neuroendocrinology 61(1):51–56, 1995.
580. Ghigo E, et al: Arginine enhances the growth hormone-releasing activity of a synthetic hexapeptide (GHRP-6) in elderly but not in young subjects after oral administration, J Endocrinol Invest 17(3):157–162, 1994.
581. Ghigo E, et al: Growth hormone-releasing peptides, Eur J Endocrinol 136(5):445–460, 1997.
582. Laron Z, et al: Growth hormone-releasing activity of growth hormone-releasing peptide-1 (a synthetic heptapeptide) in children and adolescents, Acta Endocrinol 129(5):424–426, 1993.
583. Bellone J, et al: Growth hormone-releasing effect of hexarelin, a new synthetic hexapeptide, before and during puberty, J Clin Endocrinol Metab 80(8):1090–1094, 1995.
584. Loche S, et al: The growth hormone-releasing activity of hexarelin, a new synthetic hexapeptide, in short normal and obese children and in hypopituitary subjects, J Clin Endocrinol Metab 80(2):674–678, 1995.
585. Ghigo E, et al: Growth hormone-releasing activity of growth hormone-releasing peptide-6 is maintained after short-term oral pretreatment with the hexapeptide in normal aging, Eur J Endocrinol 131(5):499–503, 1994.
586. Penalva A, et al: Influence of sex, age and adrenergic pathways on the growth hormone response to GHRP-6, Clin Endocrinol 38(1):87–91, 1993.
587. Veldhuis JD, et al: Estradiol potentiates ghrelin-stimulated pulsatile growth hormone secretion in postmenopausal women, J Clin Endocrinol Metab 91(9):3559–3565, 2006.
588. Villa P, et al: Estro-progestin supplementation enhances the growth hormone secretory responsiveness to ghrelin infusion in postmenopausal women, Fertil Steril 89(2):398–403, 2008.
589. Ghigo E, Aimaretti G, Corneli G: Diagnosis of adult GH deficiency, Growth Horm IGF Res 18(1):1–16, 2008.
590. Gasperi M, et al: Low dose hexarelin and growth hormone (GH)-releasing hormone as a diagnostic tool for the diagnosis of GH deficiency in adults: comparison with insulin-induced hypoglycemia test, J Clin Endocrinol Metab 84(8):2633–2637, 1999.
591. Peino R, et al: The use of growth hormone (GH) secretagogues in the diagnosis of GH deficiency in humans, Growth Horm IGF Res 9:101–105, 1999.
592. Chihara K, et al: A simple diagnostic test using GH-releasing peptide-2 in adult GH deficiency, Eur J Endocrinol 157(1):19–27, 2007.
593. Aimaretti G, et al: Endocrine responses to ghrelin in adult patients with isolated childhood-onset growth hormone deficiency, Clin Endocrinol (Oxf) 56(6):765–771, 2002.
594. Casanueva FF, Dieguez C: Interaction between body composition, leptin and growth hormone status, Baillieres Clin Endocrinol Metab 12(2):297–314, 1998.
595. Makimura H, et al: The effects of central adiposity on growth hormone (GH) response to GH-releasing hormone-arginine stimulation testing in men, J Clin Endocrinol Metab 93(11):4254–4260, 2008.
596. Cordido F, et al: Massive growth hormone (GH) discharge in obese subjects after the combined administration of GH-releasing hormone and GHRP-6: evidence for a marked somatotroph secretory capability in obesity [see comments], J Clin Endocrinol Metab 76(4):819–823, 1993.
597. Rahim A, O'Neill PA, Shalet SM: The effect of body composition on hexarelin-induced growth hormone release in normal elderly subjects, Clin Endocrinol 49(5):659–664, 1998.
598. Ghigo E, et al: Arginine potentiates but does not restore the blunted growth hormone response to growth hormone-releasing hormone in obesity, Metab Clin Exp 41(5):560–563, 1992.
599. Casanueva FF, et al: Depending on the time of administration, dexamethasone potentiates or blocks growth hormone-releasing hormone-induced growth hormone release in man, Neuroendocrinology 47:46–49, 1988.

600. Trainer PJ, et al: Pyridostigmine partially reverses dexamethasone-induced inhibition of the growth hormone response to growth hormone-releasing hormone, J Endocrinol 134(3):513–517, 1992.

601. Frantz AG, Rabkin MT: Human growth hormone: clinical measurement, response to hypoglycaemia and suppression by corticosteroids, N Engl J Med 271:1375–1381, 1964.

602. Magiakou MA, et al: Suppressed spontaneous and stimulated growth hormone secretion in patients with Cushing's disease before and after surgical cure, J Clin Endocrinol Metab 78(1):131–137, 1994.

603. Leal-Cerro A, et al: Inhibition of growth hormone release after the combined administration of GHRH and GHRP-6 in patients with Cushing's syndrome, Clin Endocrinol 41(5):649–654, 1994.

604. Leal-Cerro A, et al: Ghrelin is no longer able to stimulate growth hormone secretion in patients with Cushing's syndrome but instead induces exaggerated corticotropin and cortisol responses, Neuroendocrinology 76:390–396, 2002.

605. Giordano R, Picu A, Broglio F, et al: Ghrelin, hypothalamus-pituitary-adrenal (HPA) axis and Cushing's syndrome, Pituitary 7(4):243–248, 2004.

606. Leal-Cerro A, et al: Growth hormone releasing hormone priming increases growth hormone secretion in patients with Cushing's syndrome, Clin Endocrinol 38(4):399–403, 1993.

607. Nascif SO, et al: Decreased ghrelin-induced GH release in thyrotoxicosis: comparison with GH-releasing peptide-6 (GHRP-6) and GHRH, Pituitary 10(1):27–33, 2007.

608. Momany FA, et al: Conformational energy studies and in vitro and in vivo activity data on growth hormone-releasing peptides, Endocrinology 114(5):1531–1536, 1984.

609. Smith RG, et al: Modulation of pulsatile GH release through a novel receptor in hypothalamus and pituitary gland, Recent Prog Horm Res 51:261–285, 1996; discussion 285–286.

610. McDowell RS, et al: Growth hormone secretagogues: characterization, efficacy, and minimal bioactive conformation, Proc Natl Acad Sci U S A 92(24):11165–11169, 1995.

611. Patchett AA, et al: Design and biological activities of L-163,191 (MK-0677): a potent, orally active growth hormone secretagogue, Proc Natl Acad Sci U S A 92(15):7001–7005, 1995.

612. Elias KA, et al: In vitro characterization of four novel classes of growth hormone-releasing peptide, Endocrinology 136(12):5694–5699, 1995.

613. Smith RG, et al: Growth hormone releasing substances: types and their receptors, Horm Res 51(suppl 3):1–8, 1999.

614. Rahim A, O'Neill PA, Shalet SM: Growth hormone status during long-term hexarelin therapy, J Clin Endocrinol Metab 83(5):1644–1649, 1998.

615. Svensson J, et al: Two-month treatment of obese subjects with the oral growth hormone (GH) secretagogue MK-677 increases GH secretion, fat-free mass, and energy expenditure, J Clin Endocrinol Metab 83(2):362–369, 1998.

616. Loche S, et al: The growth hormone response to hexarelin in children: reproducibility and effect of sex steroids, J Clin Endocrinol Metab 82(3):861–864, 1997.

617. Mericq V, et al: Effects of eight months treatment with graded doses of a growth hormone (GH)-releasing peptide in GH-deficient children, J Clin Endocrinol Metab 83(7):2355–2360, 1998.

618. Yu H, et al: A double blind placebo-controlled efficacy trial of an oral growth hormone (GH) secretagogue (MK-0677) in GH deficient (GHD) children, Proceedings of the 80th Annual Meeting of the Endocrine Society, New Orleans, LA, 1998. Abstract OR24-6.

619. Codner E, et al: Effects of oral administration of ibutamoren mesylate, a nonpeptide growth hormone secretagogue, on the growth hormone-insulin-like growth factor I axis in growth hormone-deficient children, Clin Pharmacol Ther 70(1):91–98, 2001.

620. Laron Z, et al: Intranasal administration of the GHRP hexarelin accelerates growth in short children, Clin Endocrinol 43(5):631–635, 1995.

621. Schambelan M, et al: Recombinant human growth hormone in patients with HIV-associated wasting: a randomized, placebo-controlled trial, Serostim Study Group, Ann Intern Med 125(11):873–882, 1996.

622. Chapman IM, et al: Oral administration of growth hormone (GH) releasing peptide-mimetic MK-677 stimulates the GH/insulin-like growth factor-I axis in selected GH-deficient adults, J Clin Endocrinol Metab 82(10):3455–3463, 1997.

623. Svensson J, et al: Oral administration of the growth hormone secretagogue NN703 in adult patients with growth hormone deficiency, Clin Endocrinol (Oxf) 58(5):572–580, 2003.

624. Falutz J, et al: Metabolic effects of a growth hormone-releasing factor in patients with HIV, N Engl J Med 357(23):2359–2370, 2007.

625. Falutz J, et al: Long-term safety and effects of tesamorelin, a growth hormone-releasing factor analogue, in HIV patients with abdominal fat accumulation, AIDS 22(14):1719–1728, 2008.

626. Van den Berghe G, deZegher F, Bouillon R: The somatotrophic axis in critical illness: effects of growth hormone secretagogues, Growth Horm IGF Res 8:153–155, 1998.

627. Van den Berghe G, et al: Pituitary responsiveness to GH-releasing hormone, GH-releasing peptide-2 and thyrotrophin-releasing hormone in critical illness, Clin Endocrinol 45(3):341–351, 1996.

628. Van den Berghe G, et al: The somatotropic axis in critical illness: effect of continuous growth hormone (GH)-releasing hormone and GH-releasing peptide-2 infusion, J Clin Endocrinol Metab 82(2):590–599, 1997.

629. Van den Berghe G, et al: Reactivation of pituitary hormone release and metabolic improvement by infusion of growth hormone-releasing peptide and thyrotropin-releasing hormone in patients with protracted critical illness, J Clin Endocrinol Metab 84(4):1311–1323, 1999.

630. Murphy MG, et al: MK-677, an orally active growth hormone secretagogue, reverses diet-induced catabolism, J Clin Endocrinol Metab 83(2):320–325, 1998.

631. Neary NM, et al: Ghrelin increases energy intake in cancer patients with impaired appetite: acute, randomized, placebo-controlled trial, J Clin Endocrinol Metab 89(6):2832–2836, 2004.

632. Hanada T, et al: Anti-cachectic effect of ghrelin in nude mice bearing human melanoma cells, Biochem Biophys Res Commun 301(2):275–279, 2003.

633. Nagaya N, et al: Treatment of cachexia with ghrelin in patients with COPD, Chest 128(3):1187–1193, 2005.

634. Nagaya N, et al: Effects of ghrelin administration on left ventricular function, exercise capacity, and muscle wasting in patients with chronic heart failure, Circulation 110(24):3674–3679, 2004.

635. Jenkins RC, et al: The effects of dose, nutrition, and age on hexarelin-induced anterior pituitary hormone secretion in adult patients on maintenance hemodialysis, J Clin Endocrinol Metab 84(4):1220–1225, 1999.

636. Takala J, et al: Increased mortality associated with growth hormone treatment in critically ill adults, N Engl J Med 341:785–792, 1999.

637. Rudman D, et al: Effects of human growth hormone in men over 60 years old, N Engl J Med 323(1):1–6, 1990.

638. Murphy MG, et al: Effect of alendronate and MK-677 (a growth hormone secretagogue), individually and in combination, on markers of bone turnover and bone mineral density in postmenopausal osteoporotic women, J Clin Endocrinol Metab 86(3):1116–1125, 2001.

639. Bach MA, et al: The effects of MK-0677, an oral growth hormone secretagogue, in patients with hip fracture, J Am Geriatr Soc 52(4):516–523, 2004.

640. Kirk SE, et al: Effect of obesity and feeding on the growth hormone (GH) response to the GH secretagogue L-692,429 in young men, J Clin Endocrinol Metab 82(5):1154–1159, 1997.

641. Lasseter KC, et al: Ghrelin agonist (TZP-101): safety, pharmacokinetics and pharmacodynamic evaluation in healthy volunteers: a phase I, first-in-human study, J Clin Pharmacol 48(2):193–202, 2008.

642. Garcia JM, Polvino WJ: Effect on body weight and safety of RC-1291, a novel, orally available ghrelin mimetic and growth hormone secretagogue: results of a phase I, randomized, placebo-controlled, multiple-dose study in healthy volunteers, Oncologist 12(5):594–600, 2007.

643. Koo GC, et al: Immune enhancing effect of a growth hormone secretagogue, J Immunol 166(6):4195–4201, 2001.

644. Piccoli F, et al: Pharmacokinetics and pharmacodynamic effects of an oral ghrelin agonist in healthy subjects, J Clin Endocrinol Metab 92(5):1814–1820, 2007.

645. Date Y, et al: The role of the gastric afferent vagal nerve in ghrelin-induced feeding and growth hormone secretion in rats, Gastroenterology 123:1120–1128, 2003.

Chapter 17

INSULIN-LIKE GROWTH FACTOR-1 AND ITS BINDING PROTEINS

DAVID R. CLEMMONS

The family of insulin-like growth factors (IGFs) is unusual when considered in the context of traditional hormones. Although like classically defined hormones, these substances are secreted into extracellular fluids and act on cells within tissues at distal target sites, they also act on cells that are adjacent to cells of origin and on the cells of origin themselves, processes that have been termed *autocrine* and *paracrine growth stimulation*. Therefore, these substances can be viewed as either traditional hormones or as locally produced growth factors. The ability to genetically manipulate animals has resulted in a greater understanding of the role of locally produced and systemically transported IGF-1 in regulating growth in vivo. Although knowledge is still evolving in this area, it is clear that the full understanding of the mechanism of action of polypeptide growth factors, such as IGF-1, cannot be elucidated without an appreciation for both their systemic endocrine effects, which can be demonstrated in classic in-vivo infusion experiments, or these local actions which require tissue-specific gene knock-out experiments, wherein local production is attenuated. Clearly, both of these sources of peptide, autocrine produced and endocrine transported, are important for regulation of growth. Attempts to manipulate growth factors' actions, such as in treating cancers that are growth-factor dependent, will have to consider not only ablation of circulating IGFs but also ablation of local tissue production. Thus complete understanding of the physiologic mechanisms that regulate both types of production is necessary.

The IGFs belong to a family of polypeptides that evolved from a common ancestral precursor into IGF-1, IGF-2, and proinsulin. All three peptides evolved before the emergence of a pituitary gland, although growth hormone (GH) control of IGF-1 appeared near the time that IGF-1 and insulin diverged. Unlike insulin, both IGF-1 and IGF-2 circulate bound to high-affinity binding proteins. This results in a very different plasma half-life and differences in their target cell actions. Similarly, the IGFs have distinct cellular receptors which bind IGF-1 and 2 with much higher affinity than insulin. The insulin receptor has similar selectivity. IGF-1 or 2 are ubiquitously secreted in all tissues, and the IGF-1 receptor is present on all cell types, thus enabling them to regulate systemic growth.

IGF-1 was originally discovered because of its ability to stimulate sulfation of cartilage proteoglycans.[1] The administration of

GH to hypophysectomized animals resulted in induction of a substance in serum that was a potent stimulant of cartilage sulfation. In contrast, when GH was added to cartilage in vitro, it had minimal bioactivity. This suggested that a separate growth factor was induced in the serum of these animals. Purification of this substance showed that its amino acid sequence was similar to insulin and led to studies which showed that it could stimulate growth in vivo.[2]

Molecular technology made it possible to determine the structure of the IGF receptors, and further studies have identified the signal transduction pathways that are linked to each receptor. Both the insulin and IGF-1 receptors can activate similar signaling molecules, although in many cases, each receptor induces a subset of signaling molecules that are distinct. A more complete description of the relative roles of IGF-1, insulin, and GH in growth and metabolic regulation ultimately awaits the elucidation of all the proteins that are induced by activation of each receptor, which will lead to a better understanding of their respective target cell roles, as well as their relative hierarchical importance in growth regulation.

IGF-1 Gene and Protein Structures

The insulin-like growth factor-1 gene is a complex, multicomponent gene with 6 exons. The gene structure is shown in Fig. 17-1. The first and second exons encode the 5′ untranslated and pre-propeptide regions of IGF-1. Exon 3 encodes the distal propeptide sequence and the regions of the mature peptide that are homologous to the B chain of insulin, the region homologous

to the C peptide and to the A chain region. Exon 4 encodes a D extension peptide. The fifth and sixth exons are shuffled and can encode one of two sequences termed *IGF-1A* and *IGF-1B*. This alternative splicing occurs in multiple tissues, and both IGF-1A and IGF-1B have been found to be secreted by specific cell types in culture.

Several forms of IGF-1 mRNA are transcribed, and at least four specific transcripts have been detected in tissues.[3] The most abundant IGF-1 transcript (6 kb) contains multiple polyadenylation sites and a long 3′ untranslated sequence. The abundance of this transcript is regulated by GH. GH increases transcription of IGF-1 by inducing STAT5b which binds to an intronic region between exons 2 and 3 and initiates transcription. Several different fetal and tissue-specific promoters of IGF-1 have been identified, and they account for distinct transcript patterns in various tissues and the appearance of various forms at specific periods in development.[4] Other abundant transcripts include a 3.2 kb transcript, a 2.7 kb transcript, and a 0.9 kb transcript. Stimuli other than GH have been shown to influence the abundance of these transcripts in various tissues.[5] The small, 0.9-kb transcript is one source of the mature 70 amino acid IGF-1 peptide. This transcript is present in the liver and is an important source of the peptide that is present in the systemic circulation. Alternative processing of IGF-1 mRNA following its transcription has been shown to occur in multiple tissues and may be physiologically relevant in specific situations, such as muscle repair after injury.[6] Variable polyadenylation sites and regulation of processing of the 3′ untranslated RNA extensions have been demonstrated and can result in different-length transcripts.[7]

The polypeptide structures of three members of the IGF gene family are shown in Fig. 17-2. Mature IGF-1 and IGF-2 contain 70 and 67 amino acids, respectively. Proinsulin has a longer C peptide region compared to IGF-1 or IGF-2. The sequence in this region is not conserved. The A chain and B chain peptide regions are of similar length. The sequences in this region are 41% and 43% homologous with proinsulin. IGF-1 and 2 contain D-domain extensions of 8 and 6 amino acids, respectively. Unlike proinsulin, IGF-1 and 2 are not cleaved into two-chain polypeptides during intracellular processing, but rather they are secreted as intact single-chain proteins. Forms of IGF-1 have been isolated from serum and from cell culture supernatants that contain the E peptide extensions (e.g., both A and B), but the relative abundance of these forms in most tissues is unknown. The frequency of processing of the E peptide domains is unclear, since longer forms of IGF-1A or IGF-1B have been shown to be secreted by cells in culture. However, some cells do not secrete IGF-1 with the E peptide extension.

Specific amino acids within the IGF-1 molecule have been shown by site-directed mutagenesis to account for receptor and/ or binding protein association (Table 17-1). Specifically, tyrosine 24, tyrosine 60, and to some extent tyrosine 31 are required for IGF-1 receptor recognition.[8] The tyrosines at positions 24 and 60 are conserved within IGF-2, but tyrosine 31 is not present. The residue within the proinsulin sequence that is homologous to Tyr24 (e.g., Phe25) is important for insulin binding to its receptor. Tyrosine 60 appears to be necessary for IGF-1 to maintain a stable conformation. Studies using mutant forms of IGF-1 with large deletions indicate that the region between residues 24 and 37 contains the primary receptor binding site.[9] Mutations in this region have very little effect on binding protein affinity. More recent crystallographic[10] and NMR studies[11] have confirmed the importance of these residues for receptor binding. These studies

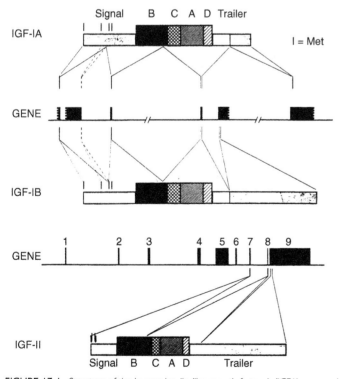

FIGURE 17-1. Structure of the human insulin-like growth factor 1 *(IGF1)* gene and the precursor proteins it encodes. The *black boxes* that are shown represent exons. The portions of each exon that encode parts of the precursor protein are shown by *lines*. The IGF-1A and IGF-1B precursor forms are represented by *boxes*. The *B, C, A,* and *D* domains of the mature peptides are noted.

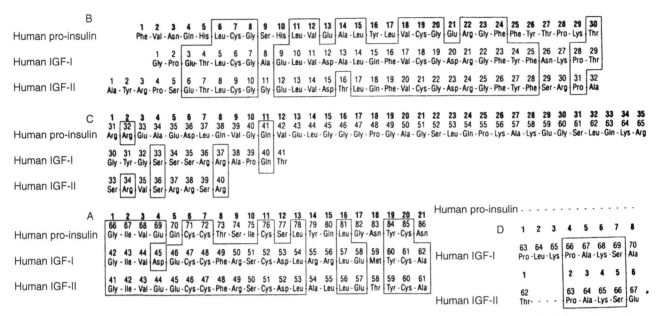

FIGURE 17-2. The sequences of proinsulin, insulin-like growth factor I (IGF-I), and IGF-2. The sequences are divided into the *B, C, A,* and *D* domains.

Table 17-1. Specific Amino Acids in Insulin-Like Growth Factor I (IGF-I) That Mediate Binding Protein and Receptor Association

Region of IGF-I	Ligand Interaction
B chain Glu3, Thr4, Gln15, Phe16	Required for binding to IGF-binding proteins (IGFBPs) 1–6
A chain Phe 49, Arg50, Ser51	Required for optimal binding to IGFBP-1, 2, 4, 5
Tyr24, Tyr31, Tyr60,	IGF-I receptor
Tyr24-Arg37	Contains the primary receptor binding site
Tyr60	Necessary for a stable conformation

highlighted the importance of Phe16 and Leu54 for ligand-induced activation and suggest they are required by full activation of the receptor kinase. These studies have also shown the importance of specific residues in the C domain, particularly Arg35 and Arg36.[12] Alanine scanning mutagenesis has confirmed the importance of Phe23 and 25, Tyr31, Arg36, Arg 37, Val44, and Tyr60, the residues that compose the binding site. These studies also identified a secondary site composed of Glu9, Asp12, Phe16, Leu54, and Glu58. Substitution for these residues resulted in a 33- to 100-fold reduction in receptor affinity.[13]

IGF-1 and IGF-2 contain 4 amino acids that are the primary determinants of their high affinity for IGF-1 binding proteins. These include the amino acids at positions 3, 4, 15, and 16 of the B chain region of IGF-1 and the homologous residues 6, 7, 18, and 19 in IGF-2.[14] These residues are critical for recognition by all six forms of IGF-binding proteins (IGFBPs). Mutant forms of IGF-1 that contain substitutions of proinsulin residues in these four positions have a nearly total loss of binding protein activity. In addition, residues at amino acids 49, 50, and 51 in the A chain are important for recognition by four of the six high-affinity binding proteins. The major exception is IGFBP-3, wherein only the B chain residues appear to be important. Recent x-ray crystallographic studies of the IGF-1/IGFBP-4 complex have confirmed the importance of these residues. They confirmed that they are the primary sites within IGF-1 that interact with IGFBP-4 and

explained how the interaction between IGF-1 and IGFBP-4 interferes with receptor binding.[15] Studies of the tertiary structures of IGF-1 and IGF-2 have shown that these residues are surface exposed. A recent NMR study showed that two of three helices that are present in IGF-1 form a surface-exposed hydrophobic patch that contains these A- and B-chain residues. A peptide that bound to this patch inhibited IGF-1/IGFBP binding. The C-peptide regions in each of the three proteins are divergent, and this accounts for most of the heterogeneity of sequence between IGF-1 and IGF-2. The three disulfide linkages are conserved in all three peptides.

The structure of IGF-1 is highly conserved across species. Bovine IGF-1 is identical to human, and rat differs by only three amino acids. IGF-1-like molecules have been detected in all vertebrates that have been analyzed, and even species as low on the phylogenetic tree as *Caenorhabditis elegans* contain IGF-1-like molecules. Computer modeling studies have indicated that the three-dimensional structure of IGF-1 is probably similar to that of insulin, which (except for the C-peptide) has been analyzed by x-ray crystallography.[10] Except for residues contained in the C-peptide, many of the IGF-1 residues that bind IGF-1 receptor are also present in insulin. The high affinity of IGF-1 for the IGF-1 receptor as compared to insulin is explained by the presence of the C-peptide.[12,13,14] In contrast, the higher affinity of the insulin receptor for insulin is accounted for by residues 4, 15, 49, and 51. If these insulin residues are substituted for those of IGF-1, this IGF-1 mutant has an affinity for the insulin receptor that is equal to insulin.[16] Different forms of IGF-1 have been found to be present in human serum and tissues. The most extensively studied form is des-1-3 IGF-1, which occurs in brain and in serum. This IGF variant has much lower affinity for IGFBPs and therefore is more biologically active.

IGF-I Receptor

The IGF-1 receptor is ubiquitously present and has been shown to be present in cell types derived from all three embryonic lineages. When animal tissues are analyzed, the receptor is

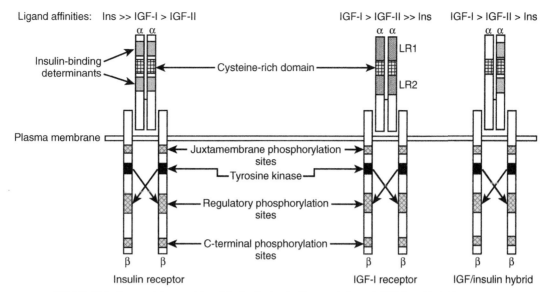

FIGURE 17-3. Structural characteristics of the insulin, insulin-like growth factor 1 (IGF-1), and hybrid receptors.

detected uniformly, thus accounting for IGF-1's ability to stimulate growth of all tissues. The receptor number per cell is tightly controlled and maintained in a narrow range of 20,000 to 35,000. This may be an important regulatory function, since cellular transformation in response to IGF-1 usually requires >1,000,000 receptors per cell,[17] whereas cells that have <100,000 receptors per cell rarely induce tumors in experimental animal models. Thus the variables that regulate IGF-1 receptor number may be important in terms of the genesis of neoplasia.

Hormones such as GH, FSH, LH, progesterone, estradiol, and thyroxine have been shown to increase IGF-1 receptor expression.[18] Similarly, PDGF, EGF, FGF, and angiotensin II upregulate receptor expression in specific cell types.[19] Following hormone binding, there is down-regulation of receptor number with internalization of receptors. However, possibly due to IGF binding proteins, the rate of internalization of IGF-1 receptors is substantially slower than that of other growth factors such as epidermal growth factor or insulin.

The biochemical structure of the receptor is similar to other polypeptide growth factor receptors (Fig. 17-3). The receptor is a heterotetrameric glycoprotein composed of two ligand binding subunits, termed *alpha subunits*, that contain 706 amino acids and two beta subunits that contain 627 amino acids. Only the beta subunits have a transmembrane domain (see Fig. 17-3). In man, the protein is translated from a single mRNA transcript derived from a gene that contains 21 exons located on chromosome 15, Q25-Q26.[20] The prepropeptide is 1367 amino acids, and the signal peptide is removed cotranslationally. The precursor is cleaved between Lys708/Arg709 to generate the alpha and beta subunits. These are linked together by disulfide bonds to form the heterotetrameric receptor. Amino acid sequence comparison with the insulin receptor reveals 46% amino acid identity.[20]

The alpha subunit contains three domains that are essential for ligand binding. These have been termed *leucine rich* (LR), *cysteine rich* (CR), and *carboxy terminal* (CT) *domains*. The receptor binds IGF-1 with a mean equilibrium dissociation constant (KD) of 10^{-9} M. IGF-2 binds with sixfold lower affinity, and insulin with a 200- to 300-fold lower affinity.[21] The composition of crystal structure of the first three domains of the alpha subunit of both the IGF-1 and insulin receptors shows that there are two important differences, one in LR1 and one in the CR1, that account for these differences in ligand binding.[22] Mutagenesis studies have shown that the residues Asp8, Tyr28, His30, Leu33, Phe58, Tyr79, and Phe90 within the LR1 domain are important for binding.[23,24] The CR region contains four residues that are essential to maintaining high affinity. A short C-terminal region (692-702) is also very important, since changes in 7 of these 10 residues reduced binding affinity 10- to 30-fold.[24,25] Following site one (LR-CR-CT) contact, the ligand becomes immobilized then cross-links through its second binding domain to a distinct site on the second monomer, thus resulting in high-affinity binding.

The beta subunit of the receptor is composed of an insert domain followed by two fibronectin repeat domains, then a transmembrane domain between positions 906 and 929 that is followed by an intracytoplasmic domain. This region contains intrinsic tyrosine kinase activity and critical sites of tyrosine and serine phosphorylation. The tyrosine kinase (TK) domain is 84% homologous with the insulin-receptor TK domain. The catalytic domain contains an ATP binding motif and a catalytic lysine at position 1003. Substitution for this lysine abolishes IGF-1-stimulated biological actions. Ligand binding to the alpha subunit triggers a conformational change that leads to autoactivation. This in turn leads to *trans* subunit autophosphorylation wherein a specific tyrosine 1135 on one beta subunit is transphosphorylated by the TK activity located on the paired beta subunit. This nonphosphorylated tyrosine is autoinhibitory, and its phosphorylation leads to kinase activation and transphosphorylation of the paired tyrosine 1135 on the corresponding subunit, followed by sustained TK activation.[26]

There are at least six important tyrosines contained within the cytoplasmic domain that are phosphorylated by the intrinsic tyrosine kinase. The most important is a triple tyrosine motif at positions 1131, 1135, and 1136. Substitutions for these tyrosines abolish IGF-1 signaling.[24,25] Crystal structure analysis has shown that phosphorylation of all three tyrosines is required to obtain the optimal conformation.[27] Following activation of the intrinsic tyrosine kinase activity, the enzyme autophosphorylates tyrosine 950 in the beta subunit, which forms a binding site for two important intracellular substrates, insulin receptor substrate 1 (IRS-1) and insulin receptor substrate 2 (IRS-2).[28] Substitution for this residue attenuates IRS-1 phosphorylation. Following IRS-1 binding to Tyr950, the IGF-1R kinase phosphorylates specific sites on IRS-1 that provide binding sites for adaptor proteins, such as Grb-2, which in turn leads to Ras activation. Other kinases, such as phosphotidylinositol-3 (PI-3) kinase are activated by binding to phosphorylated IRS-1. Mutation of tyrosine 1316 in the beta subunit abrogates the ability of IGF-1R to activate PI-3 kinase. The receptor can also directly phosphorylate other substrates, including Shc, Crk, and Grb-10.[23] Phosphorylation of beta subunit residues 1280 and 1283 is necessary for binding to 14-3-3, an additional signaling intermediate, and for mediating IGF-1's anti-apoptotic activity. The NPXY motif located near the transmembrane domain is required for internalization.

Chimeric receptors that contain heterodimers of the IGF-1 and insulin receptor have been described.[29] These dimers are disulfide linked. Receptor hybrids have been detected in several tissues and cell types. It is possible that they exist in all cells in which both IGF-1 and insulin receptors are expressed. The ligand specificity and affinity properties of hybrid receptors are much closer to those of the IGF-1 receptor as compared to the insulin receptor. Hybrid receptor activation has been shown to lead to stimulation of signal transduction in vitro[30]; however, the biological significance of hybrid receptor activation in tissues in whole animals has not been determined. Following IGF-1 activation of the receptor, it undergoes endocytosis. This is regulated in part by the adaptor protein 2 complex.[31] Following its recruitment to endosomes, the receptor is cleaved by a cysteine protease, and ligand is released.[32] Ubiquitination also regulates this process, and two E3 ligases, Nedd4 and MDM2, have been shown to play a role. Nedd4 binds to IGF-1R through Grb-10 and MDM2 through beta arrestin; thus these molecules also play a role in IGF-1R degradation.

The IGF-1 receptor has been overexpressed in several types of cells in culture. Receptor overexpression enhances growth in soft agar and tumor formation in nude mice.[17] Studies using antisense oligonucleotides to lower IGF-1 receptor number have confirmed its importance for growth and transforming activity of human tumor cells.[33] Importantly, deletion of specific tyrosines, such as tyrosines 1280 and 1281, results in a marked diminution in the transforming property of the IGF-1 receptor, although mitogenesis in vitro is still preserved.[34] Additionally, the receptor is important for IGF-1's ability to modulate the effects of other growth factors. Mouse fibroblasts containing deficient numbers of IGF-1 receptors do not undergo DNA synthesis in response to the addition of epidermal growth factor. Similarly, overexpression of the EGF and PDGF receptors does not lead to proliferation of fibroblasts in soft agar in the absence of IGF-1 receptors,[35] and reexpression of the IGF-1 receptor allows proliferation to occur. Large T-antigen induction by the cellular transforming virus SV-40 requires expression of the IGF-1 receptor, and wild-type Ras activation has less of an effect on cellular transformation if the IGF-1 receptor is absent.[36] Likewise, *Src* oncogene expression results in transforming activity only in the presence of an IGF-1 receptor.

The IGF-1 receptor has an important role in normal development and normal fetal growth. Animals that have had the IGF-1 receptor deleted by homologous recombination are born 40% of normal size.[37] These animals are not viable at birth, due to hypoplasia of diaphragmatic muscle. Defects in the development of the nervous system, skin, and bones have been noted. These developmental abnormalities apparently occur relatively late in gestation. Fibroblasts obtained from these embryos have a mark-edly attenuated growth response compared to fibroblasts from normal embryos.

The receptor is also important for prevention of apoptosis. IGF-1 and its receptor support the viability of nonproliferating cells in culture, such as neurons. The extent of apoptosis that can be induced in neurons by osmotic hyperglycemia, ischemia, or potassium shock is dependent upon normal IGF-1 receptor expression, suggesting that it is neuroprotective.[38] Hematopoietic cells that undergo apoptosis if IL-3 is withdrawn are protected by IGF-1 exposure if IGF-1 receptors are present. Plating tumor cells on a surface that does not allow ligand binding to integrins results in susceptibility to apoptosis, and this susceptibility can be reversed by incubation with IGF-1.[39] In contrast to the IGF-1 receptor, overexpression of the insulin receptor is nontransforming. Likewise, overexpression of a chimeric receptor bearing the beta subunit of the insulin receptor is nontransforming, but if the IGF-1 receptor beta subunit is expressed with the insulin receptor alpha subunit, then mitogenic activity of insulin is detected at much lower ligand concentrations, and this receptor construct allows transformation to occur.[40]

Receptor-Mediated Signal Transduction

Following activation of the intrinsic tyrosine kinase activity and phosphorylation of tyrosine 950, the docking protein IRS-1 binds directly to the receptor (Fig. 17-4). The functionally similar protein IRS-2 has been shown to bind by a similar mechanism.[41] Following binding, IRS-1 is tyrosine phosphorylated by the receptor at multiple sites, creating docking motifs that are critical for binding of intracellular proteins that contain Src homology-2

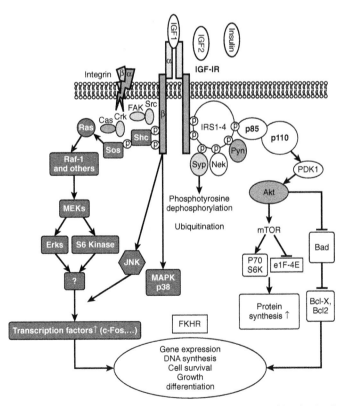

FIGURE 17-4. The two major signaling pathways that are used by the insulin-like growth factor 1 (IGF-1) receptor. These include the MAP kinase *(shaded)* and PI-3 kinase *(open)* pathways. P-110 and P-85 represent the major subunits of phosphatidylinositol-3′-kinase.

(SH-2) domains. These domains contain approximately 100 amino acids that share sequence similarity to cellular oncogene *Src*. Six of the tyrosines in IRS-1 occur within YXXM sequences, a recognition motif for some SH-2 domains. *IRS1* gene deletion in mice results in a major decrease in body weight, with proportionate reduction in liver, heart, and spleen.[42] Activation of signaling pathways that lead to enhanced IRS-1 degradation result in attenuation of IGF-1 signaling.

Signaling proteins that bind directly to the phosphorylated tyrosines on IRS-1 include the adaptor proteins Grb-2 and p85. Grb-2 forms a complex with the Ras-activating protein Son of Sevenless (SOS), and this complex leads to subsequent p21 Ras activation, which activates Raf and downstream components of the MAP kinase pathway.[43] Activation of this pathway is important for the mitogenic function of IGF-1.

IRS-1 phosphorylation also results in binding of the p85 regulatory subunit of PI-3 kinase, and this leads to binding of the catalytic subunit p110 and its activation. This results in generation of inositol triphosphate and activation of protein tyrosine kinase B.[44] This kinase activates mTOR and P70 S6 kinase, which leads to activation of protein translation. This pathway is also important for IGF-1-induced increases in cell motility and for inhibition of apoptosis. AKT also phosphorylates GSK-3 beta, leading to its inactivation, which is important for several responses that include stimulation of glucose transport.

The IGF-1 receptor can directly phosphorylate Shc, and this leads to association of Grb-2, which activates Ras and MAPK independently of IRS-1. Although Shc can be directly phosphorylated by the IGF-1 receptor, in certain situations such as following glucose-induced oxidative stress, Shc activation proceeds by a different mechanism. In vascular endothelial or smooth muscle cells, hyperglycemic stress leads to increased secretion of ligands for the $\alpha V\beta 3$ integrin. Oxidative stress also leads to activation of c-Src. $\alpha V\beta 3$ activation results in translocation of activated c-Src to a plasma membrane–associated scaffolding protein, SHPS-1. The IGF-1 receptor phosphorylates SHPS-1, which results in recruitment of activated Src, which recruits Shc and phosphorylates it.[45] Since IRS-1 signaling is markedly down-regulated by hyperglycemia, this mechanism allows full MAP kinase activation in response to IGF-1 even in the absence of IRS-1 activation. An additional signaling molecule that is activated by the receptor is Crk, a Grb-2-like protein, with SH-2 and SH-3 domains. Crk then activates Grb-2 and SOS after it is phosphorylated by the IGF-1 receptor.[21] Other signaling pathways that have been shown to be activated by IGF-1 include protein kinase-C, phospholipase-C, and direct stimulation of calcium-permeable ion channels. Activation of these proteins leads to activation of downstream signaling cascades, including G-protein activation. Additional signaling molecules that have been shown to interact with the IGF-1 receptor include RACK-1[46] and Grb-10.[47]

Since there is specificity between insulin and IGF-1 in terms of their metabolic and growth-promoting actions, it was presumed that major differences would be detected in the signal transduction pathways that each hormone utilized. However, IGF-1 and insulin-receptor kinase domains are 84% identical, and similar residues are autophosphorylated. Presumably, during normal growth or stimulation of glucose transport, either distinct domains are activated in the IRS-1 and IRS-2, or separate combinations of signaling pathways are activated. However, in pathophysiologic states such as hyperglycemia, IGF-1 receptor activation of MAP and PI-3 kinase is enhanced in some cells, whereas insulin-receptor signaling is inhibited. Other differences

in signaling have also been reported. Activation of Crk-2 is specific for the IGF-1 receptor.[21] Since Crk-2 has transforming activity, its activation may partially account for the ability of overexpression of IGF-1 receptors to be transforming. Insulin and IGF-1 receptors have been shown to utilize different G-protein signaling components.[48] Activation of Src kinase results in phosphorylation of the IGF-1 receptor but not the insulin receptor. In summary, multiple signaling events are activated in response to IGF-1 receptor stimulation. The best characterized are those that lead to MAP or PI-3 kinase activation, but other pathways may be important in specific physiologic or pathophysiologic situations.

Blocking specific functions of intracellular signaling pathways has been shown to attenuate specific IGF-1 actions. The PI 3–kinase pathway appears important for glucose transport and for cell migration, and specific inhibitors of PI-3 kinase have been shown to inhibit these IGF-1-stimulated effects.[44,49] Similarly, the MAP kinase pathway appears to be the predominant pathway for mitogenesis and rescue from apoptosis.[39] Protein kinase C also appears to be essential for IGF-1-stimulated cell migration and stimulation of the transcription of specific genes. However, the requirement of stimulation of a specific pathway for a specific function is not absolute, since the results generated using specific inhibitors of each pathway support the conclusion that there are overlapping functions. In addition to interactions between the IGF-1 and insulin receptor–linked signaling pathways, several other signaling pathways have been shown to influence IGF-1-stimulated signaling events. Several hormones and growth factors such as EGF, angiotensin II, aldosterone, and estrogen have been shown to modulate IGF-1 receptor–linked signaling events.[50-52] Conversely, cellular activation by IGF-1 has been shown to result in transactivation of the androgen receptor EGFR, VEGFR, and the chemokine receptor CXR4.[53,54] In addition, postreceptor signaling pathway cross-talk has been demonstrated for the GH receptor, estrogen receptor, progesterone receptor, glucocorticoid receptor, and multiple cytokine pathways such as TNFα,[55] which induces tissue refractoriness to IGF-1 in states of cachexia.

IGF-2 Mannose-6 Phosphate Receptor

The IGF-2/cation-independent mannose-6 phosphate receptor is a single-chain, membrane-spanning glycoprotein that contains 2451 amino acids. It binds mannose-6 phosphate residues on lysosomal enzymes as well as IGF-2. There is a large extracellular domain, a 23 amino acid transmembrane domain, and a 164 residue carboxy terminal intracytoplasmic domain. The extracellular domain is composed of 15 repeating motifs. Motifs 7 to 9 bind mannose-6 phosphate, and motif 11 contains the IGF-2 binding region.[56] Analysis of this region shows that Tyr1542, Glu1544, Phe1567, Thr1520, and Ile1572 come in close contact with IGF-2, and mutagenesis studies have confirmed its importance for binding.[57] Intracellularly, this receptor functions to translocate newly synthesized lysosomal enzymes into endosomes. On the cell surface, it binds to mannose-6 phosphate–containing extracellular glycoproteins, which are endocytosed into endosomes. The receptors are then recycled back to the cell surface. Proteins other than lysosomal enzymes shown to bind to this receptor include proliferin, thyroglobulin, and latent transforming growth factor beta (TGF-β). Binding of latent TGF-β has been shown to result in cleavage of the inactive form into active TGF-β. In adipocytes, it has been shown that insulin is a potent stimulant of redistribution of mannose-6 phosphate receptors from intracellular locations to the plasma membrane. The receptor binds IGF-2 with an affinity in the range of KD 1 to 3 nM. The affinity for IGF-1 is 80-fold lower, and the receptor does not bind insulin. Mannose-6 phosphate–containing proteins bind to a site that is distinct from IGF-1 or IGF-2, and the receptor can bind both types of ligands simultaneously. Once IGF-2 is bound, it is internalized and degraded. The extracellular portion of the receptor can be proteolytically cleaved in certain cell types, and the cleavage product is released. This soluble form has been detected in plasma; however, the physiologic significance of its release into plasma has not been determined.

The role of this receptor in IGF physiology is incompletely understood. Deletion of the receptor or mutations that result in loss of IGF-2 binding result in death of fetal mice.[58] The receptor is subject to parental imprinting, such that only the maternal allele of the IGF-2 receptor and the paternal allele of IGF-2 are expressed. Therefore, mice that inherit a receptor allele containing a mutation from the mother have functionally altered IGF-2 receptors. These mice develop severe edema in utero prior to death.[58] They are also larger than fetuses of comparable developmental age. If IGF-2 is deleted concomitantly, 50% of the fetuses survive birth; however, postnatal survival is poor. The hypothesis has been that these mice lack the putative scavenging function of the IGF-2 receptor and accumulate toxic levels of IGF-2. Although the scavenging function of the receptor is well accepted, it is clear that this receptor does not mediate the actions mediated by the IGF-1 receptor, such as growth stimulation. In most systems, inhibition of the IGF-1 receptor is sufficient to completely block the mitogenic response to IGF-1 or IGF-2 stimulation. Increases in calcium flux have been shown to occur following stimulation of 3T3 cells by IGF-2 binding to this receptor. Additionally, the receptor has been shown to activate GTP binding proteins, but the exact functional significance of these effects is undetermined. The cytoplasmic portion of the receptor encodes regions that are necessary for specific subcellular localization and endocytosis, as well as binding to GTP binding proteins.[59] Partitioning of the receptor following internalization can be hormonally regulated. Treatment with insulin was found to cause a rise in the fraction of surface receptors without a change in total number. Mannose-6 phosphate stimulates a similar increase, and this can be blocked by pretreatment with pertussis toxin, implying both stimulatory and inhibitory GTP binding protein regulation.

IGF-Binding Proteins

A characteristic of IGF-1 and IGF-2 that distinguishes them from proinsulin is the ability to bind to high-affinity IGF binding proteins (IGFBPs). The IGFBPs are a family of six proteins that each have high affinity for IGF-1 and IGF-2.[60] In each case, this affinity is greater than the affinity of the type 1 IGF receptor for IGF-1. One or more members of this family is present in all extracellular fluids. Therefore, they control the ability of IGF-1 and IGF-2 to bind to receptors. In addition to this property, the major functions of the IGFBPs include: (1) transporting the IGFs in the vasculature, (2) controlling their access to the extravascular space, (3) controlling tissue localization and distribution, and (4) controlling access to receptors and thereby modulating the biological responses of cells to IGF-1.

The gene structure of the IGFBPs shows that each of the six forms contains four exons.[61] The mRNA species range in size

Table 17-2. Affinities of Insulin-Like Binding Proteins (IGFBPs) for Insulin-Like Growth Factor 1 (IGF-1) and IGF-2

IGFBPs	Affinity ($K_a \times 10^9$) L/M	
	IGF-1	IGF-2
IGFBP-1	1.1	1.2
IGFBP-2	3.4	10.9
IGFBP-3	8.9	22.1
IGFBP-4	2.6	6.0
IGFBP-5	38	41
IGFBP-6	0.1	4.4

from 1.4 kb (IGFBP-2) to 6 kb (IGFBP-5). Their protein structures show great similarity. Of the 18 cysteines, all are conserved in 5 of the 6 binding proteins. IGFBP-4 has 2 additional cysteines, and IGFBP-6 has only 16 cysteines. If the cysteine structure is disrupted, IGF-1 binding is markedly attenuated. All are secreted proteins and contain a hydrophobic leader sequence. The affinity of each protein for IGF-1 and IGF-2 is shown in Table 17-2. The greatest difference is in IGFBP-6, which has a 40-fold higher affinity for IGF-2.

There is a high degree of sequence homology in both the N-terminal and C-terminal domains of each protein.[61] Similarly, the sequences in these regions are highly conserved across species. In contrast, the middle third sequence diverges completely. This is important functionally because this is the major site of proteolytic cleavage for IGFBPs. Two of the proteins are N-glycosylated, and glycosylation sites occur in the middle third of the sequence, thereby providing specificity for this property among the different proteins. Recent structural studies have yielded a great deal of information regarding the IGF binding sites and the specific residues that are responsible for IGF binding. Two-dimensional NMR studies of IGFBPs showed that a hydrophobic pocket in the amino terminals (residues 49 to 74) contained six amino acids that form the binding pocket R49, V50, K68, L70, L72, L74.[11] Mutagenesis studies confirmed the significance of this region for IGFBP-5 binding and showed that similar residues in IGFBP-3 had a similar function.[62] Similarly, mutagenesis of the residues in IGFBP-2 that are comparable to Leu70, 73, 74 in IGFBP-5 results in a major decrease in IGF binding. A specific domain in the C-terminus of these proteins also contributes to IGF binding. The C-terminal binding site contribution to net affinity of the entire protein is greater for IGFBP-1 and 2.[63] Recent studies have suggested there is strong cooperativity between these domains which contributes to high-affinity binding of the full-length proteins, and that covalent linkage between the N and C terminus is necessary for maximal affinity.[64] The residues in IGF-2 that bind to the C-terminal domain binding site in IGFBP-6 are similar to those that bind the IGF receptor, and this probably accounts for the ability of the IGFBPs to inhibit IGF-1 binding to its receptor.

SPECIFIC PROPERTIES OF EACH FORM OF IGFBP

IGFBP-1 contains 235 amino acids and is not glycosylated. It contains an Arg-Gly-Asp near its carboxy terminus which mediates binding to the $\alpha 5\beta 1$ integrin.[65] IGFBP-1 has been detected in multiple types of extracellular fluids. The affinities of IGFBP-1 for IGF-1 and IGF-2 are nearly equal.

IGFBP-2 contains 289 amino acids and is not glycosylated. Its sequence is highly conserved across species, especially in the C-terminus.[61] It has an Arg-Gly-Asp sequence near its carboxy terminus, and it has been shown to bind to cell surfaces. Following cleavage, its affinity for IGF-1 and 2 is greatly reduced.

IGFBP-3 contains 266 amino acids and is variably N-glycosylated.[81] This accounts for its varying molecular weight estimates between 43 and 56 kD. There are three potential N-linked glycosylation sites. Digestion within N-glycanase reduces the estimated molecular mass to 34 kD. Glycosylation does not alter the affinity of this protein. IGFBP-3 contains a highly basic region between residues 216 and 244 (in which 10 of 18 amino acids are basic). This region accounts for its heparin-binding activity and its ability to adhere to glycosaminoglycans.[66]

IGFBP-4 contains 237 amino acids. It is N-glycosylated and therefore has a mass estimate of 28 kD in the glycosylated form and 24 kD in the nonglycosylated form. Glycosylation does not affect the affinity for IGF 1 or 2. IGFBP-4 is cleaved in most physiologic fluids to 16- and 14-kD fragments that have a reduced affinity for IGF-1 and 2.[67]

IGFBP-5 has 252 amino acids and is the most highly conserved form of IGF binding protein, with 97% homology in sequence between the mouse and human forms.[68] It is most closely related in sequence to IGFBP-3 (e.g., 50% homology in the amino and carboxy terminal ends). IGFBP-5 contains the same heparin-binding domain as IGFBP-3 between amino acids 201 and 218.[69] This sequence mediates its binding to extracellular matrix, and some specific ECM proteins that bind IGFBP-5 have been defined.[69] IGFBP-5 is O-glycosylated and has size estimates between 31 and 34 kD. This protein has a high affinity for IGF-1 and IGF-2. It is proteolytically cleaved into a 22 kD fragment in physiologic fluids that has a much lower affinity for these ligands.

IGFBP-6 has 216 amino acids, and the human form has 16 cysteines. The protein is O-glycosylated. It has a high affinity for IGF-2 compared to IGF-1, but the physiologic significance of this difference has not been ascertained.[70] IGFBP-6 is proteolytically cleaved in physiologic fluids.

CONTROL OF IGF-1 CONCENTRATIONS IN SERUM

Prior to the availability of IGF-1 to administer to humans, the primary means of assessing IGF-1's effects on anabolism was to make inferences from changes in plasma or tissue IGF-1 concentrations. Correlations between IGF-1 levels and parameters of anabolism, such as growth rate, rates of total body protein synthesis, and nitrogen balance were undertaken, and inferences were drawn based on changes in IGF-1 serum levels in response to variables such as GH administration. These studies formed the basis of several principles of IGF-1 physiology that have been confirmed directly by manipulation of IGF-1 expression in transgenic animals or by infusion of IGF-1 into animals and humans and indirectly by measurements of changes in IGF-1 concentrations in states of GH deficiency or excess.

Age is an important determinant of the normal serum IGF-1 concentrations. Plasma concentrations rise from very low levels (20 to 60 ng/mL) at birth to peak values between 212 and 638 ng/mL at puberty.[71] The concentrations then fall rapidly in the second decade, reaching a mean value of 284 ng/mL by age 20 and then decline more slowly over each decade (Fig. 17-5). They are reduced to <50% of the 20-year-old value by age 60 years. A portion of this change is due to age-dependent changes in GH secretion. Although the change in GH may account for much of the decline that occurs during adulthood, it does not account for all of the major increase that occurs during childhood.

There are important genetic determinants of plasma IGF-1 concentrations. Studies in twins have shown that approximately 40% of each individual's IGF-1 variability can be accounted for

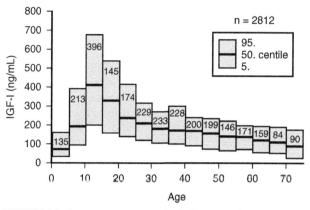

FIGURE 17-5. Serum concentrations of insulin-like growth factor 1 (IGF-1) in healthy subjects, aged birth to 75 years. The means are shown as *solid lines*, and the 95% confidence intervals are shown as *rectangles*.

on the basis of undefined genetic factors which are linked to height.[72] There is a very close correlation between IGF-1 concentrations and statural height in many different types of populations that have been studied, and these appear to be due, at least in part, to this genetic factor. This genetic determinant is independent of intrinsic GH secretion. Recently a polymorphism in the *IGF1* gene that occurs in 12% of Caucasians has been shown to be associated with a lower mean serum IGF-1 concentration (~30% reduction) and a decreased final adult height (e.g., ~2 cm). The presence of this polymorphism in individuals >60 years was associated with a twofold increase in the prevalence of type 2 diabetes and an increased incidence of heart attacks and strokes.[73]

The major hormonal determinant of plasma IGF-1 concentrations is growth hormone. Children with definitive evidence of growth hormone deficiency (GHD) usually have IGF-1 values that are below the 95% confidence interval.[74,75] Because values vary so much throughout childhood, however, age-adjusted normative data are required to interpret low plasma IGF-1 values (see Fig. 17-5). Consideration of developmental stage (skeletal age) is also important for interpreting low values.[76] In children, normal IGF-1 value is strong evidence that GH deficiency is not present. Conversely, a low IGF-1 is very suggestive of GHD, but it does not definitively prove that GHD is present.[77] Other causes of growth retardation can be associated with a low IGF-1, although causes such as constitutional growth delay are usually associated with normal levels. Administration of GH to patients with GHD results in a substantial rise in IGF-1, and this occurs during the 4 to 6 hours following an injection. The values peak at 24 hours and then begin to attenuate. Because GH also increases the plasma concentrations of IGFBP-3 and a third protein termed *acid labile subunit* (ALS), which binds both IGFBP-3 and the IGFs, the formation of this ternary complex accounts for the extended duration of the change in serum IGF-1. The IGF-1 response of a short child to GH administration has not proven to be a useful diagnostic test of GH deficiency.[78,79] In spite of these problems in interpreting low values, basal IGF-1 measurements have proven very useful for as a screening test for selecting individuals who should undergo stimulation testing to assess their GH secretory response.[74,75]

In states of GH excess, IGF-1 values are invariably increased. The mean IGF-1 for patients with acromegaly is seven times the normal age-adjusted control value.[80] The sensitivity and specificity of a single IGF-1 measurement for accurately diagnosing acromegaly in patients older than 20 years is >97%.[81] The severity of the IGF-1 abnormality appears to correlate with disease activity, and values correlate with measurement of soft tissue growth, such as heel pad thickness.[80] IGF-1 measurements are useful in monitoring the response to therapy and correlate well with residual GH secretion in these patients.[82] Generally, if 24-hour mean GH values are less than 1.6 ng/mL, then IGF-1 will be within the age-adjusted 95% confidence interval. IGF-1 values are also elevated during the last trimester of pregnancy, presumably due to increases in placental GH secretion.

Another hormonal variable that controls IGF-1 concentrations is thyroxine. Plasma IGF-1 concentrations are low in severe thyroxine deficiency and rise with thyroid hormone replacement.[83] Serum IGF-1 values are not suppressed in Turner's syndrome, and estrogen replacement results in little change. Prolactin has a weak, stimulatory effect on plasma IGF-1. In subjects who are severely growth hormone deficient, prolactin concentrations of 200 ng/mL or greater can maintain IGF-1 in the normal range.[83]

Nutritional status is an important determinant of plasma IGF-1 concentrations. Adequate caloric and protein intake have to be maintained in order to maintain an adequate serum IGF-1, both in children and adults.[84] Fasting for 3 days results in substantial reduction in total serum IGF-1 and a blunted response to the administration of GH.[85] Ten days of fasting results in a 70% decrease in plasma IGF-1. Following a 5-day fast, values decline by 53%, and subjects must be refed for at least 8 days for values to return to normal. During fasting and refeeding, the changes in IGF-1 correlate with changes in nitrogen balance.[85] These changes are due to both energy and protein deficiency. An energy intake of 20 Kcal/kg is required to maintain a normal IGF-1, whereas an intake of 0.6 gm/kg of protein is required. The energy must be supplied as at least 100 gm of carbohydrate. Similarly, the quality of the protein intake (e.g., the amount of essential amino acids) is an important determinant of IGF-1 if the protein intake is below 0.5 g/kg/day. Children with severe protein-calorie malnutrition have low IGF-1 values that respond to treatment.[85] Other catabolic conditions, such as hepatic failure, inflammatory bowel diseases, or renal failure, are associated with low serum IGF-1 concentrations.[86,87] Insulin is an important determinant of IGF-1 concentrations. Although it is difficult to differentiate between nutritional regulation and insulin action, insulin perfusion of the liver in diabetic animals results in a substantial increase in plasma IGF-1. Patients with poorly controlled type 1 diabetes mellitus have low normal IGF-1s that rise into the normal range with adequate insulin treatment.[88] Furthermore, in poorly controlled type 1 diabetes, there is a correlation between hemoglobin A_1C values and IGF-1. Similarly, patients with severe insulin resistance have low IGF-1 values.[89]

CONTROL OF IGFBP CONCENTRATIONS IN BLOOD AND EXTRACELLULAR FLUIDS

IGFBP-3 is the most abundant form of IGFBP in plasma. It has the highest affinity for IGF-1 and IGF-2. It also binds to ALS, and the ternary complex that is formed has a long half-life. These characteristics explain why IGFBP-3 accounts for most of the binding protein activity in blood.[90] The IGFBPs in plasma perform three functions. The first is to act as transport proteins for the IGFs. The second is to regulate their half-lives, and the third is to provide a specific means for transcapillary transport into extravascular fluid compartments.

The plasma concentrations of IGFBP-3 are regulated by GH. IGFBP-3 concentrations are low in patients with GHD and increase as a function of GH secretion.[91] This increase is partially due to a direct effect of GH on IGFBP-3 synthesis; however, it is also because the half-life of IGFBP-3 is prolonged by binding to the two other proteins to form a ternary complex (consisting of IGF-1 or IGF-2, IGFBP-3, and ALS). ALS is an 88-kD glycoprotein containing several leucine-rich domains that are known to facilitate protein/protein interactions, and it is this domain structure that accounts for its binding to IGFBP-3.[92] Since IGF-1 and ALS synthesis are also increased by GH, all three components are increased, and this acts to prolong the half-life of each component. The binding of IGF-1 to this complex in plasma functions to prolong its half-life from 6 minutes in the free form, which is similar to that of insulin, to 16 hours. The prolongation of the half-life of ALS-associated IGF-1/IGFBP-3 complexes is also due to the fact that this macromolecular complex (150 kD) cannot freely cross capillary barriers, and therefore it is not excreted by the kidney. If sufficient IGF-1 and IGFBP-3 are infused to exceed the binding capacity of ALS, then their half-lives are shortened substantially, indicating that it is the ternary complex that maintains the stability and prolongs their half-lives. The molar concentration of IGFBP-3 in serum is generally equal to the sum of IGF-1 and IGF-2, and therefore it is usually saturated. The affinity of IGFBP-3 for IGF-1 and IGF-2 is not lowered by binding to ALS, and its high affinity and its long half-life account for the fact that 75% of the IGF-1 and 2 in plasma is carried in this complex. The exact function of this large storage pool of IGF-1 and 2 in serum is unknown. However, it is clear that changes in the IGF-1 concentrations within this large complex correlate with the anabolic response to GH administration. Plasma IGFBP-3 levels are elevated in patients with acromegaly and low in patients with GH deficiency, as are ALS levels.[91,93,94] Age is an important determinant of IGFBP-3 concentrations, and serum IGFBP-3 varies with age in a manner similar to IGF-1.[76]

Hormones other than GH can influence the synthesis of IGFBP-3 and therefore its plasma concentration. IGFBP-3 is low in prepubertal males and increases following testosterone administration. It decreases 40% following menopause and can be increased in postmenopausal females with physiologic estrogen replacement.[95] IGFBP-3 concentrations are low in patients with hypothyroidism and increase 55% following administration of thyroxine.[96]

Insulin enhances the IGFBP-3 synthesis response to GH, but it does not appear to have a direct effect. Insulin also stimulates ALS secretion, and severe diabetes results in reduced ALS levels and reduced ternary complex formation. Although GH directly stimulates IGFBP-3 and ALS synthesis, infusion of IGF-1, while increasing serum IGFBP-3 transiently, acts to suppress its concentrations over time by suppressing GH release from the pituitary and thereby lowering ALS synthesis.[97]

IGFBP-3 abundance in serum is also regulated by protease activity.[98] Several proteases that degrade IGFBP-3 have been described, including PSA and plasmin, but the exact identity of the serum protease has not been determined. Protease concentrations are abundant in human pregnancy serum[99] and are also present in GH-resistant states such as diabetes.[100] Proteolytic cleavage reduces the affinity of IGFBP-3 greatly, and the IGF-1 that is released binds to unsaturated IGFBP-1, 2, and 4, wherein it can equilibrate much more readily with the interstitial fluids. Therefore, an important function of proteases that cleave IGFBP-3 may be to liberate IGF-1 and IGF-2 from the IGFBP-3/ALS complex and allow them to bind to lower-affinity forms of IGFBPs that can cross capillary barriers, thus facilitating a more favorable equilibrium with the extravascular space.

The next most abundant IGFBP in plasma is IGFBP-2. The affinity of IGFBP-2 for IGF-1 is less than IGFBP-3, and its plasma concentrations are substantially lower. IGFBP-2 concentrations are inversely regulated by GH; that is, they are high in GHD, suppressed with administration of GH, and reduced in acromegaly.[101] Unlike IGFBP-3, IGFBP-2 does not bind to ALS, and there is no ternary complex in plasma; therefore, its half-life when bound to IGF-1 is approximately 90 minutes. It is not saturated, and excess binding capacity exists. Intact IGFBP-2 crosses the capillary barriers. Hepatocytes appear to be the major source of serum IGFBP-2, and the abundance of its mRNA in liver is regulated in parallel with its plasma concentrations.[102] Hypophysectomy in experimental animals results in a major increase in hepatic IGFBP-2 mRNA expression. GH administration to normal or GH-deficient humans results in substantial lowering of plasma IGFBP-2.[60] IGF-1 is a major regulator of IGFBP-2 concentrations in serum. Following IGF-1 administration to GH-deficient humans or patients with diabetes, there is a three- to fourfold increase in IGFBP-2.[60] Plasma IGFBP-2 concentrations are also increased by IGF-2, and they are elevated in patients with retroperitoneal tumors that produce IGF-2.[103] Hepatic IGFBP-2 mRNA expression is significantly increased in diabetic rats and suppressed with insulin administration. Severely limiting nutrient intake in humans results in increases in plasma IGFBP-2, as does poorly controlled type 1 diabetes.[104] The response to nutrient restriction is dependent upon protein intake, since it can be mimicked with low-protein diets that contain a normal caloric content, and IGFBP-2 expression in animals is increased during protein restriction.[105,106] Since the half-life of the IGF-1 bound to IGFBP-2 is considerably less than IGF-1 bound to IGFBP-3, it has been assumed that IGF-1 that is bound to IGFBP-2 is in more rapid equilibrium with IGF-1 in the extravascular space.

The third most abundant protein in serum is IGFBP-1. IGFBP-1 also circulates in binary complexes with IGF-1 and IGF-2. Its affinity for the two growth factors is coequal (see Table 17-2). IGFBP-1 is acutely regulated by insulin.[107] Insulin-deficient states such as fasting or type 1 diabetes are associated with very high concentrations of IGFBP-1, whereas administration of insulin or ingestion of a meal results in marked suppression.[108] Major sites of synthesis of IGFBP-1 are highly restricted, and the liver is the principal site of synthesis, although kidney, maternal placenta, and uterus are other sources of this peptide. Plasma concentrations are controlled primarily by hepatic synthesis and release. Hepatic synthesis is primarily under the control of insulin.[107] IGFBP-1 in blood is unsaturated, and therefore IGFBP-1 is proposed to be a major modulator of free IGF-1 levels, particularly in response to food intake. Postprandially, changes in serum insulin result in a four- to fivefold decrease in IGFBP-1. This is due to direct suppression of hepatic synthesis. Insulin directly affects *IGFBP1* gene transcription, and there is an insulin-response element in the 5′ flanking region of the *IGFBP1* gene.[109] IGFBP-1 crosses intact capillary beds, and the amount that crosses in a fixed time period is dependent upon ambient insulin concentrations.[110]

Because IGFBP-1 can bind free IGF-1, it has been proposed to have a gluco-regulatory function, that is, since IGF-1 enhances insulin sensitivity, factors that lead to excessive IGFBP-1 could lead to reduced insulin sensitivity. In states of significant insulin resistance, there is enhanced phosphorylation of IGFBP-1, which

increases its affinity for IGF-1 and therefore results in further attenuation of IGF-1's ability to enhance insulin sensitivity.[111] Both fasting and diabetes have been shown to cause disproportionate increases in serum IGFBP-1 concentrations.[104,108] In addition, administration of glucocorticoid increases IGFBP-1 through a direct effect on *IGFBP1* gene transcription.[109] Administration of large concentrations of IGFBP-1 to hypophysectomized rats results in slight increases in glucose concentrations, suggesting that IGFBP-1 may have some role in regulating the insulin-like actions of IGF-1.[112]

The exact roles of IGFBP-1 and IGFBP-2 in controlling the distribution of the IGFs has not been determined. In catabolic states, such as nutritional deprivation, GH deficiency, or renal failure, IGFBP-1 and IGFBP-2 levels are increased. Similarly, in these conditions, the amount of IGF-1 that is bound to IGFBP-3 is decreased.[113] Therefore, they can become the major serum binding component.

IGFBP-4 concentrations in serum have been shown to correlate with changes in bone physiology. Specifically, in states of low bone turnover and in states associated with low parathyroid hormone concentrations, serum IGFBP-4 concentrations are increased. There is a correlation between sunlight exposure and IGFBP-4, suggesting that vitamin D or one of its active metabolites regulates IGFBP-4.[114]

IGFBP-5 exists in serum mostly as proteolytic fragments, and intact IGFBP-5 is present at very low concentrations. The fragments that are present have very low affinity for IGF-1 and IGF-2, and therefore their plasma concentrations are unlikely to be major regulators of IGF-1 action. IGFBP-5 in plasma binds to ALS, and its concentrations are regulated by growth hormone and IGF-1. Both intact IGFBP-5 and its major fragment increase substantially when GH is administered to GH-deficient patients.[115]

Circulating IGFBP-6 levels are lower in females than males, but estrogen does not change its concentration.[116] IGFBP-6 increases with physical stress, and serum concentrations are elevated in patients with critical illnesses.[117] Similarly, they are increased in renal failure.[118]

CONTROL OF IGF-1 SYNTHESIS IN TISSUES

While it is beyond the scope of this chapter to discuss the expression of IGF-1 in all tissues that have been studied, some general principles are important for a fundamental understanding of the autocrine/paracrine mediated actions of this growth factor. Connective tissue cells within a given tissue or organ are often the origin of IGF-1 transcripts. In-situ hybridization studies have shown that fibroblasts and other cells of mesenchymal origin are the primary extrahepatic source of IGF-1 in vivo.[119] Importantly, the abundance of this transcript in connective tissue cells is increased in response to GH, and its synthesis is also regulated by factors that are released in response to injury, such as PDGF.[120]

Cartilage and Bone

In cartilage, both GH and fibroblast growth factor have been shown to be potent stimuli of IGF-1 synthesis by prechondrocytes.[121] Its synthesis is most abundant in those cells that are actively differentiating; when chondrocytes reach the hypertrophic state, IGF-1 synthesis is diminished. Fetal chondrocytes, during development, have been shown to be an abundant source of IGF-1 mRNA.

Similar to cartilage, bone osteoblasts are a source of IGF-1 peptide, and it is synthesized in fetal calvarial tissue.[122] GH also increases IGF-1 synthesis by osteoblasts. IGF-1 synthesis rates correlate with changes in osteoblast DNA synthesis, type I collagen synthesis, and synthesis of other components of bone extracellular matrix.[123] Several bone trophic factors, such as bone morphogenic proteins, stimulate the synthesis of IGF-1.[124] In bone, IGF-1 mRNA expression is down-regulated by glucocorticoids. In contrast, estrogen stimulates the expression of IGF-1 in osteoblasts.[125] PTH also stimulates *IGF1* gene transcription, and its effect is mediated through cAMP induction, which enhances *IGF1* gene transcription.[126] In contrast, the bone growth factors, FGF, PDGF, and TGF-β, down-regulate IGF-1 expression. IGF-1 appears to be an important factor for erythropoiesis. Red cell mass is decreased in IGF-1-deficient humans and is restored to normal with IGF-1 administration.[127] Erythroid precursor cells synthesize IGF-1, and its synthesis can be stimulated in these cells both by GH and erythropoietin. Similarly, granulocyte precursor cells synthesize IGF-1 mRNA, and this is stimulated by granulocyte/macrophage colony-stimulating factor.

Reproductive Tract

IGF-1 expression is decreased in the ovary of the hypophysectomized rat, and ovarian expression increases in response to GH. Estrogen can increase ovarian IGF-1 expression, and this has been localized primarily to the granuloma cells of the early follicle.[128] IGF-1 receptors are also present in these follicular cells, indicating the possibility for an autocrine loop. Follicular fluid contains IGF-1 and IGF-2 peptides, and their concentrations are increased following FSH administration. Several studies suggest that the effects of IGF-2 predominate over IGF-1 in the ovary, and much more IGF-2 is produced in that organ. In the oviduct, IGF-1 and IGF-2 have been shown to be present in oviductal fluid. Oviductal cells express mRNAs encoding both IGF-1 and IGF-2, as well as IGF-1 receptors. Endometrium normally expresses IGF-1 mRNA, and in rats, a 20-fold increase can be induced with estradiol administration.[129] Estrogen induces IGF-1 expression primarily in the epithelium, whereas progesterone induces it in the endometrial stroma. In the late proliferative phase, IGF-1 mRNA is present almost exclusively in the stroma. Similarly, IGF-1 receptor mRNA is up-regulated during the secretory phase of the menstrual cycle. The testes express IGF-1 mRNA, and the source of origin is the Leydig cell. IGF-1 expression by Leydig cells is down-regulated by interleukin 1 and stimulated by LH.

Neural Tissue

Circulating plasma IGF-1 crosses the blood-brain barrier. However, much of the IGF-1 that is present in CSF is believed to arise from IGF-1 synthesis within the CNS. The major sites of IGF-1 mRNA are the Purkinje cells of the cerebellum, the olfactory bulb, and the hippocampus.[130] The retina is also a site of postnatal expression. Astroglial cells in the cerebellum are also an important site of IGF-1 synthesis. Immunohistochemical staining has shown that IGF-1 is transported along axons and dendrites and that IGF-1 peptide is present in the choroid plexus. Factors that regulate IGF-1 synthesis in peripheral tissues such as nutrition, thyroid hormone, and estrogen also regulate CNS IGF-1 expression.[131] TNFα down-regulates IGF-1 expression.

Skeletal Muscle

IGF-1 mRNA is expressed in the satellite cells and myoblasts of skeletal muscle.[132] Following an ischemic or toxic injury, there is a major increase in IGF-1 mRNA expression.[133] The wave of increase of expression after skeletal muscle injury coincides with the appearance of regenerating tissue and rapid cell division. Work-induced hypertrophy in muscle can also lead to an increase in expression of IGF-1 and IGF-2, indicating that this change is GH independent.[134] The IGF-1B transcript is selectively increased. Cardiac muscle is also a site of IGF-1 synthesis, and it is increased in models of cardiac hypertrophy that have been induced either by pressure or volume overload.[135] Blood vessels are also an important site of IGF-1 synthesis. Both endothelial and smooth muscle cells contain IGF-1 mRNA. Pressure overload, oxidative stress, and angiotensin II increase IGF-1 expression.[136] Following mechanical injury to blood vessels, there is an increase in IGF-1 expression by smooth muscle cells.[137]

Liver

IGF-1 expression in liver correlates extremely well with changes in plasma GH concentrations. Expression in hepatic tissue is low in hypophysectomized animals and increases after administration of GH.[138] The effect of GH has been shown to be mediated through the transcription factor STAT 5B. Likewise, nutritional deprivation results in a major decrease in IGF-1 mRNA abundance, and this can be restored with refeeding.[139] A part of this change is due to a change in transcription, and part is due to a decrease in mRNA stability.

The liver is a major site of insulin action, and insulin regulates the ability of the liver to respond to GH with IGF-1 mRNA expression.[140] Similarly, the effect of thyroxine on serum IGF-1 is mediated through its effect on hepatic IGF-1 expression.

Development

IGF-1 transcripts are easily detected in developing rats in intestine, liver, lung, and brain. Expression is present in as early as 11-day embryos, and IGF-1 mRNA abundance increases 8.6-fold by day 13.[141] In early embryos, IGF-1 is detected in yolk sac, hepatic bud, and dermal myotomes, sclerotomes, and brachial-arch mesoderm. In late fetal development, IGF-1 content is increased in muscle, precartilaginous mesenchymal condensations, perichondrium, and the immature chondrocyte periosteum, as well as ossification centers. In human fetal embryos, IGF-1 mRNA levels are relatively low at 16 weeks, and the highest levels are found in placenta and stomach. At 20 weeks, fetal kidney, lung, brain, cartilage, liver, and the placenta have detectible transcripts. The perisinusoidal cells of the liver and the perichondrium appear to be foci of intense expression in 20-week fetuses, and the cells of origin appear to be fibroblast-like. Postnatally, IGF-1 expression increases markedly in skin, nerve, and muscle.

IGF-1 Expression in Kidney

IGF-1 is expressed at low levels in the fetal kidney; however, in the adult kidney in rats, IGF-1 mRNA is abundant.[142] Immunohistochemical staining shows moderate amounts of IGF-1 in both the proximal and distal tubules of human fetuses. In adult rats, IGF-1 is localized primarily over the collecting ducts. Overexpression of IGF-1 in transgenic animal kidneys has been shown to result in renal growth, and GH administration to GH-deficient rats results in increased expression of IGF-1 in the kidney. Unilateral nephrectomy in rats results in compensatory growth of the contralateral kidney and in increased mRNA expression 24 hours after nephrectomy.[143] This increase in compensatory synthesis is partly dependent on GH, since it is reduced in hypophysectomized animals. After ischemic injury, there is increased IGF-1 immunoreactivity in the regenerating cells of the proximal tubules.

CONTROL OF IGFBP CONCENTRATIONS IN TISSUES

Since IGF-1 and IGF-2 function not only as endocrine hormones but also as paracrine regulators of growth and differentiation in tissues, the primary role of the IGFBPs in tissues may be to control the amount of locally produced IGF that is accessible to receptors. The exact regulation of each of the six binding proteins in each tissue in which they are expressed is beyond the scope of this chapter. The reader is referred to a review that comprehensively discusses this subject.[60]

Actions of the IGFs

IGF-1 ACTIONS IN VITRO

IGF-1 receptors are present in almost all cell types and mediate most of the effects of IGF-1 and IGF-2 in vitro, as well as the growth-promoting effects of insulin when it is present in sufficiently high concentrations to activate this receptor (e.g., $>10^{-7}$ M). Several biological actions of IGF-1 have been studied using cells in culture, including anabolic effects such as increases in protein synthesis and cell size; effects on carbohydrate metabolism, such as glucose transport, glucose oxidation, and lipid synthesis; and effects on cell growth, including stimulation of DNA synthesis, mitogenesis, and inhibition of cell death. Other generalized processes that have been analyzed include cell cycle progression, cell differentiation, and cellular migration. Specific events such as synthesis of individual proteins have been analyzed, as well as the ability of IGF-1 to augment specific functions of differentiated cells that are stimulated by other hormones or growth factors.

Cell Cycle Progression

One of the most commonly studied effects of IGF-1 in vitro is its ability to stimulate DNA synthesis. IGF-1 appears to act principally by stimulating entry into DNA synthesis from the latter part of the G_1 phase of the cell cycle.[144] In some systems, its presence is required for progression through all 12 hours of G_1. Compared to other growth factors, such as PDGF or FGF, IGF-1 is not as potent in stimulating quiescent cells to enter G_1, but once cells have entered the cycle, it is often sufficient to stimulate progression through to "S" phase. In some cell types, it is possible to alter this requirement by overexpressing EGF, the *c-myb* proto-oncogene, or SV40 T antigen.[145] Generally, these manipulations cause cells to secrete more autocrine-produced IGF-1 and thereby stimulate the IGF-1 receptor. Support for the hypothesis that constitutively synthesized IGF-1 is still required in such systems derives from studies in which antibodies that inhibit IGF-1 binding to its receptor block DNA synthesis, and cells that have had the IGF-1 receptor deleted grow poorly in response to stimulation by other growth factors.[146] Similarly, in some systems, enhanced expression of the IGF-1 receptor will abrogate the need for PDGF or FGF.

Other growth factors have been shown to work cooperatively with IGF system components. PDGF and FGF increase the number of IGF-1 binding sites, and FGF, EGF, angiotensin II, and aldosterone can transactivate the IGF-1 receptor tyrosine kinase.[50-52] IGF-1 is a mitogen for essentially every type of cell that possesses IGF-1 receptors. These include all mesenchymal cell types, most types of epithelial cells, including neuronal epithelium, and multiple endodermally derived cell types. Cell lines in culture that have been shown to have an increased number of IGF-1 receptors are more sensitive to IGF-1's growth-promoting actions. A factor complicating the interpretation of all of the studies that analyze IGF-1 effects on growth in vitro is the autocrine secretion of IGF-1. This autocrine-synthesized IGF-1 is capable of binding to receptors and potentiating IGF-1 action through the IGF-1 receptor.[147] Therefore, analysis of the effects of IGF-1 added to cells in culture often must take into account this confounding variable. In many of the studies in which synergism between IGF-1 and other growth factors has been analyzed, the end result is often influenced by autocrine-secreted IGF-1. Hormones such as TSH and FSH and growth factors such as PDGF and EGF may exert part of their proliferative effects by stimulating autocrine secretion of IGF-1.[148]

EFFECTS OF IGF-1 ON THE PROLIFERATION OF DIFFERENT TYPES OF CELLS

Cartilage

Many of the growth-promoting actions of GH on skeletal growth are believed to be due to the local production of IGF-1 by pre-chondrocytes or early differentiating chondrocytes within the epiphyseal growth plate. In vitro, IGF-1 stimulates cartilage cell division and size, as well as proteoglycan synthesis, which contributes to enhanced extracellular matrix synthesis.[149] IGF-1 also inhibits apoptosis in these cells.[150] Transplantation of articular chondrocytes that had been transfected with IGF-1 cDNA showed increased cell growth and matrix synthesis.[151]

Bone

IGF-1 stimulates several anabolic effects on bone cells in culture. Exposure of pre-osteoblast cells to IGF-1 results in stimulation of type I collagen synthesis, DNA and RNA synthesis, as well as total protein synthesis.[152] In addition, skeletal tissue is a rich source of stored IGF-1. Osteoblasts themselves can synthesize IGF-1, and several of the IGFBPs that bind to bone extracellular matrix can act as storage reservoirs.[124] IGF-1 expression has been shown to be stimulated by a number of hormones and cytokines that are potent trophic growth factors for bone, implying that many of their effects may be mediated locally through IGF-1 production. Genetic models in which components of the IGF system have been altered have confirmed the importance of locally synthesized IGF-1.[153] Targeted overexpression of IGF-1 in bone is associated with increased bone mineral density,[154] and targeted deletion of the IGF-1 receptor is associated with poor responsiveness to parathyroid hormone.[155] Targeted deletion of hepatic *IGF1* gene expression, which reduces serum IGF-1, results in decreased cortical bone thickness.[156]

Skin

Proliferation of primary human keratinocytes in culture has been shown to be stimulated by IGF-1, and IGF-1 is produced by dermal fibroblasts but not by skin epithelial cells. This suggests that paracrine stimulation of skin epithelium by IGF-1 that is derived from dermal fibroblasts may be the primary mechanism by which this growth factor contributes to epithelial proliferation.

Skeletal Muscle

Several types of myoblasts in culture have been shown to respond to IGF-1 addition. Both IGF-1 and IGF-2 stimulate muscle-cell protein synthesis, as well as DNA synthesis.[132] Their effects are complex, because they both stimulate differentiation in these cells (see following discussion). IGF-1 is synthesized by the satellite cells, which are pre-myoblast precursors, and its synthesis in satellite cells is controlled by the need to maximize the proliferative pool. Following stimulation of myoblast proliferation, prolonged exposure to higher concentrations of IGF-1 results in terminal differentiation. This effect is linked to the ability of IGF-1 to enhance the expression of the myogenic differentiation protein, myogenin. Muscle-specific deletion of the IGF-1 receptor results in muscle hypoplasia at birth, and IGF-1 overexpression enhances DNA synthesis during regeneration after injury.[157] Increased expression also increases muscle DNA synthesis and cell number in normal animals.[158] Cardiac muscle IGF-1 overexpression has been shown to reduce ventricular dilatation in models of cardiomyopathy.[159]

Smooth Muscle

Targeted overexpression of IGF-1 results in enhanced smooth muscle cell growth in response to balloon injury.[160] The expression of contractile proteins such as myosin heavy-chain is increased in these animals, leading to enhanced contractility. Similarly, IGF-1 overexpression in intestinal smooth muscle leads to increased growth of the muscularis.

Nervous System

The major nervous-system cell types that grow in response to IGF-1 are astrocytes and glial cell precursors.[161] In end-terminally differentiated neurons, IGF-1 has been shown to stimulate neurite outgrowth and myelin synthesis. Cells derived from the sympathetic nervous system, such as adrenal chromaffin cells, are stimulated to divide by IGF-1. IGF-1 is also a stimulant of neurite outgrowth in axons damaged by denervation.[162] In animals, IGF-1 is required for normal growth of the olfactory bulb.[163] Deletion of IGF-1 or IGF-1R results in brain growth retardation, and conversely, a localized increase in cerebellar expression was associated with increased cerebellar size.[164] Detailed analysis has shown that some of these changes are due to changes in cell number. Following injury, animals that had had IGF-1 receptor expression deleted in brain showed decreased proliferation of oligodendrocytes and reduced myelin synthesis.[165]

Other Cell Types

Other cell types that have been shown to be IGF-1 responsive include mammary epithelial cells, vascular smooth muscle cells, endothelial cells, mesangial cells, erythroid progenitor cells, oocytes, adrenal fasciculata cells, granulosa cells, promyelocytic cells, granulocyte colony-forming cells, fetal hepatocytes, pancreatic islet cells, oligodendrocytes, Sertoli cells, and spermatogonia.[148]

EFFECTS ON CELL DEATH

In many systems, IGF-1 has been shown to be a potent inhibitor of programmed cell death. The systems that have been the best characterized are hematopoietic and neuronal cell precursors. In hematopoietic cells, erythroid progenitor cells can be induced to undergo apoptosis with serum or erythropoietin deprivation, and this effect is suppressed by IGF-1.[166] IGF-1 inhibits apoptosis in myeloid precursors that occurs following the withdrawal of stimulatory cytokines, such as interleukin 3.[167] In tumor cell types, transfection with a dominant negative form of the IGF-1 receptor (a form of IGF receptor that has a tyrosine kinase–defective subunit) results in enhancement of the apoptotic effect that is induced by cytotoxic agents. During ovarian follicle development, IGF-1 stimulation by gonadotrophins may prevent apoptosis of the developing follicular cells. IGF-1 has been shown to inhibit the apoptosis that occurs during development in myoblasts, neurons, and oligodendrocytes.

EFFECTS ON CELLULAR DIFFERENTIATION

In cultured myoblasts, IGF-1 induces the expression of myogenin, a specific myoblast differentiation factor, and myogenin induction can be blocked with antisense oligonucleotides that inhibit the synthesis of autocrine-stimulated IGF-1.[168] Autocrine-produced IGF-2 may have similar effects. The programmed events that occur during differentiation in response to IGF-1 are time specific since, in L-6 myoblasts, cellular exposure to high concentrations of IGF-1 early in the differentiation program acts to inhibit differentiation, but at later time points, it is accelerated.[169] IGF-2 can inhibit apoptosis that occurs during transition from proliferation to differentiation in myoblastic cell lines. Differentiation markers have also been shown to be preferentially stimulated in response to IGF-1 or 2 in osteoclasts, chondrocytes, and neural cells. The addition of IGF-1 to different types of cultured neurons has been shown to enhance neuronal differentiation. Maintenance of neuroepithelial cultures in several model systems has been shown to be enhanced by IGF-1, probably by inhibiting apoptosis.

EFFECTS ON SPECIFIC CELLULAR FUNCTIONS

Production of steroids by ovarian granulosa cells and thecal cells has been shown to be stimulated by IGF-1 and IGF-2, and their effects are synergistic with FSH.[170] IGF-1 also stimulates steroid hormone secretion by ACTH-responsive, adrenal cortical cells.[171] IGF-1 stimulates testosterone secretion from Leydig cells and acts synergistically with LH to increase the response. Similarly, thyroglobulin production by thyroid follicular cells is synergistically enhanced with TSH plus IGF-1. GH secretion by pituitary cells is inhibited by IGF-1.[172] IGF-1 inhibits glutamate-stimulated release of gamma amino butyric acid from Purkinje cells. IGF-1 is a specific stimulant of IGFBP-5 transcription by muscle cells and fibroblasts.[173] Other proteins whose transcription is stimulated by IGF-1 include elastin by smooth muscle cells, crystallin by lens epithelial cells, and cholesterol side cleavage enzyme by adrenal cortical cells. Some proteins whose expression is increased following IGF-1 have been shown to result in specific functional changes in that cell type (e.g., the increased α actin in skeletal muscle[174] and the increased myelin in neuronal cells).[164] Microarray studies have shown that IGF-1 selectively up-regulates the expression of several genes and some, such as heparin-binding EGF and twist, may have important implications for cellular growth.[175,176]

Several metabolic processes that are stimulated by IGF-1 in a variety of cell types have been analyzed. These include glucose uptake, glycolysis, glycogen synthesis, and glucose oxidation in skeletal muscle cells.[177] These metabolic effects can be mediated by the insulin receptor if sufficient IGF-1 is added in vitro (e.g., concentrations > 10^{-8} M); however, antibody-blocking studies have indicated that IGF-1 can have direct effects on this process through its own receptor in some cell types. Similarly, the hybrid IGF-1/insulin receptor may play a role in mediating these effects in some cell types. Total protein synthesis, extracellular matrix protein synthesis, cell migration, and the synthesis of proteoglycans and collagen, in particular, have been analyzed extensively in connective tissue cells. IGF-1 often acts in concert with other growth factors to stimulate connective tissue cell protein synthesis. IGF-1 is a potent stimulant of cell migration and stimulates this process by both chemotaxis and chemokinesis.[178] IGF-1 is not directly angiogenic, but it can stimulate the synthesis of angiogenic peptides such as vascular endothelial cell growth factor.

ROLE OF IGF-1 IN MALIGNANT TUMORS

Because IGF-1 is a potent inhibitor of apoptosis, it has been proposed that it may function to enhance tumor formation in several experimental animal models. The presence of an intact IGF-1 receptor is required for propagation of several types of tumors.[179] In the absence of IGF-1 receptors, C6 glioma cells do not form tumors, and they undergo apoptosis. Often the presence of a normal IGF-1 receptor number is inadequate for tumor formation, and the IGF-1 receptors need to be overexpressed.[17] However, several processes that are necessary for tumor formation can be facilitated by IGF-1, even in the absence of enhanced receptor number, such as prevention of cell death. Deletion of the receptor results in inability of cells that would normally be tumorigenic in nude mice to form tumors, and mutation of specific tyrosine residues on the receptor and expression of these mutated receptors results in lack of tumor formation.[180] In human tumors, a direct causal role for the receptor in tumor pathogenesis has been difficult to prove. All of the data that exist are correlative. In Wilms tumor, small cell lung carcinoma, uterine cancer, and some colorectal cancers, IGF-1 receptor number is increased.[179] No mutations of the receptor have been identified as a cause of human tumors.

Several cell types that form tumors in animals have been shown to overproduce IGF-1 or IGF-2. However, in these systems, antisense IGF-1 often does not inhibit tumor formation or induce apoptosis. In contrast to the effects that are induced by blocking receptor-binding ovarian carcinomas that overexpress IGF-2 have a higher rate of metastasis.[181] Precancerous liver nodules that occur in virally-induced models of hepatic cancers overexpress IGF-2. Pancreatic tumor cells that have been transformed with SV-40 T antigen require IGF-2 for continued growth. Certain fetal tumors, such as Wilms tumor and neuroblastoma, are accompanied by loss of imprinting of the IGF-2 gene, and overproduction of IGF-2 accompanies tumor formation.[182] The IGF-2 receptor has also been implicated as a tumor suppressor in hepatocellular carcinomas, possibly through its role in the clearance and degradation of IGF-2. The only paraneoplastic syndrome that is known to be definitively linked to IGF-2 overproduction occurs with retroperitoneal sarcomas. Overproduction of IGF-2 by the tumor results in hypoglycemia.[183] The mechanism that has been proposed is that IGF-2 forms binary complexes with specific forms of IGFBPs in plasma that do not bind ALS (such as IGFBP-2), and this allows accelerated equilibration of IGF-1 and IGF-2 with extravascular fluids, thus leading to increased IGF-1 in interstitial fluids and to hypoglycemia.

Studies in mice have shown that IGF-1 overexpression is associated with mammary intraepithelial neoplasia; conversely, expression of dominant negative forms of the IGF-1 receptor is associated with decreased tumor progression.[184] Similarly, animals with low serum IGF-1 due to gene targeting of hepatic IGF-1 have delayed onset and reduced severity of many types of tumors.[180] Transgenic overexpression of IGF-1 in mouse prostate also leads to a higher prevalence of tumors at younger ages compared to control animals.[185] Recent studies have documented the important role of IGF-1/IGF receptor in immunocompromised animals having brain tumor xenografts. These studies have shown that anti-IGF-1 receptor antibody and tyrosine kinase inhibitors have potent effects in inhibiting tumor cell propagation, and they prolong mouse survival.[186,187] In addition, studies have shown that antibodies can alter the metastatic potential of the primary tumor,[188] suggesting that IGF-1/IGF-1R may play a role in tumor cell dissemination.[188]

Control of IGF-1 Actions in Cells and Tissues by IGFBPs

Since the IGFBPs are ubiquitously present in all tissues and have high affinity for IGF-1, they function to regulate IGF-1 actions by controlling access to receptors. The most important determinant of this capacity to modulate IGF-1 action is their affinity, although other variables such as binding to other cell surface proteins, internalization, or nuclear localization which lead to IGF-1-independent actions may play a role.

VARIABLES THAT REGULATE IGFBP AFFINITY

The estimates vary, but the affinity of each binding protein ranges between 2- and 50-fold greater than the affinity of the type 1 IGF receptor for IGF-1. The biological consequence of this high-affinity binding is the inhibition of IGF-1 or IGF-2 binding to cell surface receptors. Variables that lower IGFBP affinity to levels that are less than the IGF-1 receptor, such as proteolysis, function to allow an increase in the amount of receptor-associated IGF. In contrast, variables that lower IGFBP affinity into a range where it approximates that of the receptor but leaves the form of IGFBP intact may result in prolonged but enhanced diffusion of IGF-1 and IGF-2 on to receptors. Either process may result in enhancement of IGF-1 actions, but the type of effect that is enhanced may differ. Additionally, IGFBPs may function to alter the clearance rate of IGF-1 and IGF-2 in tissues and thereby provide a more stable reservoir of peptides. At present, three variables have been identified that significantly alter the affinity of one or more of the IGFBPs. These include proteolysis, phosphorylation, and adherence to cell surfaces or extracellular matrix.

Proteolysis

Proteolysis of IGFBP-3 by serum proteases has been shown to result in marked reduction in affinity for IGF-1 and a significant but less intense change in affinity for IGF-2. The principle fragment that is retained, the 32-kD fragment, has at least a 20-fold reduction in affinity for IGF-1. This protease activity is increased in pregnancy, diabetes, and nutritional deprivation. Matrix metalloproteases, such as MMP-1, MMP-2, and MMP-9, degrade several forms of IGFBPs, including IGFBP-3, and constitute part of the protease activity of pregnancy.[189] Several well-defined proteases have been shown to degrade IGFBP-3, including plasmin, cathepsin-D, and prostate-specific antigen. IGFBP-3 proteolytic activity has been noted in lymph, follicular fluid, peritoneal fluid, and amniotic fluid. The IGFBP-2 protease is also a cation-dependent serine protease and cleaves IGFBP-2 into multiple fragments. The rate of IGFBP-2 cleavage is increased by IGF-1 binding. IGFBP-5 is cleaved by proteases in a variety of physiologic fluids, including serum, and by the complement C1s that is present in cell-culture supernatants from fibroblasts, osteoblasts, and smooth muscle cells. IGFBP-5, like IGFBP-3, is also cleaved by MMP-2, MMP-9, and PAPP-A. Blocking proteolytic cleavage by incubating IGF-1 with a mutated, protease-resistant form of IGFBP-5 was shown to result in inhibition of IGF-1-stimulated cell growth. IGFBP-4 proteases are also present in several physiologic fluids. PPAP-A, a metalloprotease, has been shown to cleave IGFBP-4.[190] Like IGFBP-2, IGFBP-4 proteolytic activity is enhanced by IGF binding to IGFBP-4. There is correlative data suggesting that degradation of IGFBP-4 results in relief of inhibition of IGF-1 actions in vivo.[191]

IGFBP Phosphorylation

Three of the six forms of IGFBPs have been shown to be phosphorylated: IGFBP-1, IGFBP-3, and IGFBP-5. IGFBP-1 is phosphorylated on serine residues at positions 101, 119, and 169. Casein kinase 2 phosphorylates IGFBP-1, which increases its affinity for IGF-1 by sixfold. The form of IGFBP-1 that is increased during poorly controlled diabetes is a very highly phosphorylated form.[111] IGFBP-3 is phosphorylated at positions 111 and 113, and IGF-1 stimulates its phosphorylation. Casein kinase 2 phosphorylates IGFBP-3.

Adherence to Cell Surface, Extracellular Matrix, and Glycosaminoglycans

Both IGFBP-3 and IGFBP-5 have been shown to adhere to cell surfaces. Proteoglycans may be important cell surface–binding components for both proteins. Specific receptors have been postulated to exist for IGFBP-3. The type-V TGF-β receptor is a cell-surface protein that binds IGFBP-3.[192] IGF-1 that is bound to ECM or cell-associated IGFBP-3 is in more favorable equilibrium with receptors, since IGFBP-3 binding to cells lowers its affinity. IGFBP-5 binding to ECM or to proteoglycans causes an eightfold reduction in its affinity. In addition to proteoglycans, other types of extracellular matrix proteins bind to IGFBP-5 (e.g., plasminogen activator inhibitor-1, osteopontin, and thrombospondin).[193] Localization of IGFBP-5 within the extracellular matrix may provide an important means for focally concentrating IGF-1 or IGF-2 in the pericellular environment.[194]

EFFECTS OF SPECIFIC FORMS OF IGFBPs ON IGF-I ACTIONS

IGFBP-I

When present in concentrations that are greater than IGF-1, IGFBP-1 inhibits IGF-1 actions. If high-affinity forms of IGFBP-1 are added in a 4:1 molar excess over IGF-1, they inhibit DNA synthesis, glucose incorporation, and glucose transport.[195] IGFBP-1 has shown to block IGF-1 binding to receptors on human endometrial membranes, and it inhibits the mitogenic response of endometrial stromal cells to EGF.[60] IGFBP-1 can also enhance the cellular response to IGF-1. If the dephosphorylated form of IGFBP-1 is utilized and added in an equimolar ratio or less with IGF-1, IGFBP-1 can potentiate the in-vitro response of smooth muscle cells, keratinocytes, and fibroblasts to IGF-1.[60] It also enhances the effect of IGF-1 on adrenal steroidgenesis.[196] IGFBP-1 has been shown to directly stimulate migration of CHO cells, fibroblasts, and trophoblasts by binding to the α5β1 integrin receptor through its RGD sequence.[65] This effect does not require IGF-1 binding to IGFBP-1. In general, IGFBP-1 is induced by stresses such as insulin deficiency,[107] hypoxia,[197] and endoplasmic-reticulum stress.[198] This suggests that it functions to coordinate the IGF-1 response in these pathophysiologic conditions.

IGFBP-2

IGFBP-2 has also been shown to be inhibitory in most in-vitro experiments. Using purified IGFBP-2, it was shown to inhibit IGF-1-stimulated thymidine incorporation into chick embryo fibroblasts and rat astroglial cells, as well as a human lung carcinoma cell line. IGFBP-2 inhibited IGF-1- or IGF-2-stimulated protein synthesis in MDBK cells, and des IGF-1, a form which

does not bind to IGFBP-2, was stimulatory.[60] Overexpression in renal epithelial cells in vitro resulted in inhibition of IGF-1 actions. IGFBP-2 was shown to mediate the inhibitory effect of TGFβ on lung epithelial cell growth.[199] Conversely, IGFBP-2 has been shown to stimulate IGF-1-stimulated glucose incorporation and AIB transport in microvascular endothelial cells and DNA synthesis in smooth muscle cells.[200] IGFBP-2 contains a heparin-binding domain which has been shown to stimulate neuroblastoma bone cell proliferation; carboxy terminal fragments that contain this domain enhance chondrocyte proliferation.[201,202] IGFBP-2 enhances glioblastoma invasion and stimulates the growth of prostate cancer cells, but whether these effects are direct or mediated by enhancing IGF-1 activity has not been determined.[203] IGFBP-2 adheres to ECM through its heparin-binding domain, and the matrix-associated protein enhanced the effect of IGF-2 on osteoblast growth.[204] These effects require IGFBP-2 association with ECM through its heparin-binding domain. Recently IGFBP-2 has been shown to stimulate growth of hematopoietic stem cells, implying a direct role in precursor-cell compartment expansion.[205] Like IGFBP-1, IGFBP-2 is upregulated in response to injury, particularly in the CNS, and this is believed to be an important mechanism for targeting IGFs to sites of injury.[206]

IGFBP-3

IGFBP-3, if added in molar excess, inhibits glucose incorporation into fat cells, as well as IGF-1-stimulated DNA synthesis in human fibroblasts.[60] Maximum inhibition was noted at a 5:1 molar ratio. IGFBP-3 inhibits IGF-1-stimulated glucose incorporation. If IGFBP-3 is pre-incubated with muscle cells then removed from the medium, it can potentiate their AIB transport response to IGF-1.[60] Using this experimental paradigm, IGFBP-3 was also shown to enhance the IGF-1-stimulated DNA synthesis response of human fibroblasts, but co-incubation with IGFBP-3 was inhibitory. IGFBP-3 inhibited IGF-1-stimulated cyclic AMP generation by rat granulosa cells and inhibited IGF-1-stimulated collagen synthesis by osteoblasts. Addition of IGFBP-3 to breast epithelial cells results in growth inhibition.[207] It inhibits the growth of breast cancer cells in part by stimulating the activity of a phosphatase that down-regulates IGF-1 signaling.[208] Like IGFBP-5, IGFBP-3 has been shown to adhere to fibroblast extracellular matrix, and matrix-associated IGFBP-3 enhanced the ability of IGF-1 to stimulate MAP kinase activation.[209]

IGF-Independent Effects of IGFBP-3

IGFBP-3 has been shown to bind to the type-V TGF-β receptor. Direct addition of IGFBP-3 has been shown to attenuate the effects of several growth factors, including FGF, on cell growth. TGF-β is believed to cause part of its growth-inhibitory effect in breast carcinoma cells through induction of IGFBP-3. Increasing the expression of IGFBP-3 has been shown to inhibit the proliferative actions of several growth factors.[210] IGFBP-3 inhibited TGF-β-stimulated chrondrocyte proliferation by inducing STAT-1 phosphorylation and increasing the expression of the CDK inhibitor p21.[211] IGFBP-3 can inhibit growth of fibroblasts that do not possess IGF-1 receptors, indicating that IGFBP-3 has growth-suppressive effects that are independent of IGF-1 binding.[212] IGFBP-3 has also been shown to stimulate apoptosis in certain cell lines, including cells that do not possess IGF-1 receptors. In addition to its ability to bind to the type-V TGF-β receptor, IGFBP-3 has been shown to bind the RXRα receptor and to inhibit retinoic acid signaling.[213] This response requires nuclear translocation of IGFBP-3. The delineation of the specific amino acids that mediate IGF binding to IGFBP-3 has made it possible to prepare mutant forms that do not bind IGF-1 or IGF-2. These studies have shown that the non-IGF-binding mutants enhance cytokine-induced apoptosis. Similarly, expression of one of these mutants inhibited proliferative tumor growth in mice.[214] In contrast, the mutant accelerated the growth of esophageal cancer xenografts, whereas the wild-type protein was inhibitory, implying that it maintained its function as an inhibitor solely by inhibiting the effects of IGF-1.[215] This mutant also inhibited insulin-stimulated glucose transport in adipocytes.[216] Therefore, it appears that IGFBP-3 can have IGF-dependent *and* IGF-independent inhibitory actions. In general, the IGF-independent actions have been shown to be inhibitory, but when the IGF-dependent effects are analyzed, IGFBP-3 can enhance or inhibit IGF-1 actions, depending upon the cellular context.

IGFBP-4

IGFBP-4 has been consistently shown in in-vitro experiments to inhibit the actions of IGF-1 on cartilage and bone growth.[217] IGFBP-4 that is synthesized constitutively by intestinal carcinoma cells inhibits their growth. Several differentiated functions of IGF-1 have been shown to be inhibited by IGFBP-4, including the generation of cyclic AMP by osteoblasts, protein synthesis by prostatic cells, and glycogen synthesis by osteosarcoma cells, as well as the steroidogenic response of granulosa cells to FSH. IGFBP-4 potently inhibits smooth muscle cell replication and AIB transport.[218] A protease-resistant mutant of IGFBP-4 inhibited osteoblast proliferation. Cultured myoblasts overexpressing IGFBP-4 showed impaired proliferation and differentiation. The proteolytic cleavage of IGFBP-4 by PAPP-A has been proposed as a mechanism for releasing IGFs to bind to receptors and thus enhancing IGF actions.[219]

IGFBP-5

IGFBP-5 has been shown to potentiate the effects of IGF-1 in stimulating protein synthesis and DNA synthesis in skeletal tissue, including myoblasts, smooth muscle cells, fibroblasts, osteoblasts, and chondrocytes.[69] The potentiation of IGF-1-stimulated fibroblast and smooth muscle cell growth is believed to occur by association of IGFBP-5 with ECM.[220] ECM binding requires a specific region of basic amino acids that are located between positions 201 and 218, and mutation of specific basic residues within this motif results in the loss of ECM association and an inability of IGFBP-5 to potentiate IGF's effects.[220] IGFBP-5 binds to several specific ECM proteins, and association with these proteins has been shown to facilitate its capacity to enhance IGF-1 actions.[60] IGFBP-5 can also potentiate the effect of IGF-2 on mouse osteoblast, DNA, and protein synthesis. IGFBP-5 has been shown to have effects that are independent of IGF-1. A fragment of IGFBP-5 that does not bind IGF-1 has been shown to potentiate the effect of IGF-1 on osteoblast DNA synthesis and to stimulate mesangial cell migration. Direct injection of IGFBP-5 into bone of IGF-1-deficient mice resulted in enhanced osteoblast growth.[221] Overexpression of IGFBP-5 has been shown to activate MAP kinase independently of IGF-1.[222] Deletion of IGFBP-5 expression by osteosarcoma cells showed that it was important for cell survival. Schwann-cell differentiation that is stimulated by IGF-1 has been shown to be potentiated by IGFBP-5. In contrast, some studies have demonstrated that IGFBP-5 overexpression results in growth inhibition.[223] In mammary gland, its expression is induced during involution; inhibition of its expression reduces epithelial cell apoptosis.[224] Additionally, IGFBP-5 enhanced the proapoptotic effect of TNFα on breast carcinoma cell proliferation.[225] In skeletal myoblasts, IGFBP-5 has been shown to inhibit this proliferation and thereby facilitate differentiation.[226]

IGFBP-6

IGFBP-6 appears to preferentially inhibit the effects of IGF-2 in several tissues and cell types.[227] Addition of IGFBP-6 inhibited cartilage growth, and its overexpression in rhabdomyosarcoma or bronchial epithelial cells resulted in growth inhibition.[228] It also has been shown to inhibit cancer cell adhesion and migration.[229] It facilitated apoptosis in oligodendrocytes and inhibited the antiapoptotic effect of IGF-1. Cellular toxins have been shown to induce IGFBP-6, and blocking its induction has been associated with a reduction in toxin-induced cell death.[230]

In summary, IGFBPs are important modulators of IGF-1 and IGF-2 actions. They function to control the half-life of IGFs in blood and their distribution among tissues and extracellular fluids. In extracellular fluids, they control the ability of IGF-1 and 2 to associate with receptors. Factors that alter the affinity of IGFBPs for IGF-1 and IGF-2 can result in enhancement of IGF-1 actions. The exact role of each of these binding proteins in particular tissues in vivo is currently a major focus of research.

Actions of IGF-1 in vivo

IGF-1 was initially termed *somatomedin* because it mediated the growth-promoting actions of GH, and it was presumed to be a growth stimulant for all tissues. Several correlative types of experiments were conducted to support this hypothesis. These included hypophysectomy, which lowered serum IGF-1 and reduced growth or implantation of GH-secreting tumors, which raised serum IGF-1 and stimulated growth. Additionally, serum IGF-1 concentrations were shown to correlate with changes in GH secretion and growth rates. The initial hypothesis stated that GH-stimulated IGF-1 synthesis in the liver resulted in increased plasma IGF-1, which was transported to skeletal tissues where it acted to stimulate growth.[1] The development of cDNA probes for IGF-1 has allowed new types of experiments that led to refinement of this hypothesis. IGF-1 synthesis was demonstrated in multiple extrahepatic tissues, and paracrine-synthesized IGF-1 stimulated growth.[148] This raised the question as to what percentage of the generalized growth-promoting actions of IGF-1 is mediated by this autocrine/paracrine secretion, and what percentage is mediated by its endocrine effects.

Administration of IGF-1 to whole animals results in balanced growth, and if the animal has been hypophysectomized, the effect is enhanced.[3] A rate-limiting factor is the amount of IGF-1 that can be infused, since very high concentrations will induce hypoglycemia. IGF-1 also feeds back on the pituitary and suppresses GH. This results in a reduction in total serum IGF-1 concentrations due to suppression of ALS and IGFBP-3. If animals are made catabolic, either by nutritional deprivation[231] or administration of glucocorticoids,[232] administration of IGF-1 results in a partial reversal of catabolism. Likewise, systemic administration of IGF-1 has been shown to improve wound healing, enhance recovery of renal function after kidney injury, and stimulate whole-body protein accretion.[233] When IGF-1 is given to nutritionally compromised animal models, the increase in the weight of organs such as spleen and kidney appears to be enhanced preferentially compared to changes in skeletal growth.[233,234] In contrast, in well-nourished, hypophysectomized rats and mice, there is proportionate body growth in response to IGF-1, with skeletal tissue being stimulated in a manner nearly identical to nonskeletal tissue.[234] IGF-1 stimulates an increase in glomerular filtration rate and has a direct trophic effect on gut epithelial proliferation. Infusion of IGF-1 tends to lower IGFBP-3 and raise IGFBP-2, changes which are similar to those that occur in GH deficiency. Infusion of IGF-1 to insulin-deficient, diabetic rats results in improved growth and improvement in glucose utilization. Similarly, peripheral glucose uptake and glycerol synthesis are stimulated. Infusion of IGF-1 into the insulin-deficient BB rat results in suppression of hepatic glucose output, possibly due to a suppressive effect on glucagon and GH, and these actions led to enhanced sensitivity to insulin.[235] Diabetic animals that receive IGF-1 have less increase in body fat compared to animals that are treated with insulin.

Modulation of in-vivo Actions by IGFBPs

In-vivo studies have been performed wherein specific forms of IGFBPs have been administered with IGF-1. Administration of an equimolar amount of IGFBP-1 with IGF-1 reduced the growth response of hypophysectomized rats compared to IGF-1 alone.[236] Administration of a large, single dose of IGFBP-1 without IGF-1 resulted in a modest increase (6%) in plasma glucose concentrations. Acute increases in plasma IGFBP-1 result in decreased protein synthesis basally and in response to IGF-1. In contrast, administration of IGFBP-1 with IGF-1 (1:4 molar ratio) to wounds results in enhanced wound healing, including increases in re-epithelialization and formation of granulation tissue.[237] Similarly targeted deletion of IGFBP-1 in liver decreases hepatic regeneration after injury.[238] In addition, overexpression of IGFBP-1 in pancreas in vivo was shown to have a trophic effect on islet cells. These findings indicate that in some specialized circumstances, increased tissue expression of IGFBP-1 may enhance IGF-1 actions as compared to global inhibition that occurs when IGFBP-1 is administered systemically. Subcutaneous administration of IGFBP-2 together with IGF-2 has been shown to stimulate bone formation and inhibit the development of disuse osteoporosis in mice.[204] Administration of a complex of IGFBP-2 and IGF-2 stimulated osteoblast differentiation.[239]

Because of its role in carrying IGFs in serum, animal studies in which IGF-1 and IGFBP-3 are infused together have been important for defining the endocrine actions of IGF-1. In-vivo administration of a combination of IGF-1 and IGFBP-3 has been shown to consistently enhance of IGF-1's trophic effects.[240] Administration of an equimolar concentration of IGF-1/IGFBP-3 to hypophysectomized rats showed increased bone mineralization and increased growth rates compared to IGF-1 alone. Administration of equimolar concentrations of IGF-1/IGFBP-3 to estrogen-deficient rats resulted in 30% improvement in bone mineral density. Muscle mass was also increased in these animals. A recent study showed that IGFBP-3 induced insulin resistance when administered to rats without IGF-1[241]; however, when administered with IGF-1, it protected mice against the development of diabetes.[242] When IGFBP-3 is given without IGF-1, it can induce apoptosis.[243,244] Administration of IGFBP-4 with IGF-1 to mice resulted in increased serum IGF-1 and increased rates of bone formation.[245] This effect was dependent upon ongoing IGFBP-4 proteolysis. IGFBP-5 administration with IGF-1 to ovariectomized mice resulted in enhanced bone formation.[246]

Transgenic Animal and Gene-Targeting Studies

Several transgenic animal models of IGF-1 action have been utilized in which IGF-1 has been overexpressed. To determine if IGF-1 could substitute for GH and stimulate generalized somatic growth, GH secretion was attenuated by cytotoxic destruction of somatotrophs, and then IGF-1 replacement was affected by expressing IGF-1 mRNA in several tissues.[247] These animals grew normally, although there was some disproportionate growth of the kidneys, liver, pancreas, and spleen. Additionally, small-bowel length and mass are greater, as is villus height and crypt depth. Likewise, brain size appeared to be particularly sensitive to IGF-1 transgene overexpression. If IGF-1 is overexpressed on a background of no-growth hormone deficiency, more modest increases in somatic growth compared to control animals are noted; however, total body size can be increased by 30%. Brain size is increased disproportionately by 50%. The effect is due in part to inhibition of apoptosis.[248] Whether suppression of GH results in the inability to attain greater growth rates following IGF-1 overexpression is unknown. Interestingly, the GH-deficient mice have a somewhat hypoplastic liver, and this effect is not totally reversed by IGF-1 transgene overexpression.[247] The major conclusion from these studies was that most but not all of the growth-promoting effects of GH are mediated by IGF-1 using both autocrine/paracrine, as well as endocrine, mechanisms and that local expression of IGF-1 in tissues such as brain results in disproportionate increases in growth.

Attempts to determine the effects of IGFBPs have also utilized transgenic animals. IGFBP-1 transgenic animals show variable phenotypes, depending upon which organs express the transgene. Mice that had expression predominantly in pancreas, kidney, and brain had normal organ sizes except in brain, which was decreased in size.[249] Since IGFBP-1 is not constitutively expressed in brain, it presumably bound to IGF-1 or IGF-2, and the animals had a reduction in brain growth. In contrast, in mice with abundant hepatic expression, there was a slight growth retardation at birth and a 10% to 15% reduction in postnatal growth.[250] Hepatic overexpression during fetal life also results in growth retardation (e.g., 18% reduction in birth weight).[251] If the level of expression of IGFBP-1 in the liver is increased to a very high level, this results in more severe growth retardation and delayed skeletal maturation.[252]

Overexpression of IGFBP-2 resulted in fetal and postnatal growth retardation.[253] This effect is present even in the face of GH and IGF-1 excess. In contrast, deletion of IGFBP-2 expression showed a reduction in bone turnover and reduced bone mineral content at age 16 weeks in mice.[254] Histologic evaluation confirmed decreased bone turnover rate.[254]

In IGFBP-3 transgenic animals, there is modest (10%) fetal and postnatal reduction in growth despite a 2.8-fold increase in total serum IGF-1 concentrations. Analysis of bone showed that resorption was increased and formation was decreased.[255] Overexpression of the non-IGF binding mutant form of IGFBP-3 resulted in an increase in GH and IGF-1 levels in serum but no evidence of growth retardation.[256] Deletion of IGFBP-3 alone has not been reported, but generalized knockout of steroid receptor coactivator 3, which regulates IGFBP-3 synthesis, was associated with a 20% decrease in postnatal growth.[257] Because there are six forms of IGFBPs, following deletion of a single form of IGFBP, compensatory changes which offset the effects of the single gene deletion can occur. Mice were prepared that had deletion of

IGFBP-3, 4, and 5, and this resulted in a significant reduction (55%) in serum IGF-1 and a 38% reduction in postnatal growth rate.[258]

Targeted overexpression of IGFBP-4 in smooth muscle or in bone has been shown to attenuate IGF-1 actions. Cancellous bone formation was reduced, and this was associated with impaired growth.[259] When IGFBP-4 is overexpressed in smooth muscle, several organs (e.g., bladder and uterus) show disproportionate growth impairment. In contrast, generalized deletion of IGFBP-4 resulted in a 10% reduction in body weight.[260] Overexpression of IGFBP-5 (fourfold increase in serum concentrations) resulted in fetal growth retardation and a significant (17% to 23%) reduction in body size in the early postnatal period.[261] Overexpression of ALS resulted in modest postnatal growth restriction (e.g., 5.3% to 8.1%),[262] and deletion of ALS also resulted in modest growth retardation.[263] Taken together these studies have demonstrated that low levels of expression of the IGFBPs 2, 3, 4, and 5, as well as ALS, are necessary for normal growth. However, overexpression in which there is an imbalance between the concentration of a specific form of IGFBP and IGF-1 often results in growth retardation. This finding suggests that it is both the balance between free and bound IGF-1 and the ability of IGFBPs to prolong IGF-1's half-life and deliver the optimal amount to tissue receptors that determine how they modulate the growth response.

A great deal of information regarding the fetal and postnatal growth-promoting effects of IGF-1 has been obtained by homologous recombination experiments. In experiments in which the IGF-1 gene was deleted, the fetuses were born alive and were 60% of normal birth length and weight.[264] Homozygous animals had extremely high juvenile mortality rates, and only approximately 10% to 20% of these animals survived to adulthood. This appears to be due somewhat to the gene dosage effects, since animals that had only a partial reduction in IGF-1 expression survived into adulthood. The animals that do survive to adulthood are disproportionately short and have an abnormally slow growth rate during the juvenile period. They reach 50% of normal adult size. They also have poor Leydig cell development and small brain sizes. Skeletal abnormalities were also noted. The cause for the increased premature death is unknown. No apparent abnormalities of differentiation have been noted. Fetal growth retardation begins at day 13.5 in utero, and body size is reduced progressively at each stage up to birth.

Deletion of the IGF-1 receptor results in a much more severe phenotype. The animals are 45% of the normal size at birth.[264] All have a hypoplastic diaphragm and die at birth. Likewise, there are multiple skeletal and skin defects, indicating that the receptor is necessary for normal muscle, skin, and bone development in utero. Haploinsufficiency of the IGF-1 receptor results in survival and modest growth retardation (e.g., 8% reduction in adult size).[265] These animals tolerate oxidative stress better than controls and have a 16% to 33% increase in lifespan. Deletion of IGF-1 receptor expression in endothelium resulted in some protection against the development of neovascularization.[266]

IGF-2 gene deletion gives a very different phenotype. The animals are approximately 60% of normal size at birth, but unlike the IGF-1 mice, they grow normally postnatally and do not die in excessive numbers.[267] No differentiation defects or structural tissue defects are noted. Deletion of both IGF-1 and IGF-2 resulted in extremely small mice approximately 30% of normal size. This manipulation is lethal, since the mice cannot generate a normal inspiration. They are phenotypically similar to the mice lacking the IGF-1 receptor.

Autocrine/Paracrine Regulation of IGF-1-Mediated Growth

Experimental animal models have been useful in re-addressing the question of autocrine/paracrine effects of IGF-1. Since multiple animal studies had shown that IGF-1 mRNA transcripts were expressed in connective tissue cells, principally fibroblasts, and in the equivalent cell types in some organs such as the intestine, wherein the cells in the lamina propria express abundant IGF-1 transcripts, a major question arose: Is expression of IGF-1 in peripheral tissues regulated in a similar manner to that expressed in the liver and secreted into blood? Administration of GH to hypophysectomized rats showed that IGF-1 transcripts were increased in skeletal tissue such as cartilage, bone, muscle, and skin and in organs such as the brain, indicating that this autocrine/paracrine–produced IGF-1 could be regulated locally. This raised the important question of the extent that autocrine/paracrine–produced IGF-1 contributed to growth, as opposed to IGF-1 produced in the liver then transported through the circulation to target tissues.

An example of local control of IGF-1 is the response to injury that occurs following several types of injury models, such as freezing ear cartilage or thermal burns.[148] Fibroblast or chondrocyte precursor cells surrounding the damaged area immediately begin to synthesize IGF-1, and the peak of synthesis usually occurs between 3 and 7 days after injury. Following balloon denudation of blood vessels, the increase in IGF-1 mRNA expression coincides with an increase in the number of precursor cells that are entering the proliferative pool. Therefore, it has been assumed that local regulation of growth, particularly in response to injury but also to other stimuli such as unilateral nephrectomy, wherein the contralateral kidney makes more IGF-1 and enlarges, may be more responsive to local IGF-1 regulation.

Transgenic animals that overexpress IGF-1 in tissues (other than liver) showed normal growth rates if a high level of IGF-1 expression is maintained.[247] Another type of experiment that has reinforced the importance of tissue expression is analysis of brain growth. The blood-brain barrier provides some partitioning between blood IGF-1 and locally produced IGF-1. Transgenic animals in which there is intense expression of IGF-1 within the CNS show larger brains than animals that do not have this intense expression, indicating a paracrine regulation of growth that is probably partially independent of blood IGF-1 concentrations.[248]

A recent experimental animal model that has helped to further understanding of the relative components of autocrine/paracrine–produced IGF-1 as compared to blood-transported IGF-1 is the mouse in which hepatic IGF-1 expression has been selectively targeted.[268] This results in an 80% reduction in plasma IGF-1 concentrations. In contrast to global IGF-1 knockout animals, in which the expression of IGF-1 in peripheral tissues as well as liver is eliminated, all other tissues in these animals synthesized IGF-1 normally. These animals were normal size at birth and postnatal growth was very minimally retarded (e.g., 6%). This indicates that deletion of IGF-1 expression in the liver results in a major reduction in endocrine-produced IGF-1 and that autocrine/paracrine IGF-1 in these experimental mice is adequate to allow normal statural growth. Since peripheral tissue IGF-1 expression is also under the control of GH, this type of experiment does not distinguish between how much of the locally produced IGF-1 is regulated by factors other than GH and how much is under GH control. It does eliminate the possibility that in order to grow normally, one has to have a completely normal blood IGF-1 concentration. It also proves definitively that the major source of blood IGF-1 is the liver. Although it might not be surprising that fetal growth was normal in these animals, since IGF-2 is an important fetal growth factor, it is striking that there was no juvenile growth retardation, in spite of these low plasma IGF-1 concentrations. These studies have been extended by simultaneously deleting liver ALS expression. This dual inhibition results in a 16% reduction in growth and a more severe decrease in serum IGF-1.[269] These animals also have reduced bone mineral density. In contrast, deletion of ALS alone resulted in only mild growth retardation.[270] These findings indicate that a normal serum IGF-1 is necessary for normal growth but also that tissue IGF-1 is making a very significant contribution. In more recent studies, an animal model in which IGF-1 expression is deleted in peripheral tissues but transgenic overexpression of IGF-1 is induced in liver has been developed. These animals have a sixfold increase in serum IGF-1 which results in maintenance of normal growth. Therefore, supraphysiologic concentrations of IGF-1 in serum alone are sufficient for normal growth; however, these animals show a disproportionate increase in growth of the spleen, thymus, and kidneys.[271] In summary, these findings support the conclusion that both hepatic and extrahepatic IGF-1 synthesis are necessary for normal growth. They further support the conclusion that normal GH secretion is required for balanced organ growth and for coordination between the affects of blood-transported and locally synthesized IGF-1.

Effects of IGF-1 in Humans

The data regarding IGF-1 administration to humans as compared to administration of GH need to be reevaluated in light of recent findings regarding autocrine/paracrine actions of IGF-1. Following GH administration, IGF-1 mRNA is induced in multiple tissues in experimental animals that have been made GH-deficient, and there is a rise in serum IGF-1. This indicates that both autocrine/paracrine mechanisms and endocrine ones are activated by GH. In contrast, administration of IGF-1 alone to GH-deficient animals or humans does not result in autocrine/paracrine activation of IGF-1 gene expression. Similarly, other growth-regulatory molecules such as IGFBP-3 and ALS are regulated differentially in response to GH and IGF-1. Therefore, IGF-1 administration does not always induce the same gene-expression profiles as GH, and the changes in proteins that function coordinately with IGF-1 lead to distinctly different tissue responses.

Administration of IGF-1 to normal humans results in changes that are comparable to those noted previously in animal studies. A large bolus of rapidly administered IGF-1 (e.g., 100 mcg/kg) results in hypoglycemia.[272] When analyzed on a molar basis, IGF-1 is one twelfth as potent as insulin in reducing glucose. A continuous infusion of 24 mcg/kg/hr of IGF-1 to normal humans results in a 50% reduction in C-peptide but maintenance of euglycemia. Peripheral glucose uptake is increased at these infusion rates, and hepatic glucose production and free fatty acid levels are suppressed. Protein breakdown is also decreased. However, using lower infusion rates (5 mcg/kg/hr), which do not necessitate supplemental glucose to avoid hypoglycemia, there is no effect on protein breakdown. Insulin sensitivity is also enhanced, as assessed by insulin-to-glucose ratios measured during the IGF-1 infusion. IGF-1 has consistently suppressed insulin levels and resulted in more efficient glucose responsiveness to insulin.[273] Since GH is also suppressed, inhibition of several of the known insulin-antagonist actions of GH may contribute to this change. IGF-1 also suppresses glucagon, and such suppression probably contributes to the enhanced insulin sensitivity that is observed during IGF-1 infusions.[273]

Administration of exogenous IGF-1 to catabolic subjects results in improvement in nitrogen balance. The degree of improvement is comparable to that achieved with GH administration.[274] A study that used the same design (i.e., 6 days of a 50% caloric restriction) showed that concomitant administration of GH with a 12 mcg/kg/hr infusion of IGF-1 resulted in further enhancement of nitrogen retention compared to either treatment alone.[97] GH inhibited the development of symptomatic hypoglycemia. Infusion of IGF-1 alone resulted in suppression of IGFBP-3 concentrations and suppression of acid-labile subunit, but administration of concomitant GH resulted in maintenance of normal levels of IGFBP-3 and ALS in plasma.[97] This high level of the IGF-1/IGFBP-3 probably contributed to improved nitrogen balance. Other changes in IGFBPs also occur. IGF-1 alone increases IGFBP-2 concentrations threefold, suggesting that a larger fraction of the IGF-1 is bound to IGFBP-2 under these conditions, and thus it has a shorter half-life. A reduced anabolic response to IGF-1 alone may occur as a consequence of these changes in IGFBP profiles. Several other studies have suggested that maintenance of ternary-complex activity results in a better anabolic response. Administration of the IGF-1/IGFBP-3 complex to patients with severe burns resulted in increased protein synthesis rates.[275] The mechanism of improvement may be multifactorial, since administration of the complex to thermally injured rats results in preservation of normal gut mucosa and improved nutrient absorption.[276] Administration of IGF-1/IGFBP-3 to osteoporotic patients for 4 weeks following hip fracture showed that it was anabolic and improved bone density.[277]

Cholesterol is also lowered in response to IGF-1 infusion, as is potassium. Renal function improves, with an approximately 25% increase in glomerular filtration rate and renal blood flow. The fractional excretion of phosphate is decreased, which probably contributes to the antiphosphaturic effect noted in acromegaly. In addition to improvement in renal function, there is an improvement in the anemia that accompanies renal failure.[278]

GH selectively stimulates whole-body protein synthesis and has a lesser effect on inhibiting proteolysis. IGF-1 infusions at relatively high concentrations inhibit proteolysis but have no effect on protein synthesis. With prolonged administration of IGF-1 (e.g., 5 to 7 days given as a subcutaneous injection), there is no effect on proteolysis but a marked increase in protein synthesis, and the effects are indistinguishable from GH.[279] Therefore, the mode of administration and the actual dose of IGF-1 given are important determinants of whether IGF-1 has an acute insulin-like effect on protein synthesis (e.g., inhibiting proteolysis) or a chronic GH-like effect in preferentially stimulating protein synthesis. The combination of GH plus IGF-1 has a greater effect on decreasing protein oxidation in GH-deficient subjects compared to either substance given alone.[280] When catabolism is induced by administering high doses of glucocorticoids, IGF-1 has a significant effect on attenuating proteolysis and a small effect on increasing protein synthesis.[281] These effects are less dramatic than those with GH.[280] The effect of IGF-1 in enhancing insulin sensitivity appears to be preserved even in dexamethasone-treated patients.

BONE METABOLISM

Short-term IGF-1 administration to normal subjects increases bone turnover, with a preferential effect on bone formation.[282] Young women with anorexia nervosa and severe osteopenia also respond by increasing bone turnover, and there is a short-term anabolic effect.[283] IGF-1 is also an effective stimulant of bone formation in men with osteoporosis.[284] Patients with growth hormone deficiency also respond to IGF-1 with increased bone turnover.[285] IGF-1 has been given to elderly subjects with osteoporosis and results in increased markers of bone resorption, such as pyridinoline crosslinks in the urine. However, there are also increases in markers of bone formation, indicating that bone turnover is stimulated. Serum IGF-1 concentrations correlated with the presence of vertebral factures in diabetic postmenopausal women and predicted low bone mass in premenopausal women.[286] However, the net effect of long-term administration of IGF-1 on bone mineral content is unknown. Studies in rats have shown that administration of IGF-1 in combination with IGFBP-3 may be a potent stimulant of cortical bone formation, and a 4-month course of treatment in humans with osteoporosis with IGF-1/IGFBP-3 supported this conclusion.[277] These enhanced effects of IGF-1/IGFBP-3 compared to IGF-1 alone may be due to the inability of IGF-1 administration alone to sustain high plasma IGF-1 concentrations over prolonged time periods.

OTHER EFFECTS OF IGF-1

In addition to its effects in suppressing free fatty acids, ketone bodies, and triglycerides acutely, IGF-1 suppresses apolipoprotein B-100 levels. IGF-1 administration also suppresses plasminogen activator inhibitor-I levels, and this has the potential to lower the risk of thrombosis in patients with atherosclerosis. IGF-1 has been shown to be neurotrophic in humans, and trials in amyotrophic lateral sclerosis have shown some improvement in nerve regeneration and a slight prolongation of survival, indicating improved muscle function; however, significant improvement could not be demonstrated in a placebo controlled trial.

IGF-1 in Diabetes

Studies in mice have shown that overexpression of IGFBP-3 results in reduced insulin action in muscle and fat. Similarly, deletion of IGF-1 expression in liver results in increased GH secretion and reduced insulin sensitivity.[287] In contrast, overexpression of IGFBP-2 results in enhanced insulin sensitivity. This effect is probably direct, since the animals are refractory to the development of glucose intolerance even when fed a high-fat diet.[288] When insulin sensitivity is assessed formally with the euglycemic hyperinsulinemic clamp method, IGF-1 administration to type 2 diabetics results in a substantial improvement in sensitivity to insulin.[289] This also occurs in insulin-deficient diabetics and patients with extreme insulin resistance syndromes, including those involving mutations of the insulin receptor. IGF-1 infusion into type 1 diabetics lowers hepatic glucose output and increases peripheral glucose utlization.[290] Preliminary studies have indicated that administration of IGF-1 to patients with severe insulin resistance results in long-term lowering of glucose and improved insulin sensitivity.[291] Adolescents with type 1 diabetes who were treated for 4 weeks with subcutaneously administered IGF-1 had reduced insulin requirements and improved their metabolic control. These effects were attributed to suppression of the "dawn phenomenon."[292] Administration of IGF-1 to patients with type A extreme insulin resistance has resulted in improved metabolic control. Some studies, however, have not seen the same degree of improvement in patients with type A insulin resistance. Administration of IGF-1 to subjects with type 2 diabetes shows that it results in a 3.4-fold improvement in insulin resistance as assessed by direct measurement. More importantly, IGF-1 lowers hemoglobin A1C by 1.7% and improves glucose tolerance.[293] Insulin concentrations are lowered in these patients, suggesting that a change in insulin sensitivity is the primary mechanism accounting for this improvement. Similarly, in type 1 diabetics, the requirement for exogenous insulin can be lowered by IGF-1 while maintaining good glycemic control.[291-294] In a large ($n = 208$) group of type 2 diabetics who were treated with 4 different doses of IGF-1 for 3 months, the groups that received the two highest doses had a 1.6% reduction in hemoglobin A1C, indicating that long-term improvement in diabetic control is achievable with IGF-1.

Side effects have been noted both in normal subjects and in diabetics who have received high concentrations of IGF-1 for several weeks. These include parotid gland tenderness, subcutaneous edema, and a 10% increase in heart rate. In rare subjects, there is edema of the retina, and occasionally pseudotumor cerebri has been noted. Other unusual side effects include Bell's palsy and severe myalgias. All of these side effects have been noted to be reversible and remit after stopping IGF-1.[293-296] Administration of the combination of IGFBP-3 and IGF-1 to type 1 diabetics for 2 weeks resulted in a 48% reduction in insulin dosage and a 23% reduction in blood glucose, indicating improvement in insulin sensitivity.[295] This combination also improved control in patients with type 2 diabetes and was associated with a reduction in side effects.[296]

Growth Hormone Insensitivity Syndromes

The types of genetic defects that lead to the growth hormone sensitivity syndrome have been expanded to include GH receptor mutations, Stat 5b mutations, ALS mutations, and mutations in the IGF-1 gene.[297] Administration of IGF-1 to patients with GH insensitivity syndrome who had mutations of the GH receptor resulted in improvement in growth rates. Analysis of growth rates in nine such subjects who were treated for 1 year showed that they grew 7.5 cm in the first year, as compared to pretreatment growth rates of 4 cm/yr. Longer-term studies administering IGF-1 at 50 mcg/kg twice a day subcutaneously to patients with GH insensitivity syndrome have shown that the first-year growth velocity cannot be maintained in the second year, and the growth rates are reduced to 6 cm per year.[298-300] This growth rate has been maintained for periods as long as 4 years in subjects who received IGF-1, so there appears to be a growth benefit which, if projected to adulthood, would result in significant improvement in final adult stature. However, the growth rates during the second through fifth years are not as robust as those in GH-deficient subjects who received GH during a similar interval. Hypoglycemia occurs occasionally in these patients but is usually avoidable by a dosage adjustment. Other side effects that have been noted with acute, high-dose administration of IGF-1 to adults have not been observed in these children. One child with a GH insensitivity syndrome did develop pseudotumor cerebri, which resolved while treatment was continued. Another troublesome feature that has been noted, however, is a coarsening of the facial features, particularly in those subjects who are receiving the treatment during initiation of adolescence. This effect appears to be more significant than that noted with GH administration during puberty. Evaluation of these patients 1 to 2 years after stopping IGF-1 shows that their coarse facial features resolve. Whether the suboptimal growth rates and coarsening of facial features are due to stimulation by IGF-1 in the absence of the direct actions of GH that are mediated through the GH receptor is unknown. Similar growth responses have been demonstrated using the IGF-1/IGFBP-3 combination.[301]

A single patient has been described in whom there was a mutation resulting in deletion of a major portion of the *IGF1*

gene.[302] This resulted in severe growth retardation at birth that persisted into adulthood. Head circumference was also reduced. Administration of IGF-1 prior to epiphyseal fusion resulted in growth acceleration. It also resulted in improvement in insulin sensitivity. Four patients have been described with either a single allele or point mutation in the IGF-1 receptor.[303-305] All cases resulted in growth retardation. One child with two point mutations responded to high doses of GH with an increase in growth.[305]

REFERENCES

1. Salmon WD Jr, Daughaday WH: A hormonally controlled serum factor which stimulates sulfate incorporation by cartilage in vitro, J Lab Clin Med 49:825, 1957.
2. Schoenle E, Zapf J, Humbel RE, et al: Insulin-like growth factor I stimulates growth in hypophysectomized rats, Nature 296:252, 1982.
3. Murphy LJ, Freisen HG: Differential effects of estrogen and growth hormone on uterine and hepatic insulin like growth factor-I gene expression in ovariectomized and hypophysectomized rat, Endocrinology 122:325, 1988.
4. Holt EC, Van Wyk JJ, Lund PK: Tissue and development specific regulation of a complex family of insulin-like growth factor I messenger ribonucleic acids, Mol Endocrinol 2:1077, 1988.
5. Carlsson B, Carlsson L, Billig H: Estrus cycle dependent covariation of the insulin-like growth factor I (IGF-I) messenger ribonucleic acid and protein in rat ovary, Mol Cell Endocrinol 64:271, 1989.
6. Rotwein P, Bichell DP, Kikuchi K: Multifactorial regulation of IGF-I gene expression, Mol Reprod Dev 35:358, 1993.
7. Hepler JE, VanWyk JJ, Lund PK: Different half-lives of insulin-like growth factor-I mRNA that differ in length of 3′ untranslated sequence, Endocrinology 127:155, 1990.
8. Bayne ML, Applebaum J, Chicchi GG, et al: The roles of tyrosines 24, 31, and 60 in the high-affinity binding of insulin-like growth factor-I to the type 1 insulin-like growth factor receptor, J Biol Chem 265:15648, 1990.
9. Bayne ML, Applebaum J, Underwood D, et al: The C region of human insulin-like growth factor (IGF) I is required for high-affinity binding to the type I IGF receptor, J Biol Chem 264:11004, 1989.
10. Vajdos FF, Ultsch M, Schaffer ML, et al: Crystal structure of human insulin-like growth factor-1: detergent binding inhibits binding protein interactions, Biochem 40:11022, 2001.
11. Zeslawski W, Beisel HG, Kamionka M, et al: The interaction of insulin-like growth factor-I with the N-terminal domain of IGFBP-5, EMBO J 20:3638, 2001.
12. Shaffer ML, Deshayes K, Nakamura G, et al: Complex with a phage display-derived peptide provides insight into the function of insulin-like growth factor I, Biochem 42:9324, 2003.
13. Gauguin L, Delaine Ca, Alvino CL, et al: Alanine scanning of a putative receptor binding surface of insulin-like growth factor-I, J Biol Chem 283:20821, 2008.
14. Clemmons DR, Dehoff MH, Busby WH, et al: Competition for binding to insulin-like growth factor (IGF) binding protein-2, 3, 4, and 5 by the IGFs and IGF analogs, Endocrinology 131:890, 1992.
15. Siwanowicz I, Popowicz GM, Wisniewska M, et al: Structural basis for the regulation of insulin-like growth factors by IGF binding proteins, Structure (Camb) 103:155, 2005.
16. Gauguin L, Klaproth B, Sajid W, et al: Structural basis for the lower affinity of the insulin-like growth factors for the insulin receptor, J Biol Chem 283:2604, 2008.
17. Kaleko M, Rutter WJ, Miller D: Overexpression of the human insulin-like growth factor-I receptor promotes ligand dependent neoplastic transformation, Mol Cell Biol 10:464, 1990.
18. Werner H, Roberts CT Jr: The IGFI receptor gene: a molecular target for disrupted transcription factors, Genes Chrom Can 36:113, 2003.
19. Du J, Meng XP, Delafontaine P: Transcriptional regulation of the insulin-like growth factor-I receptor gene: Evidence for protein kinase C dependent and independent pathways, Endocrinology 138:1378, 1996.

20. Abbott AM, Bueno R, Pedrin MT, et al: Insulin-like growth factor-I receptor gene structure, J Biol Chem 267:10759, 1992.
21. LeRoith D, Werner H, Beitner-Johnson D, et al: Molecular and cellular aspects of the insulin-like growth factor-I receptor, Endocrine Rev 16:143, 1995.
22. Lou M, Garrett TP, McKern NM, et al: The first three domains of the insulin receptor differ structurally from the insulin-like growth factor 1 receptor in the regions governing ligand specificity, Proc Natl Acad Sci U S A 103:12429, 2006.
23. Keyhanfar M, Booker GW, Whittaker J, et al: Precise mapping of an IGF-I binding site on the IGF-1R, Biochem J 401:269, 2007.
24. Lawrence MC, McKern NM, Ward CW: Insulin receptor structure and its implications for the IGF-1 receptor, Curr Opin Struct Biol 17:699, 2007.
25. Whittaker J, Groth AV, Mynarcik DC, et al: Alanine scanning mutagenesis of a type I insulin-like growth factor receptor ligand binding site, J Biol Chem 276:43980, 2001.
26. Wu J, Li W, Craddock BP, et al: Small-molecule inhibition and activation-loop trans-phosphorylation of the IGF1 receptor, EMBO J 27:1985, 2008.
27. Pautsch A, Zoephel A, Ahorn H, et al: Crystal structure of bisphosphorylated IGF-1 receptor kinase: insight into domain movements upon kinase activation, Structure 9:955, 2001.
28. Yamasaki H, Pager D, Gebremedhin S, et al: Human insulin-like growth factor-I receptor 950 tyrosine is required for somatotroph growth factor signal transduction, J Biol Chem 267:20953, 1992.
29. Soos MA, Field CE, Siddle K: Purified hybrid insulin/insulin-like growth factor-I receptors bind insulin-like growth factor-I but not insulin with high affinity, Biochem J 290:419, 1993.
30. Pandini G, Frasca F, Mineo R, et al: Insulin/insulin-like growth factor I hybrid receptors have different biological characteristics depending on the insulin receptor isoform involved, J Biol Chem 277:39684, 2002.
31. Rotem-Yehudar R, Galperin E, Horowitz M: Association of insulin-like growth factor 1 receptor with EHD1 and SNAP29, J Biol Chem 276:33054, 2001.
32. Navab R, Chevet E, Authier F, et al: Inhibition of endosomal insulin-like growth factor-I processing by cysteine proteinase inhibitors blocks receptor-mediated functions, J Biol Chem, 276:13644, 2001.
33. Bohula EA, Salibury AJ, Sohail M, et al: The efficacy of small interfering RNAs targeted to the type 1 insulin-like growth factor receptor (IGF1R) is influenced by secondary structure in the IGF1R transcript, J Biol Chem 278:15991, 2003.
34. Li S, Resnicoff M, Boneya R: Effect of mutations at serines 1280–1281 on the mitogenic and transforming activities of the IGF-I receptor, J Biol Chem 271:12254, 1996.
35. DeAngelis T, Ferber A, Baserga R: The insulin-like growth factor I receptor is a requirement for the mitogenic and transforming activities of the platelet derived growth factor receptor, J Cell Physiol 164:214, 1995.
36. Sell C, Rubini R, Rubin R, et al: Simian virus 40 large tumor antigen is unable to transform mouse embryo fibroblasts lacking type I insulin like growth factor receptor, Proc Natl Acad Sci U S A 90:11217, 1993.
37. Liu JP, Baker J, Perkins AS, et al: Mice carrying null mutations of the genes encoding insulin like growth factor I (IGF-I) and type 1 IGF receptor (IGF/r), Cell 75:73, 1993.
38. D'Mello SR, Galli C, Ciott T, et al: Induction of apoptosis in cerebellar granule neurons by low potassium:

inhibition of death by insulin-like growth factor-I and cAMP, Proc Natl Acad Sci U S A 90:10989, 1993.
39. Rubin R, Baserga R: Biology of disease: Insulin-like growth factor-I receptor: its role in cell proliferation, apoptosis, and tumorigenicity, Lab Invest 13:311, 1995.
40. Faria TN, Blakesley VA, Kato H, et al: Role of the carboxy-terminal domain of the insulin and insulin-like growth factor-I receptors in receptor function, J Biol Chem 269:13922, 1994.
41. Sun XJ, Wang LM, Zhang Y, et al: Role of IRS-2 in insulin and cytokine signaling, Nature 377:173, 1995.
42. Pete G, Fuller Cr, Oldham JM, et al: Postnatal growth responses to insulin-like growth factor I in insulin receptor substrate-1-deficient mice, Endocrinol 140:5478, 1999.
43. Myers MJ, White MF: The IRS-1 signaling system, Trends in Biological Sciences 19:289, 1994.
44. Myers MG, Sun XJ, Cheatham B, et al: IRS-I is a common element in insulin and insulin-like growth factor I signalling to the phosphatidylinositol 5′-kinase, Endocrinology 132:1421, 1993.
45. Clemmons DR, Maile LA: Interaction between insulin-like growth factor-I receptor and alphaVbeta3 integrin linked signaling pathways: cellular responses to change sin multiple signaling inputs, Mol Endocrinol 19:1, 2004.
46. Kiely PA, Sant A, O'Connor R: RACK1 is an insulin-like growth factor 1 (IGF-1) receptor-interacting protein that can regulate IGF-I mediated Akt activation and protection from cell death, J Biol Chem 277:22581, 2002.
47. Giovannone B, Lee E, Laviola L, et al: Two novel proteins that are linked to insulin-like growth factor (IGF-I) receptors by the Grb10 adapter and modulate IGF-I signaling, J Biol Chem 278:31564, 2003.
48. Dalle S, Ricketts W, Imamura T, et al: Insulin and insulin-like growth factor I receptors utilize different G protein signaling components, J Biol Chem 276:15688, 2001.
49. Myers MJ, White MF: Insulin signal transduction and the IRS proteins, Ann Rev Pharmacol 36:615, 1996.
50. Lauzier MC, Page EL, Michaud MD, et al: Differentiation regulation of hypoxia-inducible factor-1 through receptor tyrosine kinase transactivation in vascular smooth muscle cells, Endocrinol 148:4023–4031, 2007.
51. Holzman JL, Liu L, Duke BJ, et al: Transactivation of the IGF-1R aldosterone, Am J Physiol Renal Physiol 292:F1219, 2006.
52. Song RX, Zhang Z, Chen Y, et al: Estrogen signaling via a linear pathway involving insulin-like growth factor I receptor, matrix metalloproteinases, and epidermal growth factor receptor to activate mitogen-activated protein kinase in MCF-7 breast cancer cells, Endocrinol 148:4091, 2007.
53. Verras M, Sun Z: 2005 Beta-Catenin is involved in insulin-like growth factor 1-mediated transactivation of the androgen receptor, Mol Endocrinol 19:391, 2005.
54. El-Shewy HM, Kelly FL, Barki-Harrington L, et al: Ectodomain shedding-dependent transactivation of epidermal growth factor receptors in response to insulin-like growth factor type 1, Mol Endocrinol 18:2727, 2004.
55. Venters HD, Tang Q, Liu Q, et al: A new mechanism of neurodegeneration: a proinflammatory cytokine inhibits receptor signaling by a survival peptide, Proc Natl Acad Sci U S A 96:9879, 1999.

56. Brown J, Delaine C, Zaccheo OJ, et al: Structure and functional analysis of the IGF-II/IGF2R interaction, EMBO J 27:265, 2008.
57. Williams C, Rezgui D, Prince SN, et al: Structural insights into the interaction of insulin-like growth factor 2 with IGF2R domain 11, Structure 15:1065, 2007.
58. Lau MM, Stewart CHE, Liu Z, et al: Loss of imprinted IGF-II cation independent mannose 6 phosphate receptor results in fetal overgrowth and perinatal lethality, Gene Dev 8:2953, 1994.
59. McKinnon T, Chakraborty C, Gleeson L, et al: Stimulation of human extravillous trophoblast migration by IGF-II is mediated by IGF type 2 receptor involving inhibitory G protein(s) and phosphorylation, J Clin Endocrinol Metab 86:3665, 2001.
60. Jones JI, Clemmons DR: Insulin like growth factor and their binding proteins: biologic actions, Endocrine Rev 16:3, 1995.
61. Rechler MM: Insulin like growth factor binding proteins, Vitamins and Hormones 47:1, 1993.
62. Imai Y, Moralez A, Andag C, et al: Substitutions for hydrophobic amino acids in the N-terminal domains of IGFBP-3 and -5 markedly reduce IGF-I binding and alter their biologic actions, J Biol Chem 275:18188, 2000.
63. Bach LA, Headley SJ, Norton RS: IGF-binding proteins-the pieces are falling into place, Trends Endocrinol Metab 16:228, 2005.
64. Kuang Z, Yao S, McNeil KA, et al: Cooperativity of the N- and C-terminal domains of insulin-like growth factor (IGF) binding protein 2 in IGF binding, Biochem 46:13720, 2007.
65. Jones JL, Gockerman A, Busby WH Jr, et al: Insulin-like growth factor binding protein 1 stimulates cell migration and binds to the α5β1 integrin by means of its Arg-Gly-Asp sequence, Proc Natl Acad Sci U S A 90:10553, 1993.
66. Booth BA, Boes M, Dake BL, et al: Structure function relationships in the heparin binding C-terminal region of insulin-like growth factor binding protein-3, Growth Regul 6:206, 1996.
67. Durham SK, Keifer MR, Riggs BL, et al: Regulation of insulin like growth factor binding protein-4 by a specific insulin like growth factor binding protein-4 protease in normal human osteoblast like cells. Implications on human cell physiology, J Bone Mineral Res 9:111, 1994.
68. James PL, Jones SB, Busby WH, et al: IGF binding protein-5 is expressed in myoblast differentiation and is highly conserved, J Biol Chem 268:22305, 1993.
69. Clemmons DR: Insulin-like growth factor binding proteins and their role in controlling IGF actions, Cytokine Growth Factor Rev 8:45, 1997.
70. Martin JL, Willetts KE, Baxter RC: Purification and properties of a novel insulin-like growth factor-II binding protein from transformed human fibroblasts, J Biol Chem 265:4124, 1990.
71. Aimaretti G, Boschetti M, Corneli G, et al: Normal age-dependent values of serum insulin growth factor-1: results from a healthy Italian population, J Endocrinol Invest 31:455, 2008.
72. Hong Y, Pedesen NL, Brismar K, et al: Quantitative genetic analyses of insulin like growth factor I (IGF-I), IGF binding protein-1 and insulin levels in middle-aged and elderly twins, J Clin Endocrinol Metab 81:1791, 1996.
73. Vaessen N, Heutink P, Janssen JA, et al: A polymorphism in the gene for IGF-I: functional properties and risk for type 2 diabetes and myocardial infarction, Diabetes 50:637, 2001.
74. Juul A, Skakkebaek NE: Prediction of the outcome of growth hormone provocative testing in short children by measurement of serum levels of insulin-like growth factor I and insulin-like growth factor binding protein 3, J Pediatr 130:197–204, 1997.
75. Ranke MB, Schweizer R, Elmlinger MW, et al: Significance of basal IGF-I, IGFBP-3 and IGFBP-2 measurements in the diagnostics of short stature in children, Horm Res 54:60, 2000.
76. Juul A, Dalgaard P, Blum WF, et al: Serum levels of insulin-like growth factor (IGF) binding protein-3 (IGFBP-3) in healthy infants, children, and adolescents: the relation to IGF-I, IGF-II, IGFBP-1, IGFBP-2, age, sex, body mass index, and pubertal maturation, J Clin Endocrinol Metab 80:2534, 1995.
77. Mitchell H, Dattani MT, Naduri V, et al: Failure of IGF-I and IGFBP-3 to diagnose growth hormone insufficiency, Arch Dis Child 80:443, 1999.
78. Jorge AA, Souza SC, Arnhold IJ, et al: Poor reproducibility of IGF-I and IGF binding protein-3 generation test in children with short stature and normal coding region of the GH receptor gene, J Clin Endocrinol Metab 87:469, 2002.
79. Jorgensen JO, Hansen TK, Conceicaso FL, et al: Short-term tools to measure responsiveness to growth hormone replacement, Horm Res 55(suppl 2):40, 2001.
80. Clemmons DR, Underwood LE, Ridgeway EC: Evaluation of acromegaly by radioimmunoassay of somatomedin-C, N Engl J Med 301:1138, 1979.
81. Melmed S: Acromegaly, N Engl J Med 322: 966, 1990.
82. Stoffel-Wagner B, Springer W, Bidlingmaier F, et al: A comparison of different methods for diagnosing acromegaly, Clin Endocrinol 46:531, 1997.
83. Clemmons DR: Clinical utility of measurements of insulin-like growth factor 1, Nat Clin Pract Endocrinol Metab 2:436, 2006.
84. Noel M, Chevenne D, Porquet D: Utility of insulin-like growth factor-I and its binding protein assays, Curr Opin Clin Nutr Metab Care 4:399, 2001.
85. Thissen JP, Underwood LE, Ketelslegers JM: Regulation of insulin-like growth factor-I in starvation and injury, Nutr Rev 57:167, 1999.
86. Tonshoff B, Kiepe D, Ciarmatori S: Growth hormone/insulin-like growth factor system in children with chronic renal failure, Pediatr Nephrol 20:279, 2005.
87. De Palo EF, Bassanello M, Lancerin F, et al: GH/IGF system, cirrhosis and liver transplantation, Clin Chim Acta 310:31, 2001.
88. Bereket A, Lang CH, Blethen SL, et al: Effect of insulin on the insulin-like growth factor system in children with new onset insulin dependent diabetes, J Clin Endocrinol Metab 80:1312, 1995.
89. Morrow LA, O'Brien MB, Moller DE, et al: Recombinant human insulin-like growth factor-I therapy improves glycemic control and insulin action in the type A syndrome of severe insulin resistance, J Clin Endocrinol Metab 79:205, 1994.
90. Baxter RC, Martin JL: Radioimmunoassay of growth hormone dependent insulin-like growth factor binding protein in human plasma, J Clin Invest 78:1504, 1986.
91. Blum WF, Albertsson-Wikland K, Rosberg S, et al: Serum levels of insulin-like growth factor I (IGF-I) and IGF binding protein 3 reflect spontaneous growth hormone secretion, J Clin Endocrinol Metab 76:1610, 1993.
92. Leogney SR, Baxter RC, Carrerato T, et al: Structure and functional expression of acid-labile subunit of the insulin-like growth factor binding protein complex, Mol Endocrinol 6:870, 1992.
93. Grinspoon S, Clemmons DR, Swearingen B, et al: Serum insulin-like growth factor-binding protein-3 levels in the diagnosis of acromegaly, J Clin Endocrinol Metab 80:927, 1995.
94. Laursen T, Flyvbjerg A, Jorgensen JO, et al: Stimulation of the 150-kilodalton insulin-like growth factor binding protein-3 ternary complex by continuous and pulsatile patterns of growth hormone (GH) administration in GH-deficient patients, J Clin Endocrinol Metab 85:4310, 2000.
95. Pfeilschifter J, Scheidt-Nave C, Leidig-Bruckner G, et al: Relationship between circulating insulin-like growth factor components and sex hormones in a population based sample of 50- to 80-year-old men and women, J Clin Endocrinol Metab 81:2534, 1996.
96. Miell JP, Taylor AM, Zini M, et al: Effects of hypothyroidism and hyperthyroidism on insulin-like growth factors (IGFs) and growth hormone- and IGF binding proteins, J Clin Endocrinol Metab 76:950, 1993.
97. Kupfer SR, Underwood LE, Baxter RC, et al: Enhancement of the anabolic effects of growth hormone and insulin like growth factor-I by the use of both agents simultaneously, J Clin Invest 91:391, 1993.
98. Maile LA, Holly JM: Insulin-like growth factor binding protein (IGFBP) proteolysis: occurrence, identification, role and regulation, Growth Horm IGF Res 9:85–95, 1999.
99. Olausson H, Lof M, Brismar K, et al: Longitudinal study of the maternal insulin-like growth factor system before, during and after pregnancy in relation to fetal and infant weight, Horm Res 69:99, 2008.
100. Clemmons DR, Sleevi M, Busby WH Jr: Recombinant, nonglycosylated human insulin-like growth factor-binding protein-3 (IGFBP-3) is degraded preferentially after administration to type II diabetics, resulting in increased endogenous glycosylated IGFBP-3, J Clin Endocrinol Metab 90:6561, 2005.
101. Blum WF, Brier BH: Radioimmunoassays for IGFs and IGFBPs, Growth Regulation 4:11, 1994.
102. Ooi GT, Orlowski CC, Brown AL, et al: Different tissue distribution and hormonal regulation of messenger RNAs encoding rat insulin-like growth factor binding proteins-1 and 2, Mol Endocrinol 4:321, 1990.
103. Daughaday WH, Trivedi B, Baxter RC: Serum "big" insulin-like growth factor-II from patients with tumor hypoglycemia lacks normal E-domain O-linked glycosylation, a possible determinant of normal propeptide processing, Proc Natl Acad Sci U S A 90:5283, 1993.
104. Bereket A, Lang CH, Wilson TA: Alterations in the growth hormone-insulin-like growth factor axis in insulin dependent diabetes mellitus, Horm Metab Res 31:172–181, 1999.
105. Smith WJ, Underwood LE, Clemmons DR: Effects of Caloric or Protein Restriction on Insulin-Like Growth Factor-I (IGF-I) and IGF-Binding Proteins in Children and Adults, J Clin Endocrinol Metab 80:443, 1995.
106. Straus DS, Takemoto CD: Effect of dietary protein deprivation insulin-like growth factor IGF-I and II, IGF binding protein-2 and serum albumin gene expression in the rat, Endocrinology 127:1849, 1990.
107. Ooi GT, Tseng LY, Tran MQ, et al: Insulin rapidly decreases insulin-like growth factor-binding protein-1 gene transcription in streptozotocin-diabetic rats, Mol Endocrinol 6:2219, 1992.
108. Busby WH, Snyder DK, Clemmons DR: Radioimmunoassay of a 26,000 dalton plasma insulin like growth factor binding protein: control by nutritional variables, J Clin Endocrinol Metab 67:1225, 1988.
109. Gan L, Pan H, Unterman TG: Insulin response sequence-dependent and independent mechanisms mediate effects of insulin on glucocorticoid-stimulated insulin-like growth factor binding protein-1 promoter activity, Endocrinol 146:4274, 2005.
110. Bar RS, Boes M, Clemmons DR, et al: Insulin differentially alters transcapillary movement of intravascular IGFBP-1, IGFBP-2 and endothelial cell IGF binding proteins in rat heart, Endocrinology 127:497, 1990.
111. Westwood M, Gibson JM, Williams AC, et al: Hormonal regulation of circulating insulin-like growth factor-binding protein-1 phosphorylation status, J Clin Endocrinol Metab 80:3520, 1995.
112. Lewitt MS, Denyer GS, Cooney GJ, et al: Insulin-like growth factor binding protein-1 modulates blood glucose levels, Endocrinol 129:2254, 1991.
113. Davies SC, Wass JAH, Ross RJM, et al: Induction of a specific protease for insulin-like growth factor binding protein-3 in the circulation during severe illness, J Endocrinol 130:469, 1991.
114. Scharla SH, Strong DD, Rosen C, et al: 1,25-Dihydroxyvitamin D3 increases secretion of insulin-like growth factor binding protein-4 (IGFBP-4) by human osteoblast-like cells in vitro and elevates IGFBP-4 serum levels in vivo, J Clin Endocrinol Metab 77:1190–1197, 1993.
115. Ehrnborg C, Ohlsson C, Mohan S, et al: Increased serum concentration of IGFBP-4 and IGFBP-5 in healthy adults during one month's treatment with supraphysiological doses of growth hormone, Growth Horm IGF Res 17:234, 2007.
116. Rooman RP, De Beeck LO, Martin M, et al: IGF-I, IGF-II, free IGF-I and IGF-binding proteins-2 to -6 during high dose estrogen treatment in constitutionally tall girls, Eur J Endocrinol 146:823, 2002.
117. Baxter RC: Changes in the IGF-IGFBP axis in critical illness, Best Pract Res Clin Endocrinol Metab 15:421, 2001.
118. Houang M, Cabrol S, Perin L, et al: Insulin-like growth factor-I (IGF-I), insulin-like growth factor binding proteins (IGFBP) and insulin-like growth factor type I receptor in children with various status of chronic renal failure, Growth Horm IGF Res 10:332, 2000.
119. Han VKM, D'Ercole AJ, Lund PK: Cellular location of somatomedin (insulin-like growth factor) messenger RNA in the human fetus, Science 236:193, 1987.

120. Roberts CT, Lasky SR, Lowe WL, et al: Molecular coding of rat insulin-like growth factor-I complementary DNA: Differential messenger RNA processing of regulation by growth hormone in extrahepatic tissue, Mol Endocrinol 1:243, 1987.
121. Isgaard J, Nilsson A, Vikma A, et al: Growth hormone regulates the level of IGF-I mRNA in rat growth plate, Endocrinology 122:1515, 1988.
122. Grundberg E, Brandstrom H, Lam KC, et al: Systemic assessment of the human osteoblast transcriptome in resting and induced primary cells, Physiol Genomics 33:301–311, 2008.
123. Silver DM, Fudo H, Halperin D, et al: Differential expression of insulin like growth factor I (IGF-I) and IGF-II messenger ribonucleic acid in growing rat bone, Endocrinology 132:1158, 1993.
124. McCarthy TL, Ji C, Centrella M, et al: Links among growth factors. Hormones and nuclear factors with essential roles in bone formation, Crit Rev Oral Biol Med 11:409, 2000.
125. Mendez-Davila C, Garcia-Moreno C, Trubi C, et al: Effects of 17beta-estradiol, tamoxifen and raloxifene on the protein and mRNA expression of interleukin-6, transforming growth factor-beta1 and insulin-like growth factor-1 in primary human osteoblast cultures, J Endocrinol Invest 27:904, 2004.
126. Rosen CJ: The cellular and clinical parameters of anabolic therapy for osteoporosis, Crit Rev Eukaryot Gene Expr 13:25, 2003.
127. Sivan B, Lilos P, Laron Z: Effects of insulin-like growth factor-I deficiency and replacement therapy on the hematopoietic system in patients with Laron syndrome (primary growth hormone insensitivity), J Pediatr Endocrinol Metab 16:509, 2003.
128. Davidson Tr, Chamberlain CS, Bridges TS, et al: Effect of follicle size on in-vitro production of steroids and insulin-like growth factor (IGF-I), IGF-II, and the IGF binding proteins by equine ovarian granulosa cells, Biol Reprod 66:1640, 2002.
129. Moyano P, Rotwein P: Mini-review: estrogen action in the uterus and insulin-like growth factor-I, Growth Horm IGF Res 14:431, 2004.
130. D'Ercole AJ, Ye P: Expanding the mind: IGF-I and brain development, Endocrinol epub July 31, 2008.
131. Cardona-Gomez GP, Mendez P, DonCarlos LL, et al: Interactions of estrogen and insulin-like growth factor-I in the brain: molecular mechanisms and functional implications, J Steroid Biochem Mol Biol 83:211, 2002.
132. Adamo ML, Farrar RP: Resistance training, and IGF involvement in the maintenance of muscle mass during the aging process, Ageing Res Rev 5:310, 2006.
133. Edwall D, Schalling M, Jennische E, et al: Induction of insulin-like growth factor I messenger ribonucleic acid during regeneration of rat skeletal muscle, Endocrinol 124:820, 1989.
134. Paul AC, Rosenthal N: Different modes of hypertrophy in skeletal muscle fibers, J Cell Biol 156:751, 2002.
135. McMullen JR, Izumo S: Role of the insulin-like growth factor I (IGFI)/phosphoinositide-3-kinase (PI3K) pathway mediating physiological cardiac hypertrophy, Novartis Found Symp 274:90, 2006.
136. Cooper SA, Whaley-Connell A, Habibi J, et al: Renin-angiotensin-aldosterone system and oxidative stress in cardiovascular insulin resistance, Am J Physiol Heart Circ Physiol 293:2009, 2007.
137. Cercek B, Fishbein MC, Forrester JS, et al: Induction of insulin-like growth factor I messenger RNA in rat aorta after balloon denudation, Circ Res 66:1755, 1990.
138. Eleswarapu S, Gu Z, Jiang H: Growth hormone regulation of insulin-like growth factor-I gene expression may be mediated by multiple distal signal transducer and activator of transcription 5 binding sites, Endocrinol 249:2230, 2008.
139. Lowe WL, Adamo M, Werner H, et al: Regulation by fasting of insulin-like growth factor I and its receptor: Effects on gene expression and binding, J Clin Invest 84:619, 1989.
140. Butler ST, Marr AL, Pelton Sh, et al: Insulin restores GH responsiveness during lactation-induced negative energy balance in dairy cattle: effects on expression of IGF-I and GH receptor, J Endocrinol 176:205, 2003.
141. Rotwein P, Pollack KM, Watson M, et al: Insulin-like growth factor gene expression during rat embryonic development, Endocrinology 121:2141, 1987.
142. Hirschberg R: The physiology and pathophysiology of IGF-I in the kidney, Adv Exp Med Biol 343:345, 1993.
143. Flyvbjerg A, Bennett WF, Rasch R, et al: Compensatory renal growth in uninephrectomized adult mice is growth hormone dependent, Kidney Int 56:2048, 1999.
144. Dupont J, Pierre A, Froment P, et al: The insulin-like growth factor axis in cell cycle progression, Horm Metab Res 35:740, 2003.
145. Travali S, Reiss K, Ferber A, et al: Constitutively expressed c-myb abrogates the requirement for insulin-like growth factor-I in 3T3 fibroblasts, Mol Cell Biol 11:731, 1991.
146. Coppola D, Ferber A, Miura A, et al: A functional insulin-like growth factor I receptor is required for the mitogenic and transforming activities of the epidermal growth factor receptor, Mol Cell Biol 14:4588, 1994.
147. Pietrzkowski Z, Lammers R, Carpenter G, et al: Constitutive expression of insulin-like growth factor-I and insulin-like growth factor-I receptor abrogates all requirements for exogenous growth factors, Cell Growth and Differentiation 3:199, 1992.
148. Lowe WL: Biologic actions of the insulin-like growth factors. In LeRoith D, editor: Insulin-like Growth Factors: Molecular and Cellular Aspects, Boca Raton, 1991, CRC Press, p 49.
149. Nilsson O, Marino R, De Luca F, et al: Endocrine regulation of the growth plate, Horm Res 64:157, 2005.
150. Loeser RF, Shanker G: Autocrine stimulation by insulin-like growth factor 1 and insulin like growth factor 2 mediates chondrocyte survival in vitro, Arthritis Rheum 43:1552, 2000.
151. Madry H, Zurakowski D, Trippel SB: Overexpression of human insulin-like growth factor-I promotes new tissue formation in an ex vivo model of articular chrondrocyte transplantation, Gene Ther 8:1443, 2001.
152. Yakar S, Rosen C: From mouse to man: redefining the role of insulin-like growth factor-I in the acquisition of bone mass, Pro Soc Expo Biol Med 228:245, 1998.
153. Zhang M, Xuan S, Bouxsein ML, et al: Osteoblast-specific knockout of the insulin-like growth factor (IGF) receptor gene reveals an essential role of IGF signaling in bone matrix mineralization, J Biol Chem 277:44005, 2002.
154. Zhao G, Monier-Faugere MC, Langub MC, et al: Targeted overexpression of insulin-like growth factor I in osteoblasts of transgenic mice: increased trabecular bone volume without increased osteoblast proliferation, Endocrinol 141:2674, 2000.
155. Wang Y, Nishida S, Boudignon BM, et al: IGF-I receptor is required for the anabolic actions of parathyroid hormone on bone, J Bone Miner Res 22:1329, 2007.
156. Sjogren K, Sheng M, Moverare S, et al: Effects of liver-derived insulin-like growth factor I on bone metabolism in mice, J Bone Miner Res 17:1977, 2002.
157. Takahashi T, Ishida K, Itoh K, et al: IGF-I gene transfer by electroporation promotes regeneration in a muscle injury model, Gene Ther 10:612, 2003.
158. Banu J, Wang L, Kalu DN: Effects of increased muscle mass on bone in male mice overexpressing IGF-I in skeletal muscles, Calcif Tissue Int 73:196, 2003.
159. Welsh S, Plank D, Witt S, et al: Cardiac-specific IGF-1 expression attenuates dilated cardiomyopathy in tropomodulin-overexpressing transgenic mice, Circ Res 90:641, 2002.
160. Zhu B, Zhao G, Witte DP, et al: Targeted overexpression of IGF-I in smooth muscle cells of transgenic mice enhances neointimal formation through increased proliferation and cell migration after intraarterial injury, Endocrinol 142:3598, 2001.
161. Cao Y, Gunn AJ, Bennet L, et al: Insulin-like growth factor (IGF)-1 suppresses oligodendrocyte caspase-3 activation and increases glial proliferation after ischemia in near-term fetal sheep, J Cereb Blood Flow Metab 23:739, 2003.
162. Homma K, Koriyama Y, Mawatari K, et al: Early down-regulation of IGF-I decides the fate of rat retinal ganglion cells after optic nerve injury, Neurochem Int 50:741, 2007.
163. Vicario-Abejon C, Yusta-Boyo MJ, Fernandez-Moreno C, et al: Locally born olfactory bulb stem cells proliferate in response to insulin-related factors and require endogenous insulin-like growth factor-I for differentiation into neurons and glia, J Neurosci 23:895, 2003.
164. Ye P, Xing YZ, Dai ZH, et al: In vivo actions of insulin-like growth factor-I (IGF-I) on cerebellum development in transgenic mice: Evidence that IGF-I increases proliferation of granule cell progenitors, Dev Brain Res 95:44, 1996.
165. Bateman JM, McNeill H: Insulin/IGF signaling in neurogenesis, Cell Mol Life Sci 63:1701, 2006.
166. Muta K, Krontes B: Apoptosis of human erythroid colony forming cells is decreased by stem cell factor and insulin-like growth factor-I as well as erythropoietin, J Cell Physiol 156:264, 1993.
167. Rodriguez-Tarduchy G, Collins MKL, Garcia I, et al: Insulin-like growth factor I inhibits apoptosis in IL-3 dependent hematopoietic cells, J Immunol 149:535, 1992.
168. Florini JR, Ewton DZ, Root SL: IGF-I stimulates terminal myogenic differentiation by induction of myogenin gene expression, Mol Endocrinol 5:718, 1991.
169. Palmer S, Myerson G, Lindgren E, et al: Insulin-like growth factor-I shifts from promoting cell division to potentiating maturation during normal differentiation, Proc Natl Acad Sci USA 88:9994, 1991.
170. Khamsi F, Roberge S, Yavas Y, et al: Recent discoveries in physiology of insulin-like growth factor-1 and its interaction with gonadotropins in folliculogenesis, Endocrine 16:151–165, 2001.
171. Mesiano S, Jaffe RB: Role of growth factors in the developmental regulation of the human fetal adrenal cortex, Steroids 62:62, 1997.
172. Yamasaki H, Prager D, Gebremedhin S, et al: Insulin-like growth factor-I (IGF-I) attenuation of growth hormone is enhanced by overexpression of pituitary IGF-I receptors, Mol Endocrinol 5:890, 1991.
173. Duan C, Hawes S, Prevette T, et al: Insulin like growth factor-I (IGF-I) stimulates IGF binding protein-5 synthesis through transcriptional activation of the gene in aortic smooth muscle cells, J Biol Chem 271:4280, 1996.
174. Spangenburg EE, Bowles DK, Booth FW: IGF-I induced transcriptional activity of the skeletal {alpha} action gene is regulated by signaling mechanisms linked to voltage-gated calcium channels during myoblast differentiation, Endocrinol 145:2054, 2003.
175. Dupont J, Fernandez AM, Glackin CA, et al: Insulin-like growth factor 1 (IGF-1) induced twist expression is involved in the anti-apoptotic effects of the IGF-I receptor, J Biol Chem 276:26699, 2001.
176. Mulligan C, Rochford J, Denyer G, et al: Microarray analysis of insulin and insulin-like growth factor-1 (IGF-1) receptor signaling reveals the selective up-regulation of the mitogen heparin-binding EGF-like growth factor by IGF-1, J Biol Chem 277:42480, 2002.
177. Grohmann M, Foulstone E, Welsh G, et al: Isolation and validation of human prepubertal skeletal muscle cells: maturation and metabolic effects of IGF-I, IGFBP-3 and TNFalpha, J Physiol 568:229, 2005.
178. Zheng B, Clemmons DR: Blocking ligand occupancy of the $\alpha V\beta 3$ integrin inhibits IGF-I signaling in vascular smooth muscle cells, Proc Natl Acad Sci U S A 95:11217, 1998.
179. Samani AA, Yakar S, LeRoith D, et al: The role of the IGF system in cancer growth and metastasis: overview and recent insights, Endocr Rev 28:20, 2007.
180. Yakar S, LeRoith D, Brodt P: The role of the growth hormone/insulin-like growth factor axis in tumor growth and progression: lessons from animal models, Cytokine and Growth Fact Rev 16:407, 2005.
181. Sayer RA, Lancaster JM, Pittman J, et al: High insulin-like growth factor-2 (IGF-2) gene expression is an independent predictor of poor survival for patients with advanced stage serous epithelial ovarian cancer, Gynecol Oncol 96:355, 2005.
182. Haruta M, Arai Y, Sugawara W, et al: Duplication of paternal IGF2 or loss of maternal IGF2 imprinting occurs in half of Wilms tumors with various structural WT1 abnormalities, Genes Chrom Can 47:712, 2008.
183. Baxter RC, Daughaday WH: Impaired function of the ternary insulin like growth factor binding complex in patients with hypoglycemia due to non-islet cell tumors, J Clin Endocrinol Metab 73:696, 1991.
184. Sachdev D, Hartell JS, Lee AV, et al: A dominant negative type I insulin-like growth factor receptor inhibits metastasis of human cancer cells, J Biol Chem 279:5017, 2004.
185. DiGiovanni J, Kiguchi K, Frijhoff A, et al: Deregulated expression of insulin-like growth factor 1 in prostate epithelium leads to neoplasia in transgenic mice, Proc Natl Acad Sci U S A 97:3455, 2000.

186. Wu KD, Zhou L, Burtrum D, et al: Antibody targeting of the insulin-like growth factor I receptor enhances the anti-tumor response of multiple myeloma to chemotherapy through inhibition of tumor proliferation and angiogenesis, Cancer Immunol Immunother 56:343, 2007.

187. Wu JD, et al: In-vivo effects of the human type I insulin-like growth factor receptor antibody A12 on androgen-dependent and androgen-independent human prostate tumors, Clin Cancer Res 11:3065, 2005.

188. Miyamoto S, et al: Blockade of paracrine supply of insulin-like growth factors using neutralizing antibodies suppresses the liver metastasis of human colorectal cancers, Clin Cancer Res 11:3494, 2005.

189. Fowlkes J, Enghild JJ, Suzukik N, et al: Matrix metalloproteases degrade insulin like growth factor binding protein-3 in dermal fibroblast cultures, J Biol Chem 269:25742, 1994.

190. Lawrence JB, Oxvig C, Overgaard MT, et al: The insulin-like growth factor (IGF-I)-dependent IGF binding protein-4 protease secreted by human fibroblasts is pregnancy-associated plasma protein-A, Proc Natl Acad Sci USA 196:3149, 1999.

191. Nichols TC, Busby WH Jr, Merricks E, et al: Protease-resistant insulin-like growth factor (IGF) binding protein-4 inhibits IGF-I actions and neointimal expansion in a porcine model of neointimal hyperplasia, Endocrinol 148:5002, 2007.

192. Leal SM, Liu Q, Huang GS, et al: The type V transforming growth factor beta receptor is a putative insulin like growth factor binding protein 3 receptor, J Biol Chem 272:20572, 1997.

193. Clemmons DR: Use of mutagenesis to probe IGF binding protein structure/function relationships, Endocr Rev 22:800, 2001.

194. Rechler MM, Clemmons DR: Regulatory actions in insulin-like growth factor binding proteins, Trends Endocrinol Metab 9:176, 1998.

195. Burch WW, Correa J, Shaveley JE, et al: The 25 k Dalton insulin-like growth factor (IGF) binding protein inhibits both basal and IGF mediated growth in chick embryonic pelvic cartilage in vitro, J Clin Endocrinol Metab 70:173, 1990.

196. Fottner C, Spottl G, Weber MM: The divergent effect of insulin-like growth factor binding protein (IGFBP)-1 on IGF induced steroidogenesis in bovine adrenocortical cells is not due to its phosphorylation status, Exp Clin Endocrinol Diabetes 115:232, 2007.

197. Kajimura S, Aida K, Duan C: Understanding hypoxia-induced gene expression in early development: in vitro and in vivo analysis of hypoxia-inducible factor-1 regulated zebra fish insulin-like growth factor binding protein gene expression, Mol Cell Biol 26:1142, 2006.

198. Marchand A, Tomkiewicz C, Magne L, et al: Endoplasmic reticulum stress induction of insulin-like growth factor-binding protein-1 involves ATF4, J Biol Chem 281:19124, 2006.

199. Wolf E, Lahm H, Wu M, et al: Effects of IGFBP-2 overexpression in vitro and in vivo, Pediatr Nephrol 14:572, 2000.

200. Bar RS, Booth BA, Bowes M, et al: Insulin-like growth factor binding proteins from cultured endothelial cells: purification, characterization, and intrinsic biologic activities, Endocrinology 125:1910, 1989.

201. Russo VC, Schutt BS, Andaloro E, et al: Insulin-like growth factor binding protein-2 binding to extracellular matrix plays a critical role in neuroblastoma cell proliferation, migration and invasion, Endocrinol 146:4445, 2005.

202. Kiepe D, Van der Pas A, Ciarmatori S, et al: Defined carboxy-terminal fragments of insulin-like growth factor binding protein-2 exert similar mitogenic activity on cultures rat growth plate chondrocytes as IGF-I, Endocrinol 149:4901–4911, 2008.

203. Wang H, Wang H, Shen W, et al: Insulin-like growth factor binding protein 2 enhances glioblastoma invasion by activating invasion-enhancing genes, Cancer Res 63:4315, 2003.

204. Conover CA, Johnstone EW, Turner RT, et al: Subcutaneous administration of insulin-like growth factor (IGF)-II/IGF binding protein-2 complex stimulates bone formation and prevents loss of bone mineral density in a rat model of disuse osteoporosis, Growth Horm IGF Res 12:178, 2002.

205. Zhang CC, Kaba M, Iizuka S, et al: Angiopoietin-like 5 and IGFBP2 stimulate ex-vivo expansion of human cord blood hematopoietic stem cells as assayed by NOD/SCID transplantation, Blood 111:3415, 2008.

206. Chesik D, De Keyser J, Wilczak N: Insulin-like growth factor binding protein-2 as a regulator of IGF actions in CNS: implications in multiple sclerosis, Cytokine & Growth Factor Reviews 18:267, 2007.

207. Strange KS, Wilkinson D, Emerman JT: Mitogenic properties of insulin-like growth factors I and II, insulin-like growth factor binding protein-3 and epidermal growth factor on human breast carcinoma cells, Breast Cancer Res Treat 75:203, 2002.

208. Ricort JM, Binoux M: Insulin-like growth factor binding protein-3 activates a phosphotyrosine phosphatase. Effects on the insulin-like growth factor signaling pathway, J Biol Chem 277:19448, 2002.

209. Martin JL, Jambazov S: Insulin-like growth factor binding protein-3 in extracellular matrix stimulates adhesion of breast epithelial cells and activation of p44/42 mitogen-activated protein kinase, Endocrinol 147:4400, 2006.

210. Huynh H, Yang XF, Pollak M: Estradiol and antiestrogens regulate a growth-inhibitory insulin-like growth factor binding protein 3 autocrine loop in human breast cancer cells, J Biol Chem 271:1016, 1996.

211. O'Rear L, Longobardi L, Torello M, et al: Signaling cross talk between IGF-binding protein-3 and transforming growth factor (beta) in mesenchymal chondroprogenitor cell growth, J Mol Endocrinol 34:723, 2005.

212. Silha JV, Sheppard PC, Mishra S, et al: Insulin-like growth factor (IGF) binding protein-3 attenuates prostate tumor growth by IGF-dependent and IGF-independent mechanisms, Endocrinol 147:2112, 2006.

213. Liu B, Lee HY, Weinzimer SA: Direct functional interactions between insulin-like growth factor-binding protein-3 and retinoid X receptor- regulate transcriptional signaling and apoptosis, J Biol Chem 275:33607, 2000.

214. Schedlich LJ, Young TF, Fifth SM, et al: Insulin-like growth factor-binding protein (IGFBP)-3 and IGFBP-5 share a common nuclear transport pathway in T47D human breast carcinoma cells, J Biol Chem 273:18347, 1998.

215. Takaoka M, Kim SH, Okawa T, et al: IGFBP-3 regulated esophageal tumor growth through IGF-dependent and independent mechanisms, Cancer Biol Ther 6:534, 2007.

216. Chan SS, Twigg SM, Firth SM, et al: Insulin-like growth factor binding protein-3 leads to insulin resistance in adipocytes, J Clin Endocrinol Metab 90:6588, 2005.

217. Mohan S, Bautista CM, Wergedal J, et al: Isolation of inhibitory insulin-like growth factor (IGF) binding protein from bone cell conditioned medium: a potential local regulator of IGF action, Proc Natl Acad Sci U S A 86:8338, 1989.

218. Conover CA, Durham SK, Zapf J, et al: Cleavage analysis of insulin-like growth factor (IGF)-dependent IGF-binding protein-4 proteolysis and expression of protease-resistant IGF-binding protein-4 mutants, J Biol Chem 270:4395, 1995.

219. Spicer LJ: Proteolytic degradation of insulin-like growth factor binding proteins by ovarian follicles: Biol Reprod 70:1223, 2003.

220. Parker A, Rees C, Clarke JB, et al: Binding of insulin-like growth factor binding protein-5 to smooth muscle cell extracellular matrix is a major determinant of the cellular response to IGF-I, Mol Biol Cell 9:2383, 1998.

221. Miyakoshi N, Richman C, Kasukawa Y, et al: Evidence that IGF-binding protein-5 functions as a growth factor, J Clin Invest 107:71, 2001.

222. Kuemmerle JF, Zhou H: Insulin-like growth factor-binding protein-5 (IGFBP-5) stimulates growth and IGF-I secretion in human intestinal smooth muscle by Ras-dependent activation of p38 MAP kinase and Erk1/2 pathways, J Biol Chem 277:20563, 2002.

223. Butt AJ, Dickson KA, McDougall F, et al: Insulin-like growth factor-binding protein-5 inhibits the growth of human breast cancer cells in vitro and in vivo, J Biol Chem 278:29676, 2003.

224. Marshman E, Green KA, Flint DJ, et al: Insulin-like growth factor binding protein-5 and apoptosis in mammary epithelial cells, J Cell Sci 116:675, 2003.

225. Butt AJ, Dickson KA, Jambazov S, et al: Enhancement of tumor necrosis factor-alpha-induced growth inhibition by insulin-like growth factor-binding protein-5 (IGFBP-5), but not IGFBP-3 in human breast cancer cells, Endocrinol 146:3113, 2005.

226. Mukherjee A, Wilson EM, Rotwein P: Insulin-like growth factor (IGF) binding protein-5 blocks skeletal muscle differentiation by inhibiting IGF actions, Mol Endocrinol 22:206, 2008.

227. Bach LA: IGFBP-6 five years on; not so "forgotten"? Growth Horm IGF Res 15:185, 2005.

228. Kiepe D, Ulinski T, Powell DR, et al: Differential effects of insulin-like growth factor binding proteins 1, -2, -3 and -6 on cultured growth plate chondrocytes, Kidney Int 62:1591, 2002.

229. Fu P, Thomson JA, Bach LA: Promotion of cancer cell migration: an insulin-like growth factor (IGF) independent action of IGF-binding protein-6, J Biol Chem 282:22298, 2007.

230. Guo L, Zhao YY, Zhao YY, et al: Toxic effects of ICDD on osteogenesis through altering IGFBP-6 gene expression in osteoblasts, Biol Pharm Bull 30:2018, 2007.

231. Douglas RG, Gluckman PD, Ball B, et al: The effects of infusion of insulin-like growth factor I (IGF-I), IGF-II and insulin on glucose and protein metabolism in fasted lambs, J Clin Invest 88:614, 1991.

232. Chrysis D, Zhang J, Underwood LE: Divergent regulation of proteasomes by insulin-like growth factor I and growth hormone in skeletal muscle of rats made catabolic with dexamethasone, Growth Horm IGF Res 12:434, 2002.

233. Lang CH, Frost RA: Role of growth hormone, insulin-like growth factor-I and insulin-like growth factor binding proteins in the catabolic response to injury and infection, Curr Opin Nutr Metab Care 5:271, 2002.

234. Thissen JP, Underwood LE, Maiter DM, et al: Failure of IGF-I infusion to promote growth in protein-restricted rats despite normalization of serum IGF-I concentrations, Endocrinology 128:885, 1991.

235. Jacob RJ, Sherwin RS, Bowen L, et al: Metabolic effects of IGF-I and insulin in spontaneously diabetic BB/w rats, Am J Physiol 260:E262, 1991.

236. Cox GN, McDermott MJ, Merkel E, et al: Recombinant human insulin-like growth factor binding protein-1 inhibits growth stimulated by IGF-I and growth hormone in hypophysectomized rats, Endocrinol 35:1913, 1994.

237. Galiano RD, Zhao L, Clemmons DR, et al: Interaction between the insulin-like growth factor family and the integrin receptor family in tissue repair processes, J Clin Invest 98:2462, 1996.

238. Leu JI, Crissey MA, Taub R: Massive hepatic apoptosis associated with TGF-beta1 activation after Fas ligand treatment of IGF binding protein-1-deficient mice, J Clin Invest 111:129, 2003.

239. Palermo C, Manduca P, Gazzerro E, et al: Potentiating role of insulin-like growth factor binding protein (IGFBP)-2 on IGF-II-stimulated alkaline phosphatase activity in differentiating osteoblasts, Am J Physiol Endocrinol Metab 286:E648, 2004.

240. Bagi CM, Brommage R, Adams SO, et al: Benefit of systemically administered rh IGF-I and rh IGF-I/IGBP-3 on cancellous bone in oophorectomized rats, J Bone Mineral Res 9:1301, 1994.

241. Kim HS, Ali O, Shim M, et al: Insulin-like growth factor binding protein-3 induces insulin resistance in adipocytes in vitro and in rats in vivo, Pediatr Res 61:159, 2007.

242. Chen W, Salojin KV, Mi QS, et al: Insulin-like growth factor (IGF)-I/IGF-binding protein-3 complex: therapeutic efficacy and mechanism of protection against type 1 diabetes, Endocrinol 145:627, 2004.

243. Zappala G, Elbi C, Edwards J, et al: Induction of apoptosis in human prostate cancer cells by insulin-like growth factor binding protein-3 does not require binding to retinoid X receptor-alpha, Endocrinol 149:1802, 2007.

244. Fang P, Hwa V, Little BM, et al: IGFBP-3 sensitizes prostate cancer cells to interferon-gamma-induced apoptosis, Growth Horm IGF Res 18:38, 2007.

245. Miyakoshi N, Qin X, Kasukawa Y, et al: Systemic administration of insulin-like growth factor (IGF) binding protein-4 (IGFBP-4) increases bone formation parameters in mice by increasing IGF bioavailability via an IGFBP-4 protease-dependent mechanism, Endocrinol 142:2641, 2001.

246. Andress DL: IGF-binding protein-5 stimulates osteoblast activity and bone accretion in ovariectomized mice, Am J Physiol Endocrinol Metab 281:283, 2001.

247. Behringer RR, Lewin TM, Quaife CJ, et al: Expression of insulin-like growth factor I stimulates normal somatic growth in growth hormone deficient transgenic mice, Endocrinology 127:1033, 1990.

248. Chrysis D, Calikoglu AS, Ye P, et al: Insulin-like growth factor-I overexpression attenuates cerebellar apoptosis by altering the expression of Bcl family proteins in a developmentally specific manner, J Neurosci 21:1481, 2001.

249. Dai A, Xing Y, Boney CM, et al: Human insulin-like growth factor binding protein-1 (hIGFBP-1) transgenic mice: characterization and insights into the regulation of IGFBP-1 expression, Endocrinology 135:1316, 1994.

250. Rajkumar K, Barron D, Lewitt M, et al: Growth retardation and hyperglycemia in insulin-like growth factor binding protein-1 transgenic mice, Endocrinology 136:4029, 1995.

251. Watson CS, Bialek P, Anzo M, et al: Elevated circulating insulin-like growth factor binding protein-1 is sufficient to cause fetal growth restriction, Endocrinol 147:1175, 2006.

252. Ben Lagha N, Menuelle P, Seurin P, et al: Bone formation in the context of growth retardation induced by hIGFBP-1 overexpression in transgenic mice, Connect Tissue Res 43:515, 2002.

253. Eckstein F, Pavicic T, Nedbal S, et al: Insulin-like growth factor binding protein-2 (IGFBP-2) overexpression negatively regulates bone size and mass, but not density, in the absence and presence of growth hormone/IGF-I excess in transgenic mice, Anat and Embryology 206:139, 2003.

254. DeMambro VE, Clemmons DR, Horton LG, et al: Gender-specific changes in bone turnover and skeletal architecture in IGFBP-2 null mice, Endocrinol 149:2051, 2008.

255. Silha JV, Mishra S, Rosen CJ, et al: Perturbations in bone formation and resorption in insulin-like growth factor binding protein-3 transgenic mice, J Bone Miner Res 18:1834, 2003.

256. Silha JV, Gui Y, Mishra S, et al: Overexpression of gly56/gly80/gly81-mutant insulin-like growth factor binding protein-3 in transgenic mice, Endocrinol 146:1523, 2004.

257. Liao L, Chen X, Wang S, et al: Steroid receptor coactivator 3 maintains circulating insulin-like growth factor I (IGF-I) by controlling IGF-binding protein 3 expression, Mol Cell Biol 28:2460, 2008.

258. Ning Y, Schuller AG, Bradshaw S, et al: Diminished growth and enhanced glucose metabolism in triple knockout mice containing mutations of insulin-like growth factor binding protein-3, -4, and -5, Mol Endocrinol 20:2173, 2006.

259. Zhang M, Faugere MC, Malluche H, et al: Paracrine overexpression of IGFBP-4 in osteoblasts of transgenic mice decreases bone turnover and causes global growth retardation, J Bone Miner Res 18:836, 2003.

260. Ning Y, Schuller AG, Conover CA, et al: Insulin-like growth factor (IGF) binding protein-4 is both a positive and negative regulator of IGF activity in vivo, Mol Endocrinol 22:1213, 2008.

261. Salih Da, Tripathi G, Holding C, et al: Insulin-like growth factor binding protein 5 (IGFBP-5) compromises survival, growth, muscle development, and fertility in mice, Proc Natl Acad Sci U S A 101:4314, 2004.

262. Silha JV, Gui Y, Modric T, et al: Overexpression of the acid-labile subunit of the IGF ternary complex in transgenic mice, Endocrinol 142:4305, 2001.

263. Domene HM, Bengolea SV, Jasper HG, et al: Acid-labile subunit deficiency: phenotypic similarities and differences between human and mouse, J Endocrinol Invest 28:43, 2005.

264. Baker J, Liu JP, Robertson EJ, et al: Role of insulin like growth factors in embryonic and postnatal growth, Cell 75:83, 1993.

265. Holzenberger M, Leneuve P, Hamard G, et al: A targeted partial invalidation of the insulin-like growth factor receptor gene in mice causes a postnatal growth deficit, Endocrinol 141:2557, 2000.

266. Kondo T, Vicent D, Suzuma K, et al: Knockout of insulin and IGF-I receptors on vascular endothelial cells protects against retinal neovascularization, J Clin Invest 111:1835, 2003.

267. DeChiara RM, Efstratiadis A, Robertson EJ: A growth deficiency phenotype in heterozygous mice carrying an insulin-like growth factor II gene disruption, Nature 345:78, 1990.

268. Sjogren K, Liu JL, Blad K, et al: Liver-derived insulin-like growth factor I (IGF-I) is the principal source of IGF-I in blood but is not required for postnatal body growth in mice, Proc Natl Acad Sci U S A 96:7088, 1999.

269. Yakar S, Rosen CJ, Beamer WG, et al: Circulating levels of IGF-I directly regulate bone growth and density, J Clin Invest 110:771, 2002.

270. Ueki I, Ooi GT, Tremblay ML et al: Inactivation of the acid labile subunit gene in the mice results in mild retardation of postnatal growth despite profound disruptions in the circulating insulin-like growth factor system, Proc Natl Acad Sci U S A 97:6868, 2000.

271. Wu Y, Sun H, Yakar S, et al: Elevated levels of IGF-1 in serum rescue the severe growth retardation of IGF-1 null mice, Endocrinology 2009, Epub ahead of print.

272. Guler H-P, Zapf J, Froesch ER: Short-term metabolic effects of recombinant human insulin-like growth factor-I in healthy adults, N Engl J Med 317:137, 1987.

273. Kerr D, Tamborlane V, Rife F, et al: Effect of insulin-like growth factor-I on the responses to and recognition of hypoglycemia in humans. A comparison with insulin, J Clin Invest 91:141, 1993.

274. Clemmons DR, Smith-Banks A, Celniker AC, et al: Reversal of diet-induced catabolism by infusion of recombinant insulin-like growth factor-I (IGF-I) in humans, J Clin Endocrinol Metab 75:234, 1992.

275. Herndon DN, Ramzy PI, DebRoy MA, et al: Muscle protein catabolism after severe burn: effects of IGF-1/IGFBP-3 treatment, Ann Surg 229:713, 1999.

276. Jeschke MG, Bolder U, Chung DH, et al: Gut mucosal homeostasis and cellular mediators after severe thermal trauma and the effect of insulin-like growth factor-1 in combination with insulin-like growth factor binding protein-3, Endocrinol 148:354, 2007.

277. Boonen S, Rosen C, Bouillon R, et al: Musculoskeletal effects of the recombinant human IGF-I/IGF binding protein-3 complex in osteoporotic patients with proximal femoral fracture: a double-blind, placebo-controlled pilot study, J Clin Endocrinol Metab 87:1593, 2002.

278. Deicher R, Horl WH: Hormonal adjuvants for the treatment of renal anaemia, Eur J Clin Invest 35(suppl 3):75, 2005.

279. Mauras N, Martha PM Jr, Quarmby V, et al: rhIGF-I administration in humans: metabolic effects of bolus vs continuous subcutaneous delivery, Am J Physiol 272:E628, 1997.

280. Mauras N, Haymond MW: Are the metabolic effects of GH and IGF-I separable? Growth Horm IGF Res 15:19, 2005.

281. Mauras N, Beaufree B: Recombinant human insulin like growth factor I enhances whole-body protein anabolism and significantly diminishes the protein catabolic effects of prednisone in humans without a diabetogenic effect, J Clin Endocrinol Metab 80:869, 1995.

282. Ebling PR, Jones JD, O'Fallon WM, et al: Short term effects of recombinant human insulin like growth factor I on bone turnover in normal women, J Clin Endocrinol Metab 77:1384, 1993.

283. Grinspoon S, Baum HBA, Lee K, et al: Effects of short term rhIGF-I on bone turnover in osteopenic women with anorexia nervosa, J Clin Endocrinol Metab 81:3364, 1996.

284. Johansson AG, Lindh E, Blum WF, et al: Effects of growth hormone and insulin-like growth factor-I in men with osteoporosis, J Clin Endocrinol Metab 81:44, 1996.

285. Biandi T, Glatz Y, Bouillon R, et al: Effects of short term insulin-like growth factor-I (IGF-I) or growth hormone treatment on bone metabolism and on production of 1,25 dihydroxycholecalciferol in GH deficient adults, J Clin Endocrinol Metab 83:81, 1998.

286. Liu JM, Zhao HY, Ning G, et al: IGF-1 as an early marker for low bone mass or osteoporosis in premenopausal and postmenopausal women, J Bone Miner Metab 26:159, 2008.

287. Haluzik M, Yakar S, Gavrilova O, et al: Insulin resistance in the liver-specific IGF-1 gene-deleted mouse is abrogated by deletion of the acid-labile subunit of the IGF-binding protein-3 complex: relative roles of growth hormone and IGF-1 in insulin resistance, Diabetes 52:2483, 2003.

288. Ezzat VA, Duncan ER, Wheatcroft SB, et al: The role of IGF-I and its binding proteins in the development of type 2 diabetes and cardiovascular disease, Diabetes Obesity and Metab 10:198, 2008.

289. Pratipanawatr T, Pratipanawatr W, Rosen C, et al: Effect of IGF-I on FFA and glucose metabolism in control and type 2 diabetic subjects, Am J Physiol Endocrinol Metab 282:E1360, 2002.

290. Simpson HL, Jackson NC, Shojaee-Moradie F, et al: Insulin-like growth factor I has a direct effect on glucose and protein metabolism, but not effect on lipid metabolism in type 1 diabetes, J Clin Endocrinol Metab 89:425, 2004.

291. Kuzuya H, Matsuura N, Sakamoto M, et al: Trial of insulin-like growth factor-I therapy for patients with extreme insulin resistance syndromes, Diabetes 42:696, 1993.

292. Cheetham TD, Jones J, Taylor AM, et al: The effects of recombinant insulin-like growth factor I administration or growth hormone levels and insulin requirements in adolescents with type 1 insulin-dependent diabetes mellitus, Diabetologia 36:678, 1993.

293. Moses AC, Young SCJ, Morrow LA, et al: Recombinant human insulin-like growth factor I increases insulin sensitivity and improves glycemic control in Type II diabetes, Diabetes 45:95, 1996.

294. Quattrin T, Thrailkill K, Baler L, et al: Dual hormonal replacement with insulin and recombinant insulin like growth factor I in insulin dependent diabetes mellitus: effects on glycemic control, IGF-I levels, and safety profiles, Diabetes Care 20:374, 1997.

295. Clemmons DR, Moses AC, McKay MJ, et al: The combination of insulin-like growth factor I and insulin-like growth factor-binding protein-3 reduces insulin requirements in insulin-dependent type 1 diabetes: evidence for in vivo biological activity, J Clin Endocrinol Metab 85:1518, 2000.

296. Clemmons DR, Sleevi M, Allan G, et al: Effects of combined recombinant insulin-like growth factor (IGF)-I and IGF binding protein-3 in type 2 diabetic patients on glycemic control and distribution of IGF-I and IGF-II among serum binding protein complexes, J Clin Endocrinol Metab 92:2652, 2007.

297. Rosenfeld RG, Belgorosky A, Camacho-Hubner C, et al: Defects in growth hormone receptor signaling, Trends Endocrinol Metab 4:1043, 2007.

298. Guevara-Aguirre J, Vasconez O, Martinez V, et al: A randomized, double-blind, placebo-controlled trial of safety and efficacy of recombinant human insulin-like growth factor I in children with growth hormone receptor deficiency, J Clin Endocrinol Metab 80:1393, 1995.

299. Backeljaw PF, Underwood LE: Prolonged treatment with recombinant insulin-like growth factor I in children with growth hormone insensitivity syndrome: a clinical research center study, J Clin Endocrinol Metab 81:3312, 1996.

300. Chernausek SD, Backeljauw PF, Frane J, et al: Long-term treatment with recombinant insulin-like growth factor (IGF)-I in children with severe IGF-I deficiency due to growth hormone insensitivity, J Clin Endocrinol Metab 92:902, 2007.

301. Keating GM: Mecasermin, BioDrugs 22:177, 2008.

302. Camacho-Hubner C, Woods KA, Miraki-Moud F, et al: Effects of recombinant human insulin-like growth factor I (IGF-I) therapy on the growth hormone IGF system of a patient with partial IGF-I gene deletion, J Clin Endocrinol Metab 84:1611, 1999.

303. de Lacerda L, Carvalho JA, Stannard B, et al: In vitro and in vivo responses to short-term recombinant human insulin-like growth factor-1 (IGF-I) in a severely growth-retarded girl with ring chromosome 15 and deletion of a single allele for the type 1 IGF receptor gene, Clin Endocrinol 51:541, 1999.

304. Okubo Y, Siddle K, Firth H, et al: Cell proliferation activities on skin fibroblasts from a short child with absence of one copy of the type 1 insulin-like growth factor receptor (IGF1R) gene and a tall child with three copies of the IGF1R gene, J Clin Endocrinol Metab 88:5981, 2003.

305. Abuzzahab MJ, Schneider A, Goddard A, et al: IGF-I receptor mutations resulting in intrauterine and postnatal growth retardation, N Engl J Med 349:2211, 2003.

Chapter 18

SOMATIC GROWTH AND MATURATION

LEONA CUTTLER and MADHUSMITA MISRA

Growth is an inherent property of life. Normal somatic growth requires the integrated function of many of the hormonal, metabolic, and other growth factors. This chapter first briefly reviews the determinants of growth. Then it deals in detail with the overall result of these processes—normal patterns of linear growth. Finally, the differential diagnosis and the management of disorders of growth are discussed.

Determinants of Normal Growth

CELLULAR GROWTH

Normal growth requires an intrinsically normal cell that is nourished by an optimal milieu (with respect to pH, trace minerals, and substrates for structural and energy purposes) and is exposed to the necessary growth factors. It is regulated by the same molecular mechanisms that determine physiologic responses in the mature cell.

The body grows primarily through proliferation of cells by mitosis.[1,2] In contrast, increased cell size generally plays a greater role in organ growth as development approaches completion. Growth factors and other environmental signals are necessary for the entry of a quiescent cell into the cell cycle, and they affect cell division by modulating passage through the first phase of the mitotic cell cycle (G_1).[3,4] The first subphase of G_1 requires "competence factors," such as fibroblast growth factor, which induces cells to become competent to synthesize DNA. Cells then require essential amino acids to progress to a critical point in the cycle at which "progression factors" can induce completion of G_1. Progression factors are exemplified by insulin-like growth factors (IGFs), insulin, thyroxine, and hydrocortisone. Growth factors modulate the internal regulatory pathways governed by cyclins and cyclin-dependent kinases (CDKs), which are **proto-oncogenes,** and CDK inhibitors (CDKI), which are **tumor suppressors.** Specifically, growth factors lead to accumulation of the D-type cyclins, which sense and mediate growth factor stimulation in G_1. The binding of cyclin D with CDK 4/6 results in phosphorylation of "pocket" proteins (pRb, p107, and p130) and release of inhibitory control of these proteins on the E2F family transcription factors, which then drive expression of various effectors of DNA synthesis.[5] It is important to note that free E2F initiates a positive feedback loop by increasing cyclin E transcription and protein stabilization, because binding of cyclin E with CDK2 also phosphorylates pocket proteins and causes further release of E2F. The balance between cyclin, CDK, and CDKI activity therefore determines the start of DNA synthesis (S phase of the cell cycle). From this point onward, cell-cycle processes depend entirely on intracellularly triggered controls involving cyclins. After completing DNA synthesis, the cell finishes doubling its entire contents (G_2 phase) and then undergoes the M phase of the cycle, during which cell division is completed.

Reduction in growth factors leads to rapid decreases in expression of D-type cyclins and exit from the cell cycle, resulting in quiescence. In addition, "contact inhibition," or the lack of available space for cell division, can lead to an accumulation of p27, causing growth arrest without affecting expression of cyclin D.

The cell cycle to a great extent is also regulated by nuclear factor-κB (NF-κB).[6] This transcription factor is held inactive in the cytoplasm when bound to its inhibitory partner IκB. When IκB undergoes regulated serine phosphorylation, it is polyubiquinated, which targets it for degradation within the proteosome. This releases NF-κB to move to the nucleus, where it promotes cell-cycle progression and inhibits programmed cell death (apoptosis).

Cell senescence is the response of the cell to conditions such as telomere attrition, DNA damage, and oncogene activation—processes that appear to be interrelated. During each mitotic cycle, a portion of the terminal end (the telomere) of each chromosome is lost; this eventually shortens the chromosome to the point where cell proliferation becomes impossible and the cell dies.[7] The enzyme telomerase supports the synthesis of telomeric DNA, which maintains telomere length and proliferative potential. Telomerase is present in somatic cells of the fetus, permitting continued growth. With maturation of the fetus, however, telomerase levels begin to fall and decline progressively with aging, thus limiting mortality.

SOMATIC GROWTH

Prenatal Growth

Prenatal and postnatal requirements for growth differ in several respects. Embryonic growth is determined primarily by genetic programming of local sequential inductions.[8] Coordination of cell differentiation and morphogenesis requires a class of developmental genes that belong to the homeobox family.[9-11] Homeobox genes encode transcription factors that bind DNA, thereby controlling gene expression, cell differentiation, and organ development. Abnormalities of several homeobox genes are known to cause organ malformation and to affect linear growth. Fetal growth depends heavily on the delivery of nutrients, metabolic substrates, and oxygen, as well as IGFs, from the mother. The placenta regulates many of these and contributes to the fetal nutritional and hormonal milieu.[12-14] Placental size is a determinant of fetal growth, and placental growth itself is influenced by genomic factors,[14,15] growth factors, maternal weight and nutrition (perhaps via leptin),[16] parity, parental size,[17] and uterine blood flow. Placental regulation of fetal blood flow is, in turn, a determinant of growth; discordance in the size of monozygous twins has been attributed to the unequal distribution of blood flow that results from placental arteriovenous anastomoses.[18]

Both placental growth and function involve hormones. Specific deletion of placental IGF-2, which is an imprinted gene expressed from the paternal allele, sequentially reduces placental growth, decreases nutrient delivery, and restricts fetal growth.[14] The placenta also influences fetal growth through its elaboration of hormones. For example, human placental lactogen seems to influence regulation of fetal IGF-1,[19] although the role of the placental variant of GH in regulating fetal IGF-1 and growth remains unclear.[20,21] Umbilical cord leptin appears to be an index of fetal nutrition in humans and correlates with birth size independent of IGF-1.[22,23]

Familial and environmental variables that predict birth size independent of gestational age include parental heights, sibling birth weight, maternal weight, parity, glycemic status and history of smoking, altitude, gender, and uterine constraints, such as the number of fetuses carried.[17,24-30]

Some of the hormonal requirements for fetal growth differ from those that regulate postnatal growth. For example, prenatal growth is less dependent on GH and thyroxine. Individuals with congenital GH deficiency or resistance often have normal birth length despite low IGF-1 levels, although in large population studies, average birth length is reduced by 1 standard deviation (SD).[12,31,32] Similarly, newborns with congenital hypothyroidism typically have normal birth size, although their bone maturation lags during the last trimester.[33]

In contrast, the IGF system affects prenatal and postnatal growth, although specific influences and regulatory components differ according to stage of development. Immunoreactive IGF is present in most fetal tissues. Rodent models that lack IGF-1, IGF-2, or the IGF-1 receptor have reduced birth weights, suggesting a role for both IGF-1 and IGF-2 in prenatal growth.[34-37] IGF-1 and IGF-2 act through the IGF-1, insulin, and IGF-2 receptors, and IGF-2 is approximately equal in importance to IGF-1 for fetal growth, each contributing about 40%.[37,38] IGF-2 abundance in early pregnancy promotes fetal growth and viability near term, primarily through effects of IGF-2 on placental growth and differentiation.[39] IGF-1, in contrast, is important for fetal but not placental growth, and its effects are mediated by decreased release of vasoconstrictors, thus optimizing placental blood flow and nutrient delivery to the fetus. Six IGF binding proteins (IGFBPs) regulate the amount of free IGF available and are regulated in turn by IGFBP proteases. High levels of IGFBPs have been associated with fetal growth inhibition, likely from sequestration of fetally derived IGF-1.[40-43] IGFBP-3 also prolongs the half-life of IGFs in circulation, and levels are reduced in the cord serum of small for gestational age (SGA) fetuses.[44]

Pregnancy-associated plasma protein A (PAPP-A), which cleaves IGFBP-4, increases free IGF availability,[45] and low first-trimester PAPP-A levels in pregnant women are associated with lower birth weight.[46]

In contrast to fetal growth, postnatal growth is less dependent on IGF-2 than on IGF-1 levels. Whereas animals lacking IGF-2 that survive may have relatively normal postnatal growth, those with IGF-1 deficiency remain stunted. During fetal life, IGF-1 is relatively independent of GH and is regulated greatly by nutritional status (particularly glucose availability and consequent fetal insulin secretion) and placental lactogen, whereas postnatal levels are dependent on both GH and nutritional status.[8,12,19,31] Although the serum IGF level is even lower prenatally than in infancy, it rises during gestation and correlates with size at birth.[12] IGF-2 blood levels are higher than those of IGF-1 in utero, in contrast to postnatal life. Human correlates, substantiating the role of IGFs in prenatal growth, are the identification of a patient with homozygous partial deletion of the gene encoding IGF-1 and identification of patients with IGF-1 receptor mutations with severe intrauterine growth retardation, as well as postnatal growth failure.[47]

In addition to IGFs, insulin influences fetal growth. Infants of diabetic mothers and children with Beckwith-Wiedemann syndrome (with hyperinsulinism) have excessive fetal growth, and those with pancreatic agenesis have poor fetal growth. Mutations in the insulin receptor and in IRS-1, a downstream molecule in the signaling pathways of both IGF-1 and insulin receptors, are also associated with suboptimal fetal growth and insulin resistance.[48]

Sex hormones may play a subtle role in normal fetal growth: Plasma levels of testosterone, estradiol, and dehydroepiandrosterone are at or above pubertal levels by mid-gestation; estrogen promotes fetal bone development[49]; and androgen action seems to account for the greater birth weight of boys compared with girls.[8,31]

An understanding of the regulation of fetal growth has assumed particular importance because of potential links between prenatal growth and later disease. Strong experimental evidence in animal models indicates that an adverse fetal environment, as reflected in birth size, can lead to a poor health outcome in adults.[50] Diverse causes of poor fetal growth (including maternal undernutrition or glucocorticoid exposure) can have similar deleterious effects on postnatal health (including hypertension, cardiovascular disease, and glucose intolerance). Considerable human data support such a "fetal origins of adult disease" model.[36] The risks for insulin resistance, diabetes, and visceral adiposity are particularly high in SGA infants with rapid postnatal "catch-up growth."[51-53] Although the underlying mechanisms are not fully understood, evidence points to the development of a "thrifty" phenotype, with fetal metabolism adapting to undernutrition through epigenetic modifications in key genes (including the glucocorticoid receptors, peroxisome-proliferator–activated receptor [PPAR-α], Pdx1, and Glut4), which persists into adulthood.[54-56] Another proposed mechanism invokes a defect in placental inactivation of maternal cortisol due to decreased 11β-hydroxysteroid dehydrogenase activity, leading to elevated fetal cortisol and reprogramming of the hypothalamic-pituitary-adrenal axis for hyperresponsiveness to stress.[57] Dehydroepiandrosterone (DHEAS) and androstenedione levels have been reported to be higher in SGA children,[58] and early pubarche and polycystic ovary syndrome (PCOS) may be important sequelae of SGA.[59] In addition, a reduction in the total number of nephrons as a consequence of intrauterine growth retardation with compensatory effects influencing the renin-angiotensin system may predispose these individuals to subsequent hypertension.[60]

Postnatal Growth

Familial and environmental determinants of early postnatal growth include gestational age at delivery, birth size, parental heights, socioeconomic status, and breastfeeding.[17]

Genetic determinants exist for both postnatal and prenatal growth.[61] Genes on the Y chromosome seem to enhance stature commencing in antenatal life,[61,62] and the X chromosome carries genetic determinants, including the *SHOX* gene (see Skeletal Dysplasias below), which promotes linear growth and regulates body proportions.[61,63] The epigenetic process of genomic imprinting, like X-inactivation, is due to methylation of genes to silence them,[15] and clusters of autosomal "imprinted" genes also regulate growth. Although the exact nature of most imprinted genes is unknown, the genes for IGF-2 and its receptor on chromosome 15 are imprinted. The *IGF-2* gene is silenced in eggs and thus is maternally imprinted, whereas the IGF-2 receptor is paternally imprinted. Other genes that regulate height include those implicated in Noonan syndrome[64] and other genetic causes of short stature (described later). In addition, genome-wide analysis has allowed the identification of single nucleotide polymorphisms in regions that include candidate and novel genes and implicate pathways (let-7 targets, chromatin remodeling proteins, Hedgehog signaling) that may regulate height.[65,66]

The **axial and appendicular skeletons** account for the vast majority of postnatal linear growth. These bones are formed by endochondral ossification, which commences with chondrocytes of the epiphyses laying down an orderly cartilage template, which osteoblasts then convert to bone.[67-69] The cranium and some of the clavicle are formed by direct intramembranous ossification. The cycle of bone cell remodeling for structural purposes is linked closely to the overall metabolic needs for calcium

and phosphorus homeostasis, primarily through the actions of parathormone and calciferol. Chondrocyte proliferation is inhibited by parathyroid hormone–related protein (PTHrP) and fibroblast growth factor (FGF) paracrine signaling mediated through the PTH receptor and FGF receptor 3 (FGFR3). This effect is opposed by Indian hedgehog signaling, which operates in a negative feedback loop with PTHrP. The natriuretic factor system, particularly involving the C type, similarly appears to play a local role in endochondral ossification, in this case as positive regulators.[70,71]

Nutrition and metabolism must be adequate for normal growth. Adult height has been used as a marker for the nutritional status of populations during childhood and has been shown to be related to cognitive function.[72,73] Calories seem particularly critical for cell multiplication. Two percent to 13% of normal energy consumption goes into promoting growth.[1,74] Protein intake is particularly important for normal growth in cellular size. It must be adequate with respect to both amount and provision of essential amino acids or their ketoanalogues.[75-77] Essential fatty acids are necessary for normal growth in lower animals, but this may not hold true for primates.[78] Vitamins A and D are important for normal growth.[1,79] Trace metals, such as zinc and copper, are probably essential for normal growth and sexual maturation[80-83] because of their role as cofactors for enzyme function. The pH must be maintained at optimal levels to conserve mineral homeostasis.[84]

The general level of **activity** seems to promote overall body growth, just as normal muscular activity is necessary for limb growth. The mechanism is unclear; it may be related to neural trophic factors or to blood flow. The efficiency of nitrogen accretion and growth is decreased in inactive rats.[85]

Hormones are essential "catalysts" of growth. Under normal circumstances, the growth hormone (GH)-IGF system, thyroid hormone, and sex steroids are fundamental regulators of linear growth.

A complex interplay of extracellular peptides with intracellular transcription factors and signaling systems governs the development of the hypothalamic and the pituitary **Growth hormone (GH)** secretory system.[86,87] Pituitary secretion of GH is normally under the immediate control of hypothalamic hormones: somatostatin, which inhibits its release, and growth hormone-releasing hormone (GHRH). GHRH stimulates GH synthesis and secretion. Defects in GHRH synthesis or action stunt growth in mouse models, and humans with a defect in the GHRH receptor similarly show growth failure,[88] attesting to the fundamental importance of GHRH in GH secretion and growth.

The balance between GHRH and somatostatin is determined by a complex flux of input from higher cerebral centers, which mediate nutritional, metabolic, and endocrine signals (Fig. 18-1).[89-97] Diverse neurotransmitters are involved; they include acetylcholine, galanin, and neuropeptide Y. Dopamine is inhibitory to GH release in the newborn period.[98]

Endocrine input includes the endogenous GH secretagogue (GHS) ghrelin, an orexigenic peptide originating in the stomach and hypothalamus. Ghrelin stimulates GH release, primarily through promoting GHRH release, but also by acting directly on the pituitary, through specific receptors (GHSR). In addition, there is negative feedback on GH secretion by circulating IGF-1, which is primarily of hepatic origin, and glucose levels.[99,100]

GH secretion is also influenced by androgens and estrogen (which appear responsible for the rise in GH secretion during

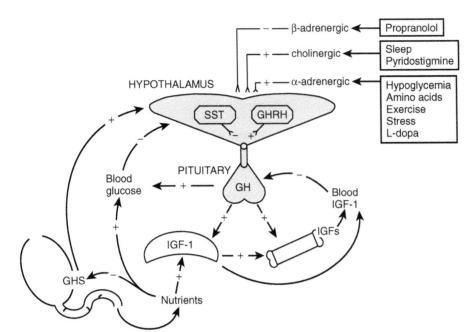

FIGURE 18-1. Growth hormone (GH) regulatory axis: Major factors regulating GH release. GH is secreted after the integration of diverse hypothalamic stimuli. It stimulates insulin-like growth factor-1 (IGF-1) production by the liver, bone, and other tissues, as well as gluconeogenesis. GH release from the pituitary gland is under tonic inhibition by hypothalamic somatostatin, and GH-releasing hormone (GHRH) stimulates GH release when somatostatin (SST) tone wanes owing to fluctuations in input from higher neural centers. Ghrelin is an endogenous GH secretagogue (GHS) and orexogenic peptide mainly secreted by the stomach in response to fasting. Its major indirect effect on GH is to antagonize SST release at the level of the hypothalamus. Small amounts of GHS are formed in the hypothalamus, however, and these weakly stimulate GHRH release directly; neonatally, GHS pituitary expression is high. SST tone is inhibited by cholinergic, dopaminergic, and α-adrenergic neuronal inputs to the hypothalamus and is stimulated by β-adrenergic ones. Negative feedback effects are exerted primarily by the long-loop actions of blood glucose and IGF-1, but also by short-loop signals between the various signal peptides of the axis. IGF-1 and blood glucose also exert negative feedback effects on GH release. Pharmacologic stimuli to GH release are shown in boxes. *Solid lines* indicate major regulatory pathways, *dotted lines* minor ones. +, Stimulator of GH, GHS, or IGF-1 release; −, inhibitor of GH, GHS, or IGF-1 release.

normal puberty), as well as by thyroxine and glucocorticoids (hypothyroidism and cortisol excess reduce GH secretion).

After secretion, GH is approximately 50% bound to GH-binding protein (GHBP). GHBP rises through childhood.[101] It is the extracellular domain of the GH receptor (GHR); its underlying alternate splicing may be differentially regulated from the intact GHR.[102] GHR is a member of the cytokine family. One molecule of GH binds to two GHR molecules, indicating receptor dimerization, which is critical for GH action. (This leads to activation of a receptor-associated Janus tyrosine kinase [JAK-2] and, in turn, transduction through a number of pathways, including the MAPK [mitogen-activated protein kinase] and STAT [signal transducers and activators of transcription] pathways.[103]) These paths result in activation of genes (including *IGF-1*) that mediate GH's biological effects. Abnormalities of the GHR and its signaling system result in GH insensitivity and growth failure (see discussion to follow).

GH appears to stimulate growth through a combination of direct effects and effects mediated by IGFs.[104] GH stimulates the production of endocrine IGF-1 and its major binding protein (IGFBP-3). It also directly induces the clonal expansion and differentiation of target stem cells (such as prechondrocytes), and these differentiating cells (chondrocytes) then respond to GH by forming IGF-1 and IGF-1 receptors, which makes them responsive to the growth-promoting effect of both endocrine IGF-1 and IGFs secreted locally (autocrine and paracrine IGFs).[105,106]

IGF-1, produced by the liver and other tissues, is a critical regulator of postnatal growth and represents a major mechanism by which GH promotes growth. Circulating IGF-binding proteins (IGFBPs) sequester IGFs, whereas at the cell surface they can promote IGF action and exert novel actions.[107] Defects in IGF-1 synthesis or action lead to growth failure in humans and laboratory animals. The effects of IGF-1 may depend on the tissue of origin. Local production of IGF-1 in peripheral tissues appears to mediate GH-induced somatic growth, whereas circulating IGF-1, which originates primarily in the liver, may not be

essential for growth, but provides negative feedback for the GH axis.[106] The free (unbound) IGF-1 is thought to be the biologically active fraction of circulating IGF-1, but the validity of current assays for this moiety is in question.[108,109] IGF-1 production is regulated primarily by GH when nutrition is normal. IGF-2 is produced by cells independently of GH and seems to be normally important only for local growth regulation.[110] IGF-2 levels seem to be modulated locally by the activity of a metabolizing receptor complex consisting of the IGF-2 receptor and glypican-3.[111]

There is more to the regulation of plasma IGF-1 concentrations and bioactivity than GH. Hepatic IGF-1, the major source of blood IGF-1, is fundamentally under broad regulation by nutrition. Undernutrition decreases plasma IGF-1 levels despite normal or elevated GH concentrations.[112] Overnutrition (i.e., obesity) has the opposite effect.[89] Studies in rats suggest that insulin plays a role in mediating nutritional effects on hepatic IGF-1 formation through its stimulation of amino acid uptake.[113,114] The increased plasma-free IGF-1 concentration in obese patients has been attributed to the suppressive effect of their insulin excess on IGFBP-1.[115] Thyroid hormone and cortisol are necessary for hepatic IGF-1 production, and prolactin has a slight effect on it.[116]

Factors other than GH and nutrition—including age—determine IGF production, and these are poorly understood. Plasma IGF-1, IGFBP-3 levels,[117] and somatomedin activity[118] rise slowly during the prepubertal years with no change in GH production (Fig. 18-2).[119] As a result, IGF-1 levels in normal children younger than 5 years of age overlap with those of GH-deficient children, making use of these tests in diagnosing GH deficiency difficult in young children. During puberty, IGF-1 levels rise further, and since IGFBP-3 levels rise to a lesser degree, free-plasma IGF-1 rises even more markedly.[117] The pubertal increase in IGF-1 is mediated by sex hormone stimulation of GH secretion,[120-122] although a separate direct effect on IGF-1 has been suggested.[123] IGF-1 levels during adolescence, therefore, corre-

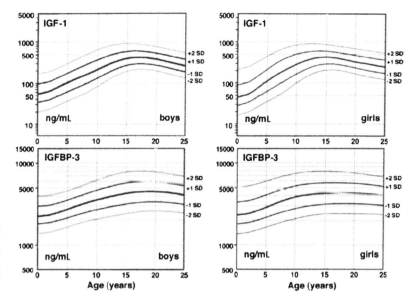

FIGURE 18-2. Plasma insulin-like growth factor-1 (IGF-1) and IGF-binding protein-3 (IGFBP-3) normal ranges from infancy to adulthood. Increases after 10 years of age are related to pubertal stage rather than to age. IGF-1 values are given in terms of the World Health Organization reference preparation 87/518, which is of low (44%) purity with respect to authentic recombinant human IGF-1, so the values shown are in excess of the true IGF-1 concentration.[41] (Data from Diagnostic Systems Laboratories, Inc., 1997, Webster, TX.)

late more with pubertal development and bone age than with chronologic age.

The relationship of plasma IGF-1 levels to normal linear growth is not a simple one. Plasma IGF-1 levels do not correlate with growth rate in childhood except during the pubertal growth spurt, when levels peak about a year after peak height velocity.[124] IGFBPs in plasma determine the unbound concentration of IGF-1, transport the IGFs to target cells, and influence the interaction of IGFs with their receptors; a tissue IGFBP-protease system modulates IGF-1 bioavailability to target cells.[105,107,125,126] IGFBPs also appear to be bioactive molecules that have IGF-independent functions.[107,126] IGF bioactivity may be influenced by circulating somatomedin inhibitory activity, which is attributable to both glucocorticoids and incompletely characterized peptides.[127,128] The cytokines interleukin-6 and tumor necrosis factor-α have direct inhibitory effects on chondrocytes.[129]

Growth may be normal with subnormal GH production in the poorly understood "growth without growth hormone syndrome."[130] Most often, this syndrome has been identified after surgical treatment for large hypothalamic and pituitary tumors, but the syndrome occasionally has been recognized in benign forms of hypopituitarism.[131] IGF-1 levels may be low, but bioactivity normal. Most such patients are obese, so insulin excess or sensitivity has been suspected to be the underlying growth factor. Individual variation in local aromatase activity and thus availability of estrogen has also been suggested.[132] Hyperprolactinemia is seldom found.

Thyroid hormone is necessary for postnatal bone growth because of both indirect effects on the GH-IGF axis and direct effects on bone growth.[133] Thyroid hormone is required for normal GH secretion in response to GHRH and for normal GH action as indexed by GHBP, IGF, and IGFBP levels. Hypothyroidism (and, to a lesser degree, mutations of the thyroid receptor-β) produces short stature and delays bone maturation.

Glucocorticoids in above-normal amounts are inhibitors of linear growth.[128,134] The mechanism is both indirect and direct. Glucocorticoid excess inhibits spontaneous GH secretion by stimulating somatostatin tone. The bioactivity of plasma IGF-1 falls during glucocorticoid therapy; this may reflect an increase in IGF-binding protein.[135,136] Glucocorticoids themselves directly

hinder cartilage growth,[137] perhaps in part by inhibiting GH and IGF-1 induction of their respective receptors.[138]

Increased secretion of **sex hormones** clearly initiates the pubertal growth spurt. The growth-promoting actions of sex hormones require adequate GH; GH-deficient children will not undergo a normal pubertal growth spurt unless GH is replaced. About half of the contribution of sex hormones to the pubertal growth spurt is due to their stimulation of the GH-IGF axis, which appears to be mediated primarily by estrogen.[91,120,121,139] The remaining effects of sex steroids on growth are direct or are mediated by a direct effect on IGF.[123,140-142]

Estrogen and androgen both stimulate bone growth, bone turnover, and epiphyseal growth.[123,143,144] Androgen appears to stimulate and estrogen to inhibit periosteal bone formation, while estrogen promotes greater cortical thickening by inhibiting endosteal bone resorption. Estrogen is particularly effective in reducing bone turnover, however, and estrogens are responsible for epiphyseal closure.[145] To some extent, these effects may be exerted prenatally, since maternal estrogen can have permanent effects on fetal bone development.[146] Differences between these actions of sex hormones account for women's bones being shorter and narrower than men's.

Early pubertal amounts of estradiol (about 0.25 mg/month) stimulate growth in girls, in contrast to inhibition of growth by high doses of estrogen.[147] Peak growth velocity of boys occurs at a testosterone production rate of about 50 to 100 mg/month.[148] Whether other sex steroids play an independent role in growth is unknown; it has been reported that dehydroepiandrosterone sulfate promotes calcification of cartilage, and subandrogenic doses of androstenedione promote growth.[49]

Patterns of Normal Somatic Growth

INTRAUTERINE GROWTH

During the first trimester, tissue patterns and organ systems develop. In the second trimester, major cellular hyperplasia occurs in the fetus and its growth velocity is maximal. During the third trimester, organ systems mature and weight gain is maximal. Weight increases relatively more than length does in the third trimester because of the accumulation of fat and muscle. Overall, fetal growth is more rapid than postnatal growth.

Standards for intrauterine growth are shown in Fig. 18-3.[149] Race, altitude, and gender cause subtle differences from these norms.[150]

Healthy infants born prematurely have weights appropriate for gestational age and continue to grow at the same rate that they would have grown in utero.[151] When corrected for postconceptional age, length and weight follow postnatal standards. Consequently, the lengths of children born prematurely remain slightly less through infancy than those of children born at term, but the differences become negligible over time. Very premature infants, however, require intensive care to survive and uniformly lose weight during the first weeks of life; it takes several years for the great majority to catch up to the weight and length of term infants, and females achieve greater catch-up growth than males.[152,153] In contrast to premature infants, 10% to 15% of those born small for gestational age prove to have persistent short stature beyond 4 years of age[154] (see discussion that follows).

POSTNATAL GROWTH

Growth is the fundamental characteristic of childhood. Patterns of childhood growth are highly predictable, and deviation from these patterns often signifies the presence of serious disorders.

Postnatal growth patterns of normal children are well characterized, resulting in several clinical parameters for assessment of growth.

1. **Linear growth** is assessed as supine **length** until 2 to 3 years of age (using a firm box with inflexible head board and movable foot board) and, thereafter, as erect **height** measured with the use of calibrated stadiometers. Stature then is plotted on growth charts. Traditionally, these linear growth standards have been derived from cross-sectional data as shown in Fig. 18-4.[155] Because differences in the timing of puberty can influence normal growth rates, longitudinal growth charts are useful in sequential assessment of individual children.[156,157] Height SD in relation to the mean for age and gender can be determined from the Centers for Disease Control and Prevention website.[155] Syndrome-specific growth charts have been developed for Turner's syndrome, Down syndrome, and achondroplasia.[158-160] There is a "secular trend" toward increasing height of populations with time associated with improvements in nutrition and health,[161] although the most recent U.S. data suggest little change in the past 25 years.

2. **Weight and body mass index** (BMI; weight [kg]/height [cm]^2) are measured and plotted on appropriate growth charts.[155] Weight is a labile parameter relative to height, being sensitive to acute illness and changes in nutrition, activity, and muscle mass. Whether weight is appropriate can be estimated by comparing a child's percentile position for weight with respect to height age or by calculating the BMI. BMI is the recommended parameter for assessing whether children over 2 years old are overweight (BMI 85th to 94th percentile for age) or obese (BMI at or above the 95th percentile for age).

3. **Growth velocity** is assessed from sequential height measurements and can be plotted on growth velocity charts (Fig. 18-5).[156,157] A minimum interval of 6 months is needed for meaningful assessments of growth velocity. Growth occurs in three phases—infantile, childhood, and pubertal—each of which has distinct characteristics.[162] Linear growth velocity is most rapid in infancy, averaging 15 cm/year in the first 2 years of life. Two thirds of infants cross percentile channels on the linear growth curves.[163] The growth of infants seems to result from an initial steep vector, which is generated by the GH- and thyroxine-independent cell proliferation that uniquely drives intrauterine growth, superimposed on a shallow vector, which is dependent on the endocrine factors that determine subsequent growth during childhood.

4. **Growth patterns:** From the end of infancy until puberty begins, growth normally proceeds along a channel that closely corresponds to a given height-attained percentile on cross-sectional growth standards. A child normally establishes this channel by 2 to 3 years of age,[163] although, on rare occasions, a gradual drift by as many as 40

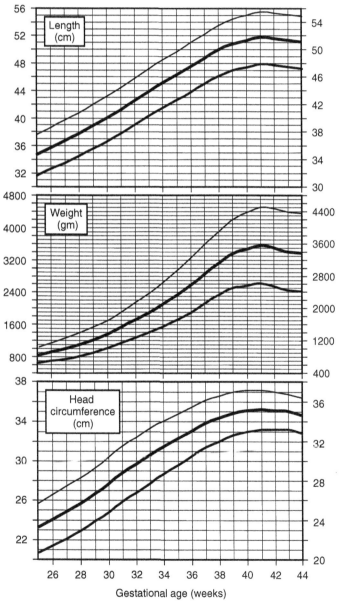

FIGURE 18-3. Intrauterine growth charts. Data represent birth weights according to gestational age of live-born Caucasian infants at sea level. Infants with major congenital malformations were excluded. (Data from Usher R, McLean F: Intrauterine growth of live-born Caucasian infants at sea level: Standards obtained from measurements in seven dimensions of infants born between 25 and 44 weeks of gestation. J Pediatr 74[6]:901–910, 1969.)

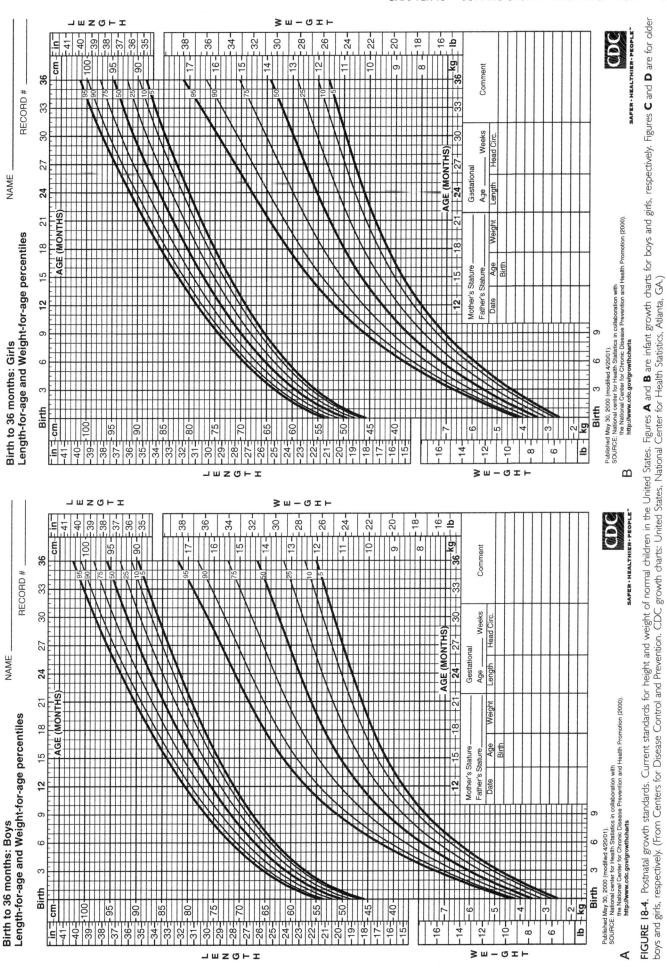

FIGURE 18-4. Postnatal growth standards. Current standards for height and weight of normal children in the United States. Figures **A** and **B** are infant growth charts for boys and girls, respectively. Figures **C** and **D** are for older boys and girls, respectively. CDC growth charts: United States, National Center for Health Statistics, Atlanta, GA.) (From Centers for Disease Control and Prevention. CDC growth charts: United States, National Center for Health Statistics, Atlanta, GA.)

Continued

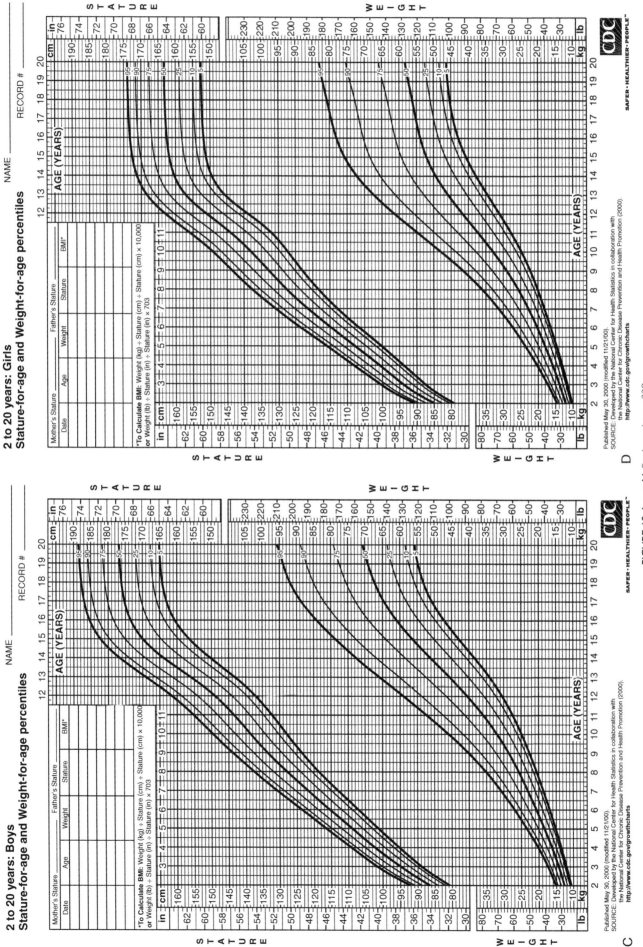

FIGURE 18-4, cont'd For legend see e339.

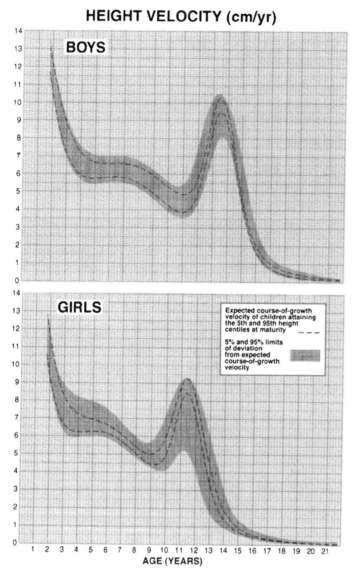

FIGURE 18-5. Longitudinal height velocity standards derived from the Fels, Berkely, and Denver growth studies.[141] (Courtesy R.D. Bock.)

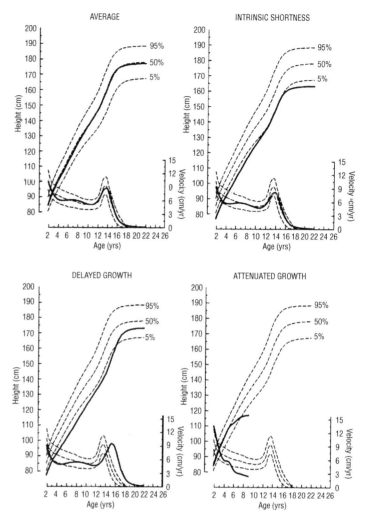

FIGURE 18-6. Linear growth curves in children with various types of growth patterns. Note that three prepubertal children of similar short stature at 9 years of age have different prognoses for growth. The growth curve of an average-size child is shown for comparison. On each chart, the upper scale shows the height attained, and the lower scale shows the height velocity. Normal percentiles are from the National Center for Health Statistics. Growth curves were generated by the TRI-FOUR program of Bock et al. (Bock RD, du Toit SHC, Thissen D: A.U.X.A.L: Auxological Analysis of Longitudinal Data, Scientific Software, 1993, Chicago, IL. Courtesy of R.D. Bock.)

percentile positions in height attained may occur over a period of several years in normal children.[164] The velocity of growth (cm per year) actually decelerates slightly during this period (see Fig. 18-5) and averages about 6 cm per year in midchildhood.[157] However, normal children cross height-velocity percentiles to maintain their height channel (Fig. 18-6).[156,165,166] A growth velocity that is consistently along the third percentile will lead to a subnormal height.

The growth channel seems to be genetically determined. Children grow as if to reach a genetically predetermined height. This **target height,** which represents the child's genetic potential, can be approximated by calculating the midparental height (the average of the parents' heights) and adding 6.5 cm for boys or subtracting 6.5 cm for girls (to adjust for the average differences between men and women). Alternative functions have been proposed for children with short parents. However, all such predictions are accurate only within a range of 7 to 10 cm.[167]

Deflections from this channel are firmly resisted, as if growth is being developmentally canalized.[168] The mechanisms by which the growth channel is maintained are unknown. They may involve recognition of cell density, which is a determinant of the cell population in culture systems.[169] In the course of a year, healthy children maintain their percentile position with respect to height attained by means of short-term fluctuations in growth velocity, termed stasis and saltation.[170] These oscillations may be marked, growth sometimes seeming nil over 3-month periods, and are a potential source of error in growth diagnosis. GH variability has been reported to increase during periods of short-term growth.[171] Variations tend to be seasonal, a "blooming" trend most often occurring in the spring.

During puberty, children may again cross height-attained percentiles because the pubertal growth spurts of individuals occur out of phase. The magnitude of this pubertal growth spurt is apparent only from growth-velocity standards based on age of menarche or longitudinal data. Peak growth velocity occurs approximately 1 year before menarche[172] in girls, and at a bone age of approximately 12 years in girls and 13 years in boys.[173] Girls on average achieve only 7 cm further growth after menarche.[174] During the course of sexual maturation, the epiphyseal cartilage plates become progressively obliterated, and growth ceases when the process is complete. Only about 1 cm of growth occurs after fusion is complete in the femur and tibia.

The causes of the decrease in growth velocity from the fetal to the neonatal and subsequent early childhood years are not known but may be a consequence of differential expression of IGF-1 versus IGF-2, their receptors, and the various IGF binding proteins in the growth plate with increasing age.[175] In addition, fibroblast growth factors may play a role.[176]

Some of the greater ultimate height of boys than of girls results from their later puberty and consequent longer period of prepubertal growth[166]; boys additionally have a slightly greater peak linear growth velocity than girls.[156] Early maturers have more brisk pubertal growth than late maturers; however, they also stop growing earlier.[156] This tendency occurs at comparable levels of bone maturation (Table 18-1).[177] The growth patterns of nonwhite American children differ from those of whites in some particulars.[178] Immigrant children go into a phase of catch-up growth in an optimum nutritional environment.[179]

5. **Body proportions** (arm span and upper-to-lower segment ratio) change in concert with growth. The limbs are relatively short in infancy. By about 11 years of age, adult proportions are reached (Figs. 18-7 and 18-8).[180,181] Occasional marked changes in segmental proportions appear during puberty.[182] Many growth disorders are characterized by abnormal body proportions (see later discussion).

6. **Head circumference** increases most rapidly during early infancy (Fig. 18-9). It is related to both skeletal and brain growth, and about half the variation is familial.[183-185]

CATCH-UP AND CATCH-DOWN GROWTH AND COMPENSATORY GROWTH

Catch-up growth occurs upon relief from any disorder that has caused a deviation from a child's genetic growth channel and restores the child to his or her original channel.[168,186-188] In classic ("type 1") catch-up growth, the rate of growth is supranormal and exceeds that expected for the age at which growth had been

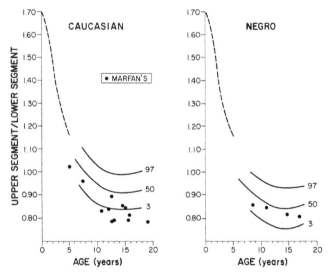

FIGURE 18-7. Normal standards for the ratio of the upper segment to the lower segment of the body. The lower segment represents the measurement from the top of the symphysis pubis to the heel; the upper segment is computed by subtracting the lower segment from height. The *dotted line* shows the average for young children in 1932. (Percentile and Marfan data from McKusick VA: Heritable Disorders of Connective Tissue, ed 4. St Louis, Mosby, 1972.)

Table 18-1. Percentage of Adult Height Achieved at Successive Bone Ages, Variation in Height Prediction From Bone Age, and Variation in Bone Age in Relation to Chronologic Age

	Bone Age, yr												
	6.0	7.0	8.0	9.0	10.0	11.0	12.0	13.0	14.0	15.0	16.0	17.0	18.0
Percentage of mature height													
Boys													
Average*		69.5	72.3	75.2	78.4	80.4	83.4	87.6	92.7	96.8	98.2	99.1	99.6
Accelerated*		67.0	69.6	72.0	74.7	76.7	80.9	85.0	90.5	95.8	98.0	99.0	
Retarded*	68.0	71.8	75.6	78.6	81.2	82.3	84.5	88.0					
Girls													
Average	72.0	75.7	79.0	82.7	86.2	90.6	92.2	95.8	98.0	99.0	99.6	99.9	100.0
Accelerated		71.2	75.0	79.0	82.8	88.3	90.1	94.5	97.2	98.6	99.3	99.8	
Retarded	73.3	77.0	80.4	84.1	87.4	91.8	93.2	96.4	98.3	99.4	99.8	100.0	

	Chronologic Age, yr												
	6.0	7.0	8.0	9.0	10.0	11.0	12.0	13.0	14.0	15.0	16.0	17.0	18.0
Height prediction standard deviation, inches													
Boys		1.47	1.27	1.33	1.14	1.09	1.21	1.21	0.88	0.49	0.41		
Girls		1.73	1.46	1.37	1.15	1.06	0.6	0.42	0.38	0.26	0.20		
Bone age standard deviation, months													
Boys	9.3	10.1	10.8	11.0	11.4	10.5	10.4	11.1	12.0	14.2	15.1	15.4	
Girls	9.0	8.3	8.8	9.3	10.8	12.3	14.0	14.6	12.6	11.2			

From Gruelich WW, Pyle SI: Radiographic Atlas of Skeletal Development of the Hand and Wrist. Palo Alto, CA, Stanford University Press, 1959.
*With respect to whether bone age is within 1 year of chronologic age.

arrested. During adolescence, it may resemble the pubertal growth spurt. This type of catch-up growth has been further subclassifed.[189] A different kind of catch-up growth ("type 2") occurs following adequate therapy for sexual precocity.[190] In this situation, restoration of height potential occurs because restitutional linear growth proceeds without bone maturation advancement, that is, height age catches up to bone age (Table 18-2). This is particularly true for sexual precocity that occurs very

early; however, suppression of pubertal progression around the lower limit of normal age for pubertal onset may not be associated with similar benefits for height potential. Complete compensation for growth failure can occur upon correction of the underlying disorder if diagnosed early. Catch-up may be incomplete, however, if the growth disorder is of many years' duration and extends into the age at which puberty normally occurs.

Growth plate physiology plays an important role in mediating "catch-up" and "catch-down" growth. The growth plate goes through a programmed pattern of senescence through childhood and adolescence, dependent on factors intrinsic to the growth plate.[191,192] Information regarding previous growth history appears to be retained in the memory of the growth plate, likely in resting zone "stem cell–like" chondrocytes, and influences future structural and functional changes in the growth plate, with effects on "catch-up" and "catch-down" growth.[193]

Endocrine deficiencies causing short stature have important effects on the growth plate. Following induced hypothyroidism

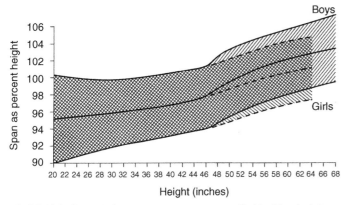

FIGURE 18-8. Standards for arm span as a percentage of height. The *shaded area* represents the normal range, smoothed. (Data from Engelbach W: Endocrine Medicine, vol 1. Springfield, IL, Charles C Thomas, 1932, p 261.)

Table 18-2. Definitions of Growth Parameters

Parameter	Definition
Bone age	Age for which bone maturation is average
Chronologic age	Calendar age
Height age	Age for which height is average
Weight age	Age for which weight is average

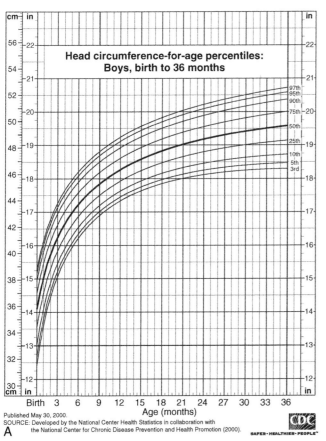

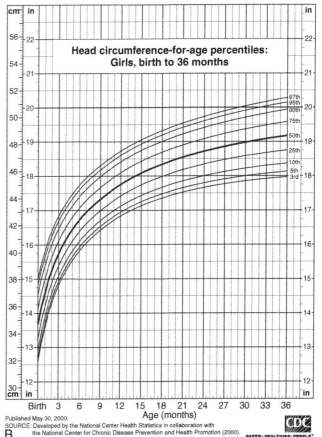

FIGURE 18-9. Head circumference standards for the infant boys **(A)** and girls **(B)**. (From Centers for Disease Control and Prevention, 2000, Atlanta, GA.)

and hypercortisolism in experimental models, growth plate chondrocyte proliferation slows down, with a slower depletion of resting zone chondrocytes, leading to preservation of proliferative capacity and slowing of senescence. With normalization of hormone levels, growth plates grow more rapidly, resulting in "catch-up" growth.[194,195] However, akin to humans, catch-up growth after correction of hypothyroidism remains incomplete, with adult height being less than in euthyroid controls. Estrogen administration accelerates growth plate senescence, and fusion occurs with exhaustion of proliferative potential.[195] The duration of estrogen exposure to induce epiphyseal fusion depends on age. A younger child requires more years of estrogen exposure than an older child, likely because a longer duration of estrogen exposure is required to exhaust the larger reserve capacity of growth plate chodrocytes in a younger child. Finally, although GH deficiency leads to marked growth deficits, provided sufficient time is available, GH replacement causes sustained "catch-up" growth sufficient to achieve target height.[196]

In contrast to situations of hormone replacement for endocrine deficiencies, "catch-up" growth in other situations of short stature is not as optimal. In SGA infants, an early increase in growth rate has been associated with an increase in IGF-1 levels after intrauterine constraints are eliminated, because high GH levels from intrauterine undernutrition and associated GH insensitivity take time to normalize.[51] However, "catch-up" does not occur in as many as 10% to 15%, and only about half of very low birth weight, SGA infants demonstrate complete "catch-up." About a third remain shorter than target height, with the initial "catch-up" being followed by "catch-down" growth.[197] In addition, following GH therapy in short children born SGA, cessation of GH therapy before epiphyseal fusion leads to a reduction in growth velocity SD score (SDS) and height SDS over a 5-year period, with maximum growth deceleration occurring during the first year after GH therapy is stopped. Another form of "catch-down" growth occurs in children born in families with a history of short stature, in whom length SDS decreases over the first 2 years of life to the familial range, and the extent of loss of length SDS is greater in appropriate for gestational age (AGA) than SGA babies.

Compensatory growth is the term used for the local organ regeneration that occurs after the mass of an organ has been reduced, as by removal or destruction of a portion of that organ.[168] Examples include the compensatory growth that occurs after partial hepatectomy or loss of a kidney. Local IGF-1 and IGF-2 are involved in this type of growth.[110]

SKELETAL MATURATION: BONE AGE IN PREDICTION OF ADULT HEIGHT AND PUBERTAL MILESTONES

Bone growth is accompanied by a predictable pattern of bone maturation. After epiphyseal ossification centers first appear, they undergo modeling in shape and then fuse with the shaft. Bone maturation is assessed as bone age (BA, skeletal age), based on x-rays of the left wrist (see Table 18-2). Figs. 18-10 and 18-11 schematically show the Gruelich and Pyle BA standards.[198,199] The normal range for BA is indicated in Table 18-1. The evaluation is most reliable if the maturation of each center is assessed for calculation of the average,[200] to circumvent normal variations in the epiphyseal ossification pattern.[201] Other atlas methods are available for assessing bone maturation.[202] Skeletal development of young black children is about 0.67 SD advanced over whites of comparable economic status.[203] Other ethnic differences exist

that are, to an unknown extent, nutritional.[202] Bone age is influenced by thyroid hormone, growth hormone, sex steroids, and unknown factors. In both boys and girls, estrogen is responsible for ultimate fusion of the epiphyses.

BA is a better predictor of pubertal milestones than is chronologic age. It is as if bone and neuroendocrine maturation have common genetic, nutritional, and endocrine determinants.[204] A BA of 11 to 12 years corresponds better to the onset of puberty in girls and boys, respectively, than do these chronologic ages. Peak height-velocity phase differences are 25% less when plotted against BA instead of chronologic age.[165] In girls, menarche has been demonstrated to occur at a mean skeletal age of approximately 13 years.[198,205]

Bone age can be used to predict ultimate height potential, since the degree of bone maturation is inversely proportional to the amount of epiphyseal cartilage growth remaining. It follows that if a child's BA and height age (HA; see Table 18-2) are equal, he or she has the potential to reach an average adult height. The fraction of final height achieved at each BA is known (see Table 18-1). Therefore, **predicted adult height** can be calculated by dividing a child's current height by this fraction (method of Bayley and Pinneau).[177] The error inherent in this method is less than 1.5 inches in normal children (see Table 18-1). However, spontaneous shifts by as much as 5 inches in predicted height may occur in 3% of the population for reasons that are unclear.[206] The error is not reduced by serial readings.[200] Because height prediction methods were developed based on normal children, the error is greater in children who are very short[207] or have abnormalities such as bone dysplasias.

To reduce the error in height prediction, elaborate tables have been devised that take into consideration not only a child's BA and height but also the height and weight of the genetic target.[208] Genetic influences on height predicted from bone age can be roughly accounted for by adding one-third the amount that the midparental height differs from the average.[174]

Three methods for assessing height predictions based, in part, on bone age have been developed.[177,208,209] All are based on data from normal children. The Bayley-Pinneau method can be applied simply to young children with abnormal bone ages, so it is used most frequently in children with growth disorders; however, its accuracy has not been verified in many of these.

Growth Disorders

Children who present for inadequate or excessive linear growth generally have either a genetically based, normal variant growth pattern or a disorder of the factors that control growth, as discussed previously. In some children, no cause for abnormal growth can be identified (idiopathic short stature). The following section first categorizes the disorders that cause short stature according to the factors that influence growth. Endocrinopathies are discussed here only insofar as they affect growth. Alternative categorizations of growth disorders are possible; the one presented is preferred because it follows from an understanding of factors that influence growth and avoids ambiguous terminology. Then we present an approach to the differential diagnosis of these disorders according to the clinical assessment of the growth pattern with which the patient presents, along with those clinical features and laboratory tests that discriminate among these disorders. Discussion of treatment for short stature follows. Tall stature is discussed in a parallel manner in the final section.

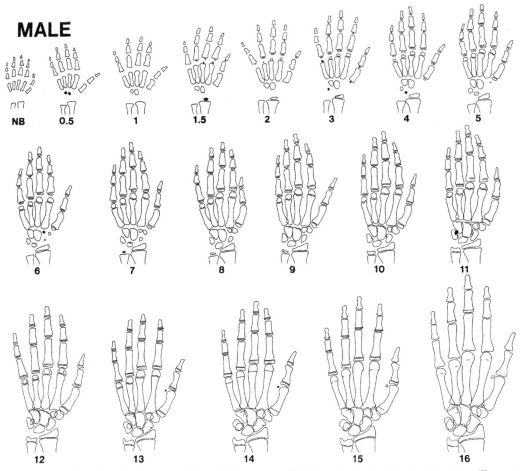

FIGURE 18-10. Progression of ossification of the hand and wrist in boys. Tracings are modified from the standards of Gruelich and Pyle,[198] according to the manner of Wilkins.[199] Newly apparent ossification centers are shown in *black*. Late perfusion is depicted as a *single line* at the junction of the epiphysis and the shaft. Bony projections, which appear as a *double contour* within the outlines of a center, are not illustrated after their appearance has matured.

SHORT STATURE

Causes of Short Stature (Table 18-3)

Genetic and Familial Conditions

Familial Variants. Conditions traditionally considered to be normal variants dominate as the most frequent causes of short stature. Two major nonpathologic familial patterns of growth cause the great majority of cases of short stature. One is **familial short stature** (sometimes termed **familial intrinsic short stature** or **genetic short stature**), in which normal children's growth approximates that of their short parents. The other is **constitutional delay in growth and pubertal development**, in which healthy children who are short (delayed puberty may be the most prominent symptom) spontaneously achieve their normal growth potential at a later than average age. Characteristically, a parent or close relative has a similar growth pattern. In both of these growth patterns, which traditionally are considered normal variants, the typical patient is of normal birth size, and length progressively crosses growth channels to fall below the fifth percentile by 2 to 3 years of age. Height age and bone age then characteristically advance at a normal rate, so that height is below but closely parallel to the fifth percentile through the prepubertal years. These two normal variants differ, however, because in the former, the bone age is normal and puberty occurs at a normal age, whereas in the latter, the bone age is delayed and there is a corresponding delay of puberty until the child reaches a pubertal bone age, at which time a growth spurt results in an adult height that generally is normal for the family target height. These diagnoses rest on the family history, growth pattern, and bone age, and exclusion of other abnormalities. Predictions of adult height are particularly prone to overestimation of growth potential in some very short children.[207] As the molecular controls of growth are elucidated, it is likely that some subgroup(s) of these children will be found to have specific diseases. Some endocrinologists now classify familial short stature and constitutional delay in growth and pubertal development as forms of idiopathic short stature (see later), although others disagree with categorizing these conditions as disorders.[210]

Skeletal Dysplasias. Osteochondrodysplasias consist of a large group of developmental disorders of chondro-osseous tissue, characterized by disproportionate growth, deformation of the skeleton or of individual bones or groups of bones, and genetic transmission; they often are associated with short stature. Osteochondrodysplasias include more than 150 mostly rare conditions, the number expanding as underlying molecular defects are characterized (Table 18-4).[211,212] Abnormal body proportions, such as upper body segment abnormally longer than lower body segment (see Fig. 18-7),[180] or arm span disproportionate to height (see Fig. 18-8),[181] are characteristic in skeletal dysplasias, which are diagnosed by these features together with specific radiologic bone abnormalities.

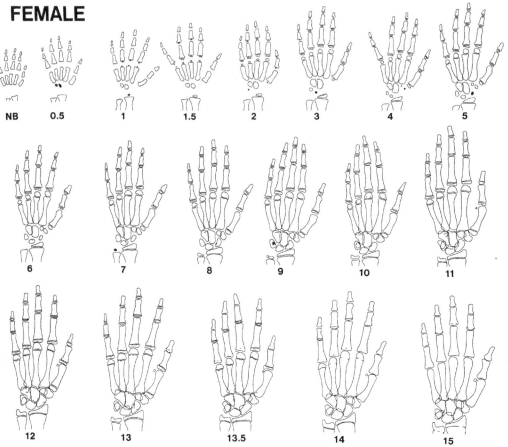

FIGURE 18-11. Progression of ossification of the hand and wrist in girls. See legend for Fig. 18-10.

Table 18-3. Factors Causing Short Stature, With Representative Clinical Conditions

Factors Affecting Height	Representative Conditions		Clinical and Laboratory Features
Genetic	"Normal variants"	Familial short stature	Family history of shortness, normal bone age; no clinical or laboratory abnormalities
		Constitutional delay in growth and development	Family history of delayed growth and pubertal development, delayed bone age; no other clinical or laboratory abnormalities
	Chromosomal aneuploidy	Turner's syndrome	Short, gonadal dysgenesis, otherwise variable phenotype, karyotype necessary to exclude X deletion
		Trisomy 13-15	Mental retardation, congenital heart disease, bilateral cleft palate and lip, microphthalmia, colobomata, holoprosencephaly, IUGR
		Trisomy 16-18	Mental retardation, congenital heart disease, foot/hand deformities, IUGR
		Down syndrome (trisomy 21)	"Mongoloid" facies, hypotonia, mental retardation
	Skeletal dysplasias	See Table 18-4	
	Dysmorphic syndromes	Noonan's syndrome	Similar to Turner's (see Table 18-5), normal karyotype, and present in both sexes, *PPN11* mutation in 50% and in *SOS1* in 20%
		Russell-Silver syndrome	IUGR, relative macrocephaly, small triangular face, asymmetry, abnormalities in chromosome 7 in 10% or 11 in 60%
		Prader-Willi syndrome	Obesity, hypogonadism, hypotonia, intellectual and behavioral deficits, chromosome 15 abnormalities
		Williams' syndrome	"Elfin facies," supravalvular aortic stenosis, ± infantile hypercalcemia, IUGR,[442] 7q11.23 deletion
		Leprechaunism mutation[199]	Congenital lipodystrophy, "puckish" facies, IUGR, insulin resistance and receptor
		Bloom syndrome	Photosensitive dermatitis with telangiectatic erythema, malar hypoplasia, small nose, DNA helicase mutation
		Smith-Lemli-Opitz syndrome	Male pseudohermaphroditism, microcephaly, syndactyly, characteristic facies, cholesterol biosynthetic defect

CBP, CREB-binding protein; *GH,* growth hormone; *IGF-1,* insulin-like growth factor-1; *IUGR,* intrauterine growth retardation.

Table 18-3. Factors Causing Short Stature, With Representative Clinical Conditions—cont'd

Factors Affecting Height	Representative Conditions		Clinical and Laboratory Features
		Fanconi's syndrome	Radial aplasia, GH deficiency, DNA instability mutations
		Rubinstein-Taybi syndrome	Broad thumbs, antimongoloid eyes, hypoplastic maxilla, mental retardation, subset with *CBP* mutations
		Cockayne's syndrome	Onset in early childhood, lipodystrophy, retinitis pigmentosa, photosensitivity, mental retardation, microcephaly, DNA repair defect
		Progeria (Hutchinson-Gilford syndrome)	Onset in infancy, characteristic facies, arteriosclerosis, lipodystrophy, mental retardation, lamin A/C mutation
		Werner's syndrome	Onset in late childhood, characteristic facies, atherosclerosis, cataract, lamin A/C or DNA helicase mutation
		Rothmund-Thomson	"Marbled" pigmentation ± photosensitivity (poikiloderma congenital), cataract, ± syndrome ectodermal dysplasia, DNA helicase mutation
		Wolcott-Rallison syndrome	Fetal growth retardation, diabetes, mental retardation, PERK mutation (affects IGF synthesis)
		IGF-1 gene mutation	Severe fetal growth retardation, sensorineural deafness, mental retardation
		IGF-1 receptor mutations	Prenatal and postnatal growth retardation, variable mental retardation, behavioral abnormalities, insulin resistance
		Insulin receptor mutations	Fetal growth retardation, mental retardation, insulin resistance
Intrauterine	Growth retardation	Small for gestational age	Ongoing growth failure in a minority of nonsyndromic cases; diverse maternal, placental and fetal disorders, most unexplained
		Fetal alcohol syndrome	Characteristic facies (short palpebral fissure length, thin upper lip, indistinct philtrum), microcephaly, mental retardation
		Fetal hydantoin syndrome	Hypertelorism, terminal digit hypoplasia, mental retardation, seizures
		Congenital rubella syndrome	Hepatosplenomegaly, pancytopenia, patent ductus arteriosus, cataract, deafness
Nutritional	Inadequate intake	Starvation	Weight generally depressed more than height
		Psychosocial feeding problems	
		Anorexia due to chronic disease	
	Vitamin/mineral deficiency	Rickets	Nutritional deficiency in vitamin D is most common cause, but there are diverse other acquired and genetic causes; alkaline phosphatase elevated in most types
		Zinc deficiency	
	Nutrient loss	Malabsorption	Symptoms of gastrointestinal, liver, or pancreatic disease; respiratory problems if due to cystic fibrosis
		Chronic vomiting	Obstruction to gastrointestinal tract, achalasia of esophagus, electrolyte disturbances, increased intracranial pressure
	Metabolic wastage	Uncontrolled diabetes mellitus	High glycohemoglobin, hepatomegaly (Mauriac syndrome); exclude other causes of poor growth; fetal diabetes causes IUGR
Psychosocial	Psychosocial dwarfism	See description under GH/IGF-1	
Hormonal	GH deficiency	Congenital	May have neonatal hypoglycemia, midline defects; may have only short stature
			Isolated or CPHD
			Associated with structural brain abnormalities and/or genetic defects, or idiopathic
			Frequent MRI abnormalities
		Acquired	May have history of trauma, CNS insult, or abnormal CNS exam
		Psychosocial deprivation	May show abnormal behavior, hyperphagia; may mimic panhypopituitarism; growth improves with better environment
	GH insensitivity	GH/IGF-1 resistance: GH receptor defects	Birth size normal or low, severe postnatal growth failure, hypoglycemia (see text)
		GH signal transduction defects	
		IGF-1 defects	
		Bioinactive GH	
	Hypothyroidism		Growth failure may be only symptom
	Glucocorticoid	Excess	Supraphysiologic levels attenuate growth. Often associated with obesity
	Pseudohypoparathyroidism	Resistance to PTH	Short, obese, round face, short metacarpals, developmental delay, subcutaneous calcification, abnormal Ca and P
	Sex steroids	Deficiency	Deficiency after 10-11 years of age impairs growth
Chronic illness			May have history or symptoms of chronic condition or short stature may be presenting feature; weight often impaired more than height
Idiopathic	Idiopathic short stature		Height more than 2 SDs below the mean, unexplained by above condiitons. Some include familial short stature and constitutional delay in growth and development in this category

CBP, CREB-binding protein; *GH,* growth hormone; *IGF-1,* insulin-like growth factor-1; *IUGR,* intrauterine growth retardation.

The most common is achondroplasia, an autosomal dominant condition that has a frequency of about 1 in approximately 20,000, with about 90% of cases representing fresh mutations.[213] It causes short stature (often apparent at birth and with deceleration of growth rate in infancy), short limbs, macrocephaly, a low nasal bridge, caudal narrowing of the spinal canal, and, occasionally, hydrocephalus (Fig. 18-12).[213] The average adult height is about 125 cm in females and 131 cm in males.[213] Growth curves for achondroplasia have been developed.[214] Achondroplasia gen-

erally is caused by a gain-of-function mutation in the *FGFR3* gene.[215,216] The inactivating mutation of Indian hedgehog leads to a similar phenotype.[217]

Hypochondroplasia is an allelic variant of achondroplasia.[215,216] Although it results from a mutation of the *FGFR3* gene (as does achondroplasia), it is a distinct condition with autosomal dominant inheritance, and the two conditions have not been found in the same family. It manifests with short stature and dysmorphic features that often are milder than achondroplasia.

Table 18-4. Representative Types of Skeletal Dysplasia of Known Genetic Basis

Dysplasia Group	Inheritance	IUGR	Genetic Basis
Achondroplasia Group			
Achondroplasia	AD	+	*FGFR3* activating mutation
Hypochondroplasia	AD	−	*FGFR3* activating mutation
Type II Collagenopathies			
Spondyloepiphyseal dysplasia (SED) congenital	AD	+	*COL2A1*
Type IX Collagenopathies			
Stickler dysplasia	AD	+	*COL11A1*
Other Spondyloepiphyseal Dysplasias			
X-linked SED tarda	XLD	−	*Xp22.2-p22.1*
Pseudoachondroplasia and Multiple Epiphyseal Dysplasias (MED)			
Pseudoachondroplasia and MED (Fairbanks type)	AD	−	*COMP*/cartilage oligomeric matrix protein
MED (other types)	?	−	*COL9A2*
Chondrodysplasia Punctata			
Zellweger syndrome	AR	+	*PEX1,2,5,6*/peroxins
Brachytelephalangic type	XLR	+	*ARSE*/arylsulfatase E
Metaphyseal Dysplasia			
Jansen type	AD	+	*PTHR*
Schmid type	AD	−	*COL10A1/COL10* α chain
Adenosine deaminase deficiency	AD	−	*ADA*/adenosine deaminase
Acromelic and Acromesomelic Dysplasias			
Trichorhinophalangeal syndrome types	AD	+	*TRPS1* ± *EXT1*
Grebe and Hunter-Thompson dysplasias	AR	+	*CDMP1*/cartilage-derived morphogenic protein
Albright hereditary osteodystrophy		−	*GNAS1*/guanine nucleotide α subunit, inactive
Dysplasias With Prominent Membranous Bone Involvement			
Cleidocranial dysplasia	AD	+	*CBFA1*/core-binding factor α subunit
Bent Bone Dysplasias			
Campomelic dysplasia	AD	+	*SOX9/SRY* box-9
Dysostosis Multiplex			
Mucopolysaccharidosis II	XLR	−	*IDS*/iduronate-2-sulfatase
Mucopolysaccharidosis, others	AR	−	Diverse
Dysplasias With Decreased Bone Density			
Osteogenesis imperfecta (diverse)	AD/AR	±	*COLA1* or 2/α (1 or 2) 1 procollagen
Dysplasias With Defective Mineralization			
Hypophosphatasia, infantile type	AR	+	*ALPL*/alkaline phosphatase
Hypophosphatemic rickets	XLD	−	*PHEX*
Increased Bone Density Without Modification of Bone Shape			
Osteopetrosis/renal tubular acidosis	AR	+	*CA2*/carbonic anhydrase II
Pyknodysostosis	AR	+	*CTSK*/cathepsin K
Disorganized Development of Cartilaginous and Fibrous Components of Skeleton			
Fibrous dysplasia (McCune-Albright syndrome)	Spmos	−	*GNAS1*, activating
Fibrodysplasia ossificans progressiva	AD	+	*BMP4*/bone morphogenetic protein 4

From International Working Group on Constitutional Diseases of Bone: International nomenclature and classification of the osteochondrodysplasias (1997). Am J Med Genet 79(5):376–382, 1998; and Superti-Furga A, Bonafe L, Rimoin DL: Molecular-pathogenetic classification of genetic disorders of the skeleton. Am J Med Genet 106(4):282–293, 2001.

AD, Autosomal dominant; AR, autosomal recessive; SPmos, sporadic mosaic; XLD, X-linked dominant; XLR, X-linked recessive.

Newborns may be slightly small, but short stature generally becomes evident by 3 years of age. Few craniofacial abnormalities are seen in hypochondroplasia. Children are minimally short limbed. The hands and feet are usually stubby, and genu varum may occur. Adult height is approximately 120 to 150 cm. The most objective radiologic finding is narrowing of the lower lumbosacral interpedicular distances.

Osteochondrodysplasias may cause specific patterns of disproportion. In spondoepiphyseal dysplasia, the spine is disproportionately affected and growth slows in midchildhood, causing an attenuated growth pattern. On the other hand, some bone dysplasias cause proportionate dwarfism. Tubular stenosis is a proportionate form of bone dysplasia that is associated with congenital hypoparathyroidism.[218] Activating mutation of the PTH/PTHrP receptor has been discovered to cause Jansen's metaphyseal dysplasia, which is associated with asymptomatic hypercalcemia.[219] Various atlases are available to distinguish among the known types of bone dysplasia.[168,213,220,221] In recent years, it has become possible to make a specific genetic diagnosis in many cases.[215]

Leri-Weil dyschondrogenesis is a dominantly inherited skeletal dysplasia that affects both sexes and is characterized by short stature, mesomelia, and Madelung wrist deformity.[222] Short stature begins in early childhood. The underlying molecular abnormality is haploinsufficiency for the gene SHOX (short stature homeobox-containing gene), located on the distal part of the X chromosome pseudoautosomal region. SHOX is highly expressed in osteogenic tissue. Langer mesomelic dysplasia (associated with severe dwarfism) is due to SHOX nullizygosity.[223] SHOX insufficiency is also considered the major cause of short stature in Turner's syndrome, and it has been suggested as a contributor to idiopathic short stature in some cases (see later). The diagnosis of SHOX haploinsufficiency should be considered in young children with short stature (more than 2 SDs below the mean), high-arched palate, increased upper-to-lower segment ratio (see later), reduced arm span for age (see later), increased carrying angle, Madelung deformity or other wrist abnormality, tibial bowing, or appearance of calf muscular hypertrophy.[222] Exposure to sex steroids may make these abnormalities more obvious. Molecular analysis for defects in the SHOX gene is available. GH treatment of short children with SHOX deficiency, some

of whom had the full Leri-Weil phenotype, appears to increase growth velocity and height SDS, although it is not clear whether those with the Leri-Weil phenotype show as much growth as those who are simply short.[224]

Chromosomal Abnormalities, Monogenic Disorders, and Syndromes

Several syndromes are associated with short stature (see Table 18-3).[213,225-233] Those in which short stature or endocrine problems are prominent are discussed here.

Turner's Syndrome. Turner's syndrome (gonadal dysgenesis), caused by deletion of X-chromosomal material, is the most common pathologic cause of short stature in girls. Haploinsufficiency for the SHOX gene,[234,235] contributes to short stature in Turner's syndrome.[234,236]

The incidence of Turner's syndrome is 1 in 2500 newborn girls.[237] The average birth size of these children is at the lower end of the normal range. Although significant variation has been noted among affected individuals, height typically drops below the third percentile by 2 to 3 years of age, and this is followed by gradual and progressive deviation from the normal growth channels.[238] Growth may become further attenuated in the teenage years and epiphyseal closure is delayed, in part because of hypogonadism.[239] The most characteristic features of Turner's syndrome are short stature and gonadal dysgenesis. The presence of pubertal development should not deter consideration of the diagnosis, because about 10% of patients have some residual ovarian tissue rather than streak gonads. Thus, these patients may have spontaneous menarche, although few sustain regular menses.[240] Additional manifestations of Turner's syndrome include lymphedema, particularly in the newborn period, and the dysmorphic features and congenital anomalies listed in Table 18-5. Although about 70% of patients with Turner's syndrome

Table 18-5. Approximate Incidence of Somatic Abnormalities in Turner's and Noonan's Syndromes[a]

Abnormality	Turner's Syndrome, %	Noonan's Syndrome, %
Short stature (<10%)	100/80[b]	90/90
Gonadal failure	99/85?	≤10/≤10[c]
Cryptorchidism	NA/33	NA/75
Hypertelorism	<25	100
High palate	80	75
Neck webbed	50	10
Neck short	68	100
Cubitus valgus	68	30
Chest deformity[d]	50	50
Coarctation of aorta	20	<1
Pulmonic stenosis	10	50[e]
Mental retardation	10[f]	25
Pigmented moles, multiple	50	<10

NA, Not applicable.

[a]Defined on the basis of the presence (Turner's) or absence (Noonan's) of a sex chromosome abnormality. Turner's syndrome in females results from deletion of genetic material on the X chromosome. Various sex chromosomal abnormalities have been reported in Turner's syndrome in males—for example, XO, XXY, XO/XY, XO/XY/XYY, XX/XXY.

[b]Female/male.

[c]The distinction between delayed puberty and hypogonadism has seldom been made.

[d]Pectus or an apparent increase in internipple distance.

[e]The high incidence of congenital heart disease in Noonan's syndrome may be due to ascertainment bias, Dr. Noonan being a cardiologist. A variety of other congenital heart defects have been reported in both syndromes.

[f]Males seem to have a greater incidence of mental retardation, although finding this may be a matter of ascertainment.

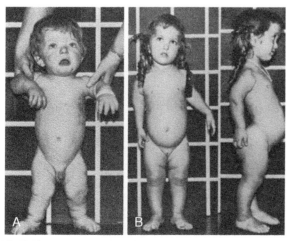

FIGURE 18-12. Achondroplasia. **A,** One-year-old boy with a height age of 4 months. **B,** Four-year-old girl with a height age of 20 months. (From Jones KL [ed]: Smith's Recognizable Patterns of Human Malformation, 4th ed. Philadelphia, WB Saunders, 1988.)

have learning disabilities that affect nonverbal perceptual motor and visuospatial skills, most are of normal intelligence, and only about 10% exhibit substantial developmental delay.[237] Variation in the physical manifestations of Turner's syndrome is illustrated in Fig. 18-13.[213] Aortic root dilatation and renal anomalies are infrequent but important.[241] The incidence of autoimmune thyroiditis and diabetes mellitus is increased. Although some correlations have been noted between karyotype and phenotype (e.g., those with 45,X/46,XX or 45,X/47,XXX are more likely to have spontaneous menarche than those with 45,X, those with isochromosome Xq are at increased risk for autoimmune disease, those with a ring chromosome are at greater risk for developmental delay[237]), phenotypic predictions based on karyotype are unreliable. Karyotype analysis is essential in the investigation of any girl with unexplained short stature. Without growth-promoting therapy, adult height averages 56.5 inches.[238]

At diagnosis, patients with Turner's syndrome require echocardiograms; renal ultrasound; hearing tests; and assessment of growth, pubertal development/ovarian function, and psychosocial issues. During childhood, they require regular reassessment for abnormalities in these areas.[237]

Although Turner's syndrome does not involve GH deficiency as a cause of the growth impairment, GH treatment (particularly in doses higher than those used for GH deficiency) appears to increase growth. Results suggest that long-term GH treatment increases adult height in many recipients by about 2 cm for each year of treatment, although reports vary in the degree of height gained with no discernible gain in some.[237,238,242-244] Variability in response to GH may reflect, in part, X-linked imprinting.[245] GH treatment is often recommended when the height of a girl with Turner's syndrome drops below the fifth percentile on the normal female growth curve, although some data suggest that earlier treatment may be beneficial.[246] In addition to increasing height, GH treatment is associated with increased lean body mass, but it does not affect bone mineral density.[247] The side effects of GH treatment are discussed later. Children with Turner's syndrome who are treated with GH appear to have an increased underlying risk for some of the adverse events associated with GH treatment.[248] To induce pubertal development in girls with ovarian failure due to Turner's syndrome, very low dose exogenous estrogen therapy (and, eventually, cycling with progesterone) is needed in adolescence and beyond.[147]

Noonan's Syndrome. Noonan's syndrome, originally called "male Turner's syndrome," is diagnosed in patients of either sex with normal external genitalia who have a Turner-like phenotype but normal sex chromosomes.[249-253] It may be transmitted as an autosomal dominant disorder. Mutations in *PTPN11,* the gene that encodes the nonreceptor-type protein tyrosine phosphatase SHP-2, account for about 50%, missense mutations in *SOS1* account for about 20%, and *KRAS* mutations account for less than 5% of cases.[254-262] Although the anomalies in an individual may resemble those in Turner's syndrome, the overall incidence of malformations is different, with predominantly right-sided cardiac lesions in Noonan's and left-sided lesions in Turner's syndrome (see Table 18-5). Patients with Noonan's syndrome have a better prognosis for gonadal function (delayed puberty rather than gonadal failure) and become somewhat taller than patients with Turner's syndrome, having adult heights that average 162.5 cm in males and 152.7 cm in females.[263] Although mild GH resistance has been found in some patients with Noonan's syndrome,[264] GH treatment can increase growth,[265,266] and the U.S. Food and Drug Administration (FDA) approved GH for short stature associated with Noonan's syndrome in 2007.

Prader-Willi Syndrome. In Prader-Willi syndrome, short stature is associated with neonatal failure to thrive and hypotonicity, obesity of onset at about 2 years of age due to development of a voracious appetite, intellectual impairment, and hypogonadism.[267,268] It is associated with lack of expression of paternally inherited genes imprinted and located in a critical region of the proximal part of the long arm of chromosome 15; 70% of cases are due to a de novo paternally derived deletion in this region, and unimaternal disomy accounts for about 25% of cases (Fig. 18-14).[269,270] Some may have GH deficiency. GH therapy increases linear growth, may decrease body fat,[271-273] and has been approved by the FDA for this condition. Some reports have described fatalities in individuals with Prader-Willi syndrome soon after the start of GH therapy.[274] Although the causes have not been completely elucidated, worsening of obstructive sleep apnea (to which individuals with Prader-Willi syndrome

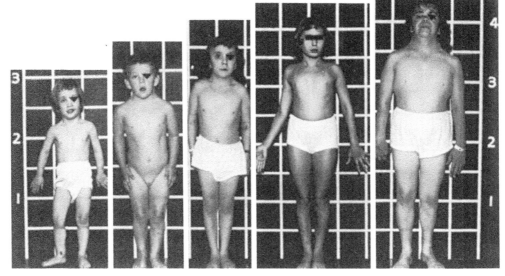

FIGURE 18-13. Variable phenotypes of Turner's syndrome: five girls with 45,X syndrome illustrating the variability of features such as webbed neck and broad chest. (From Jones KL [ed]: Smith's Recognizable Patterns of Human Malformation, 4th ed. Philadelphia, WB Saunders, 1988.)

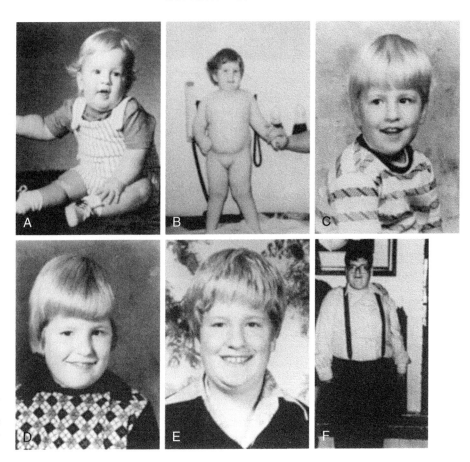

FIGURE 18-14. Evolution of the phenotype in Prader-Willi syndrome in a patient with a 15q deletion. **A,** 11 months. **B,** 2.5 years. **C,** 3.5 years. **D,** 7 years. **E,** 13 years. **F,** 27 years. (From Cassidy SB: Prader-Willi syndrome. J Med Genet 34:917–923, 1997.)

are predisposed), potentially due to IGF-1–mediated tonsillar hypertrophy, has been postulated. The FDA states that GH is contraindicated in children with Prader-Willi syndrome who are severely obese or have a history of upper respiratory obstruction or sleep apnea or severe respiratory impairment. Children with Prader-Willi syndrome should be evaluated for upper respiratory obstruction or sleep apnea before beginning GH treatment, and treatment should be discontinued if these develop. Patients should be monitored for respiratory infection, which should be diagnosed early and treated aggressively.

18q Deletions. Deletions of 18q occur in about 1 of 40,000 children. Approximately two thirds of affected children have heights greater than 2 SDs below the mean, and most have abnormal growth velocities.[275] These patients may be at increased risk for GH deficiency.[275]

Down Syndrome. Stunting of growth and cerebral dysfunction are virtually uniform features of autosomal aneuploidy. Down syndrome (trisomy 21 and variants thereof) is the most common multiple malformation syndrome in humans. Adult height averages 155 cm in affected males and 145 cm in females.[160]

Other dysmorphic syndromes associated with short stature are discussed in Table 18-3. More detailed descriptions are available in Online Mendelian Inheritance in Man (OMIM) at http://www.ncbi.nim.nih.gov/omim/.

Intrauterine Growth Retardation and Small for Gestational Age

Small for gestational age (SGA) has been variously defined as birth weight or length below the 10th percentile or 2 SDs below the mean.[149,276,277] About 10% to 15% of children born SGA have persistent growth failure beyond 2 to 3 years of age.[278] Even among those who have catch-up growth, SGA status is associated with increased long-term risk for developing insulin resistance, obesity, and type 2 diabetes mellitus. **Intrauterine growth retardation (IUGR)** is a term that sometimes is used interchangeably with SGA; however, IUGR actually implies a pathologic process that restricts fetal growth and is diagnosed through serial prenatal ultrasounds.[278]

The reason for being born SGA is multifactorial and includes intrinsic fetal abnormalities (genetic alterations and syndromes, congenital malformations, congenital infections), placental factors, and maternal factors (such as ingestion of drugs, tobacco, and alcohol; malnutrition and intercurrent illness; and uterine abnormalities) (see Tables 18-3 and 18-4). Genetic causes include chromosomal abnormalities, single gene defects, and uniparental disomy (UPD).[279,280] Congenital diabetes mellitus and insulin receptor mutations,[114] congenital IGF-1 deficiency, and IGF-1 receptor mutations in humans (as well as IGF disruption in animal models) cause IUGR and SGA.[35,47,281] However, the exact origin in any given child remains unknown in up to 60% of cases.[282]

Russell-Silver Syndrome is a term applied to some children with IUGR in association with dysmorphic features such as pseudohydrocephalus (a relatively large head with a small face), clinodactyly, and subtle body asymmetry. It is a heterogeneous condition. A clinical scoring system has been suggested to establish the diagnosis.[283] About half of patients with the syndrome have delayed puberty and reach normal adult height,[284] but the remainder may be quite short.[285] It has been suggested that approximately 10% have uniparental disomy of maternal chromosome 7,[279] and 60% have an epigenetic defect at chromosome 11p15.[283,286] In the latter group, loss of IGF-2 expression in the fetus may contribute to IUGR.[283]

Other cases of IUGR with ongoing postnatal growth failure are nonsyndromic and occur as the seemingly nonspecific result of such dissimilar disorders as maternal heroin addiction,[287] intrauterine infection,[288] placental insufficiency,[289] fetal malnutrition,[290,291] and hypoxia-related congenital anomalies.[292] A common thread to these may be a decreased endowment in total body cell number.[293] Another proposed mechanism is fetal hypercortisolism.[57] Unexplained IUGR may also have genomic roots in view of the fact that maternal uniparental disomy for chromosome 6 has been reported to be associated with IUGR only because it unmasked congenital adrenal hyperplasia, an autosomal recessive trait.[280]

The clinical management of children with short stature attributed to SGA involves attempts to ascertain and manage the underlying cause of the condition.[276] For those SGA children who fail to manifest catch-up growth in height by 2 to 3 years of age, the FDA has approved GH therapy.[294,295] GH has been found to increase growth rate in these children in a dose-dependent manner.[276,296-299] Although some data suggest reduced insulin sensitivity in short SGA children treated with GH,[300] to date long-term GH treatment has not been found to increase the risk for type 2 diabetes mellitus.[278,301]

Undernutrition and Chronic Nonendocrine Disease.
Undernutrition sufficient to reduce calorie intake to below 82% to 91% of the recommended level will arrest growth.[302,303] This degree of undernutrition is suggested by weight for height, BMI, or body fat below the 10th percentile.[304] Undernutrition may result from inadequate nutrient intake (due to psychosocial feeding or eating disorders, or poor appetite due to chronic disease), excessive nutrient output (chronic vomiting or malabsorption as in inflammatory bowel disease, celiac disease, cystic fibrosis, or hepatic disease), or metabolic wastage (as in poorly controlled diabetes mellitus).[305,306] A unique cause of malnutrition in infants is the diencephalic syndrome. This is characterized by a paucity of body fat resembling lipodystrophy in a hyperalert, otherwise healthy child. Radiosensitive brain tumors in the anterior hypothalamic area are the usual cause. Disturbance of the regulation of appetite, secretion of pituitary lipolytic hormones such as GH, and increased energy expenditure have been postulated as the mechanism.[307,308] Deficiency of trace metals such as zinc and copper also causes growth failure.[82,83]

Data indicate height attenuation in children treated with stimulants for attention deficit hyperactivity disorder[309]; although the mechanisms are not known, gastrointestinal disturbance or a change in appetite has been suggested.

Chronic nonendocrine disorders of virtually any organ system may attenuate growth.[310] Generally, weight is suppressed more than height, in contrast to primary endocrine disorders. Mechanisms of growth impairment vary according to the disease and often include undernutrition, medication effects (e.g., supraphysiologic doses of glucocorticoids), chronic acidosis, and/or secondary endocrine dysfunction. Examples include celiac disease, inflammatory bowel disease, chronic renal failure, cardiovascular disease, hematologic disorders, poorly controlled diabetes mellitus, chronic acidosis, cystic fibrosis, and chronic infections. Although the primary disorder is evident in many cases of short stature due to chronic illness, short stature is sometimes the primary presenting feature. This occurs notably in inflammatory bowel disease, celiac disease, and renal dysfunction.

Celiac disease and Crohn's disease are notorious for presenting as short stature without gastrointestinal complaints. In approximately 2% to 8% of children with short stature and no gastrointestinal symptoms, celiac disease may be the underlying cause, and if other causes of short stature are excluded, the risk for celiac disease is increased in some reports to 19% to 59%.[311]

For measurement of immunoglobulin (Ig)A tissue transglutaminase and antiendomysial antibodies is a screening test for celiac disease,[263,312] and sometimes referral to a gastroenterologist is needed.[313]

Poor growth in Crohn's disease reflects poor food intake, malabsorption, disease severity, direct effects of the inflammatory process on the growth axis (with evidence implicating tumor necrosis factor [TNF]-α, interleukin [IL]-6, and IL-1-β), the presence of jejunal disease, and perhaps genetic susceptibility factors (including IL-6 gene polymorphism and polymorphism on the TNF-α promoter gene).[129,314-317] GH deficiency has been reported,[318] but an actual link between the two conditions is uncertain. Growth in Crohn's disease can also be adversely affected by glucocorticoid therapy and may improve with nutritional intervention or surgery.[129,319] Studies to date have not demonstrated consistent benefit from GH therapy. Although a recent study indicates that many children show an increase in height SDS after beginning treatment for Crohn's and reach final heights close to target heights, about one fifth have final height significantly lower (>8 cm lower) than target height.[316] Rickets, due to vitamin D deficiency, can be due to inadequate intake, malabsorption, liver disease, or renal disease. Impaired growth is a common feature.

Chronic renal disease—including renal tubular acidosis and chronic renal insufficiency— suppresses growth. Poor growth in chronic renal insufficiency probably reflects chronic acidosis, poor intake, anemia, subnormal formation of 1,25-dihydroxycholecalciferol, renal osteodystrophy, and, at times, use of medications (e.g., glucocorticoids). In addition, serum IGF-1 is generally normal, but IGF bioactivity and free IGF-1 are low,[320,321] probably because of excessive circulating IGF-binding proteins.[322] The FDA has approved GH for the treatment of short stature due to renal failure before transplantation, and consensus guidelines have been developed.[323] GH has also been used in some studies after transplantation, with promising results.[323,324]

Metabolic disorders may affect growth. Chronic acidosis[84] or chronic alkalosis[325] may cause growth failure. Chronic anemia[326] and rickets lead to a delayed growth pattern.[327,328] A defect in zinc action has resulted in growth failure.[329] Diabetes mellitus, when poorly controlled, can lead to Mauriac syndrome, involving growth failure and hepatomegaly due to excessive glycogen deposition. In thalassemia, growth impairment may reflect not only chronic anemia, but also endocrine dysfunction due to hemosiderosis.[330]

Endocrine Disorders

GH Deficiency

GH deficiency is a key cause of short stature. It is difficult to diagnose because it may cause no phenotypic abnormalities other than slow linear growth, and diagnostic tests are controversial. If untreated, GH deficiency can result in adults with proportionate extreme short stature (formerly termed midgets). Recent advances in our understanding of molecular loci influencing GH synthesis and secretion have elucidated specific causes of previously unexplained GH-related growth failure.

GH deficiency can be congenital or acquired. Both congenital and acquired forms may be isolated or may coexist with other pituitary hormone deficiencies (panhypopituitarism or combined pituitary hormone deficiency [CPHD]).

Congenital forms of GH deficiency are due to primary hypothalamic and/or pituitary defects. They may be associated with structural brain defects, midline facial abnormalities, and/or genetic abnormalities. Among the midline defects are septo-optic dysplasia (involving varying degrees of hypoplasia of the optic nerves, chiasm, and infundibular region of the hypothalamus) and holoprosencephaly. Clues to the presence of midline defects include a cleft palate, a single central incisor, and microphallus.[331-334] Specific gene defects can disrupt pituitary development and GH secretion. Diverse patterns of pituitary hormone deficiency can result from mutations of homeodomain transcription factors, such as POU1F1 (Pit-1), Prop-1 (considered the most common genetic cause of combined pituitary hormone deficiency), LHX3, LHX4, PTX2, GLI2, SOX3, and OTX2, which are essential for pituitary development.[11,335-348] Combined pituitary hormone deficiency (CPHD) of GH, prolactin, and thyroid-stimulating hormone (TSH) is the typical outcome of inactivating mutations of both POU1F1 and PROP1, while PROP1 defects also sometimes cause follicle-stimulating hormone (FSH), luteinizing hormone (LH), and adrenocorticotropic hormone (ACTH) deficiencies, sometimes associated with pituitary enlargement preceding hypoplasia. Mutations in *HESX1* can cause a broad spectrum of phenotypes, including septo-optic dysplasia, interruption of the pituitary stalk (ectopic posterior pituitary), and isolated GH deficiency or CPHD.[349] Septo-optic dysplasia (SOD), in its complete form, involves hypoplasia or aplasia of the optic nerves and/or optic chiasm, agenesis or hypoplasia of the septum pellucidum, and defects in hypothalamic function (GH deficiency alone or CPHD); however, incomplete forms of SOD may occur. In one study, 35 of 73 subjects with CPHD, belonging to 18 unrelated families, had *PROP1* gene defects, and in another study of 195 patients with combined pituitary hormone deficiency, 20 had *PROP1* mutations.[340,350]

Other congenital primary pituitary disorders that lead to isolated GHD include defects in the GH gene,[351-356] bioactive GH,[357,358] and mutations in the GHRH-receptor gene.[359,360] It is surprising that primary genetic defects of the GHRH gene have not yet been identified.

Most GH deficiency currently is considered idiopathic, and this occurs in 1 in 3500 children.[361] Magnetic resonance imaging shows abnormalities, including a small anterior pituitary, an attenuated pituitary stalk, and/or ectopic posterior pituitary, in more than 70% of GH-deficient children.[362-364] Some believe that isolated idiopathic GH deficiency is prone to overdiagnosis.

Congenital GH deficiency may present with neonatal hypoglycemia. The combination of neonatal hypoglycemia, prolonged neonatal jaundice, and, in males, micropenis suggests panhypopituitarism.[365] Congenital GH deficiency also may present with short stature in early infancy or childhood. In addition to shortness, GH deficiency classically causes relative adiposity, reduced musculature, a cherubic appearance, and a high-pitched voice. These manifestations are not present in all children with the disorder, however. The diagnosis of GH deficiency should be considered in all children with subnormal growth velocity.

Acquired GH deficiency may result from head trauma, tumors such as craniopharyngioma, Rathke's pouch cyst, histiocytosis X and other infiltrative diseases, cranial irradiation, and surgery or chemotherapy.[366-372] These children show attenuation of growth after an initial period of normal growth. Acquired, isolated, permanent idiopathic GH deficiency is considered rare.

Functional hypopituitarism is another form of acquired GH deficiency. The prototypic cause of this is the psychosocial deprivation syndrome. This "deprivation dwarfism" may be seen in children who are not malnourished or overtly disturbed, but who show abnormal behavior patterns, including hyperphagia, food hoarding, drinking from toilets, and sleepwalking.[373-375] GH deficiency in this condition rapidly resolves in a nurturing environment. In one study, initial catch-up growth did not correlate with final height, and the mean final height attained was significantly lower than the midparental target height.[376] Some short children who initially meet criteria for the diagnosis of isolated GHD, on later retesting appear to have GH sufficiency; this may reflect, in part, vagaries in current diagnostic tools and/or the existence of transient forms of functional GHD.[377]

The diagnosis of GH deficiency classically rests on the demonstration of subnormal GH responses to two or more provocative pharmacologic tests of GH reserve (i.e., a GH peak less than 5 ng/mL, indicative of complete deficiency, and 5 to 10 ng/dL, indicative of partial deficiency when a polyclonal GH assay is used[378]; some use 7 ng/mL as the cutoff point between complete and partial GH deficiency in a child with slow growth velocity, a delayed bone age, and no other disorder that accounts for slow growth. Monoclonal antibodies yield GH values that are about half the values of assays using polyclonal antisera.[379] The development of assays to measure free GH[380] may alter diagnostic criteria in the future, and a new GH reference standard is being introduced that may require a downward adjustment of the lower limit of normal. Provocative tests of GH reserve include arginine, L-dopa, clonidine, glucagon, and insulin-induced hypoglycemia.[381,382] Two pharmacologic tests are used traditionally because approximately 15% to 20% of apparently normal children have a poor response to a given single test of GH reserve. Untreated hypothyroidism, obesity, and glucocorticoid treatment may falsely lower GH levels. Sex steroid priming with estrogen or androgen for 1 to 7 days before the GH provocative test sometimes is utilized to distinguish GH deficiency from constitutional delay in growth and development.[383-385] Although this classic definition continues to have support, concern has been raised because of potential false-positive and false-negative diagnoses when this approach is used, and because of inconsistencies among GH assays.[383,386-388] Some have considered the false-positive rate to be related to evolving cutoff points in the diagnosis of GH deficiency and to inconsistencies in how GH tests have been used.[389] Alternative approaches have been proposed to diagnose forms of GH deficiency, such as neurosecretory defects and bioactive GH. These include 12- to 24-hour measurement of spontaneous GH secretion, but such tests are not used commonly today. Measurement of IGF-1 and/or IGFBP-3 has been suggested for the diagnosis; however, IGF-1 and IGFBP-3 levels are affected by undernutrition, chronic systemic diseases, and delayed puberty, and they must be interpreted in terms of age and pubertal stage (see Fig. 18-2).[390,391] Combination testing with GHRH and a somatostatin suppressor such as arginine has been suggested[90] as an alternative diagnostic procedure.[392] Because GH levels are higher in newborns than in infants and children, the diagnosis of GH deficiency has been made in neonates by demonstrating a random GH level of less than 20 ng/mL in the appropriate clinical situation (e.g., microphallus, hypoglycemia). Therapeutic trials of GH have also been suggested as a means to assess GH deficiency by examining the growth response to GH, but their interpretation is difficult (see later discussion). Overall, no single method has yet emerged as a gold standard alternative to the classical definition. Following the diagnosis of GH deficiency, magnetic resonance imaging is indicated to determine whether the hypopituitarism is due to structural lesions or tumors, and assessment of other potential pituitary deficiencies is needed.

Recombinant GH therapy (usually in a dose of 0.3 mg/kg/week subcutaneously, divided daily or 6 days/week) is the standard treatment for GH deficiency and is remarkably successful for treatment of this condition (Fig. 18-15). Alternate doses have been used, and higher ones have been approved for adolescents in puberty; the relative cost-benefit of higher doses is not clear. In GH-deficient children treated with GH daily, the growth rate during the first year of treatment is, on average, 11.5 cm.[393] Although it declines somewhat thereafter, the growth rate remains markedly above pretreatment growth velocity. Recombinant GH therapy begun early is effective in bringing adult height into the normal range.[394-396] Factors that influence adult height in GH-treated children with GHD include age at diagnosis, adequacy of GH replacement, appropriate treatment for other coexisting pituitary hormone deficits, and pubertal development. Height SDS at baseline and change in height SDS in the first year of treatment also may be predictive.[397] Data on the role of GH receptor variants in the growth response to GH treatment are inconsistent.[398,399] GH treatment also increases bone mass and lean tissue mass in children with GH deficiency.[400] Although some have advocated titration of GH dose to attain target IGF-1 levels in the high-normal range, substantive reasons exist for maintaining weight-based dosing and monitoring IGF-1 levels for safety purposes.[401]

Potential adverse effects of recombinant GH include fluid retention (sometimes with cerebral edema), pancreatitis, glucose intolerance and/or insulin resistance, transient gynecomastia, slipped capital femoral epiphysis, and growth of nevi.[402-405] Concerns about leukemia and second tumors have not been con-firmed among children who do not have other predisposing factors, although ongoing surveillance continues and discussion with families is appropriate.[406-410] Cancer survivors, particularly those treated with radiotherapy, appear to be at increased risk for developing secondary neoplasms if subsequently treated with GH, although the risk appears to diminish over time.[411] Growth deceleration associated with high-affinity, high-capacity antibodies to GH has been reported but appears very rare. Retinopathy has been described in patients with renal failure receiving GH to improve growth.[412] Some adverse effects seem specific to children with underlying predispositions; for example, some children with Prader-Willi syndrome treated with GH have died of respiratory causes.[413]

The long-term risk for cancer from childhood GH therapy appears low, but exact risk is not known.[414,415] As noted earlier, risk may be increased in children previously treated for cancer. A systematic review, however, found that circulating concentrations of IGF-1 and IGFBP-3 are associated with an increased risk for common cancers, although associations are modest.[416]

In addition to GH treatment, those children with GH deficiency associated with other pituitary hormone deficiencies (i.e., panhypopituitarism) require adequate replacement of these hormones. A review of the Canadian experience suggests that adrenal insufficiency represents a potentially avoidable cause of death in children with panhypopituitarism.[417]

Other aspects of treatment include the importance of having a pediatric endocrinologist monitor children on GH therapy at 3- to 4-month intervals to assess clinical progress and of having treated patients undergo screening for adverse effects (including annual measurement of IGF-1 and IGFBP-3, glucose/hemoglobin A1C, and thyroid function), assessment for adherence, and review of therapeutic targets. Monitoring allows dose adjustments to ensure that IGF-1 and IGFBP-3 levels are within the normal range.

Whether to discontinue GH therapy in adolescents with GHD is an important decision. It is important not to discontinue GH therapy before secondary sex characteristics are advanced because GH potentiates sex hormone effects.[142,418,419] Traditionally, GH therapy for GH-deficient children has been stopped after adult height has been reached and epiphyses have fused. However, low-dose GH improves metabolic status, body composition, and well-being in adults with GH deficiency.[383] Therefore, after linear growth has ended or an adequate adult height has been reached, GHD individuals should be retested to ascertain whether GHD persists, and for those with persistent GHD, low-dose GH treatment is recommended to maintain metabolic function.[420,421]

Alternatives to standard GH therapy, including new GH delivery systems (such as dermal patch, depot GH preparations), oral GH secretagogues, IGF-1, and GH-releasing factor, are under study or are under development.[422-426]

GH Insensitivity Syndromes

Whereas GH deficiency causes secondary IGF-1 deficiency, a growing class of disorders is known to cause primary defects in IGF-1 production or action.[427] These are termed **GH insensitivity (GHI) syndromes.** In these conditions, patients tend to have clinical manifestations similar to children with GH deficiency; however, in GHI, GH secretion is adequate, but peripheral tissues are incapable of responding normally to GH. GHI can be subdivided into primary and secondary forms. Primary GHI includes hereditary defects in (1) the GH receptor (the defects initially described by Laron and often termed **Laron dwarfism**), (2) the GH signal transduction system (i.e., postreceptor defects),

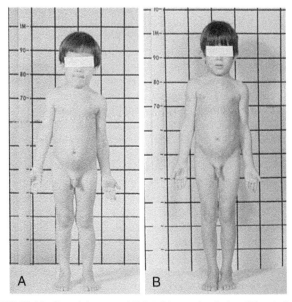

FIGURE 18-15. Growth hormone (GH)-deficient patient before **(A)** and after **(B)** treatment with GH for 1 year. Note that the growth spurt is accompanied by normal maturation of body proportions.

(3) the synthesis or action of IGF-1, and (4) bioinactive GH molecules.[357,428-433] Large kindreds with GH receptor defects have been described in the Mediterranean region and in Ecuador. Several different point mutations of the GH receptor have been described.[434,435] Postreceptor defects, such as in STAT5b, have been identified.[103,432,436,437] Growth failure due to defects of IGF-1 synthesis and to defects of the IGF-1 receptor have also been reported.[47,281,438,439] In general, the clinical phenotype associated with GHI includes severe postnatal growth failure, small face and frontal bossing, high-pitched voice, premature aging, delayed bone age, and additional features common to severe GH deficiency.[431,433] Blue sclera and limited extensibility at the elbow have been variably described. In addition to postnatal growth failure, IGF-1 gene defects can be associated with intrauterine growth failure, mental retardation, sensorineural deafness, and insulin resistance. The manifestations of GHI are heterogeneous. It has been suggested that mild forms of GHI exist,[47,433,440] and that some children with idiopathic short stature will be found to have forms of GHI.[441]

The diagnosis of GHI is suggested by extreme short stature, decreased serum concentrations of IGF-1 (and sometimes IGF-2 and IGFBP-3), and increased serum concentrations of GH. Decreased serum concentrations of GHBP are highly suggestive of a GH receptor defect but normal and high concentrations of GHBP have also been reported.[442] Inability to adequately generate IGF-1 in response to GH administration is an important aspect of demonstrating GHI, although diagnostic criteria that distinguish mild GHI from a normal state are currently imprecise.[441,443-445] Treatment with recombinant IGF-1 seems effective in some of these conditions.[428,429,446-449] However most patients have not experienced catch-up growth sufficient to bring their height into the normal range, they appear to have gained height over that predicted by natural history.[449]

Biosynthetic IGF-1 was approved by the FDA in 2005 for use in conditions of severe primary IGF-1 deficiency due to genetic GH resistance or insensitivity (GHI) and GH gene deletions with development of neutralizing antibodies to GH. Adverse effects include hypoglycemia, increased BMI, growth of lymphatic tissue (including tonsils and adenoids), lipohypertrophy at injection sites, and benign intracranial hypertension.[449] Although some have suggested that IGF-1 should be used in other conditions, others do not believe this is the case,[450] and the Drugs and Therapeutics Committee of the Lawson Wilkins Pediatric Endocrine Society, after evaluating the evidence, recommends that IGF-1 be used only in conditions approved by the FDA.[451]

GH resistance may be secondary to a variety of illnesses, malnutrition, or inhibitors of GH action, such as glucocorticoids.

Hypothyroidism

Hypothyroidism in childhood is characterized by slow linear growth velocity and if chronic may cause short stature and may retard bone age. Acquired hypothyroidism, most commonly due to autoimmune thyroiditis, may have few clear clinical features aside from growth impairment. Pubertal delay is characteristic, and precocious puberty and premature menarche occur less commonly. Congenital hypothyroidism, if untreated, can stunt growth and often causes profound mental retardation if not treated within the first few months of life. Fortunately, neonatal screening programs in many countries enable early detection and treatment in most cases. Hypothyroidism is diagnosed by measurement of free thyroxine (T_4) and TSH versus age-related norms; additional studies such as measurement of thyroid anti-

bodies can help to establish the origin of hypothyroidism. It has been suggested that mild central hypothyroidism may contribute to 10% of idiopathic short stature.[452] The replacement dose of thyroid hormone in children averages 100 mcg/m²/d.[453] Skeletal age usually (and sometimes markedly) is delayed. Catch-up growth is expected after treatment is provided for juvenile hypothyroidism if the diagnosis was made early.[168] However, once treatment is begun, skeletal maturation may accelerate unduly, resulting in patients not reaching their expected adult height.[454]

Glucocorticoid Excess

Glucocorticoid excess, whether endogenous or exogenous, profoundly slows growth. Doses of cortisol greater than about 12 to 15 mg/m²/d (prednisone 3 to 5 mg/m²/d) may impair growth in normal prepubertal children.[128] Growth failure may be the only clear clinical sign of glucocorticoid excess in children.[455,456] Cushing's syndrome is usually iatrogenic, resulting from supraphysiologic doses of glucocorticoid treatment given by any route, including topically. Endogenous glucocorticoid excess may be due to adrenal tumors (particularly in infants), primary pigmented nodular adrenocortical disease, bilateral adrenal hyperplasia secondary to ACTH-producing pituitary adenoma (Cushing's disease), or ectopic ACTH or corticotropin-releasing hormone (CRH) production. The growth attenuation seen with Cushing's syndrome of any cause contrasts with exogenous obesity, in which height velocity is normal. Significant virilization also occurs with adrenal tumors that secrete androgen and glucocorticoids, and growth inhibition may be counteracted by androgen.[457] The diagnosis of endogenous glucocorticoid excess is based on clinical evidence, assessment of suppressibility of endogenous glucocorticoids by exogenous glucocorticoid (dexamethasone suppression test), and radiologic studies undertaken to attempt localization of the lesion. Treatment for endogenous glucocorticoid excess focuses on removal or ablation of the underlying lesion (transsphenoidal removal of pituitary microadenoma in the case of Cushing's disease).[458-461] Early and effective treatment for glucocorticoid excess enables catch-up growth.[168,462]

In cases in which growth inhibition is attributable to glucocorticoid treatment for nonendocrine disease, four possible alternatives are available: (1) use of another form of therapy; (2) lowering of the daily steroid dose if the underlying disease can be controlled in this way; (3) switching the patient to alternate-morning glucocorticoid therapy[463]; or (4) switching the patient to topical (e.g., inhaled) steroid therapy.[464] Alternate-day "pulses" of prednisone or topical administration often results in preservation of the desired therapeutic effect while unwanted cushingoid changes are avoided, but neither approach provides a certain solution to the dilemma. GH therapy may partially counterbalance growth suppression due to moderate doses of glucocorticoid, with considerable variability of response.[134]

Pseudohypoparathyroidism

Pseudohypoparathyroidism is discussed is characterized by short stature, truncal obesity, short metacarpals, round face, mental retardation, and subcutaneous calcifications. Hypocalcemia and hyperphosphatemia due to end-organ resistance to parathyroid hormone can occur.

Idiopathic Short Stature (ISS)

The term **idiopathic short stature** (short stature of unknown cause; short, otherwise normal children) is used traditionally for children with heights greater than 2 SD below the mean for age and gender, and who have none of the previously described conditions. However, it is increasingly applied to also include children with familial short stature and constitutional delay in growth and development.[210,465-467] ISS accounts for the majority of children with short stature. It is likely that some subgroups of children now considered to have ISS will be found to have specific molecular defects in *GH, GH-receptor, SHOX, IGF-1,* or new genes that influence growth. However, investigations to date have revealed such abnormalities in only a minority of children with ISS.[468-470] Because stature is a normally distributed characteristic, and the definition of short stature is based on statistical criteria, most children with ISS may well continue without an identified molecular abnormality as the cause for their shortness. Some have advocated therapeutic trials of GH in individual children with idiopathic short stature to discern whether individuals should have continuing GH treatment; however, the robust growth response of many children with idiopathic short stature to short-term GH therapy suggests that short-term trials may not be particularly useful.[471] Long-term GH treatment can increase adult height by 3.5 to 7.5 cm in children with idiopathic short stature, although considerable variability in response is noted. In 2003, the U.S. FDA approved GH at a dose of 0.37 mg/kg/wk for the "long-term treatment of idiopathic short stature, also called non-growth hormone deficient short stature, defined by height SDS ≤2.25, and associated with growth rates unlikely to permit attainment of adult height in the normal range, in patients whose epiphyses are not closed and for whom diagnostic evaluation excludes other causes associated with short stature that should be observed or treated by other means."[471,472] Thus, depending on how this criterion is applied, 1.2% of all U.S. children are potentially eligible for GH treatment, with substantial implications for policy and practice.[473-477]

Monitoring of GH treatment for children with ISS is similar to that for children with GH deficiency. An additional point, however, involves discussion and planning for the target and ultimate goal of treatment. Some endocrinologists aim to maximize height, whereas others seek to alleviate disability and end treatment when a child has reached a reasonable height in the normal adult range. Given the costs and policy implications, these divergent approaches are important to consider with families as well.

Functional outcome and quality of life have not been found to be influenced by GH treatment[465,478]; this should be put in the context of ISS generally not being associated with psychopathology, although it can be associated with stress. To date, GH appears to have a similar safety profile in ISS as in other conditions.[479-481]

Alternative or supplementary treatments such as aromatase inhibitors to delay epiphyseal closure) and gonadotropin-releasing hormone (GnRH) agonists to prolong growth by suppressing puberty have sometimes been suggested; however, they are not approved by the FDA for ISS, and recent consensus statements did not advocate their use for this condition.[210,482]

Differential Diagnosis of Short Stature by Growth Pattern

To individualize the workup of short stature, it is useful to classify patients according to the relationships among **chronologic age** (CA), **height age** (HA), **weight age** (WA), **bone age** (BA), and **growth rate.** These terms are defined in Table 18-2.

Diagnostic decisions can be simplified by first categorizing the disorder of growth with regard to whether it is a primary distur-

bance of weight (undernutrition) or height by the relationship between HA and WA. If the child's WA is depressed out of proportion to the HA (e.g., weight below the 10th percentile for height), primary nutritional disorders or chronic disease should be the principal diagnostic consideration. If the height and weight are proportionately depressed (or height is depressed out of proportion to weight), genetic, endocrinologic, or metabolic disorders are more likely to be responsible.

Primary linear growth disturbances result from inherent aberrations of bone growth or of systemic factors extrinsic to bone that affect its rate of growth. Disturbances of linear growth can be understood on the basis of three general principles: (1) Normal linear growth during childhood proceeds toward a genetically determined target height by following a predictable channel that is achieved by the end of infancy; (2) normal bone growth is accompanied by a predictable rate of advance of BA; and (3) children normally enter puberty at a pubertal BA. Based on these principles, linear growth disturbances can be categorized into three growth patterns: **intrinsic** shortness, **delayed** growth, and **attenuated** growth (see Fig. 18-6; Table 18-6).[483]

Intrinsic shortness is characterized by inherent limitation of bone growth that destines affected children to be short adults. Examples of this growth pattern include familial short stature, Turner's syndrome and bone dysplasias, primary dysmorphic syndromes such as Prader-Willi syndrome and Russell-Silver syndrome, severe intrauterine growth retardation–related short stature, and impaired spinal growth secondary to irradiation. The growth curves typically fall below normal by 3 years of age. In familial short stature, growth rates generally are near the normal range, so that the child's growth curve then approximately parallels the normal curves, and those children are destined to be moderately short. In more severe disorders of bone growth, such as Turner's syndrome and achondroplasia, however, poor growth

Table 18-6. Differential Diagnosis of Short Stature by Growth Pattern

Type of Growth Pattern	Bone Age Approximates	Growth Rate	Differential Diagnostic Categories
Intrinsic shortness	Chronologic age (BA = CA > HA)	Approximates normal	Familial short stature Normal/subnormal Genetic syndromes • Chromosomal anomalies • Bone dysplasia • Dysmorphic syndromes Intrauterine growth retardation, nonspecific Spinal irradiation
Delayed growth	Height age (BA = HA < CA)	Approximates normal	Constitutional delay in growth and development Chronic disease Undernutrition
Attenuated growth	Height age (BA = HA < CA)	Subnormal	Endocrinopathies • GH deficiency • GH insensitivity • Hypothyroidism • Cushing's syndrome • Hypogonadism after 10-12 years old Acid-base disturbances Chronic disease, severe (e.g., Crohn's) Malnutrition

BA, Bone age; *CA,* chronologic age; *GH,* growth hormone; *HA,* height age.

rates lead to the growth curve deviating progressively farther below normal with time. The BA typically approximates the CA. Puberty occurs at a normal age (barring associated hypogonadism, as in Turner's syndrome). For example, a 9-year-old child with an HA of 6.5 years and a BA of 9 years will be small as an adult. Children with a **delayed** growth pattern have delayed puberty and continue to grow for longer than their peers, thus potentially reaching normal adult height. By 3 years of age, the growth curves of these children closely parallel normal growth channels, with growth rates within or close to the normal range. In contrast to children with intrinsic shortness, the bone age is significantly delayed, typically to approximately the same extent as the height age. For example, a 9-year-old child with a height age of 6.5 and a bone age of 6.5 ordinarily has normal growth potential. Constitutional delay in growth and pubertal development is by far the most common cause of a delayed growth pattern. Other examples of conditions that may be associated with a delayed growth pattern are mild undernutrition and indolent chronic disease, such as anemia and persistent poorly controlled asthma. Because familial intrinsic short stature and constitutional delay are both so common, they occur together about as often as they occur alone. When they coexist, the growth rate is likely to be slightly subnormal and to resemble the attenuated pattern.

Children with an **attenuated** growth pattern have low growth rates, resulting in their progressive deviation from normal growth channels. BA is approximately equal to HA (or even less in hypothyroidism). Delayed BA indicates that adult height potential is normal, **if** the underlying disorder is treated effectively. Beyond 3 years of age, this pattern virtually always indicates underlying pathology. The underlying disorders, unless optimally treated, preclude normal achievement of the height potential. Thus, a 9-year-old child with an HA and BA of 6.5 and subnormal growth velocity has an attenuated growth pattern; this child has an endocrine, metabolic, or systemic disease until proven otherwise. Examples of conditions that may cause this growth pattern include GH deficiency, hypothyroidism, glucocorticoid excess, severe chronic illness, and malnutrition.

Diagnostic Evaluation

Given the many potential causes of short stature, establishing a diagnosis depends on eliciting several features on history, physical examination, and laboratory studies. Children who are severely short (more than 2.5 SDs below the mean), whose growth curve shows an attenuated pattern manifesting a poor growth velocity, who are well outside their target height SD, and/or who have risk factors or clinical features suggestive of an organic cause for short stature need careful clinical and, in many cases, laboratory assessment. Documentation of the growth rate and bone age is key, as is discussed in the previous section on growth patterns.

If the child has a normal bone age, suggesting an *intrinsically short growth pattern,* it is important to seek a history of SGA, historical features suggesting Turner's syndrome (e.g., presence/absence of neonatal lymphedema or coarctation of the aorta, recurrent otitis media), a history suggestive of hypocalcemia (compatible with pseudohypoparathyroidism), and a family history of short stature. Physical examination in this group of patients should be directed toward a search for body disproportion (indicative of skeletal dysplasia) and dysmorphisms, as well as assessment of pubertal status. When the clinical assessment strongly suggests a particular diagnosis, appropriate and specific

diagnostic tests, such as karyotype, gonadotropin and calcium levels, and a skeletal survey, can proceed.

In the child with a significantly delayed bone age, indicating a *delayed or attenuated growth pattern,* review of systems should be comprehensive to assess potential systemic disease or endocrinopathy. It should focus on weight changes, appetite, food intolerance, vomiting, abdominal cramping, and stool characteristics to assess gastrointestinal disease; genitourinary symptoms, particularly polyuria and enuresis; headache and visual disturbances (suggestive of CNS lesion); lethargy or cold intolerance (suggestive but not necessarily present in hypothyroidism); and pubertal development. The past medical history and history of the use of medications, particularly glucocorticoids in any form, may be important. A classic triad for congenital hypopituitarism is perinatal hypoglycemia, prolonged jaundice, and, in boys, micropenis. The physician should seek a family history of delay of puberty or extreme short stature and should perform a careful general physical examination. Specific features on physical examination include the weight/height ratio, a search for finger clubbing or perianal sores (regarding inflammatory bowel disease), fundoscopy and examination of visual fields (to assess perichiasmatic central nervous system lesions such as craniopharyngiomas), assessment for goiter, and pubertal staging.

Constitutional delay in growth and development, which typically presents with a delayed growth pattern, is principally a diagnosis of exclusion, and in extreme cases is difficult to distinguish from isolated defects of gonadotropin or GH production. While puberty is delayed, the growth rate may fall to subnormal levels. Testing shows a delayed bone age, and the IGF-1 level remains at a prepubertal level, compatible with the bone age. Gonadotropin secretion may remain in the prepubertal range until the bone age has reached 11 to 12 years. The distinction between hypogonadism and delayed puberty sometimes can be made by determination of gonadotropin levels during sleep or in response to a gonadotropin-releasing hormone agonist test by 14 years of age.[484] GH tests may be compatible with GH deficiency unless performed after sex steroid priming.[383-385] Indeed, transient GH deficiency sometimes is associated with delayed puberty.

When the clinical assessment strongly suggests a particular diagnosis, appropriate and specific diagnostic tests should be performed. If the weight is below the 10th percentile for height, it may be difficult to distinguish undernutrition from constitutional underweight. Calorie counting, sweat test, and screening tests for occult chronic disease may be helpful. These include complete blood count, urinalysis, chemistry profile, erythrocyte sedimentation rate, and antiendomysial or antitissue transglutaminase antibodies.

If the cause of poor growth still is not clear, but the child's growth rate is subnormal (i.e., leading to an attenuated growth pattern) or the child's height is markedly below age-appropriate standards or the family target height, additional tests are indicated to assess possible hypothyroidism (free thyroxine, thyrotropin), GH deficiency (IGF-1, IGFBP-3, provocative tests of GH reserve), and, in girls, karyotype for assessment for Turner's syndrome. Controversies regarding the diagnostic tests for GH deficiency are described at the beginning of this section. Less common tests generally are based on clinical suspicion of the underlying condition (methylation analysis to diagnose Prader-Willi syndrome, SHOX protein, GH-binding protein, etc.).

Not uncommonly, previous measurements are unavailable and the child's pattern of growth is not clear, although the child seems healthy overall. In this situation, it would be reasonable to follow the child's height at regular intervals to establish a pattern of growth that dictates whether additional tests are indicated.

The diagnosis of ISS rests on exclusion of other conditions leading to short stature. In the absence of abnormalities on history, review of systems, and physical examination, laboratory tests should include screening for celiac disease, Turner's syndrome in girls, hypothyroidism, anemia, chronic inflammatory disease, renal disease, GH deficiency, and GHI.[467] Online resources such as Genetest (www.genetests.org) identify laboratories capable of performing genetic tests for specific disorders like Noonan's syndrome when such analyses are clinically indicated. *SHOX* gene analysis should be considered for patients with clinical findings compatible with *SHOX* haploinsufficiency.

Management

When at all possible, treatment should be directed at the primary cause of pathologic short stature. Examples include nutritional counseling for undernutrition, gluten-free diet for celiac disease, psychotherapy for eating disorders, thyroid hormone for hypothyroidism, and growth hormone for GH deficiency. Many of these disorders are hereditary; genetic counseling should not be overlooked.

For conditions considered normal variants (familial short stature, constitutional delay), reassurance and explanation of the wide range of normal are often very helpful. In discussing therapeutic options, the physician must advise child and family about the unknown factors (e.g., errors are inherent in height predictions). Many families often choose to forego medical intervention at this point.

Low-dose sex steroid therapy is indicated for the treatment of hypogonadism if puberty is delayed beyond 13 (girls) or 14 (boys) years of age.[485,486] In extreme cases of constitutional delay, this modality is useful for a limited time to boost self-image by advancing secondary sex characteristics gently with a mild corresponding growth spurt. To minimize the possibility of loss of growth potential, we recommend that the initial course of therapy for the induction of sexual development should consist of six monthly injections of 50 mg/m² repository testosterone in boys and 0.2 mg depot estradiol in girls.[147,486] A reasonable alternative regimen for girls begins with 5 µg ethinyl estradiol given by mouth daily.[487] Such a course of therapy has no deleterious effect on height potential and has positive effects on self-image. The patient's growth, development, and predicted height should be carefully reevaluated immediately on completion of the therapeutic regimen and again 6 months later before a second course of therapy is undertaken. Depot testosterone, 100 mg/m²/mo, and depot estradiol, 1.0 mg/mo, closely approximate midpubertal sex hormone production in boys and girls, respectively. We prefer administering injections of repository forms of sex hormones to avoid the occasional side effects of 17-alkylated steroid analogues. However, the anabolic steroid oxandrolone 0.1 mg/kg/d for 3 to 6 months has been used without compromising final height.[488] Premature use of adult replacement doses of androgen or estrogen (about twofold greater than the midpubertal doses) will cause a disproportionate advance of BA relative to linear growth and will compromise height potential. Children with delayed puberty should be followed closely from 10 years of age onward because, particularly in the most severely delayed cases with the most immature body proportions, puberty inexplicably occurs at an earlier than expected bone age, leading to children falling well short of predicted height.[207,485]

GH therapy is currently approved by the FDA for the treatment of short stature due to GH deficiency (0.18 to 0.3 mg/kg/wk, divided into daily subcutaneous doses), Turner's syndrome (up to 0.375 mg/kg/wk), chronic renal failure prior to transplantation (up to 0.35 mg/kg/wk),[271] persistent short stature after SGA status (0.48 mg/kg/wk), Prader-Willi syndrome, selected cases of idiopathic short stature (up to 0.37 mg/kg/wk), *SHOX* deficiency (up to 0.35 mg/kg/wk), and Noonan's syndrome (up to 0.34 mg/kg/wk), as described in previous sections.[294] GH is contraindicated in the presence of active malignancy or critical illness. Data are inconsistent regarding the role of GH-receptor genotypes as determinants of the growth response to GH therapy.[489-492] A higher dose for GH-deficient adolescents in puberty has also been approved. Varying lines of data suggest that long-term GH therapy may promote growth in a variety of other conditions, although inconsistencies have been noted in the findings. See References 271, 405, 473, 481, and 493 through 507 for a review of medical, ethical, and policy issues related to GH therapy for nontraditional indications. Potential adverse effects of GH and recommendations for monitoring[506,508] treatment are discussed earlier in this chapter.

Because long-term GnRH agonist therapy is successful in improving adult height of children with idiopathic sexual precocity by delaying epiphyseal fusion, attempts have been made to use this as a nonstandard method to promote growth in children with ISS. The height prognosis in isolated GH deficiency seems to be improved by adding GnRH agonist to GH therapy.[509] Although increases in adult height of normal short children have been achieved by years of GnRH agonist therapy, this has been accompanied by significantly less accretion of bone mineral density; accordingly, long-term GnRH agonist treatment is not recommended for this condition.[510,511] Adding GH to GnRH therapy is reported to yield approximately twice as much of an increase in final height; the possibility that this combination will counteract the deleterious effects of GnRH agonist alone on bone mineral density is unknown, and a recent consensus conference on the use of GnRH agonist did not recommend it for this condition.[512,513]

Aromatase inhibitors are not currently approved by the FDA for children with short stature. Data primarily from Europe suggest that they may increase height in otherwise normal short boys by delaying epiphyseal closure, and a U.S. study indicates that they can increase growth in adolescent boys with GH deficiency.[514] However, a recent analysis did not support their widespread use.[482]

Recombinant human (rh) IGF-1 was approved by the FDA in 2005 for the treatment of children with severe short stature from GH insensitivity due to genetic defects of the GH receptor, postreceptor mechanisms, or the development of GH-inactivating antibodies. Although it has been used off-label to treat children with other growth disorders, based on the evidence available to date, this practice currently is discouraged outside of experimental trials.[451,515,516]

TALL STATURE

Although tall stature (height more than 2 SDs above the mean for age and gender) is as common as short stature (more than 2 SDs below the mean for age and gender), referrals for evaluation of growth disorders are much more frequent in short than in tall children—underscoring the importance of cultural norms and societal perceptions of desired body habitus in interpretations of normal and abnormal growth.

Causes of Tall Stature

Genetic normal variants cause most cases of tall stature (Table 18-7). Two distinct familial variants, which lead to different outcomes in tall children, can be identified. One is **familial tall stature** (sometimes called *familial intrinsic tall stature* or *genetic tallness*); children are typically of normal size at birth, and a high-normal growth rate is established by 3 years of age. Thus, the child typically crosses height percentiles during the first 3 years of life and thereafter maintains a height-attained channel above and closely parallel to the 95th percentile. The other is **constitutional advancement in growth and pubertal development**, in which children grow similarly during childhood but have an advanced BA and go into puberty early, so they stop growing at a normal height. Both these groups of children have a family history of a similar growth pattern, and the child does not show clinical or biochemical features of the disorders described as follows.

Genetic and chromosomal disorders are known causes of tall stature. Hyperploidy of sex chromosomes predisposes to tall stature.[48] The most common of these disorders is *Klinefelter's syndrome* (47,XXY), which occurs in 1:500 to 1:1000 live male births. It is characterized by a decreased upper-to-lower segment ratio dating from the prepubertal years, small testes and hypogonadism, and gynecomastia; it often is associated with mild mental retardation. *XYY syndromes* are characterized by tall stature with possible behavioral abnormalities.

The prototypic genetic syndrome associated with tall stature is *Marfan syndrome,* which usually segregates with mutations in the fibrillin gene.[61,517] It is classically characterized by musculoskeletal signs (such as arachnodactyly and hyperextensibility), cardiovascular findings (such as aortic aneurysm), ocular signs (such as lens subluxation), decreased upper-to-lower body ratio, and autosomal dominant heredity. Arachnodactyly can be quantitated from the body proportions or the metacarpal index (ratio of length to midshaft breadth of metacarpals II through V; normal: male <8.0:1, female <8.7:1) on a BA. Congenital contractural arachnodactyly is a genetically closely related syndrome. *Homocystinuria* has marfanoid features but also may involve mental retardation, joint contractures, and a tendency to thromboembolism. Multiple endocrine neoplasia (MEN) type 2B also may have marfanoid features; the presence of mucosal neuromas may provide a specific clue to its presence.

Cerebral gigantism (also known as Sotos syndrome) is characterized by overgrowth during early childhood, a moderately advanced BA, macrocephaly, developmental retardation, and dysmorphisms, particularly acromegaloid facial features.[518-520] Most children are long and slender at birth; they reach an above average, occasionally excessive, adult height. A great majority of cases are due to mutation of *nuclear receptor binding SET-domain 1 (NSD1),*[520-522] sometimes in association with a chromosome **5q35** microdeletion. *Weaver syndrome,* which has somewhat different facial dysmorphisms, is sometimes an allelic variant. Sotos syndrome can be mimicked by fragile X syndrome. Disproportionate bone age advancement characterizes some other congenital overgrowth disorders, such as *Marshall-Smith syndrome,* which is characterized by poor weight gain.[213]

The prototypic congenital macrosomia syndrome is *Beckwith-Wiedemann syndrome.* The most consistent features are overgrowth, macroglossia, umbilical defects ranging from hernia to omphalocele, and earlobe pits. Hyperplasia of various visceral (especially kidney) and endocrine organs (especially pancreatic β cells) is the rule. Birth size is above average, growth velocity is high until midchildhood, and adult height is 2.5 SD above normal. Children with this syndrome are predisposed to develop embryonal intra-abdominal tumors in early childhood, most commonly Wilms tumor and adrenocortical carcinoma. The disorder is associated with loss of heterozygosity at chromosomal locus **11p15.5** due to duplications, translocation/inversion, uni-

Table 18-7. Factors Causing Tall Stature, With Representative Clinical Conditions

Factors Affecting Height	Representative Conditions		Clinical and Laboratory Features
Genetic	Normal variants	Familial intrinsic tallness	Growth parallels 95th percentile; family history of tall stature; normal physical exam, puberty, and BA
		Constitutionally advanced	Growth parallels 95th percentile; puberty and BA slightly advanced
	Chromosomal abnormalities	Klinefelter's syndrome	Hypogenitalism and hypogonadism, eunuchoid; 47,XXY
		Fragile X syndrome	Mental retardation; macro-orchidism in males
	Dysmorphic syndromes	Marfan syndrome	Arachnodactyly, hyperextensibility, lens subluxation, aortic dilation
		Beckwith-Wiedemann syndrome	Infant gigantism, macroglossia, umbilical defects, neonatal hypoglycemia due to pancreatic β cell hyperplasia, may develop embryonal tumors
		Sotos syndrome	Cerebral gigantism: dolichocephalic large head, coarse facies, cerebral dysfunction
Nutrition	Primary obesity		IGF-1 blood level nutrition driven, "growth without GH"
Hormones	GH excess		Accelerated growth, acromegaloid signs with advancing age, occasional hyperprolactinemia; may be associated with McCune-Albright syndrome
	Hyperthyroidism		Hypermetabolic features, goiter, eye abnormalities
	Sex steroid	Excess	Precocious puberty: premature secondary sexual characteristics and epiphyseal fusion, leading to compromise of adult height
		Deficiency	Deficiency beyond teenage years permits prolonged growth and may lead to eunuchoid habitus

BA, Bone age; *GH,* growth hormone; *IGF-1,* insulin-like growth factor-1.

paternal disomy, or mutations of the CDKI *p57*,[KIP2] which cause imbalance between the function of growth-promoting genes such as IGF-2 and tumor suppressor genes on this imprinted region[523]; overexpression of IGF-2 therefore has been implicated in the overgrowth. Because of the associated genetic abnormalities, it has been suggested that Beckwith-Wiedemann syndrome is the genetic opposite of Russell-Silver syndrome.[286] The *Simpson-Golabi-Behmal syndrome* is similar in consisting of macrosomia, macroglossia, omphalocele, and Wilms tumor, but it has a different pattern of associated features, such as "bulldog facies," polydactyly, fingernail hypoplasia, and even greater adult height.[111] It is caused by an X-linked mutation of glypican-3, a receptor that modulates IGF-2 action.

Lipodystrophy, particularly the total form, whether congenital or acquired, is associated with tall stature.[524] Insulin resistance frequently is so severe as to cause pseudoacromegaly, and hyperlipidemia is prominent.

Overnutrition (exogenous obesity) during childhood typically accelerates growth slightly and advances BA comparably to HA. IGF-1 levels are normal in the presence of low GH levels.[89]

Hormonal disorders of GH, sex steroids, and thyroid hormone can cause tall stature. **GH excess** is a rare but important cause of accelerated growth. This condition, termed **gigantism** during childhood, may be associated with acromegaloid features in older children (Fig. 18-16).[525,526] It usually is due to a pituitary somatotroph adenoma or to somatotroph hyperplasia. Activating mutations of G_{sa} have been described in isolated pituitary adenomas and in patients with McCune-Albright syndrome associated with hypersecretion of hormones such as GH.[527,528] Hyperprolactinemia may coexist.

Hyperthyroidism can accelerate bone growth and maturation.[524] Affected infants may have premature cranial synostosis.[529]

Sexual precocity accelerates height. Classically, BA is stimulated disproportionately, which leads to premature epiphyseal fusion. Thus, these children initially become tall but stop growing prematurely, so their adult height is stunted. Slowly progressive forms of precocious puberty do not necessarily deleteriously affect adult height, however.[530]

Sex hormone deficiency, conversely, prolongs the growing period because the epiphyses do not close. This leads to increased height and eunuchoid proportions in hypogonadal individuals.[531] Through the discovery of patients deficient in aromatase or with inactivating mutation of the estrogen receptor, estradiol has been found to be the critical hormone that brings about epiphyseal fusion.[123]

Idiopathic tall stature refers to tall stature of unknown cause. Similar to idiopathic short stature, it sometimes is defined as including the genetic normal variants of familial tall stature and constitutional advancement of growth and development.

Differential Diagnosis of Tall Stature by Growth Pattern

Because supranormal height occurs because of inherent endowment or excessive stimulation of the rate of bone growth, the diagnostic approach based on the relationships of CA, HA, BA, and growth velocity is analogous to that described for short stature. Four patterns of growth causing tall stature can be dis-

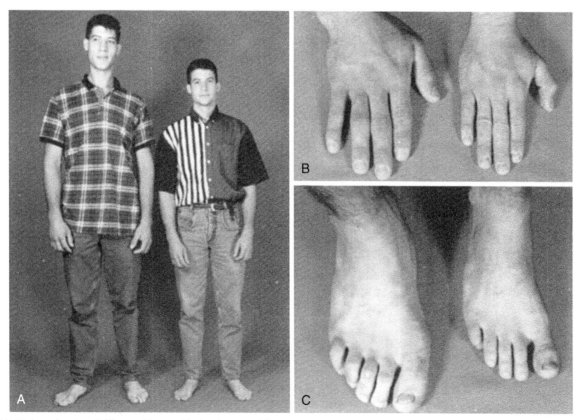

FIGURE 18-16. Pituitary gigantism. A 22-year-old-man with gigantism caused by excess growth hormone is shown to the left of his identical twin. The increased height **(A)** and enlarged hand **(B)** and foot **(C)** of the affected twin are apparent. Their height and features began to diverge at approximately 13 years of age. (From Gagel RF, McCutcheon IE: Images in clinical medicine. Pituitary gigantism. N Engl J Med 340:524, 1999.)

tinguished: intrinsic tallness, advanced growth, accelerated growth, and prolonged growth (Table 18-8 and Fig. 18-17).[483,532]

Intrinsic tallness is the term applied to literally long-boned individuals. They come to grow above, but approximately parallel to, the 95th percentile on height-attained curves. Their BA and age of puberty are normal. This usually is a normal variant (familial tall stature) but rarely is due to genetic disorders such as Marfan syndrome or homocystinuria.

Advanced growth is a pattern with similar growth in childhood, with a growth velocity that maintains them approximately parallel to the 95th percentile on height-attained curves, but

children go into puberty early to stop growing at a normal size. This pattern is indicated by a BA that is advanced in proportion to HA. Examples include normal variant (constitutional advancement of growth and development), obesity, and hyperthyroidism. Mild forms of sexual precocity also cause this growth pattern.

Accelerated growth refers to that pattern in which growth rate is excessive. Adult height is abnormal unless the underlying disorder is corrected. Adult height is subnormal in rapidly progressive sexual precocity and is excessive in GH excess.

Prolonged growth results from deficiency of sex hormones, particularly estrogen. Such patients continue growing into adulthood.

Diagnostic Evaluation

The tall child whose height parallels the 95th percentile and has tall parents, no dysmorphic features, normal pace of puberty, and a normal bone age is likely to have **intrinsic tallness** of familial origin without a pathologic basis (familial tall stature). Additional investigations often are not needed. However, chromosomal disorders, Marfan syndrome, homocystinuria, and occasionally excessive GH can simulate the clinical picture. The presence of dysmorphic features, macro-orchidism, or intellectual impairment in a tall child suggests the need for chromosome analysis, plasma amino acid assay, or genetics consultation to evaluate these possibilities.

The tall child with an **advanced growth pattern** (i.e., BA advanced in proportion to HA) is likely to have "constitutional" normal variant tallness, particularly if the height parallels the 95th percentile, family history is compatible, and the clinical examination is otherwise normal. Because hyperthyroidism may mimic this presentation, the clinical examination includes evaluation for goiter, ophthalmologic abnormalities, and hypermetabolism; thyroid function studies will provide confirmation. Exogenous obesity, in the absence of dysmorphic features or intellectual impairment, may present this pattern of tall stature. In the absence of puberty or symptoms or signs suggestive of a hypothalamic disturbance or hypoglycemia, the tall stature virtually excludes an endocrine basis for obesity.

Table 18-8. Differential Diagnosis of Tall Stature by Growth Pattern

Type of Growth Pattern	Bone Age Relationships	Growth Rate	Differential Diagnostic Categories
Intrinsic tallness	BA ≈ CA < HA	Approximates normal	Familial tallness Chromosomal disorders • XXY, fragile X, XXX • XYY • **8p** trisomy Genetic disorders • Marfanoid syndromes • Cerebral gigantism syndromes • Congenital macrosomia syndromes
Advanced growth	BA ≈ HA > CA	Approximates normal	"Constitutional" normal variant Obesity Lipodystrophy Hyperthyroidism
Accelerated growth	BA > HA > CA	Supranormal	Sexual precocity
	BA ≤ HA > CA	Supranormal	GH or IGF excess
Prolonged growth	BA < HA > CA	Normal	Hypogonadism Estrogen deficiency

BA, Bone age; *CA,* chronologic age; *GH,* growth hormone; *HA,* height age; *IGF,* insulin-like growth factor.

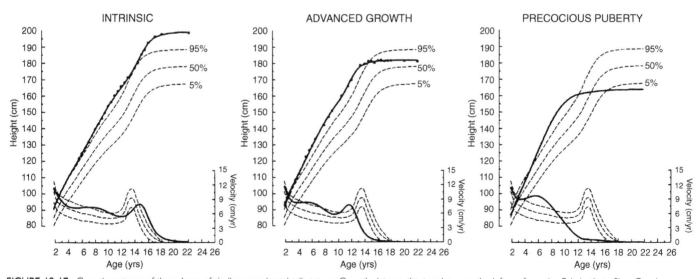

FIGURE 18-17. Growth patterns of three boys of similar prepubertal tall stature. Growth data on the two boys on the left are from the Fels Institute files. One became a tall adult (intrinsic tall stature); the other grew to be of normal adult height after undergoing an early pubertal growth spurt (advanced height). Growth data on the boy with precocious puberty are derived from the data of Thamdrup.[532] (Courtesy R.D. Bock.)

An **accelerated growth pattern** (involving progressive deviation of height above the 95th percentile and an advanced bone age) requires assessment for sexual precocity. This includes clinical assessment of primary and secondary sexual characteristics, as well as evaluation for the possibility of central nervous system disorders or abdominal masses and a search for nevi and bone deformities. If the BA is significantly advanced, screening should commence with determination of blood levels of estradiol, testosterone, dehydroepiandrosterone sulfate, gonadotropins (preferably in a third-generation assay), and possibly serum human chorionic gonadotropin (hCG). Screening for excessive GH secretion should be initiated with random GH, IGF-1, and IGFBP-3 blood levels. The definitive test for the diagnosis of GH excess is the failure of serum GH to suppress below 1 to 2 ng/mL after an oral glucose load (1.75 g/kg, maximum 100 g), although some false-positive tests have been reported.[525] Hyperprolactinemia often exists together with GH excess. If evidence of GH excess is found, serum GHRH may be measured (to assess the rare possibility of ectopic GHRH production) and appropriate imaging studies performed. In cases of GH excess, the clinician should also consider the possibilities of McCune-Albright syndrome, multiple endocrine adenomatosis type I, and carcinoid syndrome.

A **prolonged growth pattern** suggests sex hormone deficiency or resistance. Evaluation of pubertal development, sense of smell (to evaluate Kallmann's syndrome), and body proportions (eunuchoid habitus with long legs and a low upper-to-lower body segment ratio is characteristic of sex hormone deficiency) are needed. Laboratory studies include ascertainment of circulating sex hormone and gonadotropin levels, chromosome analysis, and, when indicated, imaging studies.

Management

Because familial intrinsic tall stature represents a variant of the normal, reassurance and support are needed. In certain cases (e.g., predicted adult height 3 SDs or more above the mean), familial tall stature may be particularly distressing, and treatment to curtail growth by accelerating epiphyseal fusion may be considered. Estrogen in large amounts (e.g., 0.3 mg/d of ethinyl estradiol) can be given just before or early in puberty, daily without interruption, and continued until epiphyseal fusion has occurred. A progestin (e.g., 100 mg of progesterone) taken orally daily for 10 days for the first 10 days of each month is also given to yield regular menses. Potential risks of estrogen therapy include thrombosis, hyperlipidemia, cholelithiasis, glucose intolerance, nausea, mild hypertension, and weight gain. Although evidence suggests that estrogen therapy can reduce adult height by as much as 3.5 to 7.3 cm below that predicted, the results cannot be assured[533,534] and treatment is much less effective if given in late puberty. Additional caveats include at least one report that recipients of such treatment may not express long-term satisfaction with it,[535] and that, for girls with normal variants, it may represent a form of social shaping of medicine.[536] Some authors have reported on estrogen treatment for tall stature girls with Marfan syndrome, androgen insensitivity, and other overgrowth problems.[533] Because of the potential adverse effects, relatively few endocrinologists currently offer high-dose estrogen for growth suppression.[537] Somatostatin analogue has been suggested as a treatment to reduce adult height in selected cases, but recent results suggest that findings do not justify its use.[538] Depot testosterone in highly virilizing doses (about 400 mg every 2 weeks) has been used to reduce predicted adult height in selected tall boys, but experience is limited.[533]

Hypersecretion of GH due to pituitary adenomas generally is treated by surgery and/or a somatostatin analogue. Pituitary radiation has also been utilized. More recently, a GH receptor antagonist (Pegvisomant) has been used.[539] Pituitary hyperplasia causing GH excess (as in McCune-Albright syndrome) can be treated with a somatostatin analogue. In ectopic GHRH-producing tumors, surgical removal is the treatment of choice.

The compromised height potential resulting from gonadotropin-dependent sexual precocity is treated by suppressing gonadotropins with long-acting gonadotropin-releasing hormone agonists. The most widely used agent in the United States is depot leuprolide (ordinarily given as a monthly depot intramuscular injection). The treatment is effective when started at an early age, with an average height gain above pretreatment height prediction of about 1.4 cm for each year of therapy.[540] Coincident GH deficiency must be treated for optimal growth.[541] Although GH-sufficient patients with central precocity who are started on gonadotropin-releasing hormone agonists relatively late and whose height velocity falls below the prepubertal normal range after 2 to 3 years can gain an average of 2 cm per year when GH therapy is added,[542] this approach is not fully accepted. Otherwise, premature puberty is treated by specific therapy where possible, for example, using cortisol replacement for congenital adrenal hyperplasia or inhibitors of steroidogenesis for McCune-Albright syndrome. Conversely, sex hormone deficiency can be replaced.

REFERENCES

1. Cheek D: Human Growth, Philadelphia, 1968, Lea & Febiger.
2. Winick M, Noble A: Quantitative changes in DNA, RNA, and protein during prenatal and postnatal growth in the rat, Dev Biol 12(3):451–466, Dec 1965.
3. Orlowski CC, Furlanetto RW: The mammalian cell cycle in normal and abnormal growth, Endocrinol Metab Clin North Am 25(3):491–502, Sep 1996.
4. Meredith JE Jr, Winitz S, Lewis JM, et al: The regulation of growth and intracellular signaling by integrins, Endocr Rev 17(3):207–220, Jun 1996.
5. Pajalunga D, Mazzola A, Franchitto A, et al: The logic and regulation of cell cycle exit and reentry, Cell Mol Life Sci 65(1):8–15, Jan 2008.
6. Mitchell BS: The proteasome—an emerging therapeutic target in cancer, N Engl J Med 348(26):2597–2598, Jun 26 2003.
7. Zipursky A: Telomerase, immortality, and cancer, Pediatr Res 47(2):174, Feb 2000.
8. Styne DM: Fetal growth, Clin Perinatol 25(4):917–938, vii, Dec 1998.
9. Zhao Y, Westphal H: Homeobox genes and human genetic disorders, Curr Mol Med 2(1):13–23, Feb 2002.
10. Markakis EA: Development of the neuroendocrine hypothalamus, Front Neuroendocrinol 23(3):257–291, Jul 2002.
11. Cushman LJ, Showalter AD, Rhodes SJ: Genetic defects in the development and function of the anterior pituitary gland, Ann Med 34(3):179–191, 2002.
12. Gluckman PD, Harding JE: Nutritional and hormonal regulation of fetal growth—evolving concepts, Acta Paediatr Suppl 399:60–63, Apr 1994.
13. Brooks AA, Johnson MR, Steer PJ, et al: Birth weight: nature or nurture? Early Hum Dev 42(1):29–35, May 12 1995.
14. Constancia M, Hemberger M, Hughes J, et al: Placental-specific IGF-II is a major modulator of placental and fetal growth, Nature 417(6892):945–948, Jun 27 2002.
15. Lindgren V: Genomic imprinting in disorders of growth, Endocrinol Metab Clin North Am 25(3):503–521, Sep 1996.
16. Coutant R, Boux de Casson F, Douay O, et al: Relationships between placental GH concentration and maternal smoking, newborn gender, and maternal leptin: possible implications for birth weight, J Clin Endocrinol Metab 86(10):4854–4859, Oct 2001.
17. Hindmarsh PC, Geary MP, Rodeck CH, et al: Factors predicting ante- and postnatal growth, Pediatr Res 63(1):99–102, Jan 2008.
18. Schinzel AA, Smith DW, Miller JR: Monozygotic twinning and structural defects, J Pediatr 95(6):921–930, Dec 1979.
19. Handwerger S, Freemark M: The roles of placental growth hormone and placental lactogen in the regulation of human fetal growth and

development, J Pediatr Endocrinol Metab 13(4):343–356, Apr 2000.

20. Bajoria R, Gibson MJ, Ward S, et al: Placental regulation of insulin-like growth factor axis in monochorionic twins with chronic twin-twin transfusion syndrome, J Clin Endocrinol Metab 86(7):3150–3156, Jul 2001.

21. Westwood M, Gibson JM, Sooranna SR, et al: Genes or placenta as modulator of fetal growth: evidence from the insulin-like growth factor axis in twins with discordant growth, Mol Hum Reprod 7(4):387–395, Apr 2001.

22. Christou H, Serdy S, Mantzoros CS: Leptin in relation to growth and developmental processes in the fetus, Semin Reprod Med 20(2):123–130, May 2002.

23. Vatten LJ, Nilsen ST, Odegard RA, et al: Insulin-like growth factor I and leptin in umbilical cord plasma and infant birth size at term, Pediatrics 109(6):1131–1135, Jun 2002.

24. Lubchenco LO, Hansman C, Dressler M, et al: Intrauterine Growth as estimated from liveborn birthweight data at 24 to 42 weeks of gestation, Pediatrics 32:793–800, Nov 1963.

25. Thomson AM, Billewicz WZ, Hytten FE: The assessment of fetal growth, J Obstet Gynaecol Br Commonw 75(9):903–916, Sep 1968.

26. Wingerd J, Schoen EJ: Factors influencing length at birth and height at five years, Pediatrics 53(5):737–741, May 1974.

27. Beck GJ, van den Berg BJ: The relationship of the rate of intrauterine growth of low-birth-weight infants to later growth, J Pediatr 86(4):504–511, Apr 1975.

28. Gardosi J, Chang A, Kalyan B, et al: Customised antenatal growth charts, Lancet 339(8788):283–287, Feburary 1 1992.

29. Yip R, Binkin NJ, Trowbridge FL: Altitude and childhood growth, J Pediatr 113(3):486–489, Sep 1988.

30. Knight B, Shields BM, Turner M, et al: Evidence of genetic regulation of fetal longitudinal growth, Early Hum Dev 81(10):823–831, Oct 2005.

31. de Zegher F, Francois I, van Helvoirt M, et al: Clinical review 89: small as fetus and short as child: from endogenous to exogenous growth hormone, J Clin Endocrinol Metab 82(7):2021–2026, Jul 1997.

32. Savage MO, Burren CP, Blair JC, et al: Growth hormone insensitivity: pathophysiology, diagnosis, clinical variation and future perspectives, Horm Res 55(Suppl 2):32–35, 2001.

33. Smith DW, Popich G: Large fontanels in congenital hypothyroidism: a potential clue toward earlier recognition, J Pediatr 80(5):753–756, May 1972.

34. DeChiara TM, Efstratiadis A, Robertson EJ: A growth-deficiency phenotype in heterozygous mice carrying an insulin-like growth factor II gene disrupted by targeting, Nature 345(6270):78–80, May 3 1990.

35. Liu JP, Baker J, Perkins AS, et al: Mice carrying null mutations of the genes encoding insulin-like growth factor I (Igf-1) and type 1 IGF receptor (Igf1r), Cell 75(1):59–72, Oct 8 1993.

36. Baker J, Liu JP, Robertson EJ, et al: Role of insulin-like growth factors in embryonic and postnatal growth, Cell 75(1):73–82, Oct 8 1993.

37. Louvi A, Accili D, Efstratiadis A: Growth-promoting interaction of IGF-II with the insulin receptor during mouse embryonic development, Dev Biol 189(1):33–48, Sep 1 1997.

38. Lassarre C, Hardouin S, Daffos F, et al: Serum insulin-like growth factors and insulin-like growth factor binding proteins in the human fetus. Relationships with growth in normal subjects and in subjects with intrauterine growth retardation, Pediatr Res 29(3):219–225, Mar 1991.

39. Sferruzzi-Perri AN, Owens JA, Pringle KG, et al: Maternal insulin-like growth factors-I and -II act via different pathways to promote fetal growth, Endocrinology 147(7):3344–3355, Jul 2006.

40. Randhawa R, Cohen P: The role of the insulin-like growth factor system in prenatal growth, Mol Genet Metab 86(1–2):84–90, Sep–Oct 2005.

41. Kajimura S, Aida K, Duan C: Insulin-like growth factor-binding protein-1 (IGFBP-1) mediates hypoxia-induced embryonic growth and developmental retardation, Proc Natl Acad Sci U S A 102(4):1240–1245, Jan 25 2005.

42. Modric T, Silha JV, Shi Z, et al: Phenotypic manifestations of insulin-like growth factor-binding protein-3 overexpression in transgenic mice, Endocrinology 142(5):1958–1967, May 2001.

43. Ning Y, Schuller AG, Conover CA, et al: Insulin-like growth factor (IGF) binding protein-4 is both a positive and negative regulator of IGF activity in vivo, Mol Endocrinol 22(5):1213–1225, May 2008.

44. Giudice LC, de Zegher F, Gargosky SE, et al: Insulin-like growth factors and their binding proteins in the term and preterm human fetus and neonate with normal and extremes of intrauterine growth, J Clin Endocrinol Metab 80(5):1548–1555, May 1995.

45. Conover CA, Bale LK, Overgaard MT, et al: Metalloproteinase pregnancy-associated plasma protein A is a critical growth regulatory factor during fetal development, Development 131(5):1187–1194, Mar 2004.

46. Leung TY, Sahota DS, Chan LW, et al: Prediction of birth weight by fetal crown-rump length and maternal serum levels of pregnancy-associated plasma protein-A in the first trimester, Ultrasound Obstet Gynecol 31(1):10–14, Jan 2008.

47. Woods KA, Camacho-Hubner C, Savage MO, et al: Intrauterine growth retardation and postnatal growth failure associated with deletion of the insulin-like growth factor I gene, N Engl J Med 335(18):1363–1367, Oct 31 1996.

48. Araki E, Lipes MA, Patti ME, et al: Alternative pathway of insulin signalling in mice with targeted disruption of the IRS-1 gene, Nature 372(6502):186–190, Nov 10 1994.

49. Rosenfield R: Role of androgens in growth and development of the fetus, child, and adolescent, Adv Pediatr 19:171, 1972.

50. Gluckman P: Editorial: nutrition, glucocorticoids, birth size, and adult disease, Endocrinology 142(5):1689–1691, 2001.

51. Miles HL, Hofman PL, Cutfield WS: Fetal origins of adult disease: a paediatric perspective, Rev Endocr Metab Disord 6(4):261–268, Dec 2005.

52. Ibanez L, Suarez L, Lopez-Bermejo A, et al: Early development of visceral fat excess after spontaneous catch-up growth in children with low birth weight, J Clin Endocrinol Metab 93(3):925–928, Mar 2008.

53. Ibanez L, Lopez-Bermejo A, Suarez L, et al: Visceral adiposity without overweight in children born small for gestational age, J Clin Endocrinol Metab 93(6):2079–2083, Jun 2008.

54. Park JH, Stoffers DA, Nicholls RD, et al: Development of type 2 diabetes following intrauterine growth retardation in rats is associated with progressive epigenetic silencing of Pdx1, J Clin Invest 118(6):2316–2324, Jun 2008.

55. Raychaudhuri N, Raychaudhuri S, Thamotharan M, et al: Histone code modifications repress glucose transporter 4 expression in the intrauterine growth-restricted offspring, J Biol Chem 283(20):13611–13626, May 16 2008.

56. Lillycrop KA, Phillips ES, Jackson AA, et al: Dietary protein restriction of pregnant rats induces and folic acid supplementation prevents epigenetic modification of hepatic gene expression in the offspring, J Nutr 135(6):1382–1386, Jun 2005.

57. Houang M, Morineau G, le Bouc Y, et al: The cortisol-cortisone shuttle in children born with intrauterine growth retardation, Pediatr Res 46(2):189–193, Aug 1999.

58. Ong KK, Potau N, Petry CJ, et al: Opposing influences of prenatal and postnatal weight gain on adrenarche in normal boys and girls, J Clin Endocrinol Metab 89(6):2647–2651, Jun 2004.

59. Ibanez L, Potau N, Ferrer A, et al: Anovulation in eumenorrheic, nonobese adolescent girls born small for gestational age: insulin sensitization induces ovulation, increases lean body mass, and reduces abdominal fat excess, dyslipidemia, and subclinical hyperandrogenism, J Clin Endocrinol Metab 87(12):5702–5705, Dec 2002.

60. Barker DJ, Bagby SP, Hanson MA: Mechanisms of disease: in utero programming in the pathogenesis of hypertension, Nat Clin Pract Nephrol 2(12):700–707, Dec 2006.

61. Sotos JF: Genetic disorders associated with overgrowth, Clin Pediatr (Phila) 36(1):39–49, Jan 1997.

62. Kirsch S, Weiss B, Schon K, et al: The definition of the Y chromosome growth-control gene (GCY) critical region: relevance of terminal and interstitial deletions, J Pediatr Endocrinol Metab 15(Suppl 5):1295–1300, Dec 2002.

63. Zinn AR: Growing interest in Turner syndrome, Nat Genet 16(1):3–4, May 1997.

64. Padidela R, Camacho-Hubner C, Attie KM, et al: Abnormal growth in Noonan syndrome: genetic and endocrine features and optimal treatment, Horm Res 70(3):129–136, 2008.

65. Lettre G, Jackson AU, Gieger C, et al: Identification of ten loci associated with height highlights new biological pathways in human growth, Nat Genet 40(5):584–591, May 2008.

66. Weedon MN, Lango H, Lindgren CM, et al: Genome-wide association analysis identifies 20 loci that influence adult height, Nat Genet 40(5):575–583, May 2008.

67. Baron R: General principles of bone biology. In Favus M, editor: Primer on the Metabolic Bone Disorders and Disorders of Mineral Metabolism, ed 5, Philadelphia: Lippincott, 2003, Williams & Wilkins.

68. Robson H, Siebler T, Shalet SM, et al: Interactions between GH, IGF-I, glucocorticoids, and thyroid hormones during skeletal growth, Pediatr Res 52(2):137–147, Aug 2002.

69. Horton WA: Skeletal development: insights from targeting the mouse genome, Lancet 362(9383):560–569, Aug 16 2003.

70. Matsukawa N, Grzesik WJ, Takahashi N, et al: The natriuretic peptide clearance receptor locally modulates the physiological effects of the natriuretic peptide system, Proc Natl Acad Sci U S A 96(13):7403–7408, Jun 22 1999.

71. Miyazawa T, Ogawa Y, Chusho H, et al: Cyclic GMP-dependent protein kinase II plays a critical role in C-type natriuretic peptide-mediated endochondral ossification, Endocrinology 143(9):3604–3610, Sep 2002.

72. Tanner J: Growth at Adolescence, London, 1962, Blackwell.

73. Abbott RD, White LR, Ross GW, et al: Height as a marker of childhood development and late-life cognitive function: the Honolulu-Asia Aging Study, Pediatrics 102(3 Pt 1):602–609, Sep 1998.

74. Hommes F, Drost, YM, Geraets WXM, et al: The energy requirement for growth: an application of Atkinson's metabolic price system, Pediatr Res 9:51, 1975.

75. Holt LE Jr: Some problems in dietary amino acid requirements, Am J Clin Nutr 21(5):367–375, May 1968.

76. Fisch RO, Gravem HJ, Feinberg SB: Growth and bone characteristics of phenylketonurics. Comparative analysis of treated and untreated phenylketonuric children, Am J Dis Child 112(1):3–10, Jul 1966.

77. Cahill GF Jr: Editorial: nitrogen versatility in bats, bears and man, N Engl J Med 290(12):686–687, Mar 21 1974.

78. Holman RT: Essential fatty acid deficiency, Prog Chem Fats Lipids 9:275, 1968.

79. Chesney RW: Requirements and upper limits of vitamin D intake in the term neonate, infant, and older child, J Pediatr 116(2):159–166, Feb 1990.

80. Clement D, Fomon, SJ, Forbes, GB, et al: Trace elements in infant nutrition, Pediatrics 26:715, 1960.

81. Ulmer DD: Trace elements, N Engl J Med 297(6):318–321, Aug 11 1977.

82. Nakamura T, Nishiyama S, Futagoishi-Suginohara Y, et al: Mild to moderate zinc deficiency in short children: effect of zinc supplementation on linear growth velocity, J Pediatr 123(1):65–69, Jul 1993.

83. Danks DM, Campbell PE, Walker-Smith J, et al: Menkes' kinky-hair syndrome, Lancet 1(7760):1100–1102, May 20 1972.

84. Cooke RE, Boyden DG, Haller E: The relationship of acidosis and growth retardation, J Pediatr 57:326–337, Sep 1960.

85. Viteri F: The effect of inactivity on the growth of rats fed diets adequate or restricted with respect to normal caloric intake. New Concepts about Old Aspects of Malnutrition, Academia Mexicana de Pediatria 1973.

86. Rosenfeld MG, Briata P, Dasen J, et al: Multistep signaling and transcriptional requirements for pituitary organogenesis in vivo, Recent Prog Horm Res 55:1–13; discussion 13–14, 2000.

87. Treier M, Gleiberman AS, O'Connell SM, et al: Multistep signaling requirements for pituitary organogenesis in vivo, Genes Dev 12(11):1691–1704, Jun 1 1998.

88. Mayo KE, Miller T, DeAlmeida V, et al: Regulation of the pituitary somatotroph cell by GHRH and its

receptor, Recent Prog Horm Res 55:237–266; discussion 266–267, 2000.

89. Giustina A, Veldhuis JD: Pathophysiology of the neuroregulation of growth hormone secretion in experimental animals and the human, Endocr Rev 19(6):717–797, Dec 1998.

90. Ghigo E, Aimaretti G, Arvat E, et al: Growth hormone-releasing hormone combined with arginine or growth hormone secretagogues for the diagnosis of growth hormone deficiency in adults, Endocrine 15(1):29–38, Jun 2001.

91. Veldhuis JD, Bowers CY: Three-peptide control of pulsatile and entropic feedback-sensitive modes of growth hormone secretion: modulation by estrogen and aromatizable androgen, J Pediatr Endocrinol Metab 16(Suppl 3):587–605, May 2003.

92. Tannenbaum GS, Epelbaum J, Bowers CY: Interrelationship between the novel peptide ghrelin and somatostatin/growth hormone-releasing hormone in regulation of pulsatile growth hormone secretion, Endocrinology 144(3):967–974, Mar 2003.

93. Torsello A, Scibona B, Leo G, et al: Ontogeny and tissue-specific regulation of ghrelin mRNA expression suggest that ghrelin is primarily involved in the control of extraendocrine functions in the rat, Neuroendocrinology 77(2):91–99, Feb 2003.

94. Wang G, Lee HM, Englander E, et al: Ghrelin—not just another stomach hormone, Regul Pept 105(2):75–81, May 15 2002.

95. Le Roith D, Bondy C, Yakar S, et al: The somatomedin hypothesis: 2001, Endocr Rev 22(1):53–74, Feb 2001.

96. Wallenius K, Sjogren K, Peng XD, et al: Liver-derived IGF-I regulates GH secretion at the pituitary level in mice, Endocrinology 142(11):4762–4770, Nov 2001.

97. Gasperi M, Cecconi E, Grasso L, et al: GH secretion is impaired in patients with primary hyperparathyroidism, J Clin Endocrinol Metab 87(5):1961–1964, May 2002.

98. De Zegher F, Van Den Berghe G, et al: Dopamine inhibits growth hormone and prolactin secretion in the human newborn, Pediatr Res 34(5):642–645, Nov 1993.

99. Melmed S, Yamashita S, Yamasaki H, et al: IGF-I receptor signalling: lessons from the somatotroph, Recent Prog Horm Res 51:189–215; discussion 215–216, 1996.

100. Korytko AI, Cuttler L: Regulation of GHRH receptor gene expression in the neonatal and adult rat pituitary, Growth Horm IGF Res 11(5):282–288, Oct 2001.

101. Wallis M: Growth hormone-binding proteins, Clin Endocrinol (Oxf) 35(4):291–293, Oct 1991.

102. Walker JL, Moats-Staats BM, Stiles AD, et al: Tissue-specific developmental regulation of the messenger ribonucleic acids encoding the growth hormone receptor and the growth hormone binding protein in rat fetal and postnatal tissues, Pediatr Res 31(4 Pt 1):335–339, Apr 1992.

103. Eugster EA, Pescovitz OH: New revelations about the role of STATs in stature, N Engl J Med 349(12):1110–1112, Sep 18 2003.

104. Lupu F, Terwilliger JD, Lee K, et al: Roles of growth hormone and insulin-like growth factor 1 in mouse postnatal growth, Dev Biol 229(1):141–162, Jan 1 2001.

105. Spagnoli A, Rosenfeld RG: The mechanisms by which growth hormone brings about growth. The relative contributions of growth hormone and insulin-like growth factors, Endocrinol Metab Clin North Am 25(3):615–631, Sep 1996.

106. Le Roith D, Scavo L, Butler A: What is the role of circulating IGF-I? Trends Endocrinol Metab 12(2):48–52, Mar 2001.

107. Firth SM, Baxter RC: Cellular actions of the insulin-like growth factor binding proteins, Endocr Rev 23(6):824–854, Dec 2002.

108. Daughaday WH: Free insulin-like growth factor (IGF) in disorders of IGF binding protein 3 complex formation, J Clin Endocrinol Metab 89(1):3–5, Jan 2004.

109. Domene HM, Bengolea SV, Martinez AS, et al: Deficiency of the circulating insulin-like growth factor system associated with inactivation of the acid-labile subunit gene, N Engl J Med 350(6):570–577, Feb 5 2004.

110. D'Ercole AJ: Insulin-like growth factors and their receptors in growth, Endocrinol Metab Clin North Am 25(3):573–590, Sep 1996.

111. Weksberg R, Squire JA, Templeton DM: Glypicans: a growing trend, Nat Genet 12(3):225–227, Mar 1996.

112. Misra M, Miller KK, Bjornson J, et al: Alterations in growth hormone secretory dynamics in adolescent girls with anorexia nervosa and effects on bone metabolism, J Clin Endocrinol Metab 88(12):5615–5623, Dec 2003.

113. Pao CI, Farmer PK, Begovic S, et al: Regulation of insulin-like growth factor-I (IGF-I) and IGF-binding protein 1 gene transcription by hormones and provision of amino acids in rat hepatocytes, Mol Endocrinol 7(12):1561–1568, Dec 1993.

114. Menon RK, Sperling MA: Insulin as a growth factor, Endocrinol Metab Clin North Am 25(3):633–647, Sep 1996.

115. Argente J, Caballo N, Barrios V, et al: Multiple endocrine abnormalities of the growth hormone and insulin-like growth factor axis in prepubertal children with exogenous obesity: effect of short- and long-term weight reduction, J Clin Endocrinol Metab 82(7):2076–2083, Jul 1997.

116. Schalch DS, Heinrich UE, Draznin B, et al: Role of the liver in regulating somatomedin activity: hormonal effects on the synthesis and release of insulin-like growth factor and its carrier protein by the isolated perfused rat liver, Endocrinology 104(4):1143–1151, Apr 1979.

117. Juul A, Holm K, Kastrup KW, et al: Free insulin-like growth factor I serum levels in 1430 healthy children and adults, and its diagnostic value in patients suspected of growth hormone deficiency, J Clin Endocrinol Metab 82(8):2497–2502, Aug 1997.

118. Van Den Brande J, DeCaju MVL: Plasma somatomedin activity in children with growth disturbances. In Raiti S, editor: Advances in Human Growth Hormone Research, Washington DC, 1974, US Government Printing Office, p 98.

119. Quarmby V, Quan C, Ling V, et al: How much insulin-like growth factor I (IGF-I) circulates? Impact of standardization on IGF-I assay accuracy, J Clin Endocrinol Metab 83(4):1211–1216, Apr 1998.

120. Clark PA, Rogol AD: Growth hormones and sex steroid interactions at puberty, Endocrinol Metab Clin North Am 25(3):665–681, Sep 1996.

121. Roemmich JN, Clark PA, Mai V, et al: Alterations in growth and body composition during puberty: III. Influence of maturation, gender, body composition, fat distribution, aerobic fitness, and energy expenditure on nocturnal growth hormone release, J Clin Endocrinol Metab 83(5):1440–1447, May 1998.

122. Rosenfield RL, Furlanetto R: Physiologic testosterone or estradiol induction of puberty increases plasma somatomedin-C, J Pediatr 107(3):415–417, Sep 1985.

123. Bachrach B, Smith, EP: The role of sex steroids in bone growth and development: evolving new concepts, Endocrinol 6:362–368, 1996.

124. Schaff-Blass E, Burstein S, Rosenfield RL: Advances in diagnosis and treatment of short stature, with special reference to the role of growth hormone, J Pediatr 104(6):801–813, Jun 1984.

125. Collett-Solberg PF, Cohen P: The role of the insulin-like growth factor binding proteins and the IGFBP proteases in modulating IGF action, Endocrinol Metab Clin North Am 25(3):591–614, Sep 1996.

126. Mohan S, Baylink DJ: IGF-binding proteins are multifunctional and act via IGF-dependent and -independent mechanisms, J Endocrinol 175(1):19–31, Oct 2002.

127. Phillips LS, Fusco AC, Unterman TG, et al: Somatomedin inhibitor in uremia, J Clin Endocrinol Metab 59(4):764–772, Oct 1984.

128. Allen DB: Growth suppression by glucocorticoid therapy, Endocrinol Metab Clin North Am 25(3):699–717, Sep 1996.

129. Ballinger A: Fundamental mechanisms of growth failure in inflammatory bowel disease, Horm Res 58(Suppl 1):7–10, 2002.

130. Geffner ME: The growth without growth hormone syndrome, Endocrinol Metab Clin North Am 25(3):649–663, Sep 1996.

131. Den Ouden DT, Kroon M, Hoogland PH, et al: A 43-year-old male with untreated panhypopituitarism due to absence of the pituitary stalk: from dwarf to giant, J Clin Endocrinol Metab 87(12):5430–5434, Dec 2002.

132. Faustini-Fustini M, Balestrieri A, Rochira V, et al: The apparent paradox of tall stature with hypopituitarism: new insights from an old story, J Clin Endocrinol Metab 88(8):4002–4003; author reply 4003, Aug 2003.

133. Weiss RE, Refetoff S: Effect of thyroid hormone on growth. Lessons from the syndrome of resistance to thyroid hormone, Endocrinol Metab Clin North Am 25(3):719–730, Sep 1996.

134. Allen DB, Julius JR, Breen TJ, et al: Treatment of glucocorticoid-induced growth suppression with growth hormone. National Cooperative Growth Study, J Clin Endocrinol Metab 83(8):2824–2829, Aug 1998.

135. Mehls O, Himmele R, Homme M, et al: The interaction of glucocorticoids with the growth hormone-insulin-like growth factor axis and its effects on growth plate chondrocytes and bone cells, J Pediatr Endocrinol Metab 14(Suppl 6):1475–1482, 2001.

136. Hochberg Z: Mechanisms of steroid impairment of growth, Horm Res 58(Suppl 1):33–38, 2002.

137. Baron J, Klein KO, Colli MJ, et al: Catch-up growth after glucocorticoid excess: a mechanism intrinsic to the growth plate, Endocrinology 135(4):1367–1371, Oct 1994.

138. Canalis E: Inhibitory actions of glucocorticoids on skeletal growth. Is local insulin-like growth factor I to blame? Endocrinology 139(7):3041–3042, Jul 1998.

139. Daughaday WH, Rotwein P: Insulin-like growth factors I and II. Peptide, messenger ribonucleic acid and gene structures, serum, and tissue concentrations, Endocr Rev 10(1):68–91, Feb 1989.

140. Rosenfeld RG, Rosenbloom AL, Guevara-Aguirre J: Growth hormone (GH) insensitivity due to primary GH receptor deficiency, Endocr Rev 15(3):369–390, Jun 1994.

141. Abu EO, Horner A, Kusec V, et al: The localization of androgen receptors in human bone, J Clin Endocrinol Metab 82(10):3493–3497, Oct 1997.

142. Zachmann M, Prader A, Sobel EH, et al: Pubertal growth in patients with androgen insensitivity: indirect evidence for the importance of estrogens in pubertal growth of girls, J Pediatr 108(5 Pt 1):694–697, May 1986.

143. Kousteni S, Bellido T, Plotkin LI, et al: Nongenotropic, sex-nonspecific signaling through the estrogen or androgen receptors: dissociation from transcriptional activity, Cell 104(5):719–730, Mar 9 2001.

144. Seeman E: The structural and biomechanical basis of the gain and loss of bone strength in women and men, Endocrinol Metab Clin North Am 32(1):25–38, Mar 2003.

145. Smith EP, Boyd J, Frank GR, et al: Estrogen resistance caused by a mutation in the estrogen-receptor gene in a man, N Engl J Med 331(16):1056–1061, Oct 20 1994.

146. Migliaccio S, Newbold RR, Bullock BC, et al: Alterations of maternal estrogen levels during gestation affect the skeleton of female offspring, Endocrinology 137(5):2118–2125, May 1996.

147. Rosenfield RL, Perovic N, Devine N, et al: Optimizing estrogen replacement treatment in Turner syndrome, Pediatrics 102(2 Pt 3):486–488, Aug 1998.

148. Rosenfield RL: Low-dose testosterone effect on somatic growth, Pediatrics 77(6):853–857, Jun 1986.

149. Usher R, McLean F: Intrauterine growth of live-born Caucasian infants at sea level: standards obtained from measurements in 7 dimensions of infants born between 25 and 44 weeks of gestation, J Pediatr 74(6):901–910, Jun 1969.

150. Thomas P, Peabody J, Turnier V, et al: A new look at intrauterine growth and the impact of race, altitude, and gender, Pediatrics 106(2):E21, Aug 2000.

151. Shaffer SG, Quimiro CL, Anderson JV, et al: Postnatal weight changes in low birth weight infants, Pediatrics 79(5):702–705, May 1987.

152. Niklasson A, Engstrom E, Hard AL, et al: Growth in very preterm children: a longitudinal study, Pediatr Res 54(6):899–905, Dec 2003.

153. Hack M, Schluchter M, Cartar L, et al: Growth of very low birth weight infants to age 20 years, Pediatrics 112(1 Pt 1):e30–38, Jul 2003.

154. Sas T, de Waal W, Mulder P, et al: Growth hormone treatment in children with short stature born small for gestational age: 5-year results of a randomized, double-blind, dose-response trial, J Clin Endocrinol Metab 84(9):3064–3070, Sep 1999.

155. Centers for Disease Control and Prevention: CDC growth charts: United States: National Center for Health Statistics. Available at: http://www.cdc.gov/growthcharts/html. Accessed May 30, 2000.

156. Tanner JM, Davies PS: Clinical longitudinal standards for height and height velocity for North American children, J Pediatr 107(3):317–329, Sep 1985.

157. Bock R, Rosenfield, RL: Course-of-growth norms for longitudinal height velocity, Hummanbiol (Budapest) 25:575–586, 1994.

158. Lyon AJ, Preece MA, Grant DB: Growth curve for girls with Turner syndrome, Arch Dis Child 60(10):932–935, Oct 1985.

159. Horton WA, Rotter JI, Kaitila I, et al: Growth curves in achondroplasia, Birth Defects Orig Artic Ser 13(3C):101–107, 1977.

160. Cronk C, Crocker AC, Pueschel SM, et al: Growth charts for children with Down syndrome: 1 month to 18 years of age, Pediatrics 81(1):102–110, Jan 1988.

161. Fredriks AM, van Buuren S, Burgmeijer RJ, et al: Continuing positive secular growth change in The Netherlands 1955–1997, Pediatr Res 47(3):316–323, Mar 2000.

162. Karlberg J: On the construction of the infancy-childhood-puberty growth standard, Acta Paediatr Scand Suppl 356:26–37, 1989.

163. Smith DW, Truog W, Rogers JE, et al: Shifting linear growth during infancy: illustration of genetic factors in growth from fetal life through infancy, J Pediatr 89(2):225–230, Aug 1976.

164. Reed RB, Stuart HC: Patterns of growth in height and weight from birth to eighteen years of age, Pediatrics 24:904–921, Nov 1959.

165. Tanner JM, Whitehouse RH, Takaishi M: Standards from birth to maturity for height, weight, height velocity, and weight velocity: British children, 1965. I, Arch Dis Child 41(219):454–471, Oct 1966.

166. Bock R, Thissen D: Statistical problems of fitting individual growth curves. In Johnson F, Roche, A, editors: Human Physical Growth and Maturation, New York, 1980, Plenum, 265.

167. Tanner JM, Goldstein H, Whitehouse RH: Standards for children's height at ages 2–9 years allowing for heights of parents, Arch Dis Child 45(244):755–762, Dec 1970.

168. Boersma B, Wit JM: Catch-up growth. Endocr Rev 18(5):646–661, Oct 1997.

169. Glinos A: Density dependent regulation of growth and differentiated function in suspensioin cultures of mouse fibroblasts. In Kulonen E, Pikkarainen J, editors: Biology of Fibroblast, New York, 1973, Academic, p 155.

170. Tillmann V, Thalange NK, Foster PJ, et al: The relationship between stature, growth, and short-term changes in height and weight in normal prepubertal children, Pediatr Res 44(6):882–886, Dec 1998.

171. Gill MS, Tillmann V, Veldhuis JD, et al: Patterns of GH output and their synchrony with short-term height increments influence stature and growth performance in normal children, J Clin Endocrinol Metab 86(12):5860–5863, Dec 2001.

172. Shuttleworth F: Sexual maturation and physical growth of girls age 6 to 19, Monogr Soc Res Child Dev 2:5, 1937.

173. Cara JF, Rosenfeld RL, Furlanetto RW: A longitudinal study of the relationship of plasma somatomedin-C concentration in the pubertal growth spurt, Am J Dis Child 141(5):562–564, May 1987.

174. Tanner JM, Whitehouse RH, Marshall WA, et al: Prediction of adult height from height, bone age, and occurrence of menarche, at ages 4 to 16 with allowance for midparent height, Arch Dis Child 50(1):14–26, Jan 1975.

175. Parker EA, Hegde A, Buckley M, et al: Spatial and temporal regulation of GH-IGF-related gene expression in growth plate cartilage, J Endocrinol 194(1):31–40, Jul 2007.

176. Lazarus JE, Hegde A, Andrade AC, et al: Fibroblast growth factor expression in the postnatal growth plate, Bone 40(3):577–586, Mar 2007.

177. Bayley N, Pinneau SR: Tables for predicting adult height from skeletal age: revised for use with the Greulich-Pyle hand standards, J Pediatr 40(4):423–441, Apr 1952.

178. Russell DL, Keil MF, Bonat SH, et al: The relation between skeletal maturation and adiposity in African American and Caucasian children, J Pediatr 139(6):844–848, Dec 2001.

179. Barr GD, Allen CM, Shinefield HR: Height and weight of 7,500 children of three skin colors. Pediatric multiphasic program: report no. 3, Am J Dis Child 124(6):866–872, Dec 1972.

180. McKusick V: Heritable Disorders of Connective Tissue, ed 4, St. Louis, 1972, Mosby.

181. Engelbach W: Endocrine Medicine, Vol 1, Springfield, IL, 1932, Thomas.

182. Maresh MM: Linear growth of long bones of extremities from infancy through adolescence; continuing studies, AMA Am J Dis Child 89(6):725–742, Jun 1955.

183. Weaver DD, Christian JC: Familial variation of head size and adjustment for parental head circumference, J Pediatr 96(6):990–994, Jun 1980.

184. Krieger I: Head circumference, mental retardation and growth failure, Pediatrics 37:384, 1966.

185. Cloutier MD, Stickler GB: Head circumference in children with idiopathic hypopituitarism, Pediatrics 42(1):209–210, Jul 1968.

186. Prader A: Catch-up growth. Postgrad Med J 54(Suppl 1):133–146, 1978.

187. Ranke MB: Catch-up growth: new lessons for the clinician, J Pediatr Endocrinol Metab 15(Suppl 5):1257–1266, Dec 2002.

188. Wi JM, Boersma B: Catch-up growth: definition, mechanisms, and models, J Pediatr Endocrinol Metab 15(Suppl 5):1229–1241, Dec 2002.

189. Boersma B, Houwen RH, Blum WF, et al: Catch-up growth and endocrine changes in childhood celiac disease. Endocrine changes during catch-up growth: Horm Res 58(Suppl 1):57–65, 2002.

190. Bongiovanni AM: Letter: maturational deceleration following treatment with testosterone, J Pediatr 83(6):1095, Dec 1973.

191. Kember NF, Walker KV: Control of bone growth in rats, Nature 229(5284):428–429, Feb 5 1971.

192. Schrier L, Ferns SP, Barnes KM, et al: Depletion of resting zone chondrocytes during growth plate senescence, J Endocrinol 189(1):27–36, Apr 2006.

193. Gafni RI, Weise M, Robrecht DT, et al: Catch-up growth is associated with delayed senescence of the growth plate in rabbits, Pediatr Res 50(5):618–623, Nov 2001.

194. Marino R, Hegde A, Barnes KM, et al: Catch-up growth after hypothyroidism is caused by delayed growth plate senescence, Endocrinology 149(4):1820–1828, Apr 2008.

195. Nilsson O, Baron J: Impact of growth plate senescence on catch-up growth and epiphyseal fusion, Pediatr Nephrol 20(3):319–322, Mar 2005.

196. Binder G, Iliev DI, Mullis PE, et al: Catch-up growth in autosomal dominant isolated growth hormone deficiency (IGHD type II), Growth Horm IGF Res 17(3):242–248, Jun 2007.

197. Brandt I, Sticker EJ, Gausche R, et al: Catch-up growth of supine length/height of very low birth weight, small for gestational age preterm infants to adulthood, J Pediatr 147(5):662–668, Nov 2005.

198. Greulich W, Pyle SI: Radiographic Atlas of Skeletal Development of the Hand and Wrist, Palo Alto, 1959, Stanford University Press.

199. Wilkins L: The Diagnosis and Treatment of Endocrine Disorders in Childhood and Adolescence, ed 3, Springfield, IL, 1965, Thomas.

200. Roche AF, Eyman SL, Davila GH: Skeletal age prediction, J Pediatr 78(6):997–1003, Jun 1971.

201. Baer MJ, Djrkatz J: Bilateral asymmetry in skeletal maturation of the hand and wrist: a roentgenographic analysis, Am J Phys Anthropol 15(2):181–196, Jun 1957.

202. Tanner J, Oshman D, Bahhage F, et al: Tanner-Whitehouse bone age reference values for North American children, J Pediatr 131(1 Pt 1):34–40, Jul 1997.

203. Garn SM, Sandusky ST, Nagy JM, et al: Advanced skeletal development in low-income Negro children, J Pediatr 80(6):965–969, Jun 1972.

204. Flor-Cisneros A, Leschek EW, Merke DP, et al: In boys with abnormal developmental tempo, maturation of the skeleton and the hypothalamic-pituitary-gonadal axis remains synchronous, J Clin Endocrinol Metab 89(1):236–241, Jan 2004.

205. Frisancho A, Garn, SM, Rohmann, CG: Age at menarche: a new method of prediction and retrospective assessment based on hand x-rays, Hum Biol 41:42, 1969.

206. Bayer LM, Bayley N: Growth pattern shifts in healthy children: spontaneous and induced, J Pediatr 62:631–645, May 1963.

207. Hintz RL, Attie KM, Baptista J, et al: Effect of growth hormone treatment on adult height of children with idiopathic short stature. Genentech Collaborative Group, N Engl J Med 340(7):502–507, Feb 18 1999.

208. Roche AF, Wainer H, Thissen D: The RWT method for the prediction of adult stature, Pediatrics 56(6):1027–1033, Dec 1975.

209. Tanner J, Healy, MJR, Goldstein H, et al: Assessment of Skeletal Maturity and Prediction of Adult Height (TW3 Method), 3rd ed. London, 2001, WB Saunders.

210. Cohen P, Rogol AD, Deal CL, et al: Consensus Statement on the Diagnosis and Treatment of Children with Idiopathic Short Stature: A Summary of the Growth Hormone Research Society, the Lawson Wilkins Pediatric Endocrine Society, and the European Society for Paediatric Endocrinology Workshop, J Clin Endocrinol Metab 93(11):4210–4217, Nov 2008.

211. International nomenclature and classification of the osteochondrodysplasias (1997): International Working Group on Constitutional Diseases of Bone, Am J Med Genet 79(5):376–382, Oct 12 1998.

212. Superti-Furga A, Bonafe L, Rimoin DL: Molecular-pathogenetic classification of genetic disorders of the skeleton, Am J Med Genet 106(4):282–293, Winter 2001.

213. Jones K: Smith's Recognizable Patterns of Human Malformation, Vol 4, ed 4, Philadelphia, 1988, WB Saunders.

214. Horton WA, Rotter JI, Rimoin DL, et al: Standard growth curves for achondroplasia, J Pediatr 93(3):435–438, Sep 1978.

215. Horton WA: Molecular genetic basis of the human chondrodysplasias, Endocrinol Metab Clin North Am 25(3):683–697, Sep 1996.

216. Horton WA: Fibroblast growth factor receptor 3 and the human chondrodysplasias, Curr Opin Pediatr 9(4):437–442, Aug 1997.

217. Hellemans J, Coucke PJ, Giedion A, et al: Homozygous mutations in IHH cause acrocapitofemoral dysplasia, an autosomal recessive disorder with cone-shaped epiphyses in hands and hips, Am J Hum Genet 72(4):1040–1046, Apr 2003.

218. Fanconi S, Fischer JA, Wieland P, et al: Kenny syndrome: evidence for idiopathic hypoparathyroidism in two patients and for abnormal parathyroid hormone in one, J Pediatr 109(3):469–475, Sep 1986.

219. Schipani E, Langman CB, Parfitt AM, et al: Constitutively activated receptors for parathyroid hormone and parathyroid hormone-related peptide in Jansen's metaphyseal chondrodysplasia, N Engl J Med 335(10):708–714, Sep 5 1996.

220. Silverman R: Caffey's Pediatric X-Ray Diagnosis, Vol 1, ed 8, Chicago, 1985, Year Book Medical Publications.

221. Shapiro F: Epiphyseal disorders, N Engl J Med 317(27):1702–1710, Dec 31 1987.

222. Ross JL, Kowal K, Quigley CA, et al: The phenotype of short stature homeobox gene (SHOX) deficiency in childhood: contrasting children with Leri-Weill dyschondrosteosis and Turner syndrome, J Pediatr 147(4):499–507, Oct 2005.

223. Zinn AR, Wei F, Zhang L, et al: Complete SHOX deficiency causes Langer mesomelic dysplasia, Am J Med Genet 110(2):158–163, Jun 15 2002.

224. Blum WF, Crowe BJ, Quigley CA, et al: Growth hormone is effective in treatment of short stature associated with short stature homeobox-containing gene deficiency: two-year results of a randomized, controlled, multicenter trial, J Clin Endocrinol Metab 92(1):219–228, 2007.

225. Morris CA, Mervis CB, Hobart HH, et al: GTF2I hemizygosity implicated in mental retardation in Williams syndrome: genotype-phenotype analysis of five families with deletions in the Williams syndrome region, Am J Med Genet A 123A(1):45–59, Nov 15 2003.

226. Maassen JA, Tobias ES, Kayserilli H, et al: Identification and functional assessment of novel and known insulin receptor mutations in five patients with syndromes of severe insulin resistance, J Clin Endocrinol Metab 88(9):4251–4257, Sep 2003.

227. Moebius FF, Fitzky BU, Glossmann H: Genetic defects in postsqualene cholesterol biosynthesis, Trends Endocrinol Metab 11(3):106–114, Apr 2000.

228. Dupuis-Girod S, Gluckman E, Souberbielle JC, et al: Growth hormone deficiency caused by pituitary stalk interruption in Fanconi's anemia, J Pediatr 138(1):129–133, Jan 2001.

229. Tischkowitz MD, Morgan NV, Grimwade D, et al: Deletion and reduced expression of the Fanconi anemia FANCA gene in sporadic acute myeloid leukemia, Leukemia 18(3):420–425, Mar 2004.

230. Bartsch O, Wagner A, Hinkel GK, et al: FISH studies in 45 patients with Rubinstein-Taybi syndrome: deletions associated with polysplenia, hypoplastic left heart and death in infancy. Eur J Hum Genet 7(7):748–756, Oct–Nov 1999.

231. Lehmann AR: DNA repair-deficient diseases, xeroderma pigmentosum, Cockayne syndrome and trichothiodystrophy, Biochimie 85(11):1101–1111, Nov 2003.

232. Hegele RA: Drawing the line in progeria syndromes, Lancet 362(9382):416–417, Aug 9 2003.

233. Hickson ID: RecQ helicases: caretakers of the genome, Nat Rev Cancer 3(3):169–178, Mar 2003.

234. Rao E, Weiss B, Fukami M, et al: Pseudoautosomal deletions encompassing a novel homeobox gene cause growth failure in idiopathic short stature and Turner syndrome, Nat Genet 16(1):54–63, May 1997.

235. Ogata T, Matsuo N: Sex chromosome aberrations and stature: deduction of the principal factors involved in the determination of adult height, Hum Genet 91(6):551–562, Jul 1993.

236. Ross JL, Scott C Jr, Marttila P, et al: Phenotypes Associated with SHOX Deficiency, J Clin Endocrinol Metab 86(12):5674–5680, Dec 2001.

237. Sybert VP, McCauley E: Turner's syndrome, N Engl J Med 351(12):1227–1238, Sep 16 2004.

238. Rosenfeld RG, Attie KM, Frane J, et al: Growth hormone therapy of Turner's syndrome: beneficial effect on adult height, J Pediatr 132(2):319–324, Feb 1998.

239. Saenger P: Turner's syndrome, Curr Ther Endocrinol Metab 6:239–243, 1997.

240. Pasquino AM, Passeri F, Pucarelli I, et al: Spontaneous pubertal development in Turner's syndrome. Italian Study Group for Turner's Syndrome, J Clin Endocrinol Metab 82(6):1810–1813, Jun 1997.

241. Health supervision for children with Turner syndrome: American Academy of Pediatrics. Committee on Genetics, Pediatrics 96(6):1166–1173, Dec 1995.

242. van Pareren YK, de Muinck Keizer-Schrama SM, Stijnen T, et al: Final height in girls with turner syndrome after long-term growth hormone treatment in three dosages and low dose estrogens, J Clin Endocrinol Metab 88(3):1119–1125, Mar 2003.

243. Cave CB, Bryant J, Milne R: Recombinant growth hormone in children and adolescents with Turner syndrome, Cochrane Database Syst Rev 2003(3): CD003887.

244. Quigley CA, Crowe BJ, Anglin DG, et al: Growth hormone and low dose estrogen in Turner syndrome: results of a United States multi-center trial to near-final height, J Clin Endocrinol Metab 87(5):2033–2041, May 2002.

245. Hamelin CE, Anglin G, Quigley CA, et al: Genomic imprinting in Turner syndrome: effects on response to growth hormone and on risk of sensorineural hearing loss, J Clin Endocrinol Metab 91(8):3002–3010, Aug 2006.

246. Davenport ML, Crowe BJ, Travers SH, et al: Growth hormone treatment of early growth failure in toddlers with Turner syndrome: a randomized, controlled, multicenter trial, J Clin Endocrinol Metab 92(9):3406–3416, Sep 2007.

247. Ari M, Bakalov VK, Hill S, Bondy CA: The effects of growth hormone treatment on bone mineral density and body composition in girls with turner syndrome, J Clin Endocrinol Metab 91(11):4302–4305, Nov 2006.

248. Bolar K, Hoffman AR, Maneatis T, et al: Long-term safety of recombinant human growth hormone in turner syndrome, J Clin Endocrinol Metab 93(2):344–351, Feb 2008.

249. Summitt RL: Turner syndrome and Noonan's syndrome, J Pediatr 75(4):730–731, Oct 1969.

250. Carballo EC: Turner syndrome and Noonan's syndrome, J Pediatr 75(4):729–730, Oct 1969.

251. Lo Curto F, Pucci E, Scappaticci S, et al: XO and male phenotype, Am J Dis Child 128(1):90–91, Jul 1974.

252. Heller RH: The Turner Phenotype in the Male, J Pediatr 66:48–63, Jan 1965.

253. Noonan's syndrome, Lancet 340(8810):22–23, July 4 1992.

254. Tartaglia M, Kalidas K, Shaw A, et al: PTPN11 mutations in Noonan syndrome: molecular spectrum, genotype-phenotype correlation, and phenotypic heterogeneity, Am J Hum Genet 70(6):1555–1563, Jun 2002.

255. Kosaki K, Suzuki T, Muroya K, et al: PTPN11 (protein-tyrosine phosphatase, nonreceptor-type 11) mutations in seven Japanese patients with Noonan syndrome, J Clin Endocrinol Metab 87(8):3529–3533, Aug 2002.

256. Saenger P: Editorial: Noonan syndrome–certitude replaces conjecture, J Clin Endocrinol Metab 87(8): 3527–3528, Aug 2002.

257. Tartaglia M, Gelb BD: Noonan syndrome and related disorders: genetics and pathogenesis, Annu Rev Genomics Hum Genet 6:45–68, 2005.

258. Roberts AE, Araki T, Swanson KD, et al: Germline gain-of-function mutations in SOS1 cause Noonan syndrome, Nat Genet 39(1):70–74, Jan 2007.

259. Tartaglia M, Pennacchio LA, Zhao C, et al: Gain-of-function SOS1 mutations cause a distinctive form of Noonan syndrome, Nat Genet 39(1):75–79, Jan 2007.

260. Carta C, Pantaleoni F, Bocchinfuso G, et al: Germline missense mutations affecting KRAS Isoform B are associated with a severe Noonan syndrome phenotype, Am J Hum Genet 79(1):129–135, Jul 2006.

261. Tartaglia M, Martinelli S, Stella L, et al: Diversity and functional consequences of germline and somatic PTPN11 mutations in human disease, Am J Hum Genet 78(2):279–290, Feb 2006.

262. Limal JM, Parfait B, Cabrol S, et al: Noonan syndrome: relationships between genotype, growth, and growth factors, J Clin Endocrinol Metab 91(1):300–306, Jan 2006.

263. Ranke MB, Heidemann P, Knupfer C, et al: Noonan syndrome: growth and clinical manifestations in 144 cases, Eur J Pediatr 148(3):220–227, Dec 1988.

264. Binder G, Neuer K, Ranke MB, et al: PTPN11 mutations are associated with mild growth hormone resistance in individuals with Noonan syndrome, J Clin Endocrinol Metab 90(9):5377–5381, Sep 2005.

265. Kelnar CJ: Growth hormone therapy in noonan syndrome, Horm Res 53(Suppl 1):77–81, 2000.

266. Binder G, Wittekindt, N, Ranke, MB: Noonan syndrome: genetics and responsiveness to growth hormone therapy, Horm Res 67(Suppl):45–49, 2007.

267. Bittel DC, Butler MG: Prader-Willi syndrome: clinical genetics, cytogenetics and molecular biology, Expert Rev Mol Med 7(14):1–20, July 25 2005.

268. Goldstone AP: Prader-Willi syndrome: advances in genetics, pathophysiology and treatment, Trends Endocrinol Metab 15(1):12–20, Jan–Feb 2004.

269. Holm VA, Cassidy SB, Butler MG, et al: Prader-Willi syndrome: consensus diagnostic criteria, Pediatrics 91(2):398–402, Feb 1993.

270. Cassidy SB: Prader-Willi syndrome, J Med Genet 34(11):917–923, Nov 1997.

271. Guidelines for the use of growth hormone in children with short stature: a report by the Drug and Therapeutics Committee of the Lawson Wilkins Pediatric Endocrine Society, J Pediatr 127(6):857–867, Dec 1995.

272. Carrel AL, Myers SE, Whitman BY, et al: Growth hormone improves body composition, fat utilization, physical strength and agility, and growth in Prader-Willi syndrome: a controlled study, J Pediatr 134(2):215–221, Feb 1999.

273. Lindgren AC, Hagenas L, Muller J, et al: Growth hormone treatment of children with Prader-Willi syndrome affects linear growth and body composition favourably, Acta Paediatr 87(1):28–31, Jan 1998.

274. Eiholzer U: Deaths in children with Prader-Willi syndrome. A contribution to the debate about the safety of growth hormone treatment in children with PWS, Horm Res 63(1):33–39, 2005.

275. Hale DE, Cody JD, Baillargeon J, et al: The spectrum of growth abnormalities in children with 18q deletions, J Clin Endocrinol Metab 85(12):4450–4454, Dec 2000.

276. Lee PA, Chernausek SD, Hokken-Koelega AC, et al: International Small for Gestational Age Advisory Board consensus development conference statement: management of short children born small for gestational age, April 24-October 1, 2001, Pediatrics 111(6 Pt 1):1253–1261, Jun 2003.

277. Robertson C: Catch-up growth among very-low-birth-weight preterm infants: a historical perspective, J Pediatr 143(2):145–146, Aug 2003.

278. Saenger P, Czernichow P, Hughes I, et al: Small for gestational age: short stature and beyond, Endocr Rev 28(2):219–251, Apr 2007.

279. Eggermann T, Wollmann HA, Kuner R, et al: Molecular studies in 37 Silver-Russell syndrome patients: frequency and etiology of uniparental disomy, Hum Genet 100(3–4):415–419, Sep 1997.

280. Spiro RP, Christian SL, Ledbetter DH, et al: Intrauterine growth retardation associated with maternal uniparental disomy for chromosome 6 unmasked by congenital adrenal hyperplasia, Pediatr Res 46(5):510–513, Nov 1999.

281. Abuzzahab MJ, Schneider A, Goddard A, et al: IGF-I receptor mutations resulting in intrauterine and postnatal growth retardation, N Engl J Med 349(23):2211–2222, Dec 4 2003.

282. Lin CC, Santolaya-Forgas J: Current concepts of fetal growth restriction: part I. Causes, classification, and pathophysiology, Obstet Gynecol 92(6):1044–1055, Dec 1998.

283. Rossignol S, Netchine I, Le Bouc Y, et al: Epigenetics in Silver-Russell syndrome, Best Pract Res Clin Endocrinol Metab 22(3):403–414, Jun 2008.

284. Saal HM, Pagon RA, Pepin MG: Reevaluation of Russell-Silver syndrome, J Pediatr 107(5):733–737, Nov 1985.

285. Davies PS, Valley R, Preece MA: Adolescent growth and pubertal progression in the Silver-Russell syndrome, Arch Dis Child 63(2):130–135, Feb 1988.

286. Eggerman T, Eggerman K, Schonherr N: Growth retardation versus overgrowth: Silver-Russell syndrome is genetically opposite to Beckwith-Wiedemann syndrome, Trends in Genetics 24(4):195–204, 2008.

287. Kandall SR, Albin S, Lowinson J, et al: Differential effects of maternal heroin and methadone use on birthweight, Pediatrics 58(5):681–685, Nov 1976.

288. Chiriboga-Klein S, Oberfield SE, Casullo AM, et al: Growth in congenital rubella syndrome and correlation with clinical manifestations, J Pediatr 115(2):251–255, Aug 1989.

289. Soothill PW, Nicolaides KH, Bilardo CM, et al: Relation of fetal hypoxia in growth retardation to mean blood velocity in the fetal aorta, Lancet 2(8516):1118–1120, Nov 15 1986.

290. Bergner L, Susser MW: Low birth weight and prenatal nutrition: an interpretative review, Pediatrics 46(6): 946–966, Dec 1970.

291. Naeye RL, Blanc W, Paul C: Effects of maternal nutrition on the human fetus, Pediatrics 52(4):494–503, Oct 1973.

292. Naeye RL: Organ abnormalities in a human parabiotic syndrome, Am J Pathol 46:299, 1965.

293. Medovy H: New parameters in neonatal growth–cell number and cell size, J Pediatr 71(3):459–461, Sep 1967.

294. Physician's Desk Reference, ed 57, Montvale, NJ, 2003, Thompson PDR.

295. Saenger P: US experience in evaluation and diagnosis of GH therapy of intrauterine growth retardation/small-for-gestational-age children, Horm Res 58(Suppl 3):27–29, 2002.

296. Ranke MB, Lindberg A, Cowell CT, et al: Prediction of response to growth hormone treatment in short children born small for gestational age: analysis of data from KIGS (Pharmacia International Growth Database), J Clin Endocrinol Metab 88(1):125–131, Jan 2003.

297. Pomerance JJ: Management of short children born small for gestational age, Pediatrics 112(1 Pt 1):180–182, Jul 2003.

298. Lee PA, Kendig JW, Kerrigan JR: Persistent short stature, other potential outcomes, and the effect of growth hormone treatment in children who are born small for gestational age, Pediatrics 112(1 Pt 1):150–162, Jul 2003.

299. Clayton PE, Cianfarani S, Czernichow P, et al: Management of the child born small for gestational age through to adulthood: a consensus statement of the International Societies of Pediatric Endocrinology and the Growth Hormone Research Society, J Clin Endocrinol Metab 92(3):804–810, Mar 2007.

300. Cutfield WS, Jackson WE, Jefferies C, et al: Reduced insulin sensitivity during growth hormone therapy for short children born small for gestational age, J Pediatr 142(2):113–116, Feb 2003.

301. Willemsen RH, de Kort SW, van der Kaay DC, et al: Independent effects of prematurity on metabolic and cardiovascular risk factors in short small-for-gestational-age children, J Clin Endocrinol Metab 93(2):452–458, Feb 2008.

302. Sandberg DE, Smith MM, Fornari V, et al: Nutritional dwarfing: is it a consequence of disturbed psychosocial functioning? Pediatrics 88(5):926–933, Nov 1991.

303. Pugliese MT, Lifshitz F, Grad G, et al: Fear of obesity. A cause of short stature and delayed puberty, N Engl J Med 309(9):513–518, Sep 1 1983.

304. Frisch RE, McArthur JW: Menstrual cycles: fatness as a determinant of minimum weight for height necessary for their maintenance or onset, Science 185(4155):949–951, Sep 13 1974.

305. Winter RJ, Phillips LS, Green OC, et al: Somatomedin activity in the Mauriac syndrome, J Pediatr 97(4):598–600, Oct 1980.

306. Taylor AM, Sharma AK, Avasthy N, et al: Inhibition of somatomedin-like activity by serum from streptozotocin-diabetic rats: prevention by insulin treatment and correlation with skeletal growth, Endocrinology 121(4):1360–1365, Oct 1987.

307. Addy DP, Hudson FP: Diencephalic syndrome of infantile emaciation. Analysis of literature and report of further 3 cases, Arch Dis Child 47(253):338–343, Jun 1972.

308. Vlachopapadopoulou E, Tracey KJ, Capella M, et al: Increased energy expenditure in a patient with diencephalic syndrome, J Pediatr 122(6):922–924, Jun 1993.

309. Poulton A: Growth on stimulant medication; clarifying the confusion: a review, Arch Dis Child 90(8):801–806, Aug 2005.

310. Zeitler PS, Travers S, Kappy MS: Advances in the recognition and treatment of endocrine complications in children with chronic illness, Adv Pediatr 46:101–149, 1999.

311. van Rijn JC, Grote FK, Oostdijk W, et al: Short stature and the probability of coeliac disease, in the absence of gastrointestinal symptoms, Arch Dis Child 89(9):882–883, Sep 2004.

312. Maki M, Mustalahti K, Kokkonen J, et al: Prevalence of Celiac disease among children in Finland, N Engl J Med 348(25):2517–2524, Jun 19 2003.

313. Setty M, Hormaza L, Guandalini S: Celiac disease: risk assessment, diagnosis, and monitoring, Mol Diagn Ther 12(5):289–298, 2008.

314. Sawczenko A, Ballinger AB, Croft NM, et al: Adult height in patients with early onset of Crohn's disease, Gut 52(3):454–455; author reply 455, Mar 2003.

315. Alemzadeh N, Rekers-Mombarg LT, Mearin ML, et al: Adult height in patients with early onset of Crohn's disease, Gut 51(1):26–29, Jul 2002.

316. Sawczenko A, Ballinger AB, Savage MO, et al: Clinical features affecting final adult height in patients with pediatric-onset Crohn's disease, Pediatrics 118(1):124–129, Jul 2006.

317. Shamir R, Phillip M, Levine A: Growth retardation in pediatric Crohn's disease: pathogenesis and interventions, Inflamm Bowel Dis 13(5):620–628, May 2007.

318. Bozzola M, Giovenale D, Bozzola E, et al: Growth hormone deficiency and coeliac disease: an unusual association? Clin Endocrinol (Oxf) 62(3):372–375, Mar 2005.

319. Sentongo TA, Stettler N, Christian A, et al: Growth after intestinal resection for Crohn's disease in children, adolescents, and young adults, Inflamm Bowel Dis 6(4):265–269, Nov 2000.

320. Kapila P, Jones J, Rees L: Effect of chronic renal failure and prednisolone on the growth hormone-insulin-like growth factor axis, Pediatr Nephrol 16(12):1099–1104, Dec 2001.

321. Frystyk J, Ivarsen P, Skjaerbaek C, et al: Serum-free insulin-like growth factor I correlates with clearance in patients with chronic renal failure, Kidney Int 56(6):2076–2084, Dec 1999.

322. Tonshoff B, Blum WF, Wingen AM, et al: Serum insulin-like growth factors (IGFs) and IGF binding proteins 1, 2, and 3 in children with chronic renal failure: relationship to height and glomerular filtration rate. The European Study Group for Nutritional Treatment of Chronic Renal Failure in Childhood, J Clin Endocrinol Metab 80(9):2684–2691, Sep 1995.

323. Mahan JD, Warady BA: Assessment and treatment of short stature in pediatric patients with chronic kidney disease: a consensus statement, Pediatr Nephrol 21(7):917–930, Jul 2006.

324. Fine RN, Stablein D, Cohen AH, et al: Recombinant human growth hormone post-renal transplantation in children: a randomized controlled study of the NAPRTCS, Kidney Int 62(2):688–696, Aug 2002.

325. Simopoulos AP, Bartter FC: Growth characteristics and factors influencing growth in Bartter's syndrome, J Pediatr 81(1):56–65, Jul 1972.

326. Platt OS, Rosenstock W, Espeland MA: Influence of sickle hemoglobinopathies on growth and development, N Engl J Med 311(1):7–12, Jul 5 1984.

327. Glorieux FH: Rickets, the continuing challenge, N Engl J Med 325(26):1875–1877, Dec 26 1991.

328. Alon U, Donaldson DL, Hellerstein S, et al: Metabolic and histologic investigation of the nature of nephrocalcinosis in children with hypophosphatemic rickets and in the Hyp mouse, J Pediatr 120(6):899–905, Jun 1992.

329. Sampson B, Kovar IZ, Rauscher A, et al: A case of hyperzincemia with functional zinc depletion: a new disorder? Pediatr Res 42(2):219–225, Aug 1997.

330. Multicentre study on prevalence of endocrine complications in thalassaemia major: Italian working group on endocrine complications in non-endocrine diseases, Clin Endocrinol (Oxf) 42(6):581–586, Jun 1995.

331. Ellenberger C Jr, Runyan TE: Holoprosencephaly with hypoplasia of the optic nerves, dwarfism, and agenesis of the septum pellucidum, Am J Ophthalmol 70(6):960–967, Dec 1970.

332. Rudman D, Davis T, Priest JH, et al: Prevalence of growth hormone deficiency in children with cleft lip or palate, J Pediatr 93(3):378–382, Sep 1978.

333. Roessler E, Belloni E, Gaudenz K, et al: Mutations in the human Sonic Hedgehog gene cause holoprosencephaly, Nat Genet 14(3):357–360, Nov 1996.

334. Berry SA, Pierpont ME, Gorlin RJ: Single central incisor in familial holoprosencephaly, J Pediatr 104(6):877–880, Jun 1984.

335. Cohen LE, Wondisford FE, Radovick S: Role of Pit-1 in the gene expression of growth hormone, prolactin, and thyrotropin, Endocrinol Metab Clin North Am 25(3):523–540, Sep 1996.

336. Mendonca BB, Osorio MG, Latronico AC, et al: Longitudinal hormonal and pituitary imaging changes in two females with combined pituitary hormone deficiency due to deletion of A301,G302 in the PROP1 gene, J Clin Endocrinol Metab 84(3):942–945, Mar 1999.

337. Dattani ML, Martinez-Barbera J, Thomas PQ, et al: Molecular genetics of septo-optic dysplasia, Horm Res 53(Suppl 1):26–33, 2000.

338. Parks JS, Brown MR, Hurley DL, et al: Heritable disorders of pituitary development, J Clin Endocrinol Metab 84(12):4362–4370, Dec 1999.

339. Brickman JM, Clements M, Tyrell R, et al: Molecular effects of novel mutations in Hesx1/HESX1 associated with human pituitary disorders, Development 128(24):5189–5199, Dec 2001.

340. Deladoey J, Fluck C, Buyukgebiz A, et al: "Hot spot" in the PROP1 gene responsible for combined pituitary hormone deficiency, J Clin Endocrinol Metab 84(5):1645–1650, May 1999.

341. Paracchini R, Giordano M, Corrias A, et al: Two new PROP1 gene mutations responsible for compound pituitary hormone deficiency, Clin Genet 64(2):142–147, Aug 2003.

342. Vieira TC, Dias da Silva MR, Cerutti JM, et al: Familial combined pituitary hormone deficiency due to a novel mutation R99Q in the hot spot region of Prophet of Pit-1 presenting as constitutional growth delay, J Clin Endocrinol Metab 88(1):38–44, Jan 2003.

343. Netchine I, Sobrier ML, Krude H, et al: Mutations in LHX3 result in a new syndrome revealed by combined pituitary hormone deficiency, Nat Genet 25(2):182–186, Jun 2000.

344. Sloop KW, Parker GE, Hanna KR, et al: LHX3 transcription factor mutations associated with combined pituitary hormone deficiency impair the activation of pituitary target genes, Gene 265(1–2):61–69, Mar 7 2001.

345. Raetzman LT, Ward R, Camper SA: Lhx4 and Prop1 are required for cell survival and expansion of the pituitary primordia, Development 129(18):4229–4239, Sep 2002.

346. Dattani MT: DNA testing in patients with GH deficiency at the time of transition, Growth Horm IGF Res 13(Suppl A):S122–S129, Aug 2003.

347. Baumann G: Genetic characterization of growth hormone deficiency and resistance: implications for treatment with recombinant growth hormone, Am J Pharmacogenomics 2(2):93–111, 2002.

348. Drouin J, Lamolet B, Lamonerie T, et al: The PTX family of homeodomain transcription factors during pituitary developments, Mol Cell Endocrinol 140(1–2):31–36, May 25 1998.

349. Carvalho LR, Woods KS, Mendonca BB, et al: A homozygous mutation in HESX1 is associated with evolving hypopituitarism due to impaired repressor-corepressor interaction, J Clin Invest 112(8):1192–1201, Oct 2003.

350. Reynaud R, Gueydan M, Saveanu A, et al: Genetic screening of combined pituitary hormone deficiency: experience in 195 patients, J Clin Endocrinol Metab 91(9):3329–3336, Sep 2006.

351. Wagner JK, Eble A, Hindmarsh PC, et al: Prevalence of human GH-1 gene alterations in patients with isolated growth hormone deficiency, Pediatr Res 43(1):105–110, Jan 1998.

352. Phillips JA 3rd: Mutations of the GH gene, J Pediatr Endocrinol Metab 15(Suppl 5):1435–1436, Dec 2002.

353. Millar DS, Lewis MD, Horan M, et al: Novel mutations of the growth hormone 1 (GH1) gene disclosed by modulation of the clinical selection criteria for individuals with short stature, Hum Mutat 21(4):424–440, Apr 2003.

354. Moseley CT, Phillips JA 3rd: Pituitary gene mutations and the growth hormone pathway, Semin Reprod Med 18(1):21–29, 2000.

355. Hess O, Hujeirat Y, Wajnrajch MP, et al: Variable phenotypes in familial isolated growth hormone deficiency caused by a G6664A mutation in the GH-1 gene, J Clin Endocrinol Metab 92(11):4387–4393, Nov 2007.

356. Petkovic V, Lochmatter D, Turton J, et al: Exon splice enhancer mutation (GH-E32A) causes autosomal dominant growth hormone deficiency, J Clin Endocrinol Metab 92(11):4427–4435, Nov 2007.

357. Takahashi Y, Kaji H, Okimura Y, et al: Short stature caused by a mutant growth hormone with an antagonistic effect, Endocr J 43(Suppl):S27–S32, Oct 1996.

358. Besson A, Salemi S, Deladoey J, et al: Short stature caused by a biologically inactive mutant growth hormone (GH-C53S), J Clin Endocrinol Metab 90(5):2493–2499, May 2005.

359. Gertner JM, Wajnrajch MP, Leibel RL: Genetic defects in the control of growth hormone secretion, Horm Res 49(Suppl 1):9–14, 1998.

360. Carakushansky M, Whatmore AJ, Clayton PE, et al: A new missense mutation in the growth hormone-releasing hormone receptor gene in familial isolated GH deficiency, Eur J Endocrinol 148(1):25–30, Jan 2003.

361. Lindsay R, Feldkamp M, Harris D, Robertson J, et al: Utah Growth Study: growth standards and the prevalence of growth hormone deficiency, J Pediatr 125(1):29–35, Jul 1994.

362. Hamilton J, Blaser S, Daneman D: MR imaging in idiopathic growth hormone deficiency, AJNR Am J Neuroradiol 19(9):1609–1615, Oct 1998.

363. Kornreich L, Horev G, Lazar L, et al: MR findings in growth hormone deficiency: correlation with severity of hypopituitarism, AJNR Am J Neuroradiol 19(8):1495–1499, Sep 1998.

364. Meszaros F, Vergesslich K, Riedl S, et al: Posterior pituitary ectopy in children with idiopathic growth hormone deficiency, J Pediatr Endocrinol Metab 13(6):629–635, Jun 2000.

365. Choo-Kang LR, Sun CC, Counts DR: Cholestasis and hypoglycemia: manifestations of congenital anterior hypopituitarism, J Clin Endocrinol Metab 81(8):2786–2789, Aug 1996.

366. Newman CB, Levine LS, New MI: Endocrine function in children with intrasellar and suprasellar neoplasms: before and after therapy, Am J Dis Child 135(3):259–266, Mar 1981.

367. Thomsett MJ, Conte FA, Kaplan SL, et al: Endocrine and neurologic outcome in childhood craniopharyngioma: review of effect of treatment in 42 patients, J Pediatr 97(5):728–735, Nov 1980.

368. Sklar CA, Grumbach MM, Kaplan SL, et al: Hormonal and metabolic abnormalities associated with central nervous system germinoma in children and adolescents and the effect of therapy: report of 10 patients, J Clin Endocrinol Metab 52(1):9–16, Jan 1981.
369. Roman J, Villaizan CJ, Garcia-Foncillas J, et al: Growth and growth hormone secretion in children with cancer treated with chemotherapy, J Pediatr 131(1 Pt 1):105–112, Jul 1997.
370. Adan L, Trivin C, Sainte-Rose C, et al: GH deficiency caused by cranial irradiation during childhood: factors and markers in young adults, J Clin Endocrinol Metab 86(11):5245–5251, Nov 2001.
371. Matsuno A, Nagashima T, Teramoto, A, et al: Endocrinologic aspects of 23 patients with Rathke's cleft cyst, Endocrinologist 11:245–246, 2001.
372. De Bellis A, Salerno M, Conte M, et al: Antipituitary antibodies recognizing growth hormone (GH)-producing cells in children with idiopathic GH deficiency and in children with idiopathic short stature, J Clin Endocrinol Metab 91(7):2484–2489, Jul 2006.
373. Silver HK, Finkelstein M: Deprivation dwarfism, J Pediatr 70(3):317–324, Mar 1967.
374. Powell GF, Brasel JA, Blizzard RM: Emotional deprivation and growth retardation simulating idiopathic hypopituitarism. I. Clinical evaluation of the syndrome, N Engl J Med 276(23):1271–1278, Jun 8 1967.
375. Skuse D, Albanese A, Stanhope R, et al: A new stress-related syndrome of growth failure and hyperphagia in children, associated with reversibility of growth-hormone insufficiency, Lancet 348(9024):353–358, Aug 10 1996.
376. Gohlke BC, Stanhope R: Final height in psychosocial short stature: is there complete catch-up? Acta Paediatr 91(9):961–965, 2002.
377. Zucchini S, Pirazzoli P, Baronio F, et al: Effect on adult height of pubertal growth hormone retesting and withdrawal of therapy in patients with previously diagnosed growth hormone deficiency, J Clin Endocrinol Metab 91(11):4271–4276, Nov 2006.
378. Porter BA, Rosenfield RL, Lawrence AM: The levodopa test of growth hormone reserve in children, Am J Dis Child 126(5):589–592, Nov 1973.
379. Blethen SL, Chasalow FI: Use of a two-site immunoradiometric assay for growth hormone (GH) in identifying children with GH-dependent growth failure, J Clin Endocrinol Metab 57(5):1031–1035, Nov 1983.
380. Frystyk J, Andreasen CM, Fisker S: Determination of free growth hormone, J Clin Endocrinol Metab 93(8):3008–3014, Aug 2008.
381. Frasier SD: A preview of growth hormone stimulation tests in children, Pediatrics 53(6):929–937, Jun 1974.
382. Cara JF, Johanson AJ: Growth hormone for short stature not due to classic growth hormone deficiency, Pediatr Clin North Am 37(6):1229–1254, Dec 1990.
383. Shalet SM, Toogood A, Rahim A, et al: The diagnosis of growth hormone deficiency in children and adults, Endocr Rev 19(2):203–223, Apr 1998.
384. Moll GW Jr, Rosenfield RL, Fang VS: Administration of low-dose estrogen rapidly and directly stimulates growth hormone production, Am J Dis Child 140(2):124–127, Feb 1986.
385. Marin G, Domene HM, Barnes KM, et al: The effects of estrogen priming and puberty on the growth hormone response to standardized treadmill exercise and arginine-insulin in normal girls and boys, J Clin Endocrinol Metab 79(2):537–541, Aug 1994.
386. Rosenfeld RG, Albertsson-Wikland K, Cassorla F, et al: Diagnostic controversy: the diagnosis of childhood growth hormone deficiency revisited, J Clin Endocrinol Metab 80(5):1532–1540, May 1995.
387. Ghigo E, Bellone J, Aimaretti G, et al: Reliability of provocative tests to assess growth hormone secretory status. Study in 472 normally growing children, J Clin Endocrinol Metab 81(9):3323–3327, Sep 1996.
388. Carel JC, Tresca JP, Letrait M, et al: Growth hormone testing for the diagnosis of growth hormone deficiency in childhood: a population register-based study, J Clin Endocrinol Metab 82(7):2117–2121, Jul 1997.
389. Guyda HJ: Growth hormone testing and the short child, Pediatr Res 48(5):579–580, Nov 2000.
390. Juul A, Dalgaard P, Blum WF, et al: Serum levels of insulin-like growth factor (IGF)-binding protein-3 (IGFBP-3) in healthy infants, children, and adolescents: the relation to IGF-I, IGF-II, IGFBP-1, IGFBP-2, age, sex, body mass index, and pubertal maturation, J Clin Endocrinol Metab 80(8):2534–2542, Aug 1995.
391. Andrade Olivie MA, Garcia-Mayor RV, Gonzalez Leston D, et al: Serum insulin-like growth factor (IGF) binding protein-3 and IGF-I levels during childhood and adolescence. A cross-sectional study, Pediatr Res 38(2):149–155, Aug 1995.
392. Maghnie M, Salati B, Bianchi S, et al: Relationship between the morphological evaluation of the pituitary and the growth hormone (GH) response to GH-releasing hormone plus arginine in children and adults with congenital hypopituitarism, J Clin Endocrinol Metab 86(4):1574–1579, Apr 2001.
393. MacGillivray MH, Baptista J, Johanson A: Outcome of a four-year randomized study of daily versus three times weekly somatropin treatment in prepubertal naive growth hormone-deficient children. Genentech Study Group, J Clin Endocrinol Metab 81(5):1806–1809, May 1996.
394. Blethen SL, Baptista J, Kuntze J, et al: Adult height in growth hormone (GH)-deficient children treated with biosynthetic GH. The Genentech Growth Study Group, J Clin Endocrinol Metab 82(2):418–420, Feb 1997.
395. Reiter EO, Price DA, Wilton P, et al: Effect of growth hormone (GH) treatment on the near-final height of 1258 patients with idiopathic GH deficiency: analysis of a large international database, J Clin Endocrinol Metab 91(6):2047–2054, Jun 2006.
396. Maghnie M, Ambrosini L, Cappa M, et al: Adult height in patients with permanent growth hormone deficiency with and without multiple pituitary hormone deficiencies, J Clin Endocrinol Metab 91(8):2900–2905, Aug 2006.
397. de Ridder MA, Stijnen T, Hokken-Koelega AC: Prediction of adult height in growth-hormone-treated children with growth hormone deficiency, J Clin Endocrinol Metab 92(3):925–931, Mar 2007.
398. Raz B, Janner M, Petkovic V, et al: Influence of growth hormone (GH) receptor deletion of exon 3 and full-length isoforms on GH response and final height in patients with severe GH deficiency, J Clin Endocrinol Metab 93(3):974–980, Mar 2008.
399. Pilotta A, Mella P, Filisetti M, et al: Common polymorphisms of the growth hormone (GH) receptor do not correlate with the growth response to exogenous recombinant human GH in GH-deficient children, J Clin Endocrinol Metab 91(3):1178–1180, Mar 2006.
400. Boot AM, Engels MA, Boerma GJ, et al: Changes in bone mineral density, body composition, and lipid metabolism during growth hormone (GH) treatment in children with GH deficiency, J Clin Endocrinol Metab 82(8):2423–2428, Aug 1997.
401. Baron J: Editorial: growth hormone therapy in childhood: titration versus weight-based dosing? J Clin Endocrinol Metab 92(7):2436–2438, Jul 2007.
402. Blethen SL, Allen DB, Graves D, et al: Safety of recombinant deoxyribonucleic acid-derived growth hormone: the National Cooperative Growth Study experience, J Clin Endocrinol Metab 81(5):1704–1710, May 1996.
403. Malozowski S, Tanner LA, Wysowski D, et al: Growth hormone, insulin-like growth factor I, and benign intracranial hypertension, N Engl J Med 329(9):665–666, Aug 26 1993.
404. Bramnert M, Segerlantz M, Laurila E, et al: Growth hormone replacement therapy induces insulin resistance by activating the glucose-fatty acid cycle, J Clin Endocrinol Metab 88(4):1455–1463, Apr 2003.
405. Wilson TA, Rose SR, Cohen P, et al: Update of guidelines for the use of growth hormone in children: the Lawson Wilkins Pediatric Endocrinology Society Drug and Therapeutics Committee, J Pediatr 143(4):415–421, Oct 2003.
406. Fradkin JE, Mills JL, Schonberger LB, et al: Risk of leukemia after treatment with pituitary growth hormone, Jama 270(23):2829–2832, Dec 15 1993.
407. Leukaemia in patients treated with growth hormone, Lancet 1(8595):1159–1160, May 21 1988.
408. Shalet SM, Brennan BM, Reddingius RE: Growth hormone therapy and malignancy, Horm Res 48(Suppl 4):29–32, 1997.
409. Moshang T Jr, Grimberg A: The effects of irradiation and chemotherapy on growth, Endocrinol Metab Clin North Am 25(3):731–741, Sep 1996.
410. Moshang T Jr, Rundle AC, Graves DA, et al: Brain tumor recurrence in children treated with growth hormone: the National Cooperative Growth Study experience, J Pediatr 128(5 Pt 2):S4–S7, May 1996.
411. Ergun-Longmire B, Mertens AC, Mitby P, et al: Growth hormone treatment and risk of second neoplasms in the childhood cancer survivor, J Clin Endocrinol Metab 91(9):3494–3498, Sep 2006.
412. Koller EA, Green L, Gertner JM, et al: Retinal changes mimicking diabetic retinopathy in two nondiabetic, growth hormone-treated patients, J Clin Endocrinol Metab 83(7):2380–2383, Jul 1998.
413. Van Vliet G, Deal CL, Crock PA, et al: Sudden death in growth hormone-treated children with Prader-Willi syndrome, J Pediatr 144(1):129–131, Jan 2004.
414. Swerdlow AJ, Higgins CD, Adlard P, et al: Risk of cancer in patients treated with human pituitary growth hormone in the UK, 1959–85: a cohort study, Lancet 360(9329):273–277, Jul 27 2002.
415. Sperling MA, Saenger PH, Ray H, et al: Growth hormone treatment and neoplasia-coincidence or consequence? J Clin Endocrinol Metab 87(12):5351–5352, Dec 2002.
416. Renehan AG, Zwahlen M, Minder C, et al: Insulin-like growth factor (IGF)-I, IGF binding protein-3, and cancer risk: systematic review and meta-regression analysis, Lancet 363(9418):1346–1353, Apr 24 2004.
417. Taback SP, Dean HJ: Mortality in Canadian children with growth hormone (GH) deficiency receiving GH therapy 1967–1992. The Canadian Growth Hormone Advisory Committee, J Clin Endocrinol Metab 81(5):1693–1696, May 1996.
418. Zachmann M, Prader A: Anabolic and androgenic affect of testosterone in sexually immature boys and its dependency on growth hormone, J Clin Endocrinol Metab 30(1):85–95, Jan 1970.
419. Rillema JA: Development of the mammary gland and lactation, Trends Endocrinol Metab 5(4):149–154, May–Jun 1994.
420. Molitch ME, Clemmons DR, Malozowski S, et al: Evaluation and treatment of adult growth hormone deficiency: an Endocrine Society Clinical Practice Guideline, J Clin Endocrinol Metab 91(5):1621–1634, May 2006.
421. Radovick S, DiVall S: Approach to the growth hormone-deficient child during transition to adulthood, J Clin Endocrinol Metab 92(4):1195–1200, Apr 2007.
422. Johnson OL, Cleland JL, Lee HJ, et al: A month-long effect from a single injection of microencapsulated human growth hormone, Nat Med 2(7):795–799, Jul 1996.
423. Smith RG, Van der Ploeg LH, Howard AD, et al: Peptidomimetic regulation of growth hormone secretion, Endocr Rev 18(5):621–645, Oct 1997.
424. Pihoker C, Badger TM, Reynolds GA, et al: Treatment effects of intranasal growth hormone releasing peptide-2 in children with short stature, J Endocrinol 155(1):79–86, Oct 1997.
425. Thorner M, Rochiccioli P, Colle M, et al: Once daily subcutaneous growth hormone-releasing hormone therapy accelerates growth in growth hormone-deficient children during the first year of therapy. Geref International Study Group, J Clin Endocrinol Metab 81(3):1189 1196, Mar 1996.
426. Bidlingmaier M, Kim J, Savoy C, et al: Comparative pharmacokinetics and pharmacodynamics of a new sustained-release growth hormone (GH), LB03002, versus daily GH in adults with GH deficiency, J Clin Endocrinol Metab 91(8):2926–2930, Aug 2006.
427. David A, Metherell LA, Clark AJ, et al: Diagnostic and therapeutic advances in growth hormone insensitivity, Endocrinol Metab Clin North Am 34(3):581–595, viii, Sep 2005.
428. Rosenbloom AL, Rosenfeld RG, Guevara-Aguirre J: Growth hormone insensitivity, Pediatr Clin North Am 44(2):423–442, Apr 1997.
429. Sobrier ML, Dastot F, Duquesnoy P, et al: Nine novel growth hormone receptor gene mutations in patients with Laron syndrome, J Clin Endocrinol Metab 82(2):435–437, Feb 1997.
430. Heath-Monnig E, Wohltmann HJ, Mills-Dunlap B, et al: Measurement of insulin-like growth factor I (IGF-I) responsiveness of fibroblasts of children with short stature: identification of a patient with IGF-I resistance, J Clin Endocrinol Metab 64(3):501–507, Mar 1987.

431. Laron Z: Growth hormone insensitivity (Laron syndrome), Rev Endocr Metab Disord 3(4):347–355, Dec 2002.

432. Kofoed EM, Hwa V, Little B, et al: Growth hormone insensitivity associated with a STAT5b mutation, N Engl J Med 349(12):1139–1147, Sep 18 2003.

433. Burren CP, Woods KA, Rose SJ, et al: Clinical and endocrine characteristics in atypical and classical growth hormone insensitivity syndrome, Horm Res 55(3):125–130, 2001.

434. Bougneres P, Goffin V: The growth hormone receptor in growth, Endocrinol Metab Clin North Am 36(1):1–16, Mar 2007.

435. Rosenfeld RG, Belgorosky A, Camacho-Hubner C, et al: Defects in growth hormone receptor signaling, Trends Endocrinol Metab 18(4):134–141, May–Jun 2007.

436. Milward A, Metherell L, Maamra M, et al: Growth hormone (GH) insensitivity syndrome due to a GH receptor truncated after Box1, resulting in isolated failure of STAT 5 signal transduction, J Clin Endocrinol Metab 89(3):1259–1266, Mar 2004.

437. Hwa V, Little B, Adiyaman P, et al: Severe growth hormone insensitivity resulting from total absence of signal transducer and activator of transcription 5b, J Clin Endocrinol Metab 90(7):4260–4266, Jul 2005.

438. Woods KA, Camacho-Hubner C, Bergman RN, et al: Effects of insulin-like growth factor I (IGF-I) therapy on body composition and insulin resistance in IGF-I gene deletion, J Clin Endocrinol Metab 85(4):1407–1411, Apr 2000.

439. Inagaki K, Tiulpakov A, Rubtsov P, et al: A familial insulin-like growth factor-I receptor mutant leads to short stature: clinical and biochemical characterization, J Clin Endocrinol Metab 92(4):1542–1548, Apr 2007.

440. Woods KA, Dastot F, Preece MA, et al: Phenotype: genotype relationships in growth hormone insensitivity syndrome, J Clin Endocrinol Metab 82(11):3529–3535, Nov 1997.

441. Blair JC, Savage MO: The GH-IGF-I axis in children with idiopathic short stature, Trends Endocrinol Metab 13(8):325–330, Oct 2002.

442. Attie KM, Carlsson LM, Rundle AC, et al: Evidence for partial growth hormone insensitivity among patients with idiopathic short stature. The National Cooperative Growth Study, J Pediatr 127(2):244–250, Aug 1995.

443. Buckway CK, Selva KA, Burren CP, et al: IGF generation in short stature, J Pediatr Endocrinol Metab 15(Suppl 5):1453–1454, Dec 2002.

444. Buckway CK, Selva KA, Pratt KL, et al: Insulin-like growth factor binding protein-3 generation as a measure of GH sensitivity, J Clin Endocrinol Metab 87(10):4754–4765, Oct 2002.

445. Ranke MB, Lindberg A, Price DA, et al: Age at growth hormone therapy start and first-year responsiveness to growth hormone are major determinants of height outcome in idiopathic short stature, Horm Res 68(2):53–62, 2007.

446. Guevara-Aguirre J, Rosenbloom AL, Vasconez O, et al: Two-year treatment of growth hormone (GH) receptor deficiency with recombinant insulin-like growth factor I in 22 children: comparison of two dosage levels and to GH-treated GH deficiency, J Clin Endocrinol Metab 82(2):629–633, Feb 1997.

447. Backeljauw PF, Underwood LE: Prolonged treatment with recombinant insulin-like growth factor-I in children with growth hormone insensitivity syndrome—a clinical research center study. GHIS Collaborative Group, J Clin Endocrinol Metab 81(9):3312–3317, Sep 1996.

448. Backeljauw PF, Underwood LE: Therapy for 6.5–7.5 years with recombinant insulin-like growth factor I in children with growth hormone insensitivity syndrome: a clinical research center study, J Clin Endocrinol Metab 86(4):1504–1510, Apr 2001.

449. Chernausek SD, Backeljauw PF, Frane J, et al: Long-term treatment with recombinant insulin-like growth factor (IGF)-I in children with severe IGF-I deficiency due to growth hormone insensitivity, J Clin Endocrinol Metab 92(3):902–910, Mar 2007.

450. Levitsky LL: Defining the role of IGF-I therapy for short children, J Clin Endocrinol Metab 92(3):813–814, Mar 2007.

451. Collett-Solberg PF, Misra M: The role of recombinant human insulin-like growth factor-I in treating children with short stature, J Clin Endocrinol Metab 93(1):10–18, Jan 2008.

452. Pitukcheewanont P, Rose SR: Nocturnal TSH surge: a sensitive diagnostic test for central hypothyroidism in children, Endocrinologist 7:226–232, 1997.

453. Rezvani I, DiGeorge AM: Reassessment of the daily dose of oral thyroxine for replacement therapy in hypothyroid children, J Pediatr 90(2):291–297, Feb 1977.

454. Rivkees SA, Bode HH, Crawford JD: Long-term growth in juvenile acquired hypothyroidism: the failure to achieve normal adult stature, N Engl J Med 318(10):599–602, Mar 10 1988.

455. Lee PA, Weldon VV, Migeon CJ: Short stature as the only clinical sign of Cushing's syndrome, J Pediatr 86(1):89–91, Jan 1975.

456. McArthur RG, Hayles AB, Salassa RM: Childhood Cushing disease: results of bilateral adrenalectomy, J Pediatr 95(2):214–219, Aug 1979.

457. Shahidi NT, Crigler JF Jr: Evaluation of growth and of endocrine systems in testosterone-corticosteroid-treated patients with aplastic anemia, J Pediatr 70(2):233–242, Feb 1967.

458. Leinung MC, Zimmerman D: Cushing's disease in children, Endocrinol Metab Clin North Am 23(3):629–639, Sep 1994.

459. Leinung MC, Kane LA, Scheithauer BW, et al: Long term follow-up of transsphenoidal surgery for the treatment of Cushing's disease in childhood, J Clin Endocrinol Metab 80(8):2475–2479, Aug 1995.

460. Styne DM, Grumbach MM, Kaplan SL, et al: Treatment of Cushing's disease in childhood and adolescence by transsphenoidal microadenomectomy, N Engl J Med 310(14):889–893, Apr 5 1984.

461. Lebrethon MC, Grossman AB, Afshar F, et al: Linear growth and final height after treatment for Cushing's disease in childhood, J Clin Endocrinol Metab 85(9):3262–3265, Sep 2000.

462. Davies JH, Storr HL, Davies K, et al: Final adult height and body mass index after cure of paediatric Cushing's disease, Clin Endocrinol (Oxf) 62(4):466–472, Apr 2005.

463. Soyka L: Alternate-day corticosteroid therapy, Adv Pediatr 19:47, 1972.

464. Hollman GA, Allen DB: Overt glucocorticoid excess due to inhaled corticosteroid therapy, Pediatrics 81(3):452–455, Mar 1988.

465. Lee MM: Clinical practice. Idiopathic short stature, N Engl J Med 354(24):2576–2582, Jun 15 2006.

466. Gubitosi-Klug RA, Cuttler L: Idiopathic short stature, Endocrinol Metab Clin North Am 34(3):565–580, viii, Sep 2005.

467. Wit JM, Clayton PE, Rogol AD, et al: Idiopathic short stature: definition, epidemiology, and diagnostic evaluation, Growth Horm IGF Res 18(2):89–110, Apr 2008.

468. Bonioli E, Taro M, Rosa CL, et al: Heterozygous mutations of growth hormone receptor gene in children with idiopathic short stature, Growth Horm IGF Res 15(6):405–410, Dec 2005.

469. Hujeirat Y, Hess O, Shalev S, et al: Growth hormone receptor sequence changes do not play a role in determining height in children with idiopathic short stature, Horm Res 65(4):210–216, 2006.

470. Schneider KU, Sabherwal N, Jantz K, et al: Identification of a major recombination hotspot in patients with short stature and SHOX deficiency, Am J Hum Genet 77(1):89–96, Jul 2005.

471. Finkelstein BS, Imperiale TF, Speroff T, et al: Effect of growth hormone therapy on height in children with idiopathic short stature: a meta-analysis, Arch Pediatr Adolesc Med 156(3):230–240, Mar 2002.

472. FDA Talk Paper: FDA approves Humatrope for short stature. Available at: http://www.fda.gov/bbs/topics/ANSWERS/2003/ANS01242.html. Accessed August 26, 2003.

473. Cuttler L, Silvers JB: Growth hormone treatment for idiopathic short stature: implications for practice and policy, Arch Pediatr Adolesc Med 158(2):108–110, Feb 2004.

474. Angier N: Ideas and Trends: Short Men, Short Shrift. Are Drugs the Answer? New York Times (22):12, Jun 2003.

475. Kaufman M: FDA approves wider use of growth hormone, Washington Post (July 26):A12, 2003.

476. Que V, Prakash S: Human Growth Hormone: FDA approves drug for use in healthy, short children. National Public Radio. Available at: http://discover.npr.org/features/feature.jhtml?wfld=1392897. Accessed August 14, 2003.

477. Wit JM, Reiter EO, Ross JL, et al: Idiopathic short stature: management and growth hormone treatment, Growth Horm IGF Res 18(2):111–135, Apr 2008.

478. Bryant J, Baxter L, Cave CB, et al: Recombinant growth hormone for idiopathic short stature in children and adolescents, Cochrane Database Syst Rev 2007(3):CD004440.

479. Quigley CA, Gill AM, Crowe BJ, et al: Safety of growth hormone treatment in pediatric patients with idiopathic short stature, J Clin Endocrinol Metab 90(9):5188–5196, Sep 2005.

480. Kemp SF, Kuntze J, Attie KM, et al: Efficacy and safety results of long-term growth hormone treatment of idiopathic short stature, J Clin Endocrinol Metab 90(9):5247–5253, Sep 2005.

481. Cuttler L: Safety and efficacy of growth hormone treatment for idiopathic short stature, J Clin Endocrinol Metab 90(9):5502–5504, Sep 2005.

482. Shulman DI, Francis GL, Palmert MR, et al: Use of aromatase inhibitors in children and adolescents with disorders of growth and adolescent development, Pediatrics 121(4):e975–e983, Apr 2008.

483. Rosenfield RL: Essentials of growth diagnosis, Endocrinol Metab Clin North Am 25(3):743–758, Sep 1996.

484. Ghai K, Cara JF, Rosenfield RL: Gonadotropin releasing hormone agonist (nafarelin) test to differentiate gonadotropin deficiency from constitutionally delayed puberty in teen-age boys–a clinical research center study, J Clin Endocrinol Metab 80(10):2980–2986, Oct 1995.

485. Albanese A, Stanhope R: Predictive factors in the determination of final height in boys with constitutional delay of growth and puberty, J Pediatr 126(4):545–550, Apr 1995.

486. Rosenfield RL: Clinical review 6: Diagnosis and management of delayed puberty, J Clin Endocrinol Metab 70(3):559–562, Mar 1990.

487. Ross JL, Long LM, Skerda M, et al: Effect of low doses of estradiol on 6-month growth rates and predicted height in patients with Turner syndrome, J Pediatr 109(6):950–953, Dec 1986.

488. Tse WY, Buyukgebiz A, Hindmarsh PC, et al: Long-term outcome of oxandrolone treatment in boys with constitutional delay of growth and puberty, J Pediatr 117(4):588–591, Oct 1990.

489. Blum WF, Machinis K, Shavrikova EP, et al: The growth response to growth hormone (GH) treatment in children with isolated GH deficiency is independent of the presence of the exon 3-minus isoform of the GH receptor, J Clin Endocrinol Metab 91(10):4171–4174, Oct 2006.

490. Jorge AA, Marchisotti FG, Montenegro LR, et al: Growth hormone (GH) pharmacogenetics: influence of GH receptor exon 3 retention or deletion on first-year growth response and final height in patients with severe GH deficiency, J Clin Endocrinol Metab 91(3):1076–1080, Mar 2006.

491. Binder G, Baur F, Schweizer R, et al: The d3-growth hormone (GH) receptor polymorphism is associated with increased responsiveness to GH in Turner syndrome and short small-for-gestational-age children, J Clin Endocrinol Metab 91(2):659–664, Feb 2006.

492. Carrascosa A, Esteban C, Espadero R, et al: The d3/fl-growth hormone (GH) receptor polymorphism does not influence the effect of GH treatment (66 microg/kg per day) or the spontaneous growth in short non-GH-deficient small-for-gestational-age children: results from a two-year controlled prospective study in 170 Spanish patients, J Clin Endocrinol Metab 91(9):3281–3286, Sep 2006.

493. Lantos J, Siegler M, Cuttler L: Ethical issues in growth hormone therapy, JAMA 261(7):1020–1024, Feb 17 1989.

494. Underwood LE: Growth hormone therapy for short stature: yes or no? Hosp Pract (Off Ed) 27(4):192–196, 198, Apr 15 1992.

495. Sandberg DE: Should short children who are not deficient in growth hormone be treated? West J Med 172(3):186–189, Mar 2000.

496. Finkelstein BS, Silvers JB, Marrero U, et al: Insurance coverage, physician recommendations, and access to

emerging treatments: growth hormone therapy for childhood short stature, JAMA 279(9):663–668, Mar 4 1998.

497. Zimet GD, Cutler M, Litvene M, et al: Psychological adjustment of children evaluated for short stature: a preliminary report, J Dev Behav Pediatr 16(4):264–270, Aug 1995.

498. Zimet GD, Owens R, Dahms W, et al: Psychosocial outcome of children evaluated for short stature, Arch Pediatr Adolesc Med 151(10):1017–1023, Oct 1997.

499. Kodish E, Cuttler L: Ethical issues in emerging new treatments such as growth hormone therapy for children with Down syndrome and Prader-Willi syndrome, Curr Opin Pediatr 8(4):401–405, Aug 1996.

500. Downie AB, Mulligan J, McCaughey ES, et al: Psychological response to growth hormone treatment in short normal children, Arch Dis Child 75(1):32–35, Jul 1996.

501. Lippe BM, Nakamoto JM: Conventional and nonconventional uses of growth hormone, Recent Prog Horm Res 48:179–235, 1993.

502. Allen DB, Fost NC: Growth hormone therapy for short stature: panacea or Pandora's box? J Pediatr 117(1 Pt 1):16–21, Jul 1990.

503. Voss LD: Growth hormone therapy for the short normal child: who needs it and who wants it? The case against growth hormone therapy, J Pediatr 136(1):103–106, Jan 2000.

504. Saenger P: The case in support of Gh therapy, J Pediatr 136(1):106–109; discussion 109–110, Jan 2000.

505. Cuttler L, Silvers JB, Singh J, et al: Short stature and growth hormone therapy. A national study of physician recommendation patterns, JAMA 276(7):531–537, Aug 21 1996.

506. Das U, Whatmore AJ, Khosravi J, et al: IGF-I and IGF-binding protein-3 measurements on filter paper blood spots in children and adolescents on GH treatment: use in monitoring and as markers of growth performance, Eur J Endocrinol 149(3):179–185, Sep 2003.

507. Allen DB: Growth hormone therapy for short stature: is the benefit worth the burden? Pediatrics 118(1):343–348, Jul 2006.

508. Ranke MB, Schweizer R, Elmlinger MW, et al: Relevance of IGF-I, IGFBP-3, and IGFBP-2 measurements during GH treatment of GH-deficient and non-GH-deficient children and adolescents, Horm Res 55(3):115–124, 2001.

509. Mul D, Wit JM, Oostdijk W, et al: The effect of pubertal delay by GnRH agonist in GH-deficient children on final height, J Clin Endocrinol Metab 86(10):4655–4656, Oct 2001.

510. Lee MM: Is treatment with a luteinizing hormone-releasing hormone agonist justified in short adolescents? N Engl J Med 348(10):942–945, Mar 6 2003.

511. Yanovski JA, Rose SR, Municchi G, et al: Treatment with a luteinizing hormone-releasing hormone agonist in adolescents with short stature, N Engl J Med 348(10):908–917, Mar 6 2003.

512. Pasquino AM, Pucarelli I, Roggini M, et al: Adult height in short normal girls treated with gonadotropin-releasing hormone analogs and growth hormone, J Clin Endocrinol Metab 85(2):619–622, Feb 2000.

513. Carel J, Eugster EA, Rogol A, et al: Consensus Statement on the Use of GnRH Analogs in Children. Paper presented at: GnRH Analogs Consensus Conference Group 6, In Press.

514. Mauras N, Gonzalez de Pijem L, Hsiang HY, et al: Anastrozole increases predicted adult height of short adolescent males treated with growth hormone: a randomized, placebo-controlled, multicenter trial for one to three years, J Clin Endocrinol Metab 93(3):823–831, Mar 2008.

515. Rosenbloom AL: Is there a role for recombinant insulin-like growth factor-I in the treatment of idiopathic short stature? Lancet 368(9535):612–616, Aug 12 2006.

516. Rosenbloom AL: The role of recombinant insulin-like growth factor I in the treatment of the short child, Curr Opin Pediatr 19(4):458–464, Aug 2007.

517. Pereira L, Levran O, Ramirez F, et al: A molecular approach to the stratification of cardiovascular risk in families with Marfan's syndrome, N Engl J Med 331(3):148–153, Jul 21 1994.

518. Sotos JF: Overgrowth. Section V: Syndromes and other disorders associated with overgrowth, Clin Pediatr (Phila) 36(2):89–103, Feb 1997.

519. Douglas J, Hanks S, Temple IK, et al: NSD1 mutations are the major cause of Sotos syndrome and occur in some cases of Weaver syndrome but are rare in other overgrowth phenotypes, Am J Hum Genet 72(1):132–143, Jan 2003.

520. Visser R, Matsumoto N: Genetics of Sotos syndrome, Curr Opin Pediatr 15(6):598–606, Dec 2003.

521. Kurotaki N, Imaizumi K, Harada N, et al: Haploinsufficiency of NSD1 causes Sotos syndrome, Nat Genet 30(4):365–366, Apr 2002.

522. Tatton-Brown K, Rahman N: Sotos syndrome, Eur J Hum Genet 15(3):264–271, Mar 2007.

523. Li M, Squire JA, Weksberg R: Molecular genetics of Wiedemann-Beckwith syndrome, Am J Med Genet 79(4):253–259, Oct 2 1998.

524. Sotos JF: Section III other hormonal causes, Clin Pediatr (Phila) 35(12):637–648, Dec 1996.

525. Sotos JF: Overgrowth. Hormonal causes, Clin Pediatr (Phila) 35(11):579–590, Nov 1996.

526. Gagel RF, McCutcheon IE: Images in clinical medicine. Pituitary gigantism, N Engl J Med 340(7):524, Feb 18 1999.

527. Cuttler L: The regulation of growth hormone secretion, Endocrinol Metab Clin North Am 25(3):541–571, Sep 1996.

528. Dotsch J, Kiess W, Hanze J, et al: Gs alpha mutation at codon 201 in pituitary adenoma causing gigantism in a 6-year-old boy with McCune-Albright syndrome, J Clin Endocrinol Metab 81(11):3839–3842, Nov 1996.

529. Wilroy RS Jr, Etteldorf JN: Familial hyperthyroidism including two siblings with neonatal Graves' disease, J Pediatr 78(4):625–632, Apr 1971.

530. Brauner R, Adan L, Malandry F, et al: Adult height in girls with idiopathic true precocious puberty, J Clin Endocrinol Metab 79(2):415–420, Aug 1994.

531. Uriarte MM, Baron J, Garcia HB, et al: The effect of pubertal delay on adult height in men with isolated hypogonadotropic hypogonadism, J Clin Endocrinol Metab 74(2):436–440, Feb 1992.

532. Thamdrup E: Precocious Sexual Development, Springfield, IL, 1961, Thomas.

533. Sotos JF: Overgrowth disorders, Clin Pediatr (Phila) 35(10):517–529, Oct 1996.

534. Drop SL, De Waal WJ, De Muinck Keizer-Schrama SM: Sex steroid treatment of constitutionally tall stature, Endocr Rev 19(5):540–558, Oct 1998.

535. Pyett P, Rayner J, Venn A, et al: Using hormone treatment to reduce the adult height of tall girls: are women satisfied with the decision in later years? Soc Sci Med 61(8):1629–1639, Oct 2005.

536. Lee JM, Howell JD: Tall girls: the social shaping of a medical therapy, Arch Pediatr Adolesc Med 160(10):1035–1039, Oct 2006.

537. Barnard ND, Scialli AR, Bobela S: The current use of estrogens for growth-suppressant therapy in adolescent girls, J Pediatr Adolesc Gynecol 15(1):23–26, Feb 2002.

538. Noordam C, van Daalen S, Otten BJ: Treatment of tall stature in boys with somatostatin analogue 201–995: effect on final height, Eur J Endocrinol 154(2):253–257, Feb 2006.

539. Goldenberg N, Racine MS, Thomas P, et al: Treatment of pituitary gigantism with the growth hormone receptor antagonist pegvisomant, J Clin Endocrinol Metab 93(8):2953–2956, Aug 2008.

540. Paul D, Conte FA, Grumbach MM, et al: Long-term effect of gonadotropin-releasing hormone agonist therapy on final and near-final height in 26 children with true precocious puberty treated at a median age of less than 5 years, J Clin Endocrinol Metab 80(2):546–551, Feb 1995.

541. Adan L, Souberbielle JC, Zucker JM, et al: Adult height in 24 patients treated for growth hormone deficiency and early puberty, J Clin Endocrinol Metab 82(1):229–233, Jan 1997.

542. Pasquino AM, Pucarelli I, Segni M, et al: Adult height in girls with central precocious puberty treated with gonadotropin-releasing hormone analogues and growth hormone, J Clin Endocrinol Metab 84(2):449–452, Feb 1999.

Chapter 19

GROWTH HORMONE DEFICIENCY IN CHILDREN

MEHUL DATTANI and PETER HINDMARSH

The height of an individual is the culmination of a complex process that results from an interaction between genes, nutritional status, hormonal milieu, and environmental factors. In terms of adult height, fetal growth is critical and has major implications for the ultimate stature of an individual. Birth length is approximately 30% of final height, and with a crown-rump length velocity of 50 to 60 cm/year this period represents the fastest rate of growth achieved by an individual. This growth is mediated by maternal nutrition and a number of growth factors such as insulin-like growth factor-I (IGF-I), IGF-II, fibroblast growth factor, epidermal growth factor, transforming growth factors α and β, and insulin. Any compromise in maternal nutrition or in the production of these growth factors is associated with intrauterine growth restriction.

Postnatal growth is best described by the ICP (infancy-childhood-pubertal) model of growth.[1] These three phases are regulated by different components of the endocrine system. During the infancy phase, growth is rapid but at a sharply decelerating rate. Growth at this stage is principally dependent on nutrition, although endocrine factors in the form of the growth hormone (GH)-IGF axis play an increasingly important role during the first year of life. Over the first 2 years, a period of "catch-up" or "catch down" growth commonly occurs while the infant establishes his/her own growth trajectory, with a marked increase in the correlation between current height and final height ($r = 0.8$) by 3 years of age. As a result, growth along a predictable channel is a hallmark of the healthy child. Poor growth may be a manifestation of any underlying illness reflecting a wide variety of genetic, constitutional, and pathologic conditions, of which GH deficiency (GHD) is but one cause. Stature itself is merely an indication of a potential abnormal physical state and not a diagnosis. That comes from the answer to the question, what is the explanation for this abnormality?

By 4 years of age, average height velocity has declined to 7 cm/year, with a further decline to a rate of 5 to 5.5 cm/year at 8 years of age (Fig. 19-1). The onset of the childhood phase of growth is apparent from the age of 6 months, when there is overlap between the childhood and infancy phases of growth. This childhood growth is dependent mainly on endocrine factors such as GH and thyroxine.[2] The third phase of postnatal growth, the pubertal phase, is dependent upon the normal secretion of GH and sex steroids. It is extremely variable in terms of timing, with marked sexual dimorphism that gives rise to the average difference of 12.5 cm in adult height between the sexes.

Growth hormone is the main mediator of postnatal growth,[2] and virtually any chronic childhood illness will modify secretion. As such, care needs to be exercised in the evaluation of GH secretion in these situations. Although GH deficiency (GHD) may be considered a form of IGF deficiency,[3] this approach may be limited. Since GH receptor and post-receptor issues and GHD in adults are considered elsewhere, this chapter will focus primarily on GHD as related to disorders of the hypothalamo-pituitary axis in children.

History

The history of GHD starts with the pursuit of therapeutic interventions which antedate attempts to measure serum concentra-

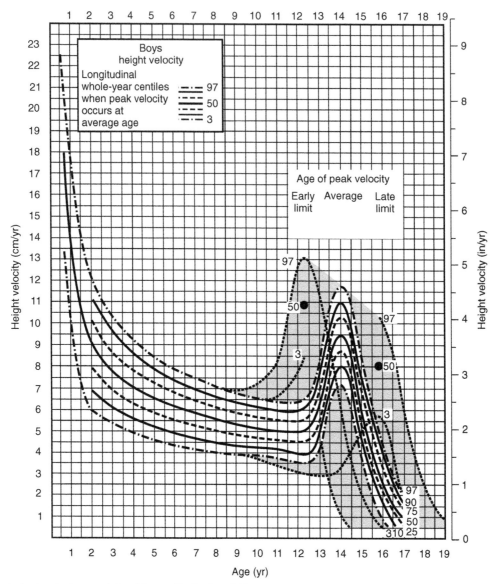

FIGURE 19-1. Height velocity chart for boys aged 0 to 19 years. Centiles 3 to 97 illustrated with 50th centile in bold. *Shaded zone,* Variation in timing of pubertal growth spurt. Visually, the chart depicts the rapid but rapidly decelerating growth during the first 4 years of life followed by a much slower declination until the onset of the pubertal growth spurt. (Copyright Castlemead Publications.)

tions of GH. In 1932, a treatment to promote growth with a crude anterior pituitary extract was reported,[4] but it was not until Raben's observations of 1958[5] and the general availability of methods of GH extraction that large studies could be conducted. These larger studies showed a beneficial effect of human GH in promoting growth in children with clear physical signs suggestive of GH deficiency.[6-9]

Growth hormone immunoassays postdated the initial therapeutic studies of GH.[10] The advent of radioimmunoassay allowed the measurement of the concentration of GH in blood in response to a variety of pharmacologic stimuli, thereby paving the way to a better understanding of which children might benefit from the then limited supplies of GH. This limitation in supply largely dictated clinical research until the advent of unlimited supplies of biosynthetic human GH (r-hGH) resulting from bioengineering technology in the late 1970s and early 1980s.

Our understanding of the physiology of GH secretion stemmed from the pioneering work of Geoffrey Harris and his group in Oxford, who suggested that release of GH from the pituitary was under the control of a releasing factor secreted from the hypothalamus. The demonstration by Brazeau et al.[11] of a GH release-inhibiting factor (somatostatin) led to a radical change in the thinking around the control of GH secretion. The final demonstration of a GH stimulating factor came in 1982 when GH releasing hormone was isolated and characterized from two pancreatic tumors.[12,13] During the search for the releasing factor, little was made of a further stimulating factor described by Bowers et al., which although synthetic in nature formed the basis from which GH releasing substances and their receptors were identified. Finally the natural ligand, ghrelin, was isolated from the stomach.[14]

For a considerable period of time, GH was believed to act via the generation of a further endocrine factor from the liver, somatomedin-C or IGF-I.[15] Further work led to the realization that liver was not the only source of IGF-I, and in a series of classic experiments, Green[16] and Isaksson[17] demonstrated in adipose tissue and cartilage, respectively, that IGF-I was generated locally and acted in a paracrine manner to promote clonal expansion of the cell population.

Epidemiology

The reported incidence of GHD is to a large extent dependent on the criteria employed to establish the diagnosis and reflects the wide variation in the stringency of diagnostic testing. In one U.K. study, an incidence of 1 in 60,000 live births was reported,[18] although a survey of Scottish schoolchildren led to a calculated prevalence of 1 per 4000 live births,[19] a value similar to that of the Utah Growth Study (1 in 3480 live births).[20]

Several large surveys have indicated that approximately 25% of children diagnosed with GHD have an underlying "organic" cause for their condition, such as trauma, CNS tumors, inflammation, irradiation, or anatomic abnormalities of the hypothalamus or pituitary.[21,22] The remainder are labeled as "idiopathic" GHD. Such surveys are likely to overestimate the number of true cases of idiopathic GHD because of variation in the diagnosis of GHD. Recent advances in developmental endocrinology suggest that many patients labeled previously as idiopathic GHD have genetic abnormalities or subtle anatomic abnormalities affecting the hypothalamus, pituitary, or both.

Pathogenesis

A list of causes of GHD is provided in Table 19-1. As mentioned already, "idiopathic" GHD constitutes by far the largest group of patients, although advances in developmental biology are forcing a rethink in this area.

GENETIC AND STRUCTURAL ABNORMALITIES

Pituitary Development

The pituitary gland, which consists of anterior, intermediate, and posterior lobes, is a central regulator of growth, metabolism, and development. Its complex functions are mediated via hormone-signaling pathways that act to regulate the finely balanced homeostatic control in vertebrates by coordinating signals from the hypothalamus to peripheral endocrine organs (thyroid, adrenals, and gonads). The mature anterior pituitary gland is populated by five neuroendocrine cell types defined by the hormone produced: corticotropes (corticotropin [formerly adrenocorticotropic hormone, ACTH]), thyrotropes (thyroid-stimulating hormone [TSH]), gonadotropes (luteinizing hormone [LH], follicle-stimulating hormone [FSH]), somatotropes (GH) and lactotropes (prolactin [PrL]).[23] The posterior gland secretes vasopressin and oxytocin. The origins of the anterior and posterior lobes of the pituitary gland are embryologically distinct. Rathke's pouch, the primordium of the anterior pituitary, arises from the oral ectoderm, whereas the posterior pituitary derives from neural ectoderm. Development of the anterior gland follows a similar pattern in a number of different species but has been best studied in rodents.

In the mouse, anterior pituitary development occurs in four distinct stages: pituitary placode formation; the development of a rudimentary Rathke's pouch; the formation of a definitive pouch; and finally the terminal differentiation of the various cell types in a temporally and spatially regulated manner (Fig. 19-2). The apposition of Rathke's pouch and the diencephalon, which

later develops into the hypothalamus, is maintained throughout the early stages of pituitary organogenesis[24] and appears to be critical for normal anterior pituitary development. A number of signaling molecules—fibroblast growth factor-8 (Fgf8),[24-26] bone morphogenetic protein 4 (Bmp4),[24,25] and Nkx2.1[26]—that are expressed in the neural ectoderm and not in Rathke's pouch are thought to play a significant role in normal anterior pituitary development, as illustrated by the phenotype of mouse mutants that are either null or hypomorphic for these alleles. These signaling molecules activate or repress key regulatory genes encoding transcription factors such as Hesx1, LIM homeobox 3 (Lhx3), and LIM homeobox 4 (Lhx4) within the developing Rathke's pouch that are essential for subsequent development of the pituitary.[23,24]

The final stage of pituitary gland development entails the terminal differentiation of the progenitor cells into the distinct cell types found within the mature pituitary gland. This process is tightly regulated by extrinsic factors (Fgf8, Bmp2, Bmp4, and Bmp7) that emanate from the surrounding infundibulum and the juxtapituitary mesenchyme. These then establish gradients of transcription factors (Lhx3, Six3, prophet of Pit1 [Prop1], Pit1, Nkx3.1, Islet-1 [Isl1], Lhx4, Six1, Brain-4 [Brn4], and pituitary forkhead [Pfrk]).[25,26] These genetic gradients lead to a wave of cell differentiation. Each of the five anterior pituitary cell types differentiates in a temporally and spatially regulated manner (Fig. 19-3),[29-32] and this process is dependent upon a number of transcription factors such as Pit1, T-pit, and steroidogenic factor 1 (Sf1).[33,34]

Table 19-1. Causes of GH Deficiency

Congenital

Genetic:
See Table 19-2

Associated With Structural Defects of the Brain:
Agenesis of the corpus callosum
Septo-optic dysplasia
Holoprosencephaly
Encephalocele
Hydrocephalus

Associated With Midline Facial Defects:
Cleft lip/palate
Single central incisor

Idiopathic

Acquired

Trauma:
Perinatal trauma
Postnatal trauma

Infection:
Meningitis/encephalitis

CNS tumors:
Craniopharyngioma
Pituitary germinoma
Histiocytosis

Following Cranial Irradiation

Following Chemotherapy

Pituitary Infarction

Neurosecretory Dysfunction

Transient:
Peripubertal
Psychosocial deprivation
Hypothyroidism

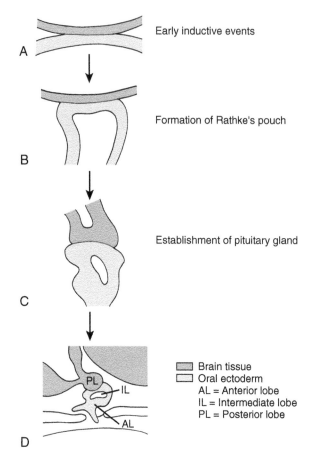

A — Early inductive events

B — Formation of Rathke's pouch

C — Establishment of pituitary gland

D

PL
IL
AL

Brain tissue
Oral ectoderm
AL = Anterior lobe
IL = Intermediate lobe
PL = Posterior lobe

FIGURE 19-2. Formation of the pituitary gland. Four-stage process commencing with early inductive events as the infundibulum of the diencephalon abuts the roof of the oral cavity. Pituitary established with signaling gradients generating spatial defined patterns of gene expression and specific cell lineages in the definitive gland. (Reproduced from Valette-Kasic and Enjalbert, Topical Endocrinology, February 2003.)

Less is known about pituitary development in humans, but it appears to mirror that in the rodent. Spontaneous or artificially induced mutations in the mouse have led to significant insights into human pituitary disease, and identification of mutations associated with human pituitary disease have in turn been invaluable in defining the genetic cascade responsible for the development of this complex structure.

Disorders of Pituitary and Extra-Pituitary Development in Humans

A number of genetic abnormalities have been identified in children who were previously thought to have idiopathic GHD or combined pituitary hormone deficiency (CPHD)[35-37] (Table 19-2). In some cases, extra-pituitary manifestations may be associated. Mutations within the paired-like homeobox gene *HESX1* are associated with the phenotypes of GHD, CPHD, and septo-optic dysplasia, a condition characterized by forebrain, pituitary, and eye abnormalities such as optic nerve hypoplasia.[38,39] The inheritance and phenotypes are variable, with both dominant and recessive modes of inheritance described. Intriguingly, *HESX1* mutations are classically associated with anterior pituitary hypoplasia with an undescended posterior pituitary and an absent or thin infundibulum.[40]

Mutations within the LIM-domain genes *LHX3* and *LHX4* are associated with CPHD with extrapituitary manifestations such as a short neck and steep cervical spine in the case of *LHX3*[41] and an abnormal cerebellum in the case of *LHX4*.[42] The inheritance of *LHX3* mutations is recessive, whereas that associated with *LHX4* mutations is dominant, unlike the murine phenotype.

Mutations within the gene encoding the transcription factor Sox2 is associated with hypopituitarism in the mouse and humans. *SOX2* is one of the earliest known genes to be expressed in embryonic stem cells and neural progenitors. Although mutations in the mouse are associated with a generalized reduction in all pituitary cell types, in the human, the most frequent pituitary defect is hypogonadotropic hypogonadism, with GHD less

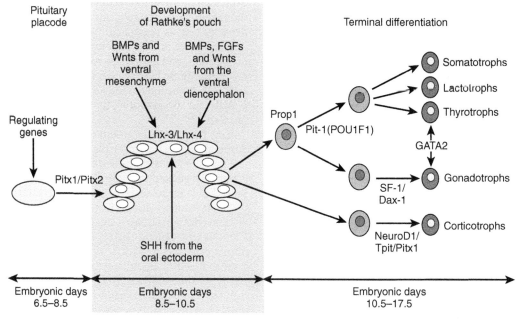

Pituitary placode

Development of Rathke's pouch

Terminal differentiation

BMPs and Wnts from ventral mesenchyme

BMPs, FGFs and Wnts from the ventral diencephalon

Regulating genes

Pitx1/Pitx2

Lhx-3/Lhx-4

SHH from the oral ectoderm

Prop1

Pit-1(POU1F1)

Somatotrophs
Lactotrophs
Thyrotrophs

GATA2

SF-1/Dax-1

Gonadotrophs

NeuroD1/Tpit/Pitx1

Corticotrophs

Embryonic days 6.5–8.5

Embryonic days 8.5–10.5

Embryonic days 10.5–17.5

FIGURE 19-3. Temporal sequence of events of pituitary development in the mouse. (Reproduced from Valette-Kasic and Enjalbert, Topical Endocrinology, February 2003.)

Table 19-2. Genes Implicated in Isolated Growth Hormone Deficiency and Combined Pituitary Hormone Deficiencies

Gene (Murine/Human)	Protein (Murine/Human)	Murine Loss of Function Phenotype	Human Phenotype	Inheritance Murine/Human
Hesx1/HESX1	Hesx1/HESX1	Anophthalmia or microphthalmia, agenesis of corpus callosum, absence of septum pellucidum, pituitary dysgenesis or aplasia	Variable: SOD, CPHD, IGHD with EPP/dominant or recessive	Dominant or recessive in both
Sox3/SOX3	Sox3/SOX3	Unknown	Isolated GHD with mental retardation	Unknown in mouse; X-linked in man
Lhx3/LHX3	Lhx3/LHX3	Hypoplasia of Rathke's pouch	GH, TSH, gonadotropin deficiency with pituitary hypoplasia Corticotrophs spared. Short, rigid cervical spine with limited rotation	Recessive in both
Lhx4/LHX4	Lhx4/LHX4	Mild hypoplasia of anterior pituitary	GH, TSH, cortisol deficiency, persistent craniopharyngeal canal, and abnormal cerebellar tonsils	Recessive in mouse, dominant in humans
Prop1/PROP1	Prop1/PROP1	Hypoplasia of anterior pituitary with reduced somatotrophs, lactotrophs, thyrotrophs, and gonadotrophs	GH, TSH, prolactin, and gonadotropin deficiency. Evolving ACTH deficiency. Enlarged pituitary with later involution	Recessive in both
Pit1/POU1F1 (PIT1)	Pou1f1/POU1F1	Anterior pituitary hypoplasia with reduced somatotrophs, lactotrophs, and thyrotrophs	Variable anterior pituitary hypoplasia with GH, TSH, and prolactin deficiencies	Recessive in mouse, dominant/recessive in man
Ghrhr/GHRHR	Ghrhr/GHRHR	Reduced somatotrophs with anterior pituitary hypoplasia	GH deficiency with anterior pituitary hypoplasia	Recessive
Gh-1/GH-1	Growth hormone (GH)		GH deficiency	Recessive, dominant, or X-linked in man

ACTH, Adrenocorticotropic hormone; *CPHD*, combined pituitary hormone deficiency; *EPP*, ectopic posterior pituitary; *GHD*, growth hormone deficiency; *IGHD*, isolated GH deficiency; *SOD*, septo-optic dysplasia; *TSH*, thyroid-stimulating hormone.

frequent. Other features include severe eye defects, esophageal atresia, hypothalamic hamartomata, learning difficulties, and sensorineural hearing loss.[43,44]

Recent studies with *SOX3* suggest a possible explanation for the predominance of males in many series of GHD. *SOX3* is sited on the X chromosome (Xq26-27) and appears not only to be important in pituitary development but is also associated with mental retardation.[45] These observations of GHD and brain developmental abnormalities are particularly important because neurodevelopmental handicap has often been ascribed to untreated neonatal hypoglycemia, whereas structural developmental problems may be a more pertinent explanation.

It is clear that our understanding of the etiology of hypopituitarism is rudimentary. The mechanisms whereby mutations in the genes that have been identified to date lead to a particular phenotype are largely unknown. Additionally, many cases of hypopituitarism may be due to changes in regulatory regions of known genes or perhaps within novel genes that have yet to be identified.

Growth Hormone–Releasing Hormone and Its Receptor

Because growth hormone–releasing hormone (GHRH) and its receptor (GHRHR; GHD Type 1B) are critical to somatotroph population expansion, abnormalities in either are likely to be associated with severe GHD. No mutations of the human *GHRH* gene have been identified, but mutations in *GHRHR* have been identified in a number of pedigrees.[46] Two large pedigrees have been identified in Pakistan (Glu72Stop mutation)[47] and in northeastern Brazil (donor splice mutation in position 1 of intron 1; IVS1, G-A, +1).[48] All patients reported to date have been either homozygous or compound heterozygous for mutations of the *GHRHR* gene. Serum GH concentrations fail to rise following standard provocative testing, as well as after GHRH administra-

tion. The patients resemble the *little* mouse (lit/lit), which has a mutation of the GHRH receptor gene affecting the ligand-binding domain (Asp60Gly; D60G).[49]

Somatotroph Development

A number of mouse models exist in which somatotrope development has been impaired. These include the Ames, the Jackson, and the Snell dwarf mice. A missense point mutation within the prophet of Pit1, or *PROP1* gene (S83P), has been shown to be responsible for the Ames dwarf mouse.[50] The phenotype results from a failure of initial determination of the Pit1 lineage required for production of GH, PrL, and TSH. The Ames pituitary gland contains less than 1% of the normal complement of somatotrophs and decreased numbers of lactotrophs and thyrotrophs. In humans, mutations within the transcription factor Prop1 are associated with CPHD in the form of GH, prolactin, TSH, and gonadotropin deficiency.[51,52] A proportion of individuals with *PROP1* mutations will develop cortisol deficiency.[53] Additionally, a number of individuals with mutations within *PROP1* develop transient pituitary masses with subsequent involution (Fig. 19-4).[54] The exact mechanism underlying this phenomenon remains unclear, but it is clearly important to exclude mutations within *PROP1* in patients with pituitary "tumors" especially the nonfunctional variety. There is considerable variability in the timing of the endocrinopathy, and a number of patients will actually commence puberty but then arrest halfway through. Recently, a mutation within *PROP1* was identified in a patient who actually achieved a normal final height without receiving any GH treatment. *PROP1* mutations are thought to be the commonest cause of familial CPHD and are usually recessive.

Pit1 (now known as Pou1f1)[55,56] is a member of the POU family of homeodomain proteins and contains a highly conserved bipartite DNA-binding domain consisting of the POU

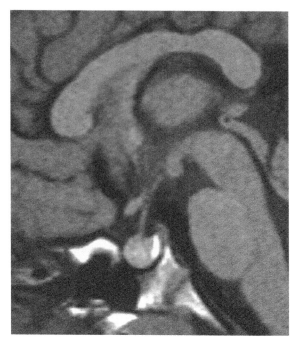

FIGURE 19-4. Pituitary "tumor" in patient with *PROP-1* mutation. Saggital MRI scan of the pituitary revealing a large, globular anterior pituitary with normal posterior pituitary enhancement. Subsequent scans revealed involution of the mass and resultant empty sella.

Table 19-3. Genetic Abnormalities in GH1

A.	Type 1	Type 1A. Autosomal recessive GHD due to total absence of GH synthesis. Type 1B. Autosomal recessive GHD due to splicing defects in *GH1* or defects in *GHRHR* genes.
B.	Type 2	Autosomal dominant GHD due to splice-site and missense mutations in the *GH1* gene, resulting in dominant negative expression of the *GH1* gene. Abnormal folding of mutant interferes with storage and secretion.
C.	Type 3	X-linked GHD. Xq21-q22 with X-linked agammaglobulinemia and Xq22-q27 with X-linked mental retardation.

homeodomain, required for low-affinity DNA binding, and a POU-specific domain, responsible for the specificity of DNA binding and potential interactions with other proteins. The Snell dwarf mouse, characterized by pituitary hypoplasia and GH, PrL, and TSH deficiencies, has a point mutation (W261C) within the Pit1 gene, affecting the third helix of the POU homeodomain. This abrogates binding of Pit1 to its target promoter sequences. Several mutations and deletions of the *POU1F1* gene have been identified in humans with CPHD, characterized by the combination of GH, PrL, and TSH deficiency.[57,58] Mutations have been described which separately affect the DNA-binding capacity of *POU1F1* or its transactivation properties. Autosomal dominant transmission, resulting from a dominant negative effect, has been observed in mutations affecting dimerization of *POU1F1*, transactivation (P24L), or in the relatively common R271W mutation, which results in increased binding to promoter elements and disruption of transcriptional activation.[59] Autosomal recessive transmission is found with other mutations, such as A172stop, E250stop, R143G, A158P, and P239S.[60] Variability in phenotype has been reported, although most patients exhibit growth retardation during the first year of life. GH and PrL deficiency is complete; TSH secretion may be observed during infancy but declines progressively during the early months of life. Magnetic resonance imaging (MRI) scanning revealed a marked variability in the size of the anterior pituitary, with some patients demonstrating a normal pituitary and others having a hypoplastic pituitary. After appropriate GH and thyroxine replacement, patients appear to enter puberty normally and have normal fertility. Lactation may be impaired. In some patients, TSH secretion may be normal.[61]

GH1 Gene

The *GH1* gene, located at chromosome 17q22-24, is part of a cluster of five structurally related genes: *GH1*, *CSHP* (chorionic somatomammotropin pseudogene), *CSH* (chorionic somatomammotropin), *GH2* (or placental variant), and *CSH2*. Mutations within the *GH1* gene are associated with isolated GH deficiency (Table 19-3). Large, recessive, inherited deletions are associated with absence of GH protein (Type 1A GHD). Complete loss of pituitary GH secretion occurs secondary to deletions resulting from nonhomologous crossing over at different sites in the GH and chorionic somatomammotropin (CS) gene cluster. The most common deletion is 6.7 kb, but deletions of 7.0, 7.6, and greater than 45 kb have also been observed.[62] Wagner et al.[63] have also described the GHD 1A phenotype in a patient with a point mutation in the GH signal peptide, E23X, resulting in premature termination of translation. Patients typically have an excellent initial response to GH therapy, but because of the absence of a normal GH molecule in fetal life, an attenuation of the growth response to exogenous GH may result from the development of anti-GH antibodies,[64] although this event has been described less frequently with newer GH preparations.

Type 1B GHD is due to homozygous splice-site mutations within the GH1 gene or homozygous mutations within the GHRHR. It is associated with an excellent response to GH treatment, with no formation of antibodies.

Type II GHD is autosomal dominant and associated with splice-site mutations.[65] These mutations lead to the production of two alternatively spliced GH molecules, 20 and 17.5 kD hGH. Mutations in an exon splice enhancer within exon 3 of the *GH1* gene have also been associated with autosomal dominant GHD.[66] The generation of the 17.5 kD form of hGH has a dominant negative effect and prevents the secretion of the normal wild-type 22kD hGH, with a consequent deleterious effect on pituitary somatotropes. In a murine model of this dominant negative mutation, there is loss of somatotroph number[67] and progressive damage to adjacent pituitary cells (with later failure of PrL, TSH, and gonadotropin secretion).[68]

Seven different splice-site mutations have been reported to date. In addition, three missense mutations (R183H, P89L, and V110F) were also recently implicated in IGHD Type II. These patients have a normal *GH1* allele but are unable to secrete the normal form of GH in appropriate concentrations. The mutant protein therefore exerts a dominant negative effect. As in the mouse evolution of other hormonal deficiencies, including ACTH, TSH, and gonadotropin, deficiencies have been described in patients with some dominant *GH1* mutations.[69]

GHD Type III, an X-linked form of isolated GH deficiency (IGHD), has been reported in patients with hypogammaglobulinemia. To date, no alteration in the *GH1* gene has been identified in this condition, and the genetic mechanisms remain unknown. Recently a polyalanine expansion within the transcription factor Sox3, which lies at Xq26-27, has been associated with X-linked GHD and mental retardation.[45] Intriguingly, duplications of this region of the X chromosome have been associated with X-linked panhypopituitarism, and *SOX3* has been implicated as the gene associated with this phenotype.[70,71]

Bioinactive Growth Hormone Molecule

Since the GH molecule exists in multiple molecular forms resulting from alternative splicing or posttranslational processing, some cases of short stature have been hypothesized to be the consequence of abnormal ratios of the various GH forms.[72] The first report of two individuals heterozygous for point mutations in the GH gene was described by Takahashi et al. and detailed the biochemistry and molecular genetics.[73] The mutant GH molecules (R77C and D112G) were capable of binding to the GH receptor, perhaps even with increased affinity, but were unable to stimulate tyrosine phosphorylation of GH-activated intracellular signaling intermediates in a normal manner. The ability of the R77C mutant to behave in a dominant negative manner was demonstrated by its ability to inhibit the in vitro actions of wild-type GH.

Structural Abnormalities

In addition to the structural abnormalities associated with the genetic problems described above, GHD can occur in the setting of other cranial or midline abnormalities such as holoprosencephaly, nasal encephalocele, single central incisor, and cleft lip and palate.

As methods of radiologic evaluation of the CNS have improved, an increasing percentage of patients with idiopathic GHD have been identified to have structural abnormalities.[74-80] Many of these are associated with some of the genetic abnormalities described above, but the findings are worthy of separate consideration. In particular, the finding on MRI of an undescended (erroneously called "ectopic") posterior pituitary (PPE) was commoner in males than females (3:1 when PPE present versus 1:1 if normal anatomy) in patients with CPHD as compared with IGHD (49% versus 12%), breech delivery (32% versus 7%), and associated congenital brain anomalies (12% versus 7%).

These findings appear to be best explained by a defect in induction of the mediobasal structure of the brain in the early embryo rather than the product of birth trauma, as previously suggested.[77] Whether pituitary insufficiency is the result of hypothalamic or pituitary dysgenesis or the product of hypoplasia or sectioning of the pituitary stalk is not always clear. Perinatal problems, however, including breech presentation, may prove to be the consequence rather than the cause of underlying CNS abnormality. The concept that PPE, stalk section or hypoplasia, and pituitary hypoplasia may represent abnormal embryonic development rather than the consequences of birth trauma is supported by the finding of similar anatomic abnormalities in patients with septo-optic dysplasia, type I Arnold-Chiari syndrome, holoprosencephaly, and increasingly in patients with mutations in the genes controlling pituitary development.

In the empty sella syndrome, abnormalities of the sellar diaphragm allow herniation of the suprasellar subarachnoid space into the region of the sella turcica.[81] This may result in damage to the sella, including the pituitary. Empty sella syndrome may be the consequence of surgery or irradiation, or may be idiopathic. It is often found in patients with mutations in *PROP-1*, when it may have been preceded by a pituitary mass.

ACQUIRED DEFECTS

Destructive Lesions of the Hypothalamus and Pituitary

A wide range of destructive lesions involving the hypothalamus or pituitary may present with isolated GHD or CPHD. Birth trauma, associated with abrupt delivery, prolonged labor, or extensive use of forceps, has been associated frequently with subsequent hypothalamic or pituitary dysfunction.[82,83] An increased incidence of GHD has been reported in breech deliveries, although it is still unclear whether such deliveries lead to acquisition of pituitary dysfunction or, on the other hand, whether preexisting CNS abnormalities result in higher rates of abnormal birth presentations.

Tumors

Central nervous system tumors are an important cause of isolated GHD and CPHD and must be excluded in every child with GHD who does not have an obvious alternative explanation for growth failure. Midline brain tumors include germinomas, meningiomas, gliomas, colloid cysts of the third ventricle, ependymomas, and optic nerve gliomas. GHD or CPHD may also occur from local extension of tumors affecting the head or neck, such as craniopharyngeal carcinomas and lymphomas.

The major pediatric tumor involving the pituitary is craniopharyngioma, which is probably an evolving congenital malformation which develops from remnants of Rathke's pouch.[84] It accounts for 5% to 15% of intracranial tumors in childhood and 80% of tumors in the hypothalamo-pituitary region. Arising from rests of squamous cells at the embryonic junction of the adenohypophysis and neurohypophysis, it forms an enlarging cyst filled with degenerating cells, leading to cyst fluid or calcification but never to malignant degeneration (Fig. 19-5). These calcifications may be seen at times on skull films and constitute an important diagnostic sign. Although craniopharyngiomas represent the consequences of a congenital malformation, they may present clinically at any age. Significant growth failure may be observed at the time of diagnosis, but patients most commonly present with complaints of increased intracranial pressure, such as headaches, vomiting, and oculomotor disturbances; visual field defects are frequently noted at the time of diagnosis.[84] Deficiency of at least one pituitary hormone, most commonly GH or gonadotropin, is present in 50% to 80% of patients. Diabetes insipidus is reported in 25% to 50% of patients at diagnosis.[84,85]

Langerhans cell histiocytosis may also present at any age. Langerhans cell histiocytosis (LCH) is characterized by clonal proliferation and accumulation of abnormal dendritic cells that can affect either a single site or many systems, causing multiorgan dysfunction. In children, the median age of diagnosis ranges between 1.8 and 3.4 years.[86] LCH infiltrates the hypothalamo-pituitary area in 15% to 35% of patients, with subsequent development of at least one pituitary hormone deficiency.[87] In a multicenter French national study of 589 pediatric patients with LCH, 145 patients (25%) had pituitary dysfunction. In 60 patients, pituitary involvement was already present at the time of diagnosis, and in 20 of them, it was the first manifestation of the disease. Patients at high risk of pituitary involvement seem to be those with multi-system disease involving skull and facial bones, mastoid, sinuses, and mucous membranes (i.e., gums, ear, nose, and throat region). Furthermore, compared to patients without pituitary involvement, patients with pituitary involvement have a higher rate of relapse (10% at 5 years versus

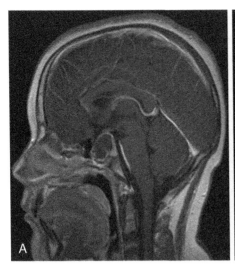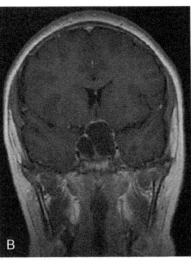

FIGURE 19-5. MRI of cystic craniopharyngioma. Saggital MRI scan **(A)** revealing large multicystic craniopharyngioma arising from the pituitary fossa and extending up to hypothalamus. Coronal section **(B)** of same lesion delineating upward and lateral spread. Both images are T-1 weighted, gadolinium-enhanced scans.

4.8% at 5 years) and a higher incidence of neurodegenerative LCH.[88]

Diabetes insipidus is the most frequently reported permanent consequence of LCH and the commonest endocrinopathy; almost all patients with pituitary involvement have DI. The second commonest endocrinopathy is GHD, which occurs in 14% of all patients with LCH and in more than 40% of patients who have pituitary involvement.[87] In the vast majority of patients, GHD is associated with DI, with a median interval of 2.9 to 3.5 years between the diagnosis of DI and development of GHD. Isolated GHD, or the association of GHD with other anterior pituitary hormone deficiencies, occurs less commonly.

Pituitary MRI findings in patients with LCH include thickening of the pituitary stalk, suggestive of the infiltrative process enhancing changes in the pituitary gland and hypothalamus, and absence of the bright signal of the posterior pituitary in T1-weighted images, caused by the loss of the phospholipid-rich ADH secretory granules. The latter is an invariable feature of patients who develop DI.[89] Although at the time of diagnosis of DI, 75% show a thickened pituitary stalk, only 24% have persistent stalk thickening after 5 years. These changes are variable and do not correlate with treatment or with clinical recovery; DI persists in all cases.

Long-term follow-up of patients with LCH has shown that the already established hormone deficiencies cannot be reversed by treatment.[89] Recently, however, isolated case reports have suggested that treatment with the purine analogue 2-chlorodeoxy-adenosine (2-CDA) may reverse established DI.[90] Subsequent studies of this form of therapy, used in refractory cases of LCH involving the CNS, showed that 2-CDA may result in partial or complete radiologic improvement of the mass lesion, but the endocrine consequences of the disease, including DI and panhypopituitarism, do not reverse.[91] Patients treated with the JLSG-96 protocol who have been followed up for 5 years developed DI with an incidence of 3.1% to 8.9%, depending on the extension of the disease (single system multisite versus multisystem).[92]

Radiotherapy used for the treatment of LCH is within the dose range of 10 to 15 Gy, which is known to be unlikely to cause GHI. However, radiotherapy has been associated with an increased risk of GHD despite the fact that the dose was less than 15 Gy, a finding that may reflect the severity and extent of the disease rather than the direct effect of radiotherapy.

Irradiation of the Central Nervous System

Cranial irradiation used for the therapy of solid brain tumors and as prophylaxis for leukemia can lead to abnormal hypothalamo-pituitary function. The sensitivity of the HP axis to radiation depends upon the dose, fractionation, tissue location, and the age of the patient.[93] Such damage is typically difficult to assess precisely, since the hypothalamus and pituitary may differ in the extent of involvement, and the loss of function may evolve with time. Sensitivity to CNS radiation may differ among patients, although the majority of children will experience some degree of hypothalamic or pituitary dysfunction within 5 years of receiving 30 Gy.[94] GHD also occurs with doses of 18-24 Gy,[95] and subtle dysfunction may be observed at even lower doses. GH secretion generally appears to be the most sensitive to irradiation, followed by TSH, gonadotropins, and finally ACTH. This may relate to the unique position of the GHRH neurons on the surface of the hypothalamus and not deep within the structure as previously thought.[96]

Pituitary dysfunction evolves over several years following irradiation, so such children should be monitored for growth deceleration. Provocative GH testing may be within normal limits, but measures of spontaneous GH secretion frequently demonstrate abnormalities.[97] Serum concentrations of IGF-1 or insulin-like growth factor–binding protein-3 (IGFBP-3) may not be reduced in the early years following cranial irradiation.[98]

Cranial irradiation may also result in precocious puberty, leading to an early pubertal growth spurt, advanced skeletal maturation, and ultimately reduced stature. This may be superimposed upon any growth restriction that results from the spinal irradiation for the primary problem.[99] Low-dose irradiation is frequently associated with a precocious onset of puberty; higher doses may result in gonadotropin deficiency and pubertal delay. In the irradiated child with early puberty, therapy with gonadotropin-releasing hormone (GnRH) analogues should be considered, with or without GH treatment, to delay epiphyseal fusion.

Lower doses of radiation (24 Gy) are also associated with GHD in approximately 30% to 60% of cases. Craniospinal irradiation used in the treatment of posterior fossa tumors and total body irradiation used in conditioning regimens for bone marrow transplant are also associated with damage to the epiphyses, with subsequent disproportionate short stature.

Traumatic Brain Injury

Traumatic brain injury (TBI) has been recognized as a cause of acquired hypopituitarism in a number of adult studies. Data on pediatric patients are sporadic, but TBI is probably underdiagnosed.[100] These effects may be significant, considering the scale of the problem. In the United Kingdom, 180 children per 100,000 population per year sustain a head injury, with 5.6 per 100,000 requiring intensive care and almost one third of those admitted to ICU undergoing neurosurgery.

Although the pituitary gland is protected within the bony cavity of the sella turcica, the rich vascular network of the hypothalamus and pituitary and the structure of the pituitary stalk make it vulnerable to the effects of traumatic brain injury. The hypothalamus and pituitary have a complex vascular supply consisting of an arterial supply via the superior and inferior hypophyseal arteries from the internal carotid artery, as well as long hypophyseal vessels and a rich network of portal capillaries that surround the pituitary and infundibulum. The pathophysiology of hypopituitarism related to TBI is not clearly defined, but it is thought that it is the result of direct trauma or of vascular injury resulting in ischemia and infarction,[101] an observation supported by the anatomical findings of autopsies following head trauma which include anterior lobe necrosis, pituitary fibrosis, hemorrhage, infarction, or necrosis of the pituitary stalk.[102]

Hormone deficiencies may be identified in the first days to weeks posttrauma (acute phase) or may develop over time (late effect). Because there is overlap between the symptoms and signs of hypopituitarism and those of neurologic/psychologic sequelae of TBI, it is possible that late evolving or partial deficiencies can remain undiagnosed for extended periods.

In the acute phase, alterations in the endocrine function may reflect an adaptive response to acute illness. The clinically significant alterations involve mainly the regulation of fluid and electrolyte balance (diabetes insipidus, SIADH, cerebral salt wasting) and the hypothalamo-pituitary adrenal axis. Most of the pituitary hormone changes observed in the acute phase are transient, and their development cannot predict the development of permanent hypopituitarism.[103]

Pituitary hormone deficiencies present in the acute phase are usually transient, but they may persist or appear and evolve over time. In adults, the incidence of permanent hypopituitarism ranges between 23% to 69%, depending on the study. The GH axis is the most frequently affected (10% to 33%), followed by the gonadal (8% to 23%), adrenal (5% to 23%), and thyroid (2% to 22%) axis. The prevalence of permanent DI varies between 0% and 6%.

Until recently, there were only sporadic reports of hypopituitarism following TBI in children, but prospective studies designed to address the problem in the pediatric and adolescent population are in progress. The incidence of hypopituitarism is reported to range from 10% to 60%, and although this is lower in children as compared with adults, it is not uncommon.[104] In general, the long-term outcome of TBI seems to be more favorable in children, although quality-of-life issues and minor disability may persist. The extent to which endocrine dysfunction contributes to these outcomes has yet to be defined.

Growth hormone deficiency appears to be the main endocrine manifestation, followed by gonadotropin deficiency. GHD can present as growth failure, whereas delayed or arrested puberty and secondary amenorrhea may present in adolescents and in patients in the transition phase. In a number of case reports, central precocious puberty has also been described in association with head injury, presenting 0.4 to 1.6 years after the event.[105]

Patients with hypopituitarism after head injury may have no clinical signs and symptoms suggestive of this disorder; its correct identification requires a high degree of suspicion. A consensus guideline on the screening of patients post TBI suggests that all patients who had TBI, regardless of its severity, should undergo baseline endocrine evaluation 3 and 12 months after the event or discharge from ITU.[106]

Infiltrative and Inflammatory Disorders

Infiltrative diseases are uncommon causes of GHD in the pediatric population, but pituitary insufficiency may be observed secondary to CNS involvement in tuberculosis,[107] sarcoidosis,[108] or toxoplasmosis. Inflammation associated with bacterial, viral, fungal, or parasitic disease may also result in hypothalamic-pituitary dysfunction. Lymphadenoid hypophysitis has also been reported.

Thalassemia is a hereditary disorder characterized by quantitative defects in synthesis of globin chains that result in ineffective erythropoiesis and, in its more severe forms, transfusion dependence. The majority of complications are the consequence of the toxic effects of iron which is deposited in organs of the reticuloendothelial system, the heart, and all target organs of the endocrine system, including the pituitary.[109] The anterior pituitary is very sensitive to iron overload, resulting in defective GH secretion, reduced responsiveness of GH to GHRH, and hypogonadotropic hypogonadism. The gonadotroph cells seem to be particularly vulnerable to the toxic effects of iron deposition, which may be related to the way iron is transported in cells. Failure of pubertal development and growth impairment are the most prominent endocrine complications and may occur despite early initiation of chelation therapy. It is estimated that 56% of thalassemic patients have at least one endocrinopathy; almost half have hypogonadism (40% to 59%), and 33% to 36% manifest growth failure.[110] The growth impairment is the result of a number of factors that include chronic anemia and tissue hypoxia, overchelation due to the toxic effects of desferrioxamine on spinal cartilage, GH insufficiency, and possible GH insensitivity.

Vascular Lesions

Aneurysms may behave as space-occupying lesions and cause hypothalamic or pituitary destruction.

Psychosocial Dwarfism

Psychosocial dwarfism is a form of poor growth associated with bizarre eating and drinking behavior, social withdrawal, delayed speech, and on occasion other evidence of developmental delay.[111] Periodic hyperphagia is associated with decreased GH responsiveness to standard provocative stimuli but also with subnormal responses to exogenous GH therapy. Removal from the stressful environment, which usually involves removal from the home, is accompanied by a restoration of normal GH secretion, typically within weeks, and a period of catch-up growth.[112,113] The mechanisms for this reversible form of GHD are unclear, but it is of note that a variety of psychiatric conditions in adults may be associated with decreased spontaneous and provocative GH secretion. Establishing the diagnosis of psychosocial dwarfism requires documentation of catch-up growth and restoration of normal GH secretion following correction of the environmental situation.

Clinical Features

THE HYPOTHALAMO-PITUITARY-SOMATOTROPH AXIS

Growth hormone is secreted by somatotropes in the anterior pituitary gland. The secretory pattern is pulsatile, with discrete pulses of GH every 3 to 4 hours and virtually undetectable GH concentrations in between. Secretion of GH varies considerably with age[114] and shows a sexually dimorphic pattern,[115] with a greater average daily GH output in women. This pattern is the result of an interaction between the hypothalamic peptides GHRH and somatostatin (SS). The amplitude of the GH peak is determined by GHRH that stimulates the pituitary somatotrophs to increase both the secretion of stored GH and GH gene transcription. SS determines trough levels of GH by inhibition of GHRH release from the hypothalamus and GH release from the pituitary. Withdrawal of SS, on the other hand, determines the timing of a GH pulse.

More recently, the use of synthetic GH-releasing peptides (GHRP) has led to the identification of a GH secretagogue (GHS) receptor (GHS-R type 1a). The receptor is strongly expressed in the hypothalamus, but specific binding sites for GHRP have also been identified in other regions of the CNS and peripheral endocrine and nonendocrine tissues in both humans and other organisms.[116,117] The endogenous ligand for the GHS receptor, ghrelin, was isolated from the stomach and is an octynylated peptide consisting of 28 amino acids.[118] It is expressed predominantly in the stomach, but lower amounts are present within the bowel, pancreas, kidney, immune system, placenta, pituitary, testis, ovary, and hypothalamus.[119] Ghrelin not only leads to the secretion of GH but also stimulates prolactin and ACTH secretion. Additionally, it influences endocrine pancreatic function and glucose metabolism, gonadal function, appetite, and behavior. It can also control gastric motility and acid secretion and has cardiovascular and antiproliferative effects. The role of endogenous ghrelin in normal growth during childhood remains unclear. Both ghrelin and GHRPs release GH synergistically with GHRH.

The expression of the human GH gene is regulated not only by a proximal promoter but also by a locus control region (LCR) 15 to 32 kb upstream of the *GH-1* gene. The LCR confers pituitary-specific, high-level expression of GH.[120,121] The full-length transcript from the *GH1* gene encodes a 191-amino-acid, 22-kD protein that accounts for 85% to 90% of circulating GH. Alternative splicing of the mRNA transcript generates a 20-kD form of GH that accounts for the remaining 10% to 15%. Within both the proximal promoter and the LCR are located binding sites for the pituitary-specific transcription factor Pit1. Additional binding sites for the transcription factor Zn15 are also located within the proximal promoter.

In the circulation, GH binds to two binding proteins, high-affinity GHBP and low-affinity GHBP.[122] Little is known about the low-affinity GHBP, which accounts for approximately 10% to 15% of GH binding, with a preference for binding to 20-kD hGH. The high-affinity GHBP is a 61-kD, glycosylated protein that represents a soluble form of the extracellular domain of the GH receptor that can bind to both 20 and 22 kD hGH and thereby prolong the half-life of GH. In-vivo studies that have co-administered GH and GHBP to hypophysectomized and GH-deficient rats have demonstrated a potentiation of weight gain and bone growth, although similar studies have not as yet been performed in man.[123]

The GH receptor (GHR) is present in a number of tissues. The hormone sequentially dimerizes its receptor, activating a receptor-associated tyrosine kinase JAK2 that in turn is auto-phosphorylated and also phosphorylates the GHR. This then leads to signal transduction using the MAPK, STAT, and PI3 kinase pathways. The end result is activation of a number of genes that mediate the effects of GH. These include early-response genes encoding transcription factors such as c-jun, c-fos, and c-myc—implicated in cell growth, proliferation, and differentiation—and IGF-I, which mediates the growth-promoting effects of GH.[124,125]

IGF-I and IGF-II are single-chain polypeptide hormones that are widely expressed. Together with a family of specific binding proteins, they are believed to mediate most of the actions of GH.

NEONATAL PRESENTATION

Recent studies in humans and in animal models have demonstrated marked similarities but also critical differences between the clinical features of GHD and various forms of IGF deficiency.[126-128] In GHD, prenatal growth is near normal, although mild reductions in birth length and weight have been observed. GHD does not cause severe IUGR, whereas loss of placental GH does.[129] However, loss of IGF-I in utero results in severe intrauterine growth restriction in both humans and mice,[130,131] suggesting that IGF-I and the IGF-I receptor are critically involved in intrauterine growth. IGF-I synthesis and secretion in utero are not regulated primarily by pituitary GH.

IGF-I production comes under GH regulation either in the last few months of fetal life or shortly after birth and is well established by 6 months of age. Growth failure is greater for skeletal growth than for body weight, so infants and young children have an appearance of relative adiposity. Neonates may present with hypoglycemia, and this suggests the possibility of other pituitary hormone deficiencies, especially ACTH. Normoglycemia is only maintained when cortisol replacement therapy is commenced, suggesting that ACTH (and consequently cortisol) secretion is critical for glucose homeostasis. However, the GH-IGF-I axis also plays a role in maintaining glucose homeostasis, although IGHD is rarely associated with neonatal hypoglycemia. A diagnostic fast may be required to dissect CPHD from other causes of hypoglycemia, although the distinguishing feature from hyperinsulinism is the absence of ketone body formation in the latter.

The presence of concomitant gonadotropin deficiency is suggested by the presence of microphallus, cryptorchidism, and scrotal hypoplasia. Genital ambiguity would not be expected, owing to placental production of hCG. Prolonged jaundice with conjugated hyperbilirubinemia and cholestasis may also be observed, typically in patients with CPHD. The relative contributions of GH, ACTH, and TSH deficiency to this presentation are unclear. It is imperative that the diagnosis of pituitary insufficiency be considered in any infant (especially term) with hypoglycemia, cryptorchidism, and microphallus, or conjugated hyperbilirubinemia. Associated features that might indicate more widespread problems (midline defects of the face, a single central incisor, nystagmus, and/or optic nerve hypoplasia) should be looked for and MRI undertaken.

INFANT AND CHILDHOOD YEARS

After the perinatal period, the defining feature of GHD is growth failure. Reduced skeletal growth may be observed during the first 6 months of life in congenital GHD, but by 6 to 12 months of age, early growth failure is almost inevitable.[132-134] Height velocity is usually between −2 and −5 standard deviations (SD) from the mean, leading to progressive height centile crossing. In patients with acquired GHD, the critical feature is a change in growth rate. Between the age of 2 years and the onset of puberty, children maintain their height percentile with remarkable integrity. Deviation from this channel (either acceleration or deceleration) needs investigation. Thus a child who has been growing along the 75th percentile but moves across to the 25th percentile warrants evaluation, even though his/her height may still be within the normal range.

Bone age is often delayed in patients with GHD, but this may not be so in acquired GHD. The close proximity of time to the growth failure or acquired GHD accompanied by accelerated puberty is occasionally seen in patients with intracranial tumors, when bone age may be accelerated.[93,94] Delayed dentition may be observed, but in the absence of midline craniofacial abnormalities is otherwise normal. Other skeletal appearances include hypoplasia of facial bones, hypoplastic nasal bridge, frontal bossing, and delayed closure of sutures. Head circumference is usually at the lower limits of normal, indicating normal brain growth.

An increase in adiposity, particularly central adiposity, can be detected by careful measurement of skinfold thicknesses. Genital growth prior to the onset of puberty is usually proportional to body size. Puberty may be delayed, but in the absence of other endocrine deficiencies is otherwise normal.

Limited data are available on the adult height of untreated GHD patients. These results are often difficult to interpret because of (1) heterogeneity in the timing of GHD, (2) heterogeneity in the severity of GHD, (3) the presence or absence of other pituitary deficiencies, and (4) delay in puberty, resulting in late epiphyseal fusion. Wit et al.[135] summarized the results from studies of 22 untreated men and 14 untreated women with severe isolated GHD and reported a mean adult height of −4.7 SD. In patients with untreated autosomal recessive GHD, Rimoin and colleagues reported mean adult heights of −7.4 SD.[136] In patients with CPHD, adult height is often not as severely affected as in IGHD, presumably reflecting pubertal delay and late epiphyseal fusion.[137]

Diagnosis of Growth Hormone Deficiency in Childhood

The diagnostic evaluation of children with growth failure is complex because there are multiple causes for short stature (Table 19-4). In the pursuit of the diagnosis of GHD, other causes for short stature need to be considered and excluded. This is because the diagnosis of GHD is one of exclusion.[138] GH is the final common pathway for postnatal growth, and many causes of poor growth may secondarily affect GH secretion.[139] There are a number of tests available for assessing GH status. Considerable attention has been paid to the underlying mechanisms assessed by the tests, how the samples should be collected, and what type of measurement should be performed. Less attention has been paid to the statistical assumptions underlying the performance of diagnostic tests. The statistical theory behind many tests is complex because the results do not follow an all-or-none law. Rather than being left with a clear-cut answer to the initial diagnostic question, the clinician is more likely to be left with a series of probabilities as to whether or not the patient is likely to have GHD.

Table 19-4. Causes of Short Stature

Nonpathogenic
Constitutional delay of growth and puberty
Familial short stature
Nutritional

Low Birth Weight

Systemic Disorders
Cardiovascular disease (e.g., congenital heart disease)
Renal (e.g., chronic renal failure, renal tubular disease)
Respiratory (e.g., cystic fibrosis, asthma)
Gastrointestinal disease (e.g., Crohn's disease)
Neurologic (e.g., brain tumor)
Psychologic (e.g., anorexia nervosa, child abuse)

Endocrine Causes
GH-related causes
Growth hormone (GH) deficiency: isolated or combined with other hormone deficiencies
Resistance to GH
IGFI deficiency
Hypothyroidism
Pseudohypoparathyroidism
Glucocorticoid excess
Cushing's syndrome
Congenital adrenal hyperplasia
Exogenous administration

Genetic Causes
Turner's syndrome
Noonan's syndrome
Down syndrome
Skeletal dysplasias: hypochondroplasia, achondroplasia, spondylo-epiphyseal dysplasia
Russell-Silver syndrome
Seckel's syndrome
Prader-Willi syndrome
Miscellaneous other syndromes (e.g., Rothmund-Thompson syndrome, Leri-Weill syndrome, progeria, mucopolysaccharidoses)

GUIDANCE DERIVED FROM CLINICAL ASSESSMENT
Neonatal Period

Several pointers to the diagnosis of GHD have already been considered in this discussion, but in the neonatal period, GHD may be isolated or associated with other pituitary hormone deficiencies. Small genitalia may point to associated gonadotropin deficiency. Hypoglycemia in the newborn period is often a feature of ACTH deficiency, although on an arbitrary basis, a serum GH of less than 10 ng/mL is considered consistent with a diagnosis of GHD under these circumstances.[140] This is not universal, however, and caution needs to be exercised in interpreting the GH response to hypoglycemia under different circumstances.[141] Prolonged neonatal jaundice raises the question of thyroxine (unconjugated) or cortisol (conjugated hyperbilirubinemia) deficiency. Given these features, it might be possible on the basis of pattern recognition to ascribe the diagnosis of GHD to a patient with a high degree of certainty. MRI of the brain should be obtained to look for an undescended posterior pituitary, anterior pituitary hypoplasia, hypoplasia or absence of the pituitary stalk, hypoplasia of the optic chiasm, and absence or hypoplasia of the corpus callosum and septum pellucidum.[74-80]

Infancy and Childhood

Diagnostic evaluation in children must be based upon auxology. Although there are a number of clinical features of GHD which are said to be classic, none is specific. For example, obesity is listed as a clinical feature of GHD, but if we simply restricted biochemical evaluation to patients with obesity as the main feature, testing the GH axis would yield a large number of individuals with a poor GH response, because obesity per se is associated with blunted GH responses to various stimuli.[142] Individuals who are GHD are often obese, but the converse is clearly not the case.

Little is known of the sensitivity and specificity of many of the clinical observations, either alone or in combination. The prevalence of many of the clinical features within the general population is unknown, which heightens the problem. Even the presence of specific features or a combination of features will increase only slightly the likelihood of disease if they are relatively insensitive.

The manifestation of GHD as a result of a GH gene deletion is early, and poor growth can be detected as early as the sixth month of postnatal life. With advancing age, more GH has to be secreted to maintain concentrations of GH sufficient for growth, so idiopathic isolated pituitary GHD may present at any time. It is the degree of deficiency that dictates when the individual comes to medical attention. Table 19-5 provides general clinical rules that are a useful aid when selecting patients for further study of the GH axis.

PRINCIPLES OF TESTING

The aim of any diagnostic test is to progress the clinical history and examination to the point where the care of the patient is altered. No test will ever benefit a patient. It is only when subsequent treatment has to differ depending on the test result that patients will be better off. There is a vast and bewildering literature on GH testing, but the clinician can be guided by asking the questions detailed in Table 19-6. It is important to remember that a diagnostic test is not just about whether a disease is present or not. It might also be important in determining severity and prognosis, responsiveness to and monitoring of therapy, and as a screening tool. As such, how the test performs under one circumstance may not be the same in another. Measuring serum IGF-1 concentrations may be unhelpful in screening for GHD but may be excellent as a marker of response to therapy.

Two points deserve special mention. First, it is unusual in endocrinology for there to be a diagnostic gold standard. The anterior pituitary is not accessible, and molecular biology is not sufficiently advanced to give definitive answers. Second, care needs to be taken in ascribing the role of a gold standard. It may change with time, and the test must be well validated by application to large numbers of individuals with and without the condition. The temptation is to use the extremes, but this may lead to a considerable overestimate of sensitivity and specificity[144] which may not be borne out in field studies.[145,146]

Two principles operate when using diagnostic tests.[147] First, probability is a useful marker of diagnostic uncertainty. This is when the sensitivity (ability to detect a target disorder when present or true positive rate) and specificity (ability to identify correctly the absence of the disorder or true negative rate) become important. If both were 85%, 15% of patients with disease would have a negative result (false negative) and 15% without disease would have a positive result (false positive). Abnormal results would occur in patients with and without disease. Whatever the result, new information has been generated that may or may not influence decision making. Second, diagnostic tests should be obtained only when they can alter the management of the case—that is, if the test result alters the probability of the disease.

Pre- and Post-test Probability

The relationship between the probability of disease after the results of diagnostic tests are known (the post-test probability) and pretest probability of disease depends on the sensitivity and specificity of the test as shown in Figure 19-6. There are two important points to note: the first is that the more certain the clinician is of the diagnosis before the test is performed, the less effect the confirmatory test has on the probability of disease. The obverse is also true. The second point is that tests will have major effects on probability of disease in the intermediate zone. Testing is not likely to be beneficial if the pretest probability is very high or low. This is one reason why screening for GH problems in short children on the basis of biochemical tests is unhelpful; the pretest probability is 1 in 3000 or 0.003%.

Clinicians are often faced with the situation where they feel really sure the patient has the condition, but the test does not confirm this. Table 19-7 analyzes this concept. Here, specificity and sensitivity have been fixed, and the effects on post-test probability are considered. In the situation where there is a 90% pretest probability that the patient is GH-deficient, then even if the test is negative in the individual, there is still a 67% probability (reduced by 23%) that they have the condition, so treatment would still be justified. When the pretest probability was 5% (very certain that the patient does not have GHD) and the test is positive, all the result says is that the patient has a 1 in 4 chance of having the condition, so we would probably not treat. In the

Table 19-5. Clinical Indicators for Further Evaluation of the GH Axis

1. Height, at any age, below the 0.4th centile on the U.K. Reference Charts.[143] The 0.4th level is chosen to improve diagnostic return from evaluation. The previous cutoff (3rd or 5th centile) lacks sensitivity and specificity.
2. Crossing of one or more height centiles on the U.K. Reference Charts over a period of 1 or more years. Centiles are equispaced (0.7 SD), allowing general rules to be applied at all ages.
3. A height that is inappropriately low for the heights of the parents.
4. Predisposing condition (tumor, radiation, etc.) or features suggestive of an underlying syndrome.
5. Neonatal signs consistent with pituitary hormone deficiencies.

Table 19-6. Underlying Principles of Assessing Tests

1. Has there been an independent blind comparison with the diagnostic "gold standard"?
2. Was the test conducted in a wide range of patients with and without the condition?
3. Is the test reproducible?
4. What was the definition of "normal" in the test situation?
5. How might the test interact with others in a diagnostic sequence?
6. Does the test entail risk or reduce risk for the patient?

Table 19-7. Effect on Post-test Probability of Differing Pre-test Certainty, Assuming Constant Sensitivity and Specificity

Pre-test Probability (%)	Post-test Probability (%)	
	Test Positive	**Test Negative**
90	98 (+8)	67 (−23)
50	87 (+37)	19 (−31)
5	25 (+20)	1 (−4)

Change from pretest probability in parenthesis.

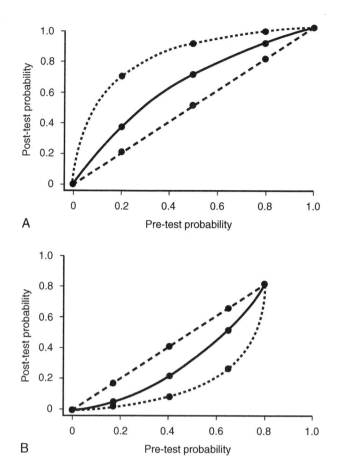

FIGURE 19-6. The relation between pre-test and post-test probability of disease. The data were constructed by using Bayes' theorem with a test sensitivity and specificity of either 70% *(solid line)* or 90% *(dashed line)*. **A,** The post-test probability if the test were positive; **B,** the post-test probability if the test were negative. If the post-test probability were the same as the pre-test probability, then the relation would be given by the line of identity. (Reproduced from Brook CGD, Hindmarsh PC, Jacobs HS [eds]: Clinical Pediatric Endocrinology, 4th ed. London: Blackwell Publishers, 2001.)

middle ground, certainty in either direction is dramatically improved.

Multiple Tests

Table 19-7 could have been made much larger by introducing any number of pretreatment probabilities. There comes a point, however, when post-test probability changes to a level where a decision has to be made to stop and either accept or reject the proposal that the condition is present. The decision to stop investigation and to treat or not depends on how convinced the clinician is of the diagnosis, the benefits and risks of the therapy, and the potential yield and risks of further tests. There are two ways to assist this situation: conduct another test or use a more sophisticated analysis rather than a simple positive or negative.

This is problematic in the GH field because the methodology assumes that the results of the two tests are independent. In normal individuals undergoing repeat GHRH tests, dependence cannot be assumed.[148] Where repeat tests have been performed in children, concordance was observed 50% of the time, a value close to that calculated for independent events using a test with 70% to 85% efficiency. If all tests are treated as independent, there is a risk of over- or underestimating the presence of the condition. Another important issue is whether the test might change in individuals as they age. There is evidence that the clonidine test is less effective in releasing GH in young adults

compared with children.[149] Whether the magnitude of the response to other stimuli can be assumed to remain unchanged is unknown.

Assuming that the two tests are performed (on different days) and that they are dependent, then if both tests need to be positive for diagnosis, this maximizes specificity and avoids falsely labeling normal children, but it misses many treatable individuals. Insisting that both tests are negative maximizes sensitivity, minimizes misdiagnoses, but falsely labels a lot more normal children.

One special area of two-tests is the question of re-testing after completion of GH therapy. Several recent publications have suggested that individuals who were originally diagnosed with GHD do not appear to have the biochemical abnormality when the test is repeated later.[150] This has led to statements being made that these individuals are no longer GHD. However, such statements reflect a subtle mind shift that has taken place. The clinicians have shifted from wishing to make a diagnosis to one of excluding a diagnosis, without taking into account the laws of probability. Two issues are worth considering: The first is that the population studied during the second test is not the same as that during the first. Those thought unlikely to have the condition have been excluded. The second point also relates to some extent to the original diagnosis. It is worth rehearsing the scenario that has led to the second test. The child was initially evaluated because of concerns over short stature and poor growth. At that point, a test was conducted because the clinician required an answer with which to rule in or rule out the diagnosis, and the result was sufficient in terms of post-test probability for therapy to be offered. If the post-test probability of the child having the condition was 87%, then this value now forms the pretest probability for the second test, not the 50:50 situation the clinician faced prior to the original investigation.

DIAGNOSIS OF GROWTH HORMONE DEFICIENCY

Assessment of GH secretion is problematic, in part because of the pulsatile nature of GH secretion.[151] The most consistent GH surges accompany slow-wave electroencephalographic rhythms during phases 3 and 4 of sleep. Although this rhythmicity is characteristic of GH secretion at all ages, the size of the amplitudes and the total integrated GH secretion varies with sex, age, pubertal status, and nutrition.[152,153] Between pulses, serum GH concentrations are extremely low, often less than 0.1 ng/mL. Consequently, measurement of random serum GH concentrations is of no value in the diagnosis of GHD. Measurement of spontaneous GH secretion requires multiple sampling, typically every 15 minutes over a 12- to 24-hour period.[151-155] Such methodologies are inconvenient and expensive, and while they allow identification of the patient with severe GHD, it is not clear that they can discriminate between partial GHD and normal secretory variation.[156] However, even the reproducibility of GH secretory patterns in children from day to day is uncertain. Rose and colleagues[156] reported that measurement of spontaneous GH secretion identified only 57% of children diagnosed as GHD by provocative testing. Lanes[157] reported that approximately 25% of normally growing children have low overnight GH concentrations. A longitudinal study of GH secretion in normal boys during puberty indicated wide intersubject variation,[152,153] and day-to-day variation has been noted among normal subjects.[158]

An alternative approach has been the measurement of urinary GH concentrations.[159-163] This methodology requires a timed urinary collection and a GH assay of high sensitivity because urinary GH concentrations are low. The theoretic advantages of

Table 19-8. Growth Hormone Stimulation Tests

Stimulus	Dose	Sampling Protocol (min)	Notes
Exercise	Cycle for 10-15 min	15 min for 90 min	Variable response, highly dependent on degree of exercise
Levodopa	<15 kg, 125 mg 15-30 kg, 250 mg >30 kg, 500 mg	15 min for 90 min	Nausea
Clonidine	0.15 mg/m²	30 min for 90 min	Tiredness; postural hypotension
Arginine HCl	0.5 g/kg (max, 30 g) IV, given as 10% arginine HCl in 0.9% NaCl over 30 min	15 min for 90 min	May cause insulin release
Insulin	0.05-0.1 units/kg IV	15 min for 120 min	Hypoglycemia; requires supervision. Can also measure cortisol reliably
Glucagon	0.1 mg/kg IM (max, 1 mg)	30 min for 180 min	Nausea
GHRH	1 µg/kg IV	15 min for 120 min	Flushing. Only assesses pituitary reserve, not whole H-P axis
GHRH-Arginine			Needs further work to assess value in Pediatrics

Tests should be performed after an overnight fast.
Patients should be documented to be euthyroid.
Prepubertal children should be primed with gonadal steroids.
GHRH, Growth hormone–releasing hormone; *IM*, intramuscular; *IV*, intravenous.

this approach include its relative ease of performance and non-invasive nature, as well as the requirement for only a single GH measurement. This must be balanced, however, by the need to assess the effects of renal function, the wide interindividual variation, and the lack of adequate age- and sex-related reference ranges.

As a result of these difficulties, the standard for the diagnosis of GHD has been provocative testing of GH "secretory reserve"[140] (Table 19-8). Physiologic stimuli for such tests have included sleep[164] and exercise,[165,166] and pharmacologic stimuli have included a wide variety of agents.[167-175] None of these tests truly mimics normal GH secretory physiology, and none has been evaluated adequately in normal children and normal short children. The limitations of provocative GH testing in the diagnosis of GHD are described below and need to be considered in the light of statistical theory (see above):

1. Provocative testing by its nature is nonphysiologic. None of the commonly used stimuli truly mimics normal regulation of GH secretion.
2. The definition of a "normal" response to stimulation is arbitrary. Normal values are difficult to obtain in pediatric practice, and reference ranges would be needed for tall, normal, and short children, because their GH secretion differs.[176] In addition, both age and pubertal stage influence GH secretion,[152,153,176] as does body composition.[142] Values for these would also have to be included.

The classic approach of defining normal data in terms of a Gaussian distribution does not come without hazard. Endocrine testing rarely fits this distribution; even if it did, it would imply that the lowest and highest 2.5% of values are abnormal and that all diseases have the same frequency—clearly unlikely. Creating upper and lower limits does not help either. It is more appropriate to identify a range of diagnostic test results beyond which the disorder of GHD is likely.

Most decisions on placing the value have been empirical rather than statistical. In practice, cutoff values could be chosen at an absolute extreme. If 100 short children were studied, and GH sufficiency or deficiency was defined by a peak response of less than 3 ng/mL, only 3% to 5% might have a response at this level. When testing the next 100 children, one or two normal indi-

Table 19-9. Considerations to Give to Test and Control Populations

1. What is the population from which patients are drawn?
2. How have patients been filtered before joining the study?
3. Test properties may differ in subpopulations within the sample.
4. Recruit consecutive patients with the problem.
5. Can the findings be generalized?

viduals might have such a response. They will be outliers, but they are important because the more patients studied, the greater the chance of finding outliers.

Moving the cutoff to more extreme values to exclude these patients restricts the population of treatable individuals. Relaxing the criteria interposes normal individuals into the diagnosis zone. Placing the cutoff is based partly on clinical judgment. Since there is no disadvantage apart from financial cost in falsely labeling someone with GHD and treating them, a relaxed cutoff would be acceptable.

The question of cutoff points for use in tests becomes more important as individuals with differing severities of the disorder are considered. In constructing normal ranges, it is clearly best if large sample sizes are chosen. Choosing populations of disease positive and disease negative is unwise, either for this task or assessing test performance, since it is unlikely that in the less severe cases the test will perform as well.[177] In the assessment of studies, some useful points are outlined in Table 19-9. Referral bias remains a major issue in many studies. In studies emanating from referral centers, the strength of a factor such as short stature may appear to be less important in that patients are already selected for this in the referral. Changes in prevalence of a condition do not change test properties, whereas changes in the spectrum of the disorder do.[178]

3. The dependence of GH secretion on other factors needs to be taken into account. Marin and colleagues[179] demonstrated that when exercise and arginine stimulation tests were performed on normal-stature children without sex steroid priming, the lower-limits-of-normal (−2 SD) peak serum GH concentration for prepubertal children

was as low as 1.9 ng/mL and rose to 7.2 ng/mL on estrogen priming. Thyroxine and cortisol, which directly alter gene transcription, influence the results obtained, and these need to be controlled before undertaking a diagnostic study. Similarly, the presence of high levels of glucose or free fatty acids may influence the response obtained.[180]

4. GH assays may measure a variety of immunoreactive molecular forms of GH.[181] These GH variants do not necessarily possess equivalent growth-promoting actions. Furthermore, considerable interassay variability exists in the measurement of these GH molecular variants.[182,183] Individual standards need to be established for each laboratory.[184] Assay precision, accuracy, and sensitivity play an important role in determining the success or failure of the diagnostic test. For example, assays for IGF-1—despite having good standardization from the technical aspect (elimination of interference of IGF-I-binding proteins [IGFBP] and the use of high affinity, high specificity antisera)—may have different performance characteristics when concentrations are either above or below the normal range.[185]

5. Most endocrine tests are conducted over short periods of time, and results are extrapolated to longer time frames. GH provocation tests take 2 hours to perform, and the results are then compared with height velocity measurements obtained over a longer period of time, often 1 year. That there is a relationship is perhaps surprising; that there are high false-positive and false-negative rates probably not.

6. Hormone pulsatility may also influence diagnostic tests if the test itself is influenced by oscillations (e.g., the stimulus applied) within the system under study. The GH response at any point in time is going to be heavily dependent on the interplay between the hypothalamic regulatory peptides involved in GH release, namely GHRH and somatostatin.[186] Somatostatin, in particular, is a key determinant of the amount of GH released as a result of GHRH stimulation. Attempts have been made to take control of this variable[187] by pretreatment with somatostatin. GHRH combined with arginine is an alternative approach.[188] It was hoped that the ghrelin-like agents would be an advance in this area because of their potent GH-releasing qualities, but they appear to suffer the same problems of reproducibility.[189]

7. Endocrine systems are also subject to feedback from target tissues, and this is an issue not only in the interpretation of single provocation tests but also where second tests are performed in rapid succession to the first. A diminished response to GHRH can be observed if the second stimulus is applied 1, 2, or 3 hours after the first.[147] The implication of doing two tests on the same day, often following each other, are immense; the cutoff that might be implied to determine normality or not may not be the same for the second test as for the first, especially if the second stimulus is different from the first.

8. Provocative testing fails to give any consideration to the effect of negative feedback by serum IGF-1.[190-193] It probably makes more sense to interpret serum GH concentrations in the light of serum IGF concentrations, much as TSH concentrations are best assessed with a knowledge of circulating thyroxine concentrations.

9. In assessing the results of endocrine evaluations, it is generally assumed that the single or multiple samples measured are relatively stable, at least over short periods. When important changes are postulated to be taking place, for example in a disease process, some knowledge of the inherent variability within the measurement system is required. In the short term, a number of studies have demonstrated variability within and between individuals in terms of GH tests.[158,194] Group data are usually reproducible, but problems can arise if it is assumed that individual oscillatory profiles are consistent from day to day.

10. In considering provocative tests, the situation may arise where no response is observed. A possible explanation is that the strength of the stimulus was insufficient to provoke hormone release. In such a situation, it is valuable to have an independent marker of stimulus application. In the insulin induced hypoglycemia test, this marker is glucose and the attainment of adequate hypoglycemia. In the glucagon test, it may be the release of glucose. In other tests, there may be no independent markers, so doubt may be cast on the reliability of the nonresponse.

11. Careful consideration needs to be given to the age of the child under study. Not only might the cutoff point criteria differ at different ages, but the likelihood of disease presence will change with age. It is highly unlikely that GHD will manifest itself during puberty. It is possible, but it is more likely that any growth or GH secretory problems at this age relate more to delayed puberty rather than an abnormality in the GH axis. Even in childhood, the return in terms of diagnosis of GHD is not high if height screening is undertaken at school entry so that with increasing age there is a diminishing diagnostic return.

12. Provocative GH testing is expensive, uncomfortable, and has risk. Insulin-induced hypoglycemia should only be performed in a supervised setting. Deaths have been documented in patients rendered hypoglycemic and corrected in an overly vigorous manner.

Of the provocative tests listed in Table 19-8, it should be noted that stimulation with GHRH is not designed to document whether a patient has GHD but rather whether GHD, established by other methodologies, is the result of pituitary or hypothalamic dysfunction.[195] Failure to respond to GHRH suggests that the abnormality is at the pituitary level. This test may be enhanced by the addition of arginine or pyridostigmine.[196]

PRACTICAL APPROACH TO DIAGNOSTIC EVALUATION

A practical approach to the diagnosis of a child with GHD is grounded on clinical assessment with allocation of pretest probability of disease presence. In the prepubertal child with abnormal growth, serum concentrations of IGF-1, IGFBP-3, and/or ALS provide a means for excluding a diagnosis of GHD. Provocative GH testing with appropriate sex steroid priming will provide information on GH secretory capability, and GHRH stimulation, with or without arginine or pyridostigmine, will allow determination of whether the defect is at the hypothalamic or pituitary level. All data need to be interpreted together with known test performances and integrated with the pretest probability to generate a posttest probability that would then lead to a decision as to whether intervention is required. The interpretation of second tests of GH secretion is problematic from both the physiologic and statistical standpoints and should be analyzed with extreme caution.

Documentation of GHD also requires that other pituitary functions be assessed periodically, including TSH, ACTH, and gonadotropin status. Other pituitary deficiencies may not be evident upon initial assessment but may develop over time. MRI of the hypothalamus and pituitary should be performed initially to determine if there is evidence of intracranial tumors, pituitary hypoplasia, or midline defects. Even if the baseline MRI is normal, in the absence of an alternative explanation for GHD or CPHD, the possibility of tumors or structural defects should not be dismissed permanently. With increasing knowledge of the genetics of pituitary disorders, these should be looked for because they have an impact on the likelihood of other pituitary hormone deficiencies evolving with time and allow genetic counseling to be undertaken.

Treatment

GROWTH HORMONE

The first successful treatment of human GHD with human pituitary–derived GH (hGH) was in the 1950s, and this was followed by a series of publications that documented the efficacy of GH in patients with GHD.[6-9] Treatment utilized human cadaver pituitary–derived hGH, which brought with it a series of problems surrounding supply. Limited supplies mandated the use of suboptimal dosages, interrupted treatment periods, and frequent cessation of therapy before maximal height had been attained. The use of human pituitary–derived hGH was halted in 1985 following the discovery of several cases of Creutzfeldt-Jakob disease associated with its use. Pituitary-derived hGH was replaced with recombinant DNA–derived rhGH, which allowed for potentially unlimited supplies, obviating the need for low-dose usage and interrupted therapeutic regimens. The initial rhGH preparation was an N-terminal methionine, met-rhGH, which was fully active biologically but was ultimately replaced by the mature 191–amino acid protein. The biopotency of current preparations of rhGH, expressed as International Units per milligram of the new World Health Organization (WHO) rhGH reference reagent for somatropin (88/624), is 3 IU/mg.

Dose Studies

Investigations of optimal dosing of rhGH have been complicated by the use of heterogeneous study populations, so studies frequently include patients with unequivocal and complete GHD together with patients with partial GHD. Several studies have demonstrated a dose-response relationship for hGH, but the slope of the response is relatively shallow.[197] MacGillivray and colleagues[198] compared the growth responses of 99 children treated with pituitary hGH at a mean dosage of 0.1 mg/kg/week with those of 77 children treated with rhGH at a dosage of 0.3 mg/kg/week. The mean time required to reach normal height (greater than −2 SD) was 48 months for the low-dose group and 27 months for the high-dose group. Fifty-one percent of the low-dose group never reached this point compared with 23% in the high-dose group. Cohen et al.[199] compared the growth responses of prepubertal, naive patients randomized to rhGH at a dosage of 0.175, 0.35, or 0.7 mg/kg/week for the first 2 years

of treatment. Significantly greater height velocities and gains in height SD resulted from the 0.35 mg/kg/week versus 0.175 mg/kg/week, but no further significant improvement was observed with the 0.7 mg/kg/week dosage. Ultimately, the issues that should determine dosage in the child with GHD are (1) how best to return the GHD child to the normal growth curve, (2) how best to ensure that the child attains his or her genetic height potential, (3) risks, and (4) cost. For the child with severe GHD, weekly dosages of 0.175 mg/kg, administered in seven daily doses either by a subcutaneous or intramuscular route, are usually sufficient to increase growth rates from 3 to 4 cm/year to more than 10 cm/year.

Response to GH therapy varies even when the diagnosis is homogeneous. This probably reflects differences in tissue responsivity which may relate in part to the function of the GH receptor. A polymorphism in the GH receptor (GHR) gene leading to retention (full length [fl]) or deletion of exon 3 (d3), which encodes a 22–amino acid (aa) residue sequence in the extracellular domain,[200,201] has been associated with the degree of height increase in response to GH replacement in children born short for gestational age (SGA), those with idiopathic short stature (ISS),[202] and in a GHD population.[203] Patients with at least one d3 allele had a significantly better first-year response leading to an improved adult height on GH treatment than patients with homozygosity for GHR-fl. However, reported studies are not all consistent, which may reflect differing populations and conditions.[204-208] False-positive findings are more likely with small sample sizes, and for quantitative trait loci, phenotypic variations tend to be overestimated with small sample sizes.[209,210]

Weight- or body-size-based dosing is common practice in pediatrics; whether it is better to dose on the basis of growth response and serum IGF-1 concentration is worth consideration. Current data suggest that upwards of 2.5 times the standard dose of r-hGH is required to attain serum IGF-1 concentrations in the upper zone of the normal distribution, although the benefit in terms of height improvement was minimal.[211]

Frequency of Administration

Several studies have compared the short-term effects of administering hGH either daily or thrice weekly.[212] Generally, daily injections are more effective, but increasing the frequency more than this makes little difference.[213] Sustained-release rhGH preparations, which may be administered as infrequently as every 2 to 4 weeks,[214] are unlikely to be effective and have potentially greater side effects due to the pulsatile nature of GH physiology.

Prediction Models

A series of models have been derived[8,215] that describe factors that might influence response, but none have gone on to test these in formal randomized control trials. Further problems arise when large multicontributor databases are used because of the accuracy of the data entered; when prognosis is considered, factors that may be important may not have been recorded. It has been reported that in children with GHD, auxologic parameters, such as chronologic age (the younger the patient, the better the response) and the difference between target height and actual height (the smaller the patient, the better the response), are better predictors of growth response than the cumulative weekly GH dosage. There are several problems with these types of models:

1. Although prediction models are useful to give an average effect, they are not individualizable.

Table 19-10. Specific Issues With Prediction Models of Response to Growth Hormone Treatment Development

1. Regression to the mean
2. Prediction gives average effect; how to apply to individuals for prognosis
3. Predictors may not be independent of each other; assumptions made in linear and multiple-regression modeling
4. Assumptions about uniformity of response
5. Spurious correlations involving time

2. They often only focus on one outcome, usually short-term growth, whereas interest may be more centered on final height. The two need not necessarily be related, and the factors that influence response in the first year of treatment may differ totally from those that lead to prediction of the individual's final height.

3. Very few prediction models have been constructed from an a-priori hypothesis, and care needs to be taken that there has been no interference from other factors accompanying the disease that might affect prognosis. The problem is that importance can be ascribed to factors that are merely markers for other factors of real importance. Examples of this can be seen in models which demonstrate that individuals who are extremely short, growing very poorly, and whose heights are subsequently further away from their genetic height respond best to treatment. All these factors are simply a marker of "how bad the disease is" and could perhaps be more easily summarized by a similar single factor that actually describes the severity of the condition.

4. Rules derived from one data set may reflect associations that have occurred by chance and often result from overfitting of the data.

5. There is always the possibility that the predictors are idiosyncratic to the population, the setting, to the clinicians, or to other aspects of the original study. Specific issues associated with growth-response models are summarized in Table 19-10.

   a. The first problem relates to the method by which response to GH is defined. In several studies, acceleration in growth rate or the difference between the pretreatment growth rate and that observed during the year of treatment is used. Using either, however, leads potentially to the generation of artifact. This is because if difference (e.g., change in height velocity) is plotted against pretreatment states (e.g., pretreatment height velocity), then a good relationship will always be demonstrated purely and simply because pretreatment height velocity is contributing to both variables.[216,217] Examination of the association between change in a variable and its initial value is complicated. It is possible, for example, that if high values are recorded at one stage and the same measure is performed at a later date, low values may be recorded even in the absence of treatment. This effect, "regression to the mean," will be most marked in those with highest or lowest initial recorded values and will induce a spurious association between change and initial value. Several methods are available to overcome this problem.[217]

   b. The prediction gives the average effect, and the confidence interval of the response is smallest at the average value of the independent variable. The difficulty comes in applying this information to the individual. Simply stating the average expected improvement is not much help. To convey this information, consideration needs to be given to the patient's perception of what they think the treatment can do. If the patient wishes a growth response that will put them into the upper half of the normal height distribution, then disappointment might ensue. It is far better to provide the individual with an understanding of the chance of a successful outcome, and the concept "number needed to treat" is useful.[218]

   c. If the treatment effect varies among individuals with the same initial height value, then spurious trends may emerge in the overall model prediction. Even though it is clear that most treatments will not affect all individuals equally, this is not well understood. Whether a child with GHD with a tall or a short parent will have a better or worse response than a child with average-height parents is difficult to determine, because at present there are no easy markers of GH sensitivity.

   d. There are inherent problems with making predictions from previous data (e.g., how does year 1 influence year 2) or from the original data set. If we are looking at serial effects on height, it is important to recognize that the data going into such analyses are highly correlated. A person who is taller than average after 1 year will also tend to be taller than average after 2 years of follow up. It is important to realize that any two quantities changing over time will show a statistical association. Methods are available to assist in this area, but of necessity the time component needs to be removed.[219]

Height Outcomes and the Influence of Puberty

Early initiation of therapy, combined with careful attention to dosage adjustments and compliance, is the best predictor of cumulative growth response in patients with GHD. Final height correlates with height at the initiation of puberty, so it is important to maximize growth during the prepubertal period, within the limits of safety and economy.[220-225] Analysis of data on final heights of rhGH-treated GHD is complicated by the heterogeneity of patient groups and dosage, but the most common observation is a general failure of children to reach their full genetic height potential, especially in the case of IGHD and particularly in females. Price and Ranke[226] have reported final heights of −1.26 SD and −1.45 SD from the mean in males and females, respectively, with IGHD, and −0.22 SD and −0.52 SD from the mean in males and females, respectively, with CPHD. In patients with longer durations of treatment and higher dosages of rhGH, adult heights tended to be greater, although still failing to achieve full genetic height potential.

It is clear that the timing of puberty has a significant impact on adult height of rhGH-treated GHD.[223-225] The duration of rhGH treatment and the height gained prepubertally are typically greater when puberty is induced rather than spontaneous. In the study by Ranke and colleagues,[227] final height was attained at 17.8 and 19.2 years in boys and at 16.0 and 17.0 years in girls following spontaneous and induced puberty, respectively. Final heights were greater after induced puberty compared with spontaneous puberty in boys (171.3 versus 166.0 cm) and in girls (157.0 versus 155.0 cm). Therapy designed at delaying the onset of puberty (both normal and precocious) may augment the cumulative growth response to rhGH.

Burns et al.[224] reported that final height in GHD patients who enter puberty spontaneously is less than in patients in whom puberty needs to be induced because of gonadotropin deficiency. Final height gain can be particularly variable in children who have had treatment for malignancies. The GHD is often complicated by skeletal damage following TBI or craniospinal irradiation, early puberty, hypothyroidism, gonadotropin deficiency, malnutrition, and concomitant chemotherapy. Gonadotropin releasing hormone analogue (GnRHa) therapy to arrest early puberty has been used in conjunction with GH treatment in this group of patients, with encouraging results. The use of GnRHa reduces the concentration of sex steroid, with a consequent delay in epiphyseal fusion. However, the use of GH and GnRHa combination therapy in children with GHD[228] is not widely used at present. It may be beneficial under certain circumstances—for example, where the diagnosis of GHD has been delayed. The effects of GnRHa in the long term are unknown; additionally, the cost of this combination therapy would need to be weighed against the benefits.

Although considerable attention has been paid to growth, it is important to realize that GH treatment in childhood can also normalize body composition, with a reduction in body fat, although effects on lean body mass are less evident. It is also associated with reversible insulin insensitivity and an increase in the ratio of high-density lipoprotein (HDL) to total cholesterol. Glomerular filtration rate (GFR) is increased and bone remodeling accelerated, with a marked increase in bone mineral mass.[229]

Adverse Effects of Human Growth Hormone

Treatment with rhGH has had an excellent safety record.[230,231] Reports of anti-GH antibodies in patients receiving rhGH have been few, with no untoward effect on the growth response. Fluid retention and carpal tunnel syndrome are observed in adults but are seldom significant in children. Whereas the incidence of type 1 diabetes mellitus is not higher in patients with idiopathic GHD than in the general population, the incidence of type 2 diabetes mellitus is greater in those patients treated with GH, although this tends to be in those predisposed to developing the condition.[232] Idiopathic intracranial hypertension (pseudotumor cerebri) has been observed occasionally but resolves with cessation of treatment and then a gradual reintroduction of rhGH but commencing at a lower dose.[231] Slipped capital femoral epiphysis

has been reported, but it is not clear that the incidence is greater than that observed in normal children during rapid periods of growth. Other possible rare and still unproven complications include acute pancreatitis, increased growth of pigmented nevi, and prepubertal gynecomastia.

The most important theoretical risk that has been raised with rhGH therapy has been that of malignancy.[230,231,233-239] Epidemiologic assessment has been complicated by the fact that many rhGH recipients are at increased risk of malignancy because of chromosomal abnormalities, prior malignancies, or prior histories of chemotherapy or irradiation. Additionally, it has been suggested that in some cases, GH deficiency itself may predispose to development of malignancy. Although a number of early reports suggested a link between hGH treatment and leukemia, Blethen and colleagues[230] reported that an analysis of 47,000 patient-years of treatment in greater than 19,000 children indicated that in children without known risk factors, rhGH therapy was not associated with an increased occurrence of tumors or recurrence rate of leukemia or CNS tumors. Despite these assurances, it is customary to delay rhGH treatment in children with treated brain tumors until they have been shown to be tumor free for at least 1 to 2 years.

More recently, the long-term follow up of these patients has revealed a higher than expected incidence and mortality of colonic cancer and Hodgkin's disease.[239] However, these data need to be put in context. The affected patients had been treated with high GH doses given two to three times a week. Hence one could speculate that the IGF-I concentrations generated by this mode of GH therapy may be excessive. IGF-I concentrations at the upper end of the normal range (top quartile for colon and prostate and top tertile for breast) have been associated with colon, breast, and prostatic cancer.[240-243] Given that lower doses of GH are given on a daily basis, it would be incorrect—at this stage at least—to extrapolate the data from the earlier studies to the present treatment regimens.

End-Points of Therapy

Given the discussion outlined above in terms of efficacy, safety, and clinical governance, Table 19-11 illustrates some suggested outcomes that can be monitored and used as a basis of short- and long-term audit, as well as safety monitoring.

Table 19-11. Short-, Medium-, and Long-Term End Points of Growth Hormone Therapy in GHD Children

	End Point	Rationale	Measure
Short Term	1. Growth acceleration	1. Assess response	1. Minimum response of greater than 2 cm/yr
	2. Reduction in adipose mass	2. Assess response	2. Skinfold thickness
	3. Correct dose	3. Optimize therapy	3. IGF-I and growth
	4. Vision and headaches	4. Raised intracranial pressure	4. Fundoscopy
	5. Assessment of limp	5. Slipped femoral epiphysis	5. X-ray
Medium Term	1. Bone maturation	1. Rate of skeletal maturation	1. Yearly bone age
	2. Pubertal status	2. Early puberty or rapid progression	2. 6-monthly Tanner staging
	3. Correct dose	3. Optimize therapy	3. IGF-I and growth response; return to target height within 6 years of therapy
	4. Thyroid status	4. Altered status or evolving endocrinopathy	4. Yearly thyroid function tests
	5. Other hormones	5. Evolving endocrinopathy	5. Gonadotroph and corticotroph function
	6. Metabolic status	6. Insulin insensitivity	6. Fasting glucose and insulin
Long Term	1. Growth	1. Outcome	1. Final height within target height of parents
	2. Bone mineralization	2. GH effect on bone	2. DEXA Scan
	3. Malignancy risk	3. ? GH cancer link	3. Cancer registry
	4. Cardiovascular risk	4. Hyperinsulinism or GH effect (? long-term GHD)	4. Fasting glucose and insulin, blood pressure, fasting lipids

DEXA, Dual-energy x-ray absorptiometry; *GHD,* growth hormone deficiency; *IGF,* insulin-like growth factor.

GROWTH HORMONE–RELEASING HORMONE

In children whose GHD is due to a hypothalamic abnormality, treatment with GHRH would appear to be an appropriate therapeutic option.[244,245] Both GHRH$_{1-44}$ and GHRH$_{1-29}$ are biologically active in humans. Unfortunately, although GHRH can be absorbed nasally, this route of administration has not proved to be effective,[246] and treatment must be via subcutaneous or intramuscular injection, as is the case with rhGH. Direct comparisons of rhGH and GHRH have not been performed, but a number of studies indicate that GHRH administered once or twice daily can increase the growth rates of children with GHD. No specific therapeutic advantage of GHRH over rhGH has been demonstrated to date, although further studies are warranted to investigate optimization of dosage and frequency of administration.

GROWTH HORMONE–RELEASING PEPTIDES AND NONPEPTIDYL GROWTH HORMONE SECRETAGOGUES

Since the discovery of growth hormone–releasing peptides (GHRPs) by Bowers et al. in the 1980s,[14] a variety of small GHRPs and nonpeptidyl small-molecule GH secretagogues have been manufactured.[247] These molecules are potent stimulators of GH release, especially when administered together with GHRH, and may be active when administered by intravenous, intramuscular, subcutaneous, nasal, and oral routes. These potential advantages must be balanced by the likelihood that normal GHRH production is required to see maximal benefit from such agents.[248,249] Clinical trials have proven disappointing however.

TRANSITION TO ADULT CARE

It has been suggested that at the end of statural growth, GH secretion should be reassessed in all patients after a wash-out period of at least 1 to 3 months.[250-252] The investigation of choice is an insulin tolerance test (ITT),[253] although the arginine + GHRH test has recently been proposed as a safer alternative, particularly in patients who have a contraindication to an ITT.[254] For between 25% to 75% of patients, the GH response to provocation is in the normal range, as would be expected from the previous discussion on testing, and probability theory needs to be employed to determine whether therapy should be continued or not.[255] In the remainder, continuation of GH therapy should be considered in those with a peak GH less than 3 µg/L, who can be described as having severe GHD. Patients with a peak GH between 3 and 7 µg/L have moderate GHD and should be followed up by an adult endocrinologist. In these individuals, adverse changes in body composition, quality of life, and bone mineral density may be an indication to recommence GH treatment,[256] although it is less likely that these individuals will develop adult GHD syndrome.[255] In those patients with multiple pituitary hormone deficiency, GHD due to a congenital lesion, and GHD secondary to radiotherapy, surgery, or a mass lesion, the GHD is highly unlikely to reverse.[257]

REFERENCES

1. Karlberg J: On the modelling of human growth, Stat Med 6:185–192, 1987.
2. Hindmarsh PC, Smith PJ, Brook CGD, et al: The relationship between growth velocity and growth hormone secretion in short prepubertal children, Clin Endocrinol 27:581–591, 1987.
3. Rosenfeld RG: Disorders of growth hormone/IGF secretion and action. In Sperling M, editor: Pediatric Endocrinology, Philadelphia, 1996, WB Saunders, pp 117–169.
4. White P: Diabetes in Childhood and Adolescence. Philadelphia, 1932, Lea and Febiger.
5. Raben MS: Treatment of a pituitary dwarf with human growth hormone, J Clin Endocrinol Metab 18:901–903, 1958.
6. Soyka ZF, Ziskind A, Crawford JD: Treatment of short stature in children and adolescents with human pituitary growth hormone (Raben). Experience with 35 cases, N Engl J Med 271:754–764, 1964.
7. Prader A, Zachmann M, Poley JR, et al: Long term treatment with human growth hormone (Raben) in small doses. Evaluation of 18 hypopituitary patients, Helv Paediatr Acta 22:423–439, 1967.
8. Tanner JM, Whitehouse RH, Hughes PCR, et al: Effect of human growth hormone treatment for 1 to 7 years on growth of 100 children with growth hormone deficiency, low birth weight, inherited smallness, Turner Syndrome and other complaints, Arch Dis Child 45:745–779, 1971.
9. Aceto T, Frasier SD, Hayles AB, et al: Collaborative study of the effects of human growth hormone in growth hormone deficiency. 1. First year of therapy, J Clin Endocrinol Metab 35:483–496, 1972.
10. Hunter WM, Greenwood FC: Preparation of iodine-131 labelled human growth hormone of high specific activity, Nature 194:495–496, 1962.
11. Brazeau P, Vale W, Burgus R, et al: Hypothalamic polypeptide that inhibits the secretion of immunoreactive pituitary growth hormone, Science 178:77–79, 1973.
12. Guillemin R, Brazeau P, Bohien P, et al: Growth hormone releasing factor from a human pancreatic tumour that caused acromegaly, Science 218:585–587, 1982.
13. Rivier J, Spiess J, Thorner MO, et al: Characterisation of a growth hormone-releasing factor from a human pancreatic islet tumour, Nature 300:276–278, 1982.
14. Bowers CY, Momany F, Reynolds GA, et al: Structure-activity relationships of a synthetic pentapeptide that specifically releases growth hormone in vitro, Endocrinology 106:663–667, 1980.
15. Salmon WD, Daughaday WH: A hormonally controlled serum factor which stimulates sulphate incorporation by cartilage in vivo, J Lab Clin Med 49:825–836, 1957.
16. Zezulak KM, Green H: The generation of insulin-like growth factor 1 sensitive cells by growth hormone action, Science 233:551–553, 1986.
17. Isgaard J, Nilsson A, Lindahl A, et al: Effects of local administration of GH and IGF-1 on longitudinal bone growth in rats, Am J Physiol 250:E367–E372, 1986.
18. Parkin JM: Incidence of growth hormone deficiency, Arch Dis Child 49:904–905, 1974.
19. Vimpani GV, Vimpani AF, Lidgard GP, et al: Prevalence of severe growth hormone deficiency, BMJ 2:427–430, 1977.
20. Lindsay R, Feldkamp M, Harris D, et al: Utah Growth Study. Growth standards and the prevalence of growth hormone deficiency, J Pediatr 125:29–35, 1994.
21. Wilton P: Progress in Growth Hormone Therapy—5 Years of KIGS, Mannheim, Germany, 1994, JJ Verlag, pp 62–66.
22. Genentech National Cooperative Growth Study Summary Report 18. San Francisco, 1994, Genentech, pp 6–13.
23. Dasen JS, Rosenfeld MG: Signaling and transcriptional mechanisms in pituitary development, Annu Rev Neurosci 24:327–355, 2001.
24. Takuma N, Sheng HZ, Furuta Y, et al: Formation of Rathke's pouch requires dual induction from the diencephalon, Development 125:4835–4840, 1998.
25. Ericson J, Norlin S, Jessell TM, et al: Integrated FGF and BMP signaling controls the progression of progenitor cell differentiation and the emergence of pattern in the embryonic anterior pituitary, Development 125:1005–1015, 1998.
26. Lazzaro D, Price M, De Felice M, et al: The transcription factor TTF-1 is expressed at the onset of thyroid and lung morphogenesis and in restricted regions of the foetal brain, Development 113:1093–1104, 1991.
27. Sheng HZ, Moriyama K, Yamashita T, et al: Multistep control of pituitary organogenesis, Science 278:1809–1812, 1997.
28. Treier M, Gleiberman AS, O'Connell SM, et al: Multi-step signaling requirements for pituitary organogenesis in vivo, Genes Dev 12:1691–1704, 1998.
29. Rosenfeld MG, Briata P, Dasen J, et al: Multistep signaling and transcriptional mechanisms for pituitary organogenesis in vivo, Recent Prog Horm Res 55:1–13, 2000.
30. Sheng HZ, Westphal H: Early steps in pituitary organogenesis, Trends Genet 15:236–240, 1999.
31. Simmons DM, Voss JW, Ingraham HA, et al: Pituitary cell phenotypes involve cell-specific Pit-1 mRNA translation and synergistic interactions with other classes of transcription factors, Genes Dev 4:695–711, 1990.
32. Japon MA, Rubinstein M, Low MJ: In situ hybridization analysis of anterior pituitary hormone gene expression during fetal mouse development, J Histochem Cytochem 42:1117–1125, 1994.
33. Li S, Crenshaw EB III, Rawson EJ, et al: Dwarf locus mutants lacking three pituitary cell types result from mutations in the POU-domain gene pit-1, Nature 347:528–533, 1990.
34. Lamolet B, Pulichino AM, Lamonerie T, et al: A pituitary cell-restricted T box factor, Tpit, activates POMC transcription in cooperation with Pitx homeoproteins, Cell 104(6):849–859, 2001.
35. Dattani MT, Robinson ICAF: The molecular basis for developmental disorders of the pituitary gland in man, Clin Genet 57:337–346, 2000.
36. Cohen LE, Wondisford FE, Salvatoni A, et al: A "hot spot" in the PIT1 gene responsible for combined pituitary hormone deficiency: clinical and molecular correlates, J Clin Endocrinol Metab 80:679–684, 1995.
37. Cohen LE, Radovick S: Molecular basis of combined pituitary hormone deficiencies, Endocr Rev 23:431–442, 2002.
38. Dattani MT, Martinez-Barbera JP, Thomas PQ, et al: Mutations in the homeobox gene HESX1/Hesx1 associated with septo-optic dysplasia in human and mouse, Nat Genet 19:125–133, 1998.
39. Thomas PQ, Dattani MT, Brickman JM, et al: Heterozygous HESX1 mutations associated with isolated

congenital pituitary hypoplasia and septo-optic dysplasia, Hum Mol Genet 10:39–45, 2001.

40. Carvalho LR, Woods KS, Mendonca BB, et al: A homozygous mutation in HESX1 is associated with evolving hypopituitarism due to impaired repressor-corepressor interaction, J Clin Invest 112(8):1192–1201, 2003.
41. Netchine I, Sobrier ML, Krude H, et al: Mutations in LHX3 result in a new syndrome revealed by combined pituitary hormone deficiency, Nat Genet 25:182–186, 2000.
42. Machinis K, Pantel J, Netchine I, et al: Syndromic short stature in patients with a germline mutation in the LIM homeobox LHX4, Am J Hum Genet 69:961–968, 2001.
43. Kelberman D, Rizzoti K, Avilion A, et al: Mutations within Sox2/SOX2 are associated with abnormalities in the hypothalamo-pituitary-gonadal axis in mice and humans, J Clin Invest 116(9):2442–2455, 2006.
44. Kelberman D, de Castro SC, Huang S, et al: SOX2 plays a critical role in the pituitary, forebrain and eye during human embryonic development, J Clin Endocrinol Metab 93(5):1865–1873, 2008.
45. Laumonnier F, Ronce N, Hamel BC, et al: Transcription factor SOX3 is involved in X-linked mental retardation with growth hormone deficiency, Am J Hum Genet 71:1450–1455, 2002.
46. Wajnrajch MP, Gertner JM, Harbison MD, et al: Nonsense mutations of the human growth hormone releasing hormone receptor (GHRHR) causes growth failure analogous to that of the little (lit) mouse, Nat Genet 12:88–90, 1996.
47. Baumann G, Maheshwari H: Severe growth hormone (GH) deficiency caused by a mutation in the GH-releasing hormone receptor gene, Acta Paediatr Suppl 423:33–38, 1997.
48. Salvatori R, Hagashida CY, Aguiar-Olivera MH, et al: Familial dwarfism due to a novel mutation of the growth hormone–releasing hormone receptor gene, J Clin Endocrinol Metab 84:917–923, 1999.
49. Godfrey P, Rahal JO, Beamer WG, et al: GHRH receptor of little mouse contains missense mutation in the extracellular domain that disrupts receptor function, Nat Genet 4:227–432, 1993.
50. Sornson MW, Wu W, Daser JS, et al: Pituitary lineage determination by the Prophet of Pit-1 homeodomain factor defective in Ames dwarfism, Nature 384:327–333, 1996.
51. Wu W, Cogan JD, Pfaffle RW, et al: Mutations in PROP1 cause familial combined pituitary hormone deficiency, Nat Genet 18:147–149, 1998.
52. Deladoey J, Fluck C, Buyukgebiz A, et al: "Hot spot" in the PROP1 gene responsible for combined pituitary hormone deficiency, J Clin Endocrinol Metab 84:1645–1650, 1999.
53. Pernasetti F, Toledo SP, Vasilyev VV, et al: Impaired adrenocorticotropin-adrenal axis in combined pituitary hormone deficiency caused by a two-base pair deletion (301–302delAG) in the prophet of PIT1 gene, J Clin Endocrinol Metab 85:390–397, 2000.
54. Mendonca BB, Osorio MG, Latronico AC, et al: Longitudinal hormonal and pituitary imaging changes in two females with combined pituitary hormone deficiency due to deletion of A301,G302 in the PROP1 gene, J Clin Endocrinol Metab 84:942–945, 1999.
55. Bodner M, Castrillo J-L, Theill LE, et al: The pituitary-specific transcription factor GHF-1 is a homeobox-containing protein, Cell 55:505–518, 1988.
56. Mangalam HJ, Albert VR, Ingraham HA, et al: A pituitary POU domain protein, Pit-1, activates both growth hormone and prolactin promoters transcriptionally, Genes Dev 3:946–958, 1989.
57. Li S, Crenshaw EB, Rawson EJ, et al: Dwarf locus mutants lacking three pituitary cell types result from mutations in the POU-domain gene, Nature 347:528–533, 1990.
58. Radovick S, Nations M, Du Y, et al: A mutation in the POV-homeodomain of Pit-1 responsible for combined pituitary hormone deficiency, Science 257:1115–1118, 1992.
59. Pfaffle R, Kim C, Otten B, et al: Pit-1: Clinical aspects, Horm Res 45(suppl 1):25–28, 1996.
60. Pernasetti F, Milner RDG, Al Ashwal AAL, et al: Pro239Ser: A novel recessive mutation of the PIT1 gene in seven Middle Eastern children with growth hormone, prolactin, and thyrotropin deficiency, J Clin Endocrinol Metab 83:2079–2083, 1998.
61. Turton JP, Reynaud R, Mehta A, et al: Novel mutations within the POU1F1 gene associated with variable Combined Pituitary Hormone Deficiency (CPHD), J Clin Endocrinol Metab 90(8):4762–4770, 2005.
62. Procter A, Phillips III JA, Cogan J: The molecular genetics of growth hormone deficiency, Hum Genet 103:255–272, 1998.
63. Wagner JK, Eble A, Hindmarsh PC, et al: Prevalence of human GH1 gene alterations in patients with isolated growth hormone deficiency, Pediatr Res 43:105–110, 1998.
64. Illig R, Prader A, Ferrandez A, et al: Hereditary prenatal growth hormone deficiency with increased tendency to growth hormone antibody formation ("A-type" of isolated growth hormone deficiency), Acta Paediatr Scand 60:607, 1971.
65. Phillips III JA, Cogan J: Genetic basis of endocrine disease. 6. Molecular basis of familial human growth hormone deficiency, J Clin Endocrinol Metab 78:11–16, 1994.
66. Moseley C, Mullis P, Prince M, et al: An exon splice enhancer mutation causes autosomal dominant GH deficiency, J Clin Endocrinol Metab 87:847–852, 2002.
67. McGuiness L, Magoulas C, Mathers K, et al: Autosomal dominant growth hormone deficiency disrupts secretory vesicles: in vitro and in vivo studies in transgenic mice, Endocrinology 144:720–731, 2003.
68. Ryther RCC, McGuiness LM, Phillips JA III, et al: Disruption of exon definition produces a dominant-negative growth hormone isoform that causes somatotroph death and IGHD II, Hum Genet 113:140–148, 2003.
69. Mullis PE, Robinson IC, Salemi S, et al: Isolated autosomal dominant growth hormone deficiency: an evolving pituitary deficit? A multicenter follow-up study, J Clin Endocrinol Metab 90(Apr (4)):2089–2096, 2005.
70. Solomon NM, Nouri S, Warne GL, et al: Increased gene dosage at Xq26-q27 is associated with X-linked hypopituitarism, Genomics 79(Apr (4):553–559, 2002.
71. Woods KS, Cundall M, Turton J, et al: Over- and underdosage of SOX3 is associated with infundibular hypoplasia and hypopituitarism, American Journal of Human Genetics 76(May (5)):833–849, 2005.
72. Kowarski AA, Schneider J, Ben-Galim E, et al: Growth failure with normal serum RIA-GH and low somatomedin activity: Somatomedin restoration and growth acceleration after exogenous GH, J Clin Endocrinol Metab 47:461–464, 1978.
73. Takahashi Y, Shirono H, Arisaka O, et al: Biologically inactive growth hormone caused by an amino acid substitution, J Clin Invest 100:1159–1165, 1997.
74. Fujisawa I, Kikuchi K, Nishimura K, et al: Transection of the pituitary stalk: Development of an ectopic posterior lobe assessed with MR imaging, Radiology 165:487–489, 1987.
75. Abrahams JJ, Trefelner E, Boulware SD: Idiopathic growth hormone deficiency MR findings in 35 patients, Am J Neuroradiol 12:155–160, 1991.
76. Cacciari E, Zucchini S, Carla G, et al: Endocrine function and morphological findings in patients with disorders of the hypothalamo-pituitary area: A study with magnetic resonance, Arch Dis Child 65:1199–1202, 1990.
77. Maghnie M, Larizza D, Triulzi F, et al: Hypopituitarism and stalk agenesis: A congenital syndrome worsened by breech delivery? Horm Res 35:104–108, 1991.
78. Root AW, Martinez CR: Magnetic resonance imaging in patients with hypopituitarism, Trends Endocrinol Metab 3:283–287, 1992.
79. Argyopoulou M, Perignon F, Brauner R, et al: Magnetic resonance imaging in the diagnosis of growth hormone deficiency, J Pediatr 120:886–891, 1992.
80. Triulzi F, Scotti G, diNatale B, et al: Evidence of a congenital midline brain anomaly in pituitary dwarfs: A magnetic resonance imaging study in 101 patients, Pediatrics 93:409–416, 1994.
81. Wilkinson IA, Duck SC, Gager WE, et al: Empty sella syndrome. Occurrence in childhood, Am J Dis Child 136:245–248, 1982.
82. Albertsson-Wikland K, Niklasson A, Karlberg P: Birth data for patients who later develop growth hormone deficiency: Preliminary analysis of a national register, Acta Paediatr Suppl 370:115–120, 1990.
83. Craft WH, Underwood LE, Van Wyk JJ: High incidence of perinatal insult in children with idiopathic hypopituitarism, J Pediatr 96:397–402, 1980.
84. DeVile CJ, Grant DB, Hayward RD, et al: Growth and endocrine sequelae of craniopharyngioma, Arch Dis Child 75:108–114, 1996.
85. Tiulpakov AN, Mazerkina NA, Brook CG, et al: Growth in children with craniopharyngioma following surgery, Clin Endocrinol (Oxf) 49:733–738, 1998.
86. Howarth DM, Gilchrist GS, Mullan BP, et al: Langerhans cell histiocytosis: diagnosis, natural history, management, and outcome, Cancer 85(10):2278–2290, 1999.
87. Nanduri VR, Bareille P, Pritchard J, et al: Growth and endocrine disorders in multisystem Langerhans' cell histiocytosis, Clin Endocrinol (Oxf) 53:509–515, 2000.
88. Donadieu J, Rolon MA, Thomas C, et al: Endocrine involvement in pediatric-onset Langerhans' cell histiocytosis: a population-based study, J Pediatr 144(3):344–350, 2004.
89. Kaltsas GA, Powles TB, Evanson J, et al: Hypothalamo-pituitary abnormalities in adult patients with Langerhans cell histiocytosis: clinical, endocrinological, and radiological features and response to treatment, J Clin Endocrinol Metab 85(4):1370–1376, 2000.
90. Ottaviano F, Finlay JL: Diabetes insipidus and Langerhans cell histiocytosis: a case report of reversibility with 2-chlorodeoxyadenosine, J Pediatr Hematol Oncol 25(7):575–577, 2003.
91. Dhall G, Finlay JL, Dunkel IJ, et al: Analysis of outcome for patients with mass lesions of the central nervous system due to Langerhans cell histiocytosis treated with 2-chlorodeoxyadenosine, Pediatr Blood Cancer 50(1):72–79, 2008.
92. Morimoto A, Ikushima S, Kinugawa N, et al: Improved outcome in the treatment of pediatric multifocal Langerhans cell histiocytosis: Results from the Japan Langerhans Cell Histiocytosis Study Group-96 protocol study, Cancer 107(3):613–619, 2006.
93. Ogilvy-Stuart AL, Clark DJ, Wallace WH, et al: Endocrine deficit after fractionated total body irradiation, Arch Dis Child 67:1107–1110, 1992.
94. Rappaport R, Brauner R: Growth and endocrine disorders secondary to cranial irradiation, Pediatr Res 25:561–567, 1989.
95. Sklar C, Mertens A, Walter A, et al: Final height after treatment for childhood acute lymphoblastic leukemia: Comparison of no cranial irradiation with 1800 and 2400 centigrays of cranial irradiation, J Pediatr 123:56–64, 1993.
96. Balthasar N, Mery PF, Magoulas CB, et al: Growth hormone-releasing hormone (GHRH) neurons in GHRH-enhanced green fluorescent protein transgenic mice: a ventral hypothalamic network, Endocrinology 144:2728–2740, 2003.
97. Blatt J, Bercu BB, Gillin JC, et al: Reduced pulsatile growth hormone secretion in children after therapy for acute lymphoblastic leukemia, J Pediatr 104:182–186, 1984.
98. Sklar CA, Sarafoglou K, Whittam E: Effects of insulin-like growth factor binding protein 3 in predicting the growth hormone response to provocative testing in children treated with cranial irradiation, Acta Endocrinol 129:511–515, 1993.
99. Quigley C, Cowell C, Jimenez M, et al: Normal or early development of puberty despite gonadal damage in children treated for acute lymphoblastic leukemia, N Engl J Med 321:143–151, 1989.
100. Acerini CL, Tasker RC, Bellone S, et al: Hypopituitarism in childhood and adolescence following traumatic brain injury: the case for prospective endocrine investigation, Eur J Endocrinol 155(5):663–669, 2006.
101. Oertel M, Boscardin WJ, Obrist WD, et al: Posttraumatic vasospasm: the epidemiology, severity, and time course of an underestimated phenomenon: a prospective study performed in 299 patients, J Neurosurg 103(5):812–824, 2005.
102. Agha A, Thompson CJ: Anterior pituitary dysfunction following traumatic brain injury (TBI), Clin Endocrinol (Oxf) 64(5):481–488, 2006.
103. Tanriverdi F, Senyurek H, Unluhizarci K, et al: High risk of hypopituitarism after traumatic brain injury: a prospective investigation of anterior pituitary function in the acute phase and 12 months after trauma, J Clin Endocrinol Metab 91(6):2105–2111, 2006.
104. Niederland T, Makovi H, Gal V, et al: Abnormalities of pituitary function after traumatic brain injury in children, J Neurotrauma 24(1):119–127, 2007.

105. Einaudi S, Bondone C: The effects of head trauma on hypothalamic-pituitary function in children and adolescents, Curr Opin Pediatr 19(4):465–470, 2007.
106. Ghigo E, Masel B, Aimaretti G, et al: Consensus guidelines on screening for hypopituitarism following traumatic brain injury, Brain Inj 19(9):711–724, 2005.
107. Bartsocas CS, Pantelakis SN: Human growth hormone therapy in hypopituitarism due to tuberculous meningitis, Acta Paediatr Scand 62:304–306, 1973.
108. Stuart CA, Neelon FA, Lebovitz HE: Hypothalamic insufficiency: The cause of hypopituitarism in sarcoidosis, Ann Intern Med 88:589–594, 1978.
109. Rund D, Rachmilewitz E: Beta-thalassemia, N Engl J Med 353(11):1135–1146, 2005.
110. Fung EB, Harmatz PR, Lee PD, et al: Increased prevalence of iron-overload associated endocrinopathy in thalassaemia versus sickle-cell disease, Br J Haematol 135(4):574–582, 2006.
111. Powell GF, Brasel JA, Blizzard RM: Emotional deprivation and growth retardation simulating idiopathic hypopituitarism, N Engl J Med 276:1271–1278, 1967.
112. Skuse D, Albanese A, Stanhope R: A new stress-related syndrome of growth failure and hyperphagia in children, associated with reversibility of growth-hormone insufficiency, Lancet 348:353–358, 1996.
113. Albanese A, Hamill G, Jones J, et al: Reversibility of physiological growth hormone secretion in children with psychosocial dwarfism, Clin Endocrinol 40:687–692, 1994.
114. Hindmarsh PC, Matthews DR, Brook CGD: Growth hormone secretion in children determined by time series analysis, Clin Endocrinol (Oxf) 29:35–44, 1988.
115. Jaffe CA, Ocampo-Lim B, Guo W, et al: Regulatory mechanisms of growth hormone secretion are sexually dimorphic, J Clin Invest 102:153–164, 1998.
116. Papotti M, Ghe C, Cassoni P, et al: Growth hormone secretagogue binding sites in peripheral human tissues, J Clin Endocrinol Metab 85:3803–3807, 2000.
117. Gnanapavan S, Kola B, Bustin SA, et al: The tissue distribution of the mRNA of ghrelin and subtypes of its receptor, GHS-R, in humans, J Clin Endocrinol Metab 87:2988, 2002.
118. Kojima M, Hosoda H, Date Y, et al: Ghrelin is a growth-hormone-releasing acylated peptide from stomach, Nature 402:656–660, 1999.
119. Smith RG, Palyha OC, Feighner SD, et al: Growth hormone releasing substances: types and their receptors, Horm Res 51(Suppl 3):1–8, 1999.
120. Bennani-Baiti IM, Asa SL, Song D, et al: DNase-I hypersensitive sites I and II of the human growth hormone locus control region are a major developmental activator of somatotrope gene expression, Proc Natl Acad Sci U S A 95:10655–10660, 1998.
121. Shewchuk BM, Asa SL, Cooke NE, et al: Pit-1 binding sites at the somatotrope-specific DNase-I hypersensitive sites I, II of the human growth hormone locus control region are essential for in-vivo hGH-N gene activation, J Biol Chem 274:35725–35733, 1999.
122. Baumann G: Growth hormone heterogeneity: genes, isohormones, variants, and binding proteins, Endocr Rev 12:424–449, 1991.
123. Clark RG, Mortensen DL, Carlsson LM, et al: Recombinant human growth hormone (GH)-binding protein enhances the growth-promoting activity of human GH in the rat, Endocrinology 137:4308–4315, 1996.
124. Carter-Su C, Schwartz J, Smit LS: Molecular mechanism of growth hormone action, Annu Rev Physiol 58:187–207, 1996.
125. Smit LS, Meyer DJ, Billestrup N, et al: The role of the growth hormone (GH) receptor and JAK1 and JAK2 kinases in the activation of Stats 1, 3, and 5 by GH, Mol Endocrinol 10:519–533, 1996.
126. Rosenfeld RG, Rosenbloom AL, Guevara-Aguirre J: Growth hormone (GH) insensitivity due to primary GH receptor deficiency, Endocr Rev 15:369–390, 1994.
127. Rosenfeld RG, Rosenbloom AL, Guevara-Aguirre J: Abnormalities of growth hormone action. In Kelnar CJH, Savage MO, Stirling HF, et al: Growth Disorders. Pathophysiology and Treatment, London, 1998, Chapman & Hall, pp 549–564.
128. Woods KA, Dastot F, Preece MA, et al: Phenotype-genotype relationships in growth hormone insensitivity syndrome, J Clin Endocrinol Metab 82:3529–3535, 1997.
129. Rygaard K, Revol A, Esquivel-Escobedo D, et al: Absence of human placental lactogen and placental growth hormone (hGH-V) during pregnancy: PCR analysis of the deletion, Hum Genet 102:87–92, 1998.
130. DeChiara TM, Efstratiadis A, Robertson EJ: A growth-deficiency phenotype in heterozygous mice carrying an insulin-like growth factor II gene disrupted by targeting, Nature 345:78–80, 1990.
131. Liu JP, Baker J, Perkins AS, et al: Mice carrying null mutations of the genes encoding insulin-like growth factor I (Igf-1) and type 1 IGF receptor (Igf1r), Cell 75:73–82, 1993.
132. Goossens M, Brauner R, Czernichow P, et al: Isolated growth hormone deficiency Type 1A associated with a double deletion in the human growth hormone gene cluster, J Clin Endocrinol Metab 62:712–716, 1986.
133. Wit JM, Van Unen H: Growth of infants with neonatal growth hormone deficiency, Arch Dis Child 67:920–924, 1982.
134. Gluckman PD, Gunn A-J, Wray A: Congenital idiopathic growth hormone deficiency associated with early postnatal growth failure, J Pediatr 121:920–923, 1992.
135. Wit JM, Kamp G, Rikken B: Spontaneous growth and response to growth hormone treatment in children with growth hormone deficiency and idiopathic short stature, Pediatr Res 39:295–302, 1996.
136. Rimoin DL, Merimee TJ, Rabinowitz D, et al: Genetic aspects of clinical endocrinology, Recent Prog Horm Res 24:365–437, 1968.
137. van der Werff ten Bosch JJ, Bot A: Growth of males with idiopathic hypopituitarism without growth hormone treatment, Clin Endocrinol (Oxf) 32:707–717, 1990.
138. Milner RDG, Russell-Fraser T, Brook CGD, et al: Experience with human growth hormone in Great Britain: the report of the MRC working Party. Clin Endocrinol 11:15–38, 1979.
139. Vanderschuren-Lodeweyckx M, Wolter R, Mulla A, et al: Plasma growth hormone in coeliac disease, Acta Pediatr (Helv) 28:349–357, 1973.
140. Rosenfeld RG, Albertsson-Wikland K, Cassorla F, et al: The diagnosis of childhood growth hormone deficiency revisited, J Clin Endocrinol Metab 80:1532–1540, 1995.
141. Hussain K, Hindmarsh P, Aynsley_Green A: Spontaneous hypoglycemia in childhood is accompanied by paradoxically low serum growth hormone and appropriate cortisol counterregulatory hormonal responses, J Clin Endocrinol Metab 88:3715–3723, 2003.
142. Iranmanesh A, Lizaralde G, Veldhuis JD: Age and relative adiposity are specific negative determinants of the pregnancy and amplitude of growth hormone (GH) secretory bursts and the half-life of endogenous GH in healthy men, J Clin Endocrinol Metab 73:1081–1088, 1991.
143. Freeman JV, Cole TJ, Chinn S, et al: Cross sectional stature and weight reference curves for the UK, 1990. Arch Dis Child 73:17–24, 1995.
144. Blum WF, Ranke MB, Kietzmann K, et al: A specific radioimmunoassay for the growth hormone (GH)-dependent somatomedin-binding protein: its use for diagnosis of GH deficiency, J Clin Endocrinol Metab 70:1292–1298, 1990.
145. Tillman V, Buckler JM, Kibirge MS, et al: Biochemical tests in the diagnosis of childhood growth hormone deficiency, J Clin Endocrinol Metab 82:531–535, 1997.
146. Mitchell H, Dattani MT, Nanduri V, et al: Failure of IGF-1 and IGFBP-3 to diagnose growth hormone insufficiency, Arch Dis Child 80:443–447, 1999.
147. Sox HC Jr: Probability theory in the use of diagnostic tests, Ann Int Med 104:60–66, 1986.
148. Suri D, Hindmarsh PC, Matthews DR, et al: The pituitary gland is capable of responding to two successive doses of growth hormone–releasing hormone (GHRH), Clin Endocrinol 34:13–17, 1991.
149. Rahim A, Toogood A, Shalet SM: The assessment of growth hormone status in normal young adult males using a variety of provocative tests, Clin Endocrinol 45:557–562, 1996.
150. Tauber M, Houlin P, Pienkowski C, et al: Growth Hormone (GH) retesting and auxological data in 131 GH-deficient patients after completion of treatment, J Clin Endocrinol Metab 82:352–356, 1997.
151. Thomas GB, Robinson ICAF: Central regulation of growth hormone secretion. In Kelnar CJH, Savage MO, Stirling HF, et al: Growth Disorders. Pathophysiology and Treatment, London, 1998, Chapman & Hall, pp 99–125.
152. Martha PM Jr, Rogol AD, Veldhuis JD, et al: Alterations in the pulsatile properties of circulating growth hormone concentrations during puberty in boys, J Clin Endocrinol Metab 69:563–570, 1989.
153. Martha PM, Gorman KM, Blizzard RM, et al: Endogenous growth hormone secretion and clearance rates in normal boys as determined by deconvolution analysis: Relationship to age, pubertal status and body mass, J Clin Endocrinol Metab 74:336–344, 1992.
154. Spiliotis BE, August GP, Hung W, et al: Growth hormone neurosecretory dysfunction: A treatable cause of short stature, JAMA 252:2223–2230, 1984.
155. Bercu BB, Shulman D, Root AW, et al: Growth hormone (GH) provocative testing frequently does not reflect endogenous GH secretion, J Clin Endocrinol Metab 86:709–716, 1986.
156. Rose SR, Ross JL, Uriarte M, et al: The advantage of measuring stimulated as compared with spontaneous growth hormone levels in the diagnosis of growth hormone deficiency, N Engl J Med 319:201–207, 1988.
157. Lanes R: Diagnostic limitations of spontaneous growth hormone measurements in normally growing prepubertal children, Am J Dis Child 143:1284–1286, 1989.
158. Donaldson DL, Hollowell JG, Pan F, et al: Growth hormone secretory profiles: Variation on consecutive nights, J Pediatr 115:51–56, 1989.
159. Hourd P, Edwards R: Current methods for the measurement of growth hormone in urine, Clin Endocrinol (Oxf) 40:155–170, 1994.
160. Albini CH, Quattrin T, Vandlen RL, et al: Quantitation of urinary growth hormone in children with normal and subnormal growth, Pediatr Res 23:89–92, 1988.
161. Granada ML, Sanmarti ALA, et al: Clinical usefulness of urinary growth hormone measurements in normal and short children according to different expressions of urinary growth hormone data, Pediatr Res 32:73–76, 1992.
162. Phillip M, Chalew SA, Stene MA, et al: The value of urinary growth hormone determination for assessment of growth hormone deficiency and compliance with growth hormone therapy, Am J Dis Child 147:553–557, 1993.
163. Skinner AM, Clayton PE, Price DA, et al: Urinary growth hormone excretion in the assessment of children with disorders of growth, Clin Endocrinol (Oxf) 39:201–206, 1993.
164. Underwood LE, Azumi K, Voina SJ, et al: Growth hormone levels during sleep in normal and growth hormone deficient children, Pediatrics 48:946–954, 1971.
165. Buckler JMH: Plasma growth hormone response to exercise as a diagnostic aid, Arch Dis Child 48:565–567, 1973.
166. Lacey KA, Hewison A, Parkin JM: Exercise as a screening test for growth hormone deficiency in children, Arch Dis Child 1973:48:508–512,
167. Coller R, Leboeuf G, Letarte J: Stimulation of growth hormone secretion by levodopa propranolol in children and adolescents, Pediatrics 56:262–266, 1975.
168. Youlton R, Kaplan SL, Grumbach MM: Growth and growth hormone. IV limitations of the growth hormone response to insulin and arginine in the assessment of growth hormone deficiency in children, Pediatrics 43:989–1004, 1969.
169. Lanes R, Hurtado E: Oral clonidine: an effective growth hormone–releasing agent in prepubertal subjects, J Pediatr 100:710–714, 1982.
170. Mitchell ML, Bryne MJ, Sanchez Y, et al: Detection of growth deficiency. The glucagon simulation test, N Engl J Med 282:539–541, 1970.
171. Merimee TJ, Rabinowitz D, Fineberg SE: Arginine-initiated release of human growth hormone, N Engl J Med 280:1434–1438, 1969.
172. Fass B, Lippe BM, Kaplan SA: Relative usefulness of three growth hormone stimulation screening tests, Am J Dis Child 133:931–933, 1979.
173. Weldon VV, Gupta SK, Klingensmith G: Evaluation of growth hormone release in children using arginine and L-dopa in combination, J Pediatr 87:540–544, 1975.
174. Reiter EO, Martha PM Jr: Pharmacological testing of growth hormone secretion, Horm Res 33:121–127, 1990.

175. Raiti S, Davis WT, Blizzard RM: A comparison of the effects of insulin hypoglycemia and arginine infusion on release of human growth hormone, Lancet 2:1182–1183, 1967.
176. Albertsson-Wikland K, Rosberg S: Analysis of 24-hour growth hormone profiles in children: relation to growth, J Clin Endocrinol Metab 67:493–500, 1988.
177. Lijmer JG, Mol BW, Heisterkamp S, et al: Empirical evidence of design-related bias in studies of diagnostic tests, JAMA 282:1061–1066, 1999.
178. Ware J: The limitations of risk factors as prognostic tools, N Engl J Med 355:2615–2617, 2006.
179. Marin G, Domene HM, Barnes KM, et al: The effects of estrogen priming and puberty on the growth hormone response to standardized treadmill exercise and arginine-insulin in normal girls and boys, J Clin Endocrinol Metab 79:537–541, 1994.
180. Cordido F, Fernandez T, Martinez T, et al: Effect of acute pharmacological reduction of plasma free fatty acids on growth hormone (GH) releasing hormone—induced GH secretion in obese adults with and without hypopituitarism, J Clin Endocrinol Metab 83:4350–4354, 1998.
181. Lewis UJ, Singh RNP, Tutwiler GH, et al: Human growth hormone: A complex of proteins, Recent Prog Horm Res 36:477–508, 1980.
182. Celniker AC, Chem AB, Wert RM Jr, et al: Variability in the quantitation of circulating growth hormone using commercial immunoassays, J Clin Endocrinol Metab 68:469–476, 1989.
183. Barth JH, Smith JH, Clarkson P: Wide diversity in measurements of growth hormone after stimulation tests in short children are due to assay variability, Ann Clin Biochem 32:369–372, 1995.
184. Dattani MT, Pringle PJ, Hindmarsh PC, et al: What is a normal stimulated growth hormone concentration? J Endocr 133:447–450, 1992.
185. Clemmons DR: IGF-1 assays: Current assay methodologies and their limitations, Pituitary 10:121–128, 2007.
186. Devesa J, Lima L, Lois N, et al: Reasons for the variability in growth hormone (GH) responses to GHRH challenge: the endogenous hypothalamic—somatotroph rhythm (HSR), Clin Endocrinol 30:367–377, 1989.
187. Tzanela M, Guyda H, Van Vliet G, et al: Somatostatin pretreatment enhances growth hormone responsiveness to GH-releasing hormone: a potential new diagnostic approach to GH deficiency, J Clin Endocrinol Metab 81:2487–2494, 1996.
188. Bernasconi S, Volta C, Cozzini A, et al: GH response to GHRH, insulin, clonidine and arginine after GHRH pretreatment in children, Acta Endocrinol 126:105–108, 1992.
189. Massoud AF, Hindmarsh PC, Matthews DR, et al: The effect of repeated administration of hexarelin, a growth hormone releasing peptide, and growth hormone releasing hormone (GHRH) on growth hormone (GH) responsivity, Clin Endocrinol 44:555–562, 1996.
190. Berelowitz M, Szabo M, Frohman LA, et al: Somatomedin-C mediates growth hormone negative feedback by effects on both the hypothalamus and pituitary, Science 212:1279–1281, 1981.
191. Yamashita S, Melmed S: Insulin-like growth factor I action on rat anterior pituitary cells: Suppression of growth hormone secretion and messenger ribonucleic acid levels, Endocrinology 118:176–182, 1986.
192. Abe H, Molitch M, Van Wyk JJ, et al: Human growth hormone and somatomedin-C suppress the spontaneous release of growth hormone in unanesthetized rats, Endocrinology 113:1319–1324, 1983.
193. Ceda GP, Davis WT, Rosenfeld RG, et al: The growth hormone (GH) releasing hormone (GHRH)-GH-somatomedin axis: Evidence for rapid inhibition of GHRH-elicited GH release by insulin-like growth factors I and II, Endocrinology 120:1658–1662, 1987.
194. Saini S, Hindmarsh PC, Matthews DR, et al: Reproducibility of 24hour serum growth hormone profiles in man, Clin Endocrinol 34:455–462, 1991.
195. Shriock EA, Hulse JA, Harris DA, et al: Evaluation of hypothalamic dysfunction in growth hormone (GH)–deficient patients using single versus multiple doses of growth hormone–releasing hormone (GHRH-44) and evidence for diurnal variation in somatotroph responsiveness to GHRH in GH deficient patients, J Clin Endocrinol Metab 65:1177–1182, 1987.
196. Ghigo E, Bellone J, Aimasetti G, et al: Reliability of provocative tests to assess growth hormone secretory status. Study in 472 normally growing children, J Clin Endocrinol Metab 81:3323–3327, 1996.
197. Frasier SD: Human pituitary growth hormone (hGH) therapy in growth hormone deficiency, Endocr Rev 4:155–170, 1983.
198. MacGillivray MH, Baptista J, Johanson A, et al: Outcome of a four year randomized study of daily versus three times weekly somatropin treatment in prepubertal naive growth hormone deficient children, J Clin Endocrinol Metab 81:1806–1809, 1996.
199. Cohen P, Bright GM, Rogol AD, et al: Effects of dose and gender on the growth and growth factor response to GH in GH-deficient children: implications for efficacy and safety, J Clin Endocrinol Metab 87:90–98, 2002.
200. Pantel J, Machinis K, Sobrier ML, et al: Species-specific alternative splice mimicry at the growth hormone receptor locus revealed by the lineage of retroelements during primate evolution, J Biol Chem 275:18664–18669, 2000.
201. Pantel J, Grulich-Henn J, Bettendorf M, et al: Heterozygous nonsense mutation in exon 3 of the growth hormone receptor (GHR) in severe GH insensitivity (Laron syndrome) and the issue of the origin and function of the GHRd3 isoform, J Clin Endocrinol Metab 88:1705–1710, 2003.
202. Dos Santos C, Essioux L, Teinturier C, et al: A common polymorphism of the growth hormone receptor is associated with increased responsiveness to growth hormone, Nat Genet 36:720–724, 2004.
203. Jorge AA, Marchisotti FG, Montenegro LR, et al: Growth hormone (GH) pharmacogenetics: influence of GH receptor exon 3 retention or deletion on first-year growth response and final height in patients with severe GH deficiency, J Clin Endocrinol Metab 91:1076–1080, 2006.
204. Pilotta A, Mella P, Filisetti M, et al: Common polymorphisms of the growth hormone (GH) receptor do not correlate with the growth response to exogenous recombinant human GH in GH-deficient children, J Clin Endocrinol Metab 91:1178–1180, 2006.
205. Carrascosa A, Esteban C, Espadero R, et al: The d3/fl-growth hormone (GH) receptor polymorphism does not influence the effect of GH treatment (66 microg/kg per day) or the spontaneous growth in short non-GH-deficient small-for-gestational-age children: results from a two-year controlled prospective study in 170 Spanish patients, J Clin Endocrinol Metab 91:3281–3286, 2006.
206. Audi L, Esteban C, Carrascosa A, et al: Exon 3-deleted/full-length growth hormone receptor polymorphism genotype frequencies in Spanish short small-for-gestational-age (SGA) children and adolescents (n = 247) and in an adult control population (n = 289) show increased fl/fl in short SGA, J Clin Endocrinol Metab 91:5038–5043, 2006.
207. Blum WF, Machinis K, Shavrikova EP, et al: The growth response to growth hormone (GH) treatment in children with isolated GH deficiency is independent of the presence of the exon 3-minus isoform of the GH receptor, J Clin Endocrinol Metab 91:4171–4174, 2006.
208. Ràz B, Janner M, Petkovic V, et al: Influence of growth hormone (GH) receptor deletion of exon 3 and full-length isoforms on GH response and final height in patients with severe GH deficiency, J Clin Endocrinol Metab 93:974–980, 2008.
209. Beavis WD: QTL analyses: power, precision and accuracy. In Paterson AH, editor: Molecular Analysis of Complex Traits, New York, 1998, CRC Press, pp 145–161.
210. Xu S: Theoretical basis of the Beavis effect, Genetics 165:2259–2268, 2003.
211. Cohen P, Rogol AD, Howard CP, et al: Insulin growth factor–based dosing of growth hormone therapy in children: a randomized controlled study, J Clin Endocrinol Metab 92:2480–2486, 2007.
212. Albertsson-Wikland K: The effect of human growth hormone injection frequency on linear growth rate, Acta Paediatr Scand Suppl 337:110–116, 1987.
213. Hakeem V, Hindmarsh PC, Brook CGD: Intermittent versus continuous administration of growth hormone treatment, Arch Dis Child 68:783–784, 1993.
214. Johnson OL, Cleleand TL, Lee HJ, et al: A month-long effect from a single injection of microencapsulated human growth hormone, Nat Med 2:795–799, 1996.
215. Ranke MB, Lindberg A, Guilbaud O: Prediction of growth in response to treatment with growth hormone. In Ranke MB, Gunnarsson R, editors: Progress in Growth Hormone Therapy: 5 Years of KIGS, Mannheim, Germany, 1994, JJ Verlag, pp 97–111.
216. Blomqvist N: On the bias caused by regression to the mean in studying the relation between change and initial value, J Clin Periodontol 13:34–37, 1986.
217. Hayes RJ: Methods for assessing whether change depends on initial value, Stat Med 7:915–927, 1988.
218. Taback SP, Van Vliet G: Managing the short stature of Turner syndrome: an evidence-based approval to the suggestion of growth hormone supplementation. In Hindmarsh PC, editor: Current Indications for Growth Hormone Therapy, Basel, 1999, Karger, pp 102–117.
219. Matthews JNS, Altman DG, Campbell MJ, et al: Analysis of serial measurements in medical research, BMJ 300:230–235, 1990.
220. Bramswig JH, Schlosser H, Kiese K: Final height in children with growth hormone deficiency, Horm Res 43:126–128, 1995.
221. Frisch H, Birnbacher R: Final height and pubertal development in children with growth hormone deficiency after long-term treatment, Horm Res 43:132–134, 1995.
222. Severi F: Final height in children with growth hormone deficiency, Horm Res 43:138–140, 1995.
223. Blethen SL, Compton P, Lippe BM, et al: Factors predicting the response to growth hormone (GH) therapy in prepubertal children with GH deficiency, J Clin Endocrinol Metab 74:574–579, 1993.
224. Burns EC, Tanner JM, Preece MA, et al: Final height and pubertal development in 55 children with idiopathic growth hormone deficiency, treated for between 2 and 15 years with human growth hormone, Eur J Pediatr 137:155–164, 1981.
225. Bourguignon JP, Vandeweghe M, Vanderschuren-Lodeweyckx M, et al: Pubertal growth and final height in hypopituitary boys: A minor role of bone age at onset of puberty, J Clin Endocrinol Metab 63:376–382, 1986.
226. Price DA, Ranke MB: Final height following growth hormone treatment. In Ranke MB, Gunnarsson R, editors: Progress in Growth Hormone Therapy: 5 Years of KIGS, Mannheim, Germany, 1994, JJ Verlag, pp 574–579.
227. Ranke MB, Price DA, Albertsson-Wikland K, et al: Factors determining pubertal growth and final height in growth hormone treatment of idiopathic growth hormone deficiency, Horm Res 48:62–71, 1997.
228. Tanaka T, Satoh M, Yasunaga T, et al: GH and GnRH analog treatment in children who enter puberty at short stature, J Pediatr Endocrinol Metab 10:623–628, 1997.
229. Saggese G, Baroncelli GI, Bertelloni S, et al: The effect of long-term growth hormone (GH) treatment on bone mineral density in children with GH deficiency. Role of GH in the attainment of peak bone mass, J Clin Endocrinol Metab 81:3077–3083, 1996.
230. Blethen SL, Alster DK, Graves D, et al: Safety of recombinant DNA–derived growth hormone (rhGH): The National Cooperative Growth Study experience, J Clin Endocrinol Metab 81:1704–1710, 1996.
231. Wilton P: Adverse events during growth hormone treatment: 5 years' experience. In Ranke B, Gunnarsson R, editors: Progress in Growth Hormone Therapy: 5 Years of KIGS, Mannheim, Germany, 1994, JJ Verlag, pp 291–307.
232. Cutfield WS, Wilton P, Bennmarker H, et al: Incidence of diabetes mellitus and impaired glucose tolerance in children and adolescents receiving growth-hormone treatment, Lancet 355:610–613, 2000.
233. Watanabe S, Yamagucki N, Tsunematsu Y, et al: Risk factors for leukemia occurrence among growth hormone users, Jpn J Cancer 80:822–825, 1989.
234. Fisher DA, Job J, Preece M, et al: Leukemia in patients treated with growth hormone, Lancet 1:1159–1160, 1988.
235. Fradkin JE, Mills JL, Schonberger LB, et al: Risk of leukemia after treatment with pituitary growth hormone, JAMA 270:2829–2832, 1993.
236. Oglivy-Stuart AL, Ryder WD, Gattamaneni HR, et al: Growth hormone and tumor recurrence, BMJ 304:1601–1605, 1992.

237. Moshang T, Rundle AC, Graves DA, et al: Brain tumor recurrence in children treated with growth hormone: The National Cooperative Growth Study experience, J Pediatr 128: S4–S7, 1996.

238. Swerdlow AJ, Reddingius RE, Higgins CD, et al: Growth hormone treatment of children with brain tumors and risk of tumor recurrence, J Clin Endocrinol Metab 85(12):4444–4449, 2000.

239. Swerdlow AJ, Higgins CD, Adlard P, et al: Risk of cancer in patients treated with human pituitary growth hormone in the UK, 1959–1985: a cohort study, Lancet 360:273–277, 2002.

240. Ma J, Pollak MN, Giovannucci E, et al: Prospective study of colorectal cancer risk in men and plasma levels of insulin-like growth factor (IGF)-I and IGF-binding protein-3, J Natl Cancer Inst 91:620–625, 1999.

241. Hankinson SE, Willett WC, Colditz GA, et al: Circulating concentrations of insulin-like growth factor-I and risk of breast cancer, Lancet 351:1393–1396, 1998.

242. Chan JM, Stampfer MJ, Giovannucci E, et al: Plasma insulin-like growth factor-I and prostate cancer risk: a prospective study, Science 279:563–566, 1998.

243. Palmqvist R, Hallmans G, Rinaldi S, et al: Plasma insulin-like growth factor 1, insulin-like growth factor binding protein 3, and risk of colorectal cancer: a prospective study in northern Sweden, Gut 50:642–646, 2002.

244. Thorner MO, Rogol AD, Blizzard RM, et al: Acceleration of growth rate in growth hormone–deficient children treated with human growth hormone–releasing hormone, Pediatr Res 24:145–151, 1988.

245. Thorner MO, Rochiccioli P, Colle M, et al: Geraf International Study Group. Once-daily subcutaneous growth hormone–releasing hormone therapy accelerates growth in growth hormone–deficient children during the first year of therapy, J Clin Endocrinol Metab 81:1189–1196, 1996.

246. Hummelink R, Sippell WG, Benoit KG: Intranasal administration of growth hormone–releasing hormone (1–29)-NH$_2$ in children with growth hormone deficiency: effects on growth hormone secretion and growth, Acta Paediatr Suppl 388:23–26, 1993.

247. Bowers CY, Alster DK, Frentz JM: The growth hormone–releasing activity of a synthetic hexapeptide in normal men and short stature children after oral administration, J Clin Endocrinol Metab 74:292–298, 1992.

248. Bowers CY: On a peptidomimetic growth hormone-releasing peptide, J Clin Endocrinol Metab 79:940–942, 1994.

249. Smith RG, van der Ploey LHT, Howard AD, et al: Peptidomimetic regulation of growth hormone secretion, Endocr Rev 18:621–645, 1997.

250. Allen DB: Issues in the transition from childhood to adult growth hormone therapy, Pediatrics 104:1004–1010, 1999.

251. Monson JP, Hindmarsh P: The assessment of growth hormone deficiency in children and adults with particular reference to the transitional period, Clin Endocrinol (Oxf) 53:545–547, 2000.

252. Rosenfeld RG: Transitioning patients with childhood-onset growth hormone deficiency to treatment in adulthood, J Pediatr Endocrinol Metab 15:1361–1365, 2002.

253. GH Research Society: Consensus guidelines for the diagnosis and treatment of growth hormone (GH) deficiency in childhood and adolescence: summary statement of the GH Research Society, J Clin Endocrinol Metab 85:3990–3993, 2000.

254. Donaubauer J, Kiess W, Kratzsch J, et al: Re-assessment of growth hormone secretion in young adult patients with childhood-onset growth hormone deficiency, Clin Endocrinol (Oxf) 58:456–463, 2003.

255. de Boer H, van der Veen EA: Why retest young adults with childhood-onset growth hormone deficiency? J Clin Endocrinol Metab 82:2032–2036, 1997.

256. Saggese G, Ranke MB, Saenger P, et al: Diagnosis and treatment of growth hormone deficiency in children and adolescents: towards a consensus. Ten years after the Availability of Recombinant Human Growth Hormone Workshop held in Pisa, Italy, 27–28 March 1998, Horm Res 50:320–340, 1998.

257. Shalet SM, Toogood A, Rahim A, et al: The diagnosis of growth hormone deficiency in children and adults, Endocr Rev 19:203–223, 1998.

Index

A

Accelerated growth pattern, e361–e362
Achondroplasia, e345–e348, e348t,
　e349f
Acid labile subunit, e315
Acidophil stem cell adenomas,
　e117–e119, e190–e192
Acromegaloidism, e119
Acromegaly
　acral overgrowth associated with,
　　e123
　algorithm for, e123f
　candidate genes associated with,
　　e120–e121, e120t
　cardiovascular findings, e124
　characteristics of, e117
　clinical
　　manifestations of, e122–e125
　colonic polyp risks, e125
　colonoscopic
　　monitoring in, e132–e133
　cortisol hypersecretion in, e68
　diabetes mellitus associated with,
　　e125
　diagnosis of, e121–e126, e121t,
　　e123f
　epidemiology of, e121
　familial syndromes associated with,
　　e121
　fertility concerns, e132–e133
　follow-up, e132
　ghrelin levels in, e293–e294
　gonadal function in, e125
　growth hormone hypersecretion in,
　　e117–e119, e118f, e121–e122,
　　e126, e132
　growth hormone-releasing hormone
　　in
　　description of, e282
　　ectopic, e119
　　hypersecretion, e119
　hyperprolactinemia
　　in, e125, e191–e192
　hypothalamus' role in, e119–e120
　insulin-like growth factor-1 levels as
　　screening
　　test for, e121, e315–e316
　joint arthralgias in, e124
　laboratory findings, e125
　maxillofacial disorders associated
　　with, e132–e133
　in McCune-Albright syndrome,
　　e117–e119
　mortality rate for, e125–e126,
　　e125f–e126f, e126t
　neoplasms caused by, e125
　nonpituitary, e122
　onset of, e122
　pathogenesis of, e117–e121, e119f
　patient counseling, e132–e133
　pituitary lesions, e120, e120t
　rheumatologic
　　features of, e123–e124
　skin findings in, e124
　sleep apnea in, e124–e125
　somatotroph adenoma as cause of,
　　e117–e119
　thyroid findings in, e124

Acromegaly (Continued)
　treatment of, e126–e131
　　dopamine agonists, e130
　　goals for, e126, e127t
　　growth hormone-receptor
　　　antagonist, e130–e131, e133
　　integrated approach, e131–e133
　　octreotide, e128, e130f
　　pegvisomant, e130–e131
　　pharmacologic, e127t, e128–
　　　e131, e129f
　　pituitary irradiation, e127–e128
　　radiotherapy, e127–e128
　　somatostatin-receptor ligands,
　　　e127t, e128–e130, e133
　　surgery, e126–e127, e127t,
　　　e131–e132
ACTH. See Adrenocorticotropic
　hormone
Acyl-ghrelin, e66–e67, e287–e289
Ad4BP. See Steroidogenic factor 1
Adenohypophysis, e1
Adenoma. See also Macroadenomas;
　Microadenomas
　adrenal. See Adrenal adenomas
　gonadotroph. See Gonadotroph
　　adenomas
　growth hormone-cell, e120, e120t
　lactotroph, e25, e173
　pituitary. See Pituitary adenomas
　somatotroph, e117–e119, e122,
　　e170–e173
　thyrotropin-producing. See
　　Thyrotropin-producing
　　adenomas
Adenosine deaminase deficiency, e348t
Adiponectin, e74
Adipose tissue
　growth hormone effects on
　　distribution of, e268–e269
Adiposity
　growth hormone release and, e68
Adipsic diabetes insipidus, e248,
　e248t
Adipsic hypernatremia, e87–e88
Adolescents. See also Children
　growth hormone therapy in, e354
Adrenal adenomas
　adrenalectomy for, e154
　definition of, e139
　glucocorticoid
　　production by, e137–e138
Adrenal cancer, e160. See also
　Adrenocortical carcinoma
Adrenal gland(s)
　adrenocorticotropic hormone effects
　　on, e44
Adrenal masses
　pheochromocytoma. See
　　Pheochromocytoma
Adrenal steroidogenesis
　adrenocorticotropic hormone
　　stimulation of, e43–e44
　agents that inhibit, e156–e157
Adrenal tumors.
　adenoma. See Adrenal adenoma
Adrenalectomy
　Cushing's syndrome treated with,
　　e154–e155, e159

Adrenocortical carcinoma
　cortisol production in, e145
Adrenocorticotropic hormone
　adrenal gland effects
　　description of, e44
　corticotrope cell production of, e1
　cortisol and, e65
　in Cushing's disease, e65
　deficiency of
　　anorexia caused by, e102
　　diagnostic evaluations, e104
　　hypoglycemia and, e381
　　hyponatremia associated with,
　　　e103, e251
　　hypopituitarism secondary to,
　　　e103
　　isolated, e101–e102
　　lymphocytic hypophysitis, e102
　　in neonates, e381
　　signs and symptoms of, e103,
　　　e103t
　　treatment of, e105t, e106
　differential regulation of, e47
　excess, skin pigmentation caused by,
　　e44
　GABA effects on, e46
　glucocorticoids effect on, e38,
　　e45–e46, e45f
　history of, e34
　hypothalamic, e46
　insufficiency of, e234
　measurement of, e48–e49
　melanocortin-2 receptor binding of,
　　e44
　overexpression of, e43–e44
　oxytocin effects on, e46
　precursors of, e44–e46, e48–e49
　processing of, e42–e43
　　anterior pituitary, e42
　　enzymes involved in, e41–e42
　　hypothalamus, e42–e43
　　intermediate lobe, e42
　　N-glycosylation, e42
　　pathways, e41–e42, e42f
　　pro-opiomelanocortin binding,
　　　e44–e45
　rhythmic release of, e64–e66
　secretion of
　　agents that modulate, e157
　　atrial natriuretic peptide effects
　　　on, e46
　　circadian rhythmicity effects on,
　　　e47, e48f
　　corticotropin-releasing hormone,
　　　e34, e46
　　cytokines that affect, e46–e47
　　glucocorticoids effect on, e45–
　　　e46, e45f
　　integrated control of, e47
　　interleukin-1 effects on, e46
　　L-dopa effects on, e46
　　leukemia inhibitory factor effects
　　　on, e47
　　mechanisms that regulate, e47–
　　　e48, e48f
　　pituitary adenylate cyclase-
　　　activating polypeptide effects
　　　on, e46
　　pulsatile, e47–e48, e65

Adrenocorticotropic hormone
　(Continued)
　regulation of, e45–e48, e48f
　retinoic acid effects on, e158
　rosiglitazone effects on, e158
　serotonin effects on, e46
　stress effects, e48
　vasoactive intestinal polypeptide
　　effects on, e46
　vasopressin, e46
　steroidogenesis, stimulated by,
　　e43–e44
　structure of, e41
　syndrome of ectopic, e138–e139
　　Cushing's disease vs., e150–e151
　　definition of, e138
　　epidemiology of, e140–e141
　　extrapituitary tumors as cause of,
　　　e43
　　gender distribution of, e140–e141
　　history of, e138
　　hypokalemic metabolic alkalosis
　　　in, e144
　　incidence of, e140
　　metyrapone for, e156
　　prognosis for, e160
　　pro-opiomelanocortin expression,
　　　e37
　　small cell lung cancer as cause of,
　　　e138, e140
　　somatostatin analogue testing,
　　　e152
　　surgery for, e155
　　treatment of, e155
　　tumors that cause, e138t
　synthesis of
　　corticotropin-releasing hormone's
　　　role in, e34, e46
　　description of, e34
　　24-hour profile of, e76
Adrenocorticotropic hormone receptors
　description of, e44
Advanced growth pattern, e361
Aging. See also Elderly
　follicle-stimulating hormone levels,
　　e69–e70
　growth hormone levels affected by,
　　e68
　insulin-like growth factor-1 levels
　　and, e315
　luteinizing hormone levels,
　　e69–e70
　slow-wave sleep affected by, e61,
　　e62f
　thyroid-stimulating hormone levels,
　　e71
Ahumada-Argonz-del Castillo
　syndrome, e188–e189
Albright hereditary osteodystrophy. See
　also Pseudohypoparathyroidism
Alström syndrome, e94
Amenorrhea, e25, e29
　growth hormone levels in, e68
　prolactin-secreting pituitary
　　adenomas and, e193–e194
Amine precursor uptake and
　decarboxylation cells
　description of, e138
Anabolism, e315

Page numbers followed by 'f' indicate figures and 't' indicate tables

Printed and bound by CPI Group (UK) Ltd, Croydon, CR0 4YY

03/10/2024

01040364-0014